九十初度
Life at Ninety

陈可冀医学选集
Selected Medical Works of Ke-ji Chen

（2000 ~ 2019 选集）

下　册
Volume Ⅲ

主　　编　陈维养

编辑小组　（按姓氏笔画排序）

于子凯　田　琳　白　霞
付长庚　刘龙涛　汤　静
邱　禹　赵芳芳　姜众会
袁　琳　黄明艳

科 学 出 版 社
北　京

内 容 简 介

本书是在陈可冀院士从医70周年之际，对2000～2019年期间陈可冀院士作为第一作者和通讯作者公开发表的中英文学术论文进行了系统的整理和筛选，编辑成册（1954～1999年的论著已在《陈可冀医学选集——七十初度》一书刊载）。全书共入选文章332篇，其中中文文章271篇，英文文章61篇，分为心迹、临床及基础研究、医论、泛著、英文著述等5个章节。本书较为系统的展示了陈可冀院士和他的团队近20年来基础和临床研究的成果，也是2000年以来我国中西医结合医学发展轨迹的缩影。

本书适用于全国中西医结合工作者参考阅读。

图书在版编目（CIP）数据

陈可冀医学选集：九十初度（2000～2019选集）：上中下册/陈维养主编.—北京：科学出版社，2020.1

ISBN 978-7-03-062445-1

Ⅰ.①陈… Ⅱ.①陈… Ⅲ.①医学-文集 Ⅳ.①R-53

中国版本图书馆CIP数据核字（2019）第205689号

责任编辑：鲍 燕 曹丽英/责任校对：王晓茜

责任印制：肖 兴/封面设计：北京图阅盛世文化传媒有限公司

科学出版社 出版

北京东黄城根北街16号

邮政编码：100717

http://www.sciencep.com

三河市春园印刷有限公司 印刷

科学出版社发行 各地新华书店经销

*

2020年1月第 一 版 开本：889×1194 1/16

2020年1月第一次印刷 印张：99 插页：29

字数：3 206 000

定价：698.00元（上中下册）

（如有印装质量问题，我社负责调换）

目　　录

上　册

第一篇　心　　迹

第二篇　临床及基础研究

心脑血管疾病研究

临床研究

基础研究

进展及述评

中 册

血瘀证与活血化瘀研究

老年医学研究

清宫医药档案研究

第三篇　医　　论

第四篇 泛 著

下　册

第五篇　英文著述

附录

图录

第五篇　英文著述

Ethnic Chinese Medicine, Borderless Civilization —On the Identity of Humane and Scientific Nature of Chinese and Western Medicines

CHEN Ke-ji

The identity of Eastern and Western cultures should include aspects such as its concepts of societal development and science and technology. Though this is related to issues like history of the culture and regional cultural psychologies, the essence lies in the identity of social values at its core.

Into the 21st century, contemporary scientific and cultural identity has its distinctive imprints of the time and modernity. The direction and progress of China's economic globalization is inevitably accompanied by issues of global exchanges and identity of its science and technology. From a broader perspective, medical science is no exception. Chinese medicine (CM), whilst continuing the confirmation and enhancement of its core values, needs necessarily to follow the direction that takes advantages of complementation between Chinese and Western medicine, promotes two-way communication, identifies and integrates the strengths of Chinese and Western medicines. Of course, without doubt, we must also realize that there will be issues arising from long-existing differences in regional cultural and ethical understandings. In short, my belief is that CM has its ethnic origin yet civilization is without borders. Hence, practitioners of Chinese or integrative medicines (IM)should have the kindred spirit to carry on the lineage of knowledge from generation to generation, caring for the well-being of general public and at the same time with eyes and hearts open to the world, to take in the excellent cultural concepts and science and technology from abroad.

IM is a process of mutual communication through practice and gradual complementation and fusion which the public has recognized and come to identify with. It results from continuous communication and fusion between Chinese and modern medicines on aspects of oriental and occidental humanistic care concepts, spiritual and material cultures, local and foreign, mainstream and non-mainstream, macro-and microscopic, multi-sector and multi-level, as well as the superficial and essential. In the implementation of society medicine in China, people are free to consult a diverse selection of Chinese, Western, ethnic or IM in accordance to their needs. This is a fine illustration of the practical fusion of science, technology as well as cultural and rational ethical values. Of course, we should accord CM its due identity as a matter of fact of its thousands of years of practice history and its empirical clinical values, to foster and improve the ethnic confidence of the general public on CM. For whatever that is ethnic, it belongs essentially to the world.

“To inherit well, to develop well, to use well” .We must first enhance the ethnic self-confidence, and simultaneously fostering progress which is innovation driven. Chinese traditional culture affects deeply the clinical practice of CM, as it attaches great importance to the “Doctrine of the Mean” which upholds moderation. Of primary importance of the eight laws of treatment is the law of harmony, which focuses on the issue of “over or under” treatment as it advocates the principle of achieving “state of equilibrium and harmony” [refer to edicts in the “Book of Rites (Li Ji)” or “Analects of Confucius (Lun Yu)”].Likewise, CM practice calls for rational measures following the principle of “yin yang ebb and flow” to correct the deviated and save the inadequate, to reach a state of “yin and yang in equilibrium” as dictated in “Yellow Emperor's Internal Medicine Classics (Huang Di Nei Jing)” .This theory is in congruence and very consistent with modern medicine which advocates the concepts of “balance of internal and external environments” and “internal stability” , including internal environment stability of neuroendocrine and immune systems. As such, I have repeatedly advocated in academic exchanges in many occasions both in China and overseas that integration of Chinese and Western medicines can assume many forms as in "seeking the common to be together", "seeking difference to be together", and of course "together while different". The matter here is to enhance the standard of clinical diagnosis and overall therapeutic effectiveness.

Chinese traditional culture and traditional medical ethics has always emphasized the value of medical ethics, calling the practice of medicine an act of benevolence. Master SUN Si-miao's (Tang Dynasty)is the most representative of this concept. The forewords of LI Shi-zhen's (Ming Dynasty) "Compendium of Materia Medica (Ben Cao Gang Mu)" offers that "one takes the practice of medicine as the way, use it to defend life, promote it to save the world, this is the act of benevolence". The motto of my mentor Prof. YUE Mei-zhong is "nurture a heart that is unselfish, for without it, skills alone could be harmful". Chinese and Western medicines should respect each other, work together, be receptive and inclusive, and complement each other's strengths, in such a way that both the humanistic and scientific natures are attended to. We should advocate a diversified model where we could inherit and innovate to carry forward the excellence of CM, and further improve the context of communication to meet the needs of local and overseas exchanges. Always have ideals and visions in heart and be brave to take on responsibilities and when faced with adversities, be positive and diligent and accomplish the task with sincerity and credibility. It should also point out here that we should have an attitude of patience and preparedness to cope with the situation. In our mind we should always keep the light of our ideals aglow.

I first studied CM in the fifties of last century. Master PU Fu-zhou taught us WU Ju-tong's "Febrile Disease Differentiation (Wen Bing Tiao Bian)" and WANG Meng-ying's "Compendium on Epidemic Febrile Diseases (Wen Re Jing Wei)", illustrated by his own clinical experiences. Master Pu in great patience went through each point of the principles, explaining to us that the five evolutive phases and six climatic factors rule the diseases. At the time I just went from Western medicine to learn CM and was not able to well comprehend the lecture. Now I have come to age and have more clinical experience and looking back, it is very clear the impacts of seasons, climates, days and nights have on human body and diseases. It reflects the doctrine of "correspondence between heaven and man". Nowadays, there are not much in-depth studies on the occurrence of the six excesses and the patterns of these external factors in inducing disease. Through all these, I have come to realize with great humility the truth of respect for the teachers and that the ocean of knowledge is boundless. If we were to be in the ancient times where one was to expose to learning of ceremonies and rites, music, astrology, poetry, literature, history, arts and crafts, maybe this would help us to have greater enthusiasm in understanding and learning traditional culture and science.

In our long clinical practice of treating cardiovascular disease with the principle of "Activating blood to remove stasis", we came to the conclusion that the teachings of "Xin (Heart)rules the blood of body" [*Plain Questions: Wei Conditions* (Su Wen: Wei Lun)] is in such consistency with modern medicine understandings. Other teachings such as "treat symptoms when in haste, treat cause when at ease" [*Medical Edicts of Times: On Disease Etiologies* (Gu Jin Yi Jian: Bing Ji Fu)by GONG Xin], "once symptoms and cause are known, all measures are appropriate, otherwise, all measures are futile" [*Plain Questions: On Symptoms and Cause of Diseases* (Su Wen: Biao Ben Bing Chuan Lun)], "flow then there be no pain, when there is pain it is blocked" [*Medical Inventions* (Yi Xue Fa Ming)by LI Gao], all have great clinical values in the field of cardio-cerebrovascular medicine.

In the practice of geriatric diseases, we also come to realize the rationality of teachings such as "self-healing results when yin and yang come to harmony[Treatise on Diagnosis: Tai Yang Meridian Disease *Differentiation and Treatment*—Clause 58" (Shang Han Lun: Bian Tai Yang Bing Mai Zheng Bing Zhi)], and "replenish Shen (Kidney)to replenish Pi (Spleen)and vice versa" [Jifeng Prescriptions for *Universal Relief* (Ji Feng Pu Ji Fang)—Volume 12 of Song Dynasty], "six fu-organs must be open to be useful" [*Plain Questions: On Five Zang* (Su Wen: Wu Zang Bie Lun)], and "solutions for the elderlies are in the Fu-organs"

(*Plain Questions: Shi Cong Rong Lun*).

From insights and ideas of other teachings such as "fire to be dispersed, wood dredged, earth removed, gold discharged and water diverted" [*Plain Questions: Six Primes Records* (Su Wen: Liu Yuan Zheng Ji Da Lun)], "wind, cold and dampness mingled to cause disease" [*Plain Questions: Bi Conditions* (Su Wen: Bi Lun)], and "sweet and warm herbs to remove high fever" [Differentiation on Endogenous and Exogenous Diseases (Nei Wai Shang Za Bing Lun)by LI Gao, we also find these theories sound and rational in our daily clinical practices.

As a result of occupation preferences and psychological inclinations, different professionals may have their in-group and out-group preferences with signs of incompleteness in each. However, through amassing social and healthcare experience, I believe that it will eventually reach the cognitive consensus where the realization is all undertakings should be driven by patients' interests. We need to be open and inclusive, put to practice in complementing each other's strengths and in certain degree gradually working towards integration, to realize mutual adaptation between the so-called traditional culture and scientific culture, and to materialize thousands of years of Chinese traditional culture that advocates the concept of "differences co-existing in harmony" . We really have to put our feet on the ground, inherit and at the same time strive for innovative development, seek truth through facts, make new contribution and achievement in both theories and actual therapeutic effects.

The growth and progress of scientific knowledge is inevitably closely related and inseparable from people's ideal, mindset, emotion, knowledge, experience, time and space. Progressing on the pace of the era, modern medicine, with its advances in omics and precision medicine, is changing every day and these impacts can not be ignored. As years go by I am now in my senior years and with it I have enhanced my rationality, enhanced the mutual recognition and equal importance of humanistic and scientific nature of Chinese and Western medicines, and enhanced my perception and determination to further promote and accelerate the development of IM.

First published: CHEN Ke-ji. Ethnic Chinese medicine, borderless civilization-On the identity of humane and scientific nature of Chinese and Western medicines.[J].Chin J Integr Med, 2017, 23 (8): 563-565.

Thanks for Your Accompanying in the Journey of Integrative Medicine —Strength and Confidence from the Predecessors of Chinese Medical Association

CHEN Ke-ji

After graduation from Fujian Medical College (now named Fujian Medical University)in 1954, I had my residency training at the Department of Internal Medicine of University Hospital. In early 1956, I came to China Academy of Traditional Chinese Medicine (now named China Academy of Chinese Medical Sciences) and worked at the Division of Senior Officials and Foreign Guests. I joined the Chinese Medical Association in October 1956. At the same year the 18th Annual Conference of the Chinese Medical Association was held at its old address in Dong Si, Beijing, China. It was my first time to attend the Chinese Medical Association's annual conference, where Dr. FU Lian-zhang was re-elected as the president. In the morning of the first conference day, the final presentation was a research report titled "Bezoar's Anticonvulsant Effect" by Prof. ZHOU Jin-huang and Dr. ZHU Yan. I believe this report was very edificatory for my future research directions and ideas, because it made me realize that for Chinese medicine research, beyond the clinical progress, the mechanism of action should be clarified. Dr. Zhu once was criticized for talking about that "Chinese medicine research must have mouse's nod", and he was transferred from the Institute of Chinese Medicine to Xiyuan Hospital's Hematology Lab as a research director. Working in the same hospital, we had a lot of communications. He attended most of weekly case discussions in the Department of Internal Medicine. Prof. ZHOU Jin-huang also invited me to his home many times to exchange the methodological ideas about integrative medicine. He was particularly interested in tonics, and I learned a lot from talking with him.

In 1956, the Eighth Congress of Chinese Communist was held in Beijing. Dr. FU Lian-zhang, Deputy Minister of Ministry of Health and President of the Chinese Medical Association, was responsible for health care of the attendees. At a pre-meeting for health care, he seriously criticized a few physicians who prescribed expensive and valuable Chinese medicine (e.g., deer heart)during the registration time. His voice was very high with a strong Fujian Changting accent. I deeply felt that a good doctor should have responsibility, professional competence, and morality. Although many years passed by, I always bear Dr. Fu's words in mind. Two years ago when I had an opportunity to western Fujian, I specially visited Changting, Dr. Fu's hometown. Staying at the Tingzhou Christian Hospital where Dr. Fu worked, I was very emotional.

In May 1992, Academician WU Jie-ping was to give an academic report in a medical assembly for the celebration of the 20th anniversary of diplomatic relationship between China and Japan. I was assigned to draft the report. Dr. WU Jie-ping, the 19th President of Chinese Medical Association, made several phone calls to explain the key points for this report. The title of the report is "Clinical Features and Progress of Traditional Chinese Medicine." The English translation was published in Chinese Medical Journal in 1993. The original title in the English version was "Clinical Features and Research of Traditional Chinese Medicine." Academician WU Jie-ping called me, asking me to change "Research" to "Investigation", the word contains a more practical and profound meaning. Consequently, later I was very interested in reading *Journal of Clinical Investigation* (JCI), which often presents high quality clinical trials and research.

Academician WU Jie-ping was very interested in integrative medicine. He was two-term vice-chairman of the China Association of Science and Technology, while I was a member in the Executive Council for three terms. At each quarterly meeting we discussed integrative medicine and its significance to Chinese medicine. He shared a very deep friendship with my mentor, Dr. YUE Mei-zhong, who was very famous in Chinese medicine. Dr. Yue was the member of the Fifth National People's Congress Standing Committee and Vice President of the Chinese Medical Association. In 1957, Drs. Wu and Yue visited Japan together. From 1962, at the request of Premier ZHOU En-lai, they went to Indonesian many times to provide medical care to President Sukarno together with Prof. FANG Qi and HU Mao-hua. In 1969, together with Prof. TAO Shou-qi, Drs. Wu and Yue went to Vietnam to treat Mr. Ho Chi Minh who suffered from acute myocardial infarction. Dr. WU Jie-ping appreciated Dr. Yue for his professional Chinese medicine and his open mind to the complementary advantage with Western medicine. In addition to the Vice President of the Chinese Medical Association, Dr. Yue also served as President of the Chinese Association of Traditional Chinese Medicine and advisor of the Chinese Association of Integrative Medicine. In 1997, the First World Integrative Medicine Congress was held in Beijing with approximately 1000 foreign guests. Academician WU Jie-ping attended the meeting and announced the official opening of the General Assembly. Academician CHEN Zhu was also invited to the conference for an excellent lecture about the treatment of myeloid leukemia with arsenic trioxide.

My belief in integrative medicine came from teachings and friendship of my predecessors. One of them is Dr. FANG Qi, former executive council member of Chinese Medical Association. He presided over a thesis defense for one of my graduate students. The thesis was entitled "Clinical Study of Fumaric Alkali in the Treatment of Premature Beats." His comments were profound and pertinent. This graduate student has been a professor at UCLA for many years. The thesis was later published in Chinese Journal of Cardiovascular Diseases in 1983. From 1979 to 2009, I had been invited to serve as the Traditional Medicine Consultant at World Health Organization. Coincidentally, in 1983 I participated in a World Health Organization meeting together with Prof. FANG Qi and Prof. MAO Shou-bai. Prof. Fang also provided guidance on my presentation about the progress of integrative medicine, which was presented at another meeting of the World Health Organization Western Pacific Region.

I miss several distinguished medical scientists who helped and supported my career development, including KUANG An-kun, WU Ying-kai, TAO Shou-qi, HUANG Wan, QIAN Yi-jian, ZHANG Xi-jun, and WENG Xin-zhi. Academician WU Ying-kai was a cardiothoracic surgeon, but he was an extremely comprehensive clinician, knowing the health policy well and willing to support the cause of integrative medicine and its academic progress. In 1959, he organized the First National Conference on Cardiovascular Diseases in Xi'an, China. On the first day morning three academic reports were presented in the General Assembly, including Prof. HUANG Wan's research progress of atherosclerosis, Prof. KUANG An-kun's non-drug treatment of hypertension, and my Chinese medicine classification and treatment prospects of hypertension. At that time I was 29 years old, but Academician WU Ying-kai encouraged me and asked me to give the presentation.

In 1978, the Cardiovascular Disease Branch of Chinese Medical Association was established in Taiyuan, Shanxi Province, during the National Conference on Cardiovascular Diseases of the Chinese Medical Association. Academician WU Ying-kai was elected as chairman, and I was elected as executive council member. Dr. WU Ying-kai designated me to serve as the branch secretary, and deputy chief editor of Chinese Journal of Cardiovascular Diseases for the first four terms. The following scientists have been served as Chief Editors: WU Ying-kai, TAO Shou-qi, FANG Qi, and GU Fu-sheng. I remember two weeks before the Taiyuan meeting, Academician WU Ying-kai organized a small scale meeting at Fuwai Hospital to prepare launching the *Chinese Journal of Cardiovascular Diseases*. I attended the meeting with Professors HUANG Wan, FANG Qi, CAI Ru-sheng, Mr. ZHU Li from Fuwai Hospital Office. Dr. WU Ying-kai showed us the handwriting journal title by Mr. HUANG Shu-ze, Deputy Minister, Department of Health. Dr. WU Ying-kai looked very satisfied. The handwriting title of the journal is still in use. Academician WU Ying-kai had a strong career ambition. Under his leadership, the Beijing Coronary Heart Disease Collaborative Group operated effectively with brilliant achievements. I myself also learned a lot. Dr. Wu had personally followed Mr. PU Fu-zhou, a famous doctor of

Chinese medicine, to learn the treatment for esophageal cancer using Chinese medicine.

When the Geriatrics Branch of Chinese Medical Association was established, the first chairman was HUANG Shu-ze, Deputy Minister, and I was elected as the member of the executive council. Mr. Huang encouraged the younger generation. He wrote a prelude for the revised gerontology book "Yang Lao Feng Qin Shu" which was made in Song Dynasty and was corrected and annotated by Prof. LI Chun-sheng and me. Persuaded by Professors MOU Shan-chu and WANG Xin-de, I agreed to be elected as the fifth and sixth chairman and seventh honorary chairman of the Geriatrics Branch of Chinese Medical Association. I hosted three Xiangshan Science Conferences related to geriatrics and gerontology.

Professors HUANG Wan and CHEN Zai-jia were very supportive for the research and development of Guanxin No. 2 Compound (冠心二号方). In February 1982, we jointly published an article "Guanxin No. 2, case analysis of double-blind treatment in 112 patients with angina pectoris" in *Chinese Journal of Cardiovascular Diseases*. The article was generally considered by the medical professional community as the first article that met the clinical requirements of evidence-based medicine in the field of integrative medicine related to the research of cardiovascular diseases.

Prof. WENG Xin-zhi was a member of the executive council of Chinese Medical Association. He served as editor-in-chief of the *Chinese Journal of Internal Medicine* for a long period. He was intelligent and his writing was fast. When launching the *Chinese Journal of Integrated Traditional and Western Medicine* in 1981, I needed expert opinions from some well-known specialists. While someone advised him that integrative medicine was a "dangerous place" and he should avoid writing anything, Dr. Weng actively wrote articles to discuss research methods and support the integrative medicine career.

In 1970's, Prof. QIAN Yi-jian and I joined the Beijing Medical Team and stayed in Wuwei, Gansu for one year. Both of us were medical team leaders, and sometimes we were roommates, getting along very well and forming a close friendship. For many years he served as the editor-in-chief of *Chinese Medical Journa*l, and was responsible for the clinical care tasks at Beijing Hospital. He often invited me to go to Beijing Hospital for consultation. Inspired by the older generation of expert wisdom, I founded the English version of "Chinese Journal of Integrative Medicine" in 1995 to promote the development of integrative medicine internationally. The journal has domestic and foreign editors in a 50% to 50% ratio (SCI-IF: 1.401). The journal had Dr. WU Jie-ping as the honorary editor-in-chief. After Dr. Wu passed away, the journal invited the Honorary President of Chinese Medical Association HAN Qi-de and President CHEN Zhu as honorary editors-in-chief.

Prof. TAO Shou-qi once cooperated with us in research to observe heart-rate increasing effect of higenamine, a component of *Radix Aconiti lateralis*. He could stare at the screen to observe the positive effect for more than one hour. He was a down-to-earth person and I admired him very much. This research was published in the *Chinese Journal of Cardiovascular Diseases* in 1980.

My book "Complete Collection of Qing Court Medical Cases" which was based on the research of original medical archives in Qing palace won the Chinese Government Publication Award in 2012. At the beginning of the publication, Prof. KUANG An-kun enthusiastically wrote a preface. He mentioned that he had discussed medical sciences with me when we were roommates during a medical conference, and that he was assigned by Premier ZHOU En-lai and Minister of Foreign Affair CHEN Yi to treat foreign officials. He felt such heritage work was very significant. He noticed a foreign book "Ces malades qui nous gouvernent" which recorded the medical experiences of Mr. Roosevelt, Mr. Churchill and other foreign officials. He encouraged me to continue my studies in the original medicine archives of Qing Dynasty. I appreciate these physician mentors of older generation very much.

In 2007, the opening assembly of the Traditional Chinese and Western Medicine Branch, Chinese Medical Doctor Association was held in Beijing Friendship Hotel. Dr. HAN Qi-de, Vice-Chairman of the Standing Committee of the National People's Congress, Honorary President of the Chinese Medical Association participated in the meeting. He said that integrative medicine is unique to China, it is the inevitable development of Chinese medicine, and it is a breakthrough point for Chinese medicine. However, it is also a very complex and difficult task. His speech greatly encouraged us.

In 2013, at the National Conference of Traditional Chinese and Western Medicine in Beijing Jingxi Hotel, Prof. ZHANG Yan-ling, Vice President of the Chinese Medical Association and President of the Chinese Medical Doctor Association, stressed the necessity of integrative medicine and its important role in health care reform. His speech was also inspiring.

On March 23, 2014, the Nobel Laureate Lectures and Academician Forum was held in National Conference Center. Academician CHEN Zhu, Vice Chairman of the Standing Committee of the National People's Congress, and President of the Chinese Medical Association presented a speech entitled "Building A Modern Chinese Medical System with A Combination of Chinese and Western Medicine." His presentation indicated the bright prospects of fusion of Chinese and Western medicine. My presentation in the general assembly emphasized the clinical complementary advantages of integrative medicine. Academician WANG Chen, executive council member of the Chinese Medical Association, introduced the research progress of integrative medicine in influenza and respiratory diseases. We responded to President CHEN Zhu, and will strive to further develop integrated medicine and our country's medical science and technology.

Whenever I cherish the memory of the older generation of the eminent medical scientists of Chinese Medical Association who helped me grow, my mood cannot be calm and my heart always feels grateful. Although I am getting old, I would like to use all my life, trying to learn from their patriotic spirit, professional dedication, and their love to the Chinese Medical Association. I will try to face the challenge, push the cooperation between Chinese and Western medicine, and serve the public.

(This article was made to commemorate the centenary of the Chinese Medical Association. Please see the Chinese Medical Association website in Chinese)

First published: CHEN Ke-ji. Thanks for your accompanying in the journey of integrative medicine: Strength and confidence from the predecessors of Chinese medical association[J]. Chin J Integr Med, 2016, 22 (9): 643-646.

Historical Responsibility and Great Trust of the Times
—Review and Outlook of 60 Years of Integrative Medicine Clinical Sciences

CHEN Ke-ji

The founding of China Institute of Chinese Medicine, known now as the China Academy of Chinese Medical Sciences, was proclaimed in December 1955 in Beijing. Premier ZHOU En-lai commemorated the occasion with his inscription extolling "to carry forward the heritage of Chinese medicine" . Just before and after its establishment, the Academy recruited numbers of famous Chinese and Western medicine specialists all over the country to participate in this endeavour. The first "Western Medicine Doctors Learning Chinese Medicine" class was opened by the Ministry of Health and held at Xiyuan Hospital, China Institute of Chinese Medicine. A tremendous amount of work was dedicated to the organization and building of the scientific and medical research team and its reserves. In addition, a large number of young Chinese and Western medicine doctors with recognized academic and clinical abilities were also organized to enter into apprenticeship with famous Chinese medicine masters dedicated to inherit the academic thoughts and to systematically record and study the clinical experiences of these masters. The "Western Medicine Doctors Learning Chinese Medicine" undertaking followed the central government guidelines "to study systematically, to master completely, to record and to improve" and created such a great impact resulting in a nationwide following of outstanding outcome. It greatly promoted the development of the realm of Chinese medicine and brought forth even greater strides in fostering the science of integrative Chinese and Western medicines with favorable responses internationally. China's persistent efforts and outstanding achievement in inheriting and improving traditional medical sciences have repeatedly earned praises from the World Health Organization (WHO).

Chinese medicine enjoys thousands of years of brilliant history. It has made indelible contributions to assurance and protection of people's wellbeing, as well as to social progress of the nation. As Western medicine gradually makes its inroad to China, Chinese and Western medicine professionals were able to have increased exposure, communication and exchanges where it was realized that both medicines have their strengths and shortcomings, and it would be of mutual benefits to enhance unity and cooperation between the two, to complement each other with advantages while avoiding the defects, all for the good of people's health. Undoubtedly, this is a responsibility entrusted by history to generations of us medical practitioners, and it is also a great trust of the times bestowed upon us. We must keep pace with the times, to author a new chapter in the history of Chinese and Western medicines to contribute to humanity.

When New China was first founded, the State advocated the "unity of Chinese and Western medicine" approach. Article 21 of the "Constitution of People's Republic of China" states that "The State is to develop medical and health services and to develop modern medicine and traditional medicine of China" . In 1978, China restored its graduate school system and integrative medicine as a discipline was classified a Class Ⅰ Discipline. For more than 30 years, a great number of graduate students and successor talents of Chinese and Western medicines, both of clinical and basic sciences, have been nurtured and trained. In 1981, Chinese Society of Integrative Medicine (later renamed the Chinese Association of Integrative Medicine sanctioned by China Association of Sciences and Technology)was established which actively promoted academic exchange, and has so far convened four World Integrative Medicine Congress to foster academic exchanges and influences at home and overseas. In the same year, the Association founded the *Chinese Journal of Integrated Traditional and Western Medicine* and in 1995 an English version of the *Chinese Journal of Integrative Medicine* was published which is a SCI-source journal with 50% each of the editorial board taken up by Chinese and overseas experts. A great number of those who have published articles on these journals are now eminent scientists and experts in the fields of integrative medicine and Chinese medicine serving in positions as lead scientists, professors and chief physicians with impeccable track records. Numerous Chinese medicine universities in Beijing, Guangzhou, Shanghai and Hunan offer 5-year undergraduate or 7-year continuous graduate degrees in integrative medicine which play a significant role in strengthening and developing both the integrative medicine and Chinese medicine disciplines.

In 2003, China State Council promulgated the "Chinese Medicine Regulations of the People's Republic of China" and its Article 3 states: "to promote an organic integration of two different Chinese and Western medicine systems to develop fully the Chinese medicine enterprise" . Meeting WHO Director General, Dr. Margaret Chan in June 2013, Chinese President XI Jin-ping stressed the need to "promote integrative medicine and Chinese medicine development in foreign countries" . This further illustrates that integrative medicine have gradually been recognized and appreciated by the State, the society and the general public. Many cities of China have integrative medicine hospitals where Chinese and Western medicine techniques complement each other to improve both disease diagnosis and treatment which in turn better serves the society and assures health of the general public. Today, in most of the general hospitals of the country, an integrative medicine or Chinese medicine specialty ward is commonly present. This is especially true at the community level where this practice is applied flexibly providing greater convenience in disease prevention and treatment.

Over the past 60 years, integrative medicine has made huge clinical progress and attained great achievements. Academic Chinese medicine concepts such as attention to the relation between people and nature, the "correspondence between human and universe" concept, and the Chinese medicine healing edicts of "eight principles" and "eight laws" are put under comprehensive studies together with clinical application to develop coordination and integration as well as macro-and micro-integration of disease syndrome integration concept and syndrome differentiation and treatment concept. This not only improves the levels of diagnosis and treatment, but also brings about a new concept in clinical diagnosis and treatment from a philosophical level of understanding.

Inspired by the teaching of "qi blood equilibrium" emphasized in Huangdi's Internal Classic (Huang Di Nei Jing), Xiyuan Hospital of China Academy of Chinese Medical Sciences developed the modern activating blood circulation and removing stasis (ABCRS)school. It applies the ABCRS principle in preventing and treating different types of coronary diseases and care of post-vascularization reconstructions, and makes use of randomized controlled trial (RCT)research method in obtaining evidence-based medical results of higher standards. This undertaking was able to be propagated nationwide leading to the birth of a series of proprietary Chinese medications developed based on modern pharmacology and molecular biological mechanisms of action. Various institutes of China Academy of Chinese Medical Sciences also obtained outstanding achievements, including international clinical application of artemisinin and its derivatives, and the inventor Prof. Youyou Tu won the Nobel prize for physiology and medicine in 2015. Cure for infectious diseases including severe acute respiratory syndrome, and research on influenza treatment, application of dynamic and static integration principle in fracture treatment, application of strengthening vital qi and consolidating the constitution principle in the treatment of cancer treatment and its medications for maintenance application, phased syndrome differentiation and treatment for diabetes, studies on the mechanism of cold heat syndrome differentiation and treatment and its therapeutic efficacy for rheumatoid arthritis, study of coronary heart disease symptom complex and syndrome differentiation and treatment, study of Shen (Kidney)replenishing, stasis removing and detoxifying medications for aplastic anemia, syndrome differentiation and treatment for functional dyspepsia, cognitive dysfunction treatment research, research on the effect of acupuncture on functional diseases, study of adverse effect of Chinese medicine in clinical applications, etc., and these studies all have wide influence all over the country.

Other institutes in the country focus on clinical application research of integrative medicine also gain admirable results. We have multi-center RCT study on Xuezhikang (血脂康)by Fuwai Hospital, study of syndrome differentiation and treatment and medications for brain diseases by Beijing University of Chinese Medicine, the application of "Fu Purging and Toxin Removing" medication in acute abdomen cases including peritoneal infection by Tianjin Nankai Hospital, studies on anti-platelet effect of Qi Replenishing and Blood Activating Compounds by Tianjin University of Traditional Chinese Medicine, the development of injectable medications for acute disease with stasis and toxin by Tianjin First Central Hospital. It is also notable that there are researches in Shanghai and Harbin on effect of arsenic trioxide in the treatment of myeloid leukemia, development of Chinese medicines for treatment of hepatic fibrosis and for prevention and treatment of degenerative diseases in Shanghai, as well as the use of Shen replenishing principle in delaying ageing, research on cardiocerebral diseases medications based on collateral disease theory in Hebei Province, and research studies into the effect of acupuncture as an ancillary means to enhance in vitro reproductive function by the Medical Department of Beijing Medical University. There are so many outstanding achievements on the horizon of integrative medicine, and this is truly amazing.

Recently, the Integrative Medicine Committee of China Medical Doctor Association together with Evidence-Based Medical Professional Committee of Chinese Association of Integrative Medicine issued "Guidelines to Clinical Research Methods for Chinese and Integrative Medicine" which was published by the People's Medical Publishing House. Committees of various disciplines of the Association as well as other academic bodies all contributed to the establishment of research method guidelines compliant with Chinese medical theories and at the same time in correlation to modern clinical, medical and scientific practices. These guidelines are based on consensus of experts' recommendations and it is believed that on this foundation of clinical studies methodology improvement, clinical integrative medicine will advance further to the next level. Institutes affiliated with China Academy of Chinese Medical Sciences taking various clinical disciplines in stride have conducted multifaceted, multi-disciplinary in-depth basic medical science research studies on Chinese medicine pharmacology, genomics, proteomics, metabolomics as well as molecular biology with most outstanding results. What the China Academy of Chinese Medical Sciences set down in the 50's as the research and development direction which is 'to confirm efficacy, to consolidate patterns and to investigate the mechanisms of action' shall continue to serve as the guiding light leading us moving forward with prudence to bring forth greater achievement.

First published: Chen KJ. Historical responsibility and great trust of the times—review and outlook of 60 years of integrative medicine clinical sciences[J].Chin J Integr Med, 2015, 21 (11): 804-806.

Reflections on Human Longevity and Chinese Medicine Prevention and Treatment of Chronic Diseases

CHEN Ke-ji

1 Life Expectancy Study

International geriatric life science community, including medical and scientific communities, currently considers human life expectancy to be about 120 years. This is in congruence with recordings from "Hong Fan–Book of Documents (Shang Shu • Hong Fan)" , and is also in general agreement with teachings from "Longevity–Yellow Emperor's Canon of Internal Medicine (Huang Di Nei Jing • Tian Nian)" where it is said "a man is to die at age of a hundred years" meaning "passing away after living a hundred years" . Recently there is a report of people dying at the age of 150 years in England, I am afraid this is misinformed.

Good health and longevity are people's ultimate dreams. There are many such legends in ancient China, such as that of Sichuan's Pengshan legend which claims that Pen-Tsu lived to a ripe old age of 880, and there are many legends of the like. In the West, legends similar to those from the East abound. In the Bible Methuselah is said to live for 969 years. Both the West and the East are on the same page here. The truth is, life is really short. If one were to live for 100 years, it is a mere 36, 500 days, and this is indeed too short. That's why all of us harbor great expectation and desire for better health and longevity. With today's social progress, technology improvement and medical advance, it is apparent that we are already looking at an extended average life span that is much longer than that of our ancestors. I visited the 'Three Su House' several times in Meishan City in Sichuan Province of China where one finds the great late literati SU Dong-po (1037–1101 AD)of the late Song Dynasty, who lived to be 64 years old and was considered to have a long life. Su was banished to Hangzhou in 1080, and returned to Chibi in 1082, where he wrote the eternally favorite collection Fu of the Tang Dynasty (712–770 AD)lived to be 59 and when he was just 50 years of age, he was already 'deaf in the ears and numb at the shoulders' and reeked with chronic diseases. DU Fu claimed himself in his own poems as 'weakness and illness turned me an old man' , as well as exclamations expressed as 'old and sickly, in my solitary boat' and many other emotional outpours. BAI Ju-yi (772–846 AD), a famous poet from the late Tang Dynasty, in poor moods because of many chronic diseases, expressed in "Early Spring in South Lake" that 'not that spring in Southern China is of no good, it is just that weakness and illness year after year dampens one's mood' . The famous Ci-Fu master SIMA Xiang-ru (179–118 BC)of the West Han Dynasty, a native of Chengdu, Sichuan, was known to be a patient of the emaciation-thirst disease (Xiao Ke)with polydipsia and polyuria, apparently suffering from outright manifestations of the three elimination syndrome. At the time, emaciation-thirst disease was also known in his namesake as Xiangru disease. Medical historians have thus confirmed that Xiangru disease is what in modern day known as diabetes mellitus. Chronic diseases such as diabetes and its complications are in reality the causes of early death and shortened life-span.

Chronobiology is receiving ever more attention from gerontologists and geriatric physicians, in aspects ranging from basic science to real social life. The focus now is to how to adopt further measures to seek a healthy long life-span for all. This is also being advocated by the World Health Organization (WHO)in the pursue of an active ageing for the general population.

2 Prevention and Treatment of Chronic Diseases

It has been confirmed, and is the consensus now, that individual life-span is closely related to one's "Nian Nu Jiao–Memories of Past at Red Cliff" that have passed down through the times. In it one finds the famous lines lamenting 'my heart overflowing, surely a figure of fun, a man gray before his time' and 'this life is a dream' . At that time Su was about 45 to 47 years old and already had white hair. The famous realist poet DU genetic composition as well as one's lifestyle. It is also recognized that timely prevention and treatment of chronic diseases in the middle and old age population are of extreme importance. Data of the Sixth Chinese National Census show a total of 178 million of China's population (13.3%)are people 60 years old or above, while there are 119 million (8.9%)who are 65 years or above. Of people aged 60 and above, 53.2% of the urban sector are chronic disease ridden against 38.5% in the rural sector, and 4.2% of this urban sector suffer from dementia while 4.4% of the same from depression. Statistically, common old age diseases in descending order of occurrence are hypertension, cerebrovascular disease, diabetes, chronic obstructive pulmonary disease, rheumatoid arthritis and ischemic cardiovascular disease. However, from our actual clinical experience, of the chronic diseases, those actually affecting survival and quality of life and hence most deserving of timely treatment are cognitive disorders, neoplastic and cardiocerebrovascular diseases, metabolic disorders such as diabetes, bone and joint disorders, prostate disease, cataracts and deafness, among others.

A vast majority of older population suffers from a variety chronic diseases and it is very common for them to take a lot of medication each day. It is hence of great importance to have a concise and simple treatment and medication regimen to avoid overtreatment. Prof. YUE Mei-zhong, based on his lifelong clinical observations, used very lifelike and vivid phrases to succinctly describe common chronic diseases observed in the aged:

"Remember only things afar, but never the recent, tears come with laugher but not from crying, fond of grandchildren yet not the sons, prefer hard food but not the soft ones, eyes blurry unable see the near, ears deaf yet inquisitive of gossips, loquacious even in the company of strangers, want to pee far yet the drops fall on the shoes. "

These simple phrases encompass problems faced by the elderly, from cognitive impairment, psychological disorders, oral and denture problems, personality changes, degeneration in vision and hearing, to prostate disease and a weak bladder.

In a broad stroke, experts summarize the signs of good health in the elderly: (1)eyes brimming with radiance, (2)voice in consonance, (3)liberal in the front (ease of urination), (4)constraint at the back (no incontinence), (5)a trimmed shape (not plumb nor full), (6)strong dentures, (7)agile waist and appendages, pulse configuration defined. I think this is an excellent generalization of health in the elderly. The Chinese Association of Gerontology of the Chinese Medical Association in 2013 established a set of health standards for the aged and this could be used as a reference for clinical treatment and studies. [1]

2.1 Chinese Standards for the Healthy Aged

(1)Changes in vital organs secondary to increase in age do not cause functional impairment, absence of major diseases, related risk factors controlled within the standard range and age-appropriate, possess resistance to diseases, (2)cognitive function normal, able to adapt to the environment, with optimistic and positive attitude, good degree of self-satisfaction or self-evaluation, (3)can deal properly with family and social relationships, actively participate in family and social activities, (4)normal daily living activities, able to self-care and provide basic cares, (5)of good nutritional constitution, with appropriate body weight and maintains a good lifestyle. [1]

2.2 Chinese Medicine Differentiation and Understanding of Pathogenesis of Chronic Diseases

Based on Chinese medicine (CM), ten principles of syndrome differentiation (eight principles plus qi and blood differentiations), chronic diseases common to the elderly can generally be attributed to "yin and yang imbalance, disharmony between Ying and Wei, weakness of Zang and Fu, and multiple organ impairment" caused by advance of age, leading to manifestations such as "vulnerability to deficiency and excess, vulnerability to cold and heat, and intermingled deficiency and excess" . Generally, the most commonly seen are Ying deficiencies, yet not uncommon are qi, blood and yang deficiencies. These manifestations are accompanied often than not by blood stasis, turbid resistance, and wind illness. These cases are complicated as a rule with poor compliance and poor responsiveness.

Based on these observations, clinical treatment options should be weighed cautiously. With diminished renal and liver functions, the elderly population is prone to adverse reactions hence medication dosages should be halved beyond the age of eighty. As a rule the dosage of symptomatic relief medicines should not be more than 10 g, and those of laxative nature 3 to 6 g. Since qi and yang deficiencies are common occurrence in the elderly, dosages of *Astragalus membranaceus* (Fisch.)Bunge and *Radix Aconiti lateralis preparata* could be slightly larger. Although *Fructus Jujubae* and *Radix Glycyrrhizae* do act to replenish the Pi (Spleen)and tonify the Middle, their dosages should not be too large in fear of causing qi stasis with Middle distension. Dosages of *Radix Scutellariae*, *Rhizoma Coptidis* and other bitter and cold medicines should also be slightly less in the elderly. It not only is important to prescribe rationally, it also calls for timely modification of the dosages in order to optimize the effect. For the "old old population" (the elderly over 90 years of age), particular attention should be paid to an integrated maintenance of the quality of life. The same should be applied when integrated medicine measures are used, such as prescription of antihypertensive, hypoglycemic, lipid-lowering drugs, as well as the application of anti-platelet drugs, with strict reference to patients 'age, presence of other diseases and the patients' subjective feelings, to arrive as much as possible at a balanced and individualized treatment regimen.

2.3 Geriatric Treatment Considerations

Aside from want of efficacy, the treatment approach needs to be mild and steer clear from falsehoods. During the course of treatment the attention must be laid in mediating the patient's bodily constitution. Measures should be timely and on the mark in such a way that it 'sweat but not hurt' , 'warm but not dry' , 'discharge but not damage' , 'cool but not congeal' , 'replenish but not stagnate' , and 'eliminate but not eiminish' . As much as possible avoid using highly poisonous medicines the likes of *Fructus Crotonis, Semen Strychni, Radix Euphorbiae pekinensis, Flos Genkwa, Radix Kansui, Epicautagorhami Marseul* and *Lytta vesicatoria*.

Of these treatment considerations, the need to regulate the Pi and Wei (Stomach)is of utmost importance. CM theory emphasizes on the approach 'to use the acquired to nourish the inherited' and as such it is very important to be able to digest food well and to channel away stasis, as well as to keep patent the two bodily elimination processes. Caution is to be called on greasy and sticky foods which could lead to phlegm generation and hence dampness. In order to enhance qi to help digest the food, appropriate application of aromatic and turbidity-removing medicines are beneficial. In addition, one should seek to reach a rational balance of practical issues such as the complementary and synergistic effects of CM and Western medicines. The conventional recipes commonly cited are listed in Table 1.

Table 1 Conventional Recipes Commonly Used for Geriatric Diseases

Formula	Origin	Effect
Modified Shenling Baizhu Powder (参苓白术散)	Prescriptions of the Bureau of Taiping People's Welfare Pharmacy (Taiping Huimin Heji Ju Fang)	Regulates the Pi and Wei, more of yang nursing effect than yin nursing
Wendan Decoction (温胆汤)	Invaluable Prescriptions for Ready reference (Qian Jin Yao Fang)	Eliminates phlegm and removes irritation
Xiaoyao Powder (逍遥散)	Prescriptions of the Bureau of Taiping People's Welfare Pharmacy	Removes depression and promotes qi
Zisheng Pill (资生丸)	Medical Notes of Xianxing Studio (Xian Xing Zhai Yi Xue Guang Bi Ji)	Replenishes accompanied by regulation. When WANG Ken-tang first met and saw MIAO Xi-yong partook this prescription at will, commented "Those who are hungry have an eyeful, those who are full will be made hungry"
Yiguan Decoction (一贯煎)	Liu Zhou Discourse on Medicine (Liu Zhou Yi Hua)	Yin deficiency and qi stasis
Erzhi Pill (二至丸)	Collection of Prescriptions with Notes (Yi Fang Ji Jie)	Replenishes the Gan (Liver)and Shen (Kidney)
Jiaotai Pill (交泰丸)	Han's Medical Recipe Collection (Han Shi Yi Tong)	Promotes Xin (Heart)to Shen circulations
Kuanxiong Pills (宽胸丸)and Kuanxiong Aerosol (宽胸气雾剂)	Based on traditional pain relief recipe Kulai Xiaoqu Powder (哭来笑去散)	An aromatic recipe for qi promotion and pain relief
Guanxin Ⅱ Recipe (冠心2号方)	An Ancient Blood Invigorating and Stasis Removing Recipe (活血化瘀祖方)	Refined coronary drops (Lemai Granules, 乐脉颗粒)
Yu Xin Tong Recipe (愈心痛方)	Proprietary	Blood and qi invigorating compound recipe
Yugeng Tongyu Recipe (愈梗通瘀方)	Proprietary	Compound recipe to promote qi, invigorate blood, eliminate turbidity and regulate qi and relieve pain
Xuefu Zhuyu Decoction (血府逐瘀汤)	Correction on Errors in Medical Classics (Yi Lin Gai Cuo)	Promotes qi, invigorates blood circulation and relieve pain
Buyang Huanwu Decoction (补阳还五汤)	Correction on Errors in Medical Classics	Replenishes qi to promote blood circulation to remove meridian obstruction
Buzhong Yiqi Decoction (补中益气汤)	Treatise on the Spleen and Stomach (Pi Wei Lun)	Regulates and replenishes Pi and Wei, to enhance yang and benefit the qi
Linggui Zhugan Decoction (苓桂术甘汤)	Treatise on Febrile Diseases (Shang Han Lun)	Replenishes the Spleen to eliminate dampness
Zhishi Xiebai Guizhi Decoction (枳实薤白桂枝汤)	Synopsis of the Golden Chamber (Jin Kui Yao Lue)	Circulates the qi and activates yang
Qingxuan Drops (清眩颗粒)	Proprietary	Nourishes yin to suppress hyperactive yang
New Buxin Pill (新补心丹)	Proprietary	Nourishes the yin and calms the mind
Guben Pill (固本丸)	YUE Mei-zhong Complete Works	Nourishes the yin to replenish qi, clears the Lung (Fei) to suppress fire
Sanzi Yangqin Decoction (三子养亲汤)	Han's Medical Recipe Collection (Han Shi Yi Tong)	Promotes qi and depresses regurgitating qi, eliminates phlegm to remove stasis
Ganlu Decoction (甘露饮)	Prescriptions of the Bureau of Taiping People's Welfare Pharmacy	For food stagnation and resistance in the middle
Zhisou Powder (止嗽散)	Medicine Comprehended (Yi Xue Xin Wu)	For adverse exogenous affectations leading to hindered expectoration
Xingsu Powder (杏苏散)	Detailed Analysis of Epidemic Warm Diseases (Wen Bing Tiao Bian)	Ventilates the Fei (Lung)to eliminate phlegm
Xianfang Huoming Decoction (仙方活命饮)	Standards of Diagnosis and Treatment (Zheng Zhi Zhun Sheng)	Clears the heat to detoxify, activates the blood circulation to relieve pain
Roucongrong Pill (肉苁蓉丸)	Holy Benevolent Prescriptions (Shen Hui Fang)	For exhaustion with low back and leg pains
Modified Juanbi Decoction (蠲痹汤)	Yang's Home Collections (Yang Shi Jia Cang Fang)	Expels wind to eliminate cold and to promote blood circulation

3 Original Representative Works and Persons of the Science of Health Preservation and Self-Health Preservation

- The Medical School
  Yellow Emperor's Canon of Internal Medicine and Prescriptions Worth Thousand Golds
- The Confucian School
  Rich Dew of Spring and Autumn (Chun Qiu Fan Lu)
- The Taoist School
  The Book of Dao (Tao De Jing)
- The Buddhist School
  Sutra in Forty-Two Sections (Si Shi Er Zhang Jing)
- The Alimentation School
  Lao Lao Heng Yan
- The Martial School
  The Classics of Tendon Changing (Yi Jin Jing)
- The Miscellaneous Schools
  Eight Treatises on Nurturing Life (Zun Sheng Ba Jian), Book of Health for the Aged (Yang Lao Feng Qin Shu)

4 Three Outstanding Forms to Extend Life-Span

4.1 Life of primitive form

mere survival in its primordial biological form (if not short-lived then it is yours, response to what is yours?).

4.2 Life of quality

the sum of all there is in life culminating in a state of quality (quality of living to the age of a hundred years without losing one's mind).

4.3 Life of mission

a life of responsibility and commitment (together through thick and thin, when all is well, one is well).

"To know one's strength and shortcomings, we feel humbled and inadequate. There are things in this world that we can do, and there are those we do not need to do" .

Our lives are just like candles in the wind. We shall get away from the myth of health preservation as had Mencius who lived to be 83 and advocated 'the benevolent shall inherit longevity' . The difference between people lies in how they make use of their spare time (Einstein). A useless life is tantamount to premature death (Goethe). To be calculating is a burden in life, one's at the loss. Not to be calculating is winning, it is not a loss. Not everything will go well in life but we need to do our utmost in all, and donot turn trivia matters between people into issues of contention.

Older people should use the "staircase" way to meet the challenges of adversity. Koran puts it the best in the famous saying, "If the hill is not coming to Muhammad, Muhammad will go to the hill. "

REFERENCE

[1] Chinese Association of Gerontology of Chinese Medical Association. Chinese standards for the healthy aged (2013)[J]. Chin J Gerontol (Chin), 2013, 32: 801.

First published: Chen Ke-ji. Reflections on human longevity and Chinese medicine prevention and treatment of chronic diseases[J]. Chin J Integr Med, 2015, 21 (9): 643-647.

Common Glory: The Traditional and the Contemporary —Complementary Nature of Chinese and Modern Medicine—A Speech at Nobel Laureate Summit and Academician Forum of Medicine (2014)

CHEN Ke-ji

I want to take this chance to talk about three points. First, I want to talk about the strength of Chinese medicine. Second, I will introduce some of the achievements of Chinese medicine in recent years. And third, let's talk about my team's researches on Chinese medicine in the treatment of coronary heart disease (CHD).

As we all know, the Great Wall is the symbol of China. It was built in 7th to 8th century B. C. Yet we might not know that the Chinese medicine has even a longer history than the Great Wall.

Dr. ZHANG Zhong-jing is the founder of Chinese medicine differentiation principles while Galen is the founder of modern medicine and the advocate of anatomy and applied medicine as well. They were both living around from 150 to 210 A.D. Practice has proved that the two medical systems have complemented mutual advantages and advanced each other, which has become a dominant feature and superiority of China's characteristic medical and health services, provided peculiar for the development of Chinese medical science, and played more and more important roles in the realization of healthy China. A Chinese philosopher once said, "If sharing challenges, the challenge will be dispersed, if sharing fruits, fruits will be times" .However, as academician CHEN Zhu pointed out previously, "There exist two contradictory attitudes towards Chinese medicine among some people even in China. Some believe that Chinese medicine is pseudoscience and should be cancelled. Others hold that Chinese medicine having thousands years of clinical practice has reached its summit, and the so-called modernization of Chinese medicine can only distort its essence. Patients and physicians sometimes fall into the two extremities. "

Prof. Ka Kit Hui from University of California at Los Angeles has summarized the Chinese medicine theory to three words— "Balance, Flow and Spirit" , which means the balance of human, nature and internal milieu (organs), to enhance the flow of qi and blood and all sorts of circulations, and to enhance the vital qi, so-called Zhengqi (正气), which is mental, vital and of immuno-regulation. In Chinese medicine theory, it is quite emphasized on self-regulating mechanisms so as to balance a harmonized body function.

China has ten thousands of works as a couple of recorded herbal resources. And many have experienced long-term applications by both East and West. For instance, Compendium of Materia Medica (Ben Cao Gang Mu)is a work authored by LI Shi-zhen (1518–1593 A.D.)in 1578, which has recorded 1, 892 different herbs for clinical practice with 374 more entries added. This collection has been translated and published in many languages, including English, Russian, German, Latin, etc., for medical use and experimental researches.

I would like to give an example. Dr. Robert Temple, the Director for Drug Policy of Food and Drug Administration (FDA), USA, once delivered a lecture at the 3rd World Conference of Integrative Medicine in Guangzhou in 2002. He said, "Facing diseases, Eastern and Western medicine are in the same boat" .That means Chinese medicine and modern medicine need to converge or integrate with each other and be applied in a complementary way for better clinical practice, better medicinal resources and better medical progress.

For my second point, I invite you to look at some achievements of Chinese medicine. As we all understand, as an interpretive clinical service, we need to be patient and sensitive to provide high level function and high-quality service, and to pursue patient satisfaction and high-level contributions.

Here I would like to introduce a well-known Chinese medicine doctor, a great Master, Dr. PU Fu-zhou. In

1956, Dr. Pu treated encephalitis B patients, now also called encephalitis B, with a Chinese formula he created according to syndromes of summer febrile disease and summer hydrosis, and got a big success. Another great Chinese medicine doctor is Master YUE Mei-zhong. I was honored to have Dr. Yue as my mentor learning Chinese medicine theories and engaging in clinical practice under his guidance from 1956. Dr. Yue prescribed Chinese herbal medicines and cured the former Indonesia President Sukarno, who once suffered from renal calculus with left kidney failure.

There is a great saying from a famous Chinese philosopher, Confucius. I would like to share with you. “Gentleman aims at harmony, but not uniformity. A common man seeks uniformity yet fails harmony. ” Chinese medicine looks quite different from modern medicine, yet in the spirit of this saying, we can develop through convergence with organization and integration.

A successful example is that Chinese experts integrate the Chinese and modern medicine treatment for cancer in order to get better treatment results and to enhance patients’ quality of life. One of common application is Fu Zheng Gu Ben (扶正固本)therapy by modulating the immune function of the cancer patients.

Artemisinin, is an outstanding fruit of the convergence with ordinary medicine. Due to its advantage, artemisinin has saved billions of lives so far. Artemisinin was extracted from Artemisia Annua L. with is the foundation of the four artemisinin-based combination therapies (ACT's)recommended by World Health Organization (WHO)as the first-line treatment for malaria. This slide showed the chemical structures of artemisinin and its derivates. This is a target of artemisinin which locates in metastatic melanoma cells in each ring stage.

Arsenic trioxide was primarily recorded in Ri Hua Zi Materia Medica, which is traditionally used for ulcer and carrion. In modern time, people use it for skin cancer and other diseases combined with calomelas and arenobufagin. The main chemical component of arsenic trioxide is As_2O_3, for treating acute promyelocytic leukemia (APL)as a Chinese herbal medicine. The mechanism of this drug for effectively treating APL lies in induction of cellular disintegration and apoptosis, demonstrated by Dr. WANG Zhen-yi and academician CHEN Zhu. Their work gives some hints to us that it is promising to develop innovative new drug by positively targeting at enhancing therapeutic efficacy.

There is an innovation that a physician from Hong Kong has demonstrated that orally taking arsenic trioxide was also effective in the treatment of APL.

My next topic is my team's work on Chinese medicine for the treatment of coronary heart disease (CHD). Chinese Health Report shows the total affected population of such disease is about 230 million. Every 10 to 12 seconds, there will be one person die of it in China. The same report also shows the incidence of sudden death is 41.84 per thousand on Chinese population of 1.3 billion. The actual number of sudden death in China is over half of million every year. Actually, such diseases must exist in ancient China. The researchers found that the lumen of the left coronary artery of this ancient female was markedly narrowed by more than 3/4. In 1972, an American famous cardiologist, Dr. Paul D. White, visited Beijing. When he knew this story he said, “I believe there should be some active herbal drugs for coronary heart disease within TCM” .In recent forty years, we have carried out some clinical trials of “ABC” (activating blood circulation)formulae to treat CHD, including CH-2 and Xuefu Zhuyu Decoction (血府逐瘀汤). “ABC” here means activating microcirculation and removing stasis. Herbs or formulae with such functions are widely used for treating CHD nowadays[1-3]

CH-2 is a Chinese herbal medicine normally named as Component of Coronary Heart No. Ⅱ (冠心二号, 精制冠心颗粒).It is a compound formula developed by my team for treating CHD, which could be used for anti-angina pectoris, anti-platelet, and prevention of restenosis after percutaneous coronary intervention (PCI) in CHD. This formula consists of five herbs, including *Ligusticum wallichii*, *Paeonia rubra*, *Salvia miltiorrhiza*, *Carthamus tinctorius* and *Dalbergia odorifera*. Our researches proved that this compound formula could reduce the frequency of myocardial ischemia attack, and prevent platelet aggregation and arthrosclerosis. Some chemical components of CH-2 can enhance the fibrinolytic activity.

Tetramethylpyrazine (ligustrazine)is one of the active compounds of CH-2. We have demonstrated its pharmacological effects and analyzed its toxicity and metabolism. The results of our work show that this drug may pass through the blood brain barrier and contribute to ABC-herbs' clinical effects by inhibiting thromboxane B2 (TXB2)production. Tetramethypyrazine has been widely applied for treating ischemic stroke nowadays.

These ABC-herbal medicines may also serve as anti-platelet agents, including *Paeoniae rubra, Salvia miltiorrhiza*, Ligusticum wallichii, etc. There are also other effective components isolated from herbal medicines with anti-platelet property, such as propylgallate, salvianic acid A and berberine.

In the past decades, great scientific progresses have been achieved using PCI with an ending to dilate the narrowed (stenotic)coronary arteries to treat acute myocardial attack. It is a very effective therapeutic method, which has cured so many patients. However, there are still patients who might occur restenosis post PCI by thrombosis.

PCI can dilate the narrowed vessels, yet some patients may suffer from restenosis 3-to 6-month. With technical consideration on Chinese and modern medicine and our experiences, we treat each patient holistically not only using several powerful assays, but also paying attention to "vulnerable patient".

What does the "vulnerable patient" mean? Vulnerable plaques are not the only culprit factor. Vulnerable blood and vulnerable myocardium play important roles in the development of acute coronary syndromes, myocardial infarction, and sudden cardiac death. "Vulnerable patient" is proposed to define subjects susceptible to an acute coronary syndrome or sudden cardiac death based on plaque, blood, and myocardial vulnerability. To prevent attack of vulnerable plaques from breaking due to the high occurrence rate and to decrease vulnerable factors such as restenosis post-PCI, we have chosen a famous Chinese medicine compound formula Xuefu Zhuyu Decoction as a treatment in accordance with its evidence of pharmacological studies. This is a typical recipe of activating blood circulation and removing stasis created by WANG Qing-ren (1768-1831 A.D.)of the Qing Dynasty. Raeoniae Paeoniae rubra and Ligusticum wallichii are the two main herbs of this formula. Based on this prescription, Ligusticum-Phenols and Paeonea-glycosides, two effective compounds, were well intermixed to make granules and enclosed into capsules (Xiongshao Capsule, 芎芍胶囊, XS0601).To obtain the efficacy evidence of XS0601, 335 cases suffering from CHD were enrolled in this study on evidence-based method study, and 308 cases completed with 147 repeated angiography.

In this multicenter clinical trial, 9 big hospitals involved including Beijing Anzhen Hospital, Beijing Xiyuan Hospital, Beijing Tongren Hospital, Guandong Provincial Hospital, China-Japan Friendship Hospital, and so on. Patients were divided into two groups, control and treatment groups. Patients of the treatment group were given XS0601 combined with standard treatment post-PCI, while patients of the control group only underwent standard treatment post-PCI. The result of the treatment group was significantly different with the control group in reducing the incidence of restenosis after a year. From a comparison of clinical ending between these two groups, there is no difference in the rates of death, nonfatal myocardial infarction (MI)and coronary artery bypass grafting (CABG)between the two groups, while the repeated PCI rate is significant different (1.91% vs. 4.6%)after a year, from the end-point events of the Chinese medicine treatment. [4]

Studies could demonstrate the mechanisms of experiments on each Chinese medicine of this formula. We found that each herbal medicine can play a role in decreasing platelet agglutination, immigration and generation of contractile fiber cells, vascular remodeling, secretion of extracellular matrix, and anti-thrombosis formation. We also established an improved method for evaluating the vascular elasticity of coronary artery.

Currently, medical scientific studies are becoming from evidence-based medicine (EBM)to value-based medicine (VBM).Academician CHEN Zhu emphasized, "Braking down the barrier between Chinese and Western medicine calls for convergence of cognitive powers of East and West. It is an inexorable trend of development and intellectual elevation leading modern medicine towards new heights."

Meanwhile, "The development of traditional Chinese medicine does not mean hostility between academic schools fighting for superiority. This development means divergent medical traditions coming together through exchange to jointly lend impetus to the progress of medical science of mankind. " said academician HAN Qi-de.

In brief, the convergence of Chinese medicine and modern medicine is a challenge full of difference, comparison, and complementation and win-win opportunities.

REFERENCES

[1] Chen KJ. Blood stasis syndrome and its treatment with activating blood circulation to remove blood stasis therapy. Chin J Integr Med 2012, 18: 891-896.

[2] Chen KJ. Certain progress in the treatment of coronary heart disease with traditional medicinal plants in China. Am J Chin Med 1981, 9: 193-196.

[3] Xiao PG, Chen KJ. Recent advances in clinical studies of Chinese medical herbs. Intern J Thytotherr Res 1987, 1 (2): 53-57.

[4] Chen KJ, Shi DZ, Xu H, et al. XS0601 reduces the incidence of restenosis: a prospective study of 335 patients undergoing percutaneous coronary intervention in China. Chin Med J 2006, 119: 6-13.

First published: Chen KJ. Common glory: the traditional and the contemporary—complementary nature of Chinese and modern medicine—A speech at Nobel Laureate Summit and Academician Forum of Medicine (2014)[J]. Chin J Integr Med, 2015, 21 (10): 723-726.

Development Track of the Modern Activating Blood Circulation and Removing Stasis (ABCRS)School on Inheritance and Innovation

CHEN Ke-ji

More than fifty years, the Research Group of Blood Stasis Syndrome (BSS)in Xiyuan Hospital, China Academy of Chinese Medical Sciences have made a systematic clinical progress on BBS research. This paper would like to introduce its brief history, contributions, formation of academic school of thoughts, the three schools of learning lineage, the uniformity of this syndrome nomenclature, BBS differentiative diagnosis and its criteria, clinical progress on ten classifications with BBS, innovation of BBS theories, the representative formulae for treating BBS patients especially applying activating blood stasis formulas for treating coronary heart disease including for the prevention of post-stenting patients and the mechanisms.

1 A Brief History

Hypertension Study Group (1956), commencement of collaborative research of cardiovascular disease with Fuwai Hospital of Chinese Academy of Medical Sciences (1959), first paper on Chinese Medicine treatment experience of atherosclerosis published (1962), Premier ZHOU En-lai's instruction to establish Coronary Heart Disease Coordination Group in Beijing area, with Academician WU Ying-kai and Professor HUANG Wan of Fuwai Hospital taking the lead and Xiyuan Hospital as deputy (16-hospital joint research on ABCRS Compound Guanxin Ⅱ[(冠心Ⅱ号), 1972], China-Japan, China-Japan-Korea International ABCRS Conferences (1992, 1994, 2000), First World Integrative Medicine Congress (1997), Cross-Strait ABCRS Symposium (1994), establishment of Cardiovascular Disease Research Laboratory, Xiyuan Hospital, China Academy of Traditional Chinese Medicine (1978), foundation of Special Committee of ABCRS, China Integrative Medicine (1981), invited to National Institutes of Health-National Center for Complementary and Alternative Medicine (NIH-NCCAM), Oxford University, University of California, Toyama Medical and Pharmaceutical University, Seoul University, Kyung Hee University, and other countries and regions to give lectures on ABCRS studies, establishment of the Cardiovascular Institute of China Academy of Chinese Medical Sciences (2013).

2 Formation of Academic School of Thoughts

The emergence of academic schools is a universal phenomenon. It covers mathematics, physics, chemistry, astrology, geology and biology, among many other disciplines. Chinese and modern medicines are no exceptions to this rule. Englishman Joseph Needham (1900–1995)asserted that "yin-yang theory is the ultimate tenet by which ancient Chinese people were able to conceive", hence it brought forth a wealth of schools, more than one thousand branches. Four generations of modern ABCRS school has journeyed the past 50 plus years of clinical practices and studies and are still making progress.

3 Three Schools of Learning Lineage

"Medical Canons of the Yellow Emperor (Huang Di Nei Jing)", "Synopsis of Golden Chamber (Jin Gui Yao Lue)" and "Correction on Errors in Medical Classics (Yi Lin Gai Cuo)".

4 Uniformity of Disease Nomenclature

The advent of ABCRS is indicated for prevention and treatment of BSS. Before the Ming Dynasty, many terms are used to describe BSS. The word 'stasis' was first seen in "The Songs of the Chu (Chu Ci)", taking the meaning of "unregulated running of blood" and "uneven or obstructed blood flow" .In "Medical Canons of the Yellow Emperor" the names take the connotations from "clotting of blood" , "obstruction of the meridian" , "clotted bleeding blood" , "foul blood" to "loss of blood" .It is depicted in "Treatise on Cold Pathogenic and Miscellaneous Diseases (Shang Han Za Bing Lun)" as "blood pooling" and "dried blood" . "Synopsis of Golden Chamber" however, has a dedicated section for Disease Pulse and Syndrome Treatment of Blood Stasis. In international conferences participated by delegates from China, Japan and Korea, we advocated the use of "BSS" as the collective nomenclature and this was acknowledged and accepted.

5 Innovation of Theories

Loss of harmony between qi and blood (representing yin and yang)will lead to blood stasis both inside and outside of the blood vessels. This teaching emphatically advocates the theories of harmony between qi and blood, and the combination of dredging and tonifying methods. In fact, WANG Qing-ren (1768–1831)of the Qing Dynasty was singularly acclaimed for his medical expertise for his creation of Xuefu Zhuyu Decoction (血府逐瘀汤), Buyang Huanwu Decoction (补阳还五汤), Shaofu Zhuyu Decoction (少腹逐瘀汤)and Tongqiao Huoxue Decoction (通窍活血汤)exactly because he possessed the similar concepts. We were able to advance this innovative development based on the theories and their inheritance.[1-3]

6 Ten Stasis Classifications

In accordance to clinical experiences and understandings, we presented the Ten Stasis Classifications, namely acute stasis, slow stasis, cold stasis, heat stasis, wound stasis, old stasis, toxic stasis, phlegm stasis, gas stasis, and prior stasis (latent stasis).[4,5]

7 Stasis Present in Many Diseases

Diseases with BSS are seen in many body systems, rising the hope that different diseases can be treated in the same way, including heart, brain, kidney, blood, digestive, respiratory, liver and gallbladder, endocrine, connective tissue, metabolic system, immune system, gynecological, pediatrics, skin, traumatology, orthopedics, EENT, cancer and others.[6,7]

8 Ten Principles Syndrome Differentiation

The eight principles syndrome differentiation plus qi and blood syndrome differentiations would make it more comprehensive. It would seem that qi and blood could take the places of the traditional yin and yang principles.[1,3]

9 Modern Classifications

Because of macro-and microscopic biological and rheological changes in amplitudes and sizes, BSS could be classified into two types, with corresponding variations in their pathogenesis and therapeutic approaches.[5]

10 Diagnostic Standards

We were able to determine macroscopically that dark-purple tongue, characteristic pain, lumps, abnormal blood vessels or veins and various bleeding as diagnostic standards of BSS, at the same time establish a standard qualitative and quantitative scoring table covering test items such as fibrinolytic activity, platelet function, in vitro thrombosis time and those generally accepted and employed in the field. Subsequently, a clinical acute coronary syndromes stasis-toxin syndrome differentiation standard was also established.

11 ABCRS Medications Classifications

These can be attributed to three major types namely blood mixing, blood activating and blood expelling, and are prescribed according to symptoms for clinical use.

12 Clinical Effects

In the treatment of coronary heart diseases using the Three Purges and Two Replenishment approaches, blood activating and stasis removing is the first focus. It has been proven of practical value in treating angina, myocardial infarction, heart failure, peri-percutaneous coronary intervention care and stroke.

13 Representative Formulae

Guanxin Ⅱ[Refined Guanxin Granules, Tablets, Capsules (精制冠心颗粒/片/胶囊)], Refined Xuefu Capsule (精制血府胶囊), Yugeng Tongyu Decoction (愈梗通瘀汤), Yuxintong Preparation (愈心痛方), ligustrazine injection and tablets, propyl gallate, Xiongshao Preparation (芎芍方).

14 Systematic Studies of BSS Pathogenesis and Mechanisms of Action of Its Medications

Systematic studies were carried out on ABCRS to activate blood and eliminate stasis treatment approach, efficacy studies of Guanxin Ⅱ, Xuefu Zhuyu Decoction, ligustrazine, propyl gallate, Yuxintong Preparation and Yugeng Tongyu Decoction on anti-platelet function, vascular endothelium protection, cardiac muscle remodeling and microcirculation improvement, and molecular biological mechanisms of action, developing a series of BSS animal models.[3,4,7]

15 Four Generations and Over 50 Years of Relentless Studies

More than two hundred doctoral students, postdoctoral researchers and successor students were trained. Graduates practicing overseas can be found in the United States, Canada, Singapore, South Korea, Australia and others.

16 Representative Works

"Blood Stasis Syndrome and Promoting Blood Circulation to Remove Blood Stasis" (CHEN Ke-ji, ZHANG Zhi-nan, Liang JZ, editors, 1987, Shanghai Science and Technology Press), "Cardiovascular Diseases and Promoting Blood Circulation to Remove Blood Stasis" (CHEN Ke-ji, 2009, Beijing Science and Technology Press), "Basic and Clinical Cardiovascular Diseases of Integrative Chinese and Western Medicine" (CHEN Ke-ji, SHI Da-zhuo, XU Hao, editors, 2014, Peking University Medical Press), and others.[8]

17 ABCRS School Representatives

Building on the promoting blood circulation to remove stasis clinical experiences of master Chinese medicine physician GUO Shi-kui, our team of over 200 persons working in unity through decades of dedicated efforts to form today's modern ABCRS School.[9-12]

18 National Awards

BSS and Research Studies on Promoting Blood Circulation to Remove Blood Stasis (National Science and Technology Progress Award First Class, 2003), Guanxin Ⅱ (Guanxin Ⅱ Formula)Pharmacodynamics Study (National Science and Technology Progress Award Second Class, 2000).

19 ABCRS Community

Doctor GUO Shi-kui is proclaimed a National Model Worker in 1980, ABCRS team of China Academy of Chinese Medical Sciences for Cardiovascular Diseases was awarded the National Outstanding Professional and Technical Advanced Team (2014)by the Organization Department of the Communist Party of China Central Committee, the Central Propaganda Department, Human Resources Ministry and Ministry of Science and Technology, and Academician CHEN Ke-ji for National Outstanding Professional and Technical Advanced Individual (2014).

20 Team Culture Motto

"Unity, inheritance, innovation and development", "opportunities of time vouchsafed by Heaven are not equal to advantages of situation afforded by the Earth, and advantages of situation afforded by the Earth are not equal to the union arising from the accord of men (Qin Mencius)".

21 Prospect

Modern ABCRS School is likened to an exotic flower in the garden of Chinese and integrative medicines confluence. ABCRS is the interface and point of integration of clinical and basic Chinese and Western medical sciences, and ABCRS contributes to the enhancement of clinical therapeutic effects.

REFERENCES

[1] Chen KJ, Zhang ZN, Liang ZJ, et al. Blood stasis syndrome and activating blood circulation to remove stasis[M]. Shanghai: Shanghai Science and Technology Press, 1987: 1-5.

[2] Chen KJ. Blood stasis syndrome and its treatment with activating blood circulation to remove stasis therapy[J]. Chin J Integ Med, 2012, 18: 891-896.

[3] Chen KJ, Guo SK, Chen ZJ, Kou WR, Wu XG Tao SQ, et al. The therapeutic effect of purified coronary heart Ⅱ tablets on 112 cases of angina pectoris by double blind method[J]. Chin J Cardiol (Chin), 1982, 10: 85-89.

[4] Chen KJ. Certain progress in the treatment of coronary heart disease with traditional medical plants in China[J]. Am Chin Med, 1981, 9: 193-196

[5] Luo J, Wang AL, Zhao W, Che FY, Fen Q, Yi DH, et al. Practical diagnostic criterion of blood stasis syndrome: introduction, reliability, and validity[J]. Chin J Integr Tradit West Med (Chin), 2015, 35: 950-956.

[6] Xiao PG, Chen KJ. Recent advances in clinical studies of Chinese medical herbs. Intern J Thytotherr Res, 1987, 1: 53-57.

[7] Lu AP, Chen KJ. Improving clinical practice guideline development in integration of traditional Chinese medicine and Western medicine[J]. Chin J Integr Med, 2015, 21: 163-165.

[8] Chen KJ, Shi DZ, Xu H, Lu SZ, Lv SZ, Li TC, et al. XS0601 reduces the incidence of restenosis: a prospective study of 335 patients undergoing percutaneous coronary intervention in China[J]. Chin Med J, 2006, 119: 6-13.

[9] Chen KJ. Reflections on human longevity and Chinese medicine prevention and treatment of chronic diseases[J]. Chin J Integr Med, 2015, 21: 643-647.

[10] Liu Y, Yin HJ, Shi DZ, Chen KJ. Chinese herb and formulas for promoting blood circulation and removing blood stasis and anti-platelet therapies[J]. Evid Based Complement Alternat Med, 2012, 2012: 184503.

[11] Xu H, Shi DZ, Chen KJ. Atherosclerosis: an integrative East-West medicine perspective[J]. Evid Based Complement Alternat, 2012, 2012: 148413.

[12] Jiao Y, Li SW, Shang QH. Multifactor dementionality reduction analysis of the correlation of Chinese medicine syndrome evolvement and cardiovascular events in patients in patients with stable coronary heart disease. Chin J Integr Med, 2014, 20: 341-346.

First published: CHEN Ke-ji. Development track of the modern activating blood circulation and removing stasis (ABCRS)school on inheritance and innovation[J]. Chin J Integr Med, 2015, 21 (12): 883-886.

Development Is A High Level Inheritance for China Time-honored Brand Products

CHEN Ke-ji

As culture is the soul of a nation, the three books, "History of Chinese Philosophy," "History of Chinese Culture" and "History of Chinese Science and Technology" have demonstrated the superiority of our great Chinese culture, and its significant impact in the field of international culture. Both core value and practical value of the Chinese culture are very clear, reflected in the views of universe, nature, life, health, disease, and therapy and related considerations, concepts, and technical methods.

The study of China Time-honored Brand products is an important part of our nation's comprehensive culture. Based on the statistics from the Committee of Ancient Book Management Commission of the State Department of China, there are more than 100, 000 copies of extant ancient books in China now, and ancient Chinese medicine books amounted to 10, 000, accounting for one tenth of the total ancient books. These books represent spiritual civilization, material, most concrete manifestation of science and technology civilization in China's medicine history, and the achievements of the Chinese medicine have been passed from generation to generation.

The culture of Chinese medicine is profound. We should inherit these precious treasures but we also should be creative. First of all, as the essence of the traditional culture and clinical practice, the Chinese medicine has a long history. About 2, 000 products of China Time-honored Brand, including about 200 Chinese herbal medicine products, have been brought together to the China National Cultural Cooperative Organization of Medicine and Pharmaceuticals. For the development of Chinese herbal medicine and pharmaceuticals, these products should be well inherited, promoted and used for public. The inheritance should not be limited to the cultural concepts, and should include in-depth study on formulation technique, clinical efficacy, and clinical indications. Only development is the high level inheritance.

Secondly, inheritance should go with innovation. The preparation techniques of Chinese medicine should be studied, and its essence should be integrated into today's latest formulation technology. The further evaluation, observation and discussion of the efficacy of Chinese medicine should be faced scientifically. We should not only take the treatment effects from previous books as the basis and support, but also be responsible and confident to have the efficacy of the China Time-honored Brand herbal medicine, the old Chinese medicine drugs further tested using clinical evidence-based medicine and biostatistics methods, and explain the actual indications of these excellent Chinese medicine comprehensively and even expand the application. This shares the same importance as the heritage of the Chinese medicine culture and specific techniques.

Thirdly, the China Time-honored Brand companies, in the development of the Chinese pharmaceuticals, should take the leading role, especially in the field of medicinal academic exchange. Traditional Chinese enterprises, especially the China Time-honored Brand companies should actively share their good practice experiences with other companies nationwide, to form a broad, good atmosphere of the traditional academic exchanges in Chinese medicine firms, with particular focus on the exchanges of classic prescriptions. In this progressing era, there should be an open attitude in scientific research and exchange. The China Time-honored Brand enterprises should not be conservative. Under appropriate conditions, the material basis of the efficacy should be studied. For the classics prescriptions, there should be a theory to explain the material properties related to the excellent efficacy. For the drug designed for long-term use, its safety and possible adverse reactions should be observed. Qualified enterprises should perform pharmacokinetic and pharmacodynamic studies.

For the heritance, innovation and development of Chinese medicine, academic and cultural exchanges are urgently needed. China National Cultural Cooperation Organization of Medicine and Pharmaceuticals has built a good platform to further implement the mechanisms of communication.

Regarding the policy of heritage and protection of Chinese medicinal culture, the Department of Commerce of China has an evaluation policy for the traditional companies. Right now the law of Chinese medicine is at the stage of public comments. The attention from the society also benefits the transmission of Chinese medicinal culture.

For the scientific popularization of the Chinese medicinal culture, the China Time-honored Brand industry employees of different companies with different education, skill levels, and consumer awareness and acceptance may have different understanding. These employees need scientific and technical guidance and policy support.

In the field of general health, I very much agree that the China Time-honored Brand herbal product has a good prospect for future development. However, the companies for these Chinese medicine must pay attention to the study and research for potential adverse reactions related to long-term use. For Chinese medicine pharmaceuticals or health care products intended for long-term use, companies should conduct pharmacokinetics and safety/toxicology studies, and pay attention to individual differences with long-term follow-up studies. We are in the information age, and the advanced data technology should be combined with the research in these China Time-honored Brand products'study.

First published: Chen KJ. Development Is A High Level Inheritance for China Time-honored Brand Products[J]. Chin J Integr Med, 2014, 20 (11): 803-804.

Blood Stasis Syndrome and Its Treatment with Activating Blood Circulation to Remove Blood Stasis Therapy

CHEN Ke-ji

1 Clinical and Practical Values in Diagnosis of Blood Stasis Syndrome

Blood Stasis Syndrome is a diagnosis that indicates a very strong sense of traditional Chinese medicine. It can relate to a lot of diseases, therefore, it has great clinical and practical values. Traditionally, chronic diseases and slow-progressing diseases mostly involve blood stasis. Severe warm diseases and trauma mostly involve acute blood stasis. Nowadays, the combined use of microscopic and macroscopic diagnoses helps us understand the variety of blood stasis. It also helps us learn about the clinical presentations of hidden blood stasis syndrome and pre-blood stasis syndrome. Recently, numerous countries that have started the clinical and experimental investigation in such topics already show some progress in their studies. American medical doctors recognize some "activating blood circulation herbs" (ABC herbs)which basically are the Chinese herbs that invigorate blood and transform blood stasis. Oketsu Syndrome, a term used by Japanese medical doctors, is found to refer to the Blood Stasis Syndrome in Chinese term.

Blood Stasis Syndrome means the circulation of blood is not smooth or blood flow is stagnant and forms stasis. This condition can be found in many ancient Chinese medical classics. The writings from Han Dynasty, which was excavated in the city of Wuwei in Gansu province, documented the use of invigorating blood and transforming stasis herbs like *Radix Angelicae Sinensis* (Dang Gui), *Cortex Moutan Radicis* (Dan Pi), and *Rhizoma Ligustici Chuanxiong* (Chuan Xiong)in the "blood stasis treatment formula" . *Divine Husbandman's Classic of the Materia Medica* (Shen Nong Ben Cao Jing)described 365 herbs. Among which 41herbs belong to the class of invigorating blood and removing stasis. In the book of *Simple Questions from the Yellow Emperor's Inner Classic* (Su Wen from Huang Di Nei Jing), explained the use of *Radix Rubiae* (Qian Cao)and others to treat "amenorrhea due to blood dryness" .Famous ancient Chinese doctor ZHANG Zhong jing even made a thesis on blood stasis.[1]

From our clinical study, blood stasis is related to the obstruction in micro-circulation, irregularity in hemorheology, abnormality in hemodynamics, abnormality in the formation of scar tissue, and etc. As a result, the following diseases are possibly related to the presentation of Blood Stasis Syndrome (Table 1).Based on different extent of the diseases, reasonable treatment plans can be developed.

Since blood stasis syndrome can be related to various diseases, the clinical use of blood-invigorating and stasis-removing herbs in associated diseases become more plausible. Their therapeutic effectiveness can be clearly shown. Thus, the "blood-invigorating and stasis-removing phenomenon" becomes more widely discussed. However, the abuse in using those herbs should be avoided. Caution should always be taken to differentiate clinical application.

2 The Establishment of Current Standards in the Diagnosis of Blood Stasis Syndrome

In October, 1988, an "International Conference on Blood Stasis Syndrome" was held in Beijing, China. In the meeting, academia from Japan, Korea, Singapore etc., recognized the following standards for diagnosing Blood Stasis Syndrome: (1)Purple tongue or blood stasis spots on tongue, (2)Typical choppy pulse or no pulse, (3)Pain occurs in a fixed, local point (or chronic pain, stabbing pain, aversion to pressure), (4)Blood stasis in abdomen, (5)Accumulation of blood stasis, (6)Bleeding out of vessels (hemorrhage, bruises due to trauma), (7)Mucosal blood stasis, abnormality in blood vessels and collecterals, (8)Dysmenorrhea with dark blood clots, amenorrhea, (9)Abnormality on skin and nails, Numbness in hemiplegia, (11)Mania due to blood stasis, and (12)Laboratory work-up shows stasis in blood circulation.

Table 1 The Diseases Possibly Related to the Presentation of Blood Stasis Syndrome in Different Systems

System	Disease
Cardiovascular system	Coronary artery disease, angina pectoris, myocardial infarction, rheumatic heart disease, heart failure, vasculitis
Digestive system	Gastric/peptic ulcer, gastritis, esophageal hemorrhage, chronic hepatitis, cirrhosis
Respiratory system	Chronic obstructive pulmonary disease, mountain sickness, altitude stress
Urological system	Acute/chronic nephritis, hematuria
Blood system	Polycythemia vera, purpura, disseminated intravascular coagulation
Nervous system	Stroke, head injury, chronic headache, schizophrenia, Parkinson's disease, peripheral neuropathy
Immune system	Psoriasis, lupus erythematosus, rheumatoid arthritis, urticaria, angioedema
Metabolic system	Hyperlipidemia, diabetic neuropathy, diabetic angiopathy
Connective tissue system	Burn, keloid tissue from trauma, corneal scar formation
Obstetrics and	Gynecology Functional uterine bleeding, dysmenorrheal, endometriosis, ectopic pregnancy, uterine leiomyoma
Pediatrics	Neonatal scleredema, neonatal hepatitis, neonatal purpura
Dermatology	Erythematous nodules, dyspigmentation, acne rosacea
Ophthalmology	Retinal angiemphraxis, immune diseases, degenerative diseases
Oral-pharyngeal	Ear, nose and throat: trigeminal neuralgia, sudden deafness
Orthopedics	Bone fractures
Surgery	Some acute abdominal pain
Oncology	Angioma, liver carcinoma, etc.
Organ transplant	Rejection of transplanted organ

Explanation: (1)The occurrence of any one of the above criteria can be diagnosed as Blood Stasis Syndrome, (2)Each medical discipline should establish their own detailed standards for blood stasis diagnosis, (3)In case of concomitant diseases, treatment should be based on the complete examination of all diseases.

The above standard on one hand presents the characteristics of traditional Chinese medicine, on the other hand, it includes the current examination in Western medicine. Therefore, this guideline is the result of a study from the combined use of macroscopic, microscopic and current perspectives.

The authors also investigated the effectiveness of using the Blood Stasis Syndrome diagnosis standards by making multi-factorial analysis, regressive analysis as well as differential analysis. They firstly suggested the use of such combined macroscopic and microscopic views in diagnosing standards to be put in clinical study. Eventually, this suggestion was widely accepted. The result is presented in Table 2.

Remarks: Grades < 19 points are categorized as non-Blood Stasis Syndrome. Grades 20–49 points are categorized as less severe Blood Stasis Syndrome. Grades > 50 points are categorized as more severe blood stasis syndrome.

The above standards and grading system will be examined in more details for further improvement.

3 Categorization of Common Blood-Invigorating and Stasis-Removing Herbs in Clinical Use

The author of this article has completed a statistical analysis on sixteen Chinese traditional medicine materia medica classics. There are 150 commonly used blood-invigorating and stasis removing herbs. But a few herbs are documented differently among the Classics. Those which share consistency in documentation in the Classics can be divided into three categories. This method of categorization has been approved in the Chinese National Academic Conference of Blood-Invigoration and Stasis-Removing. This method has been highly recommended and applied in China.[1]

3.1 Harmonizing Blood Herbs

Functions: nourish blood and regulate blood vessels

Examples: *Radix Angelicae Sinensis* (Dang Gui), *Cortex Moutan Radicis* (Dan Pi), *Radix Salviae Miltiorrhizae* (Dan Shen), *Radix Rehmanniae Recens* (Sheng Di Huang), *Radix Paeoniae Rubra* (Chi Shao Yao), and *Caulis Spatholobi* (Ji Xue Teng), total of 6 herbs.

Table 2 The Grading System in Quantifying Blood Stasis Syndrome Diagnosis Standards

Signs and symptom	Point
Purple tongue	(less severe)8, (more severe)10
Resistance to pressure in lower abdomen	(less severe)8, (more severe)10
Choppy pulse	10
Dark stool (Melena)	10
Pathogenic nodules	10
Distended veins under tongue	(less severe)8, (more severe)10
Irregular pulse	8
No pulse	10
Distended veins in abdominal wall	10
Hypodermal ecchymoses	(less severe)8, (more severe)10
Dark menstrual blood with clots	(less severe)10, (more severe)10
Persistent angina pectoris	10
General fixed pain	8
Dark red lips and gums	6
Small vessels	5
Numb extremities5	5
Surgery history	5
Mucosal membrane of palate (+)	(less severe)4, (more severe)5
Paralysis in extremities	(less severe)5, (more severe)7
Psychiatric abnormality	(Irritability)4, (Mania)8
Rough skin	(less severe)4, (more severe)5
Complete blood viscosity (+)	10

Continued

Signs and symptom	Point
Blood plasma viscosity (+)	5
External clot net weight (+)	10
External clot total weight (+)	8
Increase in platelet aggregation	10
Abnormality in blood clot elasticity	8
Microcirculation obstruction	10
Hemodynamics obstruction	10
Decrease in fiber dissolution activity	10
Resistance in platelet release	10
Pathogenic scan (+)for blood stasis	10
Blood vessel obstruction by new technology analysis	10

3.2 Invigorating Blood Herbs

Functions: invigorate blood and move blood to remove stasis

Examples: *Rhizoma Ligustici Chuanxiong* (Chuan Xiong), *Pollen Typhae* (Pu Huang), *Flos Carthami* (Hong Hua), *Artemisiae Anomalae Herba* (Liu Ji Nu), *Faeces Trogopterori* (Wu Ling Zhi), *Radix Curcumae* (Yu Jin), *Radix et Rhizoma Notoginseng* (San Qi), *Squama Manis* (Chuan Shan Jia), *Rhizoma Lignum Suberalatum* (Gui Jian Yu), *Campsitis Flos* (Zi Wei), and *Semen Vaccariae* (Wang Bu Liu Xin), total of 20herbs.

3.3 Breaking Stasis Herbs

Functions: breaking blood remove stasis, very strong action

Examples: *Radix et Rhizoma Rhei* (Da Huang), *Hirudo* (Shui Zhi), *Tabanus* (Meng Chong), *Holotrichiae Vermiculus* (Qi Cao), *Pyritum* (Zi Ran Tong), *Rhizoma Sparganii* (San Leng), *Rhizoma Curcumae* (E Zhu), *Olibanum* (Ru Xiang), *Myrrha* (Mo Yao), *Sanguis Draconis* (Xue Jie), and *Semen Persicae* (Tao Ren), total of 11 herbs.

Among the above herbs, the study examined 34 of them in 26 hemodynamic tests and comparison study was done. The result showed that the degree of strength between blood-breaking herbs and blood-invigorating herbs was actually different.

4 Comparative Study in the Effectiveness between Commonly Used Blood- Invigorating and Stasis-Removing Herbal Formula

Herbal formulae are commonly used in Traditional Chinese medicine. Based on the differentiation in Zang Fu (Viscera and Bowels), differentiation between excess and deficiency, differentiation between qi stagnation and qi deficiency, differentiation in severity of blood stasis, differentiation between cold stasis and heat toxins, differentiation between acute trauma and chronic wearing/tearing, and differentiation in wind phlegm etc., combined use of herbal formula in specific conditions can be studied. Traditionally, the Eight Principles are applied to make diagnosis in clinical use. In fact, it should be modified to become the Ten Principles to include differentiation between qi and blood.

Commonly used herbal formulae are:

Moving blood to stop pain formulae, e.g. Xuefu Zhuyu Decoction (血府逐瘀汤), Huoluo Xiaoling Pill (活络效灵丹), (2)Benefit qi to smooth out collecterals/vessels formulae e.g. Buyang Huanwu Decoction (补阳还五汤), (3)Breaking blood to remove stasis formulae e.g. Dahuang Zhechong Pill (大黄䗪虫丸), (4) Transforming stasis, clearing Heat and cooling blood formulae e.g. Taoren Chengqi Decoction (桃仁承气汤), Xianfang Huoming Decoction (仙方活命饮), (5)Removing stasis and regenerating formulae e.g. Shaofu Zhuyu

Decoction (少腑逐瘀汤), (6)Moving blood and stopping bleeding formulae e.g. Modified Sheng Yu Decoction (圣愈汤), (7)Removing stasis and regenerating formulae e.g. Taoren Chengqi Decoction (桃仁承气汤), Didang Decoction (抵当汤), (8)Transforming stasis to stop pain and connect bones/tendons formulae e.g. Qili Powder (七厘散), Dieda Pill (跌打丸), (9)Assisting pregnancy and calming fetus formulae e.g. Modified Desheng Pill (加味得生丹), (10)Dispersing cold to remove stasis formulae e.g. Wenjing Decoction (温经汤), (11)Clearing heat toxins and removing stasis formulae e.g. Xijiao Dihuang Decoction (犀角地黄汤), (12)Transforming stasis and diuretic formulae e.g Danggui Shaoyao Powder (当归芍药散), and (13)Transforming phlegm and removing stasis formulae e.g. Huoxue Fang plus Banxia Baizhu Tianma Decoction (活血方加半夏白术天麻汤), Di Tan Decoction (涤痰汤), Wen Dan Decoction (温胆汤), etc. All these formulae show effective results. Other formulae include Danshen Decoction (丹参饮), Shixiao Powder (失笑散), Simiao Yong'an Decoction (四妙勇安汤), Taohong Siwu Decoction (桃红四物汤), Huazheng Huisheng Pill (化癥回生丹), Guan Xin No. 2 Formula (冠心二号方), etc. are also handy and effective formula.

The following are the examples of using ancient Chinese doctor ZHANG Zhong-jing's blood-invigorating and stasis-removing herbal formulae in today's clinical diseases (Table 3).

In Qing Dynasty, Chinese doctor WANG Qing-ren highly recommended the method of invigorating blood and removing stasis. He recognized the importance of qi and blood. He said, "qi has excess and deficiency, blood has deficiency and stasis". "Treat exterior symptoms by treating the root problems, treat root problems by examining exterior symptoms".He invented a category of blood-invigorating and stasis-removing herbal formulae which had been wildly used.

Table 3 Using ZHANG Zhong–jing's Herbal Formulae in Today's Clinical Diseases

Herbal formulae	Modern diseases
Danggui Shaoyao Powder (当归芍药散)	Alzheimer's Disease, degenerative memory
Wenjing Decoction (温经汤)	Amenorrhea, vaginal discharge
Hong Lan Hua Wine (红蓝花酒)	Gynecological diseases, pain in chest
Biejiajian Pill (鳖甲煎丸)	Hepato-splenomegaly
Dahuang Zhechong Pill (大黄䗪虫丸)	Rhematic heart disease
Taoren Chengqi Decoction (桃仁承气汤)	Psychiatric disorders
Didang Decoction (抵当汤)	Irregular menstruation
Xiayuxue Decoction (下瘀血汤)	Abdominal pain after delivery
Wangbu Liuxin Powder (王不留行散)	Traumatic bleeding

Another study consists of 8 classical blood-invigorating and stasis-removing herbal formulae that undergo comparative analysis of effectiveness in treating cerebral vascular disorders. This study shows Chinese doctor, WANG Qing-ren's several formulae are better than other classical formulae.

5 The Clinical Effectiveness of Blood-Invigorating and Stasis-Removing Herbal Formula in Treating Cerebral Vascular Diseases

The Study in Using Blood-Invigorating and Stasis-Removing Formulae including Guan Xin No. 2 Formula and Its Ingredients to Treat Angina Pectoris and to Examine Any Anti-Platelet Function.[2]

The late prestigious Chinese clinical doctor GUO Shi-kui is famous of using blood-invigorating and stasis-removing formulae to treat coronary heart disease and cardiovascular disorders. The author had been working with him as colleague since the 50's in the last century. The author saw Dr. Guo used large dosage of modified Xuefu Zhuyu Decoction to treat a patient with angina pectoris. This patient needed to take 100 nitroglycerin tablets in one week before treatment. After treatment, his intake of nitroglycerin was reduced to about 20 tablets per week. This motivated and opened the eyes of the author in this discipline of medicine. Dr. Guo worked in Fu Wai Hospitals for a long period of time to make rounding in wards as well as to be a medical consultant. He had abundant clinical experience in treating cardiovascular diseases. In 1960, the author concluded Dr. Guo's clinical experience in using blood-invigorating and stasis-removing formulae in treating coronary heart disease and published the results in medical journals. In 1972, Beijing District Coronary Heart Disease Cooperation was established, headed by Dr. WU Ying-kai, who was the President of the Fuwai Hospital. Dr. Guo and the author were involved in developing Guan Xin No. 2 Formula. In the same year, famous doctors and professors such as Drs. HUANG Wan, CHEN Zai-jia, SHAO Geng, GU Fu-sheng, JIN Yin-chang, KOU Wen-rong, CHEN Wen-wei, etc. also participated in this study. That formula is composed of *Rhizoma Ligustici Chuanxiong* (Chuan Xiong), *Radix Salviae Miltiorrhizae* (Dan Shen), *Radix Paeoniae Rubra* (Chi Shao), *Flos Carthami* (Hong Hua), *Lignum Dalbergiae Odoriferae* (Jiang Xiang), etc. in blood-invigorating and stasis-removing herbs. More than ten hospitals joined together in the study. Thousands of patients used this formula and effectiveness was seen in greater than 80%.Later on, the formula was made in extract tablet form for coronary heart disease. It was then compared with placebo for effectiveness study. This was the first study done in the method of randomized, double-blinded, placebo controlled study in the 1970's. The results showed clinical effectiveness of the formula versus placebo 80.4% and 16.1% respectively. The *Chinese Journal of Cardiovascular Disease* added an editorial article to the study and commenced that the study had "a strong and persuasive basis" .The authors also chose benefiting-qi and invigorating-blood herbs such as *Radix Ginseng Rubra* (Hong Shen), *Radix et Rhizoma Notoginseng* (San Qi), *Rhizoma Corydalis* (Yan Hu Suo)to treat unstable angina. Promising results were seen.

The author examined *Rhizoma Ligustici Chuanxiong* (Chuan Xiong), the main ingredient in Guan Xin No. 2 Formula, under electronic microscope, and discovered the anti-platelet aggregation effect of an organic alkaloid in tetramethylprazine (Chuanxiongzine).It was also observed the reduced formation of thromboxane A_2 (TXA_2).By coordinating the study with Beijing Pharmaceutical Industrial Laboratory and several hospitals in Beijing, the organic compound was proved effective in treating cerebral vascular diseases. This ingredient is widely and continually used in nowadays China.[3]

Later, several blood-invigorating herbs are found to possess the antiplatelet property. This opens a pathway in the future to use such herbs in treating thromboembolism. After the 1990's in last century, the use of blood-invigorating and stasis-removing herbs progresses in the treatment of cardiovascular and cerebral vascular diseases. The author is confident in the study of antiplatelet effect in Chi Shao 801 Formula.

The Study of Xuefu Zhuyu Decoction and Its Effective Ingredients in Preventing the Re-stenosis after Percutaneous Coronary Intervention (PCI)in Coronary Heart Disease. [4,5]

Applying the method in serologic pharmacology, the study showed that the formula suppressed the growing of vascular smooth muscle cells (VSMCs), and affected the mRNA expression in platelet-derived growth factor alpha and beta polypeptides (PDGF-α, PDGF-β), c-fos, ras and c-myc. In the National 8th Five-year Study, the author and his colleagues, joining Peiking University the Third Clinical Medical School and Beijing Anzhen Hospital, observed higher effectiveness in using the processed product of Xuefu Zhuyu Decoction than using Western medicines to prevent renarrowing of blood vessels and recurrent angina pectoris after successful percutaneous transluminal coronary angioplasty (PTCA), and stent placement in 265 cases. In the National 10th Five-year Study, Beijing Anzhen Hospital, Beijing Tongren Hospital, China-Japan Friendship Hospital and Guangdong Provincial Hospital of Traditional Chinese Medicine coordinated a multi-center, randomized, controlled trial of 335 cases with a follow-up study on clinical endpoints, on the effectiveness of the active ingredients of Xuefu Zhuyu Decoction (Xiong-Shao Capsule, 芎芍胶囊): the compound of Chi Shao glycoside and Chuan Xiong phenol. The study showed the capsules of the compound met the Western pharmaceutical standard. Coronary-angiography was rechecked in 47.7%.The need for second time PCI or CABG in the use of Xiong-Shao Capsule verses Western medicine plus placebo are 1.91% and 4.46% respectively. The Xuefu Zhuyu Decoction group also showed a lower mortality rate and lower blood stasis grade points. This has double meanings in clinical perspective.

REFERENCES

[1] Chen KJ, Zhang ZN. The research on blood stasis and its treatment with ABC herbs. Shanghai: Shanghai Science-Technology Press, 1987.

[2] Chen KJ, Guo SK, Kou WR, et al. The clinical double blind study on 112 cases of CHD-anginal pectoris with purified coronary No. Tablet. Chin J Cardiol (Chin)1982, 10: 85-89.

[3] Chen KJ, Shi DZ. Tetramethylpyrazine: chemistry, pharmacology and clinical application. Beijing: People's Medical Publishing House Press, 1999.

[4] Chen KJ, Shi DZ, Xu H, et al. XS0601 reduces the incidences of restenosis: a prospective study of 335 patients undergoing PCI in China. Chin Med J 2006, 119: 2-7.

[5] Chen KJ, Xu H. Integrative medicine: the experience from China. J Altern Complement Med 2008, 14: 3.

First published: CHEN Ke-ji. Blood stasis syndrome and its treatment with activating blood circulation to remove blood stasis therapy[J]. Chin J Integr Med, 2012, 18 (12): 891-896.

Foreword of *Contemporary Introduction to Chinese Medicine —In Comparison with Western Medicine*

CHEN Ke-ji

Professor Xie Zhufan，Director Emeritus of Peking University Institute of Integrated Traditional Chinese and Western Medicine，is a renowned internist and integrated traditional Chinese medicine and Western medicine specialist in China.

A distinguished，erudite scholar and a clinician par excellence of forthright character，Professor Xie is a highly respected and close friend of mine for decades. His exemplary works on basic neuroendocrinology studies of Cold & Heat Theories of traditional Chinese medicine have been leading the field with solid progresses.Over the years，Professor Xie has headed several task forces on English standardization of traditional Chinese medicine nomenclatures sponsored by World Health Organization and State Administration of Traditional Chinese Medicine of China with outstanding achievements. With his extensive proficiencies in both traditional Chinese and Western medicines，Professor Xie excels in the adaptation of traditional · Chinese medical science into English and has been universally recognized as the best in the field.Amongst his abundant translated works，"On the Standard Nomenclature of Traditional Chinese Medicine" has been the most representative.

An energetic octogenarian of highest professional standards，Professor Xie works ceaselessly and tirelessly to promote academic exchanges and international collaboration in medicine.This book，*Contemporary Introduction to Chinese Medicine in Comparison with Western Medicine* is one of his recent works in collaboration with Dr.Xie Fang.The aim of this work is to provide Western practitioners a systematic approach to study，comprehend and practice traditional Chinese medicine.In spite of the vast and all-encompassing nature of traditional Chinese medicine and considerable difficulty in technical adaptation to English，Professor Xie and Dr.Xie are able，on the one hand，to maintain Chinese cultural characteristics throughout the dissertation，and on the other，stand on the Western readers' perspectives to ensure that the essence of this work is easy to read，study，comprehend and hence，to apply.This book faithfully lays out basic theories of traditional Chinese medicine，and diagnostic and therapeutic principles，with full attention on the most updated treatment of diseases commonly seen in the West such as allergic，arthritic and gastrointestinal disorders，hypertensive，coronary heart and diabetic diseases，metabolic syndromes and tumors.Fluent in language and style，it is an extremely handy and practical tool，the best of its kind one can find nowadays.

It is indeed most rewarding，and my great pleasure，to preface this work to all.

First published：CHEN Ke-ji. Foreword of *Contemporary Introduction to Chinese Medicine -In Comparison with Western Medicine* [A]. Xie Zhu-fan，Xie Fang. Contemporary Introduction to Chinese Medicine—In Comparison with Western Medicine[M].Beijing：Foreign Languages Press，2010：Foreword.

Some Key Problems and Thinkings on Gerontological Study in China

CHEN Ke-ji

The coming age wave has been a major concern of the society. As it was said in adage that “One should think about old during young” , any one, however, will think in spare time on “How many years are left? ” As for the academic circle of gerontology, more contributions to the senior citizens who make up 10% of the total population, also to the people who are going forth to the aged should be put in consideration. Problems of various disciplines are involved there among, demographic and sociologic, also those of natural sciences and specific medical sciences. Furthermore, it is also an issue of global concern that requires global strategic planning.

1 How Long Is the Natural Lifespan of Chinese People?

How long is the natural lifespan of human individuals? There were many legendary stories in the East and the West. For instance, Dong-fang Shuo (东方朔)in ancient Chinese was learnt to live for 38, 000 years, Peng Zu (彭祖)for 880 years, and of Chen Bo (陈搏)was said to last for 1, 000 years. In the Holy Bible, it was said that the lifespan of Methuselah was 969 years, Noah 950 year, Enoch 365 years, and Abraham 175 years, etc. Obviously the extreme longevity as those is only the wish of people. Although a long lifespan of 160 years has been reported at present, it is not substantiated yet by demographers and gerontologists.

Various methods have been used to estimate the natural lifespan of human being. For example, the method of multiplying human growth period (20-25 years)by 5-7, or sexual maturation period (14-15 years)by 8-10, the method based on the times (50)and cyclic time (2.4 years)of embryonic cell division, and the method based on length of pregnancy and developmental structure changes in human being. The longest lifespan is recognized as 167 years, but around 120 years is the generally accepted span. Interestingly, this number is very close to that recorded in the Chinese famous classical literatures such as “Shang Shu-Hong Fan Section” (尚书洪范篇)and “Canon of Medicine” (黄帝内经), in which “to be survival for 120 years means longevity” and “ending their natural life, all were survival for one hundred years” were described.

The upper limit of natural human lifespan is a difficult subject to study for it requires large sized sample, cross generation, longitudinal and long-term follow-up observation. The hair turning white eventually is a natural process, but variation exists certainly in the process, as “four generations under one roof” is not uncommonly seen in China. However, the actual data of natural human lifespan of Chinese people, which was so-called as “Tian Nian” (天年)in “Canon of Medicine” , gathered from systemic scientific investigation are still wanting, and a scientific answer is needed.

2 Dispute about Longevity Genes?

Many gerontologists believe that the natural lifespan is determined genetically. If the accidental premature death is excluded, the lifespan seems to closely correlate with the individual genetic aging vanance.

The actual reason for the existence of exceptional longevity in some families has arisen dispute in gerontologic circle for quite a long time. Experimental evidence confirmed that certain regions of chromosomes and mitochondria DNA may correlate with lifespan extension, aging retardation and illness prevention. Experimental studies also pinpointed that some single genes could dramatically prolong the lifespan. These data bring up a stern and practical question, i. e., do the longevity genes and aging genes exist?

Dr. Louis M. Kunkel, a molecular gerontologist of the Children's Hospital in Boston and Dr. Thomas Perls, gerontologist of Harvard Medical School, et al. reported their analysis of genetic linkage in 137 pairs of full brother/ sister, aged over 90 years (PNAS, August 2001).By DNA identification of the 400 labeled sites set at chromasome, it was found that a long and narrow area on D4SI565 loci of chromosome 4 seems to have the function, in which several longevity genes might be included. Dr. Perls said "one or several genetic missile thruster, namely, longevity gene, distribute in this region", which might retard the aging process and decrease the age related susceptibility. Dr. Kunkel believed the existence of longevity genes though how they slow down aging process is unclear.

However, British geriatrician Thomas Kirkwood held the different opinion, he considered the above conclusion seems to be lack of statistical significance. In a disquisition entitled with "No truth to the fountain of youth" put forth by 51 famous geriatricians and bio-scientists of USA, including Drs. Leonard Hayflick, Bruce A. Carnes, and S. Jay Olshansky in "Scientific American", June 2002, it was pointed out that there is no longevity genes that could directly control aging process in either animals or human beings. They explained that after successfully propagation, the unceasing accumulation of molecular products in cells or cell product in disordered state will eventually cause death, and there is no assurance for longevity. Although genes certainly influence longevity determination, the processes of aging are not genetically programmed. From the evolution perspective, longevity determination is under genetic control only indirectly. They concluded that aging is a product of evolutionary neglect, not evolutionary intent.

Geriatric community generally considered that life style, habit, behavior and environment contribute to one's health and lifespan. Such influence may account for extra 10 years of life and extend lifespan to 85 years. Beyond this, additional 15-20 years of life may depend on genetic role.

The right and wrong of longevity genes and aging genes are still practical problems that gerontologists should face up to. It also should be studied and screened by the Chinese society of science, especially the gerontologic community, in multilayers from the levels of human genome and proteome.

3 Is It Possible to Slow Down the Aging Process?

Throughout the whole history of human civilization, men are seeking how to slow down aging process, rejuvenate and live forever, to factually strengthen the vitality. This problem has perplexed the whole human beings in the past and at present. After 1970s, Chinese and foreign geriatricians have done many animal anti-aging concerning experiments. Some experiments proved that certain treatments could increase the vitality and lifespan of fruit flies as compared with those untreated controls of the same age. Nevertheless, Dr. Michael R. Rose, the biologist of UC at Ivan, believes that, theoretically, it is capable to slow down the aging process, but there is no elixir yet for doing it. After criticizing various strange methods for stir up the fire of hope, he indicated that so-called anti-aging is merely the control of various biochemical processes in human body. Hayflick held that the progress of society and biomedicine may contribute more in improving health and prolonging lifespan, but one should not applaud for commercial lies. Nowadays, there is a dangerous trend in commercial lies and various improper advertisements, which boost about some new invention, whereas, in fact, the majority of them are harmful. He warned that biomedicine is not the tiger balm, not all-conquering as alleged. As for the application of genetic engineering to importunately prolong the lifespan, it may affect the normal process of growth and normal development. He also pointed out that the core organ of man, namely the brain, is unable to replicate and transplant, brain transplantation is but a scientific fantasy, and that the saying about antioxidant can promote anti-aging process is also lack in enough scientific evidence. Moreover, he said: "It is intolerable about restrictive diet to extend lifespan".

The scientific connotation of age retardation or anti-aging should put emphasis on uplifting the quality of life of human, i. e. Add Life to Years. The Watchword of WHO in 2002 is "Physical Activity, Move for Health", which is the reliable pathway for retarding aging and increasing vitality. One should catch correctly the meaning of this slogan and do physical exercise properly, not only pay attention to avoid accelerating aging process by fierce physical activity, but also to correctly understand such problems, as "why human's lifespan could not be as long as the tortoise's", and "why lazy people live longest"?

Any traditional or modern measures or medicines for retarding aging should have its own scientific and realistic theoretical foundation, particularly in making conclusion on a certain measure/medicine about its effect on the aging process, to raise a conclusion arbitrarily without any evidence is not allowed.

The current anti-aging drugs which meet with universal recognition are melatonin, methandrostenolone, Vit E and Vit C, these medicines have some health preservation functions, but that is not meant to have anti-aging effect. There are also many Chinese herbal preparations indicated for anti-aging, which are theoretically useful according to TCM theory, and were over-enthusiastically propagandized in the market, but most of them lack in serious scientific certification, therefore, are inadvisable for recommending blindly.

4 Do We Continue to Use Hormone Replacement Therapy (HRT)?

Estrogen has been used for half century in treating menopause symptoms, such as hot flush, dryness in vagina, and night sweat. Also it is used to prevent osteoporosis, depression, urinary incontinence, dysnoesia, coronary heart diseases, etc. By the end of the last century, about 38% of menopause women in USA received long term HRT, and it was also generally used in China, but different in doses and treatment course. HRT is proved to be effective for alleviating menopause symptoms like hot flush (it can be eliminated after 3-6 months of treatment), dryness in vagina and night sweat, as well as for decreasing the occurrence of femoral head fracture. In an article published in "New England Journal of Medicine 1975", it was indicated that the estrogen therapy could increase the morbidity of cervix cancer, and an additional progestin was recommended for eliminating the adverse reaction of estrogen. In 1998 JAMA published the result of research on relationship between heart diseases and estrogen/ progestin replacement therapy. Although it was warned in the article that the treatment cannot reduce the attack of coronary heart diseases, it is still used so far by many obesity and older women. Among the menopause women in USA who accept long term HRT, 6 million take Promoro, 8 million take Progestin, these remedies are mainly the products of Wyeth Pharmaceutical Company, the turnover of the company reached 21 billion US dollars in the year 2001.

American Women's Health Initiative (WHI)holds different opinion about this kind of therapy. In a report of research published in JAMA, June 2002, the comparative study conducted in 16, 608 manopausal women, aged 50-79 years, with complete uterus was reported. Each and all the women received daily the Prempro mixture (containing estrogen 0.625 mg and progestin 2.5 mg)or the placebo respectively, the results showed that in the women treated with Prempro, the prevalence of stroke increased by 41%, that of cardiac attack increased by 29%, of total cardiovascular diseases by 22%, of breast cancer by 26%, and the venous thrombosis rate was doubled, whilst the occurrence of femoral head fracture decreased by 1/3, that of other kinds of bone fracture totally decreased by 24%, of large intestinal cancer decreased by 37% .But the total mortality in women treated by Prempro was not significantly different to that in women received placebo treatment. Accordingly, NIH recommended on July 9, 2002, to exclude HRT from treatment, which acutely shocked the public.

British medical community took different opinion on the above issue, because through analyzing the data about risks for stroke, breast cancer, and coronary heart diseases, it found that the 95% fiducial limit is too wide, thereby, it is too early to reach a conclusion. This condition is similar to that of the improper conclusion previously announced in USA in regard to the effect of AZT in prolonging AIDS patients' lifespan, which was later proved to be wrong for its undue short period of observation by a cooperated study of British and French. The study showed AZT fails to decrease the mortality of AIDS patients. So the Woman's International Study of Long Duration Oestrogen after Menopause (WISDOM)is continuously carried out in the UK till now.

Chinese doctors deem that during the combined administration of progestin and estrogen, progestin could weaken the endothelium cell mediated coronary artery dilative effect of estrogen, which countervailed the effect of estrogen in retarding plaque formation of atherosclerosis and blood vessel reconstruction. Moreover, estrogen could increase the risk of mammary epithelium proliferation and occurrence of breast cancer. In 1996, in a study of PUMC Hospital in Beijing, the combination of estrogen and progestin was applied on the castrated female rat model. Results showed that the uterine endometrial hyperplasia could not be inhibited, when the ratio of the two hormones in the combination was 1∶8, but it did show inhibition when the ratio was 1∶4, after progestin being added for 10 days, or when the ratio was 1∶0.5. The researchers held that for human, the daily dosage of estrogen of 0.3 mg is enough to achieve its effect, no need to increase it to 0.625 mg/ day.

So they considered the risks are not so serious as a hove-mentioned, which may be caused by the improper ratio of estrogen and progestin used in USA, and should not be taken as a general condition.

Gynecologists and obstetricians in Massachusetts General Hospital held that it is of no problem for using HRT in a short period of time.

Recently, after stopping the 3-year research, NIH decided to continue the follow-up study on HRT.

About the application of HRT in males, there are also different opinions in the medical community. Some specialists proposed HRT may be used in those subjects, who have low serum testosterone level, pathologic changes of target organs or tissues, and the serum prostate antigen (PSA)level is within normal range, for improving their immunity, physical strength, hematopoiesis and sexual function, as well as for regulating the lipid metabolism. However, this proposal is also a controversial topic, further studies are necessary.

5 Applying Hitech for the Development of Geriatrics

Advancement of human genome and proteome researches will undoubtedly accelerate the development of gerontology, including such aspects as studies on the mechanism of aging, and prevention and treatment of diseases. Development of biotech, new drugs and structural engineering technique would contribute to uplift the quality of life of the aged.

PET and functional MRI have made great advancement in the early diagnosis of the mental status, memory impairment and the Aamyloid deposition in the elders, which proved that the biggest gap between elderly and young people is the difference in brain activity.

The combination of molecular biology and micro-electronic technique give us such new products as DNA chips/various protein chips, which are going to be widely used in the fields as diagnosis of the elderly diseases, pharmacological and toxicological studies. The development of bio-material and bio-engineering technique will lead to accelerating the development of biological artificial organs, including artificial blood vessel, bone, joint, lens, cornea and skin, etc. Artificial lens transplantation has brought bright to over ten million senior citizens, and the quality of artificial lens are improving continuously. The bio-engineering of stem cells may be effective for treatment of cancer and nerve degeneration such as Parkinson's disease.

Structural engineering was brought up by Wolter in 1984, specified to the intracorporeal blood vascular structure, now the concept is generalized as the theory of applying principle of cytobiology and engineering in studying, developing, repairing, improving and operating the biosubstitute of tissues and its function. This new rising subject of science with high requirements for several disciplines like cytobiology, molecular biology and materials science, is important for the modern development of life sciences, including gerontology. American NIH had established four structural engineering research centers. In China, structural engineering research was started in 1994, and there are related items in many national projects, as "863" and "963" projects, in recent years.

Excepting the advance of cartilage structure engineering, recently, the new measures applied in the intervention treatment of cardiovascular diseases including PTCA, coated stenting, and laser technique, have brought new hopes to the prevention of post-operational restenosis of coronary/carotid arteries. Besides, the intervention mini-traumatic technique for treatment of cervical or lumbar vertebral prolapse, such as collagenase colliquefaction and laser pneumatolysis has won successes with significant effect.

Aging is not a disease, but elder people are liable to suffer from sickness. Aging means the lights may be on, but the voltage is low. Aging well needs the help of new hi-tech.

6 Some Principles of Geriatrics

All clm1cal measures aimed at aging and senile diseases should be established in improving health and quality of life of the aged, preventing or reducing the occurrence of aging related diseases or disabilities, and preserving health and activity in them. Moreover, gerontology should do more contributions for enhancing the elderly, play more important role in the development of society and eliminating the isolated living state of the aged in the society.

Geriatric clinical measurement should implement the idea that prevention is predominant to treatment, to plannedly and dynamically monitor the information of health, make early diagnosis and treatment, prevent the illnesses before its happening, and reduce the complications and sequelae for the elderly.

In prevention and treatment, emphasis must be put on the protection of the brain function and health behaviors, and such often encountered senile diseases as the cerebracardiac events, infectious diseases, tumor, diabetes mellitus, prostate disease, depression, dementia, insomnia and obesity as well as the diseases of bone, muscle, joint, vision and hearing.

Diseases that concerned by the American National Institute of Aging (NIA)are: Alzheimer disease and other degenerative diseases of nerve system, weakness, tumble, delirium, urinary incontinence, insomnia, severe depression, multiple illness condition, cardiovascular diseases, tumors, diabetes mellitus, skeletal system diseases, visual and auditory sensory disorder, prostate disease, infectious diseases, which could be taken as the references for us in combination of the actual situation in China.

Improving healthy behavior includes guidance for proper nutrition, smoking abstention and alcoholic beverage temperance, care of the safety in work and living, proper physical activities, psychologic health, and proper administration of Chinese and Western medicines, which should be performed by the cooperation of official ministry of health, communities and families.

7 Application of Chinese Medicine in the Coming Age Wave

China has a long history with plentiful experiences and theories of geriatric medicine. “Feng Qing Yan Lao Shu (奉亲养老书)” is a representative work written by Chen Zhi (陈直)in Song Dynasty (1085 A. D), for which I have made a commentary, and was published by Shanghai Science and Technology Publishing House in 1980s. The Chinese famous TCM professor Yue MeiZhong (岳美中)has given a summary about the eight special symptoms of the elderly, i. e. they merely remember the past things long before, tear at laughing, are fond of grandson, prefer to solid foods, poke their nose into others'business and short range urinating, etc. It also be properly de scribed in “Canon of Medicine” that the aged is lack in original-qi, with five Viscerals damaged slowly, and many symptoms come in a continuous stream. As for the TCM Syndrome Differentiation of senile diseases, equal attention was paid on the eight principles (八纲), the Qi-blood, and the Zang-Fu differentiation methods, holding that the characteristic of the senile diseases are more in the weakened and damaged condition, and often complicated with turbidity-obstruction and blood-stasis. The therapeutic principles for them are treatment with Chinese herbs of small dose, and gentle character, put Pi-Wei (stomach and spleen)in the principal place, and use various therapeutic methods. I like to use modified Zisheng Pill (资生丸)for tonifying, and Shenling Baizhu Powder (参苓白术散), Wendan Decoction (温胆汤) and Xiaoyao Powder (逍遥散)are also the preference. For treating coronary heart disease, herbs for warming and activating blood flow, as Xintong Pill (心痛丸), Kuanxiong Pill (宽胸丸), Guanxin No. 2 Tablet (冠心2号片) and Xuefu Zhuyu Decoction (血府逐瘀汤)may be applied. The recipes often used for hypertension are Tianma

Gouteng Decoction (天麻钩藤汤), Banxia Baizhu Tianma Decoction (半夏白术天麻汤)and Wendan Decoction (温胆汤), for common cold Shensu Decoction (参苏汤)and of Buzhong Yiqi Decoction (补中益气汤)plus Su Ye (苏叶), and modified Xiaochaihu Decoction (小柴胡汤), for prevention of common cold, Yupingfeng Powder (玉屏风散)frequently taking in small division, for constipation, Buzhong Yiqi Decoction (补中益气汤)plus Herba Cistanchis, Runchang Pill (润肠丸)and Maren Pill (麻仁丸), for osteoporosis, the herbs of Shen-Tonifying, for women menopausal syndrome, Niuhuang Qingxin Pill (牛黄清心丸), Erzhi Pill (二至丸)and Erxian Decoction (二仙汤), etc. with modification according to the TCM syndrome differentiation.

8 Some Thinkings

China should have a comprehensive project for the general development of science and technology on gerontological research, which are compatible with actual situation in China, and with the schedules which items should be programmed to do or not in different stages.

The study on basic theory and the mechanism of aging process must be paid reasonable attention to by the authorities.

To complete the standard for evaluating aging and health of the aged in China.

To perfect the Chinese measurement scales on quality of life for the elderly.

To run the diffused education on proper foods intake, nutrition and physical activity of the elderly.

To study the mental status of the elderly and the intervention methods.

To develop the methodology and related product for information detection in the aged.

To develop the bio-medical material, functional bio-material and rehabilitative instruments of the elderly.

To develop the traditional Chinese medicines and new drugs for the elderly.

To further establish the center of gerontology/aging/gerontological biology/geriatrics medicine.

To spread education in the elderly of the self health care knowledge.

The health insurance projects developed by the combination of official ministry of Health/Community / Family.

To build up the geriatrics research team.

To strengthen the guarantee of international cooperation, policy and funds.

First published: CHEN Ke-ji. Some key problems and thinkings on gerontological study in China[J]. Chin J Integr Med, 2005, 11 (2): 81-86.

Complementary/Alternative Medicine in Cardiovascular Diseases 2014

CHEN Ke-ji, LEE Myeong Soo, XU Hao, and Zhang Qun-hao

Cardiovascular diseases (CVDs)are the leading cause of long-term morbidity and mortality worldwide and are on an alarming rise in populations. According to the report of World Health Organization (WHO)in 2012, an estimated 17.5 million people died of CVDs, accounting for 31% of global deaths. As the increasing significance is attached to CVDs globally, the urgency to respond to CVDs with stronger and more effective therapies is widely recognized. Despite enormous efforts, revascularization, and secondary prevention, to prevent CVDs in the past, major challenges remain to cope with repeated recurrent acute cardiovascular events, readmission to the hospital and improvement of the long-term prognosis and quality of life. In this case, complementary and alternative medicine (CAM)therapies have the potential to provide a major public health beneflt.

In this special issue, papers from different parts of the world like China, Republic of Korea, Malaysia, Columbia, Chile, and so forth, are presented. These articles provide a review of this fleld and make original contributions towards the mechanism of action and the clinical application of CAM for CVDs. In these studies, anti-atherogenesis effects of some CAM products were highlighted, including the extracts of herbal plants such as paeonol (Pae), polysaccharide of *Polygonatum sibiricum* (PPGS), or fermented mung bean and fermented red yeast rice. Their cardioprotective role in hypolipidemic, antioxidant, and anti-atherogenesis was introduced. In addition, a study on the consumption of apple peel with rich phenolic compounds concluded that it reduced several metabolic syndrome parameters and the atherogenic progression in mice.

Attention was also paid to treatment of ischemia/reperfusion (I/R)injury. Increasing evidence has indicated that traditional Chinese medicine (TCM)could signiflcantly prevent myocardial apoptosis and provide alternative options for protection of myocardial I/R injury. *Huangzhi oral liquid* was an effective treatment for arrhythmias by increasing caspase-3 and apoptosis network proteins. *Shuang Shen Ning Xin* played an important antiapoptotic role by blocking the mitochondrial apoptotic pathway. Neuroprotection of *Sanhua decoction* against focal cerebral ischemia/reperfusion injury was demonstrated in rats through a mechanism targeting aquaporin 4. Two papers about ginsenoside Rb1 (GS-Rb1)discussed how to protect hypoxia-and ischemia-induced cardiomyocytes by regulating expression of miRNAs and inhibition of the mitochondrial apoptotic pathway, respectively.

The roles of Chinese medicine and other CAM therapies in relieving symptoms of hypertension, angina pectoris, and chronic heart failure were reviewed in several articles. A systematic review of randomized controlled trials showed that Chinese herbal medicine (CHM)combined with conventional therapies was effective in controlling blood pressure variability and symptoms of hypertension. Two other papers also highlighted the roles of integrative medicine therapy, for instance, *Xuefu Zhuyu decoction* functioning together with traditional antianginal medications could relieve the clinical symptoms of angina pectoris； *Wenxin Keli* and sotalol could effectively facilitate sinus rhythm reversion from hyperthyroidism related paroxysmal atrial flbrillation. In addition, the advantage of *Dangguijagyagsan*, a Korean traditional herbal prescription, on the treatment for cardiovascular diseases of menopausal women was referred to in a study. Another three-stage, multicenter, clinical trial evaluated the effcacy, safety, feasibility, compliance, and universality of CHM in the treatment of chronic heart failure.

A variety of functional readouts of CAM may reveal new therapeutic strategies to manipulate cardio protection, which could be transferred into application of treating CVDs. However, despite the growing utility of CAM, rigorous evidence-based studies with high quality are required to reinforce the application of CAM among CVD patients, especially its clinical benefit, prognostic impact, and potential interaction when used in combination with prescription medicines. It is widely acknowledged that there should be great potential in developing CAM use based on open dialogue between mainstream medicine doctors and CAM practitioners, healthcare professionals and patients.

First published: CHEN Ke-ji, LEE Myeong Soo, XU Hao, and ZHANG Qun-hao. Complementary/Alternative Medicine in cardiovascular diseases 2014[J]. Evid Based Complement Alternat Med, 2015: 1-2.

Complementary/Alternative Medicine in Cardiovascular Diseases 2013

CHEN Ke-ji, HUI Ka-Kit, Lee Myeong Soo, and XU Hao

Cardiovascular diseases (CVDs)are the leading cause of death worldwide, and the mortality is likely to further accelerate in many developing countries. In 2008, almost one in three deaths all over the world was attributed to CVDs. It is also estimated that by 2030 over 23 million deaths from CVDs will occur each year. Despite advances in modern management of CVDs, either revascularization or medical therapy, complications related to these procedures and recurrent acute cardiovascular events still afflict patients. Meanwhile, patients with CVDs often suffer from unfavorable quality of life. In recent decades, the potential beneifit of complementary/alternative medicine (CAM)therapy in improving CVDs prognosis has drawn more and more attention, and the use of CAM by physicians and patients has also increased markedly. However, the evidence of CAM for CVDs patients and the research on mechanism of actions are still insufficient. Last year, the published special issue named "The potential beneflt of complementary/alternative medicine in cardiovascular diseases" got a great success, which facilitates the compilation of this special issue 2013. We believe that such a series can have a long-term impact, and in time gather a community around it in much the same way a successful annual conference does.

In this issue, original research papers and reviews from different parts of the world including China, Republic of Korea, USA, Germany, and Malaysia are presented. These papers are focused on the mechanism of action and the clinical application of CAM in treating CVDs. In the clinical trials, the beneflts of Chinese medicine and some other CAM therapies for CVDs patients were demonstrated. A multicenter prospective cohort study showed that heart failure, age ≥ 65 years old, and myocardial infarction were associated with therapies for CVDs patients were demonstrated. A multicenter prospective cohort study showed an increase in one-year follow-up incidence of major adverse cardiac events (MACEs)in hospitalized coronary heart disease patients, and integrative medicine showed a tendency for reducing the incidence of MACEs. The similar beneflt of integrative medicine therapy for patients with acute coronary syndrome after PCI was showed in a multicenter randomized controlled trial (RCT), 5C trial. Another RCT compared the effectiveness of Qi-shen-yi-qi dripping pills (QSYQ)with that of aspirin in the secondary prevention of myocardial infarction. This trial did not show signiflcant difference of primary and secondary outcomes between aspirin and QSYQ, which suggest QSYQ might be an alternative medication for patients' intolerance of aspirin in patients who have had an MI. Speciflcally, a new potential biomarker of "toxin syndrome" in coronary heart disease patients was proposed in a paper containing two clinical trials. The authors concluded that the new biomarker "inter-alpha-trypsin inhibitor heavy chain H4" might have a potential role in early identifying high-risk coronary heart disease patients in stable period. Most of the experiment researches in this issue were focused on Chinese medicine and Korean medicine. Two researches explored the role and mechanism of Qiliqiangxin capsule (QL), an oral Chinese proprietary medicine, for arrhythmia and heart failure, respectively. A pharmacological research showed that blocking androgen receptor could abolish the ability of *Panax ginseng* to protect the heart from myocardial ischemia reperfusion injury. The beneflt of Doinseunggitang, a Korean traditional prescription, on the treatment and prevention of diabetic vascular complications was also described in a study. A systematic review suggested that oral Panax notoginseng preparation could relieve angina pectoris related symptoms. Meanwhile, the potential beneflt of Qiju Dihuang Wan, a Chinese herbal prescription, on the treatment of essential hypertension was also reviewed. Additionally, yoga was recommended as an effective intervention for reducing blood pressure in a systematic review.

Due to indeflnite mechanism of actions and lacking of high quality evidence, traditional Chinese medicine and other traditional medicine worldwide are considered as CAM in Western countries. In this case, original researches on mechanism of actions play an important role in the modernization and internationalization of CAM and should be further strengthened in future researches. In the hierarchy of evidence-based medicine, high quality RCT is still considered as the golden standard for evaluating interventional treatment. Currently, multicenter RCTs and a prospective cohort study have been conducted to evaluate the beneflt of CAM for CVDs, and most of these researches showed positive flndings. Nevertheless, the effectiveness of CAM onthe treatment of CVDs in the real world is still unclear which limits the application of CAM. The reason is that effcacy of intervention in RCT is not equal to its effectiveness in the real world. In the future, in addition to high quality RCTs, more evidence from real world researches is warranted to support the use of CAM including traditional Chinese medicine for CVDs patients.

First published: Chen KJ, Hui KK, Lee MS, et al. Complementary/Alternative Medicinc in cardiovascular diseases 2013[J]. Evid Based Complement Alternat Med, 2013, 2013: 1-2.

The Potential Beneflt of Complementary/Alternative Medicine in Cardiovascular Diseases

CHEN Ke-ji, HUI Ka-Kit, LEE Myeong Soo, and XU Hao

Cardiovascular diseases (CVDs)prevalence continues to increase, and it is still the number one killer so far. In 2002, nearly 17 million deaths all over the world were attributable to CVDs, which accounted for almost 30% of the total deaths. Despite treatment with percutaneous coronary intervention (PCI)and many other conventional medicines, CVDs patients are still confronted with certain risk of recurrent acute cardiovascular events, readmission to the hospital, and unfavorable quality of life. In recent years, more and more clinicians have successfully applied complementary/alternative medicine (CAM)in CVDs prevention and treatment based on standardized conventional therapy. Nevertheless, the role of CAM in CVDs still needs more clinical evidence and deflnite mechanism of actions.

In this issue, a collection of several original research articles and reviews are presented that address the clinical application and the mechanism of action of CAM in the treatment of CVDs. These works were submitted by researchers from different parts of the world, including China, Japan, South Korea, Australia, and Sweden. In these studies, the effectiveness of Chinese medicine and some other alternative therapeutic methods in improving symptoms was demonstrated in patients with hypertension, chronic

stable coronary artery disease, chronic heart failure, and so forth. Speciflcally, the use of Chinese herbal medicines was reviewed for the prevention of in-stent coronary restenosis after PCI. The study of Tanshinone IIA, a diterpene quinine extracted from the root of *salvia miltiorrhiza*, a Chinese traditional herb, was presented as a promising cardioprotective agent. The positive effect of Chinese food and herbal medicines in improving certain moderate dyslipidemias was described. The usefulness of Xuezhikang, an extract from Red Yeast Rice, was reviewed in the treatment of coronary heart disease complicated by dyslipidemia. A pharmacological and mechanistic study showed Naoxintong's effect on cytochrome P450 2C19. Further, one study showed the effect of berberine on improving insulin sensitivity by inhibiting fat store and adjusting adipokines proflle in human preadipocytes and metabolic syndrome patients.

In the authors' opinion, the clinical research of Chinese medicine and other CAMs for CVDs still faces some major challenges. Issues such as overall quality of medical service and the unmet medical needs in the contemporary society are common to these medicines. A general guideline is required for practicing Chinese medicine and other CAMs, which should be developed based on solid evidence from well-designed and well-executed clinical studies. Such is the direction that the research of Chinese Medicine and other CAM should follow.

First published: Chen KJ, Hui KK, Lee MS, Xu H. The potential beneflt of Complementary/Alternative Medicine in cardiovascular diseases[J]. Evid Based Complement Alternat Med, 2012, Article ID 125029. doi: 10.1155/ 2012/125029

"Acupuncture Journey to America"—A Tale of the Marvelous

CHEN Ke-ji and CONG Wei-hong

On November 16, 2010, China's acupuncture was officially added to the list of world intangible cultural heritage of humanity by the 5th United Nations Educational, Scientific and Cultural Organization Intergovernmental Committee for Safeguarding Intangible Cultural Heritage.This declaration indicates that acupuncture, the needle therapy of Chinese medicine (CM), has received worldwide recognition by people from different cultures. As a medical therapy, acupuncture has been used to treat a wide range of medical disorders in more than 160 countries.

Despite the fact that acupuncture originated in China more than 5, 000 years ago and the earliest written record on acupuncture was found in the *Yellow Emperor's Inner Canon* (Huang Di Nei Jing)dated approximately 200 BC, it did not arrive in the United States until Chinese doctors among early immigrants landed in the America in the 1, 800 s. In the late 1, 800 s, Dr. Sir William Osler, the "father of modern medicine" , commented that acupuncture was the best treatment for lower back pain.The greatest exposure of contemporary Chinese acupuncture to American public came when the *New York Times* journalist and columnist, James Reston, received acupuncture treatment in Beijing for his post-operative abdominal pain after undergoing an emergency appendectomy with standard drug anesthesia in the summer of 1971. Intrigued and impressed by the effectiveness of his experience with acupuncture, Reston wrote about his hospitalization and acupuncture treatment and published it in the *New York Times* on July 26, 1971. It is a popular public opinion that Reston's article exposed countless Americans for the first time to Chinese acupuncture and ignited "American acupuncture fever" in early 1970s. In the following year, Chinese acupuncture gained much more public attention in the United States and the West during President Richard Nixon visit of China in the spring of 1972, as evidenced by numerous publications of acupuncture stories in national news and popular magazines.

While acupuncture "fad" gradually diminished with time in the West, the real question concerned medical community was: does acupuncture really work and, if it does, how? The federal agencies of the US government, National Institute of Health (NIH)and Food Drug Administration (FDA), launched long time investigation on the safety and efficacy of acupuncture in early 1970s, but not until late 1990s, the two authorities concluded respectively that acupuncture needle is a safe medical device (FDA, 1996) and acupuncture therapy is effective for certain medical conditions (NIH, 1997). Although the mechanism of acupuncture and its traditional theory could not be fully explained scientifically at that time, patients and public demand, as well as several thousand years of historical records supported the FDA's decision and state legislation to legalize acupuncture as medical therapy. After decades of "trick or treatment" disputation, the mechanism of acupuncture actions has been explored in all directions using a variety of scientific technology and high-tech tools, such as functional magnetic resonance imaging, Doppler ultrasound, and thermal imaging. Results from these well-designed experiments showed that acupuncture does not only work on a psychological level as a "placebo" but also has real physiological effects on the human body.

In the United States, the most common applications of acupuncture include chronic pain conditions, such as arthritis, lower back pain, and headaches, as well as chronic fatigue, anxiety, depression, and stress, especially when conventional medicine fails. Acupuncture is also a very popular complementary therapy for substance abuse, nausea and vomiting post chemotherapy or operation, cancer care, acquired immunodeficiency syndrome management, immune system disorders, stroke, and many other conditions. For most patients in the United States, acupuncture is a safe and relatively inexpensive therapy with very low rate of risk and side effect. Many patients described acupuncture treatment as a "pleasant experience" in comparing with invasive procedures commonly used in Western medicine. Reportedly, as many as 86% of acupuncture patients are satisfied with their treatment.

However, due to the different cultural backgrounds and theoretical systems in medical practices between the West and East, acupuncture is still facing various challenges in America. Sustainable development of CM acupuncture in American society needs further public recognition, more convincing research achievements, and extensive social psychological studies. Ultimately, the real advance of Western medicine, CM, and integrative medicine all depends on the development of science.

In his new book, Acupuncture Journey to America, Dr.Li described exciting legend of acupuncture journey to the United States and final acceptance of Chinese acupuncture by Western society. After 40 years efforts, acupuncture has gained wide legal recognition and 44 out of 50 states in the United States have already passed state law for acupuncture practice. Furthermore, the clinical application of acupuncture continues to expand in the West and the westernized acupuncture technique is considered as a significant advance of acupuncture development in last century. The book also tells us many amazing stories about culture exchanges and integration between the East and West. It contains 45 historical photos and illustrations, and cites more than 200 original references related to the history of American acupuncture.

As to why acupuncture journey to America was so successful, Dr. Li has concluded at the end of the book that there were at least five key factors by which acupuncture was greatly promoted in the West. They are: (1)the spread of acupuncture news and stories by Western media and public, (2)the healing nature and effectiveness of acupuncture, (3)the establishment of state laws to protest patients and practitioners, (4) the growth of independent clinics as dominant entity for acupuncture service, and lastly, (5)solid clinical and basic research on acupuncture funded mainly by federal agencies.In return, these Western experience plus the westernized acupuncture techniques, which may represent an advanced model of acupuncture practice in modernized society, could potentially provide valuable information and directions to the current medical reform in China.

The history has proven that the clinical value and scientific content of acupuncture could not be ignored or overshadowed, neither by rapid development of Western medicine or social political interferences. Acupuncture belongs not only to Chinese, but to people all over the world. We are pleased to be invited to write comment on this book and wish it could cast new light on CM acupuncture—the ancient and young healing art. We also look forward to the publishing of an English version of this informative book to fill in the gap of acupuncture history.

First published: Ke-ji Chen, Wei-hong Cong. "Acupuncture Journey to America" — A tale of the marvelous[J]. Chin J Integr Med, 2012, 18 (3): 233-234.

Recommending "Unstuck—Your Guide to the Seven-Stage Journey Out of Depression"

CHEN Ke-ji and CONG Wei-hong

Depression is a common disorder worldwide. In the West, depression is also called "the blues" informally. It is a psychological disorder characterized by an all-encompassing low mood. Slightly depressed people may behave normally, while experiencing feelings of pain at heart. In mild depression cases, people may feel gloomy or distressed, which is usually associated with memory impairment, insomnia, dreaminess, etc. People suffering from severe depression may be preoccupied with, or ruminate over, thoughts and feelings of worthlessness, inappropriate guilt, helplessness, hopelessness, hallucinations, or delusions, most often accompanied by recurrent thoughts of death, suicide attempt or a specific plan for committing suicide. With the intensifying pressure and a competition of modern society, many people become victims of depression. It brings great trouble and burden to patients, their families, and society.

The latest survey results of the World Health Organization (WHO)showed the global incidence of depression to be above 3%, and about 6% in developed countries. Available data show that the incidence of depression is approximately 3% to 5% in China. However, this disease has long been neglected by the Chinese. In fact, fewer than 20% of those affected have been diagnosed, and less than 10% have received proper medical therapy. Furthermore, due to various reasons, many of them have never bothered to see a doctor for their ailment, or even do not want their families or friends to learn that they are suffering from depression. In China, mind-body disorders and psychological obstacles have become frequently encountered diseases and common diseases. At present, neuropsychiatric diseases are the biggest health burden on society both economically and sociologically, accounting for about 1/5 of the burden of disease, which will increase to 1/4 by the year 2020 as predicted by the WHO. Even more seriously, depression leads to a high suicide rate. About 15% of depression sufferers have died from suicide. In 2009, a WHO report pointed out that almost one million people die from suicide every year around the world, about 3000 deaths every day, or one death every 40 seconds, nearly 30% of which are from India and China. Suicide has been the leading cause of death in the 15 to 34 years age group in China. Meanwhile, youth suicide and the elderly suicide have been social problems that cannot be ignored.

Dr.James Gordon, a Harvard-educated psychiatrist and one of the world's leading experts in mind-body medicine, served as Chairman of the White House Commission on Complementary and Alternative Medicine Policy for years. With over 40 years of experience in the field of psychiatry, Dr. Gordon is able to offer practical advice and help for depression patients to find their way out of the darkness of depression without antidepressants. In America, his work has been featured on The Today Show, CNN, CBS Sunday Morning, and National Public Radio, as well as The Washington Post, USA Today, Newsweek, People, American Medical News, Clinical Psychiatry News, etc. His new book, *Unstuck* is an easy-to-use and practical guide explaining the seven-stage journey out of depression and the steps we can take to exert control over our own lives and find hope and happiness.

This book is designed for anyone who is suffering from depression, from mild subclinical depression (depressed mood most of the day)to its severest forms (suicide attempt or a specific plan for committing suicide), regardless of education, economic status, age, or other therapeutic activities. Using the examples from his years of experience, Dr. Gordon explains the *Unstuck* approaches: food and nutritional supplements;

Chinese medicine; movement, exercise, and dance; psychotherapy, meditation, and guided imagery; and spiritual practice and prayer. He believes that depression is not a disease over which we have no control. On the contrary, "It is a sign that our lives are out of balance, that we are stuck" . He suggests we regard depression as "the start of a journey that can help us become whole and happy, a journey that can change and transform our lives" , and try to stop overdependence on antidepressants or other chemicals which might bring uncomfortable and sometimes disabling side effects.

This book has received favorable comments from renowned professionals since its publication in America. We hope Chinese readers will benefit from it, and get some idea of the cultural differences between China and America and the consequent characteristic treatment concepts.

Dr. Gordon and Dr. CHEN Ke-ji were appointed cochairmen of the 2nd World Integrative Medicine Congress held in Beijing in 2002. Dr. Gordon's ebullient speech on the Chinese people and Chinese medicine, delivered at the opening ceremony, was widely acclaimed by Chinese physicians present. His other book, *Manifesto for A New Medicine*, published by Addison-Wesley in America and Canada in 1996, explaining the profound with simple terms, was also praised by readers and sparked a personal revolution for many healthcare providers. Dr. Chen had recommended it in the *Chinese Journal of Integrated Traditional and Western Medicine* in July 1997[1] and was honored to be invited to write a foreword for the Chinese version of *Unstuck*.

REFERENCES

[1] Chen KJ. Manifesto for a new medicine: your guide to healing partnerships and the wise use of alternative therapies. Chin J Integr Med, 1997, 3 (2): 142-143.

First published: CHEN Ke-ji, CONG Wei-hong.Recommending "unstuck–your guide to the seven-stage journey out of depression" [J]. Chin J Integr Med, 2010, 16 (4): 364-365.

XS0601 Reduces the Incidence of Restenosis: A Prospective Study of 335 Patients Undergoing Percutaneous Coronary Intervention in China

CHEN Ke-ji, SHI Da-zhuo, XU Hao, LU Shu-zheng, LI Tian-chang, KE Yuan-nan
ZHANG Min-zhou, LU Xiao-yan, SUN Rui-yuan, and YOU Shi-jie

Restenosis is still the major limitation of the long-term success of percutaneous coronary intervention (PCI). Despite numerous trials of pharmacological adjunctive therapies, including anti-proliferative agents, [1-3] calciumantagonists, [4,5] fish oil, [6-8] heparin, [9,10] lipid-lowering drugs, [11,12] prostacycline analog, [13,14] serotonin inhibitors[15] and thromboxane inhibitors, [16,17] the frequency of restenosis has not diminished since the inception of PCI. Coronary stents are the only devices that have shown success in reducing the incidence of restenosis, though the occurrence rate still high at 22%-29%. [18] The emergence of drug-coated or drug-eluting stents have been a great breakthrough in preventing restenosis with the overall restenosis rate of 8%-9%. [19] However, the inconsistency of the results reported thus far, uncertainty of the long-term efficacy and safety, the relatively high cost call for further investigation and development of preventive agent with better cost-effectiveness ratio. [20,21]

The pathogenesis of restenosis is complex and not fully understood. According to the theory of traditional Chinese medicine (TCM), restenosis falls into the category of blood-stasis syndrome. Hence, we have been investigating the prevention of restenosis by activating blood circulation (ABC)herbal medicine since 1990. The previous studies have shown that concentrated Xuefu Zhuyu pill (a classic formula for ABC)may help prevent restenosis. [22,23] Subsequently, we selected *Ligusticum chuanxiong* Hort and Paeonia lactiflora pall, the main components in concentrated Xuefu Zhuyu pill, for further studies. Active ingredients from those two components were extracted and proportions optimized to formulate XS0601 by an orthogonal design method. *In vitro* studies demonstrated that XS0601 inhibited endothelin-induced proliferation of smooth muscle cells. [24] In a porcine coronary injury model, XS0601 was shown to inhibit intimal hyperplasia and pathological vascular remodeling after balloon dilation. [25,26] Based on these observations, a pilot study of 108 patients with coronary heart disease (CHD)was carried out, in which reductions of angiographic restenosis and recurrent angina after PCI were observed upon treatment of XS0601 for 6 months. [27] In the current study, we conducted a randomized, double-blind, placebo-controlled, multi-center trial with 335 patients to test the efficacy and safety of XS0601 in preventing restenosis following PCI.

METHODS

1 Study Design

A double-blind, placebo-controlled, randomized trial with 2 study groups was conducted at 5 medical centers. The trial was carried out according to the Declaration of Helsinki and the Guidelines for Good Clinical Practice, and the protocol was approved by the institutional review boards and ethics committees at each center. To achieve a decrease in restenosis rate from 35% to 20% (α= 0.05; β= 0.20)in 6 months with XS0601 treatment, a minimum of 136 patients in each study group were estimated to be needed to achieve a statistically significant difference. To allow exclusion of patients who failed to participate in follow-up angiography and those who drop out the trial, a goal of 396 patients (198 in each group)was set for the study.

2 Inclusion and Exclusion Criteria

Patients eligible for the study were 35 to 75 years old, had angina and/or objective evidence of myocardial ischemia or acute myocardial infarction, and at least one significant (>50%)stenosis that was documented on a recent coronary angiogram and was treated successfully with PCI. The successful PCI was defined as dilatation of the lesions with less than 50% residual stenosis and a more than 20% decrease in percent diameter stenosis with no major complications. Patients were excluded if they met any of the following criteria: presence of (1)restenosis lesion or graft vessel lesion; (2)chronic completely obstructive lesion (>3 months); (3)severe left main artery lesion; (4)severe heart failure [ejection fraction (EF)<35%]; (5)uncontrolled level III hypertension; (6)severe valvular heart disease; (7)insulin-dependent diabetes mellitus; (8)diseases of hepatic, renal, hematologic and neurologic systems, psychological abnormalities, and malignancies; (9)pregnancy or breast-feeding; (10)unable to provide written consent or expected poor compliance, and (11)participants of other clinical trials.

3 Randomization and Drug Regimens

With the aid of SAS software, 396 randomized numbers were generated. To ensure an equal distribution of treatments in each center, a block randomization procedure on a site basis was used. After the patients had given informed consent, they were randomly assigned to either the XS0601 or the placebo group. The drugs were taken as 500 mg (2 capsules)3 times per day taken after meals. The treatment was initiated one day after PCI and continued for six months. The capsules used for placebo during the entire study period were indistinguishable from the active drugs. Both the placebo and active drugs were packaged and supplied by Beijing International Biological Products Institute, China. All patients received aspirin (100 mg)daily for the entire study period; 250 mg ticlopidine/bid was administrated two days before PCI and continued for two weeks, followed by 250 mg ticlopidine/qd for another two weeks.

4 PCI Procedure and Angiographic Analysis

The choice of balloon size, inflation duration and inflation pressure was determined by cardiologists. Follow-up angiography was performed at 6 months for assessment of the restenosis. Cineangiograms were obtained before, immediately and 6 months after PCI with an adequate amount of nitrate to obtain maximal dilatation of the coronary artery. All three angiograms were performed with the same kind of catheters used at baseline, and the same projections. The imaging data collected were independently assessed in a blind fashion and analyzed with a computer-assisted quantitative coronary angiographic (QCA)analysis system (Cardio 500, Kontron Elektronik, Eching, Germany)by the core laboratory.

5 Study end Points

The primary end point of this study was restenosis on the basis of the changes in percent stenosis as determined with QCA after PCI and at follow-up examination and was evaluated both per lesion and per patient. Restenosis per lesion was defined as a residual stenosis of <50% after angioplasty and subsequent aggravations to ≥50% at follow-up. Restenosis per patient was defined as the patient having at least 1 restenotic lesion. The secondary clinical end points were the combined incidence of death, nonfatal target lesion myocardial infarction, coronary artery bypass graft surgery (CABG), or repeat target-vessel angioplasty.

6 Follow-up Evaluation

The clinical follow-up visits were scheduled at 1, 3 and 6 months after PCI to determine recurrent angina and side effects of XS0601 treatment. Additional follow-up up to 12 months after PCI was conducted to assess clinical end points efficacy. Laboratory studies included routine blood analysis, urine analysis, stool occult blood test, electrocardiogram, and hepatic [alanine aminotransferase (ALT)] and renal function tests [blood urea nitrogen (BUN)and creatine].

7 Statistical Analysis

Statistical analysis was performed by the Clinical Drugs Evaluation Center of Anhui Province in a blind fashion. For statistical evaluation, intention-to-treat and per-protocol populations were defined. Statistical analysis was performed with SAS 6.12 software. All tests were two tailed and a statistical probability of $<$ 0.05 was considered significant. *T* test was used for comparison of measurement data； χ^2 test or Fisher exact test if necessary was used for comparison of enumeration data. Ridit and Wilcoxon tests were used for interclass ranked data and in-group ranked data, respectively.

RESULTS

1 Patients' Characteristics

Between June 2002 and December 2003, 335 patients with successful PCI were enrolled in 5 centers and were randomized into two groups: 166 to receive XS0601 and 169 to receive placebo. During the course of the study, nine patients were excluded in the XS0601 group due to insufficient follow-up (3)and protocol violation, noncompliance with medications (6)； while 12 patients were excluded in the placebo group with 3 incomplete follow-up and 9 noncompliance. Thus, the per-protocol population consisted of 308 patients, with 154 patients in the XS0601 group and in the placebo group. The intention-to treat population consisted of 314 patients, with 157 patients in each group. The baseline characteristics of the intention-to-treat cohort are given in Table. The two groups were well matched with regard to baseline clinical and angiographic characteristics ($P>0.05$).

Table 1 Baseline Clinical and Angiographic Characteristics*

Variables	XS0601 group (*n*=157)	Placebo group (*n*=157)
General		
Age (years)	58.52 ± 10.30	58.74 ± 9.91
Male [*n* (%)]	124 (79.0)	123 (78.3)
Height (cm)	167.38 ± 7.21	167.66 ± 6.94
Weight (kg)	72.44 ± 10.78	71.07 ± 10.09
Heart rate (/min)	74.34 ± 9.65	74.17 ± 12.43
Systolic pressure (mmHg)	130.97 ± 18.47	130.70 ± 19.70
Diastolic pressure (mmHg)	79.81 ± 10.34	80.30 ± 11.44
Risk factors		
Hypertension [*n* (%)]	85 (54.1)	84 (53.5)
Hyperlipidemia [*n* (%)]	45 (28.7)	38 (24.2)
Diabetes [*n* (%)]	28 (17.8)	32 (20.4)
Diagnosis		
Stable angina [*n* (%)]	4 (2.5)	6 (3.8)
Unstable angina [*n* (%)]	94 (59.9)	87 (55.4)
Acute myocardial infarction[*n* (%)]	59 (37.6)	64 (40.8)
Angiographic data△		
LAD/stenosis (%)	129/87.12 ± 17.20	131/81.81 ± 16.11
LCx/stenosis (%)	78/80.11 ± 20.47	75/78.90 ± 19.13
RCA/stenosis (%)	81/78.06 ± 20.59	77/79.84 ± 17.30

Continued

Variables	XS0601 group (n=157)	Placebo group (n=157)
Lesion class#		
A[n (%)]	99 (27.4)	86 (23.9)
B1[n (%)]	148 (41.0)	168 (46.7)
B2[n (%)]	59 (16.3)	62 (17.2)
C[n (%)]	55 (15.2)	44 (12.2)

*Plus-minus values are means ± SD. None of the differences between groups were statistically significant ($P>0.05$). LAD: left anterior descending artery ; LCx: left circumflex artery ; RCA: right coronary artery. Δ Vessels involved are 288 in XS0601 group, 283 in placebo group. # Lesion class was defined according to American College of Cardiology/American Heart Association (ACC/AHA)classification. Numbers of lesions are 361 in XS0601 group, 360 in placebo group.

2 Primary End Point

Among the 308 cases who completed clinical follow-up, 145 cases (47.1%)received angiographic follow-up. The mean angiographic follow-up duration was (185.4 ± 38.9)days in the XS0601 group and (184.5 ± 42.1) days in the placebo group ($P>0.05$). As shown in Fig. 1, fewer patients who received XS0601 treatment experienced restenosis (19 of 73 patient or 26.1%)in comparison to those who received placebo (34 of 72 patients or 47.2%). The beneficial effect of XS0601 was also revealed by the significant reduction of per lesion restenosis rate (23.6% in the XS0601 vs. 39.2% in the placebo group; $P<0.05$). However, XS0601 did not appear to affect the development of new lesions (12.3% vs. 13.9% in the treatment and placebo groups, respectively; $P>0.05$).

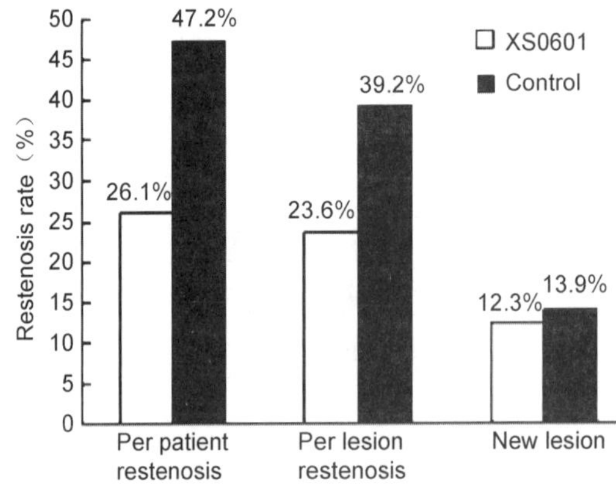

Fig. 1 Restenosis Rates per Patient and Per Lesion and Percent of New Lesion

Notes: XS0601 significantly lowered both per patient and per lesion restenosis as compared with the placebo group ($P<0.05$). As for new lesions, there was no significant difference between the two groups ($P>0.05$).

3 Sub-analysis of Restenosis Rates in Patients with Cypherstent

To understand whether XS0601 has additional benefits, we performed a subanalysis of restenosis rates in patients with either a Cypher or bare-metal stent. Among a total of 22 patients who had a Cypher stent, 7 were treated with XS0601 and 15 with placebo. No significant difference in the restenosis rate was observed between the XS0601 and placebo groups ($P>0.05$). Interestingly, in the subgroup of patients who had the bare-metal stent, a significant decrease in the restenosis rate was observed in XS0601 treated patients as compared to the placebo group (24.2% versus 50.9%, $P<0.01$). In addition, the Cypher stent did not show a significant preventive effect on restenosis as compared with general stent in either the treated or placebo group in this cohort population ($P>0.05$).

4 Serial Changes in Minimal Lumen Diameter (MLD)

There was no significant difference in the MLD before or immediately after percutaneous transluminal coronary angioplasty (PTCA)between the XS0601 group and the placebo group (0.87 mm vs. 0.88 mm and 3.00 mm vs. 2.98 mm, respectively, $P>0.05$). However, a significantly improved MLD was noted in the XS0601 group during the 6 months follow-up measurement as compared with the placebo group (2.08 mm vs. 1.73 mm; $P<0.05$), and this difference is also reflected in the quantification of cumulative percentage of MLD shown in Fig. 2.

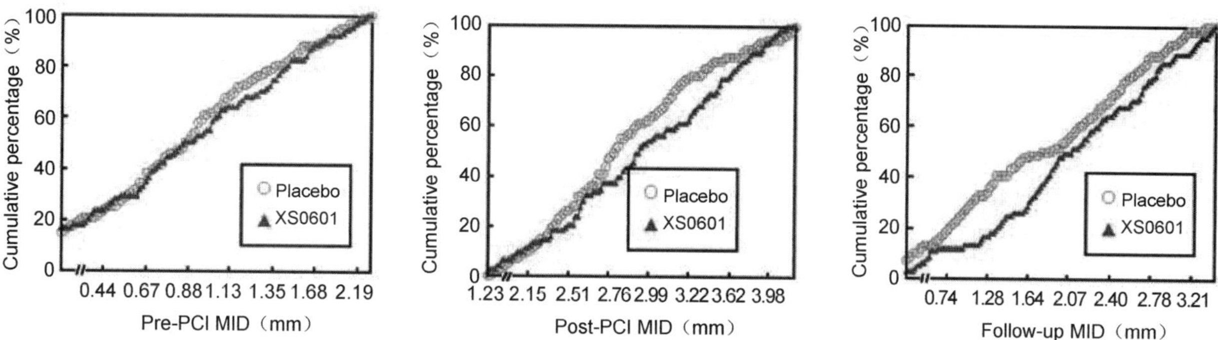

Fig. 2 Cumulative frequency distribution curves of the MLD at the target site before PCI (pre-PCI), immediately after PCI (post-PCI), and at 6-month follow-up

Notes: The pre-PCI and post-PCI curves are nearly identical, indicating very similar distribution of MLD between placebo and XS0601 groups. At follow-up, the curve for XS0601 group clearly lies to right of corresponding placebo curve as a result of larger MLD ($P<0.05$).

5 Clinical End Points

Out of the total of 308 patients evaluated, no death was found in either the treatment or the control group. One nonfatal target lesion myocardial infarction in each group was observed. No patient in the XS0601 group underwent CABG, whereas 3 patients (1.9%)in the placebo group did. Target lesion revascularization was performed in 15 patients (9.7%)in the XS0601 group and 31 patients (20.1%)in the placebo group. The resulting combined incidence was 10.4% for the XS0601 group vs 22.7% for the placebo group ($P<0.05$), indicating a significant difference. This difference is also reflected when the data are analyzed and plotted on the Kaplan-Meier curve (Fig. 3).

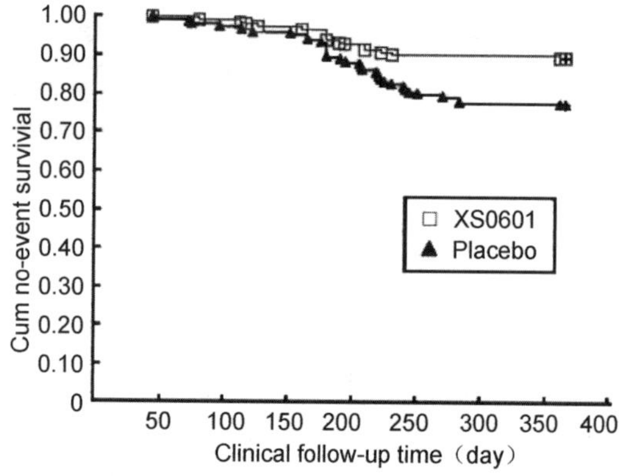

Fig. 3 Kaplan-Meier survival curve for freedom from clinical end-point events

Notes: At up to 1 year of follow-up, there was a significant difference between the XS0601 and the placebo group ($P<0.05$).

6 Recurrent Angina

Recurrent angina was evaluated at 1, 3 and 6 months after PCI. As shown in Fig. 4, one month after PCI, the incidence of recurrent angina did not differ significantly between the XS0601 group and placebo group (2.6% vs. 8.4%, $P>0.05$). However, as the follow-up time progressed, the incidence accumulated in both the XS0601 and placebo group, but with a faster pace in the latter. At three months after PCI, the incidence increased from 2.6% to 7.1% in the XS0601 group vs. 8.4% to 19.5% in the placebo group ($P < 0.01$). The significant difference continued to month 6 after PCI, where recurrent angina occurred in 17 patients (11%)in the XS0601 group compared to 66 patients (42.9%)in the placebo group ($P < 0.01$).

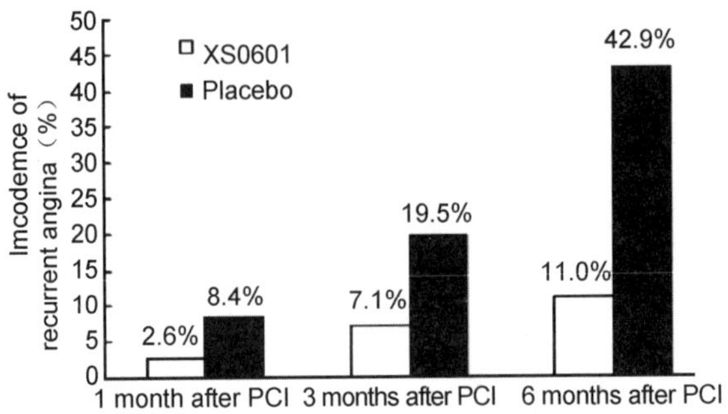

Fig. 4 The incidence of recurrent angina (RA)during the follow-up period

Notes: At 1 month after PCI, XS0601 showed the tendency to lower the incidence of RA, although there was no significant difference between the two groups ($P > 0.05$). At 3 and 6 months after PCI, the incidence of RA was significantly lowered in XS0601 group as compared with the placebo group ($P < 0.01$).

7 Side Effects

Out of the 335 patients enrolled in this study, 2 in the XS0601 group experienced gastric discomfort, which resolved without interruption of XS0601 treatment. Granulocytopenia occurred in one patient in the placebo group, which was considered to be related to concomitant administration of ticlopidine. At 6 months after PCI, in both XS0601 and placebo groups, blood pressure, heart rate, routine tests of blood, urine and stool, as well as liver and kidney functions did not differ from that measured at the beginning of the study.

DISCUSSION

The therapeutic benefit of XS0601 in preventing restenosis after PCI was assessed in the current randomized, double-blind, placebo controlled study. The results show that XS0601 could significantly reduce the incidence of angiographically demonstrated restenosis and increase MLD of target vessel. The results also show that clinically XS0601 could improve post-PCI clinical outcomes, including the incidence of recurrent angina, and the requirement of CABG or revascularization. Equally important, the results demonstrated that XS0601 was safe. Although the benefit has been clearly demonstrated in patients overall and those receiving general stents, the current study does not allow evaluation of XS0601's effect in patients undergoing Cypher stent implants due to the small sample size of patients in this study cohort. Further investigations are required to understand its efficacy in patients receiving Cypher stents.

The pathogenesis of restenosis is complex. Elastic recoil, negative arterial remodeling, and neointimal hyperplasia are recognized as sequential events occuring after PCI. [28,29] While elastic recoil and negative arterial remodeling account for the main pathogenic mechanism of restenosis after balloon angioplasty, neointimal hyperplasia remains the cause of in-stent restenosis. At the cellular and molecular levels, arterial endothelial injury caused by stents or balloon insertion initiates adhesion, activation and aggregation of platelets and induces fibrin deposition and thrombus formation. Infiltration of inflammatory cells to the arterial wall and secretion of cytokines trigger proliferation of arterial smooth muscle cells, which form neointima and replace thrombi in the lumen and result in restenosis.

The rationale for selecting XS0601 as the therapeutic candidate for the restenosis prevention study is based on the notion that the pathogenesis of stenosis as discussed above is in parallel to the theory of "obstruction of heart vessel", which is under the category of "blood-stasis syndrome" in traditional Chinese medicine (TCM). The parental medicine or prescription of XS0601, concentrated Xuefu Zhuyu pill, has been a classic formula routinely used in patients with other circulatory problems to promote blood circulation and improve blood stasis in TCM. As described in the introduction, our earlier studies have shown the potentialeffectiveness of the concentrated Xuefu Zhuyu pill and XS0601 in preventing restenosis. [23-27] The preliminary encouraging findings prompted us to initiate a larger scale investigation to further validate the efficacy and safety of XS0601 in the prevention of restenosis.

Our early studies in *in vitro* cultured cells and in animal models have demonstrated that XS0601 could hamper pathological vascular remodeling by inhibiting intimal hyperplasia after balloon angioplasty. [24-26] Results from the current study are in agreement with the early observations and confirm XS0601 as an effective oral agent in antagonising restenosis. Among different categories of drugs tested so far, two drugs, sirolimus and paclitaxel, that have shown efficacy in coated stents share similar antiproliferative effects to XS0601. However, both agents exert their effects by distinct molecular mechanisms. Sirolimus inhibits mTOR, an enzyme that is involved in transduction of extracellular mitogenic signals, whereas paclitaxel stablizes microtubules and arrests cells in the M phase of the cell cycle. The intriguing data generated in this and earlier studies strongly support additional studies to identify molecular target (s)of XS0601.

During clinical follow-up after PCI, repeat angiography was still the most reliable index to determine the occurrence of restenosis. However, due to the cultural conditions in China, most patients are reluctant to accept repeat angiography except for occurrence of typical angina. Although this clinical trial was the largest randomized, double-blind, placebo-controlled multi-center study for preventing restenosis after PCI with botanical medicine so far in China, the angiographic follow-up rate in the present study (47.1%)was relatively low as compared with some large-scale international clinical trials for preventing restenosis. Nevertheless, the effect of XS0601 in reducing clinical end-point events and recurrent angina also indicate its benefit in patients after PCI.

In conclusion, the current study demonstrated the effectiveness and safety of XS0601 as a therapeutic agent in preventing restenosis after PCI. The anatomical or vascular benefit of XS0601 also translates into improved clinical outcomes. The intriguing findings from this and earlier studies of XS0601 examplify and signify the great potential of botanical medicine and/or Chinese herbal medicine in the development of novel therapeutics.

REFERENCES

[1] Grines CL, Rizik D, Levine A, et al. Colchicine angioplasty restenosis trial (CART) (Abstr)[J]. Circulation, 1991, 84: II-365.

[2] Kent KM, William DO, Cassagneau B, et al. Double blind, controlled trial of the effect of angiopeptin on coronary restenosis following balloon angioplasty (Abstr)[J]. Circulation, 1993, 88: 1-506.

[3] Emanuelsson H, Beatt JK, Bagger JP, et al. Long-term effects of angiopeptin treatment in coronary angioplasty: Reduction of clinical events but not angiographic restenosis[J]. Circulation, 1995, 91: 1689-1696.

[4] Whitworth HB, Roubin GS, Hollmann J, Meier B. Effects of nefidipine on recurrent stenosis after percutaneous transluminal coronary angioplasty[J]. J Am Coll Cardiol, 1986, 8: 1271-1276.

[5] O'Keefe JH, Giorgi LV, Hartzler GO, et al. Effects of diltiazem on complications and restenosis after coronary angioplasty[J]. Am J Cardiol, 1991, 67: 373-376.

[6] Grigg LE, Kay TW, Valentine PA, et al. Determinants of restenosis and lack of effect of dietary supplementation with eicosapentaenoic acid in the incidence of coronary artery restenosis after angioplasty[J]. J Am Coll Cardiol, 1989, 13: 665-672.

[7] Reis GS, Sipperly ME, McCabe CH, et al. Randomised trial of fish oil for prevention of restenosis after coronary angioplasty[J]. Lancet, 1989, 2: 177-181.

[8] Bairati I, Roy L, Meyer F. Double-blind, randomised, controlled trial of fish oil supplements in prevention of recurrence of stenosis after coronary angioplasty[J]. Circulation, 1992, 85: 950-956.

[9] Ellis SG, Roubin GS, Wilentz J, et al. Effect of 18-to 24-hour heparin administration for prevention of restenosis after uncomplicated coronary angioplasty[J]. Am Heart J, 1989, 117: 777-782.

[10] Faxon D, Spiro T, Minor S, et al. Low molecular weight heparin in prevention of restenosis after angioplasty: Results of enoxaparin restenosis (ERA)trial[J]. Circulation, 1994, 90: 908-914.

[11] Weintraub WS, Boccuzzi SJ, Klein JL, et al. Lack of effect of lovastatin on restenosis after coronary angioplasty: Lovastatin restenosis trial study group[J]. N Engl J Med, 1994, 331: 1331-1337.

[12] Beigel Y, Zafrir N, Teplitzky Y, et al. The effect of lovastatin on early restenosis[J]. J Clin Pharmacol, 1995, 35: 599-605.

[13] Knudston ML, Flintoft VF, Roth DL, et al. Effect of short-term prostacyclin administration on restenosis after percutaneous transluminal coronary angioplasty[J]. J Am Coll Cardiol, 1990, 15: 691-697.

[14] Raizner AE, Hollman J, Abukhalil J, et al. Ciprostene for restenosis revisited: Quantitative analysis of angiograms (Abstr)[J]. J Am Coll Cardiol, 1993, 21: 321A.

[15] Serruys PW, Klein W, Tijssen JPG. Effect of ketanserin in the prevention of restenosis after percutaneous transluminal coronary angioplasty: A multicenter randomised double-blind placebo-controlled trial[J]. Circulation, 1993, 88: 1588-1601.

[16] Savage MP, Goldberg S, MacDonald RG, et al. Multi-Hospital Eastern Atlantic Restenosis Trial II: A placebo-controlled trial of thromboxane blockade in the prevention of restenosis following coronary angioplasty[J]. Am Heart J, 1991, 122: 1239-1243.

[17] Serruys PW, Rutsch W, Heyndricks GR, et al. Prevention of restenosis after percutaneous transluminal coronary angioplasty with thromboxane A2-receptor blockade[J]. Circulation, 1991, 84: 1568-1580.

[18] Hong MK, Mehran R, Mintz GS, et al. Restenosis after coronary angioplasty[J]. Curr Probl Cardiol, 1997, 22: 7-36.

[19] Wong A, Chan C. Drug-elutting stents: the end of restenosis? [J]. Ann Acad Med Singapore, 2004, 33: 423-431.

[20] Kereiakes DJ, Choo JK, Young JJ, et al. Thrombosis and drug-elutting stents: a critical appraisal[J]. Rev Cardiovasc Med, 2004, 5: 9-15.

[21] Bhatia V, Bhatia R, Dhindsa M. Drug-eluting stents: new era and new concerns[J]. Postgrad Med J, 2004, 80 (939): 13-18.

[22] Shi DZ, Xu FQ, Li LZ, et al. The experimental study of Xue Guan Tong on preventing restenosis after percutaneous transluminal angioplasty[J]. Chin J Integr Tradit West Med, 1995, 1: 284-287.

[23] Shi DZ, Li J, Ma XC, et al. Clinical observation of concentrated Xuefu Zhuyu Pill on preventing restenosis after percutaneous transluminal coronary angioplasty in patients of coronary heart disease[J]. Chin J TCM (Chin), 1997, 38: 27-29.

[24] Xu H, Shi DZ, Chen K, et al. Effect of Xiongshao capsule on proliferation and apoptosis of vascular smooth muscle cells in rabbits observed by serologic pharmacological method[J]. Chin J Integr Tradit West Med (Chin)2000, 20: 757-760.

[25] Xu H, Shi DZ, Chen KJ, et al. Effect of XS0601 on apoptosis and gene expression of p53 and bcl-2 in neointima of porcine coronary artery after balloon injury[J]. Chin J Intervent Cardiol (Chin), 2001, 9: 152-154.

[26] Xu H, Shi DZ, Chen KJ, et al. Effect of Xiongshao Capsule on vascular remodeling in porcine coronary balloon injury model[J]. Chin J Integr Tradit West Med, 2000, 6: 278-282.

[27] Xu H, Chen KJ, Shi DZ, et al. Clinical study of Xiongshao Capsule in preventing restenosis after coronary interventional treatment[J]. Chin J Integr Tradit West Med, 2002, 8: 162-166.

[28] Mintz GS, Popma JJ, Pichard AD, et al. Arterial remodeling after coronary angioplasty: a serial intravascular ultrasound study[J]. Circulation, 1996, 94: 35-43.

[29] Hoffmann R, Mintz GS, Dussaillant GR, et al. Patterns and mechanisms of in-stent restenosis. A serial intravascular ultrasound study[J]. Circulation, 1996, 94: 1247-1254.

First published: CHEN Ke-ji, SHI Da-zhuo, XU Hao, LU Shu-zheng, LI Tian-chang, KE Yuan-nan, ZHANG Min-zhou, LU Xiao-yan, SUN Rui-yuan, YOU Shi-jie. XS0601 reduces the incidence of restenosis: a prospective study of 335 patients undergoing percutaneous coronary intervention in China[J] . Chin Med J, 2006, 119 (1): 6-13.

Traditional Chinese Medicine And aging: Integration and Collaboration Promotes Healthy Aging

CONG Wei-hong and CHEN Ke-ji

Aging is an unavoidable law of life.Traditional Chinese medicine (TCM)has had a clear understanding of aging since very ancient times. For example, it recognizes the limit of the human life span as 100-120 years, as unequivocally stated in the ancient Huang Di Internal Classic, which is known as the "Bible of TCM." [1] On May 25, 2019, all member nations of the World Health Organization agreed to adopt the 11th revision of the *International Statistical Classification of Diseases and Related Health Problems*, which for the first time includes a chapter on traditional medicine originating from TCM.[2]

Compared with other traditional medicines, TCM is by far the most comprehensive. With a long history of practice and refinement, TCM represents the ultimate integration of humanity and natural sciences, health assessment, and herbal medicine and other means of intervention, as well as traditional Chinese culture and ancient Chinese philosophy. TCM has established unique views on life, fitness, diseases, and prevention and treatment of diseases with unique techniques, including Bian-stone, medicine, acupuncture, moxibustion, *tuina* (massage), and *daoyin* (such as tai chi and qigong)over thousands of years. Here, we introduce readers who might not be familiar with TCM and some of its key concepts in relation to human aging.

In the *Huang Di Internal Classic*, human aging is described in great detail with phenotypic features, such as graying hair and balding, dimming eyes, missing teeth, loss of ability to express oneself clearly, withered and wrinkled skin, loss of reproduction capability, crooked steps, and reduced mobility. TCM acknowledges that the main pathological changes associated with aging include degeneration and decline in functions of the viscera and organs, and that age-related problems usually occur slowly, linger together and for a long time, aggravate gradually, and resist recovery, ultimately leading to death after multiple organ failure.Dr Meizhong Yue, an outstanding 20th-century TCM geriatrician, summed up the manifestations of common age-related chronic conditions in simple terms: "Only remember distant events not recent ones; tears when laughing, no tears when crying; blurred vision; poor hearing, yet inquisitive of gossips." [3] This vivid description of age-related problems effectively portrays the complexity of aging, from cognitive impairment, psychological disorders, oral and denture problems, and personality changes, to vision and hearing loss.3 Similarly, the World Health Organization has reported that by age 60 years, the major burdens of disability and death arise from age-related vision and hearing loss, mobility difficulty, and noncommunicable diseases, including heart disease, stroke, chronic respiratory disorders, cancer, and dementia.[4]

The principle of "yin and yang" is one of the core theories of Chinese philosophy as well as of TCM. Ancient Chinese philosophy holds that everything in the universe has two sides—yin and yang—which describe the properties of both the opposites and unity of interrelated things or phenomena in nature. According to TCM theory, one's physical health depends on harmony in the functions of various bodily organs, a moderate and stable state of emotional expression, as well as adaption to different environments, of which the most vital is the dynamic balance between yin and yang. TCM deems that illnesses are fundamentally due to the disturbance of the dynamic balance between yin and yang caused by external or internal factors. When yin and yang are in a state of balance, the body is healthy. When the balance is disturbed, the body becomes unhealthy. Although yin and yang levels decline gradually during aging, yin and yang are still in a state of balance when one is healthy. However, such balance is vulnerable and will eventually change to an extreme state-an unhealthy or diseased state. The *Huang Di Internal Classic*, which first appeared around 2000 B.C., definitively pointed out that the primary cause of aging is the decrease of yin and yang, and that the yin level halves from its maximum in one's 40 s while the yang declines from its highest level at the age of 48 years. Some practical strategies on increasing life expectancy have also been described in this book, such as living in accordance with the general rule of yin and yang, and maintaining a restricted diet and a reasonable lifestyle, which helps one to reach the proclaimed life expectancy of 100-120 years.

The yin and yang concept has also been adopted in modern life science studies, helping people to understand the nature of life, aging, and illness from a different perspective. In 1986, yin and yang concepts were used for the first time to explain cell growth regulation.[5] It is accepted that the yin - yang icon symbolizes the balance and harmony between two opposing forces.[6] An "inflammation of yin and yang" picture was also taken as the cover background of the first issue of Science in 2013, indicating the opposing sides for the role of inflammation (ie, beneficial in some cases, such as in the case of acute inflammatory response to fighting against infections, but also detrimental in others, including its role in the development of neurodegenerative diseases, cardiovascular diseases, and metabolic syndrome).[7]

An holistic approach to health assessment and intervention is another key and related principle of TCM that is particularly pertinent to aging and one of the characters of geroscience research. Although geroscience is a new field of biological aging research, like TCM, it has the central theme of the health span and the primary objective of identifying the biological mechanisms and strategies that will improve the health span.[8] Modern medicine and, for that matter, the entire health-care system are based on identifying symptoms, signsz, and abnormal laboratory and imaging findings from which disease diagnosis and a treatment plan can be formulated. This approach can be effective in dealing with a single disease, but not so when dealing with issues related to aging or health conditions in older adults. Instead of focusing and treating individual symptoms, TCM approaches the whole body and its overall health condition as well as its interactions with the environment. The concept of "qi" is such an example. While there is no molecular or signaling pathway can be used to explain qi, this is a unique way, based on TCM theories and empirical experiences, to look into underlying mechanisms and potential etiology. Overall, TCM and geroscience endorse similar principles and approaches to promoting healthy aging and address the root problems of illnesses in the elderly.

TCM has also established effective strategies against specific age-related illnesses during its long history of practice managing age-related diseases. With the development of molecular biology and various advanced technological approaches, more efforts are being made to elucidate potential mechanisms and pathways for promoting healthy aging, reducing age-related risks of specific diseases, and preventing and treating age-related conditions. Results of acupuncture for chronic severe functional constipation in patients of middle and older age indicate that 8 weeks of electroacupuncture increases complete spontaneous bowel movements and is safe for the treatment of chronic severe functional constipation.[9] A study on acupuncture for urinary incontinence in elderly patients showed that electroacupuncture treatment involving the lumbosacral region resulted in less urine leakage after 6 weeks.[10] Tai chi training appears to reduce balance impairments in patients with mild-to-mod- erate Parkinson's disease (mean age = 68 ± 9 years), with additional benefits of improved functional capacity and reduced falls.[11] It may also be a useful treatment for fibromyalgia and merits long-term study in larger study populations.[12] A study of TCM's impact on age trajectories of health indicates that the TCM application has an important role in long-term health (mean age = 63.5 ± 7.7 years).[13] Furthermore, many TCM herbs have shown effects promoting anti - inflammation, anti-oxidation, anti-apoptosis, and autophagy. Treatment of bone-marrow-derived mesenchymal stem cells with astragalus polysaccharide was proved to impede mitochondrial reactive oxygen species accumulation and remarkably inhibited apoptosis, senescence, and reduction of proliferation and pluripotency of bone-marrow-derived mesenchymal stem cells caused by ferric-am-monium-citrate-induced iron overload.[14]

An ancient Chinese tale, "Blind Men and an Elephant, " warns against mistaking a part for the whole.

Likewise, life is a very complex process, and so are aging, its underpinning mechanisms, and their role in contributing to the development of age-related diseases. A one-sided view of them will only lead to judgment deviation or even major errors. An holistic view of TCM may help to gain a better understanding. As a flock of starlings relies on connectivity, dynamics, and communication, the human body is a dynamic equilibrium system with interrelated and interacting physical and mental elements.

In the past, people thought that TCM concepts might sound alien to the Western world. The integration and collaboration between TCM and modern medical research have since emerged and continue to advance at an accelerated speed. While the application of the TCM approach to geroscience research and vice versa has just begun, these two disciplines share key principles, which make it feasible and likely synergistically fruitful. This will ultimately lead to the development of novel interventional strategies for promoting healthy aging and mitigating age as a major risk for chronic diseases.

REFERENCES

[1] Huang Di Internal Classic[M]. Beijing, China: People's Medical Publishing House; 1963.

[2] https: //www.who.int/news-room/detail/25-05-2019-world- health-assembly-update. Accessed May 25, 2019.

[3] Yue M, Chen K. Meizhong Yue Collection. Beijing, China: China Press of Traditional Chinese Medicine; 2012.

[4] World Health Organization. World report on ageing and health. World Health Organization website.https: //apps.who.int/iris/handle/10665/186463. Published 2015. Accessed June 21, 2019.

[5] Marx JL. The yin and yang of cell growth control. Science.1986; 232 (4754): 1093-1095.

[6] Essence of harmony. Nat Immunol. 2005; 6 (4): 325.

[7 Mueller K. Inflammation's yin-yang. Science. 2013; 339 (6116): 155.

[8] Nikolich-Žugich J, Goldman D, Cohen P, et al. Preparing for an aging world: engaging biogerontologists, geriatricians, and the society.J Gerontol A Biol Sci Med Sci.2016; 71 (4): 435-444.

[9] Liu Z, Yan S, Wu J, et al.Acupuncture for chronic severe functional constipation: a randomized trial. Ann Intern Med. 2016; 165 (11): 761-769.

[10] Liu Z, Liu Y, Xu H, et al. Effect of electroacupuncture on urinary leakage among women with stress urinary incontinence: a randomized clinical trial. JAMA. 2017; 317 (24): 2493-2501.

[11] Li F, Harmer P, Fitzgerald K, et al. Tai chi and postural stability in patients with Parkinson's disease. N Engl J Med. 2012; 366 (6): 511-519.

[12] Wang C, Schmid C, Rones R, et al. A randomized trial of tai chi for fibromyalgia. N Engl J Med. 2010; 363 (8): 743-754.

[13] Hsu Y, Chiu C, Wray L, et al. Impact of traditional Chinese medicine on age trajectories of health: evidence from the Taiwan longitudinal study on aging. J Am Geriatr Soc. 2015; 63 (2): 351-357.

[14] Yang F, Yan G, Li Y, et al. Astragalus polysaccharide attenuated iron overload-induced dysfunction of mesenchymal stem cells via suppressing mitochondrial ROS. Cell Physiol Biochem. 2016; 39 (4): 1369-1379.

First published: Weihong Cong, Keji Chen.Traditional Chinese medicine and aging: integration and collaboration promotes healthy aging[J].Aging Medicine, 2019 (0): 1-3.

Hawthorn Extract Alleviates Atherosclerosis through Regulating Inflammation and Apoptosis Related Factors: An Experimental Study

WANG Song-zi, WU Min, CHEN Ke-ji, LIU Yue, SUN Jing, SUN Zhuo,
MA He, and LIU Long-tao

Cardiovascular and cerebrovascular diseases caused by atherosclerosis (AS)have become the leading cause of death in humans. Inflammation is among the main causes of AS. Inflammatory reactions accompany every stage of AS development. The pathological manifestations of AS also involve inflammation. [1] Apoptosis is a process in which cells automatically terminate their lives under physiological or pathological conditions regulated by an inherent genetic mechanism. Apoptosis was involved throughout the pathological process of AS, which can promote tissue resistance to endogenous or exogenous damage and influence the occurrence and development of AS. [2] Apoptotic macrophages that are not quickly eliminated induce the secretion of inflammatory factors in the intima and accelerate AS progression. The apoptosis of vascular smooth muscle cells (VSMCs)leads to the degradation of collagen components in the cells, thinning of the fibrous cap of the plaque, and formation of vulnerable plaques. [3] Therefore, regulating apoptosis and inhibiting inflammatory responses are key targets for treating AS. As a common treatment for AS, although simvastatin has shown some efficacy, statins may cause side effects, including myalgia, muscle weakness, elevated liver enzymes, hyperglycaemia, and diabetes risk. [4] Therefore, safe and effective alternative to statins are needed for treating AS. Alternative therapies, such as Chinese medicine, have attracted attention.

Hawthorn activates blood circulation to dissipate blood stasis, promote digestion to eliminate stagnation, and arrest diarrhea and treat dysentery. Recent studies showed that hawthorn flavonoids in hawthorn extract dilated the coronary artery, lowered the blood lipid and blood pressure, strengthened the heart, and excited the central nervous system. [5] A clinical study showed that hawthorn extract significantly reduced serum hypersensitive C-reactive protein (hs-CRP)and matrix metalloproteinase-9 (MMP-9)in patients with AS, suggesting that hawthorn extract can stabilize atherosclerotic plaques for treating AS. Its mechanism may be related to anti-inflammatory reactions and inhibiting extracellular matrix degradation. [6] Animal experiments also showed that hawthorn extract improved phagocytosis of the reticuloendothelial system and regulated the immune organ index as well as white blood cell count in mice. [7] Hawthorn extract inhibited the proliferation and promoted the apoptosis of HepG2 cells. [8]

The aim of this study was to investigate the effect of hawthorn extract on apoptosis and inflammation-related factors in an apolipoprotein E gene knockout (ApoE)-/-mice model of AS so as to explore the mechanism of hawthorn extract in anti-AS.

METHODS

1 Animals

Eight-week-old male ApoE-/-mice (n=36)and C57BL/6 mice (n=12), weighing 19–21 g, were obtained from the Jackson Laboratory (Bar Harbor, ME, USA)and bred by the Laboratory Animal Center of Beijing University. ApoE-/-mice were fed a high-fat diet containing 21% saturated fat and 0.15% cholesterol, while C57BL/6 mice were fed a basic diet. Mice were raised in a specific pathogen-free laboratory at a temperature of 18 ± 1 ℃, relative humidity of 40%–50%, and free access to food and water. Experiments were conducted in accordance with the Guiding Opinions on Treating Experimental Animals and the Guidelines of the Animal Investigation Committee of Peking University.

2 Drug Preparation

A total of 5 g hawthorn extract (No. AKH12-2, Linyi Aikang Pharmaceutical Co., Ltd., Shandong, China) containing 30% total flavonoids of hawthorn was dissolved in 1L distilled water, 0.5 g simvastatin tablet (No. 100601-201003, Merck Pharmaceutical, Billerica, MA, USA)was smashed into powder and dissolved in 1L distilled water. The above solution was ready for use.

3 Grouping and Administration

Thirty-six ApoE-/-mice were randomly divided into 3 groups by a random number table including model group, hawthorn extract group and simvastatin group, 12 mice in each group. Twelve C57BL/6 mice were used as a control. The mice in the hawthorn extract group was administered 50 mg/kg hawthorn extract daily and the simvastatin group was administered 5 mg/kg simvastatin (equal to 20 times of the clinical dose), and the control and model groups were administered 0.2 mL saline per day. All mice were raised for 16 weeks.

4 Plasma Lipids Analysis

After 16 weeks, mice were fasted for 12 h before sacrifice. Intraperitoneal injection of pentobarbital was administered to the mice to minimize pain and 2 mL blood samples were collected from the retroorbital plexus. After allowing the blood samples to stand for 30 min, they were centrifuged for 10 min at 3, 000 r/min and the serum was stored at –80 ℃. Total cholesterol (TC), triglyceride (TG), low-density lipoprotein cholesterol (LDL-C)and high-density lipoprotein cholesterol (HDL-C)were tested using an enzymatic assay with an AD2700 automatic biochemical detector (Olympus, Tokyo, Japan).

5 Inflammatory Mediators in Plasma

The concentrations of monocyte chemoattractant protein-1 (MCP-1), interleukin-1β (IL-1β), adiponectin (APN)and hypersensitive C-reactive protein (hs-CRP)in plasma were measured by enzyme-linked immunosorbent assay (ELISA)using the mice serum samples. ELISA kits were purchased from Shanghai Senxiong Biological Co., Ltd. (China). A standard curve was drawn according to standard serum A_{492} value of different concentrations used to calculate inflammatory factor concentrations.

6 Hematoxylin and Eosin Staining

A piece of the tissue block prepared from the aorta was separated and placed in 10% formalin. The tissue was gradually dehydrated in different concentrations of ethanol and placed in xylene to make the sample transparent. The tissue was immersed in melted paraffin and fixed in a wax-embedded block. The paraffin block was cut into a 5-μm-thick sheet, placed on a glass slide, and incubated at 45 ℃. At last it was stained with Harris hematoxylin and eosin (HE)and the sample was sealed with gum.

7 Image Analysis of HE Slice

Lesion images were captured with a CK40-32ph microscope (Olympus, Tokyo, Japan)equipped with Image-Pro 6.0 software (Media Cybernetics, Rockville, MD, USA). HE slices were scanned by tissue slicing scanners (Pannoramic MIDI, 3D HISTECH Ltd, Budapest, Hungary). Slices were placed under the scanner lens and scanned into images. Then a file containing all the tissue information on the slice was formed and could be opened by Pannoramic viewer software. After the scopes of plaque and vascular lumen were selected by the researcher, the area of the plaque and vascular lumen and their ratio could be calculated by QuantCenter Software. All slices were scanned and analyzed.

8 Aorta Lesion Examination by Scanning Electron Microscopy

The glutaraldehyde settled vascular segments was stained with 1% osmium tetroxide and then was dehydrated using a gradient series of ethanol. After drying, the sample was fractured with liquid nitrogen, dehydrated and dried with a CO_2 critical point dryer. Samples were sprayed onto the sample holder with conductive adhesive for metal spray plating. The samples were observed and photographed under an acceleration voltage of 15 kV by scanning electron microscopy.

9 Aorta Lesion Examination by Transmission Electron Microscopy

After washing with physiological saline, the isolated aortic vascular tissue was immersed in 3% glutaraldehyde and dehydrated with gradient ethanol acetone. Ultrastructural changes in the aortic vascular were observed by transmission electron microscopy (TEM)after epoxy resin embedding, positioning, repairing, slicing by ultramicrocutting, and lead citrate staining.

10 Protein Expressions of Bax and Bcl-2 by Western Blotting

Five pieces of aortic vascular tissue of 2 cm in length preserved in liquid nitrogen were homogenized by adding an appropriate amount of cell lysates and the supernatant was collected. Using a tissue protein extraction kit (1: 200； Abcam, Cambridge, UK), protein was extracted from the aortic vascular tissue. The protein concentration was measured by the Bicinchoninic acid (BCA)method. Next, 20 μg denatured protein was separated by sodium dodecyl sulfate polyacrylamide gel electropheresis (SDS-PAGE)gel and wet-transferred onto a polyvinylidene fluoride (PVDF)membrane. After blocking in skimmed milk powder for 1 h, anti-mouse Bax and Bcl-2 polyclonal antibodies were added to each membrane independently to detect the target protein and the corresponding reference overnight at 4 ℃. On the next day, the membranes were rinsed 3 times in Tris-buffered saline (TBS)containing Tween-20 for 5 min each time. A secondary anti-rabbit IgG antibody labelled with horseradish peroxidase was added and incubated for 1 h at room temperature. After rinsing the membrane 3 times in TBS containing Tween-20 for 5 min each time, protein was visualized by using the enhanced chemiluminescence system (ECL, Scientific Instrument Limited Company, Shanghai, China). β-actin (1: 200, Abcam bioscience, Cambridge, USA)was used as an internal reference, and the grey level ratio of target protein to β-actin protein was calculated by semi-quantitative analysis.

11 mRNA Expression Levels of Bax and Bcl-2 by Quantitative Real-Time Fluorescence Polymerase Chain Reaction

Bax and Bcl-2 mRNA expressions in the aortic vascular tissue were detected by quantitative real-time fluorescence polymerase chain reaction (qRT-PCR). Aortic vascular tissue (20 mg)was weighed, total RNA was extracted with Trizol, and the concentration and purity of total RNA were determined. Reverse transcription cDNAs were prepared from 1 μg of total RNA using a two-step method (DNA removal and reverse transcription). Using cDNA as a template, qRT-PCR reaction was conducted using SYBR Green. β-actin was used as an internal reference for analysis. The reaction conditions were as follows: predenaturation at 95 ℃ for 30 s, denaturation at 95 ℃ for 5 s, annealing at 60 ℃ for 20 s with a total of 40 cycles. The sequences of the mRNA primers were as follows: β-actin (266 bp): sense 5'-GTCCCTCACCCTCCCAAAAG-3', anti-sense 5'-GCTGCCTCAACACCTCAACCC-3'； Bcl-2 (230 bp): sense 5'-AGGAGCAGGTGCCTACAAGA-3', anti-sense 5'-GCATTTTCCCACCACTGTCT-3'； Bax (230bp): sense 5'-AGGAGCAGGTGCCTACAAGA-3'； anti-sense 5'-GCATTTTCCCACCACTGTCT-3'. mRNA primers were entrusted to Beijing Huatai Boao Biotechnology Co., Ltd. to synthesize and purify. The PCR samples contained the following: 12.5 μL Maxima SYBR Green/ROX qRT-PCR Master Mix, 0.75 μL sense and antisense primers, 2 μL cDNA, and 9-25 μL nuclease-free water. An ABI7500 fluorescent qRT-PCR instrument (Applied Biosystems, Foster City, CA, USA) was used for the analysis. The Ct value was obtained from the amplification curve.

12 Statistical Analysis

Statistical analysis was performed by t-test for 2 groups or analysis of variance (ANOVA)for 3 or more subgroups using SPSS19.0 statistics software (SPSS Inc. Chicago, IL, USA). $P < 0.05$ was considered significant in all analyses. All values were expressed as mean ± standard error of mean.

RESULTS

1 Modulations of Plasma Lipid Levels

Compared to the control group, the plasma levels of TC, TG and LDL-C were significantly increased and HDL-C was decreased in the model group ($P < 0.01$). Compared to the model group, treatment with hawthorn extract or simvastatin significantly decreased the levels of TC, TG and LDL-C ($P < 0.01$). In contrast, the HDL-C level was significantly increased in mice treated with hawthorn extract or simvastatin. There were no significant differences between the hawthorn extract and simvastatin groups ($P > 0.05$, Figure 1).

2 Assessment of Aortic Atherosclerotic Lesions by Light Microscopy

No evidence of AS was detected in the aortas in the control group, endothelial cells were continuous and intact, the intima was not thickened, and the internal elastic membrane structure was clear and continuous with no stratification and rupture. The thickness of the vascular wall was uniform and the cells were arranged in order (Figures 2A and B). In the model group, endothelial cells were irregular and discontinuous. The internal elastic membrane was broken and unclear. Smooth muscle cells proliferated, and plaques protruded into the lumen of the vessel (Figures 2C and D). In the hawthorn extract and simvastatin groups, endothelial cells were morphologically intact, smooth muscle cells slightly proliferated, and the plaque protruded slightly into the vessel lumen (Figures 2 E–H). After calculating by QuantCenter software, the percentage of plaque area in the model group was 61.2%, compared to the model group, the percentage of plaque area decreased in the hawthorn extract group (20.3%)and the simvastatin group (24.8%, $P < 0.05$).

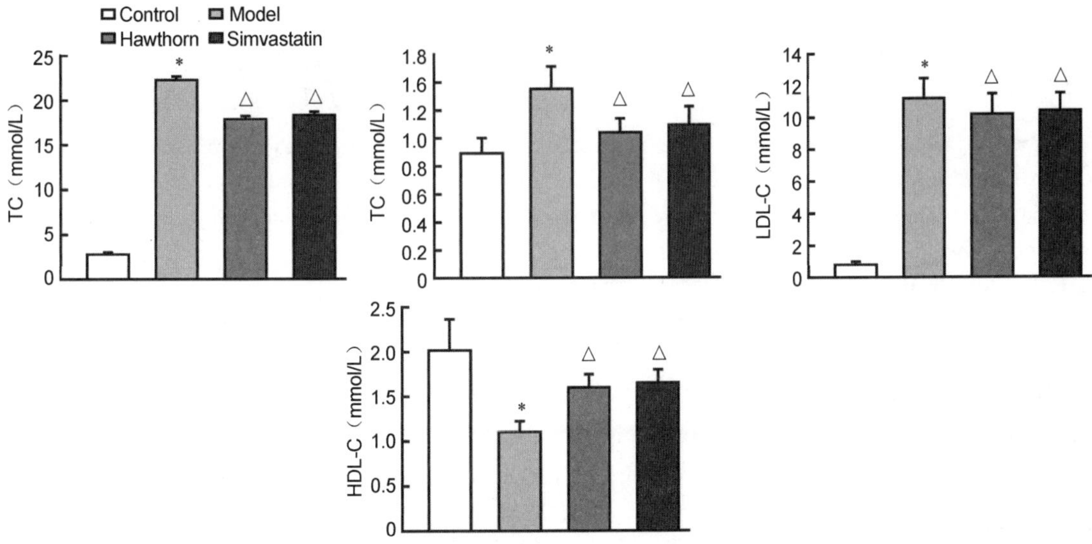

Figure 1 Modulations of Plasma Lipid Levels of Mice

Notes: $^{*}P < 0.01$, *vs.* control group; $^{\triangle}P < 0.01$, *vs.* model group.

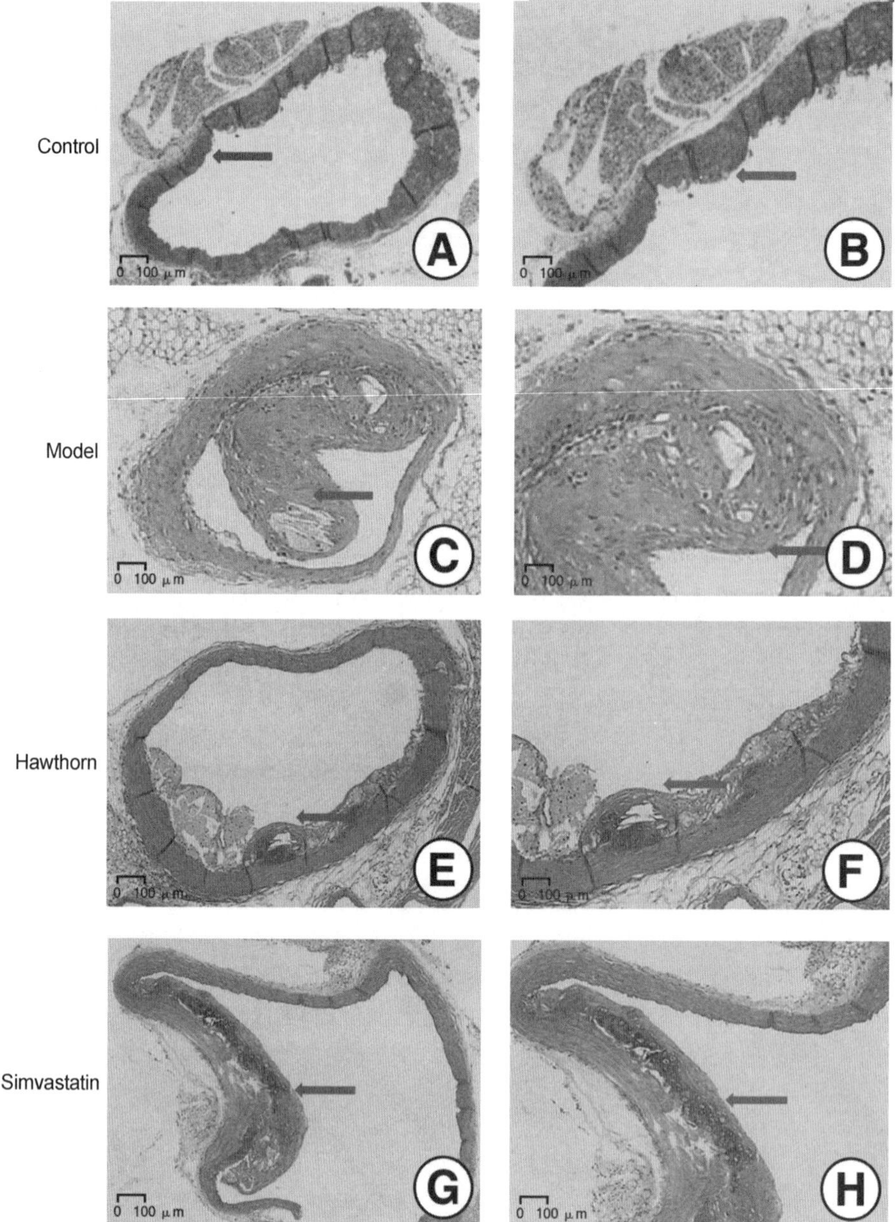

Figure 2　ssessment of Aortic Atherosclerotic Lesions by Light Microscope of Mice

Notes: A, B: smooth aortic lumen in the control group, the arrows indicate the vessel wall; C, D: arrows indicate the atherosclerotic plaque on the inner wall of the aortic in the model group; E, F: arrows indicate the plaque on the inner wall of the aortic in the hawthorn extract group; G, H: arrows indicate the plaque on the inner wall of the aorta in the simvastatin group; A, C, E, G, ×100 magnification; B, D, F, H, ×200 magnification.

3 Assessment of Aortic AS by Scanning Electron Microscopy

In the control group, the aortic intima was smooth and endothelial cells showed a regular shape and were closely connected to each other (Figure 3A). Atherosclerotic plaques appeared in the aortic arch intima in the model group. Some large plaques surfaces were not covered with endothelial cells, while other endothelial cells were withered, proliferative, or caducous. Endothelial cell lesions in the non-plaque area were similar to those area around the plaque (Figure 3B). The intima of the aorta was smooth in the hawthorn extract and simvastatin groups. Endothelial cells were tightly bound together in regular shapes. Small quantity of sediment was identified on them (Figures 3C and D).

Figure 3 sessment of Aortic AS in Mice with Scanning Electron Microscope (× 1, 000)

Notes: A: smooth inner wall of aorta in the control group, the arrow indicates the inner wall of aorta; B: plaque on the inner wall of the aorta in the model group, arrow indicates the plaque; C: adhesive substance in the hawthorn extract group, arrow indicates the adhesive substance on the inner wall of the aorta; D: adhesive substance in the simvastatin group, arrow indicates the adhesive substance on the inner wall of the aorta.

4 Assessment of Aortic AS by Transmission Electron Microscopy

Endothelial cells and smooth muscle cells of the aorta in the control group exhibited a normal shape. The elastic plates were clear and arranged in rule with no lipid droplets and calcium deposits (Figure 4A).

In the model group, most of the small plaques were covered with endothelial cells. These cells lost their normal morphology and showed a smooth surface and no villi. The cell body became thinner and the electron density of the nucleus decreased. Organelles in the cytoplasm were decreased and contained lipid droplets and lysosomes of different sizes. Smooth muscle cells and macrophages containing lipids were detected in the vascular wall. Calcium salt deposition was also observed in some areas, and most vascular smooth muscle cells showed a contractile phenotype (Figure 4B). In the hawthorn extract group and simvastatin group, lipid droplets and lysosomes in vascular cells of mice were decreased and minimal calcium salt was deposited (Figures 4C and D).

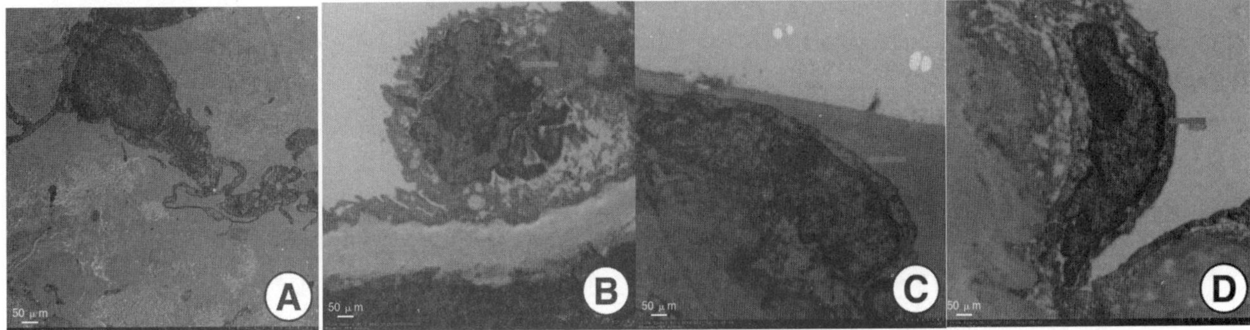

Figure 4 sessment of Aortic AS in Mice with Transmission Electron Microscope (× 4, 500)

Notes: A: normal endothelial cell in the control group, the arrow indicates the endothelia cell; B: nuclear chromatin condensation and wrinkled nuclear membrane in the model group, arrow indicates the endothelia cell; C: endothelial cell with normal nuclear and cellular structure in the hawthorn extract group, arrow indicates nuclear chromatin condensation; D: endothelial cell with normal nuclear and cellular structure in the simvastatin group, arrow indicates nuclear chromatin condensation.

5 Levels of Inflammatory Factors in Plasma

Compared to the control group, the levels of MCP-1, hs-CRP and IL-1β were significantly increased and APN was decreased in the model group (all $P < 0.01$). Compared to the model group, treatment with hawthorn extract and simvastatin decreased the levels of MCP-1, hs-CRP and IL-1β ($P < 0.01$). In contrast, the APN level significantly increased in mice treated with hawthorn extract or simvastatin. However, there were no differences on effects between the hawthorn extract and simvastatin groups ($P > 0.05$, Figure 5).

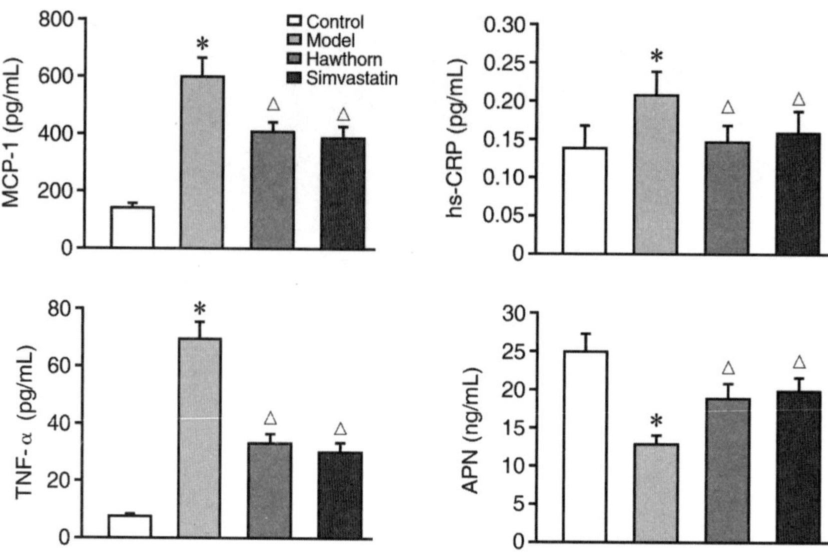

Figure 5　vels of Inflammatory Factors in Mice Plasma among Different Groups

Notes: *$P < 0.01$, vs. control group; △$P < 0.01$, vs. model group.

6 Bcl-2 and Bax Protein and mRNA Expression in Mice Aorta

Compared to the control group, the protein and mRNA expression of Bax increased, while Bcl-2 expression decreased ($P < 0.01$). Comparison to the model group, the protein and mRNA expression of Bax decreased in the hawthorn extract and simvastatin groups ($P < 0.01$). In contrast, Bcl-2 protein and mRNA expression levels were significantly increased in mice treated with hawthorn extract or simvastatin ($P < 0.01$). However, there were no differences on the effects between the hawthorn extract and simvastatin groups ($P > 0.05$, Figure 6).

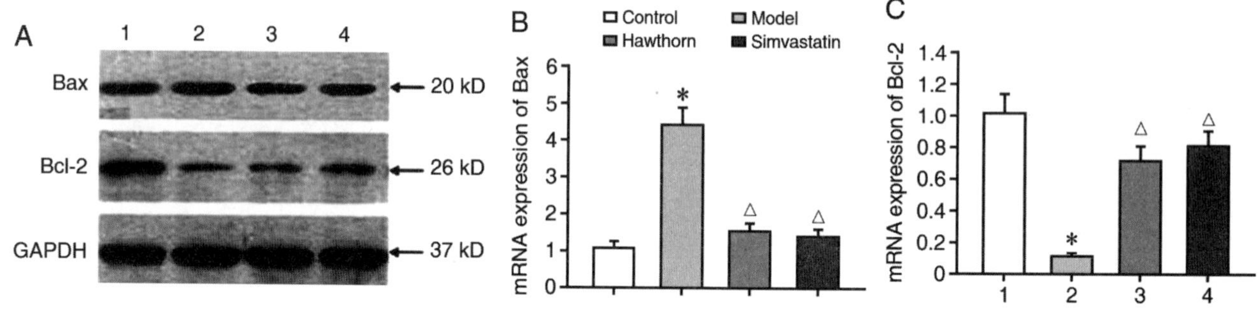

Figure 6　Bax and Bcl-2 Protein and mRNA

Notes: Expression in Mice AortaNotes: A: Bax and Bcl-2 protein expression by Western-blot, 1: control group, 2: model group, 3: hawthorn extract group, 4: simvastatin group; B: Bax mRNA expression by qRT-PCR; C: Bcl-2 mRNA expression by qRT-PCR; *$P < 0.01$, vs. control group; △$P < 0.01$, vs. model group.

DISCUSSION

The pathogenesis of AS is very complex and due to its aetiology varies, mainly including injury or apoptosis of the endothelium, abnormal lipid metabolism, hemodynamic damage, and physical and chemical damage, among other effects. Multiple complex factors acting on vascular wall lead to the occurrence of chronic inflammation of the vascular wall, resulting in AS. [9] Although a previous study showed that statins significantly reduce the size of lipid-rich plaque in patients with AS, statins are only effective in 15%–30% of AS patients[10] and some patients continue to have atherosclerotic plaques, plaque rupture, and stroke. [11]

Additionally, statins had several severe side effects, such as myotoxity, hepatotoxicity and kidney damage. [12-15] Therefore, it is very important to find more safe and effective drugs for treating patients with AS.

Hawthorn is a common natural plant for both medicine and food which is safe with no side effects reported. At present, compositions found and extracted from hawthorn mainly include: flavonoids, flavanes and their polymers, organic acids, triterpenoids and steroids. [16] Hawthorn has strong pharmacological effects on cardiovascular immune and digestive systems. [17] Pharmacological studies have shown that flavonoids composition in hawthorn extract could lower blood lipids, protect liver and treat experimental atherosclerosis, [18] lower blood pressure, increase coronary flow, and improve arrhythmia. [19] Triterpenic acid in hawthorn extract could also improve circulation and increase coronary flow. [20,21] Ursolic acid could significantly enhance the phagocytic function of peritoneal macrophages in immunosuppressive mice, increase the number of peripheral blood leukocytes, promote the proliferation of splenic lymphocytes and increase the spleen index. [22] Organic acid in hawthorn extract could increase the secretion of digestive enzymes in the stomach, enhance the activity of lipase and protease, promote intestinal peristalsis and have obvious bidirectional regulation on intestinal dysfunction, which is helpful to mechanical and chemical digestion. [23,24] Other studies showed that Shanzha Xiaozhi Capsule (山楂消脂胶囊)significantly reduced the level of serum hs-CRP in patients with non-acute coronary heart disease with phlegm and stasis syndrome. [25] In our study, the levels of TC, TG, and LDL-C in the serum were increased and HDL-C decreased in the model group. Hawthorn extract and simvastatin reduced the levels of TC, TG, and LDL-C and increased HDL-C level in the serum.

Meanwhile, we examined the effects of hawthorn extract by light microscopy and electron microscopy. The results showed that hawthorn extract protected the endothelial cells of the aorta, decreased the number of lesions of endothelial cells, and reduced lipid and calcium salt deposition in smooth muscle cells and macrophages. The size of the atherosclerotic plaque was also reduced.

MCP-1 is involved in the lipid stripe formation, plaque instability, and plaque rupture periods of AS. It combines with its receptor CC-chemokine receptor 2 to induce the expression of adhesion factors in monocytes and endothelial cells, thereby inflammatory cells migrate to the lesion and lead to inflammation during AS development. [26] Hs-CRP induces endothelial cells to secrete and express adhesion factors and chemokines. [27]The role of IL-1β in the AS inflammatory pathological mechanism are well-known. When an inflammatory reaction occurs, inflammatory corpuscles induce the secretion and maturation of downstream IL-1β, and IL-1β affects the development of AS. [28,29]APN protects the endothelium by exerting complex anti-inflammatory effects in AS. APN terminates the signal transduction pathway mediated by lipopolysaccharide, tumor necrosis factor-α, and IL-6 in macrophages and induces the expression of anti-inflammatory genes in macrophages. [30] We found that the levels of MCP-1, hs-CRP, and IL-1β in the serum were increased and APN in the serum was decreased in the model group. Hawthorn extract and simvastatin reduced the levels of MCP-1, hs-CRP, and IL-1β and increased the APN level in the serum.

An imbalance between the proliferation and apoptosis of VSMCs leads to the formation of AS plaques. In AS injury, VSMCs proliferation is dominant and apoptosis is reduced. [31,32] Apoptosis is strictly regulated by apoptosis genes. Bcl-2 is the most common antiapoptotic gene and is expressed in macrophages, VSMCs, and foam cells. Bcl-2 expression is increased in areas where inflammatory cells gather. Bax is also an essential signal for initiating apoptosis, which can resist the anti-apoptotic effect of Bcl-2 and promote apoptosis. In this study, we found that hawthorn extract and simvastatin reduced the protein and mRNA expression of Bax and increased Bcl-2 expressions.

In conclusion, our study suggests that hawthorn extract regulates lipids, inhibits proliferation, lipidosis, and calcium deposition of VSMCs, and resists inflammation and apoptosis and thus is useful for treating AS. Additionally, hawthorn extract decreased the levels of MCP-1, hs-CRP and IL-1β increased the level of APN in the serum, reduced the protein and mRNA expression of Bax, and increased the protein and mRNA expression of Bcl-2 in the aorta, suggesting that it functions by inhibiting inflammatory and apoptosis signalling pathways.

REFERENCES

[1] Wang X, Li CY, Su LP, Zhou Y. Progress of pathogenesis and treatment of atherosclerosis[J]. Pract J Card Cereb Pneum Vas Dis (Chin), 2017, 25 (2): 1-4.

[2] Libby P, Ridker PM, Hansson GK. Progress and challenges in translating the biology of atherosclerosis[J]. Nature, 2011, 473 (7347): 317-325.

[3] Martinet W, De Meyer I, Verheye S, Schrijvers DM, Timmermans JP, De Meyer GRY. Drug-induced macrophage autophagy in atherosclerosis: for better or worse? [J]. Basic Res Cardiol, 2013, 108 (1): 321.

[4] Mancini GB, Baker S, Bergeron J, Fitchett D, Frohlich J, et al. Diagnosis, prevention, and management of statin adverse effects and intolerance: Canadian Consensus Working Group update (2016)[J]. Can J Cardiol, 2016, 32 (7): S35-S65.

[5] Yu BB, Yan XS, Sun DD. Advances in pharmacological action and mechanism study of Hawthorn[J]. Central South Pharm (Chin), 2015, 13 (7): 745-748.

[6] Liu LT, Zheng GJ, Zhang WG, Guo G, Wu M. Study on treatment of carotid atherosclerosis with extraction of Polygoni Cuspidati Rhizoma et Radix and Crataegi Fructus: a randomized controlled trial[J]. Chin J Chin Mater Med (Chin), 2014, 39 (6): 1115-1119.

[7] Liu CL. Studies on the immunomodulation and cardioprotective effects of Hawthorn extract on mice[dissertation]. Xi'an: Fourth Military Medical University；2006.

[8] Peng FH, Ma X, Hu XY. Effects of Hawthorn extract on apoptosis and related factors of HepG2 cells[J]. Chin J Exp Tradit Med Form (Chin), 2016, 22 (7): 169-172.

[9] Fredman G, Tabas I. Boosting inflammation resolution in atherosclerosis: the next frontier for therapy[J]. Am J Pathol, 2017, 187 (6): 1211-1221.

[10] Zhao YK, Liu ZH, Mo ZQ. Absorptive effect and separating effect of macroporous adsorption resin on polydatin from Polygonum cuspidatum[J]. Hunan Agricul Sci (Chin), 2011, 41 (9): 123-126.

[11] Kernan WN, Ovbiagele B, Black HR, Bravata DM, Chimowitz MI, Ezekowitz MD, et al. Guidelines for the prevention of stroke in patients with stroke and transient ischemic attack: a guideline for healthcare professionals from the American Heart Association/ American Stroke Association[J]. Stroke, 2014, 45 (7): 2160-2236.

[12] Yin YJ, Zhang Q, Jia ZH, Zhang JF, Wang HT, Wei C, et al. Protective effect and its mechanism of Tongxinluo on vascular endothelial function in hyperlipidemic rabbits[J]. Chin J Integr Tradit West Med (Chin), 2018, 38 (3): 325-330.

[13] Wang Q, Liu WX. A case of drug-induced myositis caused by simvastatin in intensive lipid-lowering therapy[J]. J Cardiovasc Pulmon Dis (Chin), 2006, 25 (3): 175.

[14] Zhang B, Wang LL. Clinical application of statins and their major adverse effects[J]. J Int Pharm Res (Chin), 2013, 40 (5): 560-564+572.

[15] Xu TJ. The effect of rosuvastatin on liver color ultrasound, ALT, AST and γ-GGT of nonalcoholic fatty liver disease[J]. Chin J Integr Tradit West Med Dig (Chin), 2018, 26 (7): 582-585.

[16] Lou LJ, Luo JX, Gao Y. Overview of chemical compositions and pharmacological action of Grataegus pinnatifida Bunge[J]. China Pharm (Chin)2014, 23 (3): 92-94.

[17] Jurikova T, Sochor J, Rop O, Mlcek J, Balla S, Szekeres L, et al. Polyphenolic profile and biological activity of Chinese hawthorn (Crataegus pinnatifida Bunge)fruits[J]. Molecules, 2012, 17 (12): 14490-14509.

[18] Yang YJ, Lin J, Wang CM, Guo JJ. Experimental study on early intervention of total flavonoids from hawthorn leaves on hyperlipidemia in rats[J]. Chin Tradit Herb Drugs (Chin), 2008, 39 (12): 1848-1850.

[19] Huang K, Yang XB, Huang ZM. Advances in pharmacological action of hyperin[J]. Herald Med (Chin), 2009, 28 (8): 1046-1048.

[20] Li HZ, Huang QS, Chen WQ, Huang SX. Inhibitory effect of hawthorn extract on mutagenicity of human peripheral blood lymphocytes induced by hexavalent chromium[J]. J Mathemat Med (Chin), 2005, (6): 80-82.

[21] Lin Y, Vermeer MA, Trautwein EA. Triterpenic acids present in hawthorn lower plasma cholesterol by inhibiting intestinal ACAT activity in hamsters[J]. Evid Based Complment Alterm, 2011, 2011: 801272.

[22] Lin K, Zhang TP, Zhu S, Wu C, Zhang HY. Immunological effects of ursolic acid from hawthorn fruits on hepatocellular carcinoma HepS cell in mice[J]. Chin J Biochem Pharm (Chin), 2007 (5), 28: 308-311.

[23] Shen YJ, ed. Pharmacology of Chinese materia medica[M]. Beijing: People’s Medical Publishing House；2000: 574.

[24] Li JH, Hu JL. Pharmacological effect and clinical application of Hawthorn[J]. Chin J Drug Abus Prev Treat (Chin), 2011, 17 (6): 334-338.

[25] Wang WH, Zhao HY, Chen WQ, Luo ZX, Yu XL, He QJ, et al. Effect of Shanzha Xiaozhi Capsule on high-sensitivity C-reactive protein and matrix metalloproteinases in patients with non-acute phase coronary heart disease of phlegm and blood stasis syndrome[J]. Chin J Inf Tradit Chin Med (Chin), 2012, 19 (1): 13-15.

[26] Kuper C, Beck FX, Neuhofer W. Autocrine MCP-1/CCR2 signaling stimulates proliferation and migration of renal carcinoma cells[J]. Oncol Lett 2016, 12 (3): 2201-2209.

[27] Li Q. Effects of different doses of risuvastatin on the level of SAA hs-CRP in atherosclerotic rats[J]. Contemp Med (Chin), 2012, 18 (5): 131-132.

[28] Wu YH, Sun JW, Chi TH. Mechanism of NLRP3/ Casepase-1/IL-1 beta signaling pathway in pathogenesis of atherosclerosis in rats[J]. Chin Heart J (Chin)2018, 30 (2): 141-145.

[29] i Q, Li Y, Guo ZH, Liu L, Zhang JY, Ren X, et al. Effects of Xin Tong-tai on blood lipid, ox-LDL and IL-1β in aorta of rabbits with atherosclerosis[J]. Chin J Atheroscler (Chin), 2016, 24 (1): 39-43.

[30] Kyriazi E, Tsiotra PC, Boutati E, Ikonomidis I, Fountoulaki K, Maratou E, et al. Effects of adiponectin in TNF-α, IL-6 and IL-10 cytokine production from coronary artery disease macrophages[J]. Horm Metab Res 2011, 43 (8): 537-544.

[31] Zhang ZJ, Jia SB, Hou JJ, Liu J, Wang H, Li L. The expression of Bcl-2 and Bax in aorta of rats with hyperhomocysteinemia[J]. Guangdong Med J (Chin), 2013, 34 (8): 1160-1162.

[32] Bao XM, Zheng HC. Effect of homocysteine on proliferation and migration of rat vascular smooth muscle cells and its possible mechanism[J]. Shandong Med J (Chin), 2015, 55 (44): 25-27.

First published: WANG Song-zi, WU Min, CHEN Ke-ji, LIU Yue, SUN Jing, SUN Zhuo, MA He, LIU Long-tao. Hawthorn extract alleviates atherosclerosis through regulating Inflammation and apoptosis related factors: an experimental study[J]. Chin J Integr Med, 2019, 25 (2): 108-115.

Ligustrazine Inhibits Platelet Activation via Suppression of the Akt Pathway

LI Li, CHEN Hong-wei, SHEN A-ling, LI Qiong-yu, CHEN You-qin, CHU Jian-feng
LIU Li-ya, PENG Jun, and CHEN Ke-ji

Platelet activation is an essential process to repair injured blood vessels, restoring blood vascular integrity, which is fundamental for the maintenance of vascular function. However, aberrant platelet activation or hyperactivation of platelets may give rise to thrombosis and result in thrombotic vascular events, including atherosclerosis, arterial throm-bosis and myocardial infarction [1-5]. Under physiological conditions, platelets circulate through vessels with an intact and healthy endothelium, remaining in an inactivated state. However, when the endothelium is broken, the von Willebrand factor on the injured vascular wall interacts with its receptor located on the surface of platelets, which in turn induces platelet adhesion to extracellular matrix [6]. Platelet activation results in the release of secondary mediators, including adenosine diphosphate (ADP), thromboxane A_2 (TXA_2)and thrombin [7]. These molecules promote further adhesion, activation and aggregation of platelets, eventually forming a platelet plug to stop bleeding and to repair injured endothelium. The process of platelet activation is strongly associated with multiple intracellular signaling pathways, including the phosphoinositide 3-kinase (PI3K)/AKT serine/threoninekinase (Akt)pathway. Following activation by extracellular stimuli, PI3K is able to phosphorylate PI (4)P and PI (4, 5)P2 to generate PI (3, 4)P2 and PI (3, 4, 5)P3, respectively [8]. Akt is recruited by PIP3 to the platelet plasma membrane with the PIP3-binding domain, and phosphorylated/activated by 3-phosphoinositide dependent protein kinase 1 (PDPK1, additionally termed PDK1)and mammalian target of rapamycin complex 2 (mTORC2) [9-11]. Activated Akt has critical roles in platelet function by mediating various cellular responses, including granule secretion, platelet aggregation and thrombus formation [12-15]. Therefore, inhibition of platelet activation by suppressing the PI3K/Akt pathway may be a promising strategy to treat thrombotic vascular diseases.

A variety of antiplatelet drugs (including aspirin and clopidelgrel)demonstrate significant antiplatelet efficacy for treatment of thrombotic vascular diseases. However, the administration of most currently-used platelet activation inhibitors frequently results in bleeding complications and drug resistance [16, 17]. Recently, an increasing number of studies are focusing on medicinal herbs, in order to discover complementary and alternative compounds with relatively fewer side-effects. *Rhizoma Ligusticum Wallichii* (RLW)is a well-known medicinal herb, which has long been used in china to clinically treat various cardiovascular disor-ders [18]. Ligustrazine is one of the most pharmacologically active compounds of RLW, which has been used for anti-cardiovascular [19], antiplatelet [20], ischemic stroke [21], anti-Alzheimer's [22], neuroprotective [23]and anticancer [24] treatment. In cardiovascular and cerebrovascular diseases, ligustrazine exhibits significant therapeutic activity and may improve the microcirculation, by expanding small arteries, removing blood stasis, and by additionally having effects on antiplatelet aggregation, antioxidation, calcium antagonists and antifibrosis [18, 25-29]. However, the molecular mechanism of its mode of action has not been thoroughly elucidated. A preliminary study from our group identified that treatment with ligustrazine significantly inhibited ADP-induced platelet aggregation and Akt phosphorylation (Li et al, unpublished data). Therefore, it was hypothesized that ligustrazine hydro-chloride (LH; the clinical-grade form of ligustrazine)may exhibit antiplatelet activities by suppressing the Akt signaling pathway. To confirm this hypothesis, the present study used *in vitro* and *ex vivo* platelet activation models, established by stimulating rat platelet-rich plasma (PRP)either with the platelet activator ADP or with the specific Akt pathway activator insulin-like growth factor-1 (IGF-1). The effects of LH on platelet activation and the underlying molecular mechanisms were investigated.

MATERIALS AND METHODS

1 Materials and Reagents

Adrenaline hydrochloride was purchased from Fuyao Group (Fuzhou, china). A thromboxane B_2 (TXB_2) enzyme immunoassay kit was obtained from Enzo Life Sciences, Inc. (Farmingdale, NY, USA). Antibodies against phosphorylated (p-)Akt, Akt, β-actin, and horseradish peroxidase (HRP)-conjugated secondary antibodies were purchased from cell Signaling Technology, Inc. (Danvers, MA, USA). ADP, fluo-4-acetoxymethyl ester (Fluo-4 AM), IGF-1 and other unstated chemicals were purchased from Sigma-Aldrich (Merck KGaA, Darmstadt, Germany).

2 Preparation of LH

LH (>99.0%)was purchased from Beijing Putian Tongchuang biotechnology Co., Ltd. (Beijing, China). LH was dissolved in saline at a concentration of 20 mg/ml for *ex vivo* experiments or 180 mM for *in vitro* experiments. The chemical structures of ligustrazine and LH are presented in Fig. 1.

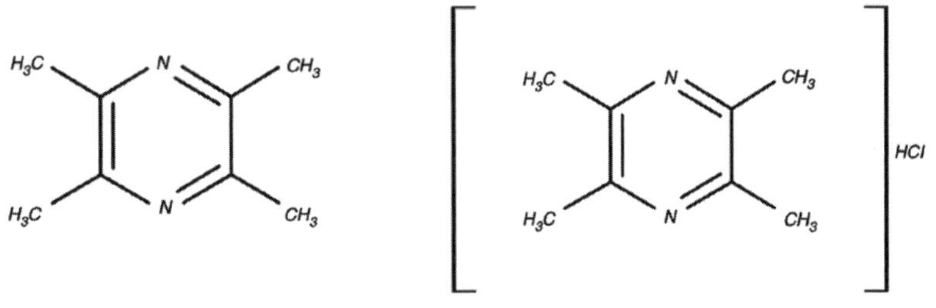

H_3C N CH_3 H_3C N CH_3

Chemical structure of ligustrazine

H_3C N CH_3 H_3C N CH_3 HCl

Chemical structure of ligustrazine hydrochloride (LH)

Figure 1 Chemical structure of Ligustrazine and Ligustrazine HCL
Notes: HCL, hydrochloride.

3 Animals and Treatment with LH

Male Sprague-dawley (SD)rats of 6-8 weeks of age (200-250 g)were purchased from Shanghai SLAC Laboratory Animal Co., Ltd. (Shanghai, China). All animals were housed in a specific pathogen-free environment with food and water supplied *ad libitum* throughout the experiment. The environment was maintained at 22 ˚C with a 12-h light/dark cycle and humidity of 55±5%. All the animal treatments were performed in compliance with international ethical guidelines and the National Institutes of Health Guidelines for the Care and Use of Laboratory Animals (Bethesda, MD, USA). The experiments were approved by the Institutional Animal care and Use committee of Fujian University of Traditional chinese Medicine (Fuzhou, China).

For the *ex vivo* experiment, 24 SD rats were randomly divided into the following three groups (n=8/group): Control, Adrenaline and Adrenaline + LH. The Adrenaline + LH group was administered LH (80 mg/kg; based on the clinical dosage and transformation between human and rat)by intraperitoneal injection daily for 7 days, while the other two groups received an equal volume of saline. At the end of the treatment, the rats in the Adrenaline + LH and Adrenaline groups were subcutaneously injected with adrenaline hydrochloride at a dose of 1 mg/kg, whereas, the rats in the Control group were subcutaneously injected with an equal volume of saline. At 1 h following the injection, the bleeding risk of SD rats from each group was evaluated and the blood samples were collected for further ex vivo experiments (including assays of platelet aggregation, analysis of intracellular Ca^{2+} mobilization and TXB_2 levels, in addition to expression of associated proteins).

4 Blood Collection and Preparation of Rat Platelets

Blood was collected from SD rats with or without LH treatment. Rats were anesthetized with sodium pentobarbital (45 mg/kg)and blood was collected from the abdominal aorta and anticoagu-lated with 3.8% sodium citrate solution (9: 1, v/v). The obtained blood samples (8-10 mL blood for each rat)were centrifuged at room temperature for 15 min at 150 *x g* to obtain PRP, which were centrifuged again at room temperature for 15 min at 150 *x g* to remove residual erythrocytes. The platelet-poor plasma (PPP)was obtained by centrifugation of blood samples at room temperature for 10 min at 1, 000 *x g*. The final concentration of platelets was adjusted to $3x10^8$/mL with the PPP, which was used as a reference solution for aggregation assays.

5 Assay of Platelet Aggregation

Platelet aggregation analysis was performed as previously described [21]. For the *in vitro* experiment, subsequent to the preparation of PRP as aforementioned, 330 μL rat PRP was incubated with 5.5 μM AdP or 300 μM IGF-1 for 5 min at 37°C, following pretreatment with various concentrations of LH (0-3 mM)for 5 min at 37 °C. For the *ex vivo* experiment, an equal volume of PRP was collected from rats in each group and incubated in 5.5 μM ADP for 5 min at 37 °C. Following incubation, aggregation of platelets in each group was monitored by measuring light transmission via a platelet aggregometer (LBY-NJ4; Pulisheng Instrument Co., Ltd., Beijing, China), and the% maximum platelet aggre-gation was recorded.

6 Measurement of Platelet Intracellular Ca^{2+} Mobilization

For the in vitro experiment, 1 mL prepared PRP ($3x10^8$ platelets/ml)was pretreated with LH (0, 1, 2 and 3 mM)in the presence of $Cacl_2$ (1 μM)for 5 min at 37 °C. For the *ex vivo* experiment, 1 mL prepared PRP ($3x10^8$ platelets/ml)from the Control, Adrenaline and Adrenaline + LH rat groups were suspended in $Cacl_2$ (1 mM)for 5 min at 37°C. Subsequently, the platelets from *in vitro* and *ex vivo* incubations were stimulated with ADP (5.5 μM)or IGF-1 (300 μM)for 5 min at 37 °C. The platelets were incubated with Fluo-4/AM (20 μM) for 60 min at 37 °C in the dark and subsequently centrifuged at room temperature for 15 min at 500 *x g*. The fluorescence intensity of 100, 000 platelets/sample was examined using a flow cytometer (BD Biosciences, San Jose, CA, USA)and analyzed via Bd CellQuest™ Pro (Version 6.0; BD Biosciences, San Jose, CA, USA).

7 Measurement of TXB_2 Expression Levels

For the *in vitro* experiment, 1 ml prepared PRP ($3x10^8$ platelets/ml)was pretreated with LH (0, 1, 2 and 3 mM)for 5 min at 37 °C. Subsequently, the platelets were stimulated with ADP (5.5 μM)or IGF-1 (300 μM) for 5 min at 37°C. The PRP was centrifuged at 1, 000 *x g* for 15 min at 4 °C. The supernatant was collected and TXB_2 levels were determined using an ELISA kit (cat. no. ADI-900-002; Enzo Life Sciences, Inc.)and expressed as pg/mL. For the *ex vivo* experiment, blood was drawn from the control, Adrenaline and Adrenaline + LH groups at the end of the experiment. Plasma was prepared by centrifuging for 15 min at 4 °C at 1, 600 *x g*, and the levels of TXB_2 in plasma were measured by ELISA, similarly to the *in vitro* experiment.

8 Tail Bleeding Assay

To evaluate the bleeding risk of LH, a modified tail cutting method was used [30]. Following adrenaline hydrochloride or saline injection for 1 h, the rats in each group were anesthetized using sodium pentobarbital (45 mg/kg). Subsequently, the tail was pre-warmed for 3 min in saline solution at 37 °C. Bleeding was induced by precise transection of the mouse tail at 3 mm from the tip. The distal portion of the tail (3 cm)was immersed vertically into saline solution at 37 °C. The time between the start of transection to bleeding cessation was recorded as the bleeding time.

9 Western Blot AnAlysis

The expression levels of associated proteins in PRP from *in vitro* and *ex vivo* experiments were determined by western blot analysis. PRP from each group was lysed with mammalian cell radioimmunoprecipitation assay lysis buffer (cat. no. P0013; Beyotime Institute of Biotechnology; Haimen, China)containing protease and phosphatase inhibitor cocktails. Total protein concentrations were determined by a bicinchoninic acid assay. Equal amounts of total proteins (50 μg)were resolved in 12% SDS-PAGE and electroblotted. The nitrocellulose membranes were blocked with 5% skimmed milk at room temperature for 2 h and incubated with primary antibodies targeting p-Akt (1 : 1, 000; cat. no. 4060), Akt (1 : 1, 000; cat no. 4685)or β-actin (1 : 1, 000; cat. no. 4967)overnight at 4°C. Subsequently, the membranes were incubated with the appropriate HRP-conjugated anti-rabbit antibody (1 : 5, 000; cat. no. 7074)at room temperature for 1 h, followed by enhanced chemiluminescence detection (Thermo Fisher Scientific, Inc., Waltham, MA, USA). β-actin was used as a loading control.

10 Statistical Analysis

All experiments were performed at least three times and presented as the mean ± standard deviation. Statistical analyses were performed using SPSS for Windows (version 18.0; SPSS, Inc., Chicago, IL, USA). Analysis of three or more groups was performed by one-way analysis of variance, followed by the least-significant difference test. Values obtained in a number of experiments were converted into% for comparison of controls with treated samples. $P < 0.05$ was considered to indicate a statistically significant difference.

Results

1 LH Inhibits Platelet Aggregation *in vitro* and *ex vivo*

To examine the potential therapeutic effects of ligustrazine on platelet activation, rat PRP was incubated with LH, followed by stimulation with ADP. As illustrated in Fig. 2A, ADP stimulation markedly induced platelet aggregation *in vitro*, and this was significantly inhibited by treatment with LH in a dose-dependent manner ($P < 0.05$ *vs*. untreated PRP; $P < 0.05$ *vs*. ADP-stimulated PRP). To verify the antiplatelet effect of LH, an ex vivo platelet activation model was employed, where the rats were pretreated with LH for 7 days followed by subcu-taneous injection of adrenaline hydrochloride for 1 h. Rat PRP from each group was collected and stimulated with ADP (used as stimulation for detection of platelet aggregation). As illustrated in Fig. 2B, treatment with LH significantly inhibited adrenaline-induced platelet aggregation ($P < 0.05$ *vs*. Control group; $P < 0.05$ *vs*. Adrenaline group). Taken together, these results suggested that ligustrazine possesses potent properties of suppressing platelet aggregation *in vitro* and *ex vivo*.

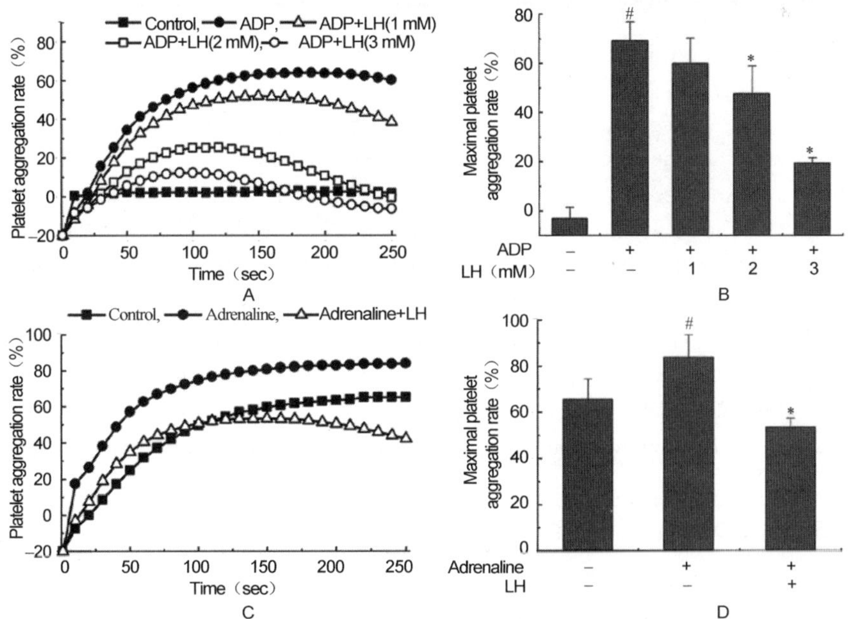

Figure 2 Effect of LH on ADP-Induced Platelet Aggregation.

Notes: (A)*In vitro* experiment. PRP was incubated with 5.5 μM ADP following pretreatment with various concentrations of LH (0-3 mM). (B)*Ex vivo* experiment. PRP collected from rats in each group was stimulated with ADP (5.5 μM). The platelet aggregation of PRP *in vitro* and *ex vivo* was determined by platelet aggregometer (left panel)and the% maximum platelet aggregation was determined at 250 sec (right panel). Data are presented as mean±standard deviation from at least three repetitions. $^{\#}P < 0.05$ vs. untreated PRP or rats in Control group; $^{*}P < 0.05$ vs. ADP-stimulated PRP or rats in the Adrenaline group. LH, ligustrazine hydrochloride; ADP, adenosine diphosphate; PRP, platelet-rich plasma.

2 LH Inhibits Intracellular Ca^{2+} Mobilization and TXA_2 Formation *in vitro* and *ex vivo*

To further determine the anti-platelet activity of LH, its effect on Ca^{2+}mobilization and TXA2 secretion was investigated. As presented in Fig. 3A and C, LH significantly and dose-dependently inhibited ADP-induced Ca^{2+} mobilization and TXB_2 secretion in platelets *in vitro* ($P < 0.05$ *vs.* untreated PRP; $P < 0.05$ *vs.* ADP-stimulated PRP). Furthermore, similar results were observed in the ex vivo platelet activation model (Fig. 3B and d; $P < 0.05$ *vs.* Control group; $P < 0.05$ *vs.* Adrenaline group), suggesting that the anti-platelet activity of ligustrazine may be mediated by the inhibition of Ca^{2+} mobilization and TXA_2 formation.

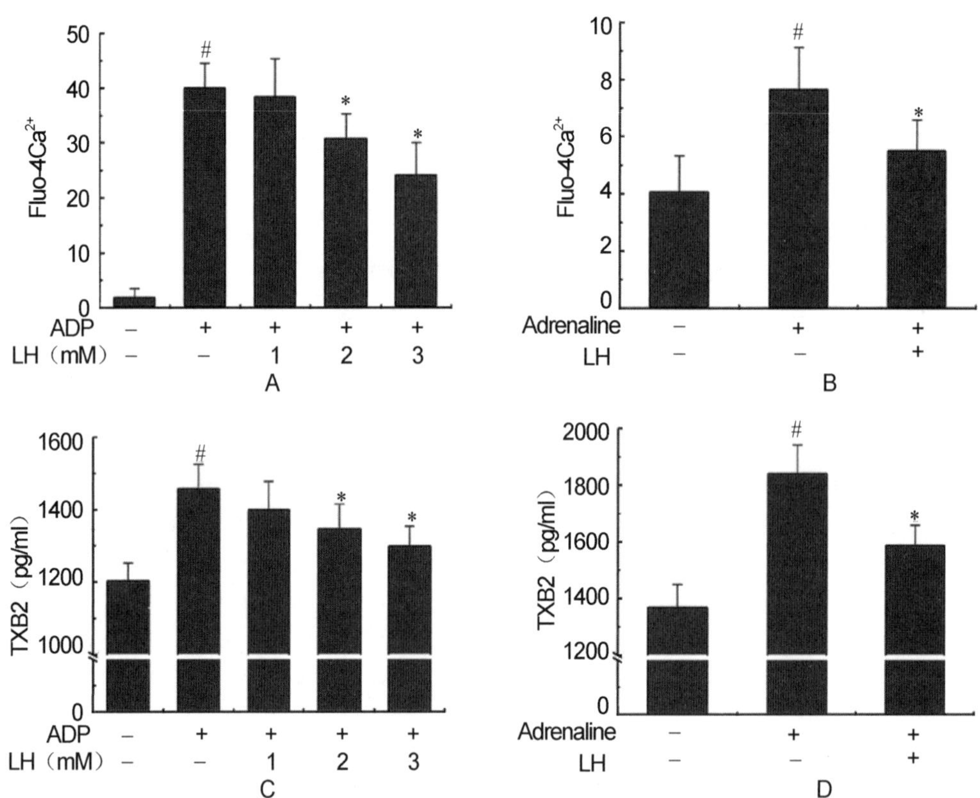

Figure 3　Effect of LH on Intracellular Ca^{2+} Mobilization and TXA_2 Formation

Notes: (A)PRP was pre-treated with various concentrations of LH (0-3 mM)in the presence of Cacl2 (1 mM). (B)PRP collected from rats in each group was suspended in $Cacl_2$ (1 mM). The platelets from *in vitro* (A)and *ex vivo* (B)experiments were stimulated with ADP (5.5μM). The intracellular Ca^{2+} concentration in PRP was determined by Fluo-4/AM (20 μM)staining, followed by flow cytometry analysis. (C)Supernatant was collected following pretreatment of PRP with various concentrations of LH (0-3 mM)followed by ADP (5.5 μM)stimulation. (D)Plasma from rats in each group was collected. TXB_2 levels in supernatants from the *in vitro* (C)and in plasma from the *ex vivo* (D)experiments were determined using an ELISA kit and expressed as pg/ml. Data are presented as mean±standard deviation from at least three repetitions. $^{\#}P < 0.05$ *vs.* untreated PRP or rats in Control group; $^{*}P < 0.05$ *vs.* ADP-stimulated PRP or rats in the Adrenaline group. LH, ligustrazine hydrochloride; TXA_2, thromboxane A_2; PRP, platelet-rich plasma; ADP, adenosine diphosphate; TXB_2, thromboxane B_2; Fluo-4/AM, fluo-4-acetoxymethyl ester.

3 LH Suppresses Phosphorylation of Akt *in vitro* and *ex vivo*

To examine the molecular mechanism of the antiplatelet effects of LH, its effect on the phosphorylation/activation of Akt was investigated. As presented in Fig. 4, ADP markedly increased the phosphorylation of Akt *in vitro* and *ex vivo*, compared with the control group; this effect was however significantly suppressed by treatment with LH. To further verify the inhibitory effect of LH on Akt signaling, a specific Akt pathway activator, IGF-1, was employed. The results in Fig. 5A demonstrated that LH treatment profoundly and dose-dependently suppressed IGF-1-induced Akt phosphorylation. The levels of total Akt were unaltered during the experiment. In addition, LH significantly inhibited IGF-1-induced platelet aggregation, Ca^{2+} mobilization and

TXB2 secretion in platelets (Fig. 5B-D; $P < 0.05$ *vs*. untreated PRP; $P < 0.05$ *vs*. IGF-1-stimulated PRP). Collectively, these results suggested that ligustrazine exerts its inhibitory effects on platelet activation at least partly via suppression of the Akt signaling pathway.

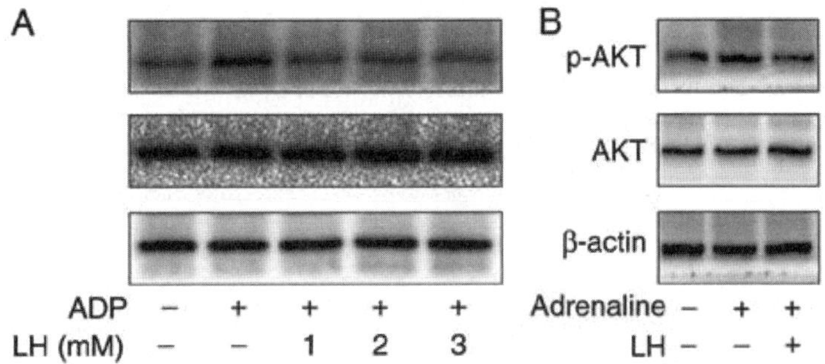

Figure 4 Effect of LH on Phosphorylation of Akt

Notes: (A)PRP was incubated with 5.5 μM ADP following pretreatment with various concentrations of LH (0-3 mM). (B)PRP collected from rats in each group was stimulated with ADP (5.5 μM). The expression levels of Akt and p-Akt were determined by western blot analysis. β-actin was used as the internal control. Images are representative of three independent experiments. LH, ligustrazine hydrochloride; Akt, AKT serine/threonine kinase; PRP, platelet-rich plasma; ADP, adenosine diphosphate; p-, phosphorylated.

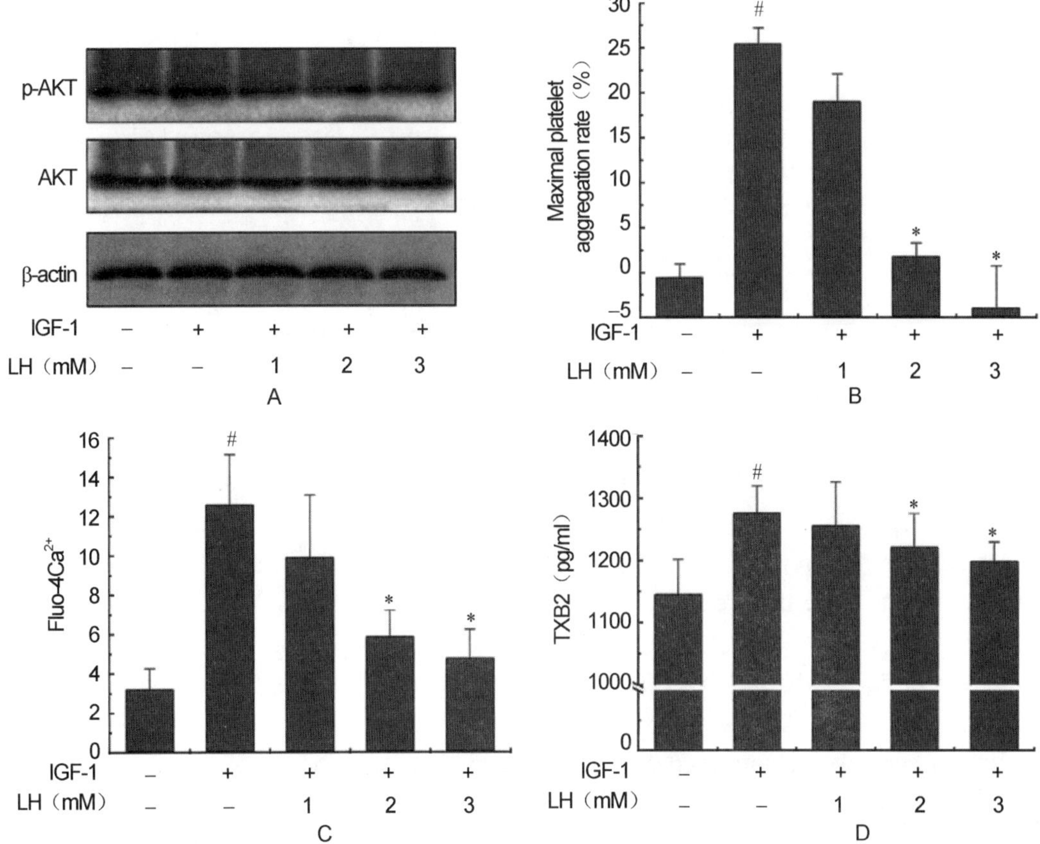

Figure 5 Effect of LH on IGF-1-induced Activation of the Akt Signaling Pathway

Notes: PRP were stimulated with IGF-1 (300μM), following pretreatment with various concentrations of LH (0-3 mM). (A) Protein expression levels of Akt and p-Akt in PRP were determined by western blot analysis. β-actin was used as the internal control. (B)Platelet aggregation was measured using a platelet aggregometer and the% of maximum platelet aggregation was determined at 250 sec. (C)The intracellular Ca^{2+} concentration in PRP was determined by Fluo-4/AM (20 μM)staining, followed by flow cytometry analysis. (D)Levels of TXB_2 in the supernatants of PRP was determined by ELISA and expressed as pg/ml. Experiments were performed at least three independent times. $^{\#}P < 0.05$ vs. untreated PRP; $^{*}P < 0.05$ vs. IGF-1-stimulated PRP. LH, ligustrazine hydrochloride; IGF-1, insulin-like growth factor-1; Akt, AKT serine/threonine kinase; PRP, platelet-rich plasma; TXB_2, thromboxane B_2; p, phosphorylated; Fluo-4/AM, fluo-4-acetoxymethyl ester.

4 LH Displays Low Risk of Hemorrhage *in vivo*

Multiple currently-used antithrombotic agents have adverse effects, including impaired blood coagulation or prolonged bleeding time. Therefore, the effect of LH on bleeding time was investigated *in vivo* in rats using a cutting tail method (30). As presented in Fig. 6, the bleeding time in the Adrenaline-treated group was shorter compared with the control group, while the bleeding time in the LH-pretreated group for 7 days was increased ($P < 0.05$ *vs*. Control group; $P < 0.05$ *vs*. Adrenaline group). However, LH did not significantly prolong the bleeding time compared with the control group, suggesting that ligustrazine may have low bleeding risk.

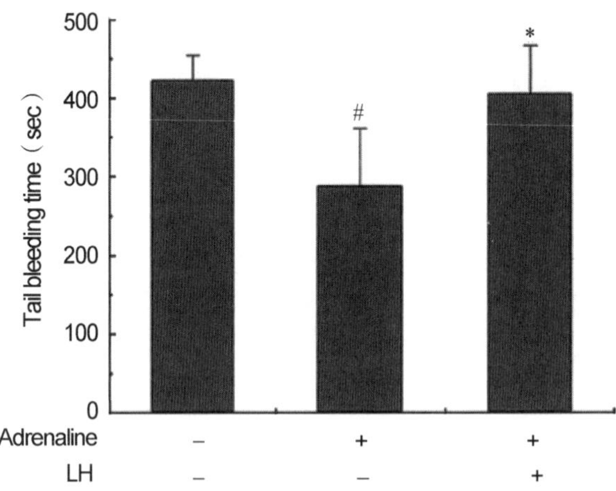

Figure 6　Effect of LH on Bleeding Time

Notes: Following administration of LH or saline for 7 days, the rats were injected with adrenaline hydrochloride or saline for 1 h. Bleeding risk was evaluated using a modified tail cutting method. The accumulated bleeding time was recorded within 600 sec. n=5 rats from each group were used in this experiment. $^{\#}P < 0.05$ *vs*. control group; $^{*}P < 0.05$ *vs*. Adrenaline group. LH, ligustrazine hydrochloride.

DISCUSSION

Due to the critical role of hyper-activation of platelets in the development of thrombotic vascular diseases, the process of platelet activation has become an attractive therapeutic target. Numerous antiplatelet chemical drugs are used to prevent or treat thrombosis. However, the currently available drugs have specific clinical disadvantages, including gastrointestinal side-effects and hemorrhage[16, 17]. Therefore, there is an urgent requirement for safer and more effective antiplatelet agents without these adverse effects. In recent years, novel therapeutic agents have been derived from Chinese medicinal herbs and there is growing interest in this area. Ligustrazine, one of the natural alkaloids isolated from RLW that is commonly used to clinically treat cardiac-cerebral diseases, has been demonstrated to possess antiplatelet activity[19-22]. However, the precise mechanism of its potential therapeutic effects remains to be further elucidated. Using in vitro and ex vivo platelet activation models, established by stimulating rat PRP with the platelet activator ADP, the present study demonstrated that LH (the clinical-grade form of ligustrazine)was able to significantly inhibit platelet aggregation. In addition, LH was able to reverse adrenaline-induced shortening of bleeding time, indicating the low bleeding risk of ligustrazine. However, the rapid metabolism and short half-life of ligustrazine severely limits its clinical application. Therefore, novel chemical forms of ligustrazine with a longer half-life require development in further studies. Additionally, a comparison of LH with other antiplatelet medicines (including aspirin and clopidelgrel)and their potential combinations require further assessment.

Platelet activation may be induced by a variety of agonists, including ADP and TXA_2, which are released from the gran-ules of activated platelets. TXA_2 exerts its function through interaction with the thromboxane receptor, contributing to the amplification of the initial platelet activation, which therefore is a principal target for most currently-used antiplatelet agents[31-33]. Although different agonists induce platelet activation through different mechanisms by respectively binding to their specific receptors, they all result in an elevation of intracellular Ca^{2+} concentration [$(Ca^{2+})i$], an event termed Ca^{2+} mobilization[34]. Ca^{2+} is an important second messenger that is critical for various cellular processes, including platelet acti-vation[35]. Therefore, the present study verified the antiplatelet activity of LH by examining Ca^{2+} mobilization and TXA_2 secretion, and the results demonstrated that LH significantly and dose-dependently inhibited ADP-induced Ca^{2+} mobiliza-tion and TXB_2 secretion in platelets *in vitro* and *ex vivo*. These results suggested that the antiplatelet activity of ligustrazine may be mediated by the inhibition of Ca^{2+} mobilization and TXA2 formation.

It is well documented that the process of platelet activation is highly regulated by multiple pathways, including the PI3K/Akt signaling pathway. Activation of the PI3K/Akt pathway results in granule secretion and the second wave of platelet aggrega-tion[9, 36-40]. To examine the mechanism of the antiplatelet activities of ligustrazine, its effect on the phosphorylation/acti-vation of Akt was determined. The present study demonstrated that treatment with LH significantly suppressed ADP-induced Akt phosphorylation *in vitro* and *ex vivo*. Notably, using the specific Akt pathway activator IGF-1, the present study further confirmed that LH significantly and specifically suppressed the activation of Akt signaling. Consequently, treatment with LH markedly inhibited IGF-1-induced platelet aggregation, Ca^{2+} mobilization and TXB_2 secretion in platelets. However, as phosphorylation of Akt is regulated by upstream regulators (including PI3K, PH domain and leucine rich repeat protein phosphatase 1, phosphatase and tensin homolog and associated microRNAs)[41-43] and exerts its function by regulating the expression of downstream molecules (including mammalian target of rapamycin)[44], the effect of LH upstream and downstream of Akt requires further assessment.

In conclusion, the present study proposed that ligustrazine possesses a broad range of antiplatelet activities, without apparent hemorrhagic side-effects. Suppression of Akt signaling may be one of the mechanisms by which ligustrazine exerts its antiplatelet function. The present results provide further preliminary evidence to support that ligustrazine may be considered a potent therapeutic agent against thrombotic vascular diseases.

REFERENCES

[1] Smith T, Dhunnoo G, Mohan I, et al. A pilot study showing an association between platelet hyperactivity and the severity of peripheral arterial disease[J]. Platelets, 2007, 18: 245-248.

[2] Georgescu A, Alexandru N, Andrei E, et al. Effects of transplanted circulating endothelial progenitor cells and platelet microparticles in atherosclerosis development[J]. Biol cell, 2016, 108: 219-243.

[3] Alexandru N, Popov D and Georgescu A. Platelet dysfunction in vascular pathologies and how can it be treated[J]. Thromb Res, 2012, 129: 116-126.

[4] Sharma G and Berger JS. Platelet activity and cardiovascular risk in apparently healthy individuals: A review of the data[J]. J Thromb Thrombolysis. 2011, 32: 201-208.

[5] Angiolillo DJ. The evolution of antiplatelet therapy in the treatment of acute coronary syndromes: From aspirin to the present day[J]. drugs, 2012, 72: 2087-2116.

[6] Spiel AO, Gilbert JC and Jilma B. von Willebrand factor in cardiovascular disease: Focus on acute coronary syndromes[J]. circulation, 2008, 117: 1449-1459.

[7] Brass LF, Manning DR, Cichowski K, et al. Signaling through G proteins in platelets: To the integrins and beyond[J]. Thromb Haemost. 1997, 78: 581-589.

[8] Franke TF, Kaplan DR, Cantley Lc, et al. Direct regulation of the Akt proto-oncogene product by phosphati-dylinositol-3, 4-bisphosphate[J]. Science, 1997, 275: 665-668.

[9] Guidetti GF, Canobbio I and Torti M. PI3K/Akt in platelet integrin signaling and implications in thrombosis[J]. Adv Biol Regul. 2015, 59: 36-52, .

[10] Moore SF, van den Bosch MT, Hunter RW, et al. Dual regulation of glycogen synthase kinase 3 (GSK3)α/β by protein kinase C (PKC)α and Akt promotes thrombin-mediated integrin $\alpha_{IIb}\beta_3$ activation and granule secretion in platelets[J]. J Biol chem., 2013, 288: 3918-3928, .

[11] Chen X, Zhang Y, Wang Y, et al. PDK1 regulates platelet activation and arterial thrombosis[J]. Blood, 2013, 121: 3718-3726.

[12] Yin H, Stojanovic A, Hay N, et al. The role of Akt in the signaling pathway of the glycoprotein Ib-IX induced platelet activation[J]. Blood, 2008, 111: 658-665.

[13] Kim S, Mangin P, Dangelmaier C, et al. Role of phosphoinositide 3-kinase beta in glycoprotein VI-mediated Akt activation in platelets[J]. J Biol chem, 2009, 284: 33763-33772.

[14] Reséndiz JC, Kroll MH and Lassila R. Protease-activated receptor-induced Akt activation-regulation and possible fun tion[J]. J Thromb Haemost,

2007, 5: 2484-2493.

[15] Chen J, De S, damron DS, et al. Impaired platelet responses to thrombin and collagen in AKT-1-deficient mice[J]. Blood, 2004, 104: 1703-1710.

[16] Di Minno MN, Lupoli R, Palmieri NM, et al. Aspirin resistance, platelet turnover, and diabetic angiopathy: A 2011 update[J]. Thromb Res, 2012, 129: 341-344.

[17] Uchiyama S. Clopidogrel resistance: Identifying and overcoming a barrier to effective antiplatelet treatment[J]. Cardiovasc Ther, 2011, 29: e100-e111.

[18] Beijing Institute of Pharmaceutical Industry. Studies of active components of Ligusticum Wallichii Franch. I. Extraction, isolation and structure identification of tetramethylpyrazine[J]. Chin, 1977, 7: 420-421.

[19] Li Z, Li D, Huang J, et al. Preparation of cardiovascular disease-related genes microarray and its application in exploring ligustrazine-induced changes in endothelial gene expression[J]. Pol J Pharmacol, 2004, 56: 427-433.

[20] Zhang F, Ni C, Kong D, et al. Ligustrazine attenuates oxidative stress-induced activation of hepatic stellate cells by interrupting platelet-derived growth factor-β receptor-mediated ERK and p38 pathways[J]. Toxicol Appl Pharmacol, 2012, 265: 51-60.

[21] Li S, Chen H, Wang X, et al. Pharmacokinetic study of a novel stroke therapeutic, 2-[[(1, 1-dimethyl-ethyl)oxidoimino]methyl]-3, 5, 6-trimethylpyrazine, by a simple HPLC-UV method in rats[J]. Eur J drug Metab Pharmacokinet, 2011, 36: 95-101.

[22] Wu W, Yu X, Luo XP, et al. Tetramethylpyrazine protects against scopolamine-induced memory impairments in rats by reversing the cAMP/PKA/CREB pathway[J]. Behav Brain Res, 2013, 253: 212-216.

[23] Cheng XR, Zhang L, Hu JJ, et al. Neuroprotective effects of tetramethylpyrazine on hydrogen peroxide-induced apoptosis in PC12 cells[J]. Cell Biol Int, 2007, 31: 438-443.

[24] Han J, Song J, Li X, et al. Ligustrazine suppresses the growth of HRPC cells through the inhibition of cap-dependent translation via both the mTOR and the MEK/ERK pathways[J]. Anticancer Agents Med Chem, 2015, 15: 764-772.

[25] Wang GJ. Changes of nail fold microcirculation in patients with acute cerebral thrombosis treated with ligustrazine[J]. Chin J Neurol Psychiatry, 1984, 17: 121-124.

[26] Sheu JR, Kan YC, Hung Wc, et al. Mechanisms involved in the antiplatelet activity of tetramethylpyrazine in human platelets[J]. Thromb Res, 1997, 88: 259-270.

[27] Lin CI, Wu SL, Tao PL, et al. The role of cyclic AMP and phosphodiesterase activity in the mechanism of action of tetramethylpyrazine on human and dog cardiac and dog coronary arterial tissues[J]. J Pharm Pharmacol, 1993, 45: 963-966.

[28] Liu SF, Cai YN, Evans TW, et al. Ligustrazine is a vasodilator of human pulmonary and bronchial arteries[J]. Eur J Pharmacol, 1990, 191: 345-350.

[29] Peng W, Hucks D, Priest RM, et al. Ligustrazine-induced endothelium-dependent relaxation in pulmonary arteries via an NO-mediated and exogenous L-arginine-dependent mechanism[J]. Br J Pharmacol, 1996, 119: 1063-1071.

[30] Alshbool FZ, Karim ZA, Vemana HP, et al. The regulator of G-protein signaling 18 regulates platelet aggregation, hemostasis and thrombosis[J]. Biochem Biophys Res Commun, 2015, 462: 378-382.

[31] Su XL, Su W, Wang Y, et al. The pyrrolidinoindoline alkaloid Psm2 inhibits platelet aggregation and thrombus formation by affecting PI3K/Akt signaling[J]. Acta Pharmacol Sin, 2016, 37: 1208-1217.

[32] Sakariassen KS, Alberts P, Fontana P, et al. Effect of pharmaceutical interventions targeting thromboxane receptors and thromboxane synthase in cardiovascular and renal diseases[J]. Future cardiol, 2009, 5: 479-493.

[33] Fontana P, Zufferey A, Daali Y, et al. Antiplatelet therapy: Targeting the TxA_2 pathway[J]. J cardiovasc Transl Res, 2014, 7: 29-38.

[34] Varga-Szabo d, Braun A and Nieswandt B. Calcium signaling in platelets[J]. J Thromb Haemost, 2009, 7: 1057-1066.

[35] Berridge MJ, Bootman MD and Roderick HL. Calcium signalling: Dynamics, homeostasis and remodelling[J] Nat Rev Mol Cell Biol, 2003, 4: 517-529.

[36] Heraud JM, Racaud-Sultan C, Gironcel D, et al. Lipid products of phosphoinositide 3-kinase and phosphatidylinositol 4', 5'-bisphosphate are both required for ADP-dependent platelet spreading[J]. J Biol chem, 1998, 273: 17817-17823.

[37] Canobbio I, Stefanini L, Cipolla L, et al. Genetic evidence for a predominant role of PI3Kbeta catalytic activity in ITAM-and integrin-mediated signaling in platelets[J]. Blood, 2009, 114: 2193-2196.

[38] Woulfe DS. Akt signaling in platelets and thrombosis[J. Expert Rev Hematol, 2010, 3: 81-91.

[39] O'Brien KA, Stojanovic-Terpo A, Hay N, et al. An important role for Akt3 in platelet activation and thrombosis[J]. Blood, 2011, 118: 4215-4223.

[40] Stojanovic A, Marjanovic JA, Brovkovych VM, et al. A phosphoinositide 3-kinase-AKT-nitric oxide-cGMP signaling pathway in stimulating platelet secretion and aggregation[J]. J Biol chem, 2006, 281: 16333-16339.

[41] Laurent PA, Severin S, Gratacap MP, et al. Class I PI 3-kinases signaling in platelet activation and thrombosis: PdK1/Akt/GSK3 axis and impact of PTEN and SHIP1[J]. Adv Biol Regul, 2014, 54: 162-174.

[42] Meuillet EJ: Novel inhibitors of AKT. Assessment of a different approach targeting the pleckstrin homology domain[J]. Curr Med chem, 2011, 18: 2727-2742.

[43] Ishibashi O, Akagi I, Ogawa Y, et al. MiR-141-3p is upregulated in esophageal squamous cell carcinoma and targets pleckstrin homology domain leucine-rich repeat protein phosphatase-2, a negative regulator of the PI3K/AKT pathway[J]. Biochem Biophys Res commun, 2018, 501: 507-513.

[44] Razmara M, Heldin cH and Lennartsson J. Platelet-derived growth factor-induced Akt phosphorylation requires mTOR/Rictor and phospholipase c-γ 1, whereas S6 phosphorylation depends on mTOR/Raptor and phospholipase D[J]. Cell Commun Signal, 2013, 11: 3.

First Published: LI Li, CHEN Hong-wei, SHEN A-ling, LI Qiong-yu, CHEN You-qin, CHU Jian-feng, LIU Li-ya, PENG Jun, CHEN Ke-ji. Ligustrazine inhibits platelet activation via suppression of the Akt pathway[J] . Int J Mol Med, 2019, 43: 575-582.

Puerarin Reduces Blood Pressure in Spontaneously Hypertensive Rats by Targeting eNOS

Shi Weili, Yuan Rong, CHEN Xun, Xin Qi-qi, Wang Yan,
Shang Xiao-hong, Cong Wei-hong, and CHEN Ke-ji

Essential hypertension, one of the major causes of cardiovascular disease in aging populations, is a chronic and lifetime disease characterized by persistent rise in systolic or diastolic blood pressure levels[1]. Long-term elevation or instability of blood pressure increases risk of series vascular related complications, including stroke, ischemic heart disease, renal disease, congestive heart failure and ocular fundus abnormalities. Hypertension has led to global increases in morbidity and mortality[2].

Renin-angiotensin-aldosterone system activation, hyperactivity of the sympathetic nervous system, and retention of renal sodium are involved in the occurrence of hypertension. But the existing pathogenesis of hypertension has not yet been fully elucidated. Hypertension is also closely related to endothelial dysfunction, which is characterized by an imbalance of endothelium-dependent relaxation and contraction[3]. Endothelium is an essential part of the vasculature and plays a key role in regulation of vascular tone by releasing of NO[4]. Reduction of NO, caused by decreased eNOS activity, is an underlying pathway of vascular endothelial dysfunction[5].

Puerariae lobata is widely known as Gegen (Chinese name)in Traditional Chinese Medicine (TCM). Puerarin is one of the main active ingredients extracted from the root of *Pueraria lobata*. Its chemical name is 8-C-β-D-Glucopyranosyl-7, 4-hydroxy-isoflavone, and molecular weight is 416.382. Puerarin plays an important role in the treatment of angina pectoris, myocardial ischemia reperfusion injury, hypertension and other cardiovascular diseases[6-8]. Its popularity may be related to the effect of vasodilatation, antioxidant activity, anti-inflammatory activity and promoting microcirculation [9]. However, the molecular mechanism underlying the antihypertensive effects of puerarin is still not well understood. Here, to provide the basis for the clinical application of puerarin, this study aimed to investigate the effect and mechanism of puerarin on blood pressure in spontaneously hypertensive rats (SHR)by qPCR array and network pharmacology.

MATERIALS

1 Experimental Animals

Sixty male SHR and ten Wistar Kyoto (WKY)rats, both at nine weeks old and of specific-pathogen-free (SPF)class, were purchased from Beijing Weitong Lihua experimental animal Co. Ltd. The animal certificate number was SYXK (Beijing)2012-0012. The rats were kept in the SPF class animal room in Xiyuan Hospital of China Academy of Chinese Medical Sciences and were provided food and water before and during the experiment. I promise that the study was performed according to the international, national and institutional rules considering animal experiments and biodiversity right.

2 Medications

Puerarin for injection (freeze-dried powder, 200 mg/bottle)was provided by Reyang Pharmaceutical Co. Ltd., and the batch number was 16041618. Losartan potassium tablets (100 mg/tablet)were provided by Hangzhou Moshadong Pharmaceutical Co. Ltd., and the batch number was L016172.

3 Reagents

The RNA extraction kit (Roche: 11667165001), All-in-One™ First-Strand cDNA synthesis kit (GeneCopoeia: AORT-0050), All-in-One™ qPCR Mix (GeneCopoeia: AOPR-0200), All-in-One™ qPCR primers (GeneCopoeia). Endothelial nitric oxide synthase (eNOS)ELISA kit (02/2017), One-step nitric oxide (NO) Kit (A013-2), malondialdehyde (MDA)kit (20160804), superoxide dismutase (SOD)kit (A001-3)and Cyclic guanosine monophosphate (cGMP)kit (03/2017)were all purchased from Nanjing Jiancheng Bioengineering Institute. Angiotensin II clia micropariticles kits (20171212, Auto Bio)were offered by department of clinical laboratory of Xiyuan Hospital, China Academy of Chinese Medical Sciences. Antibody of eNOS (AB66127), eNOS of phospho S1177 (p-eNOS)antibody (AB195944)and angiotensin Ⅱ type 2-receptor (AT2) (AB92445) were purchased from Abcam. Caveolin-1 (Cav1)antibody (16447-1-AP)and angiotensin Ⅱ type 1-receptor (AT1) (25343-1-AP)purchased from Proteintech Group and anti-beta actin antibody from Cell Signaling Technology.

4 Instruments

The intelligent and non-invasive instrument for rat tail pressure measurement (Japan, BP98AWU), automatic biochemical analyzer (Hitachi, Japan, 7600), dehydrator (Wuhan Junjie Electronics Co. Ltd., JJ-12J, China), embedding machine (Wuhan Junjie Electronics Co. Ltd. China, JB-P5), pathological microtome (Shanghai Leica Instrument Co. Ltd., China, RM2016), spreading machine (Kedi Instrument Equipment Co. Ltd., China, KD-P), roaster (Shanghai Huitai Instrument Manufacturing Co. Ltd., China, DHG-9140A), optical microscope (Nikon, Japan, ECLIPSE CI), NanoDrop® Lite UV spectrophotometer (Thermo Fisher, USA), and LightCycler480 PCR instrument (Roche, USA).

METHODS

1 Group and Administration Methods

After one week of adaptive feeding, SHR were randomly divided into the model group, losartan potassium group, high-dose puerarin group and normal-dose puerarin group, with fifteen rats in each group. WKY rats served as the normal control group. Losartan potassium tablets were given daily by intragastric administration (31.5 mg · kg^{-1}). High-dose puerarin was given by intraperitoneal injection of 80 mg•kg^{-1} per day and normal-dose puerarin (also meidium dose)was given by intraperitoneal injection of 40 mg•kg^{-1} per day. Rats in the model group and control group were injected with equal volumes of physiological saline. This method of intraperitoneal administration was carried out in accordance with the reference literature[10]. The duration of administration lasted nine weeks. Systolic blood pressure (SBP), diastolic pressure (DBP)and heart rate were measured once a week using a tail-cuff method in conscious rats. The final measured value for each rat is a mean of at least three successive readings.

2 Pathomorphological Observations of Aortic Tissues

Thoracic aortas were fixed with formalin, embedded in paraffin and sliced sequentially. Then, pathological changes in aortas were observed by Hematoxylin and eosin (HE)and Masson staining.

3 Ultrasonic Examination of Aortic Diameter

Rats were anesthetized with 8 ml · kg^{-1} one percent pentobarbital sodium. Hairs on the chest were removed with a razor blade, and detection was carried out after the coupling gel was applied. The probe was placed on the left chest and directed to the right side to achieve a long-axis view of the left ventricle. In the horizontal position of the mitral valve, images in the short-axis view of the sternum were acquired. The mean values of three consecutive cardiac cycles were measured in each rat. The diameter of the aortic root in the left ventricular outflow tract was measured by a ruler.

4 NO, SOD, MDA, cGMP and Angiotensin II

NO in serum was determined by the nitrate reductase, SOD activity was determined by the xanthine oxidase method, and MDA was detected by the thiobarbituric acid method. Serum cGMP concentration was detected by enzyme-linked immunosorbent assay. Ang II was examined by chemiluminescence of magnetic particle. Experimental procedures were all performed according to the kit instructions. In addition, concentration and vitality were calculated according to the absorbance of all samples.

5 qPCR array

Five aortic tissue samples were collected from the control group, model group and high-dose puerarin group. The All-in-One™ qPCR mix was mixed with cDNA template. The mixture was applied into the hole of the qPCR array and reacted in the real-time PCR apparatus. Raw data were analyzed with the GeneCopoeia online tool.

Results of the model group vs. the control group and the high-dose puerarin group vs. the model group were compared and screened for a second time according to the following conditions: (1)Genes were present in all the comparison results, including the control group, the model group and the high-dose puerarin group, (2)Fold change of the genes was more than 1.5 times, and (3)Trend of regulation in the two comparisons was opposite.

6 Network Analysis of Differentially Expressed Genes (DEGs)

The STRING (http: //www. string-db. org)database was used for network analysis of the DEGs which got from qPCR array.

7 Western Blot

Pre-cooled RIPA protein extraction reagent was mixed with protease inhibitor. The tissues were homogenized with an electric homogenizer, incubated on ice for twenty minutes and then centrifuged at 14, 000 g speed. Protein concentrations of the samples were detected by the BCA method and adjusted to the lowest concentration with RIPA. Then, the protein of all tissues was denatured for five minutes at 95° C. The SDS-PAGE gel was prepared, and the samples were loaded onto the gel, electrophorized and transferred onto PVDF membranes. Then, five percent bovine serum albumin was used for blocking. Last, after incubation with a primary and secondary antibody, the membranes were imaged.

8 Data Analysis Methods

Statistical analyses were performed using SPSS software (version 20.0). Variables of normal distribution were shown as $\bar{x} \pm s$. One-way ANOVA with the least significant difference (LSD)post hoc test or rank sum test with Mann-Whitney U was performed for analysis among groups. A p value less than 0.05 was considered statistically significant, and the figures were generated with GraphPad Prism 6 and Adobe Illustrator CS6.

RESULTS

1 Blood Pressure and Heart Rate

After one week of treatment, SBP and DBP were both significantly higher in the model group than in the control group ($P < 0.001$). In contrast, the SBP and DBP of the losartan potassium group were markedly lower than those in the model group ($P < 0.001$). However, there was no significant difference between the high-dose puerarin group and the normal-dose puerarin group ($P > 0.05$). After 6 weeks, the antihypertensive effect in each drug treatment group gradually stabilized. Compared with the model group, the SBP of the losartan potassium group and high-dose puerarin group was significantly decreased ($P < 0.001$), and the SBP of the normal-dose puerarin group was also significantly lower than that of the model group ($P < 0.05$) (Table

1, Figure 1). Compared with the model group, losartan potassium and high-dose puerarin treatments had a stable antihypertensive effect on DBP until seven weeks of administration ($P < 0.01$) (Table 2, Figure 2).

Table 1　Effect of Puerarin on SBP in SHR ($\bar{x} \pm s$, mmHg)

Treatment Duration	Control	Model	Losartan	High Puerarin	Normal Puerarin
0 w	98.38 ± 13.95	136.1 ± 15.01***	140.27 ± 6.46	136.5 ± 15.52	138.61 ± 11.62
1 w	110.74 ± 18.32	145.74 ± 12.26***	127.25 ± 12.16$^{\triangle\triangle\triangle}$	144.29 ± 10.64$^{\#\#}$	143.76 ± 13.88$^{\#\#}$
2 w	112.52 ± 17.99	149.1 ± 11.63***	144.73 ± 10.13	141.88 ± 8.25	149.59 ± 8.89
3 w	114.29 ± 9.79	157.56 ± 7.26***	141.76 ± 13.64$^{\triangle\triangle\triangle}$	153.77 ± 8.53$^{\#\#}$	161.2 ± 10.18$^{\#\#\#}$
4 w	110.37 ± 9.75	156.26 ± 10.11***	142.83 ± 11.43$^{\triangle\triangle}$	151.64 ± 12.52$^{\#}$	154.08 ± 15.42$^{\#}$
5 w	119.78 ± 10.08	161.06 ± 5.91***	136.17 ± 16.27$^{\triangle\triangle\triangle}$	144.01 ± 19.95$^{\triangle\triangle}$	150.69 ± 11.1$^{\#\#}$
6 w	106.21 ± 17.02	158.4 ± 5.4***	143.14 ± 9.75$^{\triangle\triangle\triangle}$	143.7 ± 8.68$^{\triangle\triangle\triangle}$	149.19 ± 12.3$^{\triangle}$
7 w	107.58 ± 12.79	161.27 ± 7.56***	148.61 ± 10.97$^{\triangle\triangle}$	144.5 ± 16.18$^{\triangle\triangle\triangle}$	151 ± 12.13$^{\triangle}$
8 w	109.27 ± 13.78	163.24 ± 3.95***	145.01 ± 13.22$^{\triangle\triangle\triangle}$	148.27 ± 14.17$^{\triangle\triangle}$	150.92 ± 15$^{\triangle\triangle}$
9 w	109.94 ± 14.48	164.61 ± 6.55***	143.9 ± 16.27$^{\triangle\triangle\triangle}$	147.75 ± 12.01$^{\triangle\triangle\triangle}$	150.33 ± 15.34$^{\triangle\triangle}$

Notes: The table showed dynamic change of SBP after drug intervention. There showed a significant increase in SBP of SHR model group compared with control group. Compared with model group, losartan decreased SBP quickly, and high-dose puerarin also decreased SBP stably. Compared with the control group, $^{***}P < 0.001$; compared with the model group, $^{\triangle}P < 0.05$, $^{\triangle\triangle}P < 0.01$, and $^{\triangle\triangle\triangle}P < 0.001$; and compared with the losartan group, $^{\#}P < 0.05$, $^{\#\#}P < 0.01$, and $^{\#\#\#}P < 0.001$. n=10.

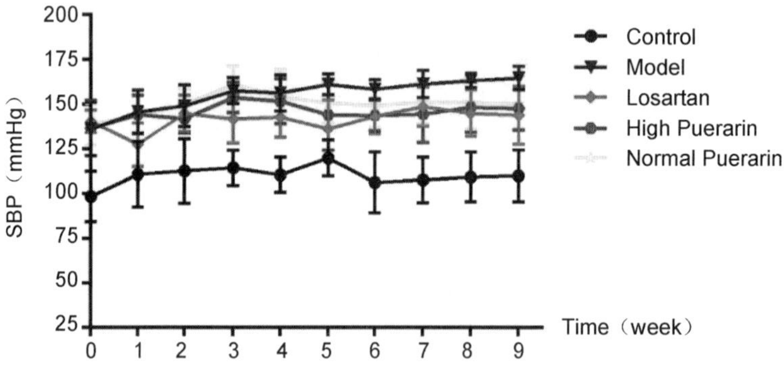

Figure 1　Effect of Puerarin on SBP in SHR

Notes: The figure showed dynamic change of SBP after drug intervention. It showed SBP of model group was the highest and SBP of control group was lowest. Compared with model group, losartan group, high-dose puerarin group and normal-dose puerarin group all decreased SBP, and high-dose puerarin group decreased SBP more stably.

Table 2　Effect of Puerarin on DBP in SHR ($\bar{x} \pm s$, mmHg)

Treatment Duration	Control	Model	Losartan	High Puerarin	Normal Puerarin
0 w	65.96 ± 8.5	104.62 ± 14.43***	108.46 ± 9.79	109.63 ± 17.47	105.8 ± 14.5
1 w	69.58 ± 18.3	103.56 ± 13.63***	83.06 ± 14.9$^{\triangle\triangle\triangle}$	98.56 ± 13.2$^{\#\#}$	103.4 ± 13.81$^{\#\#\#}$
2 w	70.29 ± 20.94	108.08 ± 12.14***	102.91 ± 8.37	97.79 ± 15.64$^{\triangle}$	104.52 ± 12.5
3 w	76.46 ± 9.48	115.86 ± 10.75***	102.59 ± 16.72$^{\triangle\triangle}$	115.02 ± 13.73$^{\#\#}$	115.18 ± 10.54$^{\#\#}$
4 w	74.53 ± 11.21	109.13 ± 15.35***	104.07 ± 8.48	112.01 ± 19.21	115.04 ± 17.24$^{\#}$
5 w	77.08 ± 13.31	118.82 ± 14.88***	98.05 ± 15.85$^{\triangle\triangle\triangle}$	99.59 ± 15.83$^{\triangle\triangle\triangle}$	106.75 ± 13.16$^{\triangle}$
6 w	70.46 ± 12.95	113.4 ± 11.81***	101.73 ± 19.87$^{\triangle}$	105.34 ± 17.58	113.23 ± 12.37$^{\#}$
7 w	72.92 ± 9.51	118.73 ± 9.85***	106.18 ± 12.78$^{\triangle\triangle}$	104.94 ± 18.02$^{\triangle\triangle}$	108.85 ± 15.4$^{\triangle}$
8 w	71.69 ± 12.1	120.47 ± 10.26***	100.02 ± 13.27$^{\triangle\triangle\triangle}$	108.4 ± 14.72$^{\triangle}$	112.44 ± 17.81$^{\#}$
9 w	76 ± 12.42	117.21 ± 15.06***	103.26 ± 14.93$^{\triangle\triangle}$	107.59 ± 15.16$^{\triangle}$	113.46 ± 11.18$^{\#}$

Notes: The table showed dynamic change of DBP after drug intervention. There showed a significant increase in DBP of SHR model group compared with control group. Compared with model group, losartan decreased DBP quickly, and high-dose puerarin decreased DBP stably. Compared with the control group, $^{**}P < 0.01$ and $^{***}P < 0.001$; compared with the model group, $^{\triangle}P < 0.05$, $^{\triangle\triangle}P < 0.01$ and $^{\triangle\triangle\triangle}P < 0.001$; and compared with the losartan group, $^{\#}P < 0.05$, $^{\#\#}P < 0.01$, and $^{\#\#\#}P < 0.001$. n=10.

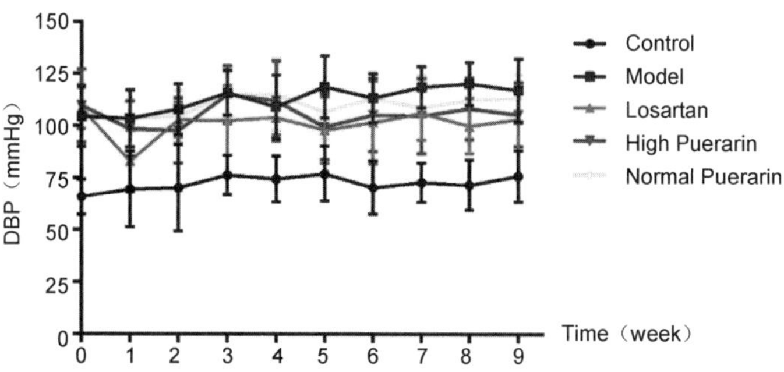

Figure 2 Effect of Puerarin on DBP in SHR

Notes: The figure showed dynamic change of DBP after drug intervention. It showed DBP of model group was the highest and DBP of control group was lowest. Compared with model group, losartan group, high-dose puerarin group and normal-dose puerarin group all decreased DBP, and losartan group and high-dose puerarin group decreased DBP effectively.

Compared with the control group, the heart rate of the model group was faster, especially after five weeks of treatment. The heart rate of the model group was significantly elevated compared to that of the control group ($P <$ 0.01). After seven weeks of administration, the heart rate of the high-dose and normal-dose puerarin groups was significantly lower than that of the model group ($P < 0.01$ or $P < 0.05$). There was no significant difference in heart rate between the losartan potassium and model groups ($P > 0.05$). Additionally, we found no significant difference in heart rate among all groups on the tenth week of drug treatment. In addition, the heart rate in all groups was higher than 400 beats per minute, which might be related to the state of anesthesia of the rats (Table 3, Figure 3).

Table 3 Effect of Puerarin on Heart Rate in SHR ($\bar{x} \pm s$, beats/min)

Treatment Duration	Control	Model	Losartan	High Puerarin	Normal Puerarin
0 w	356.54 ± 23.16	394.76 ± 30.55***	387.71 ± 23.38	387.42 ± 44.38	401.36 ± 23.34
1 w	359.39 ± 24.56	382.57 ± 29.63*	392.11 ± 25.86	373.53 ± 34.01	379.9 ± 20.44
2 w	368.2 ± 21.82	387.78 ± 23.528*	403.19 ± 31.82	387.55 ± 23.22	376.34 ± 24.4$^{\#\#}$
3 w	379.1 ± 24.27	393.05 ± 18.39	393.05 ± 29.8	393.08 ± 22.58	379.31 ± 32.81
4 w	368.17 ± 23.03	380.57 ± 25.65	382.62 ± 30.5	370.76 ± 34.31	373.85 ± 25.33
5 w	355.19 ± 27.9	383.14 ± 32.9**	381.63 ± 20.9	360.14 ± 32.75$^{\triangle\#}$	373.6 ± 15.04
6 w	358.2 ± 34.41	380.36 ± 23.03	375.98 ± 22.11	369.23 ± 29.12	372.46 ± 19.12
7 w	361.19 ± 20.94	376.8824 ± 14.77*	367.33 ± 15.45	359.04 ± 22.62$^{\triangle\triangle}$	361.4 ± 14.76$^{\triangle}$
8 w	366.27 ± 23.76	381.43 ± 14.38*	381.72 ± 17.93	364.61 ± 27.95$^{\triangle\#}$	368.42 ± 16.84
9 w	369.25 ± 18.24	384.44 ± 15.16*	374.25 ± 18.21	362.88 ± 21.83$^{\triangle\triangle}$	364.46 ± 17.95$^{\triangle\triangle}$

Notes: Compared with the control group, the heart rate of the model group was faster, especially after five weeks of treatment. There was no obvious difference between losartan group and model group for heart rate. Compared with the model group, heart rate of high-dose puerarin decreased effectively in the fifth, seventh, eighth and ninth week. Compared with the control group, $^{*}P < 0.05$, $^{**}P < 0.01$, and $^{***}P < 0.001$; compared with the model group, $^{\triangle}P < 0.05$ and $^{\triangle\triangle}P < 0.01$; and compared with the losartan group, $^{\#}P < 0.05$ and $^{\#\#}P < 0.01$. n=10.

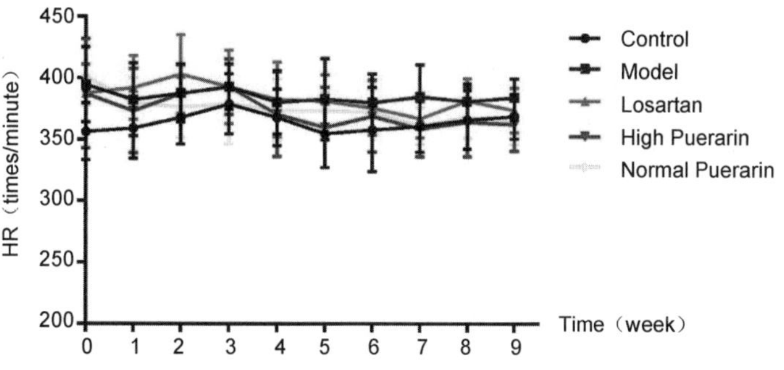

Figure 3 Effect of Puerarin on Heart Rate in SHR

Notes: The figure showed dynamic change of heart rate. It showed heart rate of model group was faster. Compared with model group, heart rate of losartan group did not decreased obviously. High-dose puerarin decreased heart rate effectively compared with model group.

2 Pathological Results

Morphological changes in aortic tissues were observed by HE staining. In the model group, the intima-media thickness (IMT)was increased, muscle fiber was thickened, and notable inflammatory cell infiltration was observed (significant increase in the number of blue nuclei) (Figure 4). The degree of aortic fibrosis was observed by Masson staining, and notable collagen fiber hyperplasia was observed (blue and green collagen fibers covering the normal red muscle fiber). Compared with the model group, the degree of collagen fiber hyperplasia in the drug group was reduced, and red muscle fibers were still clearly observed.

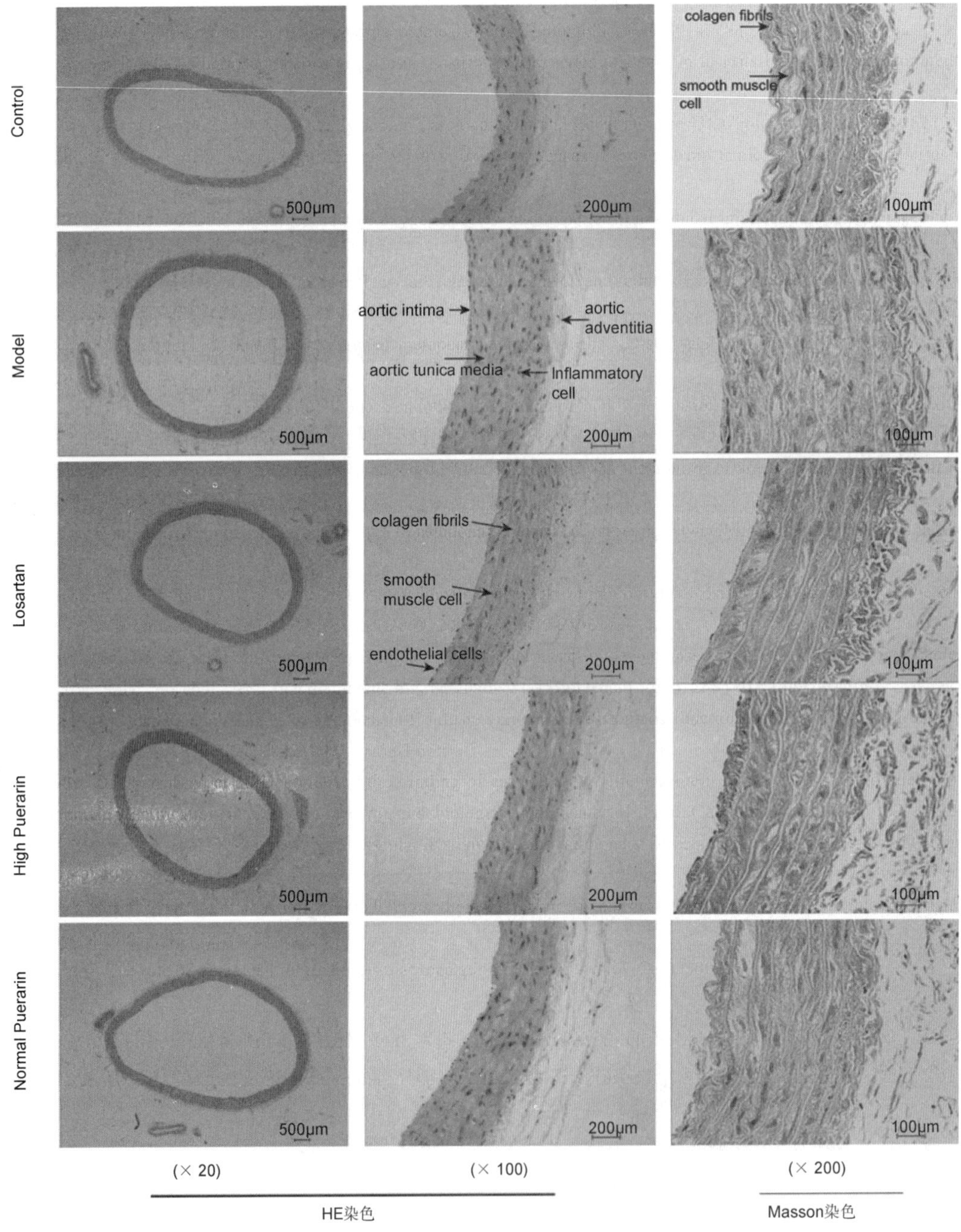

Figure 4　Pathological Morphology of The Aorta

The IMT in the model group was significantly thick than that in the control group ($P < 0.001$). After drug intervention, the aortic IMT in the losartan potassium group, high-dose puerarin group and normal-dose puerarin group were decreased compared to those in the model group ($P < 0.001$) (Figure 5).

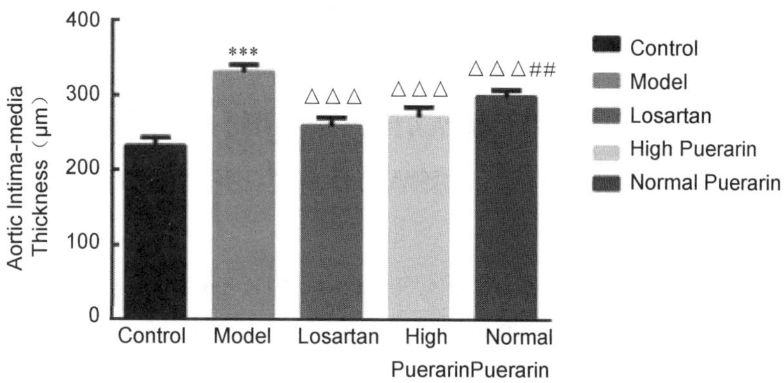

Figure 5　Effect of Puerarin on IMT in SHR

In the model group, the IMT was increased, muscle fiber was thickened, and notable inflammatory cell infiltration was observed (significant increase in the number of blue nuclei). Notable collagen fiber hyperplasia was observed (blue and green collagen fibers covering the normal red muscle fiber). Compared with the model group, the degree of collagen fiber hyperplasia in the drug group was reduced, and red muscle fibers were still clearly observed.

The IMT in the model group was significantly thick than that in the control group ($P < 0.001$). After drug intervention, the aortic IMT in the losartan potassium group, high-dose puerarin group and normal-dose puerarin group were decreased compared to those in the model group ($P < 0.001$). Compared with the control group, $^{***}P < 0.001$; compared with the model group, $^{\triangle\triangle\triangle}P < 0.001$; and compared with the losartan group, $^{\#\#}P < 0.01$. n=5.

3 Aortic Diameter Measurements

Long-term hypertension affects aortic structure as well as systolic and diastolic function. In this study, the aortic diameter of SHR was significantly wider than that of the control group ($P < 0.01$). Additionally, the aortic diameter of the drug-treated groups was decreased. Compared with the model group, the aortic diameter was significantly decreased in the losartan potassium group ($P < 0.05$)and showed a decreasing trend in the puerarin group ($P > 0.05$) (Figure 6).

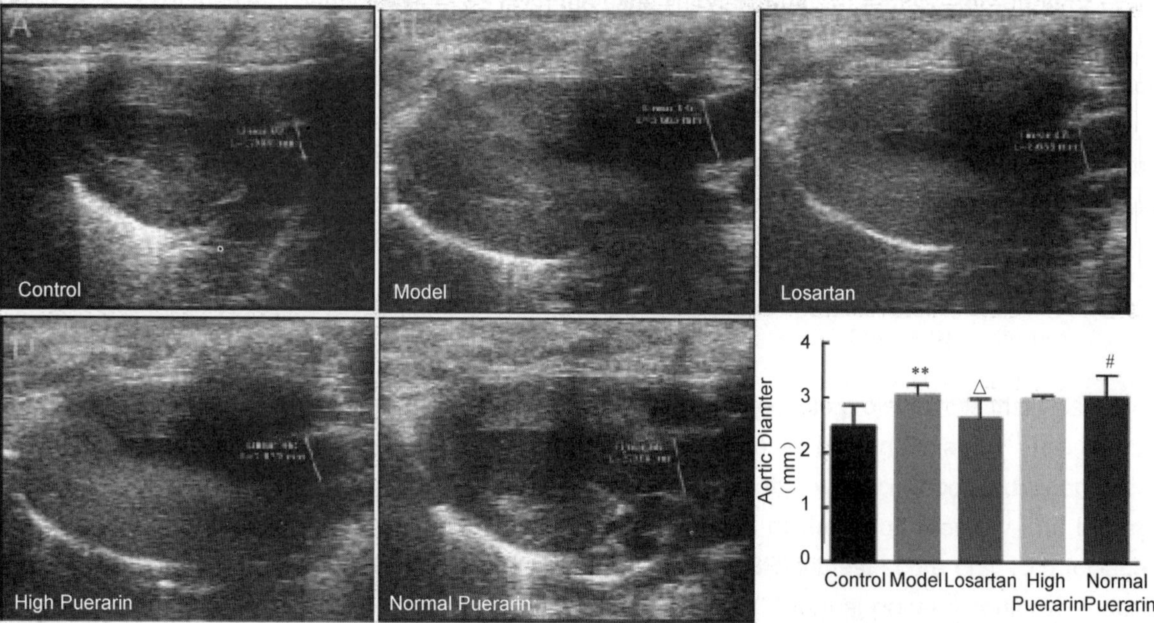

Figure 6　Effect of Puerarin on Aortic Diameter in SHR

The aortic diameter of SHR was significantly wider than that of the control group. Compared with the model group, the aortic diameter was significantly decreased in the losartan potassium group ($P < 0.05$)and aortic diameter of the puerarin group showed a decreasing trend. Compared with the control group, $^{**}P <$ 0.01; compared with the model group, $^{\triangle}P < 0.05$; and compared with the losartan group, $^{\#}P < 0.05$. n=9.

4 NO, SOD, MDA, cGMP and Ang II

After nine weeks of drug administration, the serum NO level in the model group was significantly lower than that in the control group ($P < 0.001$). Compared with the model group, the NO level of the high-dose puerarin group, normal-dose puerarin group and losartan potassium group was significantly increased ($P <$ 0.01 or $P < 0.001$). The MDA level in the model group was markedly higher than that in the control group ($P <$ 0.01). Compared with the model group, the MDA level of the high-dose puerarin group, normal-dose puerarin group and losartan potassium group was significantly decreased ($P < 0.01$ or $P < 0.001$). There was no statistically significant difference in serum SOD among all groups ($P > 0.05$). Serum cGMP level in the model group was obviously lower than that in the control group ($P < 0.05$). Compared with the model group, the cGMP level of the high-dose puerarin group, normal-dose puerarin group and losartan potassium group was significantly increased ($P < 0.01$ or $P < 0.001$). Ang II of plasma in model group had no statistical difference compared with control group ($P > 0.05$). Compared with model group, Ang II of normal and high dose puerarin decreased significantly ($P < 0.01$), and Ang II in losartan group increased ($P < 0.05$) (Figure 7).

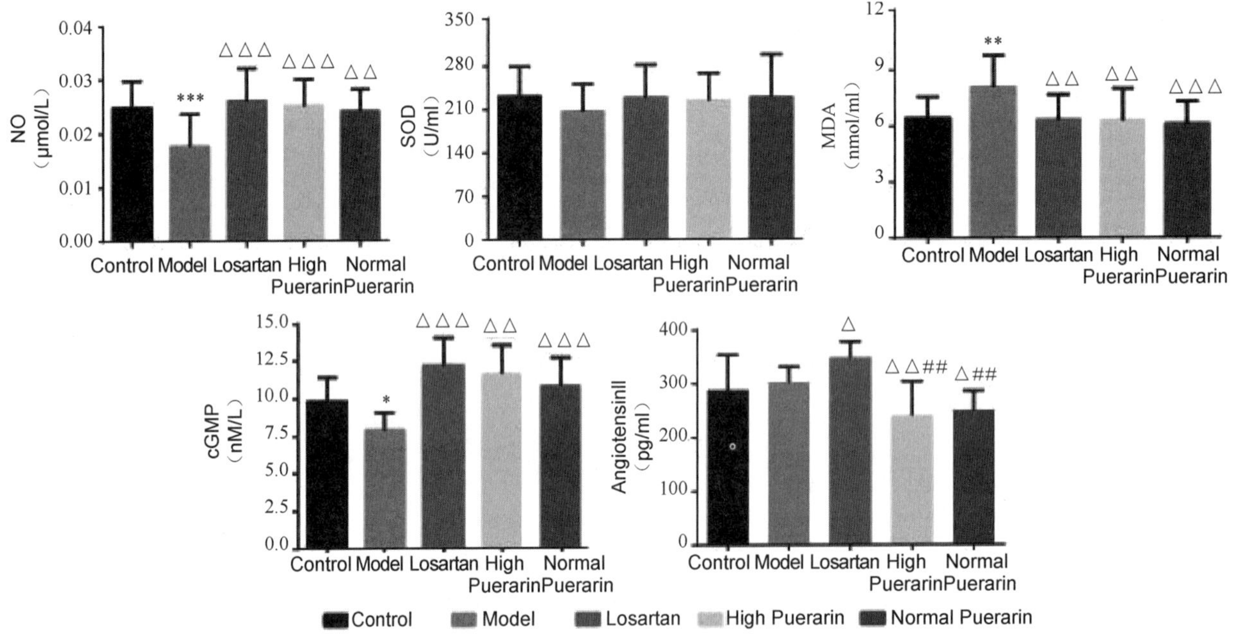

Figure 7 Effect on Oxidative Stress Related Factors and Ang II

The NO and cGMP level in serum of the model group was significantly lower than that in the control group ($P < 0.001$ or $P < 0.05$). The MDA level in the model group was markedly higher than that in the control group ($P < 0.01$). Compared with the model group, the NO and cGMP level in serum of the high-dose puerarin group, normal-dose puerarin group and losartan potassium group was significantly increased ($P < 0.01$ or $P < 0.001$), and the MDA level was significantly decreased ($P < 0.01$ or $P < 0.001$). There was no statistically significant difference in serum SOD among all groups ($P > 0.05$). Ang II of normal and high dose puerarin decreased significantly compared with model group ($P < 0.01$), and Ang II in losartan group increased ($P <$ 0.05). Compared with the control group, $^{**}P < 0.01$ and $^{***}P < 0.001$; and compared with the model group, $^{\triangle\triangle}P < 0.01$ and $^{\triangle\triangle\triangle}P < 0.001$. n=9.

5 Differentially Expressed Genes and String Network Analysis

In total, eighteen genes were identified. Compared with the model group, Gucy1b3, Ptgir, Cnga4 and eNOS were upregulated and Cav1, AT1b, Gucy1a3 and Mas1 were downregulated in the high-dose puerarin group. Results of the model group were opposite to those of the control group (Figure 8, Table 4).

As observed in Figure 9, eNOS, which is also called NOS3, was at the center of the related pathways. Additionally, eNOS was closely related to Cav1, AT1b, Gucy1a3/1b3 and Ptgs2, and Gucy1a3/1b3 was closely related to Pde5a and Pde3a. With the KEGG pathway function of the STRING network database, the pathways of target genes were analyzed. Table 5 shows that the genes affected by high-dose puerarin treatment were mainly related to the cGMP/PKG pathway.

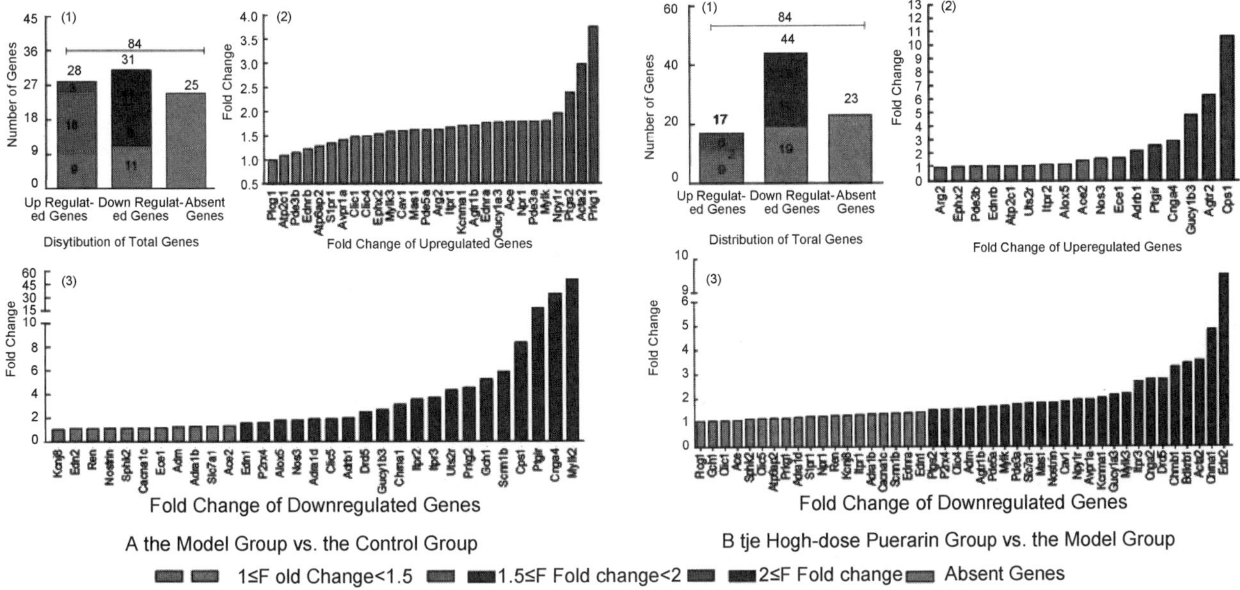

Figure 8 Comparison of Hypertension-related Genes

Notes: A: Compared with the control group, fifty-nine genes were expressed in the model group, of which 28 were up and thirty-one were downregulated. Fold change of nineteen genes was more than 1.5 in the upregulated genes, and fold change of twenty genes was more than 1.5 in the downregulated genes.

B: Compared with the model group, sixty-one genes were expressed in the high-dose group, in which seventeen were up and forty-four were downregulated. Fold change of eight genes was more than 1.5 in the upregulated genes, and fold change of twenty-five genes was more than 1.5 in the downregulated. genes.

Table 4 Comparison of Hypertension-related Genes from the Model group *vs*. the Control Group and the High-dose Puerarin *vs*. the Model Group

No	Symbol	P vs. M	FC	M vs. C	FC	Hypertension-related process
1	eNOS	Up	1.63	Down	-1.82	Vasodilation/Vasodilation/Vasotone/Blood Pressure Regulation/Nitric Oxide Metabolism/Hypoxia Response
2	Adrb1	Up	2.22	Down	-2	Smooth Muscle Contraction/Vasodilation
3	Ptgir	Up	2.63	Down	-16.67	Cyclic-GMP Synthesis & Signaling/Second-Messenger-Mediated Signaling
4	Cnga4	Up	2.96	Down	-33.33	Ion Transport
5	Gucy1b3	Up	4.84	Down	-2.7	Nitric Oxide Signaling/Cyclic-GMP Synthesis & Signaling
6	Cps1	Up	10.72	Down	-8.33	Vasodilation/Nitric Oxide Metabolism
7	Acta2	Down	-3.57	Up	2.97	Smooth Muscle Contraction/Blood Pressure Regulation
8	Mylk3	Down	-2.17	Up	1.59	Myosin Light Chain Kinases
9	Gucy1a3	Down	-2.13	Up	1.77	Smooth Muscle Relaxation/Blood Pressure Regulation/ Nitric Oxide Signaling

Continued

No	Symbol	P vs. M	FC	M vs. C	FC	Hypertension-related process
10	Kcnma1	Down	-2	Up	1.7	Smooth Muscle Contraction/Smooth Muscle Relaxation/Osmotic Shock/Hypoxia Response
11	Npy1r	Down	-1.96	Up	1.96	Blood Pressure Regulation/Vasodilation
12	Cav1	Down	-1.85	Up	1.6	Vasoconstriction/Smooth Muscle Contraction/Nitric Oxide Metabolism/Hypoxia Response
13	Mas1	Down	-1.82	Up	1.62	Renin-Angiotensin System
14	Pde3a	Down	-1.75	Up	1.79	Lipid Metabolism
15	Mylk	Down	-1.69	Up	1.8	Myosin Light Chain Kinases
16	Pde5a	Down	-1.67	Up	1.62	Vasodilation/Hypoxia Response
17	AT1b	Down	-1.64	Up	1.71	Vasodilation/Vasoconstriction/Vasotone/Renin-Angiotensin System
18	Ptgs2	Down	-1.52	Up	2.38	Vasoconstriction/Smooth Muscle Contraction/Blood Pressure Regulation

Compared with the model group, Gucy1b3, Ptgir, Cnga4 and eNOS were upregulated and Cav1, AT1b, Gucy1a3 and Mas1 were down regulated in the high-dose puerarin group. Results of the model group were opposite to those of the control group. P vs. M: the high-dose puerarin group vs. the model group; M vs. C: the model group vs. the control group; FC: fold change; eNOS (which is also called Nos3)was at the center of the related pathways. Additionally, eNOS was closely related to Cav1, AT1b, Gucy1a3/1b3 and Ptgs2, and Gucy1a3/1b3 was closely related to Pde5a and Pde3a.

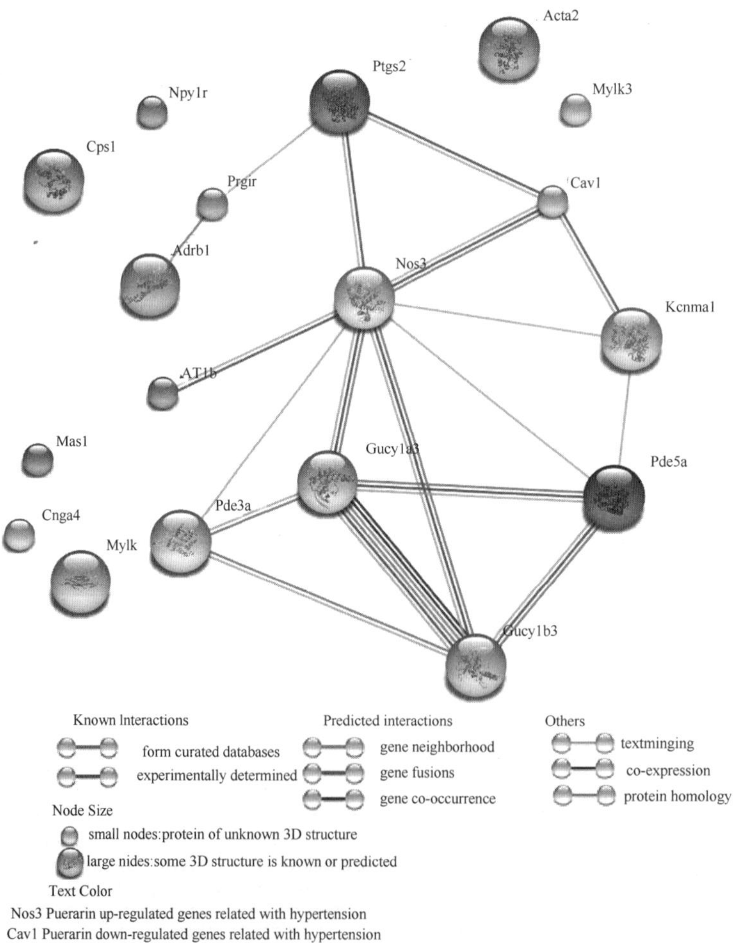

Figure 9 Network Analysis of DEGs Related to Hypertension

6 Protein Levels of eNOS, p-eNOS, AT1, AT2 and Cav1

Protein levels of major target genes were detected by western blotting. The level of p-eNOS in the model group was significantly lower than that in the control group ($P < 0.01$). Compared with the model group, the level of p-eNOS in the high-dose puerarin group was significantly increased ($P < 0.05$), whereas in the losartan potassium group, the level of p-eNOS was not significantly changed ($P > 0.05$) (Figure 10A). Moreover, there was no significant difference in the total protein expression level of eNOS among all groups ($P > 0.05$) (Figure 10B).

AT1 and AT2 are two receptors of Ang II and play different biological roles in the regulation of blood pressure. The protein expression levels of AT1 and AT2 in aortas were both detected. In addition, the level of AT1 in SHR was significantly higher than that in the control group ($P < 0.01$). AT1 levels in the losartan potassium and high-dose puerarin groups were also significantly reduced compared with those in the model group ($P < 0.01$) (Figure 10C). However, there was no significant difference in the level of AT2 among all groups ($P > 0.05$) (Figure 10D). The protein level of Cav1 in the model group was significantly higher than that in the control group ($P < 0.05$) (Figure 10E). The protein level of Cav1 in the losartan potassium group and high-dose puerarin group was significantly lower than that in the model group ($P < 0.05$ or $P < 0.001$).

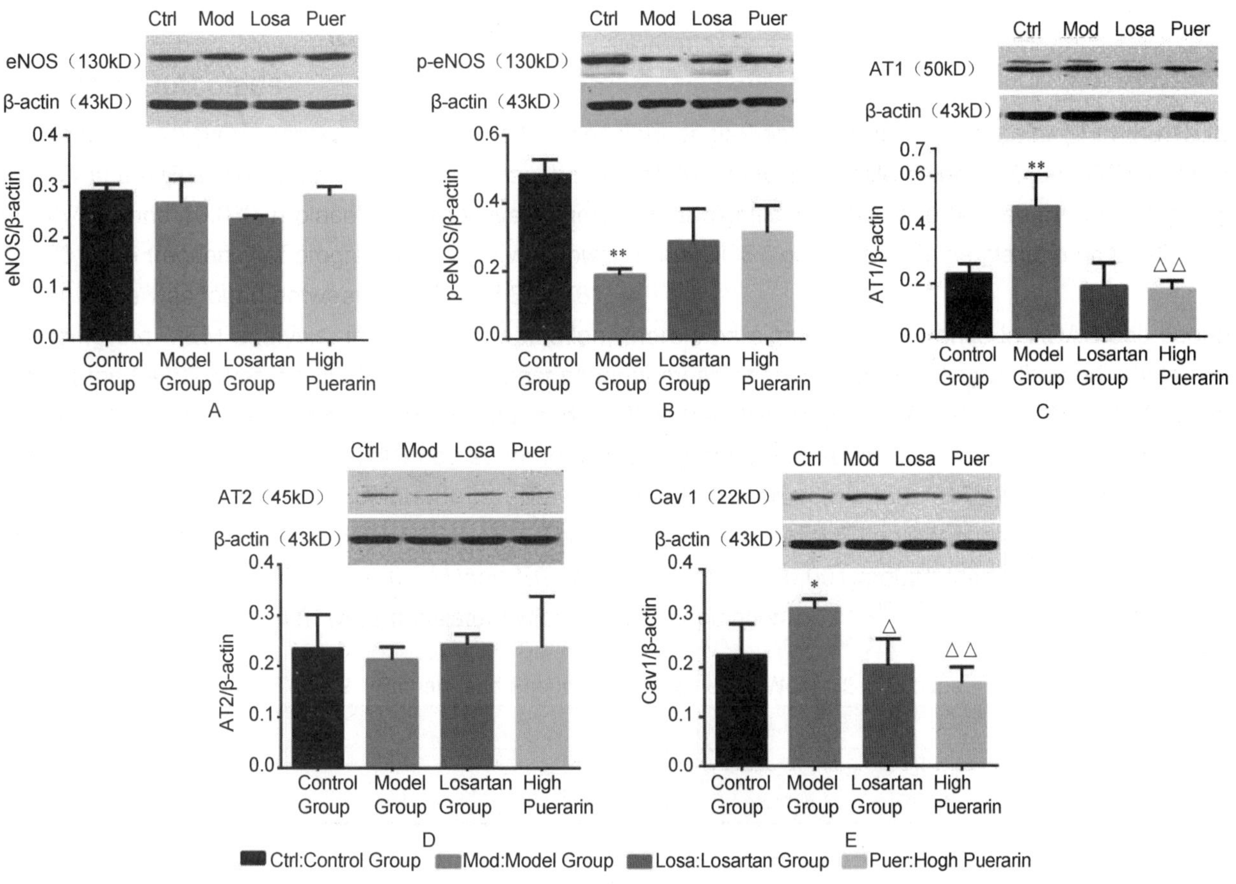

Figure 10 Effect of Puerarin on Protein of eNOS, p-eNOS, AT1 and AT2

The level of p-eNOS in the model group was significantly lower than that in the control group ($P < 0.01$). Compared with the model group, the level of p-eNOS in the high-dose puerarin group was significantly increased ($P < 0.05$). In the losartan potassium group, the level of p-eNOS was not significantly changed ($P > 0.05$) (Figure A). The AT1 and Cav1 level of model group was significantly higher than that in the control group ($P < 0.01$). AT1 and Cav1 levels in the losartan potassium group and high-dose puerarin group were also significantly reduced compared with those in the model group ($P < 0.01$) (Figure B). There was no significant difference in the level of AT2 and the total protein expression level of eNOS among all groups ($P > 0.05$) (Figure C-D). Compared with the control group, $^{**}P<0.01$; and compared with the model group, $^{\triangle}P<0.05$ and $^{\triangle\triangle}P<0.01$. n=4.

DISCUSSION

This study mainly focused on the mechanism of puerarin on blood pressure in SHR. The results showed that puerarin and losartan potassium both decreased blood pressure in SHR. Unlike losartan potassium treatment, high-dose puerarin treatment also slowed heart rate. The mechanism by which puerarin reduced blood pressure was mainly related to eNOS activation and increased NO production, which was also related to the eNOS/cGMP pathway. In addition, the increase of eNOS activity also depended on the reduction of AT1 and Cav1.

Nitric oxide synthase is a key enzyme for NO production. There are three types of nitric oxide synthases, including eNOS, inducible nitric oxide synthase and neuronal nitric oxide synthase, all of which play an important role in the development of cardiovascular diseases, such as hypertension[11,12]. ENOS is mainly distributed in vascular endothelial cells and cardiac myocytes. The activity of eNOS determines whether its substrate L-arginine is used to produce NO or superoxide anion (O2- ·). When sufficient levels of tetrahydrobiopterin are present, activated eNOS transfers the electrons provided by NADPH to L-arginine and produces NO. When eNOS activity is decreased or inhibited, the electrons provided by NADPH are received by O_2, thereby generating O2- · [13]. In a rat model of renal failure, overexpression of eNOS increased the formation of NO, decreased blood pressure, and alleviated renal injury[14]. In this study, eNOS was found to be in the center of the network affected by high-dose puerarin treatment, and the protein level of eNOS in the puerarin group was significantly higher than that in the model group ($P<0.05$), which suggested that the antihypertensive mechanism of puerarin might be closely related to eNOS activity.

The eNOS/NO/cGMP pathway plays an important role in the development of a variety of cardiovascular diseases, such as hypertension[15,16]. Activated eNOS increases NO production. cGMP is a ubiquitous intracellular second messenger and the molecular basis of many biological effects of NO. cGMP is also involved in the process of relaxing vascular smooth muscle and inhibiting platelet aggregation[15,17]. CGMP is produced from the catalysis of NO by Gucy1b3, a kind of soluble guanylate cyclase, and its activity is regulated by phosphodiesterase (PDE). For example, cGMP could be hydrolyzed by PDE5 and transformed into its inactive state 5-GMP[18]. In this study, the aortic tissue from the high-dose puerarin group exhibited significant upregulation of Gucy1b3, reduced levels of PDE5a, and increased serum levels of cGMP and NO. It was suggested that high-dose puerarin treatment induced vasodilation via increased bioavailability of cGMP, which was induced by increasing the activity of Gucy1b3 and inhibiting PDE5a. Thus, puerarin reduces blood pressure in SHR by regulating eNOS/NO/cGMP pathway (Figure11).

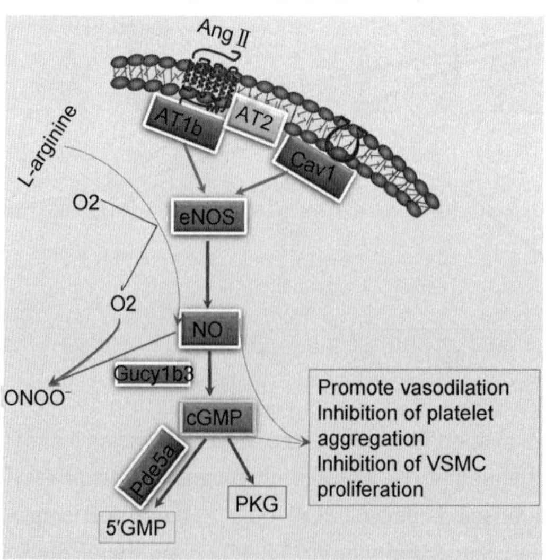

Figure 11 Possible Mechanism Underlying the Effect of High-dose Puerarin Treatment on Blood Pressure in SHR

The mechanism by which puerarin reduced blood pressure was mainly related to eNOS activation and increased NO production, which was also related to the eNOS/NO/cGMP pathway. In addition, the increase of eNOS activity also depended on the downregulation of AT1 and Cav1.

The biological activity of eNOS is affected by a lot of proteins. Ang II also reduces eNOS activity and leads to endothelial dysfunction when binds to AT1. Loot[19] found that activated endothelial Pyk2 by Ang II induced the phosphorylation of eNOS at Tyr657 and inhibited NO production to reduce endothelium- dependent vasodilatation. Under the condition of hypercholesterolemia, Ang II increase the formation of reactive oxygen species (ROS), and the phosphorylation level of eNOS at Ser-1177 decreases[20]. In addition, injection of Ang II increases the activity of NAD (P)H oxidase to promote ROS production and induces eNOS uncoupling, thus causing endothelial dysfunction[21]. In this study, the protein level of Ang II and AT1 in high-puerarin group was downregulated and eNOS was upregulated, which suggested that the mechanism underlying the promotion of NO production by puerarin may be related to downregulated Ang II and AT1 and upregulated eNOS activity (Figure11).

Cav1 is one of the key proteins involved in the formation of caveolae. Cav1 interacts with eNOS through its scaffolding domain to inhibit eNOS activity, and as a result, the formation of NO is reduced[22]. Studies with Cav1 knockout mice have shown that their basal expression levels of NO and cGMP are significantly higher than those of wild-type mice[23]. In mice lacking Cav1, blood vessels did not exhibit a stable contractile force. In addition, acetylcholine-induced vasodilatation was increased, and the response to phenylephrine was reduced, which suggested that Cav1 deficiency might decrease muscle tension and reduce whole-body blood pressure[24]. However, studies have also suggested that loss of Cav1 has no detectable effect on blood pressure. Thus, a compensatory mechanism caused by the loss of Cav1may have counteracted the increase of eNOS activity. However, this finding does not contradict the negative regulatory effect of Cav1 on eNOS activity[25]. In this study, puerarin decreased the protein level of Cav1 and increased eNOS level. This finding suggests that puerarin might reduce the expression level of Cav1 to promote the uncoupling of eNOS from Cav1 and increase the activity of eNOS, thus promoting the formation of NO to reduce blood pressure.

In summary, by means of qPCR array technology and the STRING database, this study explored the mechanism underlying the effect of puerarin on blood pressure, and the role of eNOS in this process was identified. However, the importance of eNOS in the puerarin-induced antihypertensive effects was not verified with further experiments, such as gene knockout experiments. This study also found that puerarin treatment affects heart rate and improves cardiac function in SHR. In the future, these two findings will be studied in depth to provide more comprehensive theoretical support for the application of puerarin in the clinic to treat cardiovascular diseases.

CONCLUSION

Puerarin has been widely used in the treatment of cardiovascular diseases, especially hypertension, since it was isolated in the late 1950s. This study suggested puerarin could be used as a potential antihypertensive agent. Puerarin reduced blood pressure of SHR by targeting eNOS. Activated eNOS influenced eNOS/NO/cGMP pathway and decrease of AT1 and Cav1may contributed to the activation of eNOS.

REFERENCES

[1] Lewington S, Clarke R, Qizilbash N, et al. Age-specific relevance of usual blood pressure to vascular mortality: a meta-analysis of individual data for one million adults in 61 prospective studies[J]. Lancet, 2002, 360 (9349): 1903-1913.

[2] Chockalingam A, Campbell N R, Fodor J G. Worldwide epidemic of hypertension[J]. Can J Cardiol, 2006, 22 (7): 553-555.

[3] Gkaliagkousi E, Gavriilaki E, Triantafyllou A, et al. Clinical Significance of Endothelial Dysfunction in Essential Hypertension[J]. Curr Hypertens Rep, 2015, 17 (11): 85.

[4] Gheibi S, Jeddi S, Kashfi K, et al. Regulation of vascular tone homeostasis by NO and H2S: Implications in hypertension[J]. Biochem Pharmacol, 2018, 149: 42-59.

[5] Mordi I, Mordi N, Delles C, et al. Endothelial dysfunction in human essential hypertension[J]. J Hypertens, 2016, 34 (8): 1464-1472.

[6] Tan C, Wang A, Liu C, et al. Puerarin Improves Vascular Insulin Resistance and Cardiovascular Remodeling in Salt-Sensitive Hypertension[J]. Am J Chin Med, 2017, 45 (6): 1169-1184.

[7] Yang X, Hu W, Zhang Q, et al. Puerarin Inhibits C-Reactive Protein Expression via Suppression of Nuclear Factor κB Activation in Lipopolysaccharide-Induced Peripheral Blood Mononuclear Cells of Patients with Stable Angina Pectoris[J]. Basic & Clinical Pharmacology & Toxicology, 2010, 107 (2): 637-642.

[8] Guo B Q, Xu J B, Xiao M, et al. Puerarin reduces ischemia/reperfusion-induced myocardial injury in diabetic rats via upregulation of vascular endothelial growth factor A/angiotensin-1 and suppression of apoptosis[J]. Mol Med Rep, 2018, 17 (5): 7421-7427.

[9] Zhou Y X, Zhang H, Peng C. Puerarin: a review of pharmacological effects[J]. Phytother Res, 2014, 28 (7): 961-975.

[10] Kong H, Wang X, Shi R, et al. Pharmacokinetics and Tissue Distribution Kinetics of Puerarin in Rats Using Indirect Competitive ELISA[J]. Molecules, 2017, 22 (6): 939.

[11] Lee J, Bae E H, Ma S K, et al. Altered Nitric Oxide System in Cardiovascular and Renal Diseases[J]. Chonnam Med J, 2016, 52 (2): 81-90.

[12] Tsutsui M, Tanimoto A, Tamura M, et al. Significance of nitric oxide synthases: Lessons from triple nitric oxide synthases null mice[J]. J Pharmacol Sci, 2015, 127 (1): 42-52.

[13] Paravicini T M, Touyz R M. NADPH oxidases, reactive oxygen species, and hypertension: clinical implications and therapeutic possibilities[J]. Diabetes Care, 2008, 31 Suppl 2: S170-S180.

[14] Savard S, Lavoie P, Villeneuve C, et al. eNOS gene delivery prevents hypertension and reduces renal failure and injury in rats with reduced renal mass[J]. Nephrol Dial Transplant, 2012, 27 (6): 2182-2190.

[15] Evora P R, Evora P M, Celotto A C, et al. Cardiovascular therapeutics targets on the NO-sGC-cGMP signaling pathway: a critical overview[J]. Curr Drug Targets, 2012, 13 (9): 1207-1214.

[16] Jiang J, Gan Z, Li Y, et al. REM sleep deprivation induces endothelial dysfunction and hypertension in middle-aged rats: Roles of the eNOS/NO/cGMP pathway and supplementation with L-arginine[J]. PLoS One, 2017, 12 (8): e182746.

[17] Sabino J P, Bombarda G, Da S C, et al. Role of the spinal cord NO/cGMP pathway in the control of arterial pressure and heart rate[J]. Pflugers Arch, 2011, 461 (1): 23-28.

[18] Papapetropoulos A, Hobbs A J, Topouzis S. Extending the translational potential of targeting NO/cGMP-regulated pathways in the CVS[J]. Br J Pharmacol, 2015, 172 (6): 1397-1414.

[19] Loot A E, Schreiber J G, Fisslthaler B, et al. Angiotensin II impairs endothelial function via tyrosine phosphorylation of the endothelial nitric oxide synthase[J]. The Journal of Experimental Medicine, 2009, 206 (13): 2889-2896.

[20] Amiya E, Watanabe M, Takeda N, et al. Angiotensin II impairs endothelial nitric-oxide synthase bioavailability under free cholesterol-enriched conditions via intracellular free cholesterol-rich membrane microdomains[J]. J Biol Chem, 2013, 288 (20): 14497-14509.

[21] Mollnau H, Wendt M, Szocs K, et al. Effects of angiotensin II infusion on the expression and function of NAD (P)H oxidase and components of nitric oxide/cGMP signaling[J]. Circ Res, 2002, 90 (4): E58-E65.

[22] Trane A E, Pavlov D, Sharma A, et al. Deciphering the binding of caveolin-1 to client protein endothelial nitric-oxide synthase (eNOS): scaffolding subdomain identification, interaction modeling, and biological significance[J]. J Biol Chem, 2014, 289 (19): 13273-13283.

[23] Drab M, Verkade P, Elger M, et al. Loss of caveolae, vascular dysfunction, and pulmonary defects in caveolin-1 gene-disrupted mice[J]. Science, 2001, 293 (5539): 2449-2452.

[24] Albinsson S, Shakirova Y, Rippe A, et al. Arterial remodeling and plasma volume expansion in caveolin-1-deficient mice[J]. Am J Physiol Regul Integr Comp Physiol, 2007, 293 (3): R1222-R1231.

[25] Rahman A, Sward K. The role of caveolin-1 in cardiovascular regulation[J]. Acta Physiol (Oxf), 2009, 195 (2): 231-245.

First Published: SHI Wei-li, YUAN Rong, CHEN Xun, XIN Qi-qi, YAN WANG, SHANG Xiao-hong, CONG Wei-hong, CHEN Ke-ji. Puerarin Reduces Blood Pressure in Spontaneously Hypertensive Rats by Targeting eNOS [J]. Am J Chin Med, 2019, 47: 19-38.

Chinese Herbal Medicine Qinggongshoutao for the Treatment of Amnestic Mild Cognitive Impairment: A 52-week Randomized Controlled Trial

TIAN Jin-zhou, SHI Jing, WEI Ming-qing, NI Jing-nian, FANG Zhi-yong, GAO Jin-yu, WANG Heng, YAO Hong-jun, ZHANG Jin-tao, LI Jun-tao, MIN Min, SU Li-kai, SUN Xiu-qiao, WANG Bao-ai, WANG Bao-shen, YANG Fa-ming, ZOU Yong, HU Yue-qiang, LIN Ya-ming,XU Guang-yin, LI Kang, LI Lei, ZHEN Hui, XU Jin-yan, CHEN Ke-ji, WANG Yong-yan, on behalf of the CHARM study group

As the population of older people grows, dementia is becoming a challenging issue of global health and economy.It was estimated that 35.6 million people lived with dementia worldwide in 2010, with numbers expected to almost double every 20 years[1]. Alzheimer's disease (AD)is the most popular type of dementia, AD now affects about 6.25/1000 people per year in China[2].The costs projected for care of dementias will increase over 330% by 2050 reported by Alzheimer's Association barring effective preventions or breakthrough treatments[3].However, well-studied conventional treatments for AD are generally considered to be symptom-relieving rather than disease-modifying.Mild cognitive impairment (MCI)is a transitional state between the cognitive changes of normal aging and early AD[4].Amnestic mild cognitive impairment (aMCI)is believed to be a precursor to AD and to progress to clinically diagnosable AD at a rate of approximately 10% to 15% per year, significantly higher than in the normal elderly[5].Hence, aMCI is generally recognized as a treatment target for AD[6].However, no high-quality evidence exists to support pharmacological treatments for MCI so far[7].*Ginkgo biloba* extract (EGb761)is widely used for the treatment of MCI in China.However, regarding the efficacy of EGb761 to reduce the overall incidence rate of dementia, the results were not consistent[8,9].According to traditional Chinese medicine (TCM), memory decline and dementia are believed to be caused by a deficiency of kidney essence (Shenxu in Chinese), and the treatment approach is to supplement kidney essence, as described in the *Complete Works of Jingyue (*published in 1624).Qinggongshoutao (QGST)formulation, a traditional herbal pill that was originally derived from the *Qing Dynasty Medical Archives* of Emperor Qianlong, appears to serve the function.QGST is being used to treat symptoms, such as forgetfulness, backache, knee weakness, and urinary incontinence.Experimental studies suggest that QGST have multifaceted functions, including antioxidation, neuroprotection, and improvement of memory[10].Up until now, there has been no well-controlled clinical trial to assess QGST for the treatment of dementia.The present study was designed to determine whether treatment with QGST can delay the clinical onset of AD in people with aMCI, as compared with EGb761 and placebo, and investigate further the effects of QGST on cognitive function.

METHODS

As one of Chinese Alzheimer's Disease Research on Medicinal Products projects, this trial was conducted in 17 centers in China.The patients were required to meet the diagnostic criteria for aMCI[4].The operational aMCI inclusion criteria were showed as follows: (1)memory complaints that were corroborated by an informant; (2)abnormal memory function as assessed by the Chinese version of the Adult Memory and Information Processing Battery Logical Memory Delayed Story Recall (AMIPB-DSR)subtest score of < 15.5 for age (age 50-64 years < 15.5, 65-74years < 12.5, and over 75 years < 10)[11]; (3)normal general cognitive function as determined by a clinician's judgment based on a structured interview with the patients, a Mini–Mental State Examination (MMSE)score of 24 to 30 for education[12], and Clinical Dementia Rating (CDR)Scale score 5 0.5, with the memory domain 5 0.5 or 1, and no other domain greater than 1[13]; (4)no or minimal impairments in activities of daily living as determined by a clinical interview with the patient and an informant, a score of 38 to 52 on the Alzheimer's Disease Cooperative Study–Activities of Daily Living Scale for patients with MCI (ADCS-ADL-MCI-24 items)[14]; (5)absence of dementia judged by an experienced clinician, including no impairment of cognitive function that would meet the core clinical criteria of the National Institute on Aging–Alzheimer's Association workgroups[15]; (6)the patients were required to have adequate vision and hearing to participate in the study assessments; (7)all patients and legal guardians should provide written consent;and (8)deficiency of kidney essence to be confirmed using the kidney deficiency scale from the pattern elements scale ≥ 7points[16].Detailed exclusion criteria comprised the following: (1)nonamnestic MCI; (2)meeting the diagnostic criteria for dementia; (3)cognitive impairment resulting from conditions, such as acute cerebral trauma, cerebral damage due to a lack of oxygen, epilepsy vitamin deficiency, infections such as meningitis or AIDS, significant endocrine or metabolic disease, mental retardation, a brain tumor, or drug abuse or alcohol abuse; (4)having significant psychiatric disease, depression, the Hamilton Depression Scale > 12; (5)magnetic resonance imaging scan having showed cerebral infarction, hemorrhage or focal lesions, and infections within 12 months; (6) accompanying poorly controlled diabetes or hypertension or severe arrhythmias; (7)having suffered from heart infarction within 3 months; (8)severe asthma or chronic obstructive pulmonary disease; (9)severe indigestion; (10)gastrointestinal tract obstruction or gastroduodenal ulcer; (11)use of cholinesterase inhibitors or memantine within 1 month; (12)history of hypersensitivity to the treatment drugs; (13)use of concomitant drugs with the potential to interfere with cognition, such as anticholinergics, anticonvulsants, antiparkinsonian agents, stimulants, cholinergic agents, antipsychotics, or antidepressants, or anxiolytics; (14)administration of other investigational drugs;severe impairment of the liver or kidney function;and vegetarians or contraindications for animal innards.

1 Study Design

There was a 2-week run-in period before randomization followed by a 52-week double-blind treatment period. Patients with aMCI were randomly assigned to receive (1)QGST pill (7 g per time, twice daily)and EGb761 placebo (2 tablets per time, twice daily); (2)EGb761 tablet (Ginaton) (80 mg per time, twice daily)and QGST placebo (7 g per time, twice daily);or (3)QGST placebo pill (7 g per time, twice daily)and EGb761 placebo (2 tablets per time, twice daily).QGSTwas supplied by Tianjin Zhongxin Pharmaceutical Group Co., Ltd.Darentang Pharmaceutical Factory (branch number: 141001).EGb761 was supplied by Germany's Dr.Weimar Shu Pei Pharmaceutical Factory (branch number: 5890913), and both placebos for EGb761 (branch number: 5890915)and QGST (branch number: 150101)were supplied by Tianjin Zhongxin Pharmaceutical Group Co., Ltd.The active ingredients of QGST include Ginseng (Renshen in Chinese), Radix Asparagi (Tiandong in Chinese), Radix Ophiopogonis (Maidong in Chinese), Fructus Lyczz (Gouqizi in Chinese), Radux Rehmanniae (Dihuang in Chinese), Radix Angelicae Sinensis (Danggui in Chinese), Alpinia Oxyphylla Miq (Yizhiren in Chinese), Semen Ziziphi Spinosae (Suanzaoren in Chinese), and lignum distraction (Fenxinmu in Chinese).The detailed quality control method for Chinese medicinal preparation of QGST was presented in a China Patent File (CN102048990B) (see https: //patents.google.com/patent/CN102048990B/en).To preserve blinding, the placebos of QGST and EGb761 have an identical taste and appearance to the matched drugs.Study visits took place at screening, baseline (week 0), middle points (week 4, 12, 24, 36, 48), and at the end point of treatment (week 52).

2 Randomization

This was a multicenter, randomized, double-blind, placebo-controlled, parallel group study, including a 2-week run-in period followed by a 52-week randomization period.All participants were given EGb761 placebo and QGST placebo during the run-in period, after which the patients were randomly assigned in a 5∶3∶2 ratio to QGST, EGb761, or placebo.The randomization was stratified by center using the SAS statistical software (version 9.13) (SAS Institute Inc., Cary, NC, USA).Balanced randomization generated by the SAS statistical software was carried out in three steps (in blocks of 10)by a statistician with no access to information on the patients or physicians.Patients were sequentially assigned to the lowest randomization number available at the time of each enrollment at each center.The randomized code was generated in the randomization process and sealed in an envelope.Statisticians assigned the medication group according to the randomization code.Blinding was broken only if a patient's trial medication requires specific emergency treatment.Once the blinding was broken, the patient was managed as off-trial.Patients, legal guardian, the study investigator, any other personnel involved in the study, and the investigating staff of sponsor were blinded until all patients complete the study and analysis was completed.

3 Sample Size

Previous studies showed that Alzheimer's Disease Assessment Scale–Cognition subscale (ADAS-cog) increased by 0.61 points over 12 months, with a standard deviation of 4.104.We estimated that the sample size of 360 would have 80% power to detect a difference (Cohen's d=0.5)between the treatment and placebo groups, assuming an expected rate of 20% for missed visits, at a two-sided significance level of 5%.The ratio of the QGST group, EGb761 group, and placebo group was 5: 3: 2.

4 Efficacy Measures

The primary outcome measures were the rate of progression to possible or probable AD at end point, defined according to the core clinical criteria of the National Institute on Aging–Alzheimer's Association workgroups[15] and CDR-GS score ⩾ 1.The other primary outcome was the change from baseline to 52 weeks in ADAS-cog scores[17], an 11-item scale with scores ranging from 0 to 70 and higher scores indicating more severe cognitive impairment.Secondary outcome measures included changes from baseline to 52 weeks in the MMSE scores (ranging from 0 to 30)[12], AMIPB-DSR (scores range from 0 to 56)[11], and ADCS-ADL-MCI-24 items (scores range from 0 to 69), with lower scores indicating worse function[14].In addition, the changes in the deficiency of kidney essence using Clinical Global Impression of Change of Kidney Deficiency (CGIC-KDS)was assessed[18].CGIC-KDS, based on information from a semistructured interview with the patient and the legal guardian, was designed specifically to evaluate the global assessment of changes of kidney function deficiency based on clinician and caregiver in TCM.The CGIC-KDS score ranges from 1 to 7, and the score of 1-3 indicates improvement, 4 means no change, and 5-7 indicates worse[18].

The safety assessment included (1)physical examination and vital signs; (2)electrocardiography; (3)laboratory testing, and (4)documentation of any adverse events (AEs)that occurred during the treatment period, including the severity, time of onset, duration, treatment, and relationship to the tested drugs.

5 Oversight

This study was undertaken in accordance with the principles of the Declaration of Helsinki and the International Conference on Harmonization of Technical Requirements for Registration of Pharmaceuticals for Human Use guidelines for good clinical practice.The study protocol was approved by the Medical Ethics Committee of Dongzhimen Hospital to Beijing University of Chinese Medicine and the Medical Ethics Committee of the study institutions where this study was conducted.Written informed consent was provided by the patients and their legal representatives.The sponsor (Tianjin Zhongxin Pharmaceutical Group Co., Ltd.Darentang Pharmaceutical Factory)funded the trial and provided tested drugs and placebo.The principal investigator designed the trial in consultation with the academic authors.Data were collected by the investigators, analyzed by the third party, and interpreted by all the authors.

6 Statistical Analyses

Statistical analysis of efficacy was conducted in two populations: the full-analysis set (FAS)population and the perprotocol set (PPS)population.Safety was analyzed in the safety set.The FAS included patients who received at least one dose of the trial regimen and who had both a baseline outcome measurement and at least one postrandomization outcome measurement.The PPS included patients who completed 52 weeks of the medication with good compliance and with complete data, with no major protocol violations.The ADAS-cog, MMSE, AMIPB-DSR, and ADCS-ADL-MCI-24 were analyzed using a mixed-effects model (MEM);the progression rate of AD, was analyzed using the generalized estimating equation.Both the MEM and the generalized estimating equation of repeated measurements were based on the likelihood estimation.Under the two data missing mechanisms including missing completely at random and missing at random, the missing data filling was not needed and the model could be directly fitted.Therefore, this MEM analysis did not filled in the missing data.The safety set included all patients who received at least one dose of the trial regimen and at least one safety evaluation.All *P* values were two-tailed, and all analyses were significant if the value was ≤ 0.05.

RESULTS

A total of 459 patients were screened, and 350 were randomized between May 2015 and October 2017.Of those 175 received QGST treatment, 105 received EGb761and 70 received placebo, and 1 patient in the QGST group and 1 patient in the EGb761 group did not meet the inclusion criteria and they were excluded from the FAS. Of these 348 patients,16 discontinued their treatment before week 52, and a total of 332 patients (165 of the patients in the QGST group, 98 in the EGb761 group, and 69 of those in the placebo group)completed the trial and were included in the PPS (Fig.1).The reason for discontinuing the study was showed in Fig.1.Nine patients in the QGST group discontinued research (5 patients withdrew the informed consent, 1 patient discontinued because of AEs, 2 lost to follow up, and 1 discontinued with unspecified reason);6 patients in the EGb761 group discontinued the study (2 patients withdrew the informed consent, 1 patient violated the protocol, and 3 lost to follow up);1 patient in the placebo group discontinued the study because of withdrawing the informed consent.There were no significant differences between the three groups in dropouts (*P* 5 .362).There were no significant differences between the three groups in baseline demographics and neuropsychological test performance (Table 1).

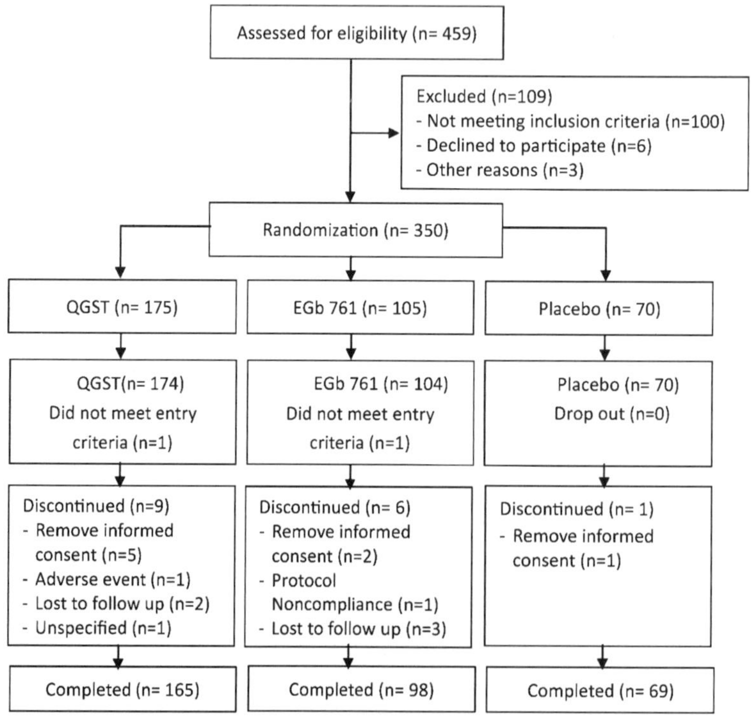

Fig.1 Flow Diagram of Enrollment, Randomization, and Follow-up

Notes: Abbreviations: QGST, Qinggongshoutao;EGb761, *Ginkgo biloba* extract.

Table 1 Baseline Characteristics of Participants by Group

Characteristic	QGST (*n*=174)	EGb761 (*n*=104)	Placebo (*n*=70)	*P*
Gender, male/female	88/86	44/60	37/33	0.2970
Age, mean (SD)	63.17 (6.59)	64.43 (7.72)	64.15 (7.25)	0.3112
Education, mean (SD)	9.14 (3.58)	9.59 (3.69)	8.91 (3.88)	0.4492
Smoking history, yes/no	45/129	20/84	18/52	0.4182
Drinking history, yes/no	46/128	20/84	18/52	0.3744
Dementia family history, yes/no	7/167	4/100	5/65	0.5236
History of stroke, yes/no	22/152	12/92	8/62	0.9471
MMSE, mean (SD)	27.60 (1.41)	27.74 (1.47)	27.51 (1.59)	0.5837
ADAS-cog, mean (SD)	12.99 (3.58)	13.07 (3.74)	13.23 (3.44)	0.8926
CDR-SB, mean (SD)	3.71 (1.19)	3.41 (1.30)	3.67 (1.29)	0.1500
AMIPB-DSR, mean (SD)	11.78 (2.46)	11.45 (2.46)	11.69 (2.08)	0.5484
ADCS-MCI-ADL-24, mean (SD)	45.72 (3.91)	45.45 (4.00)	46.53 (4.23)	0.2052
HIS, mean (SD)	2.17 (0.80)	2.14 (0.81)	2.06 (0.93)	0.6441
HAMD, mean (SD)	5.06 (2.42)	4.87 (2.43)	5.01 (2.50)	0.8142
DPES-KDS, mean (SD)	14.74 (4.02)	14.68 (4.32)	14.16 (3.79)	0.5874

1 Primary Outcomes

A total of 10 participants had progressed to possible or probable AD at the end point (2 in the QGST group, 1 in the EGb761 group, and 7 in the placebo group), the conversion rate being 1.15% in QGST, 0.96% in EGb761, and 10.0% in placebo, respectively.There was a significant difference between the three groups (*P*=0.001);the frequency of progression to AD was lower in the QGST group than in the placebo group (8.85%). No difference was found between QGST and EGb761.

Using the MEM analysis, in the FAS population, there was significant difference in ADAS-cog scores, favoring the QGST over the placebo group (least squares mean change from baseline to the end points: 2.76 in the QGST group, 2.43 in the EGb761 group, and 21.25 in the placebo group; *P*＜0.001) (Table 2).The least squares mean changes in the ADAS-cog score in all study groups and at all visits were shown in Fig.2.From the trend line at different time points, it can be seen that the improvement in ADAS-cog scores was time dependent with no difference before 36 weeks.The responder rate (ADAS-cog change ⩾ -4)was significantly higher in the QGST (29.27%, *P*＜0.001)and EGb761 (27.84%, *P*＜0.001)groups than placebo (5.80%).The results in the PPS population were consistent with the FAS population.

Table 2 Primary and Secondary Outcomes at Week 52 in Groups

Scale	Week 52 (FAS)				Week 52 (PPS)			
	QGST (*n*=174)	EGb761 (*n*=104)	Placebo (*n*=70)	P^*	QGST (*n*=165)	EGb761 (*n*=98)	Placebo (*n*=69)	P^*
ADAS-cog	2.76 (0.26)	2.43 (0.33)	21.25 (0.40)	＜0.001	2.66 (0.26)	2.45 (0.34)	21.22 (0.40)	＜ 0.001
CDR-GS＞1, n (%)	2 (1.15)	1 (0.96)	7 (10.00)	0.002	2 (1.22)	1 (1.03)	7 (10.14)	0.002
CDR-SB	0.22 (0.10)	0.25 (0.13)	20.02 (0.16)	0.064	0.20 (0.16)	0.29 (0.13)	20.01 (0.16)	0.057
MMSE	20.92 (0.14)	20.86 (0.18)	0.25 (0.22)	＜0.001	20.94 (0.14)	20.88 (0.19)	0.26 (0.22)	＜ 0.001
ADCS-ADL-MCI-24	23.02 (0.39)	22.98 (0.51)	21.35 (0.61)	0.051	22.96 (0.40)	22.97 (0.52)	1.33 (0.61)	0.053
AMIPB-DSR	23.02 (0.39)	22.98 (0.51)	21.35 (0.61)	0.196	22.96 (0.40)	22.97 (0.52)	21.33 (0.61)	0.265
CGIC-KDS	0.57 (0.08)	0.26 (0.11)	20.03 (0.14)	0.001	0.56 (0.08)	0.28 (0.12)	20.02 (0.12)	＜ 0.001

Notes:* indicates comparison between the three treatment groups.Values are in least squares mean (SE), unless otherwise specified.

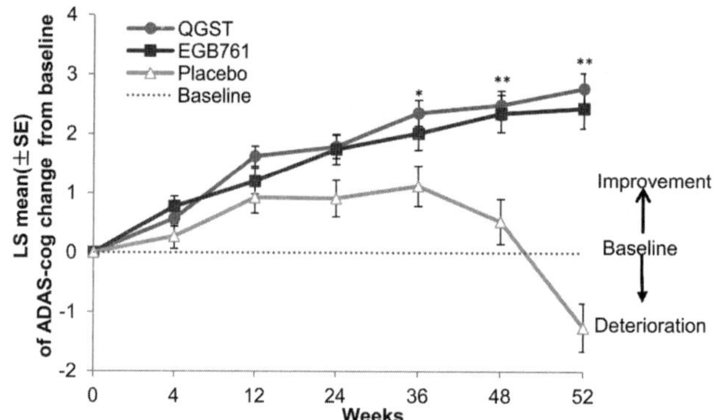

Fig.2 ADAS-cog LS Mean Change from Baseline Scores to Endpoint in the Three Groups

Notes: This figure showed the mean least squares change from baseline in the ADAS-cog score;scores range from 0 to 70, with higher scores indicating worse dementia.*$P < 0.05$ QGST versus placebo, and**$P < 0.01$ QGST versus placebo.Abbreviations: ADAS-cog, Alzheimer's Disease Assessment Scale–cognitive subscale;QGST, Qinggongshoutao;EGb761, *Ginkgo biloba* extract;LS, least squares.

2 Secondary Efficacy Outcomes

In the MEM analysis (FAS population), there were significant differences in the least squares mean change from baseline scores between the QGST and placebo groups in MMSE.After 52 weeks of treatment, the mean least squares of MMSE in the QGST group was (20.92)greater than that in the placebo group (0.25, $P < 0.001$).There was no significant difference between the QGST and EGb761 groups (20.86, P =0.792) (Fig.3).There was no significant difference in the least squares mean change from baseline to the end points between the three groups in the ADCS-ADL-MCI-24 (P=0.054).We did not observe a significant difference in AMIPB-DSR scores between the three groups.

Because QGST is a Chinese herbal medicine that enhances kidney function defined by TCM, we also examined the effect of treatment on changes in CGIC-KDS scores.After 52 weeks of treatment, the rate of improvement in kidney deficiency essence in the QGST group as measured by CGIC-KDS was 67.2% , significantly higher than the EGb761 group (49.0%)and placebo group (34.2%).Significant differences in CGIC-KDS scores between the QGST or EGb761 and placebo groups began at 12 weeks and lasted to 52 weeks;thus, the improvement in CGIC-KDS scores appeared earlier than the improvement in cognitive function (Fig.4).

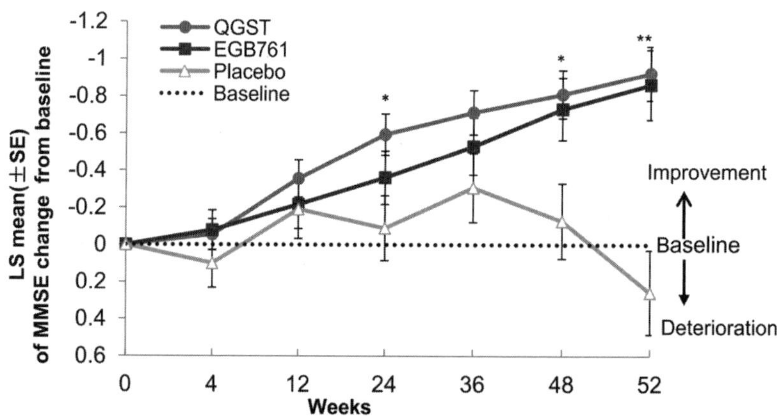

Fig.3 MMSE LS Mean Change from Baseline Scores to Endpoints in the Three Groups

Notes: This figure showed the mean least squares change from baseline to endpoints in the MMSE score;scores range from 0 to 30, with lower scores indicating worse function.*$P < 0.05$ QGST versus placebo, and **$P < 0.01$ QGST versus placebo. Abbreviations: MMSE, Mini–Mental State Examination;QGST, Qinggongshoutao;EGb761, *Ginkgo biloba* extract;LS, least squares.

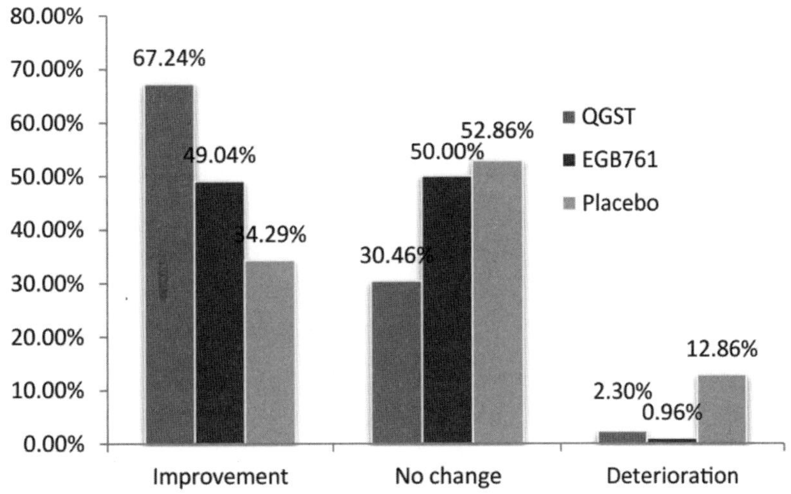

Fig.4 Between-group Comparison of the CGIC-KDS Score at 52 weeks

Notes: This figure showed changes in the CGIC-KDS score, which was designed specifically to evaluate global assessment of changes of kidney function deficiency based on clinician and caregiver in traditional Chinese medicine.The CGIC-KDS score ranges from 1 to 7, and the score of 1-3 indicates improvement, 4 means no changed, and 5-7 indicates worse.Abbreviations: CGIC-KDS, Clinical Global Impression of Change of Kidney deficiency;QGST, Qinggongshoutao;EGb761, *Ginkgo biloba* extract;LS, least squares.

3 Safety

All 348 patients in this study received at least one follow-up, and all were included in the safety analysis. A total of 87 (50%)patients in the QGST group had at least one AE during the double-blind period in the safety population, and 43 (41.35%)in the EGb761 group, 30 (42.86%)in the placebo group, with no significant differences among groups (P=0.315).The most reported AEs included upper respiratory tract infection, diarrhea, constipation, urinary tract infection, and increased blood glucose.The most frequent AEs assessed as probably related to the study medication were constipation in the QGST group (2 patients)and diarrhea in the EGb761 group, and the constipation led one patient in the QGST group to discontinue the trial.Two of 174 (1.1%)patients in the QGST group and four of 104 (3.8%)in the EGb761 group had at least one serious AE and were hospitalized during the trial.None of the serious AEs led to treatment discontinuation, and all were assessed as not related to the study medication by the investigator.No significant changes from baseline were observed in vital signs, physical examination findings, electrocardiography status, or laboratory values in all three treatment groups.

DISCUSSION

According to our previous study, insufficiency of the kidney Qi (flowing energy from kidney)is the characteristic in the early stage of dementia, stagnation of phlegm, blood stasis, and fiery are the characteristics in the middle stage, and excess of toxic heat is the characteristic in the late stage during the AD process.The therapeutic method is the nourishment of the kidney in the early stage, resolution of phlegm, blood stasis, and fiery in the middle stage, and detoxification in the late stage according to a full-course, sequential and disease-syndrome integrated treatment optimization protocol applicable to patients with AD[19]. QGST, an approved Chinese herbal drug by the China FDA, was developed from an ancient herbal prescription. The main effect of QGST pills is to nourish the kidney, and it is used to treat patients with MCI in China.

In recent years, biomarker research has made great progress in AD.However, limited progress has been made in the treatment of AD and several treatments for known pathological markers of AD have failed[20-22].Two different Ab antibodies (solanezumab and verubecestat)did not reduce cognitive or functional decline in patients with mild-to-moderate AD[23,24].As known, AD is a complex systemic disease with multiple etiologies and pathophysiology at different stage of disease[25].Herbal formulations may have advantages with multiple target regulation compared with the single target antagonist in the view of TCM[26].QGST is a compound containing multiple active components that may have an effect on multiple targets for AD.Studies have shown that QGST has ginseng-or ginsenosides-mediated neuroprotective mechanisms, including maintaining homeostasis, and antiinflammatory, antioxidant, antiapoptotic, and immune-stimulatory activities, and antiinflammatory seem contradictory;all of which may suggest a potential benefit in neurodegenerative disease, such as AD[27].Other components, such as *Angelica sinensis* and *Rehmannia glutinosa*, may also have potential neuroprotective effects and antiaging effects and reduce plasma lipid peroxide[28,29].These pharmacological findings support the clinical observation, i.e., prevent progression of AD and decline of cognition in the present study.

In this study, the rate of conversion to AD from aMCI in the placebo group was 10% at week 52 and this was consistent with a meta-analysis, which showed a cumulative dementia incidence of 14.9% in individuals with MCI older than 65 years and followed up for 2 years[7].The study finding on AD progression was also consistent with another study showing that a rate of progression from MCI to AD of 10 to 15 percent per year[5]. With the rate of ～1%, our results showed that QGST and EGb761 were effective in preventing or delaying the onset of AD in participants with aMCI.A meta-analysis has also shown that EGb761 at 240 mg/day was able to stabilize or slow the decline in cognition, function, behavior, and global change at 22-26 weeks in cognitive impairment and dementia, especially for patients with neuropsychiatric symptoms, consistent with the findings of our study[30].Another meta-analysis on effects of *Ginkgo biloba* in dementia showed that the standardized mean differences in change scores for cognition were obtained of ginkgo compared to placebo[31].However, other studies indicated an opposite conclusion on ginkgo, and it showed that long-term use of *Ginkgo biloba* extract did not reduce the risk of progression to AD compared with placebo[32].The different conclusions between different trials are possibly due to the heterogeneity of the study population.

In this study, the change in ADAS-cog scores from baseline was 2.76, 2.43, and 21.25, respectively, in QGST, EGb761, and placebo groups at the end point.Both QGST and EGb761 groups showed significant improvement after 52 weeks' treatment in global cognition and function.Compared with the placebo group, the QGST and EGb761 showed improvement in both ADAS-cog and MMSE scores from 24 weeks, and thereafter continue to improve.

At present, the cognition outcome has been suggested as a suitable and sole primary end point for the accelerated approval of a pharmaceutical treatment for MCI (FDA Draft Guidelines for Early-Stage AD)[33].In this trial, we used the ADAS-cog and MMSE as the efficacy measurements;how ever, the cognition tests used may result in unappreciated but artifactual gains because of practice effects, which means that the end point may be influenced by previous testing[34] and the practice effect may lead to false-positive findings.

QGST and EGb761 were safe and well tolerated.The frequencies of AEs in the QGST and EGb761 groups were similar to those of the placebo group.The most frequent AE assessed as probably related to the study medication in the QGST group was constipation.Because the ingredients of QGST contain honey, blood glucose was tested as a safety assessment in our study.The results showed that there was no significant difference in blood glucose after 52 weeks' treatment among the three groups.

There are some limitations in the study that should be noted.First, APOE ε 4 carrier increases the risk of aMCI to develop into AD dementia[35], but, in this study, the ApoE ε 4 carrier status was not detected in this study and we did not know whether there was a difference in the distribution of ApoE genotyping among the three groups.Second, for a preventive trial, the treatment duration and the sample size were not adequate to draw a conclusion on the longer-term (5 to 10 years)preventive effect or a disease-modifying effect.In conclusion, QGST and EGb761 may have effect on improvement of global cognition and lower the progression rate of AD in patients with aMCI.

REFERENCES

[1] Prince M, Bryce R, Albanese E, et al.The global prevalence of dementia: a systematic review and meta analysis[J].Alzheimers Dement, 2013, 9 (1): 63-75.

[2] Chan KY, Wang W, Wu JJ, et al.Epidemiology of Alzheimer's disease and other forms of dementia in China,1990-2010: a systematic review and analysis[J].Lancet, 2013, 381 (9882): 2016-23.

[3] Alzheimer's Association.Changing the trajectory of Alzheimer's disease: How a treatment by 2025 saves lives and dollars[OL].https: // www.alz.org/alzheimers_disease_trajectory.asp, 23 Jun, 2017.

[4] Petersen RC, Thomas RG, Grundman M, et al.Vitamin E and donepezil for the treatment of mild cognitive impairment[J].N Engl J Med, 2005, 352 (23): 2379-88.

[5] Petersen RC, Doody RS, Kurz A, et al.Current concepts in mild cognitive impairment[J].Arch Neurol, 2001, 58 (12): 1985-92.

[6] Petersen RC, Morris JC.Mild cognitive impairment as a clinical entity and treatment target[J].Arch Neurol, 2005, 62 (7): 1160-3.

[7] Petersen RC, Lopez O, Armstrong MJ, et al.Practice guideline update summary: Mild cognitive impairment: Report of the Guideline Development, Dissemination, and Implementation Subcommittee of the American Academy of Neurology[J].Neurology, 2018, 90 (3): 126-35.

[8] Dodge HH, Zitzelberger T, Oken BS, et al.A randomized placebo-controlled trial of Ginkgo biloba for the prevention of cognitive decline[J].Neurology, 2008, 70 (19pt2): 1809-17.

[9] DeKosky ST, Williamson JD, Fitzpatrick AL, et al.Ginkgo biloba for prevention of dementia: a randomized controlled trial[J].JAMA, 2008, 300 (19): 2253-62.

[10] Chen K, Zhou W, Li C, et al.Study on the anti-aging function of Qinggongshoutao pills[J].J Traditional Chin Med, 1985: 25-8.

[11] Shi J, Wei M, Tian J, et al.The Chinese version of story recall: a useful screening tool for mild cognitive impairment and Alzheimer's disease in the elderly[J].BMC Psychiatry, 2014, 14: 71.

[12] Folstein MF, Folstein SE, McHugh PR. 'Mini-mental state'.A practical method for grading the cognitive state of patients for the clinician[J].J Psychiatr Res, 1974, 12 (3): 189-98.

[13] Hughes CP, Berg L, Danziger W, et al.A new clinical scale for the staging of dementia[J].Br J Psychiatry, 1982, 140: 566-72.

[14] Galasko D, Bennett D, Sano M, et al.An Inventory to assess activities of daily living for clinical trials in Alzheimer's disease.The Alzheimer's disease cooperative study[J].Alzheimer Dis Assoc Disord, 1997, 11: S33-9.

[15] McKhann GM, Knopman DS, Chertkow H, et al.The diagnosis of dementia due to Alzheimer's disease: recommendations from the National Institute on Aging-Alzheimer's Association workgroups on diagnostic guidelines for Alzheimer's disease[J].Alzheimers Dement, 2011, 7 (3): 263-9.

[16] Shi J, Tian J, Long Z, et al.The pattern element scale: a brief tool of traditional medical subtyping for dementia[J].Evid Based Complement Alternat Med, 2013, 2013: 460562.

[17] Rosen WG, Mohs RC, Davis KL.A new rating scale for Alzheimer's disease[J].Am J Psychiatry , 1984, 141 (11): 1356-64.

[18] Shi J, Ni J, Wei M, et al.Association between pattern changes and cognitive outcome in Alzheimer's disease[J].J Beijing Univ Tradit Chin Med, 2017: 339-43.

[19] Joint Consensus Group (JCG)on TCM Diagnosis and Treatment of Alzheimer's Disease.Consensus on TCM diagnosis and treatment of Alzheimer's disease[J].Chin J Integr Tradit West Med, 2018, 3: 1-7.

[20] Doody RS, Thomas RG, Farlow M, et al.Phase 3 trials of solanezumab for mild-to-moderate Alzheimer's disease[J].N Engl J Med, 2014, 370 (4): 311-21.

[21] De Strooper B.Lessons from a failed g-secretase Alzheimer trial[J].Cell, 2014, 159: 721-6.

[22] Salloway S, Sperling R, Fox NC, et al.Two phase 3 trials of bapineuzumab in mild-to-moderate Alzheimer's disease[J].N Engl J Med, 2014, 370 (4): 322-33.

[23] Honig LS, Vellas B, Woodward M, et al.Trial of solanezumab for mild dementia due to Alzheimer's disease[J].N Engl J Med, 2018, 378 (4): 321-30.

[24] Egan MF, Kost J, Tariot PN, et al.Randomized trial of Verubecestat for mild-to-moderate Alzheimer's disease[J].N Engl J Med, 2018, 378 (18): 1691-703.

[25] Jack CR Jr, Knopman DS, Jagust WJ, et al.Tracking pathophysiological processes in Alzheimer's disease: an updated hypothetical model of dynamic biomarkers[J].Lancet Neurol, 2013, 12: 207-16.

[26] Tian J, Shi J, Zhang X, Wang Y.Herbal therapy: a new pathway for the treatment of Alzheimer's disease[J].Alzheimers Res Ther, 2010, 2 (5): 30.

[27] Cho I.Effects of Panax ginseng in neurodegenerative diseases[J].J Ginseng Res, 2012, 36 (4): 342-53.

[28] Zhang X, Zhang A, Jiang B, et al.Further pharmacological evidence of the neuroprotective effect of catalpol from Rehmannia glutinosa[J].Phytomedicine, 2008, 15 (6-7): 484-90.

[29] Zhou D, Li N, Zhang Y, Yan C, et al.Biotransformation of neuro-inflammation inhibitor kellerin using *Angelica sinensis* (Oliv.)Diels callus[J].RSC Adv, 2016, 6 (99): 97302-97312.

[30] Gavrilova SI, Preuss UW, Wong JW, et al.Efficacy and safety of Ginkgo biloba extract EGb 761 in mild cognitive impairment with neuropsychiatric symptoms: a randomized, placebo-controlled, double-blind, multi-center trial[J].Int J Geriatr Psychiatry, 2014, 29 (10): 1087-95.
[31] Weinmann S, Roll S, Schwarzbach C, et al.Effects of Ginkgo biloba in dementia: systematic review and meta-analysis[J].BMC Geriatr, 2010, 10: 14.
[32] Vellas B, Coley N, Ousset PJ, et al.Long-term use of standardised Ginkgo biloba extract for the prevention of Alzheimer's disease (GuidAge): a randomised placebo-controlled trial[J].Lancet Neurol, 2012, 11 (10): 851-9.
[33] Kozauer N, Katz R.Regulatory innovation and drug development for early-stage Alzheimer's disease[J].N Engl J Med, 2013, 368 (13): 1169-71.
[34] Goldberg TE, Harvey PD, Wesnes KA, et al.Practice effects due to serial cognitive assessment: implications for preclinical Alzheimer's disease randomized controlled trials[J].Alzheimers Dement (Amst), 2015, 1 (1): 103-11.
[35] Bertram L, McQueen MB, Mullin K, et al.Systematic meta-analyses of Alzheimer disease genetic association studies: the AlzGene database[J]. Nat Genet, 2007, 39 (1): 17-23.

First published: TIAN Jin-zhou, SHI Jing, WEI Ming-qing, NI Jing-nian, FANG Zhi-yong, GAO Jin-yu, WANG Heng, YAO Hong-jun, ZHANG Jin-tao, LI Jun-tao, MIN Min, SU Li-kai, SUN Xiu-qiao, WANG Bao-ai, WANG Bao-shen, YANG Fa-ming, ZOU Yong, HU Yue-qiang, LIN Ya-ming,XU Guang-yin, LI Kang, LI Lei, ZHEN Hui, XU Jin-yan, CHEN Ke-ji, WANG Yong-yan, on behalf of the CHARM study group.Chinese herbal medicine Qinggongshoutao for the treatment of amnestic mild cognitive impairment: A 52-week randomized controlled trial[J].Alzheimer's Dementia: Translational Research Clinical Interventions, 2019, (5): 441-449.

Effect of Kuanxiong Aerosol (宽胸气雾剂)on Patients with Angina Pectoris: A Non-inferiority Multi-center Randomized Controlled Trial

YANG Qiao-ning, BAI Rui-na, DONG Guo-ju, GE Chang-jiang, ZHOU Jing-min, HUANG Li, HE Yan, WANG Jun, REN Ai-hua, HUANG Zhan-quan, ZHU Guang-li, LU Shu, XIONG Shang-quan, XIAN Shao-xiang, ZHU Zhi-jun, SHI Da-zhuo, LU Shu-zheng, LI Li-zhi, and CHEN Ke-ji

Nitroglycerin preparations are widely used in clinics, and have consistently been recommended by domestic and international clinical guidelines for the treatment of angina pectoris caused by coronary heart disease (CHD). [1,2] However, nitroglycerin treatment can lead to drug tolerance, and has relatively strong vasodilative effects. As a result, nitroglycerin can lead to adverse reactions, such as headaches and hypotension. The advantages of treating angina using Chinese medicine (CM)are related to its syndrome differentiation and treatment, holistic regulation, focus on qi and blood relationship, and maintenance of the body's balance of yin and yang. However, CM dripping pill preparations that are commonly available on the market, such as Suxiao Jiuxin Pills (速效救心丸, a quick-acting drug with cardioprotective effects), have a relatively slow onset, and are unable to achieve a rapid therapeutic effect. Conversely, CM aerosols have several advantages, including rapid onset, portability, ease of use, and low toxicity. Hence, aerosols have become the preferred option for the treatment of cardiovascular emergencies.

The main treatments for angina in CM are Fangxiang Wentong (FXWT, aromatic herbs used to warm and unblock the meridian)and Xuanbi Tongyang (eliminates stagnation to activate yang). In the 1970s-1980s, 2 famous CM doctors from the China Academy of Chinese Medical Sciences, Prof. GUO Shi-kui and Academician CHEN Ke-ji, were presented with the Ministry of Health First-Grade Achievement Award for their work evaluating the clinical efficacy of Kuanxiong Aerosol (宽胸气雾剂, KA)in the treatment of angina. KA is a prescription based on the traditional principle of FXWT, and has been shown to have similar efficacy in alleviating angina to domestic nitroglycerin tablet (NT). [3-5] Subsequently, a number of clinical trials have followed, which showed that KA has valuable clinical applications in alleviating acute angina. [6-8]

Our research group has previously performed a multi-center, randomized, controlled trial (RCT)with domestic NT as control to evaluate the fast-acting effect and safety of KA. The results demonstrated that KA was not inferior to NT in rapidly relieving angina, and improving ischemic electrocardiogram (ECG) changes. Furthermore, KA had better tolerability than NT in clinical application. [9] Nevertheless, the study did not analyze the possible factors that could influence the effect of KA in the treatment of angina. Therefore, the present study employed unconditional logistic regression to further analyze the objective factors that could influence the remission rate of angina. In addition, subgroup analysis was performed to evaluate the therapeutic effect of KA for different Canadian Cardiovascular Society (CCS)classes of angina. [10]

METHODS

1 Diagnostic Criteria

1.1 Western Medicine Diagnostic Criteria

The Western medicine (WM)diagnostic criteria for stable and unstable angina were based on the "Guideline for Diagnosis and Treatment of Patients with Chronic Stable Angina" [1]and "Guideline for

Diagnosis and Treatment of Patients with Unstable Angina and Non-ST-segment Elevation Myocardial Infarction" [2]published in 2007.

1.2 CM Syndrome Differentiation Criteria

CM syndrome differentiation was referred to the "Guiding Principles for the Clinical Study of New Chinese Medicines". [11]

2 Inclusion Criteria

Patients were included if they met all the following criteria simultaneously: (1)WM diagnostic criteria and CM syndrome differentiation criteria [Xin (Heart)blood stasis syndrome or qi stagnation and blood stasis syndrome or cold-coagulation and blood-stasis syndrome]; (2)aged 30-75 years old; (3)signed the written informed consents voluntarily; (4)angina attack occurrence was at least 3 times per week before enrollment.

3 Exclusion Criteria

Patients were excluded if they met any of the following criteria: (1)pregnancy or breast-feeding women; (2)participating in other clinical subjects at the same time; (3)with alcohol allergy, nitrates prohibited and careful use; (4)with cognitive impairment, unable to cooperate; (5)with serious liver damage, kidney function or mental disorder; (6)with severe cardiopulmonary dysfunction and malignant arrhythmia.

4 Rejection Criteria

Patients were rejected if they (1)did not experience any angina attacks during the week after enrollment; (2)did not take their medication, or did not have test records.

5 Estimation of Sample Size

A statistical non-inferiority test was used to estimate the required sample size. The number of cases was based on a 1: 1 ratio of the test drug to the control. The following formula was used.

$$n=\frac{[\mu_{1-\frac{a}{2}}\sqrt{2P(1-P)}+\mu_{1-\beta}\sqrt{P_r(1-P_r)+P_c(1-P_c)}]^2}{[\triangle-(P_r-P_c)]^2}$$

Here, n is the sample size for each group, r denotes the KA group, and c the control group, P is the qualitative efficacy indicator (P= (Pr + Pc)/2), △ is the clinical non-inferiority value, and μ is the quantile of the standard normal distribution. It was assumed that α=0.025 (one-tailed test), β=0.20, and the non-inferiority standard is 8%. Based on a 5-min remission rate of 85% in the nitroglycerin and KA groups, and a dropout rate (including rejections)of 20%, the total number of cases required for both groups is 752 patients. In order to facilitate block randomization, the final number of cases selected was 780.

6 Grouping and Treatment

This study was registered in Chinese Clinical Trial Registry (registration No. ChiCTR-IPR-15007204). It was approved by the Xiyuan Hospital Ethics Committee (approval No. 2011XL030-2). SAS 9.2 statistical software was used to generate 780 random numbers, which were placed in sequentially-numbered, opaque sealed envelopes. The envelopes were randomly allocated among 13 centers, including Xiyuan Hospital of China Academy of Chinese Medical Sciences, Beijing Anzhen Hospital Affiliated to Capital Medical University, China-Japan Friendship Hospital of the Ministry of Health, Zhongshan Hospital Affiliated to Fudan University, Longhua Hospital Affiliated to Shanghai University of Traditional Chinese Medicine, Zhejiang Hospital of

Integrated Traditional Chinese and Western Medicine, Zhejiang Hospital, The First Affiliated Hospital of Zhejiang Chinese Medical University, Guangxing Hospital Affiliated to Zhejiang Chinese Medical University, Wuxi Hospital of Traditional Chinese Medicine Affiliated to Nanjing University of Chinese Medicine, The People's Hospital Affiliated to Fujian University of Traditional Chinese Medicine, The First Affiliated Hospital of Guangzhou Hospital of Chinese Medicine, and The 117th Hospital of People's Liberation Army. Each center recruited 60 cases. From November 2011 to December 2012, the eligible patients admitted to one of these 13 centers were enrolled in the study. The sealed envelopes were opened, and patients received the corresponding treatment.

All of the included patients received routine treatment according to the Chinese Society of Cardiology guidelines. [1,2] During each angina attack, the KA group received 3 sublingual sprays of KA (ingredients: Santalum oil, Piper longum oil, Asarum oil, Galangal oil, and Borneolum; 0.6 mL per spray; Nanyang Pharmaceutical Co., Ltd., China; batch No. Z20063477). The control group received 1 sublingual NT (0.5 mg/tablet; Beijing Yimin Pharmaceutical Co., Ltd., China; batch No. H11021022). The time taken for angina remission was then recorded. If the angina was not alleviated 5 min after drug administration, the patients in both groups were immediately administered 1 sublingual NT. The attending physician was informed, and the appropriate treatment was administered as recommended by the Chinese Society of Cardiology guidelines. [1,2]

Both groups were observed for 1 week. If only 1 angina attack occurred within that week, the experiment was discontinued at the end of the week. If the patient experienced more than 1 angina attack within the week, the experiment was discontinued after the second angina attack.

7 Observation and Recording of Time Taken for Angina Remission

All of the patients were equipped with a stopwatch of uniform specifications. Upon enrollment, they were given standardized instructions to calculate the time taken for angina remission. During angina attacks, measurement of the remission time began after drug administration. Patients who had 1 angina attack only recorded 1 remission time. Patients who had 2 angina attacks recorded the mean value of the 2 remission times. For patients who failed to measure the remission time using the stopwatch, a remission time was selected from 6 durations (1, 2, 3, 4, 5, or above 5 min)based on evaluation by the nursing staff or the patients themselves.

8 Primary Endpoint of Effect Evaluation for Angina Remission

Effect evaluation was performed based on the "Technique Guidelines for Chinese Medicine and Herb Clinical Research on Angina and Menonpausal Syndrome" released in 2011 by the China State Food and Drug Administration. [12] Markedly effective: angina disappeared or was essentially alleviated $\leqslant 3$ min after drug administration. Effective: angina disappeared or was essentially alleviated within 3–5 min (exclusive of 3 min) after drug administration. Not effective: angina was only slightly alleviated or did not improve >5 min after drug administration. Worsened: angina worsened after drug administration. Subgroup analysis was performed according to CCS classes of angina. [10] Safety analysis was also performed in subgroups.

9 Statistical Analyses

Statistical data was processed by the Good Clinical Practice Center of Xiyuan Hospital of China Academy of Chinese Medical Sciences, a third party that was not involved in this study. SAS 9.2 was used to perform the statistical analysis. Measurement data were analyzed using t-test and rank-sum test. Count data were analyzed using log-rank test, Kaplan-Meier estimation, χ^2-test, and Fisher's exact test. Logistic regression analysis was used to identify the factors influencing the rate of angina remission. $P < 0.05$ indicated a statistically significant difference.

RESULTS

1 Comparison of Baseline Data between Two Groups

Although 780 angina patients were included in the study, 16 were rejected as angina did not occur after enrollment, and 14 were rejected owing to incomplete data (unclear or unrecorded angina remission time). Thus, 750 patients completed the study (376 cases in the KA group, and 374 in the control group, Figure 1). There were no statistically significant differences in gender, age, height, weight, heart rate, blood pressure, complicating diseases, concurrent medications, disease duration of angina, type of angina, classification of angina, or distribution of CM syndrome between the KA and control groups ($P>0.05$, Table 1). The main type of angina included in both groups was unstable angina, the mean disease duration was about 4 years, and the angina class was predominantly CCS Ⅱ. The main CM syndromes were Xin blood stasis as well as qi stagnation and blood stasis.

2 Comparison of 3-min and 5-min Remission Rates

The 3-min angina remission rate for the KA group was 53.72% (202/376), and 47.86% (179/374)for the control group. The 5-min angina remission rate for the KA group was 94.41% (355/376), and 90.64% (339/374) for the control group. No significant difference was observed in 3-and 5-min reminssion rates between the two groups ($P>0.05$). A log-rank test and Kaplan-Meier estimation were performed to compare the angina remission rate at each time point (1, 2, 3, 4, 5, and>5 min)between the two groups (Figure 2). No significant difference was observed in the remission rates at each time point between the two groups (P=0.06).

Table 1　Comparison of Baseline Data between KA and Control Groups

Characteristic	KA group	Control group
Male (Case)	216	208
Age (Year, $\bar{x}\pm s$)	64.01 ± 9.10	64.13 ± 8.65
Height (cm, $\bar{x}\pm s$)	166.29 ± 7.50	165.81 ± 7.45
Weight (kg, $\bar{x}\pm s$)	66.72 ± 9.61	66.71 ± 10.03
Disease duration of angina (Year, $\bar{x}\pm s$)	4.32 ± 5.29	4.15 ± 4.67
Heart rate (Beat/min, $\bar{x}\pm s$)	71.47 ± 11.06	70.81 ± 9.67
Blood pressure (mm Hg, $\bar{x}\pm s$)		
Systolic blood pressure	131.62 ± 17.38	132.49 ± 16.39
Diastolic blood pressure	76.08 ± 10.57	76.85 ± 10.39
Complicating disease (Case)		
Hypertension	290	297
Diabetes	134	128
Dyslipidemia	54	72
Cerebral stroke	43	38
Type of angina (Case)		
Unstable angina	242	229
Stable angina	134	145
CCS classification of angina (Case)		
Ⅰ	52	42
Ⅱ	226	225
Ⅲ	79	91
Ⅳ	19	16

Continued

Characteristic	KA group	Control group
Distribution of CM syndrome (Case)		
Xin blood stasis	245	240
Qi stagnation and blood stasis	108	103
Cold-coagulation and blood-stasis	23	31
Concurrent medications (Case)		
Aspirin	369	352
Clopidogrel	25	29
Statins	342	321
Fibrates	17	19
Nicotinic acids	7	5
β-Blockers	243	231
Calcium channel blockers	115	129
Angiotensin Ⅱ receptor blockers	143	148
Angiotensin-converting enzyme inhibitors	92	115
Diuretics	50	38

3 Correlation Analysis of Therapeutic Efficacy

Age, gender, height, weight, disease duration, complicating diseases, concurrent medications, type of angina, class of angina, CM syndrome, heart rate, blood pressure, and group were included in the logistic regression equation. The CCS class of angina was related to the angina remission rate, and the difference was statistically significant ($P < 0.01$, Table 2).

Table 2 Logistic Regression Analysis for Factors Influencing Angina Remission Rate

Influencing factor	Odds ratio	95% CI	*P* value
Group	0.778	0.585–1.034	0.083
Gender	0.865	0.647–1.156	0.327
Age	0.989	0.973–1.005	0.192
Height	1.014	0.987–1.041	0.305
Weight	0.449	0.252–1.798	0.064
Heart rate	0.490	0.354–1.679	0.094
Blood pressure	1.048	0.605–1.815	0.867
Type of angina	0.603	0.447–1.812	0.091
Class of angina	0.598	0.483–0.740	< 0.001
Disease duration of angina	1.004	0.973–1.036	0.805
CM syndrome type	1.023	0.775–1.350	0.873
Complicating diseases	0.817	0.502–1.330	0.417
Concurrent medication	1.207	0.731–1.991	0.462

Notes: CI: confidence interval.

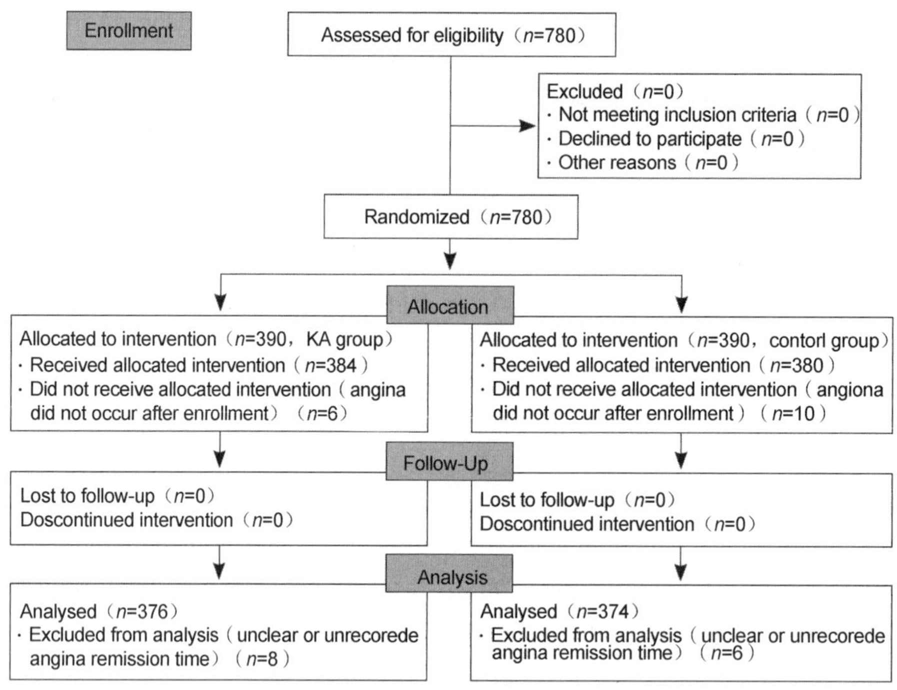

Figure 1　Flow Diagram for Study of KA on Angina Patients

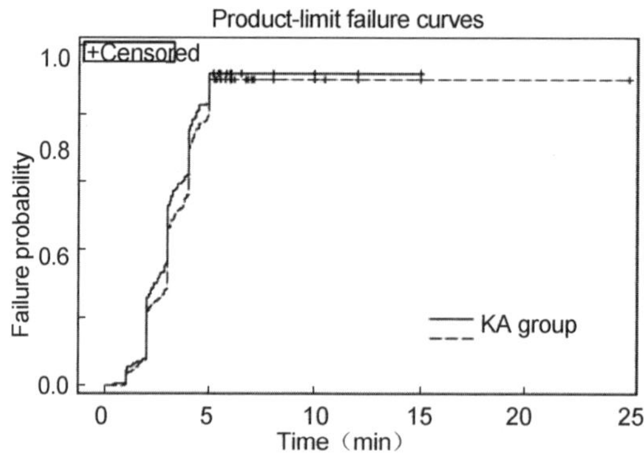

Figure 2　Kaplan-Meier Estimations of Remission Rate for Each Time Point

4 Subgroup Analysis of Angina CCS Class

As the CCS class had a significant influence on the rate of remission, a subgroup analysis was performed to compare the 3-and 5-min remission rates in the KA and control groups, within the CCS subgroups (Table 3). In the CCS Ⅰ and Ⅳ subgroups, the 3-and 5-min remission rates were not statistically significant between KA and control groups ($P>0.05$). In contrast, the differences of 3-and 5-min remission rates between KA and control groups were statistically significant in the CCS Ⅱ and Ⅲ subgroups ($P<0.05$ or $P<0.01$).

Table 3　Comparison of 3–and 5–min Angina Remission Rates between KA and Control Groups within Each CCS Subgroup [Case (%)]

Group	CCS class	case	Angina remission rate	
			with 3 min	with 5 min
KA	Ⅰ	52	36 (69.23)	49 (94.23)
	Ⅱ	226	124 (54.87)**	219 (96.90)**
	Ⅲ	79	37 (46.84)*	73 (92.41)**
	Ⅳ	19	5 (26.32)	14 (73.68)

Continued

Group	CCS class	case	Angina remission rate	
			with 3 min	with 5 min
Control	Ⅰ	42	28 (66.67)	41 (97.62)
	Ⅱ	225	112 (49.78)	212 (94.22)
	Ⅲ	91	35 (38.46)	76 (83.52)
	Ⅳ	16	4 (25)	10 (62.50)

Notes: $^{*}P < 0.05$, $^{**}P < 0.01$ vs. control group.

5 Safety Analysis of Angina CCS Class Subgroups

In the present study, adverse reactions were observed among the different CCS subgroups (Table 4). In the CCS Ⅰ and Ⅳ subgroups, there was no significant difference between KA and control groups ($P > 0.05$), while the differences in CCS Ⅱ and Ⅲ subgroups were statistically significant ($P < 0.05$ or $P < 0.01$).

Table 4 Comparison of Safety Analysis between KA and Control Groups within Different CCS Subgroups [Case (%)]

Group	CCS class	Case	Adverse reaction
KA	Ⅰ	52	0
	Ⅱ	226	21 (9.29)**
	Ⅲ	79	8 (10.13)*
	Ⅳ	19	6 (31.58)
Control	Ⅰ	42	0
	Ⅱ	225	59 (26.22)
	Ⅲ	91	19 (20.88)
	Ⅳ	16	6 (37.50)

Notes: $P < 0.05$, $^{**}P < 0.01$ vs. control group.

DISCUSSION

In this study, patients were enrolled based on the modern diagnostic criteria for CHD. We performed a prospective, multi-center RCT, which included the participations of 13 AAA hospitals (which are the highest hospitals in China)of CM, WM and integrative medicine.

The present study built on our previous work, by applying log-rank test, and Kaplan-Meier estimation to demonstrate that there were no significant differences in the angina remission rates for each time point between KA and control groups. Furthermore, logistic regression analysis was performed to examine the factors influencing the therapeutic effect of angina treatments. It was showed that CCS class of angina had a significant impact on the angina remission rate. Subsequently, a subgroup analysis based on CCS class was performed to analyze the therapeutic effect and safety of KA for treating different CCS classes. These results showed that in the CCS Ⅰ and Ⅳ subgroups, there was no significant difference in the 3-and 5-min remission rates between KA and control groups, indicating that KA was not inferior to NT in rapidly alleviating angina. In the CCS Ⅱ and Ⅲ subgroups, the 3-and 5-min remission rates were significantly better in the KA group than in the control group, indicating that KA was superior to NT.

The KA prescription originated from the Kulai Xiaoqu Powder (哭来笑去散)in Ancient and Modern Medical Guide (Gu Jin Yi Jian). Academician CHEN Ke-ji and Prof. GUO Shi-kui modified the dosage form and absorption pathway of the prescription by applying modern pharmacology and pharmaceutical technology. Among the compositions in KA, Santalum is used to regulate qi and relieve pain, [13] which is often combined with Salvia to treat blood stasis and cardiac pain. Asarum and Galangal are used to warm the Middle-jiao, dispel cold, and circulate qi. Modern study has shown that Santalum contains up to 10% volatile oils, so its aroma can permeate the body. [14]Asarum is an aromatic Chinese medicine, and the main volatile oils found in Asarum are methyl eugenol, and asarone, which have vasodilating and cardioprotective effects. [15]Galangal can rapidly open the orifices, and has analgesic effects. Borneolum is bitter, and slightly cold. The bitterness will permeate the body, and the coolness will dispel stagnation. Borneolum can also unblock the orifices, and increase mental alertness.

Previous animal experiment has shown that Kuanxin Zhitong Plaster (prescriptions were the same as KA) was able to improve microcirculation, and increase blood flow in animals. [16] KA can also effectively reduce the endothelin-1 level in the blood of angina patients, and increase the nitric oxide (NO)content and cyclic guanosine monophosphate (cGMP)levels. Hence, its mechanism of action in relieving angina attacks might be related to the NO-cGMP pathway. [17] Due to the rapid action of KA, it is the recommended drug in the CM treatment of acute angina attacks.

The severity of an angina attack is related to the degree of vascular occlusion, which reflects the coronary flow reserve. Therefore, CCS angina classification has been widely applied in the clinical evaluation of angina patients, to help guide clinical treatment, and to predict the patient prognosis.

The results of safety analysis showed that the tolerability of KA was also similar to that of NT in the CCS Ⅰ and Ⅳ subgroups. However, in the CCS Ⅱ and Ⅲ subgroups, significantly fewer patients reported adverse reactions in the KA group than in the control group, indicating that KA has higher tolerability than NT in these subgroups.

In conclusion, this study has demonstrated that KA can rapidly relieve angina pectoris. In particular, KA has superior effect, and better tolerability than NT among CCS Ⅱ and Ⅲ patients. Thus, KA will be especially useful in treating patients with these particular types of angina. The main limitation of our study is that it was not possible to implement a double-blinded design. However, our results are still credible, and can serve as a basis for using evidence-based medicine to improve the effect and safety of CM aerosols in treating angina pectoris.

REFERENCES

[1] Chinese Society of Cardiology of Chinese Medical Association. Guideline for diagnosis and treatment of patients with chronic stable angina[J]. Chin J Cardiol (Chin), 2007, 35 (3): 195-206.

[2] Chinese Society of Cardiology of Chinese Medical Association. Guideline for diagnosis and treatment of patients with unstable angina and non-ST-segment elevation myocardial infarction[J]. Chin J Cardiol (Chin), 2007, 35 (4): 295-304.

[3] Cardiovascular Disease Study Group, Xiyuan Hospital of China Academy of Chinese Medical Sciences. Observation of pain relief by Kuanxiong Aerosol in acute angina attacks[J]. J Tradit Chin Med (Chin), 1973, 23 (10): 14-16.

[4] Cardiovascular Research Laboratory and Pharmacology Group, Xiyuan Hospital of China Academy of Chinese Medical Sciences. Observations on the immediate effects of Kuanxiong Aerosol on angina attacks[J]. Chin J Integr Tradit West Med (Chin), 1981, 1 (9): 18-61.

[5] Guo SK, Chen KJ, Weng WL, et al. Immediate effect of Kuanxiong Aerosol in the treatment of angina attacks[J]. Planta Med, 1983, 47 (2): 116.

[6] Li L, Li CY, Gu H, Mao JS, Shao MJ, Li YJ, Huang L. Clinical observation of Kuanxiong Aerosol in the treatment of coronary heart disease angina[J]. Inf Tradit Chin Med (Chin), 2014, 31 (3): 131-133.

[7] Dai J, Ge CJ, Tian JF, et al. Clinical observation of Kuanxiong Aerosol in the treatment of angina[J]. Inf Tradit Chin Med (Chin), 2014, 31 (4): 135-136.

[8] Fang JY, Wang Z. Clinical observations of Kuanxiong Aerosol in the improvement of electrocardiogram changes in acute angina in patients with coronary heart disease[J]. Chin J Integr Med Cardio Cerebrovasc Dis (Chin), 2015, 13 (2): 223-224.

[9] Li LZ, Dong GJ, Ge CJ, et al. Effect of Kuanxiong Aerosol on coronary heart disease angina patients: a multicenter randomized controlled clinical study[J]. Chin J Integr Tradit West Med (Chin), 2014, 34 (4): 396-401.

[10] Campeau L. The Canadian Cardiovascular Society grading of angina pectoris revisited 30 years later[J]. Can J Cardiol, 2002, 18 (4): 371-379.

[11] Zheng XY, ed. Guiding principles for the clinical study of new Chinese medicines[M]. Beijing: Chinese Medical Science Press; 2002: 69-70.

[12] China State Food and Drug Administration. Technique guidelines for Chinese medicine and herb clinical research on angina and menonpausal syndrome. Available at http: // www. sfda. gov. cn/WS01/CL1036/64117. html.

[13] Liu LT, Chen KJ. Ancient and modern application of aromatic herbs for activating yang in preventing and treating coronary heart disease angina[J]. Chin J Integr Tradit West Med (Chin), 2013, 33 (8): 1013-1017.

[14] Chen XY, Gao Y, Li WM. CS-MS analysis of the chemical composition of commercial sandalwood volatile oils[J]. J Chin Med Mater (Chin), 2012, 35 (3): 418-421.

[15] Cheng L. Identification and pharmacological effects of Asarum[J]. Strait Pharm J (Chin), 2008, 20 (5): 68-70.

[16] Liu JG, Cui J, Liu ZQ. Effect of Kuanxin Zhitong Plaster on experimental microcirculatory disorders[J]. Chin J Microcirc (Chin), 1995, 5 (2): 43-44.

[17] Wang BJ, Dong GJ, Liu JG, et al. The relieving effects of Kuanxiong Aerosol on angina pectoris and its influences on endothelial function index in patients with coronary heart disease[J]. J Emerg Tradit Chin Med (Chin), 2015, 24 (12): 2175-2178.

First published: YANG Qiao-Ning, BAI Rui-Na, DONG Guo-Ju, GE Chang-jiang, ZHOU Jing-min, HUANG Li, HE Yan, WANG Jun, REN Ai-hua, HUANG Zhan-quan, ZHU Guang-li, LU Shu, XIONG Shang-quan, XIAN Shao-xiang, ZHU Zhi-jun, SHI Da-zhuo, LU Shu-zheng, LI Li-zhi, CHEN Ke-ji. Effect of Kuanxiong Aerosol on patients with angina pectoris: A non-inferiority multi-center randomized controlled trial[J] . Chin J Integr Med, 2018, 24 (5): 336-342.

Sodium Tanshinone IIA Aulfonate for Coronary Heart Disease: A Systematic Review of Randomized Controlled Trials

YU Mei-li, LI Si-ming, GAO Xiang, LI Jin-gen, XU Hao, and CHEN Ke-ji

Cardiovascular diseases (CVDs)are the primary cause of mortality worldwide causing 17.3 million deaths per year, and the number is estimation to reach 23.6 million in 2030, making it a critical issue for the public health system. [1,2] Coronary heart disease (CHD)is the major contributor of CVDs, which is caused by atherosclerosis, a chronic inflammatory condition of the arterial wall. [3] Though development and wide use of percutaneous coronary intervention (PCI)and optimal secondary prevention medicines have greatly reduced the incidence of adverse cardiovascular events in CHD, the residual cardiovascular risk remains high. In the FOURIER trial, [4] the four-year cardiovascular event rate in patients with atherosclerotic cardiovascular disease remained 9.8%, though the addition of evolocumab, a monoclonal antibody that inhibits proprotein convertase subtilisin-kexintype 9 (PCSK9)to the standard therapies lowered low-density lipoprotein (LDL)cholesterol levels to 0.78 mmol per liter. Therefore, how to further reduce the residual cardiovascular risk in CHD remains an urgent and critical issue. Traditional Chinese Medicine (TCM)is one of the world's most ancient medical systems and has a history of thousands of years. In recent years, several multi-center randomized clinical trials have been conducted and provided more and more evidence for the benefit of TCM in the treatment pf CHD. [5-7] *Salvia miltiorrhiza* Bunge (Danshen)has been widely used in clinical practice for more than two thousand years, with TCM property of promoting blood circulation and removing blood-stasis. Since the 1930s, Salvia's chemical composition and biological activity has been extensively studied. [8] More than 30 fat-soluble ingredients and 30 water-soluble ingredients were identified and isolated from Salvia. Tanshinone IIA is a member of the major lipophilic components extracted from the root of Salvia, which is currently used in China to treat patients suffering from CHD, ischemic stroke, etc. However, Tan IIA is not easy to be absorbed through intestinal pathway. Therefore, sodium tanshinone IIA sulfonate (STS)was developed to raise the bioavailability of the herb. In recent years, STS has indicated significant therapeutic effects and multiple pharmacological actions including vasodilative, antithrombotic, anti-inflammation, antioxidant, antiischemia, antiatherosclerosis, and lipid-lowering effect and appears to be a promising natural cardioprotective agent. [9,10]

However, there is no systematic review so far assessed effect of STS on clinical outcomes in patients with confirmed CHD treated with STS. Thus, we conducted this systematic review to evaluate the efficacy and safety of STS IIA for CHD patients.

METHODS

1 Inclusion Criteria

Randomized controlled trials (RCTs)which compared STS with placebo or no treatment with available standard therapies as basic treatment for patients with CHD were eligible for this review. Same standard therapies should be applied in both the TS and control group in each trial, and the standard therapies may be different due to different disease conditions. Patients should be clearly diagnosed with CHD, confirmed by coronary angiography showing coronary artery stenosis ≥50% or by previous myocardial infarction. No restriction was set on age, gender, race, and treatment period. Studies that included other TCM as co-intervention or as control were excluded.

The primary outcome was all-cause mortality. The secondary outcomes included major adverse cardiac events (MACE), defined as non-fatal myocardial infarction (MI), stroke, target vessel revascularization (TVR), in-stent restenosis or new lesions (without revascularization), angina pectoris episodes, duration of angina pectoris; Cardiac function evaluation, including left ventricular end-diastolic diameter (LVEDD), left ventricular ejection fraction (LVEF)and interventricular septum thickness (IVST), quality of life measured by Seattle angina questionnaire (SAQ)or 36-item short form health survey (SF-36), inflammatory factor (including C-reactive protein (CRP), interleukin-6 (IL-6), etc.), adverse events (ADEs)or adverse reactions (ADRs).

2 Searching Strategy

A comprehensive search was conducted in 2 English databases and 4 Chinese databases, including PubMed, the Cochrane Library, Chinese National Knowledge Infrastructure Databases (CNKI), Chinese Biomedical Literature Database (SinoMed), Chinese Science and Technology Periodical Database (VIP) and Wanfang Database, from inception of each database to August 2017. No language was restricted. The searching terms including: "coronary disease" "coronary artery disease" "myocardial infarction" "angina" "acute coronary syndrome" and "Tanshinone Ⅱ" "Dan Shen Ketone" "sulfotanshinone" "danshen" . Speciflc search terms and strategies were adopted for different databases.

3 Study Selection and Data Extraction

Two authors (YML and GX)independently selected the eligible studies and extract data. Full text of the articles that might be eligible after screening the titles and abstracts of the achieved citations was downloaded for further evaluation. YML and GX independently extracted data from each included trial, including characteristics, intervention/control details, clinical outcomes, etc. Disagreements between the two authors were resolved by discussion and if needed, arbitrated by a third author (XH).

4 Quality Assessment

Two authors (YML and LSM)independently assessed the methodological quality of included trials. Methodological quality of RCTs was assessed according to the risk of bias tool described in the Cochrane handbook for systematic reviews of interventions. [11] Seven elements were assessed: random sequence generation, allocation concealment, blinding of participants and personnel, blinding of outcome assessment, incomplete outcome data, selective reporting and other bias.

5 Data Analysis

All statistical analysis was performed using RevMan 5.3 software. Pooled results were presented as risk ratio (RR)with its 95% confidence interval (CI)for binary outcomes or mean difference (MD)with 95% (CI)for continuous outcomes. Statistical heterogeneity among included trials was evaluated by I^2 test. Meta-analysis was conducted, when there is no significant clinical and statistical heterogeneity ($I^2 < 75\%$)among included trials. If I^2 value is less than 25%, we used fixed effect model to pool the data. If I^2 value is between 25%-75% , we need to estimate the source of heterogeneity. If we can reduce the statistical heterogeneity ($I^2 < 25\%$)by sensitive analysis or subgroup analysis, we also used fixed effect model to pool the data. Otherwise, random effects model would be used in meta-analysis. Pooling analysis would not be conducted if there is significant statistical heterogeneity ($I^2 > 75\%$). Funnel plots was used to explore the possibility of small study effects or publication bias, if there are ten or more studies in an analysis.

RESULTS

1 Searching Results

After a primary search of 2 English databases and 4 Chinese databases, we got 1684 citations. Full-text articles of 277 trials were read, and finally, 22 RCTs were included in the review. Details of the study flow were showed in Figure 1.

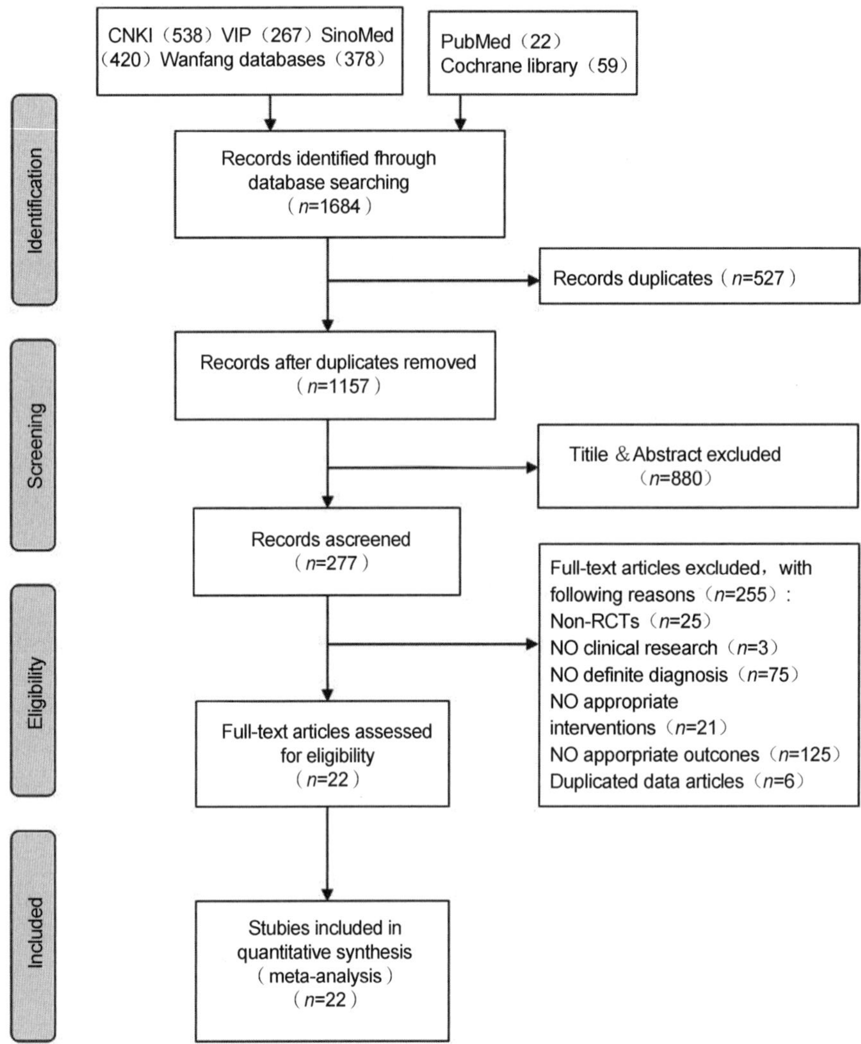

Figure 1 Flow Chart of Study Search and Selection

2 Overview on Included Studies

All of the 22 trials were parallel randomized controlled trials (RCTs)published in Chinese and conducted in China involved, and a total of 1873 participant (with 939 participants in the intervention group and 934 participants in the control group)were involved. There was a wide variation in the age of subjects (35-82 years).

In STS intervention group, besides standard therapies, 40-400 mg STS dissolved in 250 mL 0.9% sodium chloride solution or 5% glucose solution was given by intravenous drop once daily. The treatment period was between 5 days to 2 months. standard therapies varied across included trials, including TT plus conventional therapies, [12,13,16,21,30-32] PCI plus conventional therapies, [12,15,23] conventional therapies alone. [14,17-20,22,24-29,33] Among them, one trial adopted both PCI and TT[12]. The conventional therapies included standard medical treatment, psychotherapy and supportive care. The total treatment duration ranged from 7-60 days.

All-cause death as primary outcome was reported by seven trials[12,15-17,24,25,32] included in this review. Six trials [13,16,21,30-32] reported the rate of cardiac shock and heart failure. Eight trials [13,16,21,22,25,30-32] reported arrhythmia and four trials[15,16,25,32] reported vascular revascularization rate. Only one trial [25] reported rehospitalization; fourteen trials [13-15,17,20,21,23,25-29,31,33] reported inflammatory factors including CRP, IL-6, TNF-a; 5 trials [13,21,24,30,31] reported Cardiac function evaluation. One trial reported Quality of life assessed by SAQ. [15] Seven trials [15-17,20,24,27,32] mentioned the adverse events. Characteristics of the 22 included trials were listed in Appendix 1.

3 Methodology Quality Assessment

According to our predefined quality assessment criteria, all of the included trials had low methodological quality.

Only six of including trials [13,15,20,21,27,30] described the generating random sequence by random number table. No included trials described methods of allocation concealment. Only one trial[19] which used blinding was assessed as low risk of performance bias. Three trials [20,21,27] using a third party to evaluate the outcome data were assessed as low risk of detection bias. All trials reported no patents was lost to follow-up, and were assessed as low risk of attrition bias. Protocol of all included trials could not be found, but we assessed them as having low risk of reporting bias, since they all reported the important outcome measurements for CHD, which is consistent with what they described in methods section of the report. Nine trials [13,16,19,20,22,25,30-32] were assessed as low risk of other bias due to the favorable baseline comparability, adequate follow-up and compliance analysis. However, four trials [12,19,23,33] not described the details of above items, we evaluated them as having a high risk of other bias. Risk of bias graph of 22 included studies were showed in Figure 2.

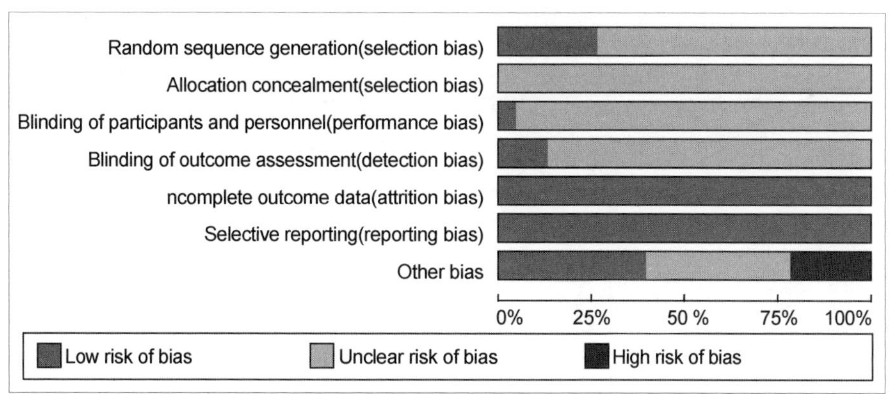

Figure 2 Risk of Bias Graph of 22 Included Studies

4 Effects of STS on All Cause Death Rate

Seven of included trials reported the all cause death rate as primary outcome and three trials [15,17,25] reported no death occurred. The rest of other four trials[12,16,24,33] reported that STS as an adjunctive therapy of conventional therapies could reduced the mortality rate by 42% (RR 0.41, 95% CI 0.18 to 0.98, *P*=0.04, I^2=0%, 242 participants, 4 trials)than conventional therapies alone.

We according the difference of intervening control measures and divided them into three subgroups as bellow. Pooled results of 3 trials[12,16,33] comparing STS with TT showed that compared with TT, STS significantly reduced all cause death rate by 25% (RR 0.25, 95% CI 0.07 to 0.87, *P*=0.03, I^2=0%, 200 participants). In the subgroup of PCI plus conventional treatment, one trial showed that STS combined with PCI reduced the mortality rate by 42% (RR 0.42, 95% CI 0.04 to 4.36)than PCI alone. One trial [24] compared STS plus conventional therapies with conventional therapies alone showed no difference between two group

(RR 1.05, 95% CI 0.20 to 5.47). The details showed in Appendix 2.

5 Effects of STS on MACE

The results of six trials[13,16,21,30-32] compared STS plus TT with TT alone showed the additional of STS to TT generated a significant reduction of cardiac shock (RR 0.35, 95%CI 0.14 to 0.86, I^2=0, P=0.02), heart failure (RR 0.41, 95% CI 0.20 to 0.83, I^2=0, P=0.01)and arrhythmia (RR 0.24, 95% CI 0.12 to 0.46, I^2=0, $P<0.0001$) (Appendix 3).

One trial[25] compared STS plus conventional therapies with conventional therapies showed significantly reduced rehospitalization (RR 0.47, 95% CI 0.23 to 0.96, 120 participants)and revascularization (RR 0.63, 95% CI 0.22 to 1.80)in the STS plus conventional therapies group. However, two trials[22,24] comparing STS plus conventional therapies with conventional therapies showed no difference on arrhythmia incidence (RR 0.98, 95% CI 0.78 to 1.25, P=0.9 123 participants)between the two groups. Another trial[15] comparing STS plus PCI with PCI showed a better effect on revascularization (RR 0.33, 95% CI 0.04 to 3.03, P=0.33 60 participants)in the STS plus PCI group.

6 Effects of STS on Cardiac Function Evaluation

Within five trials reported cardiac function evaluation, four of them[13,21,30,31] compared STS plus TT with TT showed a superior effect of STS as add-on therapy for LVEDD (MD -5.26, 95%CI -6.89 to -3.62, I^2=45%, $P<$ 0.00001, 371 participants)and IVST (MD-3.57, 95%CI -4.12 to -3.02, I^2=10%, $P<0.00001$).

However, the remaining one trial[24] showed combination of STS and conventional therapies was no better than conventional therapies alone regarding LVEF (MD 4.76, 95%CI 2.56 to 6.96, $P<0.0001$, 94 participants) and LVEDD (MD -2.16, 95%CI -4.70 to 0.38, P=0.1, 94 participants).

7 Effects of STS on Inflammatory Factor

Three trials[13,21,31] STS plus TT versus TT showed a superior effect of STS on the level CRP (MD -0.63, 95% CI -0.87 to -0.39, I^2=59%, $P<0.00001$)and TNF-a (MD -0.72, 95%CI -0.80 to -0.63, I^2=68%, $P<0.00001$) (Appendix 4).

One trial[15] compared STS plus PCI with PCI showed that additional of STS reduced the CRP levels by -0.70 mg/l (MD -0.70, 95%CI -1.10 to -0.30, I^2=68%, $P<0.0006$), the IL-6 by 0.19 pg/ml (MD -0.19, 95%CI -0.38 to 0.00)and the TNF-α pg/ml by 2.88 (MD -2.88, 95%CI -4.31 to -1.45, $P<0.00001$).

The results of other trials[14,17,20,25-29,33] compared STS as an adjunctive therapy of conventional therapies not pooled for the high heterogeneity, but each trial showed a better effect on CRP and IL-6 (Appendix 5).

8 Sensitivity Analysis

As there was high heterogeneity on the outcome of CRP in comparison of STS plus conventional therapies with conventional therapies, we did not conduct meta-analysis. For the outcome of IL-6, when removed two trials, [29,33] STS plus conventional therapies showed a better effect than conventional therapies alone (MD -3.59, 95%CI -4.46 to -2.71, I^2=39%, $P<0.00001$, 251 participants, 3 trials[17,20,28] Considering substantial heterogeneity on the outcome of TNF-α in the comparison of STS plus conventional therapies with conventional therapies, we did sensitivity analysis to analyze the source of heterogeneity and found that when two trials[17,29] were removed, the substantial heterogeneity decreased. And then, pooled results of the remaining three trials[14,20,33] showed that STS as an add-on treatment further decreased TNF-a level about 1.38 pg/ml (MD -1.38, 95%CI -1.65 to -1.10, I^2=34%, $P<0.00001$, 271 participants).

9 Safety

Seven of twenty-two included trials reported on adverse reactions. Two trials[16,32] showed STS plus TT reduce the adverse reactions (RR 0.23 95%CI 0.07 to 0.80, I^2=0%, P=0.02, 149 participants)than TT therapy alone. Adverse reactions included headache, dizziness, gastrointestinal reaction, and so on. Three trials[15,20,24] showed no significant difference about adverse reactions between the STS plus PCI or conventional therapies with PCI or conventional therapies alone. The remaining two trials[17,27] reported no adverse reactions were observed in two groups.

10 Publication Bias

As no pooled outcomes included more than ten trials, it is inappropriate to analyze publication bias by funnel plots. Therefore, this potential bias was not evaluated.

DISCUSSION

Our meta-analysis involved 22 articles with 1873 individuals. Pooled results showed combination of STS and conventional medicine treatment (TT or PCI)may have better effect on all cause death (RR 0.25/0.42), cardiac function (LVEDD average changed 2-5 mm between groups)and inflammatory factor (CRP average changed less than 1 between groups)than conventional medicine treatment alone in patients with CHD. However, the evidence was inconclusive due to poor methodological quality of the included trials and the insufficient number of trial participants. As safety of STS was rarely reported in the included trials, no firm conclusion could be drawn on this outcome.

Two similar systematic reviews and meta-analysis[34,35] were conducted in patients with unstable angina, which focused primarily on surrogate outcomes such as curative effects (mainly clinical symptoms), electrocardiogram improvement and failed to assess the more important clinical outcomes such as all cause death rate and MACEs. Another review [36] assessed effects of STS on unstable angina (UA). Similarly, the primary outcome of that review is the surrogate outcome (clinically curative effects). Thus, our review was the first systematic review that assessed effects of STS on all cause death and MACEs, which implied potential benefits on these hard outcomes.

The pharmacological and clinical effects of STS has been extensively studied. It is demonstrated that STS has diverse pharmacological effects such as antioxidant, antibacterial, anti-inflammatory, and neuroprotective effects, and it has been widely used to treat cardiovascular disease. [37,38] Among all of these effects, the anti-inflammatory effects arouse great interests. Recently, results of CANTOS trial[39] showed that anti-inflammatory therapy with canakinumab could further reduce incidence of major adverse cardiovascular events in patients with history of myocardial infarction, and reductions in the inflammatory biomarker hsCRP correlate with clinical benefits for individual patients. [39] CANTOS trial validates the inflammatory pathogenesis of atherosclerosis and usher in a new era of anti-inflammatory therapies for atherosclerosis. [40] However, potential increased fatal infection and high cost limit the clinical application of canakinumab, which call for a safer and cost-effective natural anti-inflammatory agent. Robertson et al. conducted a large-scale screening of anti-inflammatory compounds using zebrafish as an animal model and identified tanshinone IIA as one of the most potent anti-inflammatory agents among thousands of compounds screened. [41] Recently, our study demonstrates that on the basis of standard medical therapy, STS further reduce elevated hs-CRP and other circulating inflammation markers in CHD patients. [20] The diverse pharmacological effects especially anti-inflammatory effect of STS might explain the benefit on all-cause mortality or MACEs in CHD patients in this systematic review.

There were several potential limitations in this study. Firstly, there was certain heterogeneity between various studies. Although we performed subgroup analyses according to different standard therapy, other clinical characteristics such as diagnostic criteria of CHD, age, disease course, treatment duration, which all might result in heterogeneity. Secondly, the poor quality and small sample size of included original trials make results of our review less convincing. Lastly, although we extensively searched both Chinese and English databases, all of the included trials were retrieved from Chinese literature, which may limit the generalization of the evidence.

REFERENCES

[1] Dalen JE, Alpert JS, Goldberg RJ, et al. The epidemic of the 20 (th)century: coronary heart disease[J]. Am J Med, 2014, 127: 807-812.

[2] Wong ND. Epidemiological studies of CHD and the evolution of preventive cardiology[J]. Nat Rev Cardiol, 2014, 11: 276-289.

[3] Napoli C, Lerman LO, de Nigris F, et al. Rethinking primary prevention of atherosclerosis-related diseases[J]. Circulation, 2006, 114: 2517-2527.

[4] Sabatine MS, Giugliano RP, Keech AC, et al. Evolocumab and Clinical Outcomes in Patients with Cardiovascular Disease[J]. N Engl J Med, 2017, 376: 1713-1722.

[5] Chen KJ, Shi DZ, et al. XS0601 reduces the incidence of restenosis: a prospective study of 335 patients undergoing percutaneous coronary intervention in China[J]. Chin Med J, 2006, 119: 6-13.

[6] Lu Z, Kou W, Du B, et al. Effect of Xuezhikang, an extract from red yeast Chinese rice, on coronary events in a Chinese population with previous myocardial infarction[J]. Am J Cardiol, 2008, 101: 1689-93.

[7] Li X, Zhang J, Huang J, et al. A multicenter, randomized, double-blind, parallel-group, placebo-controlled study of the effects of Qili qiangxin capsules in patients with chronic heart failure[J]. J Am Coll Cardiol, 2013, 62: 1065-1072.

[8] Wang MZ, Yan FS, Gao FY. Analysis of high performance liquid chromatography on three Tanshinones from Salviamilt iorrhizae[J]. J Pharm Ana lysis, 1985, 5: 348-350.

[9] Shang Q, Xu H, Huang L. "Tanshinone IIA: A Promising Natural Cardioprotective Agent, " [J]. Evidence-Based Complementary and Alternative Medicine, 2012, 2012: 716459.

[10] Chen Z, Xu H. Anti-inflammatory and Immunomodulatory Mechanism of Tanshinone IIA for Atherosclerosis[J]. Evidence-Based Complementary and Alternative Medicine, 2014, 2014: 267976.

[11] Higgins J, Green S. Cochrane Handbook for Systematic Reviews of Interventions. Version 5.0. 2 ed. The Cochrane Collaboration, 2009.

[12] Du QM, Wang CX. Effects of sodium tanshinone ⅡA sulfonate on arrhythmia induced by myocardial ischemia-reperfusion[J]. Chinese Journal of Geriatric Heart Brain and Vessel Diseases (Chin), 2011, 13: 349-351.

[13] Fan LY, Yang J. Impact of Tanshinone ⅡA Sulfonic Acid Natrium on Blood Lipid Metabolism, Serum Inflammatory Cytokines Levels and Cardiac Function in Patients with Acute Myocardial Infarction[J]. Practical Journal of Cardiac Cerebral Pneumal and Vascular Disease (Chin), 2015, 23: 14-17.

[14] Gan SY, Rong RC, Li B. Effects Tanshinone IIA on inflammatory cytokines and oxidative stress of the patient with acute coronary syndrome[J]. Pharmacology and Clinics of Chinese Materia Medica (Chin), 2014, 30: 163-166.

[15] He Y. Efficacy and safety of Danshen injection in treating patients with unstable angina pectoris of qi deficiency and blood stasis type in perioperative period of interventional therapy: a clinical study of the efficacy and safety of IIA[J]. Xinjiang Medical University (Chin), 2016.

[16] Huang PH. Protection of Sodium Tanshinone ⅡA Sulfonate on myocardium reperfusion injury after AMI thrombolysis[J]. Medical frontier (Chin), 2012, 20: 350-351.

[17] Li CR, Gan SY, Huang HX. Study on the curative effect of Sodium Tanshinone ⅡA Sulfonate in patient with acute coronary syndrome and its influence on inflammatory cytokines[J]. Modern Journal of Integrated Traditional Chinese and Western Medicine (Chin), 2015, 24: 2284-2286.

[18] Li JC, Sun ZG. Influence of Tanshinone ⅡA Sulfonate Injection Combined with Simvastatin on Inflammatory Factor in Patients with Coronary Heart Disease[J]. Chinese Primary Health Care (Chin), 2015, 29: 111-112.

[19] Li RJ, Zhang KS. Influence of Tanshinone Ⅱ A Sulfonate Sodium Injection on Platelet Activation in Patients with Unstable Angina Pectoris of Coronary Atherosclerotic Heart Disease with Blood Stasis Syndrome[J]. China Pharmaceuticals (Chin), 2017, 29: 63-65.

[20] Li SM, Jiao Y, Wang H, et al. Sodium tanshinone IIA sulfate adjunct therapy reduces high-sensitivity C-reactive protein level in coronary artery disease patients: a randomized controlled trial[J]. Sci Rep, 2017, 7: 17451.

[21] Li Y. Effect of Tanshinone ⅡA on the cardiac function and inflammatory cytokines in patients with acute myocardial infarction[J]. Journal of Hainan Medical University (Chin), 2016, 22: 1933-1935.

[22] Liu PF, Zhang YM, Tang JW, et al. The effect and clinical significance of tanshinone injection on Plasma NT-proBNP in acute myocardial infarction[J]. Chinese Journal of Difficult and Complicated Cases (Chin), 2009, 8: 327-329.

[23] Luan T, Pan T. Effects of Tanshinone Injection on Myocardial Ischemia reperfusion Injury and Different Syndromes of TCM[J]. Chinese Journal of Integrative Medicine on Cardio-/Cerebrovascular Disease (Chin), 2012, 10: 524-526.

[24] Qi H, Zhao X, Li YF. Study on the curative effect of Sodium tanshinone IIA sulfonate Injection in treating acute myocadiac infarction[J]. China Medical Herald (Chin), 2006, 3: 22-23.

[25] Qin S. C1inical efficacy of tanshinone plus atorvastatin against CHD[J]. Clinical Journal of Chinese Medicine (Chin), 2012, 4: 25-27.

[26] Tang XJ. Clinical study of Coronary Heart Disease and Angina Pectoris with Blood Stasis Syndrome Treated by Sodium tanshinone IIA sulfonate Injection. Beijing University of Chinese Medicine (Chin), 2014.

[27] Wei Q, Shen XJ. Effects of tanshinone Ⅱ on clinical symptoms and vascular aging factor in angina pectoris of coronary heart disease patients[J].

Journal of Basic Chinese Medicine (Chin), 2014, 20: 783-785.

[28] Xie Q, Zhang XJ. 31 cases of clinical observation research of Sodium tanshinone IIA sulfonate Injection in patients with Angina After Infarction[J]. Chinese Journal of Ethnomedicine and Ethnopharmacy (Chin), 2016, 25: 126-128.

[29] Xu T, Zhang Z, Wang JP, et al. Effect of sodium tanshinone ⅡA sulfonate combined with atorvastatin on TLR4 inflammatory signal pathway and immune function of patients with coronary heart diseases[J]. Hebei Medical Journal (Chin), 2015, 37: 3365-3368.

[30] Zhang XR, Wang LJ, Liu HJ, et al. The Impact of Tan Treatment on Haemodynamics and Blood Lipid of Acute Myocardial Infarction Patients[J]. Journal of Guizhou Medical University (Chin), 2014, 39: 379-382.

[31] Chang JY, Wang SZ, and Yan JX. Impact of tanshinone ⅡA on cardiac function and hs-CRP, TNF-α, IL-6 Levels of patients with acute myocardial infarction[J]. China Medicine and Pharmac (Chin), 2016, 6: 142-145.

[32] Chen J. Influence of Sodium tanshinone IIA sulfonate Injection in Thrombolytic Therapy of Acute Myocardial Infarction patients[J]. Tianjin Pharmacy (Chin), 2007, 19: 35-36.

[33] Chu C, Tao ZG, Fan YJ. Effect of Sodium tanshinone IIA sulfonate Injection on the serum inflammatory factors in acute coronary syndrome[J]. Shandong Medical Journal (Chin), 2014, 54: 67-68.

[34] Yan GP, Zhu CL, Sun YQ. Meta-analysis of Salvianolate injection in the treatment of unstable angina pectoris[J]. J Emerg Trad Chin, Med 2015, 5: 771-4.

[35] Zhang D, Wu J, Liu S, et al. Salvianolate injection in the treatment of unstable angina pectoris: A systematic review and meta-analysis[J]. Medicine (Baltimore), 2016, 95: 1-9.

[36] Tan D, Wu JR, Zhang XM, et al. Sodium Tanshinone II A Sulfonate Injection as Adjuvant Treatment for Unstable Angina Pectoris: A Meta-Analysis of 17 Randomized Controlled Trials[J]. Chin J Integr Med, 2018, 24: 1-5.

[37] Wang X. "Progress of pharmacological research and clinical application of Tanshinone II A, " [J]. Guang Ming Journal of Chinese Medcine (Chin), 2011, 26: 1514-1517.

[38] Bai FM. "Clinical application progress of sodium tanshinone II—a sulfonate, " [J]. China Pharmacy (Chin), 2012, 23: 1770-1772.

[39] Ridker PM, MacFadyen JG, Everett BM, et al. Relationship of C-reactive protein reduction to cardiovascular event reduction following treatment with canakinumab: a secondary analysis from the CANTOS randomised controlled trial[J]. Lancet, 2018, 391: 319-328.

[40] Libby P. Interleukin-1 Beta as a target for atherosclerosis therapy: biological basis of CANTOS and beyond[J]. J Am Coll Cardiol, 2017, 70: 2278-2289.

[41] Robertson AL, Holmes GR, Bojarczuk AN, et al. A zebrafsh compound screen reveals modulation of neutrophil reverse migration as an anti-infammatory mechanism[J]. Sci Transl Med, 2014, 6: 225ra29.

First published: Yu ML, Li SM, Gao X, Li JG, Xu H, Chen KJ. Sodium Tanshinone II A Sulfonate for coronary heart disease: A systematic review of randomized controlled trials [J]. Chin J Integr Med. 2018. doi: 10.1007/s11655-018-2556-7.

Baduanjin Exercise for Patients with Ischemic Heart Failure on Phase II Cardiac Rehabilitation (BEAR Trial): Study Protocol for A Prospective Randomized Controlled Trial

YU Mei-li, LI Si-ming, LI Si-wei, LI Jin-gen, XU Hao, and CHEN Ke-ji

Chronic heart failure (CHF), a terminal stage of various cardiovascular diseases, is characterized by fatigue, chronic reduction of cardiopulmonary function and exercise tolerance with high morbidity and mortality[1-3]. Over 5.7 million Americans have been diagnosed with heart failure, and with the aging population of CAD, this number is expected to increase to 8 million by 2030 [2,3].

Cardiac rehabilitation (CR), a kind of medicine consisting of education, cognitive behavioral therapy, initiative and positive physical and psychological training, to improve cardiovascular function, is a class IA recommendation for patients with CHF [4-6]. Although the medication, cardiac resynchronization therapy defibrillator (CRT/D)intervention and conventional exercise-based CR are beneficial for CHF and have been advocated as fundamental treatment for CHF, recurrent symptomatic heart failure, high rehospitalization rates and mortality still challenge the modern medicine [7]. New approaches are urgently needed to improve quality of life and prognosis in patients with CHF.

Baduanjin exercise is a mind-body practice that combined meditation with slow, gentle, and graceful movements, as well as deep breathing and relaxation. It can regulate the vital energy (or *qi*)of collateral channels and organs in the body. As an important component of traditional Chinese *Qigong*, it has been practiced for thousands of years in China as a kind of health care method. *Baduanjin* exercise involves eight sections of simple and easy-to-learn movements, each benefiting different parts of the body [8]. Therefore, it is a popular and safe community exercise to promote health, which has been recommended by the Chinese Health Qigong Association [9].

Empirical observations have suggested that *Baduanjin* exercise may improve cardiopulmonary function and exercise tolerance [10-12]. A meta-analysis showed *Baduanjin* exercise can improve left ventricular ejection fraction (LVEF), cardiac output, stroke output and reduce resting myocardial oxygen consumption in elderly patients. Besides, it can also improve the elasticity of vascular, and regulate blood pressure, glucose, and lipid [13-16]. Compared with conventional exercise, *Baduanjin* exercise can additionally relax and ease the mind and spirit, thus improve sleep quality and unhealthy emotions [17]. These features make *Baduanjin* exercise an optimal exercise for patients with CHF, whose daily activity is greatly limited and who suffered a lot physically and mentally after a long period of medical or surgical treatment. Therefore, *Buduanjin* may be a promising exercise for cardiac rehabilitation for CHF.

However, there is a lack of high quality evidence for the effectiveness of *Baduanjin* exercise-based cardiac rehabilitation program for patients with ischemic CHF. Therefore, we conduct this randomized controlled trial to evaluate the benefits of *Baduanjin* exercise-based cardiac rehabilitation program in patients with ischemic CHF. We hypothesized that after the 12-week *Baduanjin* practice, patients would have a greater improvement in cardiopulmonary function, exercise tolerance and health-related quality-of-life scores than those practicing conventional exercise alone.

METHODS/DESIGN

1 Trial Oversight

Baduanjin exercise for patients with ischemic heart failure on phase II cardiac rehabilitation (BEAR) trial is a single-center, parallel design, prospective, randomized controlled trial, and will be conducted at Fuwai Hospital, Chinese Academy of Medical Sciences, China. 120 participants are to be recruited and the recruitment is scheduled to begin in May 2017. Participants will be randomly assigned in a 1: 1 ratio to *Baduanjin* exercise combined with conventional exercise (experiment group)or conventional exercise alone (control group)training for 12 weeks. Outcomes will be measured at baseline, 3 months and 6 months by researchers blinded to group allocation. Change on walking distance in 6-minute walk test (6MWT)[18,19] from baseline to 6 months will be served as the primary outcome parameter, whereas the change in exercise capacity index such as peak oxygen uptake (VO_2 peak), ventilatory anaerobic threshold (VAT), The minute ventilation -carbon dioxide production relationship (VE/VCO_2 slope)determined by cardiopulmonary exercise test (CPET)[20,21], LV end-diastolic volume index (LVEDVi)and left ventricular ejection fraction (LVEF)assessed using echocardiography, scores assessed using life quality of Minnesota living with heart failure questionnaire (MLHFQ) [22], amino-terminal pro-brain natriuretic peptide (NT-proBNP), high sensitivity C-reactive protein (hs-CRP), heart rate variability (HRV), major adverse cardiovascular events (MACE), NYHA classification will be served as secondary outcome parameters. The study protocol and consent documents have been reviewed and approved by the Ethics Committee of Xiyuan Hospital of China Academy of Chinese Medical Sciences (reference number: 2013XL063-1). If there is any amendment to the protocol, approval must be again sought from the Ethics Committee. The study has registered at clinicaltrials. gov (NCT03229681), and the trial will be performed in accordance with the principles of the Declaration of Helsinki and Good Clinical Practice guidelines.

Study flow of the trial is illustrated in Figure 1 and described in detail below according to the CONSORT 2010 statement[23] and Standard Protocol Items: Recommendations for Interventional Trials (SPIRIT)[see Additional file 1].

2 Diagnostic Criteria

The diagnostic criteria of heart failure according to the European Society of Cardiology (ESC)[24] require a combination of typical symptoms and signs, LVEF normal or mildly reduced, left ventricular enlargement but associated structural heart disease (eg, left ventricular hypertrophy, left atrium enlargement)and/or diastolic heart dysfunction (eg, E/e' ≥ 13 or E/A < 1).

Stable patients of CHF were defined as documented heart failure patients with LVEF ≥ 40%, NT-proBNP ≥ 125pg/ml (or BNP ≥ 35pg/ml), and with clinical typical symptoms of heart failure such as breathless, fatigue after the activity, which is similar to patient in stage C and NYHA I/II according to the ESC and the American Heart Association (AHA)/ American College of Cardiology Foundation (ACCF)guidelines [25]. Diagnosis of CAD will be based on the standard criteria established in "Nomenclature and criteria for diagnosis of ischemic heart disease," a joint report published by the International Society and Federation of Cardiology and the World Health Organization. In addition, following the current practice of CAD clinical research, we will require subjects to either have a previous history of myocardial infarction or have at least one coronary artery stenosis ≥ 50% confirmed by coronary angiography or by computed tomographic (CT)angiogram to ensure the diagnosis of CAD.

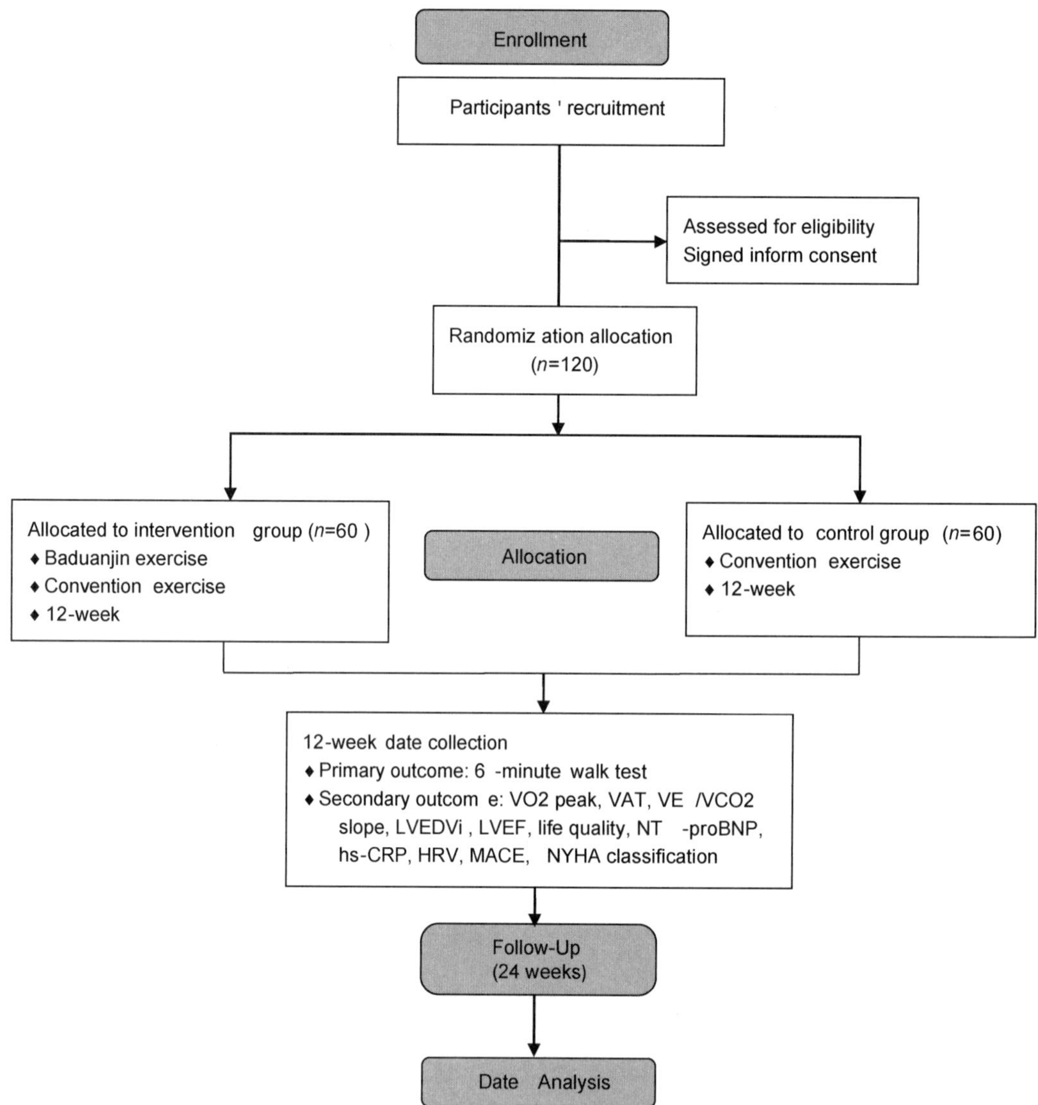

Figure 1 Flow Diagram of Study Design

3 General Inclusion Criteria

To participate in this study, subjects must be 40 to 75 years of age, meet the diagnostic criteria of stable CHF and have documented CAD.

In addition, subjects must be able to attend 2 rehabilitation courses each week at cardiac rehabilitation center of Fuwai Hospital, China Academy of Medical Sciences. All participants enrolled must provide a written informed consent before randomization (For details see Table 1).

4 General Exclusion Criteria

Patients having any of the following conditions will be excluded: with a recent acute heart failure attack (within 1 month), unable to perform rehabilitation exercises for various reasons or having practiced other traditional Chinese Qigong (such as Taijiquan)in the past three months (For details see Table 1).

Table 1 Principal Inclusion And Exclusion Criteria for the BEAR Trial

Inclusion criteria	Exclusion criteria
①Aged from 40 to 75 years	①Patient condition was too severe to exercise, or activity restrained by other diseases;
②CHF symptoms stable phase (NYHA class I or II)with CHF and with documented CAD	②Participants with poorly controlled blood pressure (SBP ≥ 180 mmHg or DBP ≥ 100 mmHg);
③Left ventricular ejection fraction ≥ 40%, NT-proBNP ≥ 125pg/ml (or BNP ≥ 35pg/ml)	③In the acute stage of chronic heart failure;
④Participants signed the informed consent.	④Resting heart rate over 120 beats per minute, or complicated with malignant arrhythmia;
	⑤Participants having contraindications to cardiopulmonary test or exercise training;
	⑥Patients complicated with other serious acute or chronic diseases or mental disorders;
	⑦Participants having practiced any kinds of traditional Chinese medicine exercises in last three months.

5 Recruitment Strategies

Inpatients and outpatients with ischemic CHF in Fuwai hospital will be screened. Every patient who is interested in and volunteers to participate in this trial will be assessed by an attending physician for eligibility. The aim, procedures, and possible side effects of the exercise will be explained in detail to the patients; all patients will be asked to sign a written informed consent form before randomization No financial incentives will be provided to the attending physicians or patients for enrollment. Eligible patients with initial compliance will proceed to be enrolled.

6 Randomization and Blinding

We generated a random sequence of 120 numbers using SAS 9.2 software, allocating the patient in a 1: 1 ratio to intervention or control group. The random sequence will be put into sealed opaque envelopes by staff not involved with the study to avoid selecting bias. Once a patient meets all the criteria, a random number determining whether the patients will receive *Baduanjin* exercise or not will be delivered to the clinical researchers (the clinical researchers will open an envelope in sequence). Patient allocation will be unblinded only after baseline data is collected for the first phase of the study.

Because *Baduanjin* exercise is an exercise training familiar to Chinese population, blinding is difficult to achieve at the physician and patient levels. In order to minimize biases as much as possible, all study participants will be discouraged from discussing with one another their practice in the trial. Finally, the clinical researchers will strictly abide by the study's protocol and will treat the patients in each group with as few differences as possible. Blinding will be maintained at the level of outcome assessment. The individuals performing data management and statistical analyses will not be involved in the clinical procedure of the trials and will not be informed of the treatment allocation.

7 Interventions

After recruitment, researchers will evaluate the cardiopulmonary function of participants, educate them about cardiac rehabilitation, and then give them exercise prescription for CR. All the participants will complete 36 CR sessions in CR center of Fuwai hospital within 12 weeks.

Participants allocated to the conventional exercise group will receive a closely supervised, group-format aerobic exercise program recommended by current guidelines [6,26] in the cardiac rehabilitation center for three months. The program includes education for diet and nutrition, medications, smoking cessation, physical and mental health and so on.

In addition to conventional exercise described above, each patient in the intervention group will also receive *Baduanjin* exercise training. Given the low-activity tolerance of CHF patients, we performed with a modified version of *Baduanjin* exercise, in which the difficult movements for CHF patient are removed according to the "Health Qigong *Baduanjin* Standard" enacted by the General Administration of Sports in 2003 and some movements beneficial to cardiopulmonary function for CHF patients are added. They will perform standard training guided by specific *Baduanjin* exercise instructors twice a week, for a total of 12 weeks. Each training session lasts for 45 min, including breathing techniques and mild warm-up (15 min), *Baduanjin* movement (25 min)and relaxation at the end (5 min).

Researchers will record the subjects' heart rate and blood pressure before and after training. During the training, exercise intensity will be assessed by Borg rating of perceived exertion scale (RPE scale)[27], which is a frequently used quantitative measure of perceived exertion during exercise. A perceived exertion of 12 or 13 which means "Somewhat hard" is considered the best and at which condition the subjects' heart rate will be recorded. Subjects will be encouraged to practice *Baduanjin* or conventional exercise at least 30 min a day at home followed the instructional DVD until finishing the follow-up at 6 months. The duration of intervention and followed-up is illustrated in Figure 2.

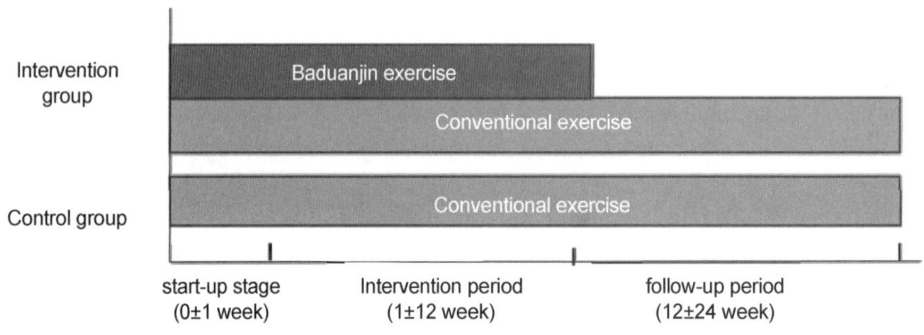

Figure 2 The Duration of Intervention and Followed-up

8 Concomitant Treatment

Participants in both groups will continue routine medications such as antiplatelet, anti-coagulation, angiotensin-converting enzyme (ACE)inhibition or beta-adrenergic block according to patients' conditions and maintain their usual treatment visits throughout the study. The doses of ACE inhibitors or angiotensin-receptor blockers and beta-blockers should be gradually increased to target dose whenever possible. All procedures as well as medication prescription will be determined by physicians following the clinical guidelines [28, 29]. The date and reasons of any medical therapy change will be recorded in the case report form (CRF).

9 Study Outcome Measures

The primary outcome is changes in 6-min walking distance assessed by the 6MWT from baseline to the end of the 12-week intervention. The 6MWT is a quick, safe, and good tolerated measure that can reflect the functional status in patient with cardiovascular disease.

Secondary outcome includes changes of VO_2 peak, PVO_2 and VAT, VE/ VCO_2 slope in cardiopulmonary exercise test (CPET)after the 12-week intervention. CPET is an objective method being increasingly used in a wide spectrum of clinical practice for assessing the functional capacity of CHF patient and has become an important tool to evaluate exercise capacity and predict outcome in patients with heart failures [20].

LVEDVi, LVEF are also to be assessed using echocardiography at baseline and at the end of the 12-week intervention.

MLHFQ, the most widely used scale for assessing the quality of life (QOL)in HF patients, will be used to assess how these two kinds of CR program will affect quality of life of patient with CHF from physical, emotional, social and mental dimensions.

The serum level of NT-proBNP, an established biomarker that can reflect the cardiac function and stability of heart failure, and hs-CRP, a factor that is independently associated with adverse cardiovascular events, will be also evaluated at baseline and at the end of the 12-week intervention.

MACE including cardiac death, nonfatal myocardial infarction, documented unstable angina requiring revascularization (bypass surgery or percutaneous coronary intervention), all-cause mortality, re-admission for acute coronary syndrome, heart failure, malignant supraventricular and ventricular arrhythmia influencing hemodynamics, ischemic stroke, and other thromboembolic events during the 6 months follow-up will also be recorded.

NYHA classification and the HRV mainly including SDANN Index and SDNN Index will also be evaluated at baseline and at the end of the 12-week intervention. Table 2 indicates the data to be collected at each phase of the study.

10 Safety / Security Assurance

Study participants are monitored weekly during the study intervention for the occurrence of adverse events defined as any undesirable experience. All adverse events during the study will be recorded on an adverse event CRF and will be evaluated for relevance to the intervention. Adverse events will also be reported to the Human Research Committee promptly in accordance with guidelines.

We will strictly follow recommendations from the consensus document of the Heart Failure Association, the European Association for cardiovascular prevention and rehabilitation as well as the exercise standard for testing and training in the consensus from the American heart association [30,31] when conducting CEPT. When screening patients, only those eligible and able to finish the test will undergo CPET. Moreover, for enrolled patients meeting the rehabilitation training standard, we stratify them according to the degree of motion risk, and then arrange proper exercise intensity and time according to the risk stratification. Before CR exercise, researchers will educate patients on rehabilitation exercises of CHF including training contraindication and notes that should be pay attention to during conventional CR exercise and *Baduanjin* exercise. Moreover, the CR center of Fuwai hospital has perfect rescue equipment and we have a thorough contingency plan and rescue procedure for cardiovascular event before the research began. Once adverse events occur during exercise, researchers will immediately start the contingency plan in case of fatal outcomes.

11 Data Management

The GCP Clinical Center of Xiyuan hospital will be responsible for randomizing subjects into different groups, monitoring research progress, managing the data, and performing statistical analyses. All investigators involved in data management and analysis will be blinded to treatment allocation. All patient data will be recorded by trained clinical researchers using a standardized, preprinted, and paper CRF. If complete, the CRF will be locked for further revision in preparation for data entry. All CRFs are kept in a secure and lock-protected location. In accordance with our study protocol, extensive procedures are in place to ensure quality control of data entry, missing data minimization, and subject confidentiality. The statistician reviews the database to ensure accurate data collection and correct data export for future analyses. For example, at the GCP Clinical Center, a data manager uninvolved with subsequent data analysis will be responsible for overseeing data entry; to ensure the reliability of the recorded data, two investigators will independently input a copy of the CRF data into a database. A third individual will check the two independently completed database to ensure that they are identical and accurately represented. If the database records are not identical, the data in question will be confirmed from the original CRF, and if any data in the CRF is unclear, the data manager will submit a clarification form to the principal investigator of the study, who will then issue an inquiry for the clinical researchers to resolve as soon as possible. After blindly checking the database and confirming the accuracy and correctness of the database, we will lock the database for further analyzing.

12 Statistical analysis

Continuous variables will be presented as the mean ± standard deviation (SD), median or interquartile range (IQR), and categorical variables as frequencies or percentages. Comparability of the baseline data between the two groups will be assessed using a two-sample Student's t test for continuous variables and the chi-square test or Wilcoxon test, for categorical variables. Questionnaire score data, known as nonnormally distributed, will be transformed or analyzed with nonparametric test.

Analysis of the primary outcome will be conducted according to the intention-to-treat (ITT)principle. The ITT set includes all patients randomized, and the per protocol set consists of all patients with no major deviation from the protocol and with an adherence rate of 80% or higher at the end of the study. The safety set consists of ITT patients excluding those who receive no CR program or who have no safety record after randomization. We will assess the effect of any missing data on the final results by sensitivity analysis. Dropouts will be included in the analysis by modern imputation methods for missing data.

For all analyses, all tests will be two tailed and a statistical probability of < 0.05 is considered statistically significant. All analyses will be conducted using SPSS 18.0 software (SPSS, Inc., Chicago, IL, USA), unless otherwise noted.

13 Adherence

During the 12-week treatment period, participants will be asked to practice according to CR training prescription strictly, and will not be allowed to take part in any new, additional exercise programs. All patients will be asked to sign a written commitment to guarantee the adherence at baseline evaluation. During the whole study period, subjects will be supervised to record the daily rehabilitation exercise time. Every week, participates will be called to the CR center to practice the conventional or *Baduanjin* exercise guiding by trained persons. Throughout the 12-week intervention period, the researchers will give patients attendance cards after each session to record total session the patients have taken part in, and patients who missed a class will be asked to attend a makeup class. The percentage of compliance will be documented in the CRF. Rate of patient compliance (total planned number of times -number of absence)/ total number of times × 100 %. Compliance greater than 80% is considered as good. Otherwise, less than 80% is considered as poor. Patients will be asked to visit the CR center regularly according to the study protocol, and researchers will inform them the visit in advance. Attendance less than 20% is considered as drop-out.

14 Sample Size calculation

Sample size is calculated based on the 6MWT according to the following superiority test formula:

$$n_c = \frac{(1+\frac{1}{k})(\mu_{1-\alpha}+\mu_{1-\beta})^2\sigma^2}{[(x_t - x_c)-\Delta]^2}$$

$n_t = kn_c$, The patients' numbers were arranged in equal proportion (k=1), a superiority one-sided test was employed. According to result of a previous study [32], x_t=512.5, x_c=436.2, δ_t=50.2, δ_c=49.8, δ is the estimated standard difference calculated as 50.0 and Δ= 0.9δ = 45.0. Setting a type I error rate of alpha at 0.05, μ_{1-a}=1.64, and setting a type II error rate of beta at 0.1 (a power of 90%), $\mu_{1-\beta}$=1.282, the calculated sample size of each group is around 49. Assuming conservatively that 20% may loss to follow-up within 6 months, the total sample size needed to detect this difference at a 5% level of significance with a power of 90% is 118 patients. For our study, we decided to recruit 120 patients for the convenience of randomization.

DISCUSSION

We conduct this trial trying to assess whether the addition of *Baduanjin* to conventional exercise of CR will further improve exercise endurance, reserve of heart function and quality of life, and if successful, this trial would provide a promising exercise for CR. As a matter of fact, the building and development of CR is still under exploration, and currently, CR mainly consists of contemporarily popular exercise. As one of traditional Chinese qigong, Baduanjin has long been practiced for health care since it has the function of regulating organs and dredging the channel and collaterals[10,11]. This exercise is especially suitable for patient with CHF complicated with CAD whose activity tolerance is poor because the action of Baduanjin exercise is simple and gentle. However, its effect hasn't been confirmed by objective evaluation.

There are several strengths of our trial. First of all, we use the objective and quantitative CEPT to assess the improvement of cardio-pulmonary function, which is reliable and convincing. Second, Baduanjin exercise is easy to master and gentle to practice for CHF patients, which guarantee the compliance. Moreover, if prove to be effective, the costless Baduanjin could be a widely welcomed exercise for CR. On the one hand, it saves time, facility for CHF patients who has poor activity tolerance. On the other hand, it may have the effect to improve prognosis for patients with ischemic CHF finally, reducing the social medical spending.

A potential limitation of the BEAR trial is that participants and exercise coaches cannot be blinded because it is difficult to conduct blinding in non-pharmacological trials[33]. It is inevitable that performance bias always exists in a practical trial. However, the exercise coaches will not participate in the procedure of recruitment, assessment and data analysis of this study which will minimize the bias.

In summary, BEAR trial will be the first RCT to evaluate the impact of Baduanjin exercise on activity tolerance in patients with ischemic CHF and results of this trial will help to establish the optimal approach for treating patients with CHF and provide reliable evidence for application of Baduanjin exercise in the cardiac rehabilitation.

REFERENCES

[1] Mozaffarian D, Benjamin EJ, Go AS, et al. Heart Disease and Stroke Statistics-2016 Update: A Report From the American Heart Association[J]. Circulation, 2016, 133 (4): e38-360.

[2] Ziaeian B, Fonarow GC. Epidemiology and aetiology of heart failure. Nat Rev Cardiol[J]. 2016, 13 (6): 368-378.

[3] Heidenreich PA, Albert NM, Allen LA, et al. Forecasting the impact of heart failure in the United States: a policy statement from the American Heart Association[J]. Circ Heart Fail, 2013, 6 (3): 606-619.

[4] Piepoli MF, Hoes AW, Agewall S, et al. 2016 European Guidelines on cardiovascular disease prevention in clinical practice: the Sixth Joint Task Force of the European Society of Cardiology and Other Societies on Cardiovascular Disease Prevention in Clinical Practice (constituted by representatives of 10 societies and by invited experts): developed with the special contribution of the European Association for Cardiovascular Prevention & Rehabilitation (EACPR)[J]. Eur Heart J, 2016, 37: 2315-2381.

[5] Yancy CW, Jessup M, Bozkurt B, et al. 2013 ACCF/AHA guideline for the management of heart failure: a report of the American College of Cardiology Foundation/American Heart Association Task Force on Practice Guidelines[J]. J Am Coll Cardiol, 2013, 62: e147-e239.

[6] American Association of Cardiovascular and Pulmonary Rehabilitation. Guidelines for Cardiac Rehabilitation and Secondary Prevention Programs (5th Revised edition)[J]. In: Williams MA, Balady GJ, Carlson RD, editors. United States, 2013.

[7] Townsend N, Nichols M, Scarborough P, et al. Cardiovascular disease in Europe: epidemiological update 2015[J]. Eur Heart J, 2015, 36: 2696-2705.

[8] Koh T. C. Baduanjin: An ancient Chinese exercise[J]. American Journal of Chinese Medicine. 1982, 10 (1-4): 14-21.

[9] The value analysis of Baduanjin in international cultural vision[J]. Chinese Medical Culture, 2016, (4): 37-40.

[10] Qin G. Effect of Qigong on cardiovascular function in College students[J]. Journal of Wuhan Institute of Physical Education, 2012, 46 (9): 97-100.

[11] Zeng YG., Zhou XQ., Wang AL. Research on the impacts of fitness Qigong Baduanjin on figure and physical function among the middle-aged and aged people[J]. Journal of Beijing Sport University, 2005, 9: 1207-1209.

[12] Wang Y. The influence of health qigong BaduanJin training on the psychological health of college students[J]. Journal of Beijing Sport University, 2011, 34 (12): 102-111.

[13] Wang XQ, Pi YL, Chen PJ, et al. Traditional Chinese exercise for cardiovascular diseases: systematic review and meta - analysis of randomized

controlled trials[J]. Journal of the American Heart Association, 2016, 5 (3).
[14] Xiong X, Wang P, Li S, et al. Effect of Baduanjin exercise for hypertension: a systematic review and meta-analysis of randomized controlled trials[J]. Maturitas, 2015, 80 (4): 370-378.
[15] Luskin FM, Newell KA, Griffith M, et al. A review of mind-body therapies in the treatment of cardiovascular disease, part 1: implications for the elderly[J]. Altern Ther Health Med, 1998, 4 (3): 46-61.
[16] Chen BL, Guo JB, Liu MS, et al. Effect of Traditional Chinese Exercise on Gait and Balance for Stroke: A Systematic Review and Meta-Analysis[J]. PLoS One, 2015, 10 (8): e0135932.
[17] Chan JSM., Ho RTH., Chung KF, et al. Qigong exercise alleviates fatigue, anxiety, and depressive symptoms, improves sleep quality, and shortens sleep latency in persons with chronic fatigue syndrome-like illness[J]. Evidence-based Complementary and Alternative Medicine, 2014, 2014: 10.
[18] Guyatt GH, Sullivan MJ, Thompson PJ, et al. The 6-minute walk: a new measure of exercise capacity in patients with chronic heart failure[J]. Can Med Assoc J, 1985, 132 (8): 919-923.
[19] Zugck C, Krüger C, Dürr S, et al. Is the 6-minute walk test a reliable substitute for peak oxygen uptake in patients with dilated cardiomyopathy?[J]. Eur Heart J, 2000, 21 (7): 540-549.
[20] Kao W, Jessup M. Exercise testing and exercise training in patients with congestive heart failure[J]. J Heart Lung Transplant, 1994, 13 (4): S117-S121.
[21] Gerardi DA, Lovett L, Benoit-Connors ML, et al. Variables related to increased mortality following out-patient pulmonary rehabilitation[J]. Eur Respir J, 1996, 9 (3): 431-435.
[22] Rector TS, Tschumperlin LK, Kubo SH, et al. Use of the Living With Heart Failure Questionnaire to ascertain patients' perspectives on improvement in quality of life versus risk of drug-induced death[J]. J Card Fail, 1995, 1 (3): 201-206.
[23] Moher D, Hopewell S, Schulz KF, et al. CONSORT 2010 explanation and elaboration: updated guidelines for reporting parallel group randomised trials[J]. BMJ, 2010, 340: c869.
[24] Catapano AL, Graham I, De Backer G, et, al. 2016 ESC/EAS Guidelines for the Management of Dyslipidaemia: The Task Force for the Management of Dyslipidaemia of the European Society of Cardiology (ESC)and European Atherosclerosis Society (EAS)Developed with the special contribution of the European Association for Cardiovascular Prevention & Rehabilitation (EACPR)[J]. Eur Heart J, 2016, 37 (29): 2315-2381.
[25] Yancy CW, Jessup M, Bozkurt B, et al. 2013 ACCF/AHA guideline for the management of heart failure: a report of the American College of Cardiology Foundation/American Heart Association Task Force on practice guidelines[J]. Circulation, 2013, 128 (16): e240-327.
[26] Haskell WL, Lee IM, Pate RR, et al. Physical activity and public health: updated recommendation for adults from the American College of Sports Medicine and the American Heart Association[J]. Circulation, 2007, 116 (9): 1081-93.
[27] Psychophysical bases of perceived exertion[J]. Borg GA Med Sci Sports Exerc, 1982, 14 (5): 377-81.
[28] Fletcher GF, Ades PA, Kligfield P, et al. Exercise standards for testing and training: a scientific statement from the American Heart Association[J]. Circulation, 2013, 128: 873-934.
[29] Piepoli MF, Conraads V, Corrà U, et al. Exercise training in heart failure: from theory to practice. A consensus document of the Heart Failure Association and the European Association for Cardiovascular Prevention and Rehabilitation[J]. Eur J Heart Fail, 2011, 13: 347-357.
[30] Piña IL, Apstein CS, Balady GJ, et al. Exercise and heart failure: A statement from the American Heart Association Committee on exercise, rehabilitation, and prevention[J]. Circulation, 2003, 107: 1210-1225.
[31] American College of Sports Medicine. ACSM'S guidelines for exercise testing and prescription[M]. 6th Ed. Philadelphia: Lippincott Williams & Wilkins, 2000: 145-149.
[32] Xiong XH, Deng X. The clinical observation of Baduanjin for chronic heart failure with CHD[J]. Modern Medicine Journal of China. 2016, 18 (5): 55-56. (in Chinese)
[33] Boutron I, Moher D, Altman DG, et al. CONSORT Group. Extending the CONSORT statement to randomized trials of nonpharmacologic treatment: explanation and elaboration[J]. Ann Intern Med, 2008, 148: 295-309.

First published: YU Mei-li, LI Si-ming, LI Si-wei, LI Jin-gen, XU Hao, CHEN Ke-ji. Baduanjin exercise for patients with ischemic heart failure on phase-II cardiac rehabilitation (BEAR trial): study protocol for a prospective randomized controlled trial. [J] . Trials, 2018, 19: 381.

Holistic Regulation of Angiogenesis with Chinese herbal Medicines as a New Option for Coronary Artery Disease

YUAN Rong, SHI Wei-li, XIN Qi-qi, CHEN Ke-ji, and CONG Wei-hong

Coronary artery disease (CAD), also known as coronary atherosclerotic heart disease, coronary heart disease and ischemic heart disease (IHD), is the most common cause of heart attacks[1]. According to the World Health Organization, CAD is the leading cause of death worldwide among all non-communicable diseases[2]. Current therapeutic options are limited to pharmacological therapy, percutaneous coronary intervention and bypass surgery. However, a large number of patients do not qualify for surgical or interventional procedures[3], and these patients mainly present with refractory angina with severe atherosclerosis in the clinic. At present, a number of studies have indicated that promoting angiogenesis is a promising approach for IHD[4], while angiogenesis in atherosclerosis induces plaque destabilization and hemorrhage[5]. Therefore, more attention should be paid to balancing the regulation of angiogenesis in myocardial ischemia and atherosclerosis.

The holistic theory of traditional Chinese medicine (TCM)aims to modulate the dynamic balance of the body. Among the different TCM therapies, activating blood circulation and removing blood stasis (ABCRS) therapy is effective in CAD treatment, with anti-platelet function, vascular endothelium protection, myocardial remodeling and microcirculation improvement[6]. Recently, an increasing number of studies have focused on the effects of Chinese herbal medicines for ABCRS on angiogenesis in myocardial ischemia and atherosclerosis. Given the double-edged role of angiogenesis, this review aims to present the recent research progress on the regulatory role of angiogenesis by Chinese herbal medicines for ABCRS, which may provide a new angle of view with regards to the prevention and treatment of CAD.

We searched the PubMed, Chinese National Knowledge Infrastructure and Chinese Scientific Journal Database with the keywords: "angiogenesis" OR "neovascularization" AND "coronary disease" OR "atherosclerosis" OR "myocardial ischemia/infarction" OR "Chinese medicine" OR "activating blood circulation and removing blood stasis" . We also searched related references.

1 The Dual Role of ANgiogenesis in CAD

1.1 Angiogenesis

Angiogenesis refers to the formation of new blood vessels from the pre-existing vasculature[7]. Under certain conditions, various angiogenic factors are produced, and vascular endothelial growth factor (VEGF), basic fibroblast growth factor (bFGF)and their receptors are the key molecular factors. The binding of VEGF/FGF to VEGF receptor (VEGFR)/FGF receptor (FGFR)induces multiple signaling networks, such as mitogen-activated protein kinase (MAPK), phosphatidylinositol 3 kinase/protein kinase B (PI3K/Akt), extracellular regulated protein kinase (ERK)and notch pathways, and the signaling cascades result in endothelial cell (EC) survival, proliferation, migration and tube formation[7-11]. A brief overview of the angiogenesis and the activation pathways is provided in Figure 1.

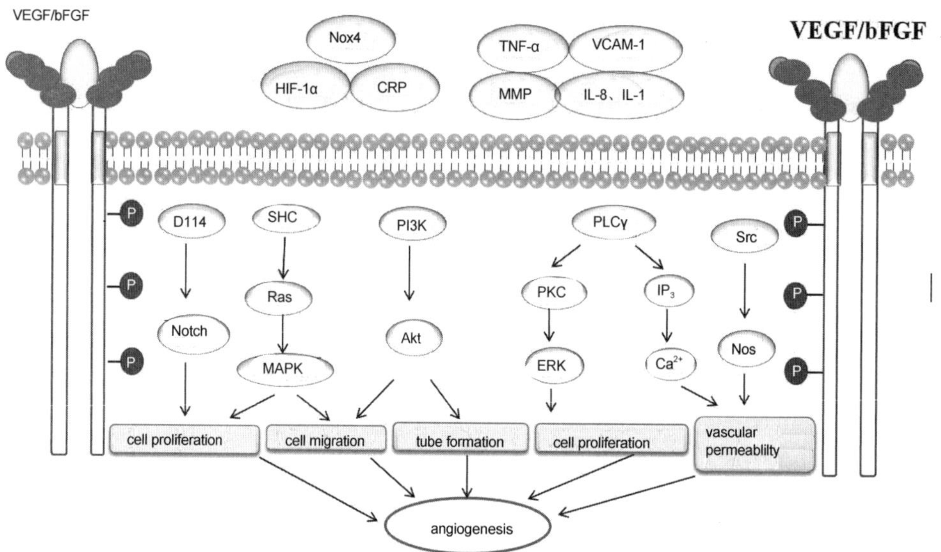

Figure 1 Schematic representation of major targets of angiogenesis. Nox4: nicotinamide adenine dinucleotide phosphate oxidase 4, HIF-1α: hypoxia-inducible factor-1α, CRP: C-reactive protein, TNF-α: tumor necrosis factor-α, VCAM-1: vascular cell adhesion molecule-1, MMPs: matrix metalloproteinases, Dll4: delta-like ligand 4, SHC: synthesized hydro carbon, PKC: protein kinase C, PLC-γ: phospholipase C-γ, IP3: inositol triphosphate 3, NOS: nitric oxide synthase

1.2 Angiogenesis in Myocardial Ischemia

Improving blood flow to the ischemic myocardium plays a critical role in the treatment of CAD, and angiogenesis is an important and promising means of increasing blood flow[12]. Numerous studies have shown that promoting angiogenesis therapy can improve myocardial ischemia by stimulating formation of collateral networks and increasing blood supply[4,13]. Nox4 alleviated hypoxia/reoxygenation injury by inhibiting apoptosis and promoting angiogenesis via upregulation of HIF-1/VEGF signaling pathway[14]. Activation of the notch1 pathway also promoted coronary neo-angiogenesis and revascularization, limited the extent of ischemic damage and improved heart function[15]. Additionally, secreted VCAM-1 induced EC migration and prevented cardiomyocyte death through activation of Akt, ERK and p38 MAPK[16]. In short, promoting angiogenesis therapy is beneficial to myocardial ischemia.

1.3 Angiogenesis in Atherosclerosis

Acute coronary syndrome may be related to atherosclerotic plaque rupture and thrombosis, while angiogenesis is a key factor in plaque destabilization leading to rupture[17]. Plaque neovascularization consists of a network of capillaries that arise from the adventitial vasa vasorum and extend into the intimal layer of atherosclerotic lesions, which promotes the growth of atherosclerotic lesions and plaque destabilization. Furthermore, excessive adventitial neovascularization is also one of the hallmarks of atherosclerotic plaque progression[18,19]. Increased IL-8, IL-1, TNF-α, CRP and MMP levels enhanced plaque progression and destabilization and caused intraplaque hemorrhage and rupture[20,21]. FGFR2 overexpression in ECs resulted in increased expression of VCAM-1, which aggravated atherosclerosis[22]. The HIF pathway was associated with angiogenesis in plaque[23]. Therefore, inhibiting plaque and adventitial angiogenesis is beneficial to atherosclerosis.

1.4 Double-edged Role of Angiogenesis

The "Janus phenomenon" illustrates the double-edged role of angiogenesis: when an intervention benefits pro-angiogenesis and collateral development, it has the potential to increase atherosclerosis, and when an intervention has anti-atherosclerotic effects, it has the potential to inhibit collateral development[20,24]. Although pro-angiogenesis therapy can improve blood supply in animal models, several clinical studies have not shown definite evidence of clinical efficacy of pro-angiogenesis in CAD, and adverse effects, including edema, inflammation and cancer, were turned up[25,26]. Although anti-angiogenesis therapy can stabilize plaques in animal models, there has been no clinical study on anti-angiogenesis therapy in atherosclerosis until now, and anti-angiogenesis therapy in cancer can lead to myocardial ischemia, hypertension and stroke[27]. Therefore, neither promotive nor inhibitory angiogenesis therapy alone is an ideal option for the treatment of CAD, and a drug that holistically regulates angiogenesis in CAD would have great potential.

2 The Holistic Regulatory Effects of Chinese Herbal Medicines for ABCRS

In TCM, myocardial ischemia and atherosclerotic plaque are collectively caused by blood stasis, and the ABCRS method is the main therapeutic method[6]. The TCM philosophy regards the ABCRS method as promoting blood circulation and dissipating stasis. Recent studies have also verified that Chinese herbal medicines for ABCRS have effects on improving microcirculation and hemorheology indices, increasing blood flow, regulating endothelial function and inhibiting the proliferation of vascular smooth muscle cells[28]. A large number of studies have indicated that Chinese herbal medicines for ABCRS can regulate angiogenesis in myocardial ischemia and atherosclerosis. Therefore, the ABCRS method might have holistic regulatory effects on angiogenesis in CAD.

2.1 Pro-angiogenic Effect

Previous studies have reported that the Xiongshao capsule and Guanxin No. 2 can promote angiogenesis in the ischemic region and increase blood supply by increasing the expression levels of VEGF and bFGF[29,30]. Tongxinluo can promote angiogenesis in the peri-infarct area and increase blood flow to the myocardium by down-regulating Nox4 and by up-regulating VEGF and endothelial NOS-mediated angiogenesis through the PI3K/Akt signaling pathway[31]. In addition, Qishen Yiqi dripping pills, Xuefu Zhuyu formula, Shu-mai-tang, Shenzhu Guanxin granules, flowers of *Panax notoginseng*, salvianolic acid B, Xuesetong soft capsules, *Radix paeoniae rubra* 801, Danhong injection and Spatholobi caulis can also protect the ischemic myocardium through the activation of VEGF and the promotion of angiogenesis[32-42] (Table 1).

Table 1 Pro–angiogenic Effects of Chinese Herbal Medicines for ABCRS

Study ID	Objects	Chinese herbs and formulae	Study design	Composition of formula	Therapeutic effect and mechanism
Chen et al. [29]	8 rats	Xiongshao capsule	Gavage for 6 weeks	*Ligusticum chuanxiong* Hort., *Radix paeoniae rubra*	Increase the expression levels of VEGF and bFGF, promote angiogenesis, enhance myocardial blood supply, improve cardiac function
Zeng et al. [30]	10 rats	Guanxin No. 2	Gavage with 20 g/kg/d for 28 days	*Ligusticum chuanxiong* Hort., *Radix paeoniae rubra*, *Salvia miltiorrhiza* Bunge, *Carthamus tinctorius* Linn., *Dalbergia odorifera* T. Chen	Increase the expression levels of VEGF and bFGF, promote angiogenesis, compensate blood supply to the heart
Wang et al. [31]	12 mice	Tongxinluo	Gavage with 0.38 g, 1.5 g/kg/d for 7/30 days	*Panax ginseng* C. A. Meyer, *Hirudo nipponia* Whitman, Scorpio, *Radix paeoniae rubra*, Periostracum Cicadae, Eupoly- phaga Seu Steleophaga, *Scolopendra subspinipes*, *Santalum album* Linn.	Increase the expression levels of VEGF, HIF-1α, eNOS, PI3K, Akt and ERK, promote angiogenesis, improve cardiac function, ameliorate cardiac remodeling
Yao [32]	ECs	Qishen Yiqi dripping pills	Drug serum for 7 days	*Salvia miltiorrhiza* Bunge, *Astragalus membranaceus* (Fisch.)Bunge, *Dalbergia odorifera* T. Chen, *Panax notoginseng* (Burk.)F. H. Chen	Increase the expression level of ERK, increase proliferation, migration and tube formation of ECs

Continued

Study ID	Objects	Chinese herbs and formulae	Study design	Composition of formula	Therapeutic effect and mechanism
Zhang et al. [33]	8 rats	Xuefu Zhuyu formula	Gavage with 13.68 g/kg/d for 7 days	*Angelica sinensis* (Oliv.)Diels, *Rehmannia glutinosa* Libosch, Semen Persicae, *Carthamus tinctorius* Linn., *Radix paeoniae rubra*, *Bupleurum chinensis* DC., *Ligusticum chuanxiong* Hort., *Achyranthes bidentata* Blume, *Platycodon grandiflorus* (Jacq.)A. DC.	Increase the expression level of VEGF, promote angiogenesis, protect myocardium
Li et al. [34]	40 patients	Xuefu Zhuyu formula	12 grains/d, po for 4 week	*Angelica sinensis* (Oliv.)Diels, *Rehmannia glutinosa* Libosch, Semen Persicae, *Carthamus tinctorius* Linn., *Radix paeoniae rubra*, *Bupleurum chinensis* DC., *Ligusticum chuanxiong* Hort., *Achyranthes bidentata* Blume, *Platycodon grandiflorus* (Jacq.)A. DC.	Increase levels of serum VEGF and bFGF, relieve angina and signs of blood stasis
Yin et al. [35]	24 rats	Shu-mai-tang	Gavage with 1.71 g/kg/d for 2, 4 weeks	*Astragalus mongholicus* Bunge, *Salvia miltiorrhiza* Bge, *Panaxpseudo-ginseng* N. Wallich, *Hirudo nipponica* Whitman, *Eupolyphaga sinensis* Walker, *Moschus berezovskii* Flerov, *Trichosanthes kirilowii* Maxim	Increase the expression levels of VEGF and platelet-derived growth factor, increase microvessels and arterioles in ischemic areas
Xu et al. [36]	30 rats	Shenzhu Guanxin granules	Gavage with 630, 1260, 3981.6 mg/kg/d for 4 weeks	*Radix Ginseng*, *Radix Panacis* quinquefolii, *Radix Notoginseng*, *Hirudo*, Rhizoma Pinelliae, Rhizoma Atractylodis, Folium Nelumbinis	Increase the expression level of VEGF, increase microvessel density, attenuate infarct size, improve cardiac hemodynamic function
Yang et al. [37]	12 rats	Panax notoginseng	Gavage with 25, 50 mg/mL/d for 2 weeks	*Panax Notoginseng* (Burk.)F. H. Chen	Increase the expression levels of HIF-1, VEGF and VEGFR2, increase blood vessel density
He et al. [38]	15 rats	Salvianolic acid B	Gavage with 100 mg/kg/d for 4 weeks	Salvianolic acid B	Increase the expression level of VEGF, promote angiogenesis, improve myocardial microcirculation
Wang et al. [39]	8 rats	Xuesetong soft capsules	Gavage with 0.4 g/kg/d for 6 weeks	Notoginseng total saponin	Increase the expression level of VEGF, increase microvessel density
Liu et al. [40]	10 rats	*Radix paeoniae rubra* 801	Gavage with 16.2 mg/kg/d for 14 days	Propyl gallate	Increase the expression levels of NO, VEGF and bFGF, increase capillary density, improve myocardial ischemia
Chen et al. [41]	25 rats	Danhong injection	Intramuscular injection with 0.76 mL/kg/d for 28 days	Radix et Rhizoma Salviae Miltiorrhizae, Flos Carthami	Increase the expression level of VEGF, increase blood vessel density, decrease ratio of infarct, improve cardiac function
Zhou et al. [42]	zebrafish embryos and ECs	Spatholobi caulis	3,10,30 and 100 μg/mL embryo m-edium for 24 h in zebrafish embr- yos; drug serum for 24 h in ECs	Caulis Spatholobi	Increase the expression levels of VEGFRs and MAPKs, increase subintestinal vessel sprouting, promote cell proliferation and migration, increase sprout intensity

2.2 Anti-angiogenesis Effect

Previous studies have determined that Tongxinluo can inhibit adventitia neovascularization and decrease microvessel density in atherosclerosis by inhibiting expression of VEGF through the p38MAPK signaling pathway[43,44]. Simiao Yongan decoction can suppress vasa vasorum neovascularization and stabilize plaques by decreasing the expression levels of HIF-1α, MEK1/2 and ERK1/2[45]. In addition, Xiongshao capsule, Huoxue capsule, Shumai capsule, modified salvia decoction, Panax notoginseng saponins, Ruanmailing, Salvianolic acid B, Guishao Tongluo and Red yeast rice can also alleviate angiogenesis and attenuate atherosclerosis by decreasing VEGF expression[46-54]. Moreover, Buyang Huanwu decoction can promote microvessel maturation and decrease the incidence of plaque rupture by increasing the expression levels of bFGF and PDGF[55] (Table 2).

Table 2 Anti-angiogenic Effect of Chinese Herbal Medicines for ABCRS

Study ID	Objects	Chinese herbs and formulae	Study design	Composition of formula	Therapeutic effect and mechanisms
Ma et al. [43]	25 apoE-/- mice	Tongxinluo	Gavage with 0.38, 0.75, 1.5 g/kg/d for 5 weeks	*Panax ginseng* C. A. Meyer, *Hirudo nipponia* Whitman, Scorpio, *Radix paeoniae rubra*, Periostracum Cicadae, *Eupolyphaga Seu Steleophaga*, *Scolopendra subspinipes*, *Santalum album* Linn.	Decrease the expression level of VEGF, inhibit vasa vasorum proliferation, decrease microvessel density, reduce plaque areas
Liu et al. [44]	15 rabbits	Tongxinluo	Gavage with 0.6 g, 0.3 g/kg/d for 4 weeks	*Panax ginseng* C. A. Meyer, *Hirudo nipponia* Whitman, Scorpio, *Radix paeoniae rubra*, Periostracum Cicadae, *Eupolyphaga Seu* Steleophaga, *Scolopendra subspinipes*, *Santalum album* Linn.	Decrease the expression level of CD31, inhibit p38MAPK pathway, inhibit adventitia neovascularization
Li et al. [45]	15 apoE-/- mice	Simiao Yongan decoction	Gavage with 11.7 mg/kg/d for 8 weeks	*Lonicera japonica* Thunb., *Scrophularia ningpoensis* Hemsl., *Angelica sinensis* (Oliv.)Diels, *Glycyrrhiza uralensis* Fisch.	Decrease the expression levels of HIF-1α, CD34, MEK1/2 and ERK1/2, suppress vasa vasorum neovascularization, stabilize plaques
Zhang et al. [46]	10 rabbits	Xiongshao capsule	Gavage with 0.24 g, 0.48 g/kg/d for 6 weeks	*Ligusticum chuanxiong* Hort., *Radix paeoniae rubra*	Decrease the expression level of VEGF in plaque, reduce plaque areas
Ren et al. [47]	16 rabbits	Huoxue capsule	Gavage with 0.5 g, 1.5 g/kg/d for 20 weeks	*Astragalus membranaceus* (Fisch.) Bunge, Semen Persicae, *Carthamus* tinctorius Linn., *Achyranthes bidentata* Blume, Spina Date Seed, *Ligusticum chuanxiong* Hort., *Radix paeoniae rubra*, *Citrus aurantium* L.	Inhibit the expression levels of VEGF and VCAM-1 in plaque, reduce intima /tunica media thickness ratio
Qiao [48]	10 apoE-/- mice	Shumai capsule	Gavage with 700 mg, 3500 mg/kg/d for 12 weeks	*Astragalus mongholicus* Bunge, *Salvia miltiorrhiza* Bge, *Panaxpseudo-ginseng* N. Wallich, *Hirudo nipponica* Whitman, *Eupolyphaga sinensis* Walker, *Moschus berezovskii* Flerov, *Trichosanthes kirilowii* Maxim	Decrease the expression levels of VEGF, VEGFR, HIF-1α and Nox4, reduce plaque areas
Pan et al. [49]	30 patients	Modified salvia decoction	22 g/d po for 6 months	*Salvia miltiorrhiza* Bunge, *Santalum album* Linn., *Ligusticum chuanxiong* Hort., *Radix paeoniae rubra*, *Angelica sinensis* (Oliv.)Diels, *Rehmannia glutinosa* Libosch, *Carthamus tinctorius* Linn.	Decrease serum levels of VEGF, MMP-9 and CRP, reduce carotid intima media thickness, reduce plaque areas
Qiao et al. [50]	10 apoE-/- mice	Panax notoginseng saponins	Gavage with 60 mg/kg/d for 12 weeks	*Panax notoginseng* (Burk.)F. H. Chen	Decrease the expression levels of VEGF, CD34 and Nox4, alleviate plaque angiogenesis, reduce plaque areas

Continued

Study ID	Objects	Chinese herbs and formulae	Study design	Composition of formula	Therapeutic effect and mechanisms
Zeng et al. [51]	10 apoE-/- mice	Ruanmailing	Gavage with 20 g/kg/d for 12 weeks	*Fallopia multiflora* (Thunb.)Harald., *Rehmannia glutinosa* (Gaetn.) Libosch. ex Fisch. et Mey, Lycium chinense Miller, *Panax ginseng* C. A. Meyer, *Salvia miltiorrhiza* Bunge, *Angelica sinensis* (Oliv.)Diels, *Ligusticum chuanxiong* Hort.	Decrease the expression levels of VEGF, bFGF and CD105, inhibit plaque angiogenesis, stabilize plaques
Zheng et al. [52]	10 apoE-/ mice	Salvianolic acid B	Gavage with 80, 160 mg /kg/d for 8 weeks	Salvianolic acid B	Decrease the expression levels of CD31, reduce neovascularization in plaque and incidence of plaque erosion, stabilize plaques
Yin et al. [53]	24 rabbits	Guishao Tongluo	Gavage with 2.08, 4.16 g /kg/d for 4 weeks	Ramulus Cinnamomi, *Radix Paeoniae Alba*, *Salvia miltiorrhiza* Bunge, *Curcuma longa* Linn.	Decrease the expression levels of VEGF, VEGFR-2, inbibit adventitial neovascularization
Yang et al. [54]	60 patients	Red yeast rice	175 mg/d po for 6 months	Fermentum rubrum	Decrease the serum level of VEGF, reduce the density and areas of carotid plaque
Pang et al. [55]	20 rabbits	Buyang Huanwu decoction	Gavage with 20 g/d for 4 weeks	Astragalus mongholicus Bunge, *Ligusticum chuanxiong* Hort., *Angelica sinensis* (Oliv.)Diels, *Radix paeoniae rubra*, Semen Persicae, *Carthamus tinctorius* Linn., Lumbricus	Increase the expression levels of bFGF and PDGF, promote microvessel maturation, decrease the incidence of plaque rupture, stabilize plaques

2.3 Holistic Regulatory Effects

Chinese herbal medicine for ABCRS has a holistic regulatory effect on angiogenesis. It has been reported that Rhodiola rosea and Shexiang Baoxin Pill can promote angiogenesis and increase myocardial microvessel density by increasing the expression levels of HIF-1α, VEGF, VEGFR2 and CD34 while inhibiting vessel growth and decreasing plaque area in atherosclerosis by reducing these indexes in the aorta[56,57]. Another study has shown that the Xuefu Zhuyu decoction inhibits cell proliferation at certain concentrations and induces tube formation to a limited degree at low concentrations over a short time frame, suggesting that the Xuefu Zhuyu decoction controls angiogenesis in a different manner from that of the continuous function of VEGF[58]. In short, these studies imply that Chinese herbal medicines for ABCRS may have effects on balancing the regulation of angiogenesis and are thus safe for the coexistence of both myocardial ischemia and atherosclerotic lesions.

3 Discussion

The relationship between angiogenesis and CAD is double-sided[4], balancing the contradictory angiogenesis effects might facilitate drug efficacy in CAD. Chinese herbal medicines have an advantage over regulating the balance of the body in different pathological states. The data reviewed here suggest that Chinese herbal medicines for ABCRS results in holistic regulatory effects and providing a new option for treating CAD. The mechanisms may be related to the multi-component nature of Chinese herbal medicines, which may exhibit different effects in different pathological tissues through multiple targets and pathways. However, the deep mechanisms are complex and have yet to be clearly elucidated.

Modern research has indicated that angiogenesis within the vasa vasorum is characterized by a network of immature and leaky vessels, which plays an important role in plaque progression. Creating a mature network and normalizing plaque vessels may potentially minimize the risk of plaque hemorrhage[59]. In addition, EC metabolism including hypoxia-related fatty acid oxidation and glycolysis has gained attention as a therapeutic target for angiogenesis[60]. Therefore, interfering with vessel normalization/maturation and EC metabolism may be new directions to study the holistic regulatory effects of Chinese herbal medicines, which will bring new ideas to the clinical prevention and treatment of CAD.

To date, numerous studies have focused on angiogenesis in a myocardial ischemia model only or an atherosclerosis model only, while studies investigating angiogenesis in the context of both pathological changes and drug interventions are rare; there are mainly a few studies in this area[3, 56, 57, 61, 62]. Therefore, a desire exists to use compound models to study the double-edged roles of angiogenesis, therapeutic interventions and mechanisms, especially of the holistic regulatory effects of Chinese herbal medicines. In addition, we can screen the drugs and active components that can both promote ischemic angiogenesis and inhibit proliferative angiogenesis by network pharmacology and pharmacodynamics and further identify the targets and signaling pathways of holistic regulation on angiogenesis.

Until now, clinical studies have mainly focused on promoting angiogenesis, while inhibiting angiogenesis in atherosclerosis is in the experimental stage and has not been applied in clinical practice. Hence, future work remains to be done to validate the clinical results. Meanwhile, diseases are complex in patients with medications and multiple risk factors. Therefore, clinical studies on long-term follow-up after angiogenesis-targeted therapy are worthy of investigation. In addition, although clinical trials have been conducted to evaluate the efficacy of Chinese herbal medicines in CAD[63], there are just a few clinical studies on the regulation of angiogenesis using Chinese herbal medicines[34,49,54]. Hence, more clinical trials will be required to study and to determine the best means of therapeutic angiogenesis.

In conclusion, future studies are needed to investigate the holistic regulatory effects of Chinese herbal medicines for ABCRS on angiogenesis in terms of both basic studies and clinical research, and the mechanisms of the herbs involved need to be uncovered.

REFERENCES

[1] Faxon DP, Creager MA, Jr Smith SC, et al. Atherosclerotic vascular disease conference: executive summary: atherosclerotic vascular disease conference proceeding for healthcare professionals from a special writing group of the American heart association[J]. Circulation, 2004, 109 (21): 2595-2604.

[2] Organization WH. World health statistics 2016. Monitoring health for the SDGs Sustainable Development Goals[J]. Geneva Switzerland WHO. 2016, 2016, 41: 293-328.

[3] Theurl M, Schgoer W, Albrecht-Schgoer K, et al. Secretoneurin gene therapy improves hind limb and cardiac ischaemia in Apo E-/-mice without influencing systemic atherosclerosis[J]. Cardiovascular Research, 2015, 105 (1): 96-106.

[4] Wu W, Li X, Zuo G, et al. The Role of Angiogenesis in Coronary Artery Disease: A Double-Edged Sword: Intraplaque Angiogenesis in Physiopathology and Therapeutic Angiogenesis for Treatment[J]. Current Pharmaceutical Design, 2017, 24 (4): 451-464.

[5] Camaré, Caroline, Pucelle, Mélanie, Nègre-Salvayre, Anne, et al. Angiogenesis in the atherosclerotic plaque[J]. Redox Biology, 2017, 12: 18-34.

[6] Chen KJ. Development track of the modern activating blood circulation and removing stasis (ABCRS)school on inheritance and innovation[J]. Chin J Integr Med, 2015, 21 (12): 883-886.

[7] Tang J, Li S, Li Z, et al. Calycosin promotes angiogenesis involving estrogen receptor and mitogen-activated protein kinase (MAPK)signaling pathway in zebrafish and HUVEC[J]. Plos One, 2010, 5 (7): e11822.

[8] Franco C A, Liebner S, Gerhardt H. Vascular morphogenesis: a Wnt for every vessel? [J]. Current Opinion in Genetics & Development, 2009, 19 (5): 0-483.

[9] Folkman J, Klagsbrun M. Angiogenic Factors[J]. Science, 1987, 235 (4787): 442-447.

[10] Olsson AK, Dimberg A, Kreuger J, et al. VEGF receptor signalling in control of vascular function[J]. Nat Rev Mol Cell Biol, 2006, 7 (5): 359-371.

[11] Chen C, Li L, Zhou H, et al. The Role of NOX4 and TRX2 in Angiogenesis and Their Potential Cross-Talk[J]. Antioxidants, 2017, 6 (2): E42.

[12] Novakova V, Sandhu G S, Dragomir-Daescu D, et al. Apelinergic system in endothelial cells and its role in angiogenesis in myocardial ischemia[J]. Vascul Pharmacol, 2016, 76: 1-10.

[13] Mitsos S, Katsanos K, Koletsis E, et al. Therapeutic angiogenesis for myocardial ischemia revisited: basic biological concepts and focus on latest clinical trials[J]. Angiogenesis, 2012, 15 (1): 1-22.

[14] Wang J, Hong Z, Zeng C, et al. NADPH oxidase 4 promotes cardiac microvascular angiogenesis after hypoxia/reoxygenation in vitro[J]. Free

Radical Biology and Medicine, 2014, 69: 278-288.

[15] Silvia N, Chiara S, Daniele B. Notch Signaling in Ischemic Damage and Fibrosis: Evidence and Clues from the Heart[J]. Frontiers in Pharmacology, 2017, 8 (373): 187.

[16] Matsuura K, Honda A, Nagai T, et al. Transplantation of cardiac progenitor cells ameliorates cardiac dysfunction after myocardial infarction in mice[J]. Journal of Clinical Investigation, 2009, 119 (8): 2204-2217.

[17] van der Hoeven NW, Hollander MR, Yıldırım C, et al. The emerging role of galectins in cardiovascular disease[J]. Vascul Pharmacol, 2016, 81: 31-41.

[18] Moulton KS. Plaque angiogenesis and atherosclerosis[J]. Current Atherosclerosis Reports, 2001, 3 (3): 225-233.

[19] Bot I, Jukema JW, Lankhuizen IM, et al. Atorvastatin inhibits plaque development and adventitial neovascularization in ApoE deficient mice independent of plasma cholesterol levels[J]. Atherosclerosis, 2011, 214 (2): 295-300.

[20] Liu MH, Tang ZH, Li GH, et al. Janus-like role of fibroblast growth factor 2 in arteriosclerotic coronary artery disease: Atherogenesis and angiogenesis[J]. Atherosclerosis, 2013, 229 (1): 10-17.

[21] Bentzon JF, Otsuka F, Virmani R, et al. Mechanisms of Plaque Formation and Rupture[J]. Circulation Research, 2014, 114 (12): 1852-1866.

[22] Che J, Okigaki M, Takahashi T, et al. Endothelial FGF receptor signaling accelerates atherosclerosis[J]. Am J Physiol Heart Circ Physiol, 2011, 300 (1): H154-161.

[23] Sluimer JC, Gasc JM, Wanroij JLV, et al. Hypoxia, Hypoxia-Inducible Transcription Factor, and Macrophages in Human Atherosclerotic Plaques Are Correlated With Intraplaque Angiogenesis[J]. Journal of the American College of Cardiology, 2008, 51 (13): 1258-1265.

[24] Epstein SE, Stabile E, Kinnaird T, et al, Janus phenomenon: the interrelated tradeoffs inherent in therapies designed to enhance collateral formation and those designed to inhibit atherogenesis[J], Circulation, 2004, 109 (23): 2826-2831.

[25] Kastrup J, Jørgensen E, Fuchs S, et al. A randomised, double-blind, placebo-controlled, multicentre study of the safety and efficacy of BIOBYPASS (AdGVVEGF121.10NH)gene therapy in patients with refractory advanced coronary artery disease: the NOVA trial[J]. Eurointervention, 2011, 6 (7): 813-818.

[26] Stewart DJ, Kutryk MJ, Fitchett D, et al. VEGF Gene Therapy Fails to Improve Perfusion of Ischemic Myocardium in Patients With Advanced Coronary Disease: Results of the NORTHERN Trial[J]. Molecular Therapy, 2009, 17 (6): 1109-1115.

[27] Deray G, Janus N, Aloy B, et al. [Renovascular effects of antiangiogenic drugs[J]. Bulletin du cancer, 2016, 103 (7-8): 662-666.

[28] Chen KJ. Practical blood stasis syndrome. People's Medical Publishing House, 2013: 120-203.

[29] Chen YN, Yan P, Lin JM, et al, The effective influence of Xiongshao capsule on ischemic myocardium in rats with ultrasonography[J] Chin J Integr Med Cardio-/Cerebrovasc Dis, 2012, 10 (2): 191-192.

[30] Zeng X, He H, Yang J, et al. Temporal effect of Guanxin No. 2 on cardiac function, blood viscosity and angiogenesis in rats after long-term occlusion of the left anterior descending coronary artery[J]. Journal of Ethnopharmacology, 2008, 118 (3): 485-494.

[31] Bai WW, Xing YF, Wang B, et al. Tongxinluo Improves Cardiac Function and Ameliorates Ventricular Remodeling in Mice Model of Myocardial Infarction through Enhancing Angiogenesis[J]. Evidence-Based Complementray and Alternative Medicine, 2013, 2013 (1): 813247.

[32] Yao J. Effect of supplementing qi and activating blood circulation on the angiogenesis of rat ischemic cardiac microvascular endothelial cells and the expression of miR-223-3p and miR-132-5p in the plasma of patients with acute myocardial infarction[D]. Shandong Univ Chin. Med, 2015: 22-25.

[33] Zhang Q Y, Wang Q L, Jian-Feng S U, et al. Angiogenesis Effects of Xuefu Zhuyu Decoction and VEGF Protein Expression of Rats with Acute Myocardial Ischemia[J]. Chin J Inform Tradit Chin Med, 2011, 18 (2): 53-54.

[34] Li J. Effect of new Xuefuzhuyu soft capsule on the signs of blood stasis and angiogenesis in coronary heart disease[D]. Shandong Univ Chin Med. 2009: 1-6.

[35] Yin H, Zhang J, Lin H, et al. Effect of traditional Chinese medicine Shu-mai-tang on angiogenesis, arteriogenesis and cardiac function in rats with myocardial ischemia[J]. Phytotherapy Research PTR, 2009, 23 (1): 92-98.

[36] Xu DP, Zou DZ, Qiu HL et al, Traditional Chinese medicine Shenzhu Guanxin granules mitigate cardiac dysfunction and promote myocardium angiogenesis in myocardial infarction rats by upregulating PECAM-1/CD31 and VEGF expression[J]. Evid Based Complement Alternat Med, 2017, 2017 (1): 5261729.

[37] Yang BR, Cheung KK, Zhou X, et al. Amelioration of acute myocardial infarction by saponins from flower buds of Panax notoginseng via pro-angiogenesis and anti-apoptosis[J]. Journal of Ethnopharmacology, 2016, 181: 50-58.

[39] He H, Shi M, Yang X, et al. Comparison of cardioprotective effects using salvianolic acid B and benazepril for the treatment of chronic myocardial infarction in rats[J]. N-S Arch Pharmacol, vol. 378, no. 3, pp. 311-322, 2008.

[39] Wang ZT, Zhang SJ, Han LH, et al. Effects of xuesetong soft capsules on angiogenesis and VEGF mRNA expression in ischemic myocardium in rats with myocardial infarction[J]. Journal of Traditional Chinese Medicine, 2012, 32 (1): 71-74.

[40] Liu JG, Zhang DW, Li J, et al, Effect of *radix paeoniae rubra* 801 on angiogenesis in rats with myocardial infarction and bearing cancer[J]. Chin Circ J, 2011, 8 (26): 52.

[41] Chen J, Cao W, Asare PF, et al. Amelioration of Cardiac Dysfunction and Ventricular Remodeling after Myocardial Infarction by Danhong Injection are Critically Contributed by Anti-TGF-β-Mediated Fibrosis and Angiogenesis Mechanisms[J]. J Ethnopharmacol, 2016, 194: 559-570.

[42] Zhou ZY, Huan LY, Zhao WR, et al. Spatholobi Caulis, extracts promote angiogenesis in HUVECs in vitro and in zebrafish embryos in vivo via

up-regulation of VEGFRs[J]. J Ethnopharmacol, 2017, 200: 74-83.

[43] Ma L, Ni M, Hao P, et al. Tongxinluo mitigates atherogenesis by regulating angiogenic factors and inhibiting vasa vasorum neovascularization in apolipoprotein E-deficient mice[J]. Oncotarget, 2016, 7 (13): 16194-16204.

[44] Meizhi L, Zhenhua J, Cong W, et al. Influence of Tongxinluo Ultrafine Powder on Early Atherosclerotic Epicardial Angiogenesis[J]. J Tradit Chin Med, 2015, 56 (3): 240-244.

[45] Li M, Zhang JP, Zhu K, et al, Experimental study of Simiao Yongan decoction regulating vasa vasorum remodeling in ApoE-/-mice with atherosclerosis vulnerable plague[J]. World Sci Technol/Mod Tradit Chin Med Mater Med, 2017, 19 (12): 1989-1997.

[46] Zhang L, Jiang YR, Guo CY, et al. Effects of active components ofRed PaeoniaandRhizoma chuanxiongon angiogenesis in atherosclerosis plaque in rabbits[J]. Chinese Journal of Integrative Medicine, 2009, 15 (5): 359-364.

[47] Ren DZ, Liu QS, Li J, et al, Effects of Huoxue capsule on expression of VEGF and VCAM-1 in rabbits with arteriosclerosis[J], Chin J Exp Tradit Med Formu, 2014, 20 (21): 167-170.

[48] Qiao Y. Effect and mechanism of Shumai capsule on atherosclerotic plaque angiogenesis[D], Shandong Univ, 2014: 70-86.

[49] Pan XP, Huang ZD, Yang WF. Effects of ultramicro-Jiawei Danshen Yin on serum VEGF, MMP-9 of patients with primary hyperlipidemia and carotid atherosclerotic[J], Guid J Tradit Chin Med Pharm, 2015, 21 (16): 21-24.

[50] Qiao Y, Zhang PJ, Lu XT, et al. Panax notoginseng saponins inhibits atherosclerotic plaque angiogenesis by down-regulating vascular endothelial growth factor and nicotinamide adenine dinucleotide phosphate oxidase subunit 4 expression[J]. Chinese Journal of Integrative Medicine, 2015, 21 (4): 259-265.

[51] Zeng XY. Effect of Ruanmailing oral liquid on angiogenesis in experimental atherosclerotic plaque[D], Fujian Med Univ, 2010: 5-6.

[52] Fang Z, Mao-Juan G, Li-Yan GU, et al. Effects of Salvianolic Acid B on Stability of Atherosclerotic Plaque in Apolipoprotein E Gene Knock-out Mice Treated with STZ and High Fat Diet[J]. Chinese Journal of Arteriosclerosis, 2011, 19 (11): 885-890.

[53] Jie YY, Yi ML, Geng W, et al. Influence of Guishaotongluo on angiogenesis of adventitial vasa vasorum and oxidative stress in early stage of atherosclerosis[J]. Chin Pharmacol Bull, 2016, 32 (3): 416-422.

[54] Yang JH, He YT, Yuan AL, et al, Effect of lipid-lowering Hongqu micropowder on serum vascular endothelial growth factor level and plaque stability in patients with carotid atherosclerosis[J], Chin J Clin Ration Drug Use, 2015, 8 (9A): 82-83.

[55] Pang XL, Yang L, Zeng WY, et al, Research the mechanism of Buyang Huanwu decoction on angiogenesis in vulnerable plaque in rabbits[J], Tianjin J Tradit Chin Med, 2015, 32 (11): 672-674.

[56] Shen W. Empirical study to compare the mechanism of angiogenesis in atherosclerosis and ischemic myocardium and to perform the medicine interventions for them[D]. Fudan Univ, 2008: 79-81.

[57] Shen W, Fan WH, Shi HM. Effects of shexiang baoxin pill on angiogenesis in atherosclerosis plaque and ischemic myocardium[J]. Zhongguo Zhong Xi Yi Jie He Za Zhi, 2010, 30 (12): 1284-1287.

[58] Fan L, Bin-Ling C, Yi-Zheng W, et al. In vitro angiogenesis effect of Xuefu Zhuyu Decoction and vascular endothelial growth factor: a comparison study[J]. Chin J Integr Med, 2015: 1-7.

[59] Goel S, Duda D G, Xu L, et al. Normalization of the Vasculature for Treatment of Cancer and Other Diseases[J]. Physiological Reviews, 2011, 91 (3): 1071-1121.

[60] Wong BW, Marsch E, Treps L, et al. Endothelial cell metabolism in health and disease: impact of hypoxia[J]. The EMBO Journal, 2017, 36 (15): 2187-2203.

[61] Shen W, Shi HM, Fan WH, et al. The effects of simvastatin on angiogenesis: studied by an original model of atherosclerosis and acute myocardial infarction in rabbit[J]. Molecular Biology Reports, 2011, 38 (6): 3821-3828.

[62] Xiao JM, Wan WH, Xu J. Effect of Rhodobryum roseum Limpr. on atherosclerosis and ischemic myocardial angiogenesis in rabbits, Chin J Mult Organ Dis Elderly, 2014, 13 (12): 935-940.

[63] Zhang J, Meng H, Zhang Y, et al. The Therapeutical Effect of Chinese Medicine for the Treatment of Atherosclerotic Coronary Heart Disease[J]. Current Pharmaceutical Design, 2017, 23 (34): 5086-5096.

First published: Yuan R, Shi WL, Xin QQ, Chen KJ, Cong WH. Holistic regulation of angiogenesis with Chinese herbal medicines as a new option for coronary artery disease[J], Evid Based Complement Alternat Med, 2018, 2018: 3725962.

Paeoniflorin Promotes Angiogenesis in A Vascular Insufficiency Model of Zebraflh in *vivo* and in Human Umbilical Vein Endothelial Cells in *vitro*

XIN Qi-qi, YANG Bin-rui, ZHOU He-feng, WANG Yan, YI Bo-wen, CONG Wei-hong, LEE Simon Ming-yuen, and CHEN Ke-ji

At present, ischemic cardio-cerebral vascular diseases remain the biggest killer worldwide.[1]Although there have been major advances in treatment during the past two decades, the mortality rates of these diseases remain high due to drug resistance, poor drug delivery, surgical contraindication and complications. As a result, it is meaningful to seek other effective treatment methods. Therapeutic angiogenesis is a treatment option for patients that opens the way for use of Chinese medicine (CM)to treat ischemic cardio-cerebral vascular disease. [2]

Angiogenesis refers to the establishment of the mature blood vessel network through expansion and remodeling of the pre-existing vascular primordium. [3]It naturally occurs during wound-healing, the female menstrual cycle and pregnancy and can be activated in ischemic diseases such as ischemic heart disease and stroke.

In ischemic pathological conditions, insufficient oxygen and nutrients is a serious threat to tissue viability and leads to poor outcome. Angiogenesis could protect ischemic tissues and improve prognosis. [4]In response to ischemia, injured tissues release angiogenic factors, including vascular endothelial growth factor (VEGF), epidermal growth factor (EGF), and fibroblast growth factor (FGF). Endothelial cells are activated by the angiogenic factors and release proteases inducing basement membrane degradation and vascular permeability increase. Then, endothelial cells proliferate and migrate into the interstitial space and assemble as solid cords that subsequently acquire a lumen. Theoretically, any changes in the process of angiogenesis will affect the formation of new blood vessels.

Paeoniae Rubra Radix, the dried root of *Paeonia lactiflora* Pallas or *Paeonia veitchii* Lynch, is one of the most commonly used traditional Chinese herbal medicines. As a herbal medicine typically used for activating blood circulation and removing blood stasis, *Paeoniae Rubra Radix* is a constituent of many CM prescriptions, such as Xuefu Zhuyu Decoction (血府逐瘀汤)and Buyang Huanwu Decoction (补阳还五汤), which have shown evidences of clinical efflcacy in treating ischemic heart disease and stroke, respectively. Previous studies showed that *Paeoniae Rubra Radix*, Xuefu Zhuyu Decoction [5, 6]and Buyang Huanwu Decoction [7]could promote angiogenesis in chick embryo chorio-allantoic membrane (CAM)and ischemic brains. It is important to identify the bioactive pro-angiogenic component of *Paeoniae Rubra Radix*.

Paeoniflorin (PF, Figure 1)is one of the principal components of *Paeoniae Rubra Radix*. Previous studies showed that PF exhibited signiflcant protective effects against ischemia in numerous experimental cardio-cerebral vascular system injuries；the protective effects involved multiple mechanisms, such as anti-apoptosis, anti-thrombosis, anti-inflammation, activation of adenosine receptor. [8-13]Although many studies have been carried out on the mechanisms underlying the beneflcial effects of PF in ischemic diseases, it is still unknown as to whether it could promote angiogenesis.

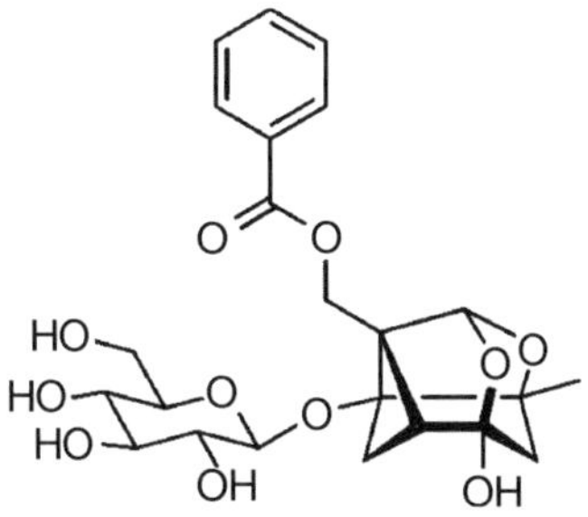

Figure 1 Chemical Structure of PF

METHODS

1 Ethics Statement

All animal experiments were conducted according to the ethical guidelines of Institute of Chinese Medical Sciences, University of Macau and Xiyuan Hospital, China Academy of Chinese Medical Sciences. The protocol was approved by Institute of Chinese Medical Sciences—Animal Ethics Committee of the University of Macau and Ethics Committee of Xiyuan Hospital of China Academy of Chinese Medical Sciences.

2 Chemicals and Reagents

Human umbilical vein endothelial cells (HUVECs)were obtained from ATCC (USA). Kaighn's modification of Ham's F12 medium (F-12 K), fetal bovine serum (FBS), 0.25% (w/v)trypsin/1 mmol/L ethylene diamine tetraacetic acid (EDTA), phosphate-buffered saline (PBS)and penicillin-streptomycin (PS)were all purchased from Invitrogen (Carlsbad, CA, USA). Endothelial cell growth supplement (ECGS), heparin and collagen were supplied by Sigma (St Louis, MO, USA). Dimethyl sulfoxide (DMSO)was obtained from Sigma (USA). VEGF receptor tyrosine kinase inhibitor Ⅱ (VRI)was purchased from Calbiochem Company (Merck KGaA, Darmstadt, Germany)and dissolved in DMSO to get a 500 μg/mL solution. PF was acquired from the Chinese National Institute for Control of Pharmaceutical and Biological Products (Beijing, China), which was dissolved in DMSO at a stock concentration of 100 mmol/L. TaqMan Universal PCR Master Mix and 250nmol/L custom TaqMan primers for zebraflsh fms-like tyrosine kinase-1 (flt-1), kinase insert domain receptor (kdr), kinase insert domain receptor like (kdrl)and von Willebrand factor (vWF)were purchased from Applied Biosystems (Indianapolis, IN, USA).

3 Maintenance of Zebraflsh and Its Embryos

Tg (fli-*1: EGFP)y1* transgenic zebraflsh were used in this study. All zebraflsh were maintained as described in the Zebraflsh Handbook.[14] Enhanced green fluorescent protein (EGFP)is expressed in all endothelial cells of *Tg* (fli-*1: EGFP)y1* zebraflsh embryos.

4 Zebraflsh Embryos Preparation

Zebraflsh were kept separately in 14 h light/10 h dark cycle water circulation system. Zebraflsh embryos were generated by natural pair-wise mating (3–12 months old)and were raised at 28.5 ℃ in embryo water. And the healthy embryos collection was performed according to the previous methods. [15]

5 Drug Treatment on Zebraflsh

VRI was used to establish vascular insufflciency model, which is a pyridinyl-anthranilamide compound that displays anti-angiogenic properties and strongly inhibits the kinase activities of both VEGF receptors 1 and 2. The 24 h post fertilization (hpf)zebrafish were treated with 300 ng/mL VRI for 3 h, and then distributed into 24-well plate (10 embryos per well). VRI was washed out and replaced with PF of different concentrations (6.25, 12.5, 25, 50 and 100 μmol/L). Embryos treated with embryo water containing 0.1% DMSO only served as vehicle control. Zebrafish embryos were raised in incubator at 28 ℃ for 24 h before morphological observation.

6 Morphological Observation of Zebraflsh

Zebrafish embryos were placed on glass slices and observed for viability and morphological changes with a fluorescence microscope (Olympus IX81 Motorized Inverted Microscope, Japan)which equipped with a digital camera (DP controller, Soft Imaging System, Olympus, Germany). To evaluate the effects of PF treatment on angiogenesis, the numbers of intact and defective intersegmental vessels (ISVs)sprouting were assessed. Images were analyzed with Adobe Photoshop 7.0.

7 Total RNA Extraction, Reverse Transcription, and Real-Time Polymerase Chain Reaction

The 24 hpf zebrafish embryos were collected, distributed to 5 groups (30 embryos per group), and subsequently treated with 300 ng/mL VRI for 3 h. VRI was washed out and replaced with PF (25, 50 and 100 μmol/L)or embryo water (with 0.1% DMSO)for 6 h. Total RNA was extracted with RNeasy mini kit (Qiagen, USA), and converted into cDNA with SuperScript™ Ⅲ flrst-strand synthesis system for real-time polymerase chain reaction (RT-PCR, Invitrogen™, USA). Then real-time PCR was performed in the ABI ViiA™ 7 PCR system (Applied Biosystems). The expression of flt-1, kdr, kdrl and vWF mRNA were normalized to the amount of β-actin 1, using the relative quantiflcation method described by the manufacturer.

The RNA primers used in this study were designed according to the database of Applied Biosystems (USA)as below: flt-1: 5'-AACTCACAGACCAGTGAACAAGATC-3'(F)and5'-GCCCTGTAACGTGTGCACTAAA-3'(R); kdrl: 5'-GACCATAAAACAAGTGAGGCAGAAG-3'(F)and5'-CTCCTGGTTTGACAGAGCGATA-3'(R); kdr: 5'-CAAGTAACTCGTTTTCTCAACCTAAGC-3'(F)and 5'-GGTCTGCTACACAACGCATTATAAC-3'(R); vWF: 5'-CTCCGTTTGACCGCAAAA-3'(F)and 5'-ACAGCAGGTGTCTCCGATCT-3'(R); β-actin1: 5'-CATCGGCAATGAGCGTTTCC-3'(F)and5'-CAAGATTCCATACCCAGGAAGGA-3'(R).

8 HUVEC Culture

HUVECs were cultured in F-12K medium with 2 mmol/L L-glutamine, 1.5 g/L sodium bicarbonate, 100 μg/mL heparin, 30 mg/mL endothelial cell growth supplement and 10% FBS at 37 ℃ in a humidified atmosphere of 5% CO_2. Tissue culture flasks and 96-well plates were pre-coated with 0.2% collagen. All experiments were conducted using HUVECs of passages 2 to 8.

9 Cell Proliferation by MTT Assay

HUVECs were seeded at 10^4 cells/well in 96-well collagen coated plates. After 24 h, cells were starved in 0.5% FBS medium for 12 h. Then HUVECs were treated with PF (0.001, 0.003, 0.01 and 0.03 μmol/L). Cells receiving DMSO (0.1%)served as vehicle control, and cells treated with 20 ng/mL VEGF served as positive control. After 30 h, cell proliferation was determined by 3- (4, 5-dimethylthiazol-2-yl)-2, 5-diphenyltetrazolium bromide (MTT)assay and the data were expressed as optical density (OD)value.

10 Wound Healing Assay

HUVECs were seeded in 48-well collagen coated plates at 10^4 cells/well. After 12 h, confluent HUVECs were scratched with a pipette tip. Images were taken as baseline with inverted microscope (In Cell Analyzer 2000, General electrics, USA). Then HUVECs were treated with PF (0.3, 1 and 10 μmol/L)for 10 h. Meanwhile, wells containing DMSO (0.1%)and 20 ng/mL VEGF served as the vehicle and positive control, respectively. Images were taken to record the invasion of HUVECs. Migration was quantifled as the difference value of the width of the area covered with cells and the area of the cell-free wound.

11 Tube Formation Assay

Confluent HUVECs were harvested and diluted (96×10^4 cells)in 500 μL low serum medium containing 0.3–10 μmol/L PF, which were then seeded on 1: 1 matrigel (v/v)coated 24-well plates in triplicate at 37 ℃ for 4 h. Cells treated by DMSO (0.1%)and 20 ng/mL VEGF were served as vehicle and positive control, respectively. The network-like structures were examined under an inverted microscope (50 × magnification). The number of branching points in 3 random fields per well was quantified by Metamorph Imaging Series software.

12 Statistical Analysis

Each experiment was repeated 3 times at least. Data were analyzed with unpaired two-tailed Student's t-tests or one-way ANOVA followed by Tukey's multiple comparison test. Chart was made with GraphPad Prism 5.0 software (San Diego, CA). All relevant data were presented as mean ± standard error of mean ($\bar{x}$ ± SEM). Differences were considered as signiflcant at $P < 0.05$.

RESULTS

1 PF Rescued VRI-Induced Blood Vessel Loss in Zebraflsh Embryos

ISVs sprouted and elongated from the dorsal aorta and posterior cardinal vein to dorsal longitudinal anastomotic vessels (DLAVs)were considered as intact vessels. As shown in Figure 2A, ISVs' growth was suppressed significantly by pretreatment with 300 ng/mL VRI for 3 h in *Tg* (*fli-1: EGFP)y1* zebrafish embryos (Figure 2A). DLAVs and ISVs growth was rescued after incubation with PF for 24 h at concentrations of 6.25, 12.5, 25, 50, and 100 μmol/L. Quantitative analysis showed that PF acted in a dose-dependent manner to rescue the VRI-induced blood vessel loss (Figure 2B).

PF Increased flt-1, kdr, kdrl and vWF Genes Expression in Zebraflsh Embryos In order to identify the molecular targets of the angiogenic effects of PF in zebrafish, real-time PCR was performed to evaluate the gene expression of flt-1, kdr, kdrl and vWF. As shown in Figure 3, flt-1, kdr, kdrl and vWF mRNA expression were signiflcantly down-regulated by VRI treatment (300 ng/mL for 3 h)and restored by PF treatment (25, 50 and 100 μmol/L for 6 h).

2 PF Promoted HUVEC Proliferation

As shown in Figure 4, treatment with PF (0.001, 0.003, 0.01 and 0.03 μmol/L)for 30 h enhanced HUVECs proliferation signiflcantly ($P < 0.01$), compared with the control group. We observed that increasing concentrations of PF from 0.001 to 0.03 μmol/L was associated with a decrease in the pro-angiogenic effect.

3 PF Promoted Wound Healing

As shown in Figure 5A, after treatment with PF (1.0 and 10 μmol/L), HUVECs showed a remarkably increased ability to migrate. Quantitative analysis showed that PF (1.0 and 10 μmol/L)promoted HUVECs invasion signiflcantly (Figure 5B). As a positive control, treatment with VEGF also enhanced HUVECs invasion significantly, conflrming the validity of the assay system.

4 PF Stimulated Capillary Tube Formation of HUVECs

Under appropriate experimental condition, HUVECs can form a tube-like structure on matrigel. In this study, VEGF strongly promoted HUVECs to form a tube-like structure, and PF (0.3 μmol/L)treatment enhanced the tube-forming ability of HUVECs (Figure 6A). Quantitative measurements showed that PF (0.3 μmol/L)significantly enhanced the number of tube branch points (Figure 6B). Thus, PF enhanced the ability of HUVECs to form tube-like structures.

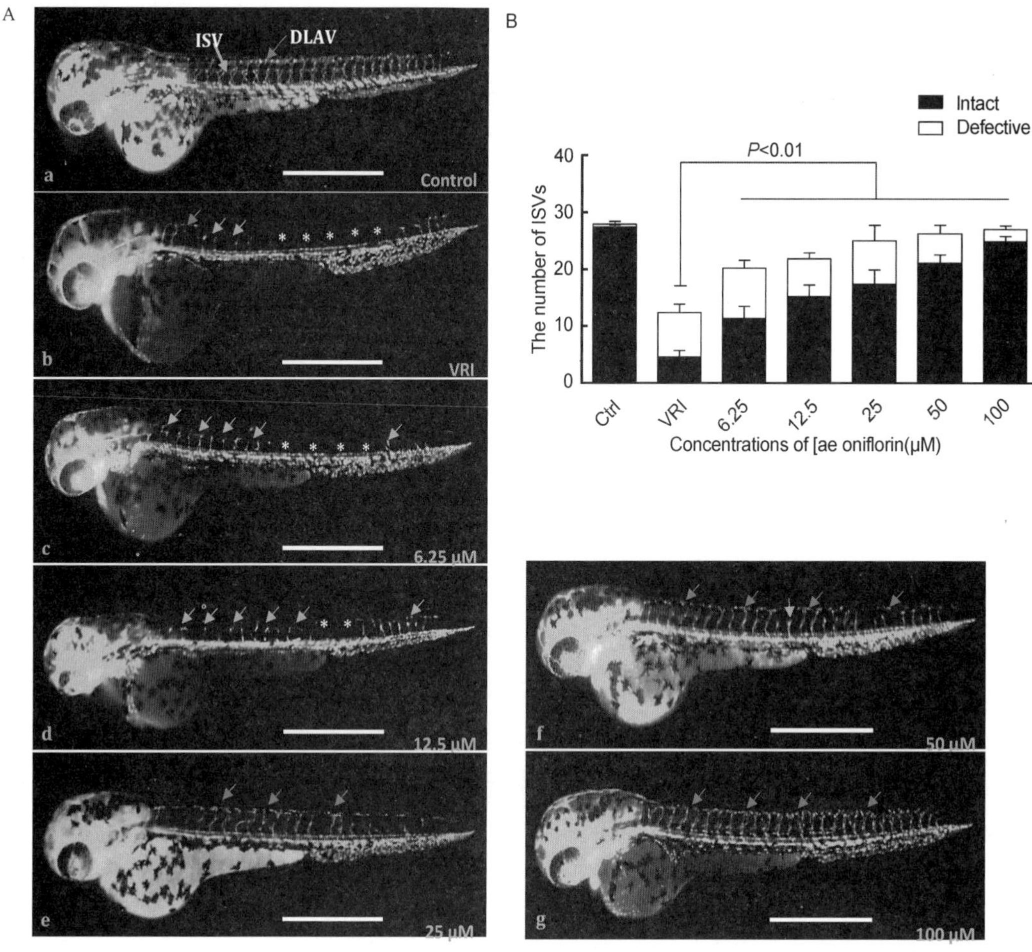

Figure 2　PF Rescued VRI-Induced Blood Vessel Loss in *Tg* (fl*i-1: EGFP)y1* Zebraflsh Embryos (n=3, $\bar{x} \pm$ SEM)

Notes: A: VRI induced ISV, DLAV loss in zebraflsh embryos. PF rescued VRI-induced blood vessel loss. Orange and blue arrows indicate ISVs and DLAVs, respectively. B: Quantitative analysis showed PF acted in a dose-dependent manner to rescued VRI-induced blood vessel loss ($P < 0.01$). White scale bar = 1.0 mm.

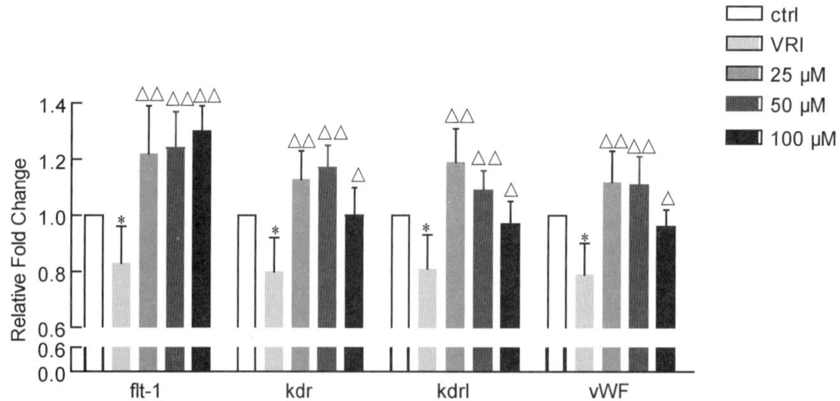

Figure 3　PF Increased flt-1, kdr, kdrl and vWF Genes Expression in Zebraflsh Embryos (n=3, $\bar{x} \pm$ SEM)

Notes: flt-1, kdr, kdrl and vWF mRNA expression were signiflcantly down regulated by VRI treatment (300 ng/mL for 3 h)and restored by PF treatment (25, 50 and 100 μmol/L for 6 h). $P < 0.05$, compared with the control group； $^{\triangle}P < 0.05$, $^{\triangle\triangle}P < 0.01$, compared with the VRI treatment group.

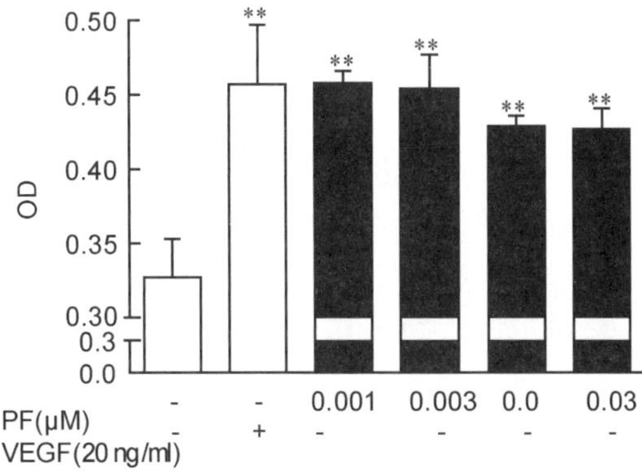

Figure 4 PF Promoted HUVECs Proliferation (n=3, $\bar{x}\pm$SEM)

Notes: MTT assay was applied for determining HUVECs proliferation. PF (0.001, 0.003, 0.01 and 0.03 μmol/L)treating for 30 h promoted HUVECs viability significantly. $P < 0.01$, compared with the control group.

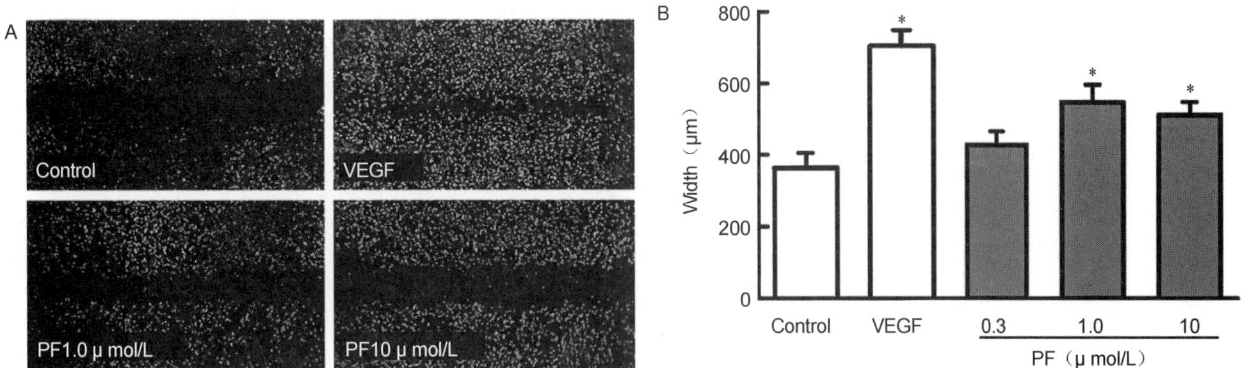

Figure 5 PF Promoted HUVECs Migration (n=3, $\bar{x}\pm$SEM)

Notes: A: Microscopic images (50×)showing the effect of PF on HUVECs migration. B: Quantitative analysis showed PF (1.0 and 10 μmol/L)promoted HUVECs migration significantly. $P < 0.01$, compared with the control group.

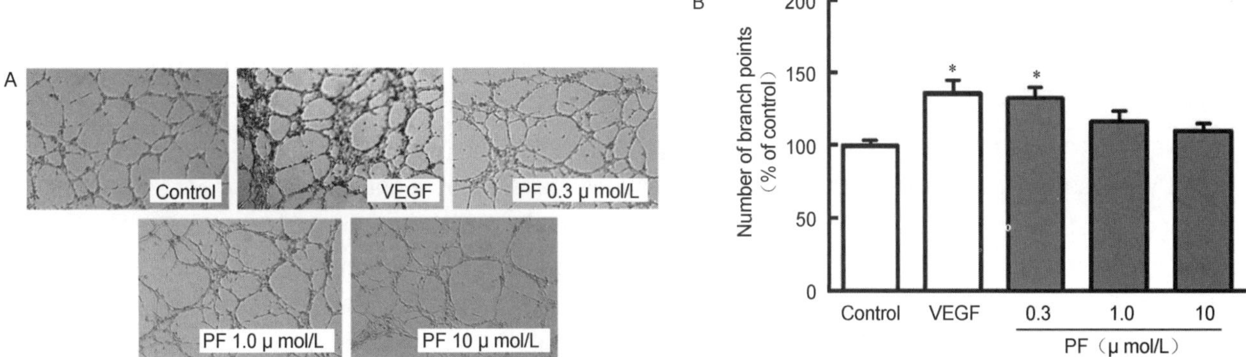

Figure 6 Effects of PF on HUVECs Tube Formation (n=3, $\bar{x}\pm$SEM)

Notes: The network like structures were examined under an inverted microscope (50×). A: VEGF strongly promoted HUVECs to form tube like structure, and PF (0.3 μmol/L)treatment enhanced the tube formation in HUVECs. B: Quantitative analysis showed that PF (0.3 μmol/L)significantly enhanced the branch point numbers in HUVECs. $P < 0.05$, compared with the control group.

DISCUSSION

Since the 1960s, Western and Chinese medicine (IWCM), especially for treating blood stasis syndrome according to the principle of activating blood circulation and removing blood stasis, has been made.[16]

According to the IWCM theory, ischemic cardio-cerebral vascular diseases are associated with blood stasis syndrome, and could be treated by activating blood circulation and ceasing blood stasis therapy. Xuefu Zhuyu Decoction and Buyang Huanwu Decoction have been the most commonly used decoctions for cardio-cerebral vascular diseases over the past two centuries and have shown significant protective effects in both clinical and experimental studies. [17, 18] Furthermore, several decoctions derived from Xuefu Zhuyu Decoction, such as Coronary Heart Ⅱ (冠心Ⅱ号方), Xueguantong (血管通), and Xiongshao Capsule (芎芍胶囊), have shown protective effects against ischemic cardio-cerebral vascular diseases, the mechanisms of which relate to anti-platelet marked progress in integrating aggregation, anti-angina, anti-atherosclerosis and improvement of cerebral blood flow. [19-22] Among the above-mentioned decoctions, *Paeoniae Rubra Radix* is the most commonly used and is a representative herb for activating blood circulation and removing blood stasis in CM. Meanwhile, several bioactive components of *Paeoniae Rubra Radix* have proven effective against ischemic cardio-cerebral vascular diseases including *Paeoniae Radix* 801, d-catechin and PF (the pharmacological mechanisms of which include anti-platelet aggregation, anti-inflammation, anti-atherosclerosis and anti-hyperlipidemia). [23-25]

During the past two decades, therapeutic angiogenesis has become a hot topic in the treatment of ischemic cardio-cerebral vascular diseases. The fact that Chinese herbal medicines for activating blood circulation and removing blood stasis exhibit strong pro-angiogenic activity provides a theoretical foundation and opens up the possibly of using such herbs to treat ischemic diseases. Earlier studies showed that *Paeoniae Rubra Radix* could promote angiogenesis, yet the effective monomer is still unclear. [6]PF is the major bioactive ingredient of *Paeoniae Rubra Radix*; therefore, we investigated whether it could promote angiogenesis in HUVECs and in a vascular insufflciency model of zebraflsh, as well as the relevant mechanisms of action.

In this study, PF was proven to promote angiogenesis, by rescuing chemical-induced vascular insufflciency in zebraflsh, and to promote proliferation, migration and tube formation in HUVECs. These results provide impetus for further research on PF for cardio-cerebral vascular diseases.

In the present study, we found that VRI could induce ISVs insufficiency and down regulate flt-1, kdr and kdrl mRNA expression in zebrafish embryos. The results are consistent with a previous study by Li, et al.[26] which proved that VRI could cause vascular insufflciency in zebraflsh embryo by inducing endothelial cell apoptosis and down-regulating the gene expression of flt-1, kdr and kdrl. Our current results showed that PF (6.25–100 μmol/L)could rescue VRI induced vascular insufficiency and PF (25–100 μmol/L), thereby restoring the mRNA expression of flt-1, kdr, kdrl and vWF genes, which are down-regulated by VRI in transgenic zebrafish. Morphological changes indicate that PF possesses pro-angiogenic activity. Furthermore, the results pertaining to mRNA expression indicate that the activation of angiogenesis-related signaling pathways is involved in the pharmacological mechanisms of the pro-angiogenic effect of PF. The flt-1 gene encodes VEGF receptor 1 in zebrafish, and the kdr and kdrl genes encodes VEGF receptor 2.[27-29]According to our real-time PCR results, PF has a tendency to upregulate expression of VEGF receptors 1 and 2. VEGF-related signaling pathways are essential in regulating endothelial angiogenesis. VEGF receptor 1 (flt-1)activation could promote endothelial cell proliferation, and VEGF receptor 2 (kdr/kdrl)plays an important role in angiogenesis in endothelial cells. [30-32] vWF is a glycoprotein produced uniquely by endothelial cells and megakaryocytes and could be an indicator of endothelial cell function and cell count. [33] The upregulation of vWF mRNA, which could be regulated by the VEGF signaling pathway, might indicate improvement of endothelial cell function. Thus, these results further support the hypothesis that the phenotypic changes occurred due to angiogenesis stimulation. Furthermore, the VEGF signaling pathway may be involved in mechanisms of action of the pro-angiogenic effect of PF.

Endothelial cells are the major target of the VEGF signaling pathway. In order to further confirm the pro-angiogenic effect of PF, we investigated our hypothesis in HUVECs. Proliferation, migration and tube formation are three major steps involved in angiogenesis in endothelial cells. Our work revealed that PF (0.001–0.03 μmol/L)could promote the proliferation of HUVECs, and it also stimulated HUVECs migration at 1.0–

10 μmol/L, and promoted tube formation at 0.3 μmol/L. Taken together, our data demonstrated that PF might promote angiogenesis by stimulating HUVECs proliferation, migration, and tube formation *in vitro*. However, the effective concentrations of PF in the three steps of angiogenesis in the present study are very different. This might be due to the different concentrations of PF activating different angiogenesis signaling pathways. Although few study has been carried out to identify bioequivalent doses between cell cultures and zebraflsh, our results suggest that PF, at least in part, exerts direct action upon endothelial cells.

Over the past few years, successful preclinical studies and promising results from early clinical trials have created great excitement regarding the potential of therapeutic angiogenesis for patients with advanced ischemic heart disease. [34] However, the results for ischemic cerebral vascular disease are not satisfactory. [35] Drug delivery remains the main challenge of central nervous system drug development, because of the generally poor diffusion through the blood-brain barrier and the blood-spinal cord barrier. PF has been reported to cross the blood-brain barrier [36, 37] and exhibit protective effects against ischemic stroke.[38] Thus, it is important to confirm if there is a protective effect of PF against ischemic stroke in humans.

PF has been reported to exhibit significant protective effects in HUVECs in an anoxia model, and against injury induced by advanced glycation end products. [13, 38] In these previous studies, the effective concentration range of PF in HUVECs was from 12.5 to 1 000 μmol/L, while in our study it was much lower, only from 0.001 to 10 μmol/L. One possible reason is that in the previous studies, HUVECs were pretreated with PF for only several hours before exposure to pathologic conditions, while in our experiments HUVECs were treated with PF for a much longer period of time under normal conditions.

One limitation of our study is that the experiments were carried out in HUVECs, a mammalian cell model *in vitro*, and zebrafish, a non-mammalian vertebrate model organism *in vivo*. Further work should be done using higher level mammalian animals, such as rat, rabbit and dog. In addition, the results of our experiments implied that the VEGF receptor signaling pathway maybe involved in the mechanisms of action of PF. However, the exact molecular targets are still unknown. As PF treatment at different concentrations exerts different effects in different periods during pathological development of ischemic diseases in laboratory experiments, it seems important to choose an appropriate PF dose and treatment time window for clinical use.

In conclusion, the present study revealed that PF could promote angiogenesis in a vascular insufflciency model of zebraflsh *in vivo* and in HUVECs *in vitro*, and that the activation of the VEGF signaling pathway was a candidate mechanism of PF's pro-angiogenic action.

REFERENCES

[1] World Health Organization. The top 10 causes of death fact sheet No 310. WHO http: //www. who. int/mediacentre/ factsheets/fs310/en/ (May 2014, date last accessed).

[2] Ferrara N, Kerbel RS. Angiogenesis as a therapeutic target. [J] Nature 2005；438: 967-974.

[3] Franco CA, Liebner S, Gerhardt H. Vascular morphogenesis: a Wnt for every vessel? Curr Opin Genet Dev 2009；19: 476-483.

[4] Krupinski J, Kaluza J, Kumar P, Kumar S, Wang JM. Role of angiogenesis in patients with cerebral ischemic stroke. Stroke 1994；25: 1794-1798.

[5] Lin F, Chen BL, Wang YZ, Gao D, Song J, Kaptchuk TJ, et al. *In vitro* angiogenesis effect of Xuefu Zhuyu Decoction and vascular endothelial growth factor: a comparison study. Chin J Integr Med 2015. [Epub ahead of print]

[6] Gao D, Song J, Hu J, Lin JM, Zheng LP, Cai J, et al. Angiogenesis promoting effects of Chinese herbal medicine for activating blood circulation to remove stasis on chick embryo chorio-allantoic membrane. Chin J Integr Tradit West Med (Chin)2005；25: 912-915.

[7] Shen J, Zhu Y, Yu H, Fan ZX, Xiao F, Wu P, et al. Buyang Huanwu decoction increases angiopoietin-1 expression and promotes angiogenesis and functional outcome after focal cerebral ischemia. J Zhejiang Univ Sci B 2014；15: 272-280.

[8] Liu DZ, Xie KQ, Ji XQ, Ye Y, Jiang CL, Zhu XZ. Neuroprotective effect of paeoniflorin on cerebral ischemic rat by activating adenosine A1 receptor in a manner different from its classical agonists. Br J Pharmacol 2005；146: 604-611.

[9] Tang NY, Liu CH, Hsieh CT, Hsieh CL. The anti-inflammatory effect of paeoniflorin on cerebral infarction induced by ischemia-reperfusion injury in Sprague-Dawley rats. Am J Chin Med 2010；38: 51-64.

[10] Nizamutdinova IT, Jin YC, Kim JS, Yean MH, Kang SS, Kim YS, et al. Paeonol and paeoniflorin, the main active principles of Paeonia albiflora, protect the heart from myocardial ischemia/reperfusion injury in rats. Planta Med 2008；74: 14-18.

[11] Zhang Y, Li H, Huang M, Huang M, Chu K, Xu W, et al. Paeoniflorin, a monoterpene glycoside, protects the brain from cerebral ischemic injury via inhibition of apoptosis. Am J Chin Med 2015； 43: 543-557.

[12] Ji QL, Yang LN, Zhou J, Lin R, Zhang JY, Lin QQ, et al. Protective effects of paeoniflorin against cobalt chloride-induced apoptosis of endothelial cells via HIF-1α pathway. Toxicol In Vitro 2012； 26: 455-461.

[13] Ye JF, Duan HL, Yang XM, Yan WM, Zheng XX. Anti-thrombosis effect of paeoniflorin: evaluated in a photochemical reaction thrombosis model *in vivo*. Planta Med 2001； 67: 766-767.

[14] Westerfield M, ed. The zebrafish book. A guide for the laboratory use of Zebraflsh (Danio rerio). 3rd ed. Eugene, OR: University of Oregon Press； 1995: 385.

[15] Tang JY, Li S, Li ZH, Zhang ZJ, Hu G, Cheang LC, et al. Calycosin promotes angiogenesis involving estrogen receptor and mitogen-activated protein kinase (MAPK)signaling pathway in zebraflsh and HUVEC. PLoS One 2010； 5: e11822.

[16] Xu H, Chen KJ. Integrative medicine: the experience from China. J Altern Compl Med 2008； 14: 3-7.

[17] Li YM, Chen KJ, Zhang XW, Wang DL, Shi ZX, Zhang TZ. Effect of Xuefu Zhuyu Pill on patients with carotid atherosclerosis by colour Doppler ultrasonography. Chin J Integr Tradit West Med (Chin)1997； 17: 152-154.

[18] Yu B, Chen KJ, Mao JM, Guo JX, Lu SZ. Clinical study on effect of concentrated Xuefu Zhuyu Pill on restenosis of 43 cases coronary heart disease after intracoronary stenting. Chin J Integr Tradit West Med (Chin)1998； 18: 585-587.

[19] Xiao PG, Chen KJ. Recent advances in clinical studies of Chinese medicinal herbs. J Phytother Res 1987； 1: 53-57.

[20] Zhou YW, Wang M, Ge ZY, Lin CR, Chen KJ. Effect of Xueguantong on plasma endothelin and calcitonin gene-related peptide in quail atherosis model. Chin J Integr Med 1997； 3: 210-211.

[21] Xu FQ, Li LZ, Xu H, Yao LF, Chen KJ, Shao NF. Effect of Xiongshao Capsule on the function of vascular endothelium of patients with cervical atherosclerosis. Chin J Integr Med 2004； 10: 14-18.

[22] Chen KJ, Shi DJ, Xu H, Lu SZ, Li TC, Ke YN, et al. XS0601 reduces the incidence of restenosis: a prospective study of 335 patients undergoing percutaneous coronary intervention in China. Chin Med J 2006； 119: 6-13.

[23] Wen C, Xu H, Huang QF, Chen KJ. Effects of drugs for promoting blood circulation on blood lipids and inflammatory reaction of atherosclerotic plaques in ApoE gene deficiency mice. Chin J Integr Tradit West Med (Chin)2005； 25: 345-349.

[24] Jiang YR, Yin HJ, Chen KJ. The research status of Peaoniae Radix 801. Chin J Integr Tradit West Med (Chin)2004； 24: 760-763.

[25] He YS, Wu YS, Lu EW, Li PL, Zhang CX, Wang YS, et al. A clinical and experimental study on anti-platelet aggregation effect of d-catechin. Chin J Integr Tradit West Med (Chin)1982； 2: 15-18.

[26] Li S, Dang YY, Che GO, Kwan YW, Chan SW, Leung GP, et al. VEGFR tyrosine kinase inhibitor Ⅱ (VRI)induced vascular insufflciency in zebraflsh as a model for studying vascular toxicity and vascular preservation. Toxicol Appl Pharmacol 2014； 280: 408-420.

[27] Shibuya M, Yamaguchi S, Yamane A, Ikeda T, Tojo A, Matsushime H, et al. Nucleotide sequence and expression of a novel human receptor-type tyrosine kinase gene (flt)closely related to the fms family. Oncogene 1990； 5: 519-524.

[28] Terman BI, Dougher-Vermazen M, Carrion ME, Dimitrov D, Armellino DC, Gospodarowicz D, et al. Identiflcation of the KDR tyrosine kinase as a receptor for vascular endothelial cell growth factor. Biochem Biophys Res Commun 1992； 187: 1579-1586.

[29] Habeck H, Odenthal J, Walderich B, Maischein HM, Schulte-Merker S. Analysis of a zebraflsh VEGF receptor mutant reveals specific disruption of angiogenesis. Curr Biol 2002； 12: 1405-1412.

[30] Ferrara N, Davis-Smyth T. The biology of vascular endothelial growth factor. Endocr Rev 1997； 18: 4-25.

[31] Klagsbrun M, D'Amore PA. Vascular endothelial growth factor and its receptors. Cytokine Growth Factor Rev 1996； 7: 259-270.

[32] Zachary I. Signaling mechanisms mediating vascular protective actions of vascular endothelial growth factor. Am J Physiol Cell Physiol 2001； 280: C1375-C1386.

[33] Zanetta L, Marcus SG, Vasile J, Dobryansky M, Cohen H, Eng K, et al. Expression of von Willebrand factor, an endothelial cell marker, is up-regulated by angiogenesis factors: a potential method for objective assessment of tumor angiogenesis. Int J Cancer 2000； 85: 281-288.

[34] Ribatti D, Baiguera S. Phase Ⅱ angiogenesis stimulators. Expert Opin Investig Drugs 2013； 22: 1157-1166.

[35] Navaratna D, Guo S, Arai K, Lo EH. Mechanisms and targets for angiogenic therapy after stroke. Cell Adh Migr 2009； 3: 216-223.

[36] He XH, Xing DM, Ding Y, Li Y, Xiang L, Wang W, et al. Determination of paeoniflorin in rat hippocampus by high performance liquid chromatography after intravenous administration of *Paeoniae Radix* extract. J Chromatogra B 2004； 802: 277-281.

[37] Liu DZ, Xie KQ, Ji XQ, Ye Y, Jiang CL, Zhu XZ. Neuroprotective effect of paeoniflorin on cerebral ischemic rat by activating adenosine A1 receptor in a manner different from its classical agonists. Br J Pharmacol 2005； 146: 604-611.

[38] Chen Y, Du X, Zhou Y, Zhang Y, Yang Y, Liu Z, et al. Paeoniflorin protects HUVECs from AGE-BSA-induced injury via an autophagic pathway by acting on the RAGE. Int J Clin Exp Pathol 2015； 8: 53-62.

First published: Xin Qi-Qi, Yang Bin-Rui, Zhou He-Feng, WANG Yan, YI Bo-wen, CONG Wei-hong, LEE Simon Ming-Yuen, CHEN Ke-ji. Paeoniflorin promotes angiogenesis in a vascular insufficiency model of zebrafish *in vivo* and in human umbilical vein endothelial cells *in vitro* [J] . Chin J Integr Med, 2018, 24 (7): 494-501.

Vascular Endothelial Growth Factor Gene Transfer Therapy for Coronary Artery Disease: A Systematic Review and Meta-Analysis

YUAN Rong, XIN Qi-qi, SHI Wei-li, LIU Wei, LEE Simon Ming-yuen, HOI Puiman, LI Lin, ZHAO Jun, CONG Wei-hong, and CHEN Ke-ji

Coronary artery disease (CAD)has become the major cause of death and illness worldwide. [1] According to the World Health Organization, CAD is the leading cause of death worldwide among all non-communicable diseases. [2] Current therapeutic options are limited to pharmacological therapy, percutaneous coronary intervention and bypass surgery; however, a large number of patients do not qualify for surgical or interventional procedures, and many patients have refractory angina despite maximal medical therapy. [3] These limitations have led to extensive research to find new treatment modalities.

CAD causes a lack of coronary blood flow, and all therapeutic interventions should aim to improve blood flow to the ischemic myocardium. [4] Therapeutic angiogenesis represents a novel treatment option for CAD patients as it can increase blood flow and repair injured and dead myocardium. [5,6] The vascular endothelial growth factor (VEGF)family includes VEGF-A, VEGF-B, VEGF-C, VEGF-D, VEGF-E and placenta growth factor (PLGF), which are key regulators of angiogenesis and lymphangiogenesis. There are two predominant isoforms of VEGF-A, VEGF-A121 and VEGF-A165, which are the most potent stimulators of angiogenic processes. VEGF-B plays a role in the maintenance of newly formed blood vessels under pathological conditions. VEGF-C and VEGF-D are primarily lymphangiogenic factors that can also induce angiogenesis. PLGF has a particular role in inflammatory responses and pathological permeability. [7-9] Currently, VEGF-A, VEGF-C, and VEGF-D are mainly used in CAD in clinical trials. [10,11]

Gene therapy is the therapeutic delivery of nucleic acid into cells to treat disease. In VEGF gene therapy, DNA encoding VEGF is transferred into cells in the ischemic myocardium, which subsequently grows new blood vessels; such therapy is a potential new treatment option. [12,13] To date, this intriguing approach to using VEGF gene therapy for CAD has been pursued in several clinical trials, but the results have been inconsistent. [14,15] Furthermore, several studies have suggested that VEGFs can accelerate the process of atherosclerosis in certain animal models and potentially destabilize coronary plaques. [16,17] These findings contradict the effect of angiogenesis therapy on CAD, since most CAD patients suffer from atherosclerosis. Hence, this therapy remains controversial, and there is no related meta-analysis. Therefore, we aimed to perform a systematic review and meta-analysis of the role of VEGF gene therapy for CAD.

METHODS

1 Search Strategy

This systematic review and meta-analysis is reported in accordance with the Preferred Reporting Items for Systematic Reviews and Meta-Analyses (PRISMA)statement. Additionally, we registered the current meta-analysis at the International Prospective Register of Systematic Reviews (number: CRD42017058430). [18]

We selected randomized controlled trials (RCTs)containing VEGF gene therapy published up to May 2018 by searching the Pubmed, Embase, and Cochrane databases and relevant references. Medical search terms included the following: 'vascular endothelial growth factor gene' OR 'VEGF gene' AND 'coronary artery disease' OR 'CAD' OR 'coronary heart disease' OR 'CHD' OR 'angina' AND 'randomized controlled trial' . We also performed a manual search. Two investigators (RY and QX)independently performed the database search and study selection.

2 Inclusion and Exclusion Criteria

We considered studies for inclusion if they met all of the following criteria: 1)RCTs comparing VEGF gene therapy and standard treatments for CAD；2)report of at least one of the outcomes of interest (mortality, serious cardiac events, follow-up left ventricular ejection fraction (LVEF), change in LVEF (ΔLVEF)and angina). Studies were excluded for the following reasons: VEGF treatment not involving gene therapy (such as VEGF protein treatment), nonrandomized study design, duplicate publication, unpublished abstracts, or no reported outcomes of interest.

3 Data Extraction and Management

Two independent investigators (RY and QX)reviewed the study and extracted the data. Any further calculations on study data were conducted by the first reviewer and checked by the second reviewer. Disagreements were resolved by consensus. Descriptive data extracted included the first author's name, year of publication, study design, total sample size, type of CAD, VEGF gene type, control treatment type, outcomes and adverse effects. The primary outcomes were mortality and serious cardiac events. Serious cardiac events included myocardial infarction, acute coronary syndrome, cardiac arrest, cardiogenic shock, heart failure, and surgical cardiac interventions. The secondary outcome measures were follow-up LVEF, ΔLVEF, Canadian Cardiovascular Society (CCS)angina class and angina frequency scores in the Seattle Angina Questionnaire.

4 Quality Assessment

The Cochrane Collaboration's tool for assessing risk of bias was used to assess the methodological quality of the included studies. The 7 items in this tool address the adequacy of randomization and allocation concealment, blinding, completeness of outcome data, selective reporting and other bias.

5 Statistical Analysis

The relative risk (RR)and 95% confidence interval (CI)were calculated to assess differences in mortality and serious cardiac events. The data represent the weighted mean difference (WMD)and 95% CI of LVEF, CCS angina class and angina frequency scores. We conducted subgroup analysis according to CAD type, VEGF gene type and delivery method and performed sensitivity analyses. We assessed publication bias by constructing a funnel plot and using Begg's and Egger's tests. A formal assessment of statistical heterogeneity was made using the I2 statistic. A fixed effects model was used when $I2 < 50\%$, and a random effects model was used when $I2 > 50\%$. Analyses were performed with Review Manager 5.3 and Stata 12.0 software.

RESULTS

1 Description of Included Studies

A total of 524 studies were identified, and 124 records were removed because they were duplicates. By screening titles and abstracts, we excluded 375 records because they were experimental studies, review articles, non-CAD studies or non-VEGF gene therapy studies. By browsing full-text articles, we excluded 11 records for not being RCTs, not involving VEGF gene therapy, or having no outcome information. Finally, a total of 14 RCTs were included. [13-15,19-29] Only one trial reported outcomes at 8 years (Hedman et al 200929), and this publication reported the same patients as Hedman et al. 2003; the other trials reported outcomes at less than 1 year. A flow chart of the study selection was generated according to the PRISMA requirements (Figure 1).

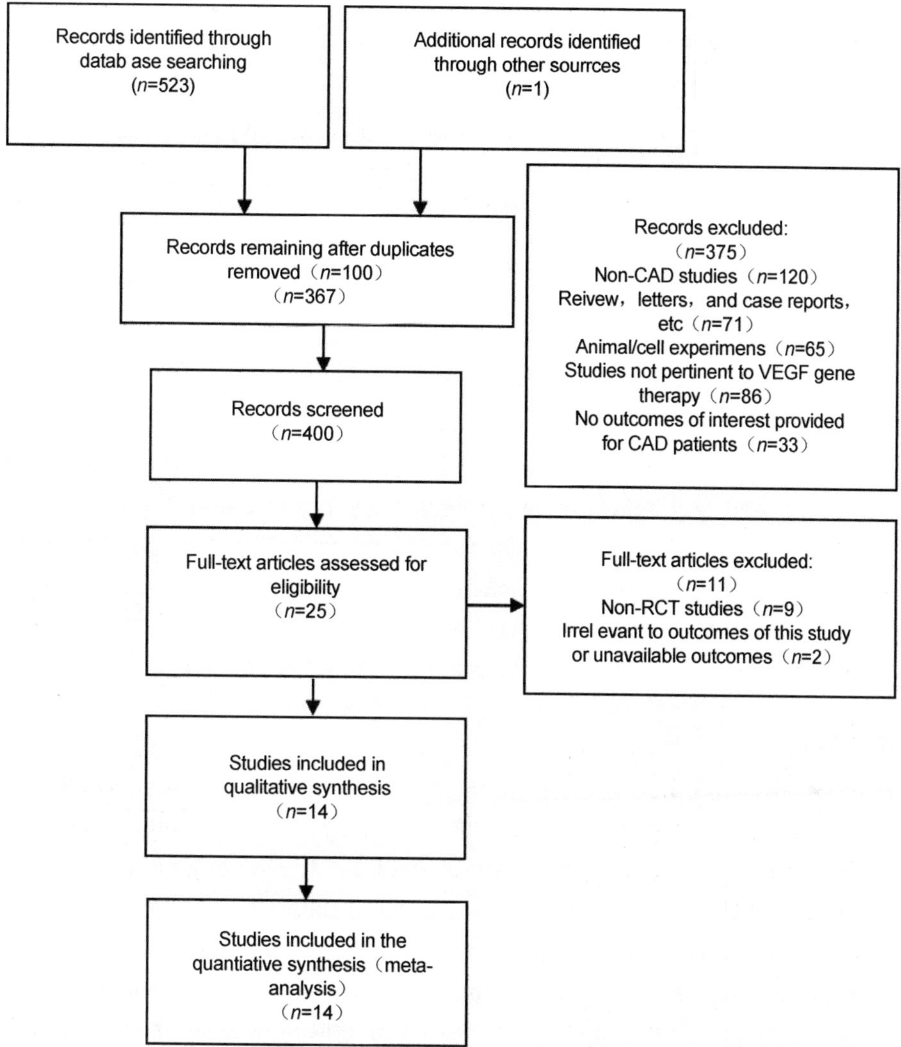

Figure 1 Search strategy and study inclusion criteria. CAD, coronary artery disease; RCT, randomized controlled trials; VEGF, vascular endothelial growth factor

2 Risk of Bias Assessment

All the included studies were RCTs. 6 trials reported the method of double-blinding, [14,15,24,26,27,29] 8 studies reported allocation concealment, [14,15,20.23.24.26.27.29] 7 trials reported complete outcome data, [14.15.19-21.24,29] and 3 trials may have had selective reporting. [22,25,27] There was an unclear risk of bias in allocation concealment, blinding of outcome assessment, incomplete outcome data and selective reporting. There was a high risk of bias in blinding (Figure 2).

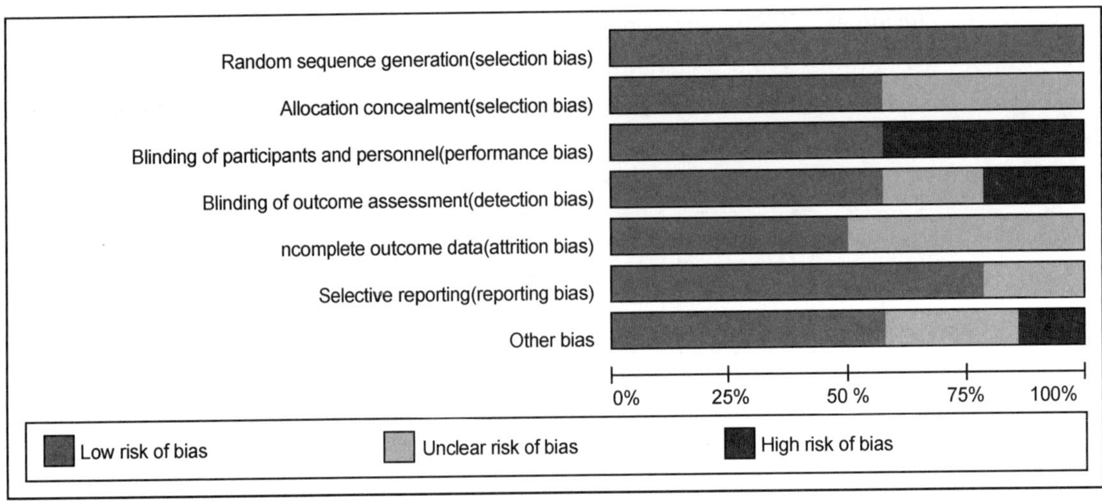

Figure 2 Diagram Showing Risk of Bias in the Included Studies

3 Study Characteristics

In this meta-analysis, 1 of the 13 articles contained 2 studies, and Hedman et al. presented the results of patients exposed to plasmid or adenovirus vector separately in one article. [26] All the clinical studies were published in English from 2001 to 2017. A final total of 550 patients (234 patients in the control group and 316 patients in the VEGF gene therapy group)were included. Subject age ranged from 56 to 71 years. The mean trial duration was 6 months (range: 3 to 12 months). Table 1 shows the distribution of these studies according to study design, patient characteristics, treatment measures, and adverse effects.

4 Primary Outcome

The outcome measures were not reported in all of the trials. In this meta-analysis, 7 studies assessed mortality. [13,14,24,19-22] There was no statistically significant difference in mortality between the VEGF gene therapy group and the control group (RR: 0.79； 95%CI: 0.29, 2.13； *P*=0.64), although the subgroup analysis was performed on different VEGF gene types and vectors. We detected no significant heterogeneity (Figure 3A). The overall sample size was relatively small, and publication bias cannot be evaluated for mortality. In addition, Hedman et al. (2009)presented the mortality at 8 years of patients grouped by vector type in one article. 29 VEGF gene therapy with an adenovirus vector tended to decrease the risk of mortality (RR: 0.75: 95%CI: 0.14, 4.05), while VEGF gene therapy with a plasmid vector did not decrease the risk of mortality (RR: 1.15: 95%CI: 0.11, 11.68)at 8 years.

In this meta-analysis, 10 studies assessed serious cardiac events. [13-15,19,20-22,24,26] Pooling data from these studies showed that VEGF gene therapy led to a significantly decreased risk of serious cardiac events (11.7 % vs 21.2%, RR: 0.56； 95%CI: 0.37, 0.84； *P*=0.005). In the subgroup analysis, the risk of serious cardiac events was significantly lower in the VEGFA-165 gene therapy group (RR: 0.52； 95%CI: 0.30, 0.91)and in the adenovirus vector group (RR: 0.55； 95%CI: 0.31, 0.96). We detected no significant heterogeneity (Figure 3B). In this analysis, there was no significant publication bias (*P*=0.94), and the funnel plot is shown in Figure 3C. In addition, Hedman et al. (2009)presented serious cardiac events over 8 years in patients grouped by vector type in one article； [29] VEGF therapy with an adenovirus vector (RR: 0.71； 95%CI: 0.34, 1.52)or a plasmid vector (RR: 0.79； 95%CI: 0.41, 1.52)tended to decrease the risk of serious cardiac events at 8 years.

Table 1 Characteristics of Randomized Controlled Trials of VEGF Gene Transfer Therapyin Coronary Artery Disease (sort by year of publication)

Study (design)	Number (T/C)	Age	Number of man (T/C)	VEGF gene treatment type	Type of CAD	Time	Control treatment	Outcomes of interest	Adverse effects
Hartikainen, J. 2017[13]	30 (24/6)	71/70	23/5	0.2mlAd-VEGF-D	refractory CAD	3, 12months	placebo injection	safe, feasible, well tolerated, increased myocardialperfusion	minor bleeding, new atrial fibrillation, pericardial effusion
Muona, K. 2013[19]	15 (12/3)	71/68	12/3	$1x10^{10}$particle units (p. u.) Ad-VEGF-D	severeCAD	3 months	placebo injection	safe, feasible, well tolerated	pyelonephritis, pericardial effusion, significant elevation in prostate-specific antigen, inflammation and immunological findings
Kukula, K. 2011[14]	52 (33/19)	62.8/61.7	24/16	0.5mgPL-VEGFA165	refractory CAD	5, 12 months	placebo plasmid	safe but did not improve myocardial perfusion, while improve symptoms	no adverse events
Kastrup, J. 2011 [15]	17 (12/5)	60.9/64.1	9/4	$4x10^{10}$ p. u. Ad-VEGF A121	refractory CAD	12, 26 weeks, 12 months	placebo infusion	safe but did not improve myocardial perfusion	vertigo, abdominal pain, influenza/rhinitis, conjunctivitis, pneumonia, hypertension, syncope, back pain, liver function abnormality, peripheral vascular disorder
Hedman, M. 2009a [29]	48 (32/16)	58/56	26/15	$2 x10^{10}$ p. u. Ad-VEGFA165	stenosis, suitable for stenting	8 years	placebo infusion	safe and does not increase the risk of major adverse cardi- ovascular events, arrhythmias, cancer, diabetes	not reported
Hedman, M. 2009b [29]	41 (26/15)	58/56	23/15	0.2 mg PL-VEGFA165					
Stewart, D. J. 2009 [20]	93 (48/45)	63/64	40/42	2 mg PL-VEGFA165	refractory CAD	3, 6 months	placebo infusion	no benefit on any of the end points	musculoskeletal pains, headache, cancer dizziness, pericardial, gastrointestinal, dermatological, retinal, peripheral edema, neurological, inflammation, hypotension
Stewart, D. J. 2006 [21]	67 (32/35)	61/60	26/32	$4x10^{10}$ p. u. Ad-VEGFA121	refractory CAD	12, 26 weeks	medication	no difference in adverse events	no adverse events
Ripa, R. S. 2006 [22]	32 (16/16)	61/62	15/14	0.5 mg PL-VEGFA165	refractory CAD	3 months	placebo infusion	safe but did not improve myocardial perfusion or clinical effects	no adverse events
Fuchs, S. 2006 [23]	10 (6/4)	61/69	61/69	$4x10^{10}$ p. u. Ad-VEGFA121	refractory CAD	3 months, 12 months	placebo infusion	practical, feasible, and potentially safe	no significant changes
Kastrup, J. 2005 [24]	80 (40/40)	61/61	33/35	0.5 mg PL-VEGFA165	severe CAD	3 months, follow-up 6 months	placebo plasmid	safe but did not improve myocardial perfusion	no serious adverse events
Tio, R. A. 2004 [25]	23 (10/13)	63/64	9/9	0.5 mg PL-VEGFA165	end-stage CAD	3 months	medication	decreased myocardial ischemia	not reported
Hedman, M. 2003a [26]	56 (37/19)	58/56	26/15	$2 x10^{10}$ p. u. Ad-VEGFA165	stenosis, suitable for stenting	6 months, follow-up 28 months	placebo infusion	safe and increase myocardial perfusion	transient fever, transient elevation of serum C-reactive protein, palindromic joint symptoms, colitis and other gastrointest-inal symptoms
Hedman, M. 2003b [26]	47 (28/19)	58/56	23/15	0.2 mg PL-VEGFA165					
Losordo, D. W. 2002 [27]	19 (12/7)	62/59	9/6	0.2 mg PL-VEGF-C	refractory CAD	12 weeks	placebo plasmid	safe and reduce angina class	no major complications
Vale, P. R. 2001 [28]	9 (6/3)	67/67	5/5	0.2 mg PL-VEGF-C	refractory CAD	3, 12 months	placebo plasmid	feasibility, safety, and improve left ventricular myocardium	no major complications

CAD= coronary artery disease; p. u. = particle units; T/C=treatment/control; VEGF= vascular endothelial growth factor; Ad= adenovirus, PL= plasmid

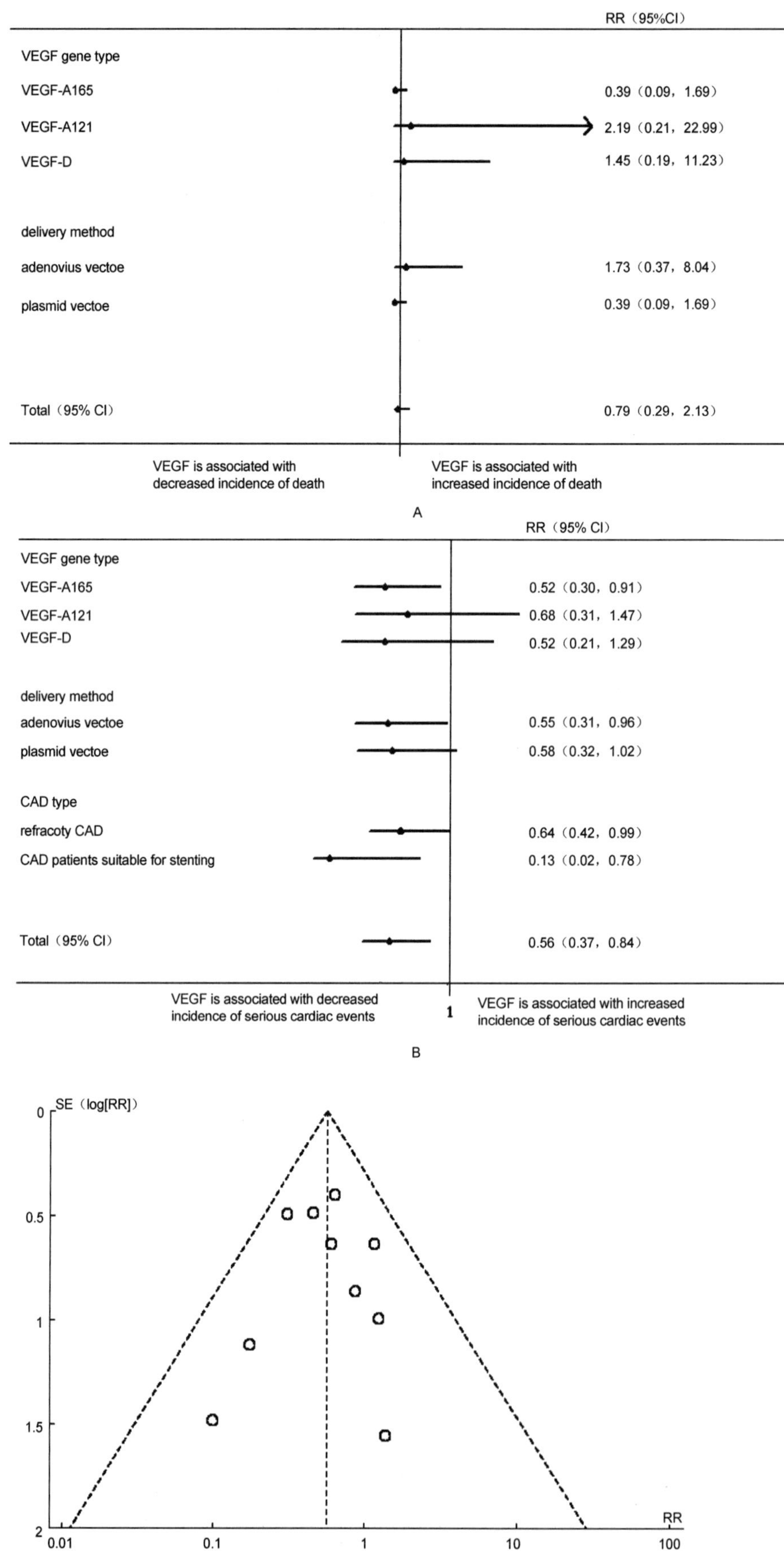

Figure 3　Meta-analyses of VEGF Gene Therapy for CAD, comparing mortality and serious cardiac events

Notes: Outcomes assessed are (A)mortality, (B)serious cardiac events. (C)Funnel plot of serious cardiac events. CI, confidence interval; CAD, coronary artery disease; VEGF, vascular endothelial growth factor.

5 Secondary Outcomes

In this meta-analysis, 7 studies (N=219 participants)assessed LVEF. [14,15,22-24,27,28] Follow-up LVEF improved in the VEGF gene therapy group (WMD: 1.95; 95%CI: 1.28, 2.62; $P < 0.00001$). In the subgroup analysis, follow-up LVEF improved in the VEGF-A165 gene therapy group (WMD: 2.03; 95% CI: 1.36, 2.70)and the plasmid vector group (WMD: 2.00; 95%CI: 1.33, 2.68). There was no statistically significant heterogeneity (Figure 4A). Then, we performed an analysis of ΔLVEF, and the overall effect on ΔLVEF was not significantly different between the two groups. In the subgroup analysis, ΔLVEF significantly increased in the VEGFA-121 gene therapy group and the adenovirus vector group (WMD: 4.74; 95%CI: 2.76, 6.71) (Figure 4B). Publication bias could not be evaluated because of the relatively small sample size.

In this meta-analysis, 7 studies assessed CCS angina class during a mean period of 6 months. [14,15,20,21,24,26] There is no significant benefit of VEGF gene therapy on CCS angina class. In the subgroup analysis, the CCS angina class was significantly lower in the adenovirus vector group (WMD: -0.92; 95%CI: -0.99, -0.86), while the opposite effect was observed in the plasmid vector group (WMD: 0.33; 95%CI: 0.27, 0.40). There was no significant difference based on VEGF gene type or CAD type (Figure 4C).

In this meta-analysis, 4 studies assessed the angina frequency scores in the Seattle Angina Questionnaire. [21.23,24,27] Pooling the data revealed no significant benefit of VEGF gene therapy (WMD: 11.97; 95%CI: -1.29, 25.23, P=0.08). In the subgroup analysis, patients treated with VEGF-A165 showed an increased angina frequency score in only one trial (Kastrup et al) (WMD: 5.00; 95%CI: 3.02, 6.98). [24] VEGF-C treatment also evoked an increased angina frequency score in only one trial (Losordo et al) (WMD: 18.00; 95%CI: 14.40, 21.60), [27] and VEGF-A121 had no effect on angina frequency scores (Figure 4D).

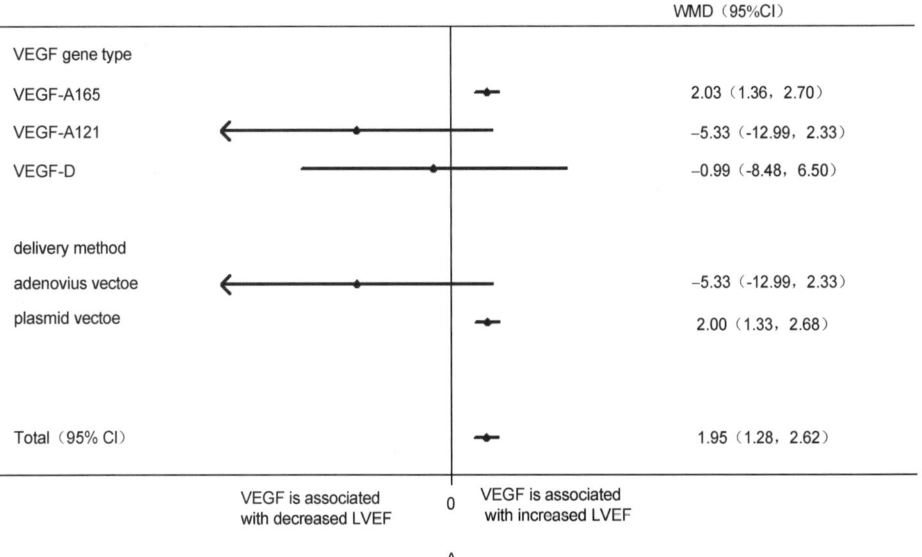

A

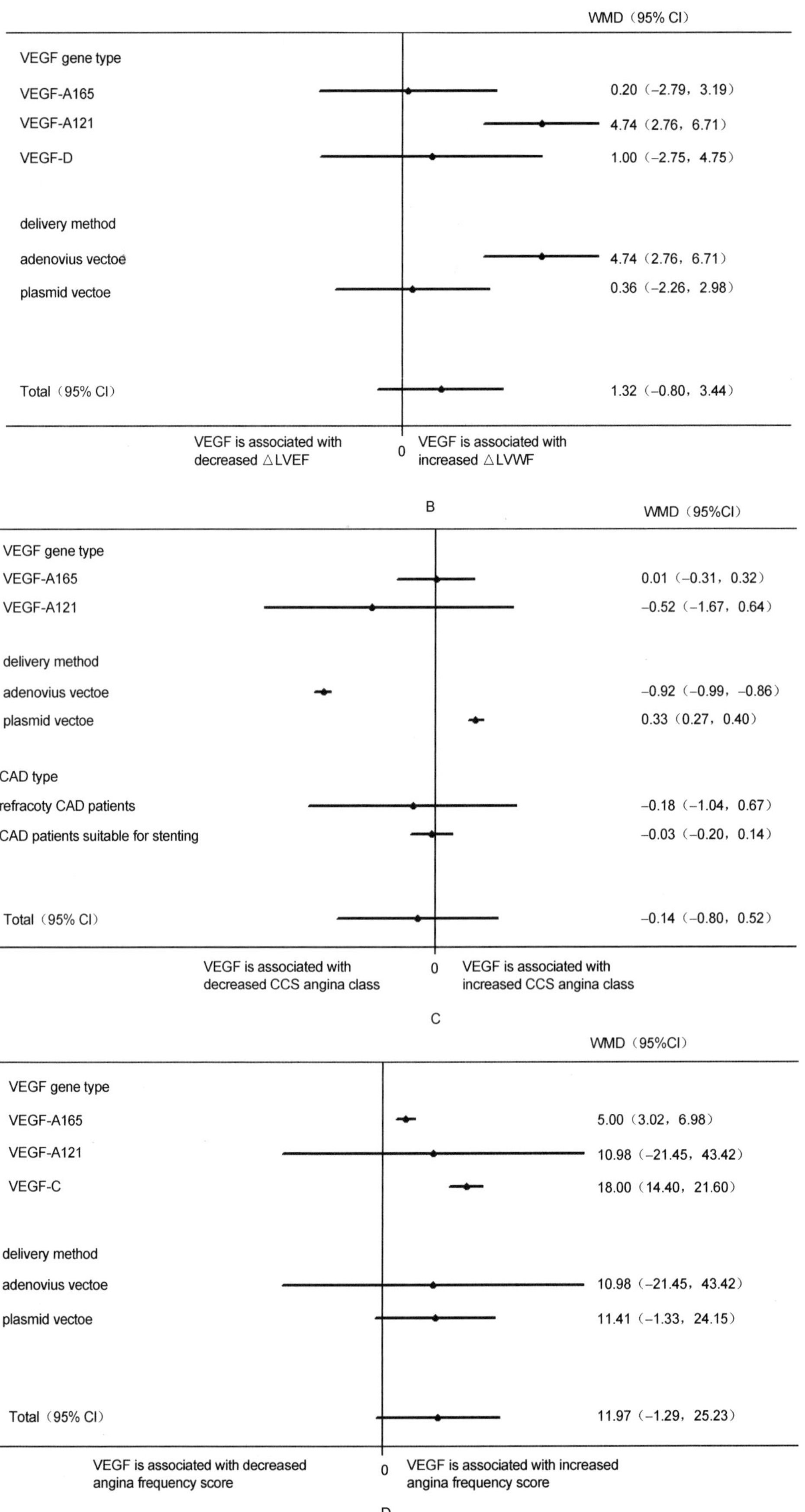

Figure 4 Meta-analyses of VEGF Gene Therapy for CAD, Comparing LVEF, △LVEF, CCS angina class, and angina frequency score

Notes: Outcomes assessed are (A)LVEF, (B)△LVEF, (C)CCS angina class, and (D)angina frequency score. CI, confidence interval; CAD, coronary artery disease; VEGF, vascular endothelial growth factor; LVEF, left ventricular ejection fraction; CCS, Canadian Cardiovascular Society.

6 Sensitivity Analyses

In sensitivity analyses, the pooled effect estimates showed no significant differences in follow-up LVEF upon excluding the study by Kastrup et al. [24], which indicated that this result was not robust. Individual study exclusion did not substantially change the pooled effect estimate of other outcomes.

7 Adverse Effects

Five trials described the adverse effects in detail, [13.155,19,20.26] and the remaining trials reported no adverse effects. The main adverse effects were peripheral vascular disorder, peripheral edema, retinal disease, musculoskeletal pain, inflammation, and pericardial effusion. Most of the adverse effects showed no difference between the two groups, except in two studies: musculoskeletal pain in the study by Stewart et al. [20] and transient fever and transient elevation of serum C-reactive protein in the study by Hedman et al. [26]

DISCUSSION

Our results showed that VEGF gene therapy could decrease the risk of serious cardiac events and slightly improve follow-up LVEF, which reflects the hopeful prospects for the treatment of CAD. In addition, VEGF gene therapy had no effect on the risk of mortality. The neutral results suggest that VEGF gene therapy for CAD is safe, but studies with longer follow-up and larger sample sizes are needed to confirm this result. Furthermore, VEGF gene therapy did not improve the angina frequency score. In the subgroup analysis, VEGF gene delivery using adenoviral vectors improved the risk of serious cardiac events, ΔLVEF, and CCS angina class, while the evidence for plasmid vectors was not sufficient. Moreover, VEGF-A165 may decrease the risk of serious cardiac events, and VEGF-A121 may increase ΔLVEF compared to other VEGF gene types. In addition, heterogeneity could not be fully investigated because of the small sample size, and the results require further validation. Overall, these data support the hypothesis that VEGF gene transfer, especially using adenoviral vectors, is a safe potential therapy for CAD that is beneficial in terms of serious cardiac events, albeit with no effect on mortality or angina frequency scores. Therefore, this meta-analysis highlights the need for further exploration in these areas.

Improving blood flow to the ischemic myocardium plays a critical role in the treatment of CAD. [4] VEGF-A165 and VEGFA-121 both induce angiogenesis and increase blood flow. VEGF-A165 is more highly expressed than VEGFA-121, while VEGFA-121 diffuse more into the ischemic milieu than VEGF-A165; VEGF-C and VEGF-D stimulate lymphatic vessel growth and do not directly stimulate inflammatory responses. [13,30-33] This meta-analysis showed that VEGF-A165 gene transfer could decrease the risk of serious cardiac events and that VEGF-A121 gene transfer could increase ΔLVEF, which indicated that VEGF-A165 may have greater potential in the prognosis of CAD, and VEGF-A121 may be more beneficial in improving cardiac function; while these results should be further investigated. Furthermore, there have been only two studies on VEGF-C (Losordo et al 2002; Vale et al 2001)and VEGF-D (Hartikainen et al 2017; Muona et al 2013), and there is no evidence of improvement; however, these issues must be further explored.

This meta-analysis showed robust and consistent findings that lend support to the safety and efficacy of VEGF gene therapy in reducing the risk of serious cardiac events while not affecting mortality. Indeed, these results were consistent across studies despite several differences, including in VEGF type, CAD type, gene delivery method and control treatment. Taken together, the results of these studies support the beneficial effects of VEGF gene therapy across clinical settings.

The results showed that VEGF gene therapy could slightly improve follow-up LVEF but not ΔLVEF, which is unlikely to be clinically important. Follow-up LVEF appeared to improve in the VEGF-A165 gene therapy group and the plasmid vector group, but these results were dominated by one study (Kastrup et al)[24] and thus not robust. In addition, findings remain controversial with respect to the effectiveness of VEGF gene therapy in improving angina. The CCS angina class was decreased by VEGF gene delivery using adenoviral vectors but increased by plasmid vectors, which may indicate that these two vector types have different effects on angina. In addition, although it seemed that VEGF-A165 and VEGF-C increased angina frequency scores, there was only one trial in each group, and more studies are needed. Regarding the high heterogeneity, CAD type, VEGF gene type, delivery method, and treatment duration were taken into account; however, the heterogeneity was not eliminated, so these results should be interpreted cautiously.

Genes encoding VEGFs can be transfected into the myocardium by plasmid DNA or adenovirus vectors. [7,34] Recently, the use of adenovirus has gained popularity due to higher cardiac tropism and promising preclinical results. Our results also showed that gene delivery using adenoviral vectors prompted improvements in serious cardiac events, ΔLVEF, and CCS angina class, which indicated that more efficient adenovirus transfection could be necessary to induce neovascularization in the ischemic myocardium.

In this meta-analysis, most of the trials reported no adverse effects, while 2 trials showed a significant difference in musculoskeletal pain, transient fever and transient elevation of serum C-reactive protein between the two groups, [20,26] which may be correlated with adverse effects of the VEGF-A gene. [36]

Moreover, adenovirus vectors may increase the risk of inflammatory activation, while most of these adverse effects alleviated after discontinuing treatment. However, more attention still should be paid to the use of VEGF gene transfer for angiogenic diseases, such as atherosclerotic disease, rheumatoid disease, retinal disease, and malignant tumors. [29,37,38]

Our meta-analysis has several limitations. First, differences in study design are likely to have introduced heterogeneity in ΔLVEF, CCS angina class and angina frequency scores. Although we performed subgroup analyses, difference remained among the studies in terms of the sample size, race, religious beliefs, and concern regarding the disease. Second, most of the included studies had a relatively small sample size and might be methodologically less robust, potentially leading to overestimation of treatment effects. Third, the long-term persistence of the treatment effects is unknown. Most of the trials ranged in duration from 3 to 12 months, and only one trial reported long-term follow-up. [29] Fourth, the publication bias could not be evaluated in all outcomes because of small sample size. In the bias evaluation, we emailed all the corresponding authors, but unfortunately, only one author replied in detail. Finally, the ideal time to begin this treatment in the clinical course of the disease is unknown. The outcomes and conclusions should be interpreted with these limitations in mind.

Therapeutic angiogenesis is still a promising new treatment for patients with CAD. However, more research, including large-scale, double-blind, randomized, placebo-controlled, multicenter trials with a standardized design, is needed to validate and verify the efficacy of VEGF gene therapy as a reliable supportive therapeutic option in CAD.

CONCLUSION

VEGF gene therapy appears to be associated with a reduction in serious cardiac events and a slight improvement in follow-up LVEF, and adenoviral vectors seem to have more benefit in terms of the risk of serious cardiac events, ΔLVEF, and CCS angina class and thus may be useful in pro-angiogenesis regimens for CAD patients. However, further clinical trials are needed to establish the optimal approach for the application of this treatment in practice.

REFERENCES

[1] Wong ND. Epidemiological studies of CHD and the evolution of preventive cardiology[J]. Nat Rev Cardiol, 2014, 11 (5): 276-289.

[2] Organization WH. World health statistics 2016. Monitoring health for the SDGs sustainable development goals[J]. Geneva Switzerland Who,

2016, 41: 293-328.

[3] Theurl M, Schgoer W, Albrecht-Schgoer K, et al. Secretoneurin gene therapy improves hind limb and cardiac ischaemia in apo e (-)/ (-)mice without influencing systemic atherosclerosis[J]. Cardiovasc Res, 2015, 105 (1): 96-106.

[4] Heusch G. Myocardial ischemia: Lack of coronary blood flow or myocardial oxygen supply/demand imbalance? [J] Circ Res, 2016, 119 (2): 194-196.

[5] Attanasio S, Schaer G. Therapeutic angiogenesis for the management of refractory angina: current concepts[J]. Cardiovasc Ther, 2011, 29 (6): 1-11.

[6] Slevin M. Therapeutic Angiogenesis for Vascular Diseases[J]. New York: Springer Netherlands, 2011: 269-270.

[7] Ylä-Herttuala S, Baker AH. Cardiovascular Gene Therapy: Past, Present, and Future[J]. Mol Ther2017, 25 (5): 1095-1106.

[8] Mitsos S, Katsanos K, Koletsis E, et al. Therapeutic angiogenesis for myocardial ischemia revisited: basic biological concepts and focus on latest clinical trials[J]. Angiogenesis, 2012, 15 (1): 1-22.

[9] Tammela T, Enholm B, Alitalo K, et al. The biology of vascular endothelial growth factors[J]. Cardiovasc Res, 2005, 65 (3): 550-563.

[10] Vuorio T, Jauhiainen S, Yläherttuala S. Pro-and anti-angiogenic therapy and atherosclerosis with special emphasis on vascular endothelial growth factors[J]. Expert Opin Biol Ther, 2012, 12 (1): 79-92.

[11] Zachary I, Morgan RD. Therapeutic angiogenesis for cardiovascular disease: biological context, challenges, prospects[J]. Heart, 2011, 97 (3): 181-189.

[12] Rissanen TT, Yla-Herttuala S. Current status of cardiovascular gene therapy[J]. Mol Ther, 2007, 15 (7): 1233-1247.

[13] Hartikainen J, Hassinen I, Hedman A, et al. Adenoviral intramyocardial VEGF-D Δ N Δ C gene transfer increases myocardial perfusion reserve in refractory angina patients: a phase I/IIa study with 1-year follow-up[J]. Eur Heart J, 2017, 38 (33): 2547-2555.

[14] Kukula K, Chojnowska L, Dabrowski M, et al. Intramyocardial plasmid-encoding human vascular endothelial growth factor A165/basic fibroblast growth factor therapy using percutaneous transcatheter approach in patients with refractory coronary artery disease (VIF-CAD)[J]. Am Heart J, 2011, 161 (3): 581-589.

[15] Kastrup J, Jorgensen E, Fuchs S, et al. A randomised, double-blind, placebo-controlled, multicentre study of the safety and efficacy of BIOBYPASS (AdGVVEGF121.10NH)gene therapy in patients with refractory advanced coronary artery disease: the NOVA trial[J]. EuroIntervention, 2011, 6 (7): 813-818.

[16] Khurana R, Simons M, Martin J, et al. Role of angiogenesis in cardiovascular disease: a critical appraisal[J]. Circulation, 2005, 112 (12): 1813-1824.

[17] Khurana R, Moons L, Shafi S, et al. Placental growth factor promotes atherosclerotic intimal thickening and macrophage accumulation[J]. Circulation, 2005, 111 (21): 2828-2836.

[18] Vrabel M. Preferred reporting items for systematic reviews and meta-analyses[J]. Oncol Nurs Forum, 2015, 42 (5): 552-554.

[19] Muona K. Intramyocardial adenovirus-mediated VEGF-D Δ N Δ C Gene transfer in patients with no-option coronary artery disease: interim safety analysis of the Kuopio Angiogenesis Trial 301[J]. Int J Cardiovasc Res, 2013, 2 (6): 1-10.

[20] Stewart DJ, Kutryk MJ, Fitchett D, et al. VEGF gene therapy fails to improve perfusion of ischemic myocardium in patients with advanced coronary disease: results of the NORTHERN trial[J]. Mol Ther, 2009, 17 (6): 1109-1115.

[21] Stewart DJ, Hilton JD, Arnold JM, et al. Angiogenic gene therapy in patients with nonrevascularizable ischemic heart disease: a phase 2 randomized, controlled trial of AdVEGF (121) (AdVEGF121)versus maximum medical treatment[J]. Gene Ther, 2006, 13 (21): 1503-1511.

[22] Ripa RS, Wang Y, Jorgensen E, et al. Intramyocardial injection of vascular endothelial growth factor-A165 plasmid followed by granulocyte-colony stimulating factor to induce angiogenesis in patients with severe chronic ischaemic heart disease[J]. Eur Heart J, 2006, 27 (15): 1785-1792.

[23] Fuchs S, Dib N, Cohen BM, et al. A randomized, double-blind, placebo-controlled, multicenter, pilot study of the safety and feasibility of catheter-based intramyocardial injection of AdVEGF121 in patients with refractory advanced coronary artery disease[J]. Catheter Cardiovasc Interv, 2006, 68 (3): 372-378.

[24] Kastrup J, Jorgensen E, Ruck A, et al. Direct intramyocardial plasmid vascular endothelial growth factor-A165 gene therapy in patients with stable severe angina pectoris A randomized double-blind placebo-controlled study: the Euroinject One trial[J]. J Am Coll Cardiol, 2005, 45 (7): 982-988.

[25] Tio RA, Tan ES, Jessurun GA, et al. PET for evaluation of differential myocardial perfusion dynamics after VEGF gene therapy and laser therapy in end-stage coronary artery disease[J]. J Nucl Med, 2004, 45 (9): 1437-1443.

[26] Hedman M, Hartikainen J, Syvanne M, et al. Safety and feasibility of catheter-based local intracoronary vascular endothelial growth factor gene transfer in the prevention of postangioplasty and in-stent restenosis and in the treatment of chronic myocardial ischemia: phase II results of the Kuopio Angiogenesis Trial (KAT)[J]. Circulation, 2003, 107 (21): 2677-2683.

[27] Losordo DW, Vale PR, Hendel RC, et al. Phase 1/2placebo-controlled, double-blind, dose-escalating trial of myocardial vascular endothelial growth factor 2 gene transfer by catheter delivery in patients with chronic myocardial ischemia[J]. Circulation, 2002, 105 (17): 2012-2018.

[28] Vale PR, Losordo DW, Milliken CE, et al. Randomized, single-blind, placebo-controlled pilot study of catheter-based myocardial gene transfer for therapeutic angiogenesis using left ventricular electromechanical mapping in patients with chronic myocardial ischemia[J]. Circulation, 2001, 103 (17): 2138-2143.

[29] Hedman M, Muona K, Hedman A, et al. Eight-year safety follow-up of coronary artery disease patients after local intracoronary VEGF gene

transfer[J]. Gene Ther, 2009, 16 (5): 629-634.

[30] Mitsos S, Katsanos K, Koletsis E, Kagadis GC, Anastasiou N, Diamantopoulos A, et al. Therapeutic angiogenesis for myocardial ischemia revisited: basic biological concepts and focus on latest clinical trials[J]. Angiogenesis, 2012, 15 (1): 1-22.

[31] Jauhiainen S, H€akkinen SK, Toivanen PI, et al. Vascular endothelial growth factor (VEGF)-D stimulates VEGF-A, stanniocalcin-1, and neuropilin-2 and has potent angiogenic effects[J]. Arterioscler Thromb Vasc Biol, 2011, 31 (7): 1617-1624.

[32] Nurro J, Halonen PJ, Kuivanen A, et al. AdVEGF-B186 and AdVEGF-D△N△C induce angiogenesis and increase perfusion in porcine myocardium[J]. Heart, 2016, 102 (21): 1716-1720.

[33] Mack CA, Patel SR, Schwarz EA, et al. Biologic bypass with the use of adenovirus-mediated gene transfer of the complementary deoxyribonucleic acid for vascular endothelial growth factor 121 improves myocardial perfusion and function in the ischemic porcine heart[J]. J Thorac Cardiovasc Surg 1998, 115 (1): 168-176.

[34] Kastrup. TherapeuticAngiogenesis in Ischemic Heart Disease: Gene or Recombinant Vascular Growth Factor Protein Therapy? [J] Current Gene Ther, 2003, 3 (3): 197-206.

[35] Chamberlain, K, Riyad, JM, et al. Cardiac gene therapy with adeno-associated virus-based vectors[J]. Curr Opin Cardiol In press, doi: 10.1097/HCO. 0000000000000386.

[36] Knod JL, Crawford K, Dusing M, et al. Angiogenesis and vascular endothelial growth factor-A expression associated with inflammation in pediatric crohn's disease[J]. J Gastrointest Surg, 2016, 20 (3): 624-630.

[37] Camarã C, Pucelle M, Nã Gre-Salvayre A, et al. Angiogenesis in the atherosclerotic plaque[J]. Redox Biol, 2017, 12: 18-34.

[38] Celletti FL, Hilfiker PR, Ghafouri P, et al. Effect of human recombinant vascular endothelial growth factor165 on progression of atherosclerotic plaque[J]. J Am Coll Cardiol, 2001, 37 (8): 2126-2130.

First published: YUAN Rong, XIN Qi-qi, SHI Wei-li, LIU Wei, LEE Simon-M, HOI Puiman, LI Lin, ZHAO Jun, CONG Weihong, CHEN Ke-ji. Vascular endothelial growth factor gene transfer therapy for coronary artery disease: A systematic review and meta-analysis[J]. Cardiovasc Ther, 2018, 36: e12461.

Comparison on Anticoagulation and Antiplatelet Aggregation Effects of Puerarin with Heparin Sodium and Tirofiban Hydrochloride: An in *Vitro* Study

LI Si-wei, FENG Xue, XU Hao, and CHEN Ke-ji

Puerarin is a flavonoid glycoside derived from the canes or roots of leguminous plant kudzu [Pueraria lobata (Willd.)*Ohwi*]. It is a vasodilator with the effects of expanding coronary artery and cerebral vessel, reducing myocardial oxygen consumption, improving microcirculation, and inhibiting platelet aggregation. Animal studies showed that puerarin could inhibit 5-hydroxytryptamine (5-HT)release in platelet-mediated by thrombin induction[1].

Sonoclot coagulation and platelet function analyzer is mainly used for the coagulation and platelet function test in vitro. At present, this instrument has gradually become an important, accurate and fast clinical hemostatic inspection tool in cardiovascular surgery, liver transplant and other surgeries of massive hemorrhage[2-4]. The parameters include activated clotting time (ACT), the liquid-remained time of blood sample, clot rate (CR), the rate of fibrin formation (indirectly reflects the level of fibrinogen), and platelet function (PF), which reflects platelet function. This study applies Sonoclot coagulationand platelet function analyzer in vitro to compare the anticoagulant/antiplatelet effects between Puerarin Injection and Heparin Sodium Injection/ Tirofiban Hydrochloride Injection, and to explore the anticoagulation and antiplatelet effects of puerarin.

METHODS

1 Source of Specimen

Twenty healthy volunteers from Beijing Fuwai Hospital were included, 9 males, 11 females, aged 25–50 years old (38 ± 6 years old). They had not taken any drug in the previous month, and there were no women who were during pregnancy, menstrual period or lactation period. All the healthy volunteers signed their informed consents and agreed to provide blood samples for experiments in March 2016 in this study.

2 Sample Collection

Fasting venous blood (3 mL)was taken from each participant in a resting state, then 0.109 mol/L sodium citrate in a ratio of 9: 1 was added to every blood sample, and each blood sample was gently mixed well. After that, 500 μL of anticoagulant blood was taken with a 1000 μL manual pipette each time and injected into a 1 mL Eppendorf tube. The lid of the tube was closed to prevent water evaporation.

3 Apparatus and Reagents

Sonoclot analyzer was purchased from the Viscell Company, UK. The 0.109 mol/L sodium citrate solution (equal to 32 g/L sodium citrate containing two molecules of water of crystallization)was purchased from Beijing Greiner Bio-one Suns Limited Company, China. Glass beads-ACT kit (gb-ACT kit)was purchased from the Sienco Company, CO, USA. The calcium chloride solution (concentration of 0.25 mol/L)was configured by our laboratory. Puerarin Injection was purchased from Baiyun Mountain in Guangzhou Tianxin Pharmaceutical Limited Company. Heparin Sodium Injection was purchased from Qianhong in Changzhou Biochemical Pharmaceutical Co., Ltd. Tirofiban Hydrochloride Injection was purchased from Iroko Cardio Australia Pty Ltd, Australia.

4 Experimental Protocol

The Eppendorf tube filled with 500 μ L anticoagulant blood was rewarmed to 37 ℃, then added with 100 μL different concentrations of each injection (puerarin, heparin sodium or tirofiban hydrochloride)respectively. After gently mixed well, 20 μL 0.25 mol/L calcium chloride solution was added for recalcification, then 360 μL blood sample was injected into a kit box with a manual pipette. Turning on the blood sample mixed button immediately, at 10 s after the lid were covered. The instrument ran automatically. The ACT, CR and PF values of glass beads coagulant was measured on blood samples spiked with increasing concentrations of the 3 different injections [puerarin (0, 2.5, 3.0, 3.2, 3.4, 3.6, 3.8 mg/600 μL), heparin sodium (0, 0.1, 0.2, 0.3, 0.4, 0.6, 0.8 IU/600 μL)or tirofiban hydrochloride (0, 0.1, 0.2, 0.3, 0.4, 0.6, 0.8 μg/600 μl)] respectively.

Based on literature[5] and preliminary experiment results, Puerarin Injection initial concentration (2.5 mg/600 μL)is roughly 5 times of the highest clinical dose, Heparin Sodium Injection initial concentration (0.1 IU/600 μL)is roughly equivalent to the highest clinical dose, and Tirofiban Hydrochloride Injection initial concentration (0.1 μg/600 μL)is roughly half of the highest clinical dose.

5 Statistical Analysis

The values of ACT, CR and PF were presented as mean and standard deviation ($\bar{x} \pm s$). All reported P values were two-sided with significance set at $P < 0.01$. All statistical analysis were performed using R (version 3.2. 3, with package stats). A correlation analysis of the values of ACT, CR and PF under different concentrations of each injection was performed and a regression equation was created. The slop of linear regression and its significance for linear relationship were used to verify the impact on the above metrics. A log-linear regression was used to model the relationship between ACT and CR for different injections to compare their CR values under the same ACT value. A paired t-test was performed to compare the impacts of two injections on PF values.

RESULTS

1 Correlation between Values of ACT, CR, PF and Concentrations of Puerarin

The values of ACT, CR, PF measured under different concentrations of puerarin are summarized in Table 1. The results showed that the values of ACT gradually increased, the values of CR and PF gradually decreased with increasing concentrations of puerarin. There was a linear relationship between ACT, CR, PF values and concentrations of puerarin ($P < 0.01$). Furthermore, corresponding to each index, a linear regression equation was obtained (Figure 1).

Table 1　Correlation Analysis between the Metrics and Concentrations of Puerarin ($\bar{x} \pm s$)

Variables	Concentrations of puerarin (mg/600 μl)							r value	*P* value
	0	2.5	3.0	3.2	3.4	3.6	3.8		
ACT (s)	165.15 ± 20.65	264.15 ± 34.61	287.75 ± 37.46	302.35 ± 40.23	315.70 ± 44.80	336.45 ± 39.99	343.63 ± 44.26	17.09	＜0.01
CR (clot signal /min)	27.60 ± 4.92	16.33 ± 6.46	12.59 ± 5.02	11.48 ± 4.05	11.50 ± 4.09	10.21 ± 3.71	9.26 ± 4.16	-14.87	＜0.01
PF	3.10 ± 1.15	2.45 ± 1.15	1.68 ± 1.11	1.38 ± 1.04	0.97 ± 1.00	0.88 ± 0.85	0.61 ± 0.65	-8.63	＜0.01

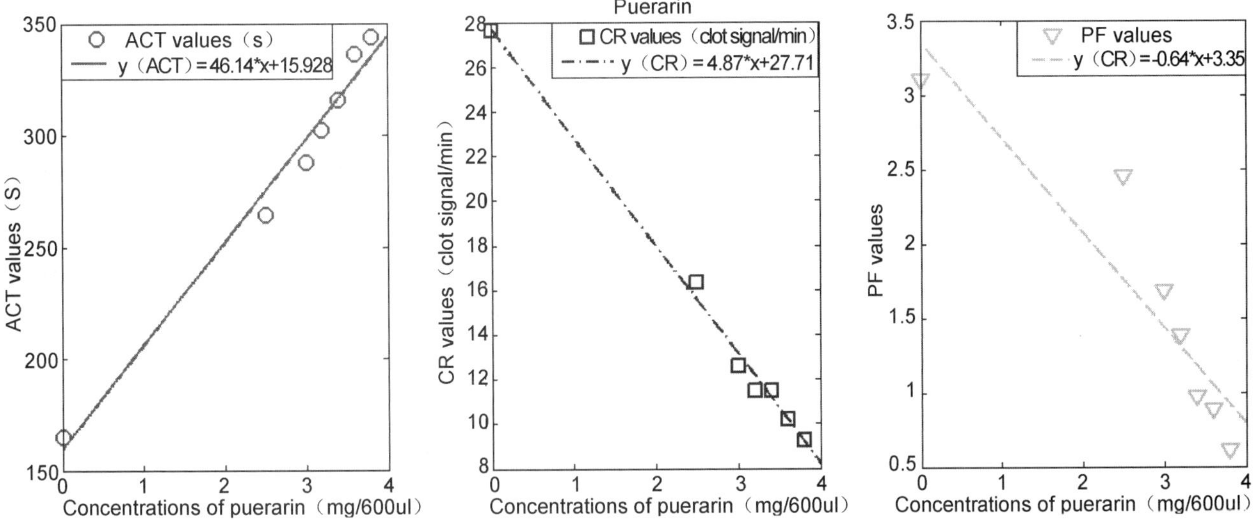

Figure 1 Linear Relationship between ACT, CR, PF Values and Concentrations of Puerarin

Notes: For each value of concentration, only mean of ACT/CR/PF values is shown for legibility.

Table 2 Correlation Analysis between the Metrics and Concentrations of Heparin Sodium ($\bar{x} \pm s$)

Variables	Concentrations of heparin sodium (IU/600 μl)							r value	*P* value
	0	0.1	0.2	0.3	0.4	0.6	0.8		
ACT (s)	165.15 ± 20.65	293.70 ± 69.62	428.30 ± 196.98	548.05 ± 232.25	665.00 ± 229.36	788.50 ± 265.50	956.18 ± 247.46	13.86	＜0.01
CR (clot signal / min)	27.60 ± 4.92	8.15 ± 2.77	4.59 ± 1.88	3.04 ± 1.74	2.62 ± 1.39	1.43 ± 0.84	0.99 ± 0.62	-10.40	＜0.01
PF	3.10 ± 1.15	1.73 ± 1.30	0.92 ± 0.66	0.87 ± 0.51	0.45 ± 0.40	0.36 ± 0.35	0.26 ± 0.24	-9.22	＜0.01

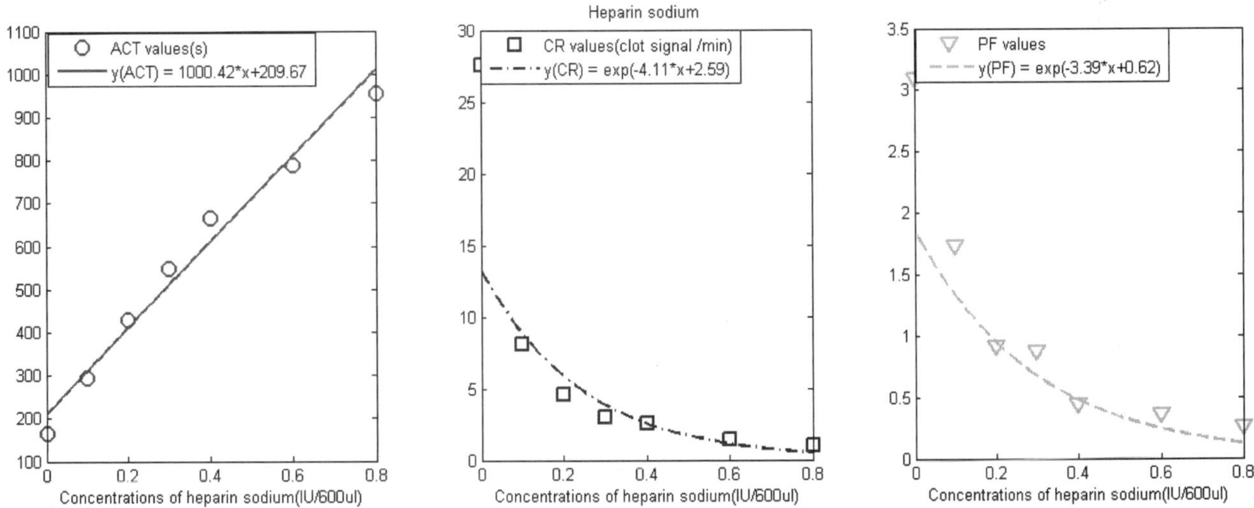

Figure 2 Linear/log-linear Relationship between ACT, CR, PF Values and Concentrations of Heparin Sodium

2 Correlation Analysis between the Values of ACT, CR, PF and Concentrations of Heparin Sodium

The values of ACT, CR, PF measured using different concentrations of heparin sodium are summarized in Table 2. The results showed that the values of ACT gradually increased, the values of CR and PF gradually decreased with the increase of concentrations of heparin sodium. There was also a linear relationship between ACT values and concentrations of heparin sodium ($P < 0.01$). For CR and PF, there was a log-linear relationship between their values and concentrations of heparin sodium ($P < 0.01$). Corresponding to each value, a regression equation was obtained (Figure 2).

Table 3 Correlation Analysis between the Metrics and Concentrations of Tirofiban Hydrochloride ($\bar{x} \pm s$)

Variables	Concentrations of tirofiban hydrochloride (ug/600 μl)							r value	P value
	0	0.1	0.2	0.3	0.4	0.6	0.8		
ACT (s)	165.15 ± 20.65	171.45 ± 21.34	167.40 ± 17.55	169.75 ± 17.71	173.25 ± 17.63	175.35 ± 22.60	175.75 ± 21.64	1.93	>0.01
CR (clot signal /min)	27.60 ± 4.92	26.05 ± 5.59	25.90 ± 5.08	25.95 ± 5.19	24.19 ± 6.62	24.45 ± 6.10	23.83 ± 5.18	-2.41	>0.01
PF	3.10 ± 1.15	1.84 ± 1.08	1.10 ± 0.73	0.97 ± 0.72	0.73 ± 0.58	0.54 ± 0.36	0.51 ± 0.45	-9.26	<0.01

3 Correlation Analysis between the Values of ACT, CR, PF and Concentrations of Tirofiban Hydrochloride

The values of ACT, CR, PF measured using different concentrations of tirofiban hydrochloride are summarized in Table 3. The results showed that there were no significant changes regarding the values of ACT and CR. But PF values gradually decreased with the increase of concentrations of tirofiban hydrochloride. There was a linear relationship between PF values and concentrations of heparin sodium ($P < 0.01$). Corresponding to each index, a linear regression equation was obtained (Figure 3). And, there is no linear relationship between ACT, CR values and concentrations of tirofiban hydrochloride.

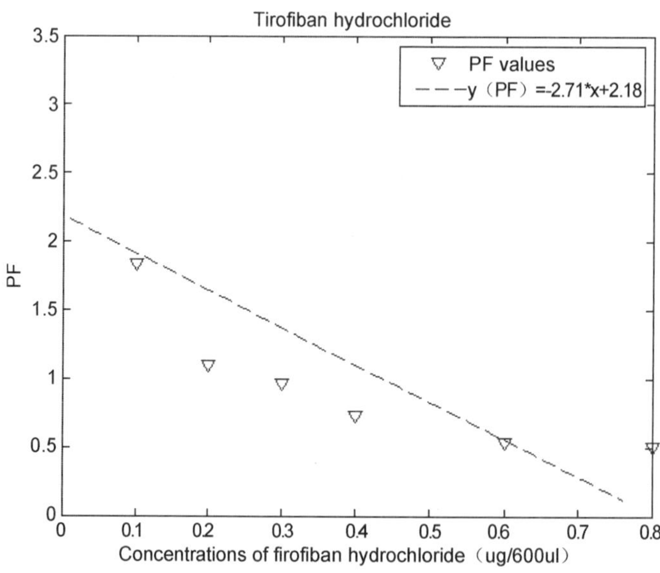

Figure 3 Linear Relationship between PF Values and Concentrations of Tirofiban Hydrochloride

4 Comparison of CR Values of Puerarin and Heparin Sodium under the Condition of the Same ACT Values

We used log-linear regression to model the relationship between CR and ACT values corresponding to the same concentration of puerarin. Their relationship can be described as equation (Ⅰ):

$CR = e^{-0.00623ACT+431}$, $P < 2.2e\text{-}16$ (Ⅰ)

The same method was used for heparin sodium. Their relationship can be described as equation (Ⅱ):

$CR = e^{-0.00281ACT+2.79}$, $P < 2.2e\text{-}16$ (Ⅱ)

Under the same ACT values, the puerarin corresponding CR values were always higher than the corresponding values of heparin sodium within the test ACT values range (Figure 4).

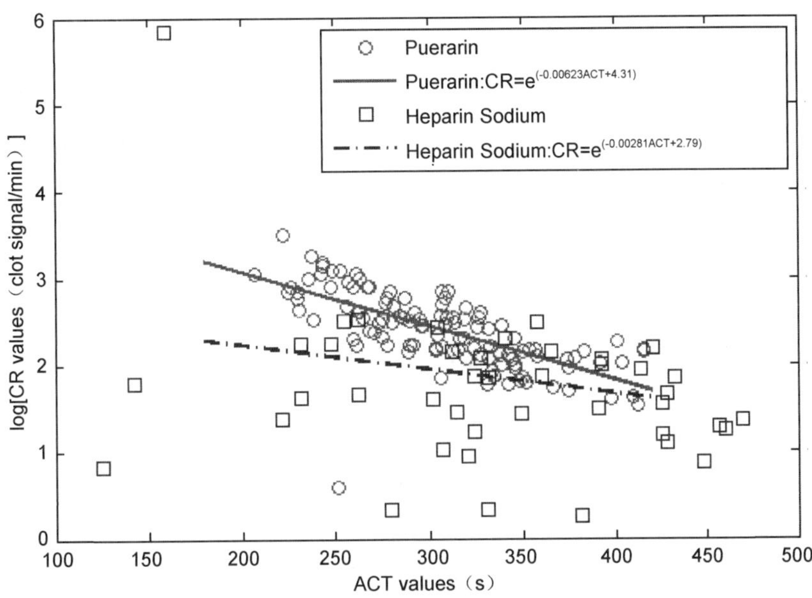

Figure 4 Linear Relationship between Log (CR Values)and ACT Values of Puerarin and Heparin Sodium

5 Comparison of PF Values of Puerarin and Tirofiban Hydrochloride

As a whole, both puerarin and tirofiban hydrochloride dropped the PF value down. The PF values decreased as the concentration increased and eventually reached to a quite low level.

For low puerarin concentrations, the PF values of puerarin were usually larger than that of all tirofiban hydrochloride concentrations. This can be verified by a paired t-test. In this test, PF value (pueraria=2.5 mg/600 μL)was significantly larger than PF value under all concentrations of tirofiban hydrochloride in our experiments ($P < 0.01$).

For high concentrations, their PF values had no significant difference [e.g, PF value (puerarin=3.8 mg/600 μL) had no significant difference with PF value (tirofiban hydrochlorid = 0.8 μg/600 μL)in paried *t*-test. However, PF values for high puerarin concentrations had a larger variance, which revealed that the individual variability for puerarin was larger than tirofiban hydrochloride (Figure 5).

DISCUSSION

Anticoagulation therapy is the basic treatment of antithrombotic therapy. Anticoagulant drugs will also increase the risk of bleeding at the same time of antithrombotic and affect platelet function. Currently, as a Chinese medicine, puerarin was only used as an adjuvant therapy of coronary heart disease, angina pectoris, retinal artery or vein occlusion, and myocardial infarction in China. It was not a common anticoagulant and antiplatelet drug. However, pharmacological study has shown that it has the strong function of anticoagulation and antiplatelet[1].

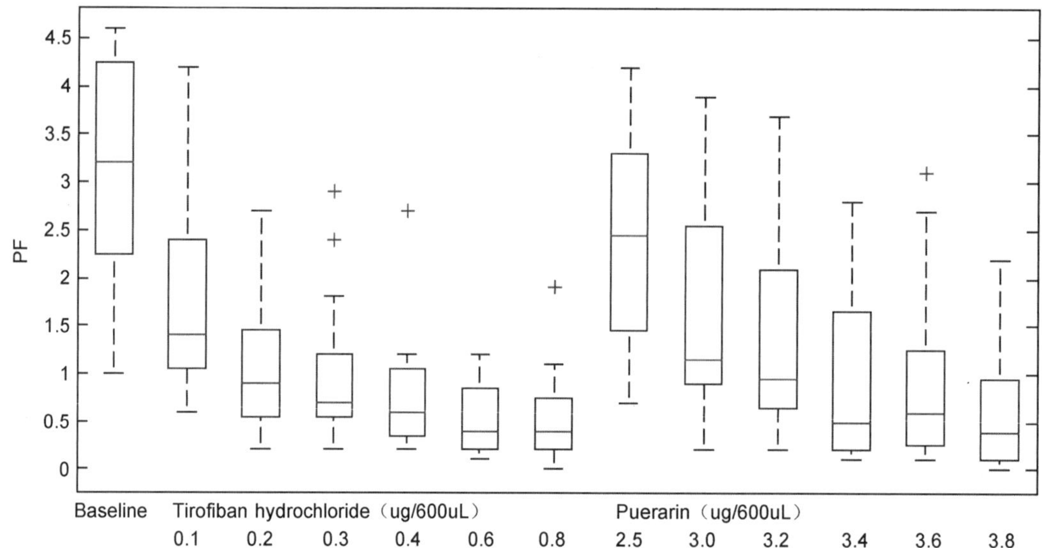

Figure 5　Box Plot of PF Values before and after Operation of Varied Concentrations of Puerarin and Tirofiban Hydrochloride

Heparin sodium is a widely used clinical anticoagulant drug, which generally does not require the regular anticoagulant monitoring. Tirofiban hydrochloride is usually used in combination with heparin in clinic. It is mainly for the prevention and treatment of cardiac ischemic complications with coronary artery sudden occlusion for coronary ischemia syndrome patients after coronary angioplasty or excision of coronary atherosclerosis plaque.

Our experiment showed that, with the increase of concentration of puerarin and heparin sodium, (1)ACT values increased gradually, which indicated that liquid-remained time of blood was extended; (2)CR values descended gradually, which suggested that its fibrin formation rate had slowed down; (3)PF values descended gradually, which indicated that its platelet function was restrained. However, for tirofiban hydrochloride, only PF value decreased as the concentration of injection increased. ACT value and CR value had no significant change as the concentration increased. It revealed that tirofiban hydrochloride had selective inhibition of platelet, with no significant impact on the fibrin formation rate and coagulation activate time.

Literature pointed out that puerarin could inhibit the 5-HT release in platelet induced by thrombin[1]. In our experiment, puerarin had strong anticoagulation and antiplatelet effects in a concentration-dependence manner, which can be also taken as an evidence. Heparin sodium is a kind of glycosaminoglycan, containing sulfate anions with large negative charges which interfered with multiple routes in the process of blood clotting. It is mainly mediated by the AT-Ⅲ. Through the combination with AT-Ⅲ, it accelerates the thrombin inactivation, inactivates serine protease, thus prevents blood coagulation from multiform anticoagulationn[6] (thrombinogenesis-preventing, thrombin activity inhibiting and platelet aggregation preventing). In our experiment, heparin sodium also showed strong anticoagulation and antiplatelet effects in a concentration-dependence manner. Tirofiban hydrochloride is a low molecular weight, non-peptide antagonist of the platelet glycoprotein Ⅱb/Ⅲa receptor (the major platelet surface receptor in platelet aggregation). It can prevent the binding interaction of fibrinogen and glycoprotein Ⅱb/Ⅲa to block platelet crosslinking and aggregation. There was a in vitro experiment which showed that tiroflban hydrochloride could inhibit the platelet aggregation induced by ADP and extend the bleeding time (BT)of both healthy people and coronary heart disease patients[7].

Based on the complexity of the clinical situation and the particularity of China's national conditions, patients may select and use a variety of anticoagulation and antiplatelet Chinese medicines (including nostrum and crude drugs etc.)by themselves at the same time. This is bound to affect the doctor's selection of anticoagulant drugs for patients.

It was shown in this study that when obtaining the same ACT value, the corresponding CR value of puerarin was obviously larger than that of heparin sodium, i. e, to get the same liquid-remained time of blood, puerarin kept a relatively higher fibrin formation rate. It was a hint that puerarin might have a lower hemorrhage risk than heparin sodium when obtaining the same anticoagulation effect in the concentration range of this experiment. Besides, for low concentration, puerarin had a weaker antiplatelet function than tirofiban hydrochloride. As concentration increased, this function of puerarin approximated tirofiban hydrochloride and eventually obtained the same effect. However, the antiplatelet effect of puerarin had a larger individual variability.

In conclusion, puerarin has strong anticoagulation and antiplatelet effects, and it may have a lower hemorrhage risk than heparin sodium when obtained the same anticoagulation effect in the concentration range of this experiment. In addition, for high concentration, puerarin has the same antiplatelet function as tirofiban hydrochloride but with a larger individual variability. The anticoagulation and antiplatelet effect of some Chinese medicine cannot be ignored. We should avoid superposition of it in the anticoagulant therapy in clinical use. The anticoagulation and antiplatelet mechanisms of puerarin still need to be further studied.

REFERENCES

[1] Yin ZZ, Zeng GY. Pharmacology of puerarin. V. Effects of puerarin on platelet aggregation and release of 5-HT from platelets[J]. Acta Acad Med Sin (Chin), 1981, 1: 44-47.

[2] Tuman KJ, Spiess BD, Mccarthy RJ, et al Comparison of viscoelastic measures of coagulation after cardiopulmonary bypass[J]. Anesth Analg, 1989: 69-75.

[3] Chapin JW, Becker GL, Hulbert BJ, et al. Comparison of thromboelastograph and Sonoclot coagulation analyzer for assessing coagulation status during orthotopic liver transplantation[J]. Transplant Proc, 1989: 3539-3539.

[4] John JD, William AL, AJ Wright. Effective hemostasis in cardiac surgery[J]. Anesthesiology, 1989: 325-326.

[5] Yang X. The study of development of purring injection[M]. Changchun: Jilin University, 2008.

[6] Chen X, Chen WZ, Zeng GY. Cardiovascular pharmacology. 3rd ed[M]. Beijing: People's Medical Publishing House, 2002: 520-523.

[7] Lynch JJ Jr, Cook JJ, Sitko GR, Holahan MA, Ramjit DR, Mellott MJ, et al. Nonpeptide glycoprotein Ⅱb/Ⅲa inhibitors. 5. Antithrombotic effects of MK-0383[J]. J Pharmacol Exp Ther, 1995: 20-32.

First Published: LI Si-wei, FENG Xue, XU Hao, CHEN Ke-ji. Comparison on anticoagulation and antiplatelet aggregation effects of puerarin with heparin sodium and tirofiban hydrochloride: an *In Vitro* study[J]. Chin J Integr Med, 2018, 24 (2): 103-108.

Ginkgo biloba Leaf Extract Protects against Myocardial Injury via Attenuation of Endoplasmic Reticulum Stress in Streptozotocin-Induced Diabetic ApoE$^{-/-}$ Mice

TIAN Jin-fan, LIU Yan-fei, LIU Yue, CHEN Ke-ji, and LYU Shu-zheng

Diabetic cardiomyopathy (DCM), one of the leading cardiovascular complications of diabetes, ultimately leads to heart failure, which increases the mortality among diabetes patients. Diabetic myocardial injuries, including cardiomyocyte apoptosis, myocardial fibrosis, and intramyocardial inflammation, are important pathological characteristics of DCM. Diabetes-induced cardiomyocyte apoptosis often occurs concomitantly with interstitial collagen deposition and myofiber disarray[1]. In addition, accumulating evidence has shown that substrate metabolic alteration, oxidative stress, and chronic inflammation contribute to DCM and diabetic myocardial injury [2,3].

Endoplasmic reticulum stress (ERS)plays a critical role in the development of diabetic myocardial injury because the sustained and uncorrected unfolded protein response (UPR)could induce cell death [4]. The UPR is mediated by three pathways, the inositol-requiring kinase-1 (IRE1), protein kinase R-like ER kinase (PERK), and activating transcription factor (ATF6)pathways. ERS-mediated cell death involves activation of c-Jun N-terminal kinase (JNK), C/EBP homologous protein (CHOP), and caspase-12, which consequently activates caspase-3.

IRE1 and JNK activation may result in upregulation of nuclear factor kappa-B (NF-κB)expression via phosphorylation of the β-subunit of IkB kinase complex (IKKβ)[5,6]. Upregulation of NF-κB expression leads to increased production of proinflammatory cytokines, such as tumor necrosis factor-α (TNF-α), interleukin-1β (IL-1β), and IL-6, which contribute to cardiomyocyte apoptosis and myocardial fibrosis [7].

Recently, herbal treatment of diabetic myocardial injury has gained much attention. Ginkgo biloba leaves have been used as a traditional herbal medicine for hundreds of years in China. The major components of Ginkgo biloba leaf extract (GBE)include two active substances, namely terpenoids (including ginkgolides and biobalide)and flavonoids (Figure 1). GBE was shown to exhibit antioxidant, free-radical scavenging, and membrane-stabilizing activities, which contributed to its beneficial effects in ischemia/reperfusion injury in diabetic rat myocardium [8]. In addition, it showed anti-inflammatory and antioxidant effects in the pancreas of streptozotocin (STZ)-induced diabetic animals [9,10]. Moreover, GBE enhanced insulin sensitivity and prevented insulin resistance by increasing insulin-induced Akt phosphorylation and insulin receptor substrate 1 expression[11]. GBE was also shown to ameliorate diabetic nephropathy in STZ-induced diabetic rats[12].

Currently, few studies have investigated the potential use of GBE for the treatment of diabetic myocardial injury. In the present study, we aimed to investigate whether GBE could protect against diabetic myocardial injury and elucidate the underlying mechanisms.

MATERIALS AND METHODS

1 Drugs

GBE powders and atorvastatin were purchased from Beijing Handian Pharmaceutical Co. Ltd. and Pfizer Pharmaceutical Co. Ltd., respectively. GBE used in the present study contains 44.9% ginkgo flavonoids, 6.3% terpenoids, and < 1ppm ginkgo acid.

2 Experimental Animals

Male ApoE-/-mice, aged 6-7 weeks and weighing 19-21 g (C57BL/6J background, introduced from Jackson Laboratory of USA by Peking University Health Science Center Laboratory Animal Science Department; quality certification number, SCXK (Beijing)2016-0012)were used in this study. The rearing condition of the mice was grade 2. Mice were maintained under controlled conditions (room temperature, 22-24 ℃; relative humidity, 50%; and lights on; from 7: 00 to 19: 00). The experimental protocol was approved by the institutional animal care and use committee of Xiyuan Hospital, China Academy of Chinese Medical Sciences. Animal experiments were carried out in accordance with the Guide for the Care and Use of Laboratory Animals published by the US National Institutes of Health.

3 Experimental Protocol

ApoE-/-mice were fed with a high-fat diet (basic diet, 78.85%; fat, 21%; cholesterol, 0.15%)for four weeks before diabetes was induced by intraperitoneal injection of 50 mg/kg/day STZ (Sigma)diluted with citrate buffer (pH 4.5; final concentration, 1%)for five consecutive days, as described in a previous study [13]. Mice exhibiting plasma glucose levels > 12 mmol/L were considered diabetic and were used in the study (n=58)[13,14]. The diabetic mice were then treated with atorvastatin [15,16] (10 mg/kg/day, Intragastric [i. g.], n=14), GBE at a low dose (200 mg/kg/day, i. g., n=16), or GBE at a high dose (400 mg/kg/day, i. g., n = 17). The doses of GBE were selected based on previous studies [17,18]. Diabetic mice treated with equal volumes of saline served as the untreated diabetic group (n=11). All ApoE-/-mice were maintained on a high-fat diet and sacrificed after 12-week treatment. C58BL/6J mice (n=20)served as the control group. The study time line is shown in Figure 2.

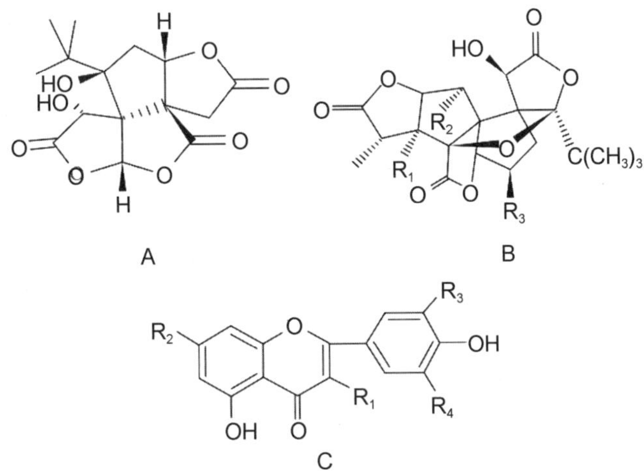

Figure 1 Chemical Structures of the Constituents of GBE.
Notes: A. Bilobalide, B. ginkgolide, and C. ginkgo flavonol glycosides.

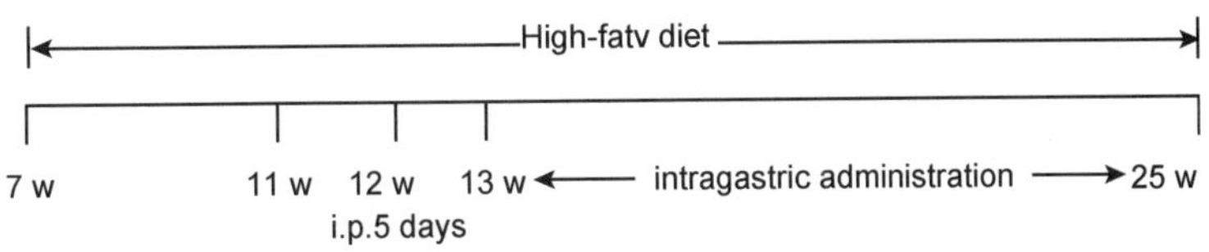

Figure 2 Timeline of the Experimental Protocol *in vivo*

4 Body Weight and Plasma Glucose Changes

The body weight and fasting plasma glucose levels were measured before the initial GBE dose and every four weeks thereafter. Plasma samples were collected by the cutting tail method, and the plasma glucose levels were measured using a glucometer (Roche).

5 Tissue Preparation and Histological Examination

All animals were euthanized, and the heart samples were collected before they were perfused with heparin saline. The specimens were transversely cut and fixed with 4% paraformaldehyde for 24 h. They were then embedded in paraffin and cut into 5-μm–thick sections for hematoxylin/eosin and Masson's staining. Immunohistochemical staining of cleaved caspase-3 was also performed (Rabbit polyclonal anti-cleaved caspase-3, CST, 1: 200 dilution). Immunohistochemical quantitative analysis was conducted on microscopic images using Image-pro plus 6.0 (Media Cybernetics, Inc., Rockville, MD, USA)software under 200 × magnification. The positive expression of cleaved caspase-3 was represented by integral optical density (IOD).

6 Western Blot Analysis

The heart tissues were removed from liquid nitrogen, weighed, and homogenized in radioimmunoprecipitation assay (RIPA)lysis buffer. Protein concentration was determined using the bicinchoninic acid method. Equal amounts of protein (40 μg)from each sample were separated by sodium dodecyl sulfate-polyacrylamide gel electrophoresis (SDS-PAGE)and transferred onto a nitrocellulose membrane. Non-specific sites were blocked by incubating the membranes with 5% non-fat milk and 0.2 % tween 20 in Tris-buffered saline for 2 h at room temperature. After washing, the membranes were incubated overnight at 4° C with the following primary antibodies: anti-CHOP (CST 2895S, 1 ∶ 2000), anti-JNK (CST9252S, 1 ∶ 3000), anti-p-JNK (CST9251S, 1 ∶ 1000), anti-caspase-12 (CST2202S, 1 ∶ 1000), anti-cleaved caspase-3 (CST 9664S, 1 ∶ 1000), and anti-NF-κB (abcam 86299, 1 ∶ 2000). The membranes were washed with TBS-T and incubated with horseradish peroxidase (HRP)-conjugated secondary antibodies. Then, the membrane was assayed using an enhanced chemiluminescence system. Glyceraldehyde 3-phosphate dehydrogenase (GADPH)was used to ensure equal sample loading. The expression levels of CHOP, caspase-12, cleaved caspase-3, and NF-κB were adjusted for GADPH, and the values were normalized over the untreated diabetic group. The expression levels of p-JNK were adjusted for total-JNK, and then normalized over the untreated diabetic group.

2.7. Quantitative Real-Time PCR. Real-time polymerase chain reaction (PCR)was performed to determine the gene expression of collagen I and III, TNF-α, and IL-1β. GADPH was used as an internal control. The primer sequences were as follows: collagen I, 5'-TGGAAACCCGAGGTATGCTT-3'and 5'-CATTGCATTGCACGTCATC G-3'; collagen III, 5'-ACTGGTGAACGTGGCTCTAA-3'and 5'-AACCTGGAGGACCTGGATTG-3'; TNF-α, 5'- CTCATGCACCACCATCAAGG-3'and 5'-ACCTGACCACTCTCCCTTTG-3'; and IL-1β, 5'-GAAGAAGAGCCCAT CCTCTG-3' and 5'-TCATCTCGGAGCCTGTAGTG-3'. Relative mRNA level was normalized over the untreated diabetic group. All experiments were repeated for at least three times.

7 Serum Lipid Proflle and Glucose Analysis

At the end of the 12-week period, all mice were fasted overnight before they were sacrificed, and blood samples were collected and centrifuged at 3000rpm for 10 min. Serum glucose, high-density lipoprotein cholesterol (HDL-c), total cholesterol (TC), triglycerides (TG), and low-density lipoprotein cholesterol (LDL-c) levels were determined using an automated system.

8 Measurement of Serum Inflammatory Cytokine Levels

Serum levels of inflammatory cytokines (IL-6, IL-1β, and TNF-α)were measured using commercially available ELISA kits, purchased from Beijing Fang Cheng Jia Hong Technology Co. Ltd. (catalog no. FU-X0850; FU-X0840; and FU-X1059, respectively). The serum was collected as previously described. Five serial dilutions of the standard were prepared according to the manufacturer's instructions. Blank and sample wells were set, respectively. Sample diluent (40 μL)was added to the sample wells in the pre-coated ELISA plates, followed by addition of the samples (10 μL). After sealing the plates with a closure plate membrane, they were incubated for 30 min at 37 ℃. HRP-conjugated reagent (50 μL)was added to all wells, except for the blank well. After incubation at 37 ℃, the liquid in the wells was removed, and the plate was washed with a wash liquid. Chromogen solution A (50 μL)and chromogen solution B (50 μL)were added to each well. The plates were incubated in dark at 37 ℃ for 15 min. The blank well was considered zero, and the absorbance of each well was measured at 450nm within 15 min after adding the stop solution.

3.0 Statistical Analysis. SPSS 17.0 was used for statistical analyses. The data were presented as the means ± standard deviation ($\bar{x} \pm s$). One-way analysis of variance (*ANOVA*)was used to perform comparisons among group means, and the least signiflcant difference (*LSD*)test was used for multiple comparisons between the untreated diabetic group and other groups. $P < 0$ 05 was considered statisti-cally signiflcant. GraphPad Prism 5.0 software was used for graphical presentation.

RESULTS

1 Body Weight and Plasma Glucose Levels

STZ resulted in a significant increase in plasma glucose levels, compared to those in the control group (14.8 ± 2.2 *vs*. 5.3 ± 0.0.8 mmol/L, $P < 0.01$). At the end of the 12-week gavage, the untreated diabetic mice showed severe hyperglycemia compared to the control group (23.4 ± 6.4 *vs*. 7.5 ± 1 mmol/L, $P < 0.01$). GBE treatment at 200 and 400 mg/kg/day suppressed the plasma glucose levels; however, only high-dose GBE resulted in a statistically significant difference (low-dose GBE group *vs*. untreated diabetic group, 18.8 ± 6.5 mmol/L *vs*. 23.4 ± 6.4 mmol/L, P=0.06; high-dose GBE group *vs*. untreated diabetic group, 15.3 ± 7.1 mmol/L *vs*. 23.4 ± 6.4 6.4 mmol/L, P=0.01).

There was significant weight loss in the diabetic mice compared to those in the control group (22.37 ± 11.67 *vs*. 26.58 ± 11.56 g, $P < 0.01$). Body weight loss was associated with hyperglycemia and polyuria. Body weight of mice in the untreated diabetic group was significantly lower than that in the control group at the end of the study course [30.01 ± 1 1.35 vs. 26.38 ± 22.72 g, $P < 0.01$). Atorvastatin and GBE treatment did not affect the body weight in diabetic mice.

2 Effect of GBE on Serum Lipid and Glucose Proflles

Serum lipid and blood glucose levels were measured before the mice were sacrificed. LDL-c, TC, TG, and blood glucose levels significantly increased in the untreated diabetic group, compared to those in the control group. Atorvastatin and GBE (200 and 400 mg/kg/day)significantly decreased LDL-c, TC, and TG levels ($P < 0.01$, Figure 3A-C). GBE at 200 mg/kg/day lowered the serum glucose levels, compared to those in the untreated diabetic group ($P < 0.05$, Figure 3E). There were no significant differences in HDL-c levels among the control, untreated diabetic, atorvastatin, low-dose GBE, and high-dose GBE groups (Figure 3D).

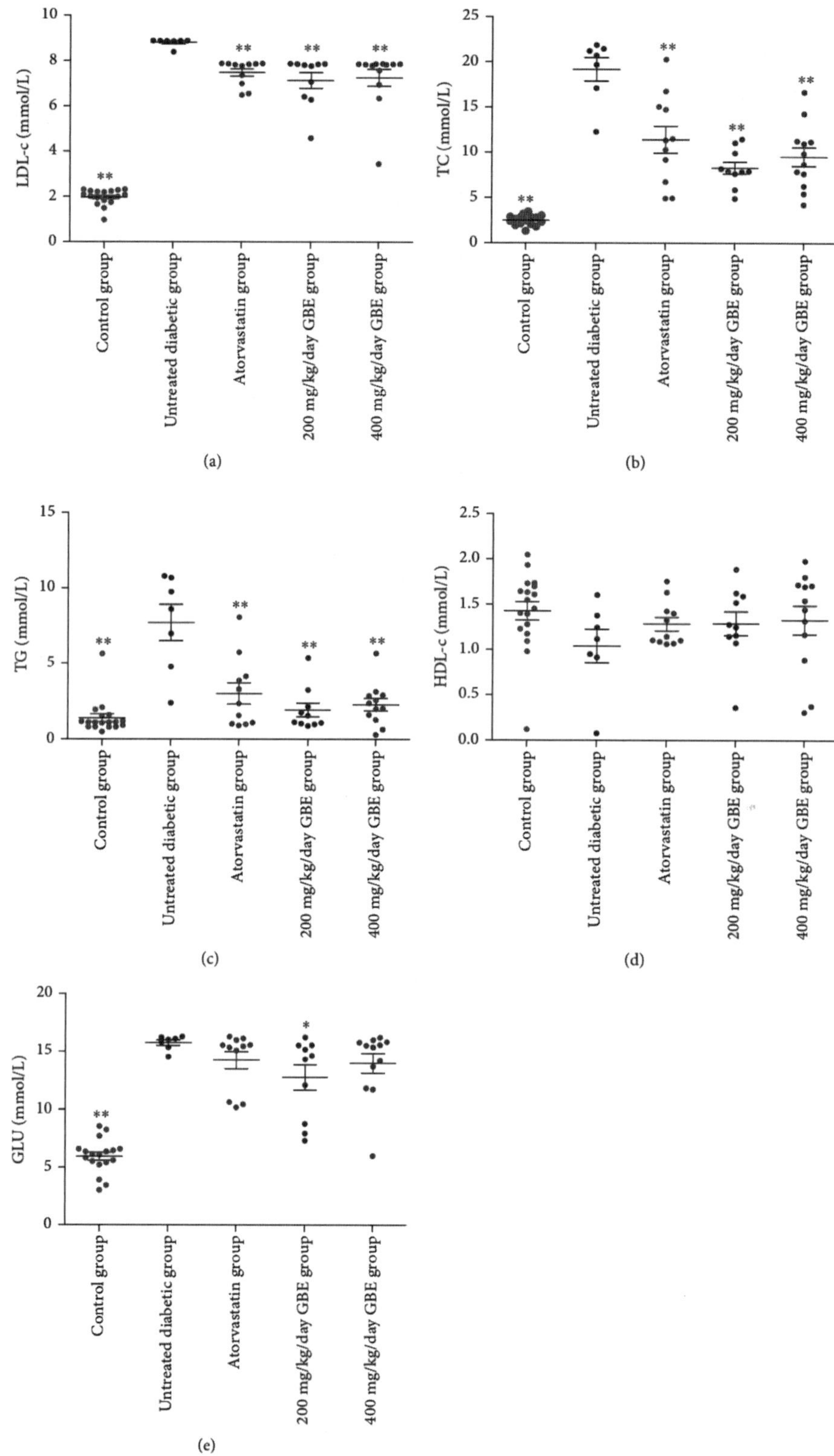

Figure 3　Serum Lipid Proflles and Glucose Levels

Notes: $^{*}P < 0.05$ and $^{**}P < 0.01$ versus the untreated diabetic group.

3 Effect of GBE on Serum Inflammatory Cytokine Levels

The levels of serum inflammatory cytokines, including IL-6, IL-1β, and TNF-α, significantly increased in the diabetic rats, compared to the control rats. GBE (200 and 400 mg/kg/day)significantly decreased serum IL-1β, TNF-α, and IL-6 levels. Moreover, high-dose GBE (400 mg/kg/day)resulted in lower levels of inflammatory cytokines, compared to those administered with low-dose GBE ($P < 0.01$, Figure 4A-C).

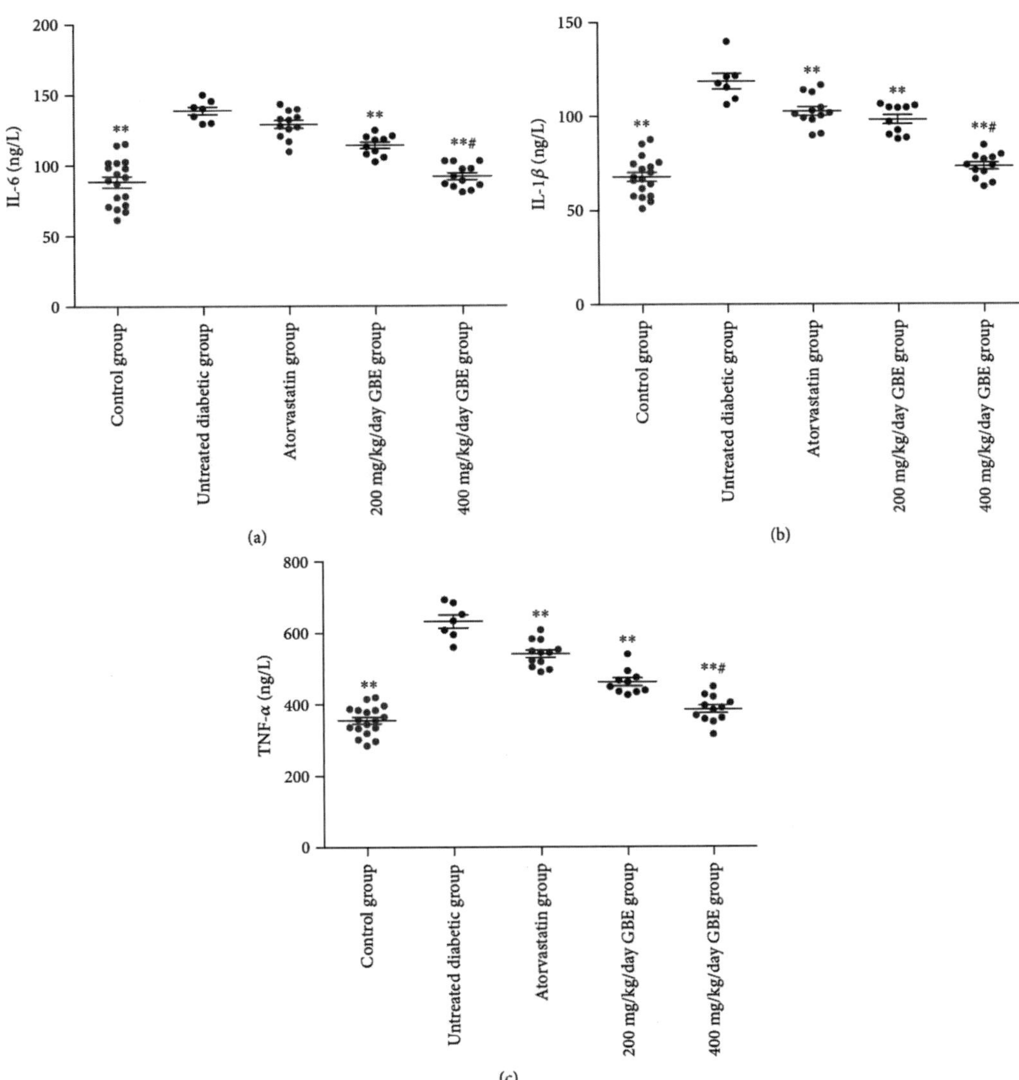

Figure 4 Serum Proinflammatory Cytokines Determined by ELISA

Notes: $^{**}P < 0.01$ versus the untreated diabetic group; $^{\#}P < 0.01$ versus the 200 mg/kg/day GBE group.

4 Effect of GBE on the Histomorphology of Diabetic Hearts

Similar to the findings reported by Abdel-Hamid et al. [19], H&E staining showed diffuse disruption of the myocardium, with fragmented and feathery appearance of DCM. Fibroblasts and inflammatory cells infiltrated the untreated diabetic myocardium, whereas atorvastatin and GBE treatment alleviated their infiltration (Figure 5A). In addition, Masson's staining showed that GBE treatment blunted the total cardiac collagen content (Figure 5B).

Immunostaining showed that cleaved caspase-3 expression significantly increased in the untreated diabetic mice, compared to that in the control group, whereas atorvastatin and GBE at 200 and 400 mg/kg/day significantly decreased the expression of cleaved caspase-3 ($P < 0.05$, Figure 5C and D). The difference between low-dose and high-dose GBE was not statistically significant.

3.5. Effect of GBE on mRNA Levels of Collagen I and III. Collagen I and III mRNA levels increased in the untreated diabetic mice. Atorvastatin and GBE (200 and 400 mg/kg/day)treatment resulted in a statistically significant decrease in collagen I and III mRNA levels ($P < 0.05$, Figure 6A and B). There was no significant difference between low-dose and high-dose GBE.

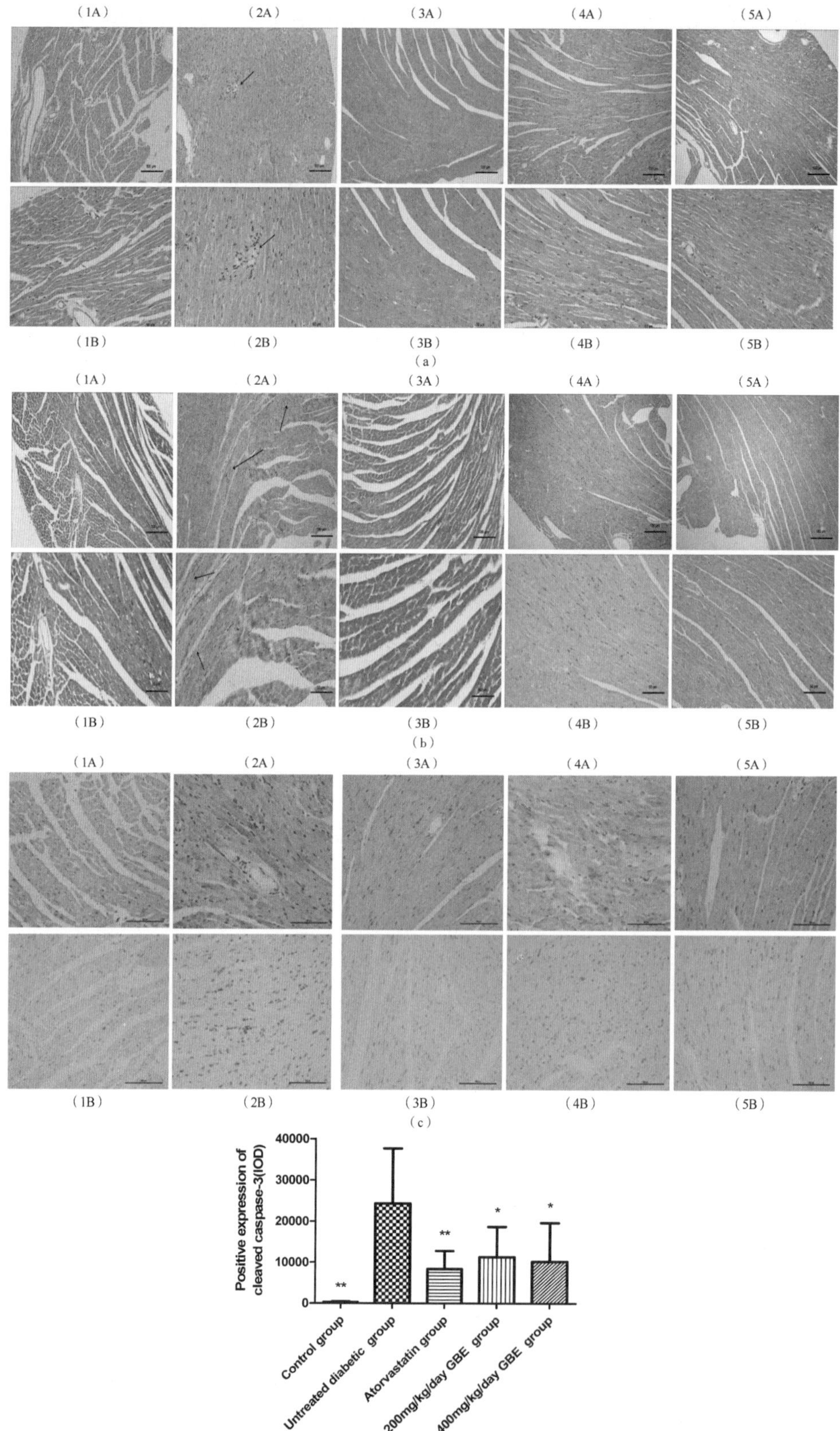

Figure 5　Effects of GBE on the Cardiac Histomorphological Changes in Diabetic ApoE$^{-/-}$ mice. (a)H&E staining of cross-sectional tissue slices of the myocardium. (b)Masson's staining of collagen in the myocardium. The blue area against the red represents collagen deposition. Arrows indicate interstitial flbers. (c, d)Immunostaining of cleaved caspase-3. The brown-yellow area represents the positive expression of cleaved caspase-3. Images of the samples incubated only with the secondary antibody were provided correspondingly. (1A, 1B)Control group; (2A, 2B)untreated diabetic group; (3A, 3B)atorvastatin group; (4A, 4B)200 mg/kg/day GBE group; and (5A, 5B)400 mg/kg/day GBE group. (A)100x magniflcation; (B)200x magniflcation. $^{*}P < 0.05$ and $^{**}P < 0.01$ versus the untreated diabetic group.

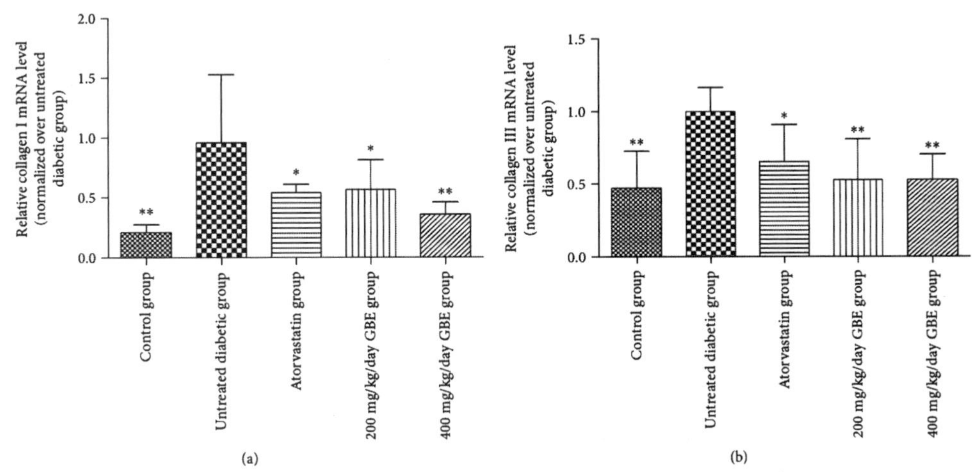

Figure 6 Relative mRNA Expression of Collagen I and III (normalized over the untreated diabetic group)

Notes: $^{*}P < 0.05$ and $^{**}P < 0.01$ versus the untreated diabetic group.

5 Effect of GBE on Intramyocardial Inflammation

NF-κB plays a crucial role in the regulation of intramyocardial inflammation in the development of DCM. The untreated diabetic mice displayed increased expression of NF-κB. Atorvastatin and GBE significantly decreased the expression of NF-κB ($P < 0.05$, Figure 7A and B). TNF-α and IL-1β mRNA levels increased in the untreated diabetic mice; however, GBE treatment at doses of 200 and 400 mg/kg/day significantly inhibited the STZ-induced increase in TNF-α and IL-1β mRNA levels ($P < 0.05$, Figure 7C and D). The difference between the findings for low-dose and high-dose GBE was not statistically significant.

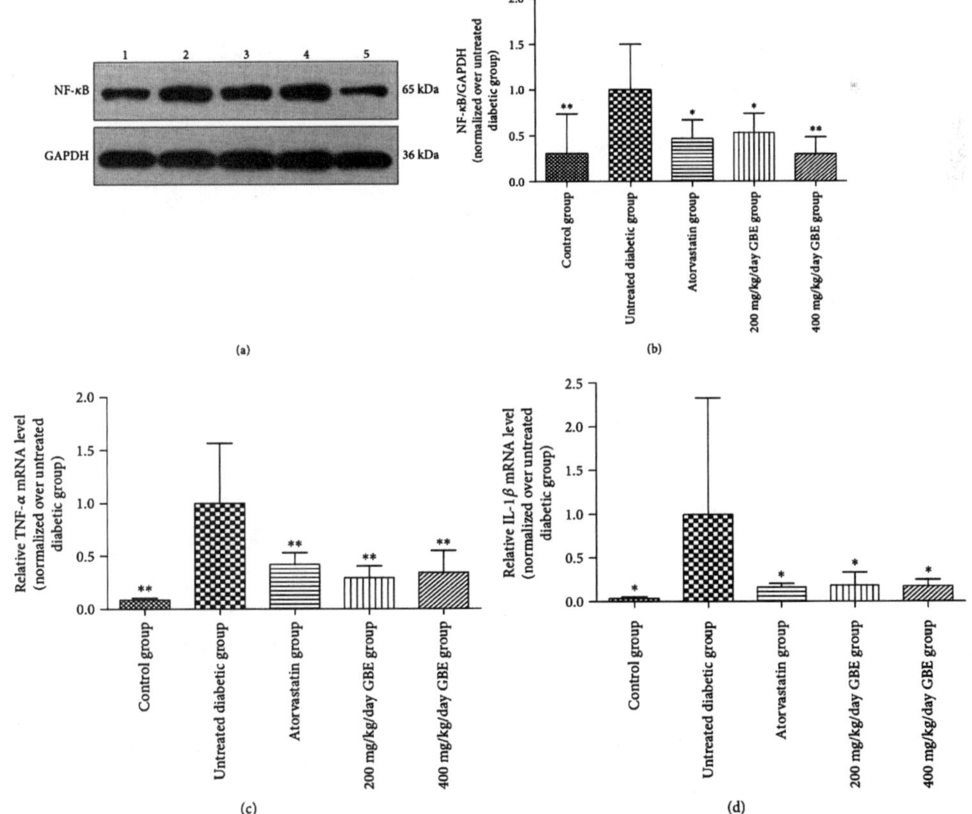

Figure 7 Effects of GBE on NF-κB-mediated Intramyocardial Inflammation

Notes: (a, b)NF-κB expression was determined by Western blotting. (c, d)Relative mRNA expression of TNF-α and IL-1β measured by real-time PCR. $^{*}P < 0.05$ and $^{**}P < 0.01$ versus the untreated diabetic group.

6 Effect of GBE on Hallmarks of ERS-Associated Apoptosis

Western blot analysis showed that the expression of the hall-marks of ERS-associated apoptosis, including p-JNK, CHOP, caspase-12, and cleaved caspase-3, signiflcantly increased in the myocardium of diabetic mice, compared to those in the normal control group. This suggested that the p-JNK, CHOP, and caspase-12 cascades were activated in the diabetic myo-cardium. Atorvastatin and GBE (200 and 400 mg/kg/day)signiflcantly decreased the expression of p-JNK, CHOP, cas-pase-12, and cleaved caspase-3 ($P < 0.05$, Figures 8 (a)–8 (h)). There were no statistical differences between the low-dose and high-dose GBE.

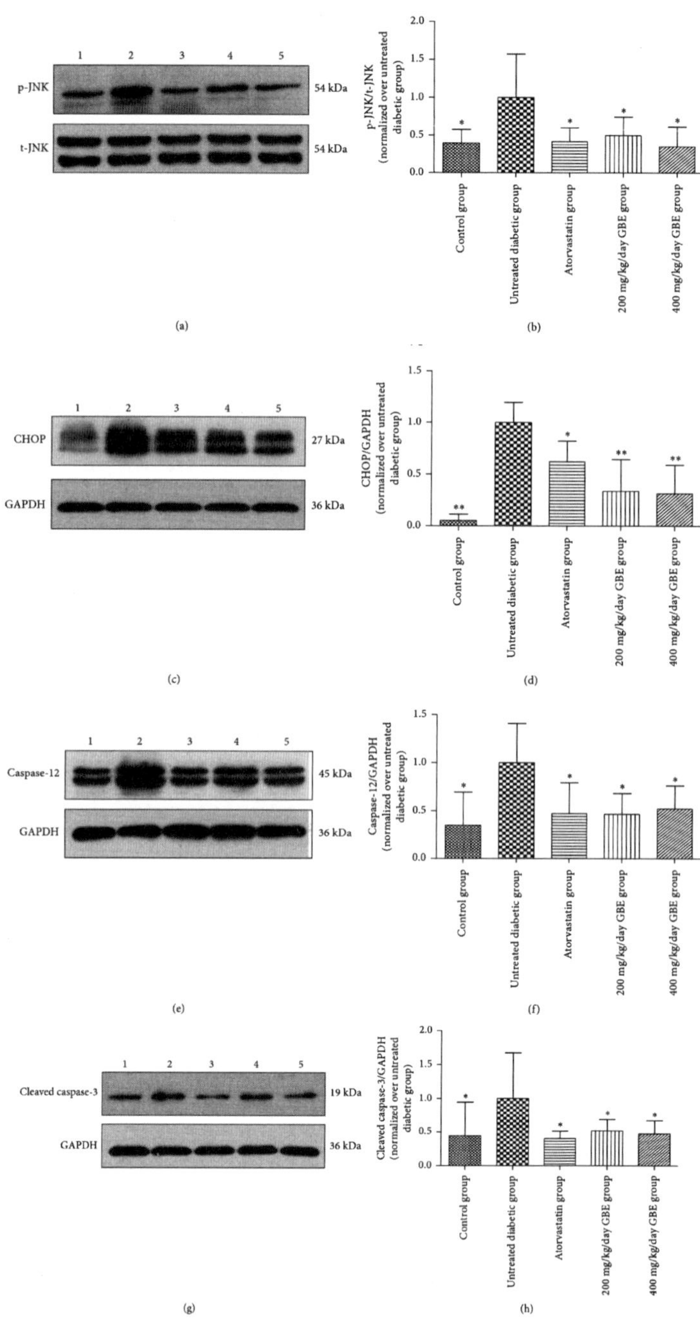

Figure 8 Effects of GBE on ERS-related Apoptosis Hallmark Expression

Notes: Expression levels of p-JNK/JNK, CHOP, caspase-12, and cleaved caspase-3 were determined by Western blotting. The expression levels of CHOP, caspase-12, and cleaved caspase-3, were adjusted for GAPDH, and the expression of p-JNK was adjusted for total JNK. These values were normalized over the untreated diabetic group. (a, b)Expression levels of p-JNK/JNK; (c, d)expression of CHOP; (e, f)expression of caspase-12; and (g, h)expression of cleaved caspase-3. $^{*}P < 0\ 05$ and $^{**}P < 0\ 01$ versus the untreated diabetic group. 1: control group; 2: untreated group; 3: atorvastatin group; 4: 200 mg/kg/day GBE group; and 5: 400 mg/kg/day GBE group.

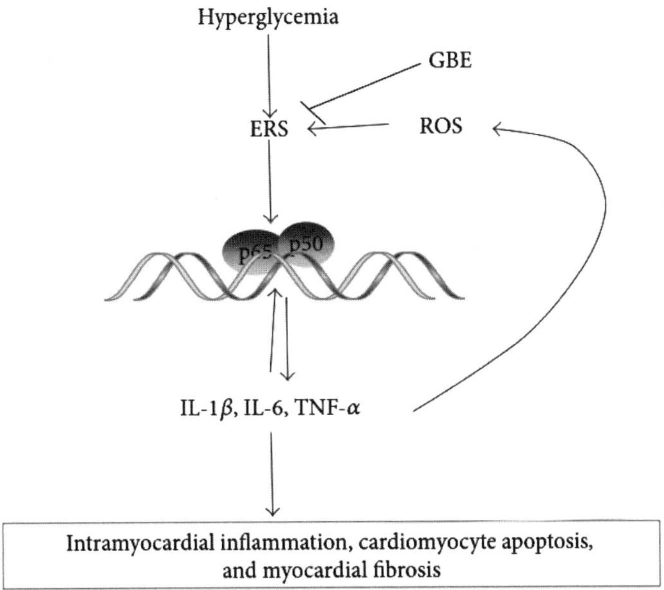

Figure 9 Mechanism Underlying the Protective Effects of GBE Against Myocardial Injury Induced by Hyperglycemia

Notes: The three pathways of UPR could activate NF-κB by phosphorylation of IKK, promoting the production of inflammation cytokines. TNF-α activates NF-κB in the presence of ROS in a positive feedback loop, resulting in the generation of more inflammatory cytokines, leading to intramyocardial inflammation, cardiomyocyte apoptosis, and myocardial fibrosis. GBE attenuated diabetic myocardial injury via blocking ERS. ROS: reactive oxygen species.

DISCUSSION

Diabetes mellitus is a worldwide metabolic disease responsible for increased morbidity and mortality. Patients with diabetes mellitus are at high risk of cardiovascular diseases, such as atherosclerosis and DCM, which are comorbidities of diabetes mellitus [20]. STZ has been frequently used to induce diabetes in experimental animals because of its toxic effects on the pancreatic β-cells and its potential to induce oxidative stress[21]. Hence, in the present study, we established a diabetic myocardial injury $ApoE^{-/-}$mouse model by STZ injection combined with high-fat diet, as previously described [22,23]. Although it was not able to distinguish between hyperlipidemia-and diabetes-induced myocardial injury, this study aimed to investigate whether GBE attenuated diabetic myocardial injury in $ApoE^{-/-}$mice, thus providing potential evidence for the treatment of diabetes patients with DCM and atherosclerosis as comorbidities. We found that collagen I and III mRNA expression was elevated in diabetic mice. TNF-α and IL-1β mRNA levels, which represent intramyocardial inflammation, increased in diabetic heart owing to increased NF-κB activation. Additionally, hallmarks of ERS-related apoptosis, including p-JNK, CHOP, caspase-12, and cleaved caspase-3 were upregulated in the diabetic heart. These indicated that interstitial collagen deposition, ERS-related apoptosis, and NF-κB-mediated inflammation were induced in diabetic $ApoE^{-/-}$. Consistent with the results of previous studies [15,16,19,24], atorvastatin treatment improved the histological abnormalities, fibrosis, and apoptosis of cardiomyocytes *via* inhibition of NF-κB-induced inflammation and cleaved caspase-3-mediated apoptosis in diabetic heart. To our knowledge, the present study is the first study to show that traditional Chinese medicine, GBE could protect against diabetic myocardial injury, particularly apoptosis, myocardial fibrosis, and NF-κB-mediated inflammation *via* inhibition of ERS-related apoptosis, as evidenced by the decrease in p-JNK, caspase-12, and cleaved caspase-3 expression. Furthermore, GBE regulated the lipid profile and blood glucose levels.

Cell death, including necrosis and apoptosis, in response to hyperglycemia has been defined as one of the important pathophysiological features of diabetic myocardial injury [1]. Cardiomyocyte loss, myocardial fibrosis, and inflammation result in myocardial remolding that leads to compromised cardiac function. In line with the results of previous studies, the present study showed that hyperglycemia triggered apoptosis of cardiomyocytes. The UPR is an adaptive process to restore the normal ER function. However, the excess and prolonged UPR in hyperglycemic conditions induces cardiomyocyte apoptosis. Three proapoptotic pathways are associated with ERS [4]. The first apoptotic pathway involves activation of JNK by the IRE-1-tumor necrosis factor receptor-associated factor 2 (TRAF2)-apoptosis signal-regulating kinase-1 (ASK1)complex. The second apoptotic pathway is the caspase-12 pathway in rodents. Clustering of caspase-12 in the endoplasmic reticulum membranes may attributable to TRAF2 recruitment by activated IRE-1 and PERK [25]. Activated caspase-12 translocates from the ER to the cytosol, where it cleaves pro-caspase 9, and subsequently activates the downstream effector caspase-3. CHOP, which is regulated by IRE1, ATF6, and particularly PERK, is the third proapoptotic pathway related to ERS. Caspase-12 and CHOP are considered specific apoptotic pathways associated with ERS [26]. The present study showed that the three proapoptotic pathways related to ERS were upregulated in the untreated diabetic ApoE$^{-/-}$mice. This was associated with increased expression of cleaved caspase-3, an effector of caspase-12. Our findings are consistent with the results of Zhenhua *et al.* [4], who showed that both the mRNA and protein levels of caspase-12 and CHOP were upregulated in STZ-induced diabetic rats. Taken together, ERS plays an important role in diabetic myocardial injury [27].

An earlier study conducted by Fitzl *et al.* [28] showed that EGb761, a standard GBE, attenuated the decrease in the volume fraction of myofibrils. According to Qiao *et al.* [17], GBE could attenuate ischemia/reperfusion-induced cardiac myocyte apoptosis by inhibiting cytochrome c release from the mitochondria and blocking the activation of caspase-3. The present study revealed that GBE downregulated the expression of p-JNK, CHOP, caspase-12, and cleaved caspase-3, indicating that GBE exerted antiapoptotic effects by attenuating ERS.

It has been reported that the IRE1α and PERK pathways of the UPR could trigger NF-κB-mediated inflammatory pathway by phosphorylation of IKKβ; in addition, the ATF6 pathway is linked to NF-κB activation, suggesting that the three pathways of the UPR could activate this inflammatory cascade [5, 6, 29]. Nuclear translocation of NF-κB results in increased expression of the downstream proinflammatory cytokines, including IL-6, IL-1β, and TNF-α. IL-1β and TNF-α further activate ERS (a positive loop), resulting in a more potent inflammatory response, myocardial interstitial fibrosis, and cardiomyocyte apoptosis. TNF-α promotes reactive oxygen species (ROS)production and inflammation [30] and mediates JNK activation leading to caspase-3 activation and cardiac cell apoptosis [14]. Therefore, inflammation can also induce ERS[31] (Figure 9). In the present study, GBE decreased collagen type I and III mRNA levels and interstitial collagen deposition, as revealed by Masson's staining. The increase in TNF-α and IL-1β mRNA levels in the diabetic heart was inhibited by GBE at 200and 400 mg/kg/day. This was associated with reduced NF-κB expression. Collectively, our findings suggest that GBE attenuated interstitial fibrosis *via* inhibition of inflammation and ERS, as well as owing to its direct radical-scavenging activity and ability to inhibit the opening of the mPTP channel[32]. Although it was not possible to establish whether GBE directly attenuated ERS or acted *via* modulation of inflammation, it was definite that GBE blocked the positive loop of ERS and inflammation *via* attenuation of ERS (Figure 9).

In the present study, we observed that GBE at 200 and 400 mg/kg/day decreased plasma glucose levels at the end of the study period. GBE at 200 mg/kg/day decreased the serum glucose level before the mice were sacrificed; additionally, GBE at 400 mg/kg/day could decrease the serum glucose levels; however, it did not reach statistical significance. Cheng *et al.* [9] showed that GBE reduced the activities of antioxidant enzymes, including superoxide dismutase (SOD), catalase (CAT), and glutathione peroxidase (GSH-Px)in the liver and pancreas of STZ-induced diabetic rats. Other studies showed that GBE could alleviate STZ-induced pancreatic damage in mice *via* inhibition of pancreatic inflammation and expression of proinflammatory cytokines, such as IL-1β, TNF-α, and IL-6 [10, 33]. The decrease in the serum levels of IL-6, IL-1β, and TNF-α by GBE treatment in our study suggested that the hypoglycemic effects were partly attributable to inhibition of inflammation.

In the present study, STZ-induced diabetic ApoE$^{-/-}$mice displayed severe hyperlipidemia, characterized by elevated serum LDL-c, TC, and TG levels, which were reversed by GBE administration, suggesting that GBE could lower lipid levels in diabetic settings. Qi *et al.* [34] reported that GBE exhibited multidirectional lipid-lowering effects in rats, including reduction of cholesterol absorption, inactivation of 3-hydroxy-3-methylglutaryl-coenzyme A (HMG-COA), and favorable regulation of the profiles of essential polyunsaturated fatty acids. Yao *et al.* [35] showed that GBE at doses of 48 and 96 mg/kg/day normalized ethanol-induced dysregulation of the lipid profiles in rats. According to the study conducted by Cheng *et al.* [9], the lipid-lowering effects were probably attributed to improvement of insulin resistance.

In conclusion, GBE attenuated diabetic myocardial injuries, including cardiomyocyte apoptosis, interstitial fibrosis, and intramyocardial inflammation in ApoE$^{-/-}$diabetic mice by inhibiting ERS. Interestingly, the cardio-protective effects of GBE in diabetic conditions were not dose-dependent, which might be because at doses of 200-400 mg/kg/day, the anti-inflammatory and antiapoptotic efficacy of GBE reached a plateau.

REFERENCES

[1] Huynh K, Bernardo BC, McMullen JR, etal. Diabetic cardiomyopathy: mechanisms and new treatment strategies targeting antioxidant signaling pathways[J]. Pharmacol Ther, 2014, 142 (3): 375-415.

[2] Palomer X, Salvadó L, Barroso E, et al. An overview of the crosstalk between inflammatory processes and metabolic dysregulation during diabetic cardiomyopathy[J]. Int J Cardiol, 2013, 168 (4): 3160-72.

[3] Falcão-Pires I, Leite-Moreira AF. Diabetic cardiomyopathy: understanding the molecular and cellular basis to progress in diagnosis and treatment[J]. Heart Fail Rev, 2012, 17 (3): 325-44.

[4] Li Z, Zhang T, Dai H, et al. Endoplasmic reticulum stress is involved in myocardial apoptosis of streptozocin-induced diabetic rats[J]. J Endocrinol, 2008, 196 (3): 565-72.

[5] Papa S, Zazzeroni F, Pham CG, et al. Linking JNK signaling to NF-kappaB: a key to survival[J]. J Cell Sci, 2004, 117 (Pt 22): 5197-208.

[6] Su J, Zhou L, Kong X, et al. Endoplasmic reticulum is at the crossroads of autophagy, inflammation, and apoptosis signaling pathways and participates in the pathogenesis of diabetes mellitus[J]. J Diabetes Res, 2013, 2013: 193461.

[7] Wen HL, Liang ZS, Zhang R, et al. Anti-inflammatory effects of triptolide improve left ventricular function in a rat model of diabetic cardiomyopathy[J]. Cardiovasc Diabetol, 2013, 12: 50.

[8] Tosaki A, Pali T, Droy-Lefaix MT. Effects of Ginkgo biloba extract and preconditioning on the diabetic rat myocardium[J]. Diabetologia, 1996, 39 (11): 1255-62.

[9] Cheng D, Liang B, Li Y. Antihyperglycemic effect of Ginkgo biloba extract in streptozotocin-induced diabetes in rats[J]. Biomed Res Int, 2013, 2013: 162724.

[10] Rhee KJ, Lee CG, Kim SW, et al. Extract of Ginkgo Biloba Ameliorates Streptozotocin-Induced Type 1 Diabetes Mellitus and High-Fat Diet-Induced Type 2 Diabetes Mellitus in Mice[J]. Int J Med Sci, 2015, 12 (12): 987-94.

[11] Banin RM, Hirata BK, Andrade IS, et al. Beneficial effects of Ginkgo biloba extract on insulin signaling cascade, dyslipidemia, and body adiposity of diet-induced obese rats[J]. Braz J Med Biol Res, 2014, 47 (9): 780-8.

[12] Lu Q, Yin XX, Wang JY, et al. Effects of Ginkgo biloba on prevention of development of experimental diabetic nephropathy in rats[J]. Acta Pharmacol Sin, 2007, 28 (6): 818-28.

[13] Geoffrion M, Du X, Irshad Z, et al. Differential effects of glyoxalase 1 overexpression on diabetic atherosclerosis and renal dysfunction in streptozotocin-treated, apolipoprotein E-deficient mice[J]. Physiol Rep, 2014, 2 (6): 6.

[14] Pan Y, Wang Y, Zhao Y, et al. Inhibition of JNK phosphorylation by a novel curcumin analog prevents high glucose-induced inflammation and apoptosis in cardiomyocytes and the development of diabetic cardiomyopathy[J]. Diabetes, 2014, 63 (10): 3497-511.

[15] Ren XM, Zuo GF, Wu W, et al. Atorvastatin Alleviates Experimental Diabetic Cardiomyopathy by Regulating the GSK-3beta-PP2Ac-NF-kappaB Signaling Axis[J]. PLoS One, 2016, 11 (11): e0166740.

[16] Quidgley J, Cruz N, Crespo MJ. Atorvastatin improves systolic function, but does not prevent the development of dilated cardiomyopathy in streptozotocin-induced diabetic rats[J]. Ther Adv Cardiovasc Dis, 2014, 8 (4): 133-144.

[17] Qiao ZY, Huang JH, Ma JW, et al. Ginkgo biloba extract reducing myocardium cells apoptosis by regulating apoptotic related proteins expression in myocardium tissues[J]. Mol Biol Rep, 2014, 41 (1): 347-53.

[18] Liu Y, Liu YF, Tian JF, et al. The effect and mechanism of extract of Ginkgo biloba (EGb)on cardiovascular protection on the rat model of type 2 diabetes after myocardial infarction. Chinese Journal of integrated traditional and Western Medicine[J]. 2017, 37 (9): 1100-1104. [Article in Chinese]

[19] Abdel-Hamid AA, Firgany Ael-D. Firgany, Atorvastatin alleviates experimental diabetic cardiomyopathy by suppressing apoptosis and oxidative stress[J]. J Mol Histol, 2015, 46 (4-5): 337-45.

[20] Packard C, Olsson AG. Management of hypercholesterolaemia in the patient with diabetes[J]. Int J Clin Pract Suppl, 2002 (130): 27-32.

[21] Wu KK, Huan Y. Diabetic atherosclerosis mouse models[J]. Atherosclerosis, 2007, 191 (2): 241-9.

[22] Huang R, Shi Z, Chen L, et al. Rutin alleviates diabetic cardiomyopathy and improves cardiac function in diabetic ApoE knockout mice[J]. Eur J Pharmacol, 2017, 814: 151-160.

[23] Li W, Fang Q, Zhong P, Chen L, et al. EGFR Inhibition Blocks Palmitic Acid-induced inflammation in cardiomyocytes and Prevents Hyperlipidemia-induced Cardiac Injury in Mice[J]. Sci Rep, 2016, 6: 24580.

[24] Van Linthout S, Riad A, Dhayat N, et al. Anti-inflammatory effects of atorvastatin improve left ventricular function in experimental diabetic cardiomyopathy[J]. Diabetologia, 2007, 50 (9): 1977-86.

[25] Yoneda T, Imaizumi K, Oono K, et al. Activation of caspase-12, an endoplastic reticulum (ER)resident caspase, through tumor necrosis factor receptor-associated factor 2-dependent mechanism in response to the ER stress[J]. J Biol Chem, 2001, 276 (17): 13935-40.

[26] Morishima N, Nakanishi K, Takenouchi H, et al. An endoplasmic reticulum stress-specific caspase cascade in apoptosis. Cytochrome c-independent activation of caspase-9 by caspase-12 [J]. J Biol Chem, 2002, 277 (37): 34287-94.

[27] Xu J, Zhou Q, Xu W, et al. Endoplasmic reticulum stress and diabetic cardiomyopathy[J]. Exp Diabetes Res, 2012, 2012: 827971.

[28] Fitzl G, Martin R, Dettmer D, et al. Protective effects of Gingko biloba extract EGb 761 on myocardium of experimentally diabetic rats. I: ultrastructural and biochemical investigation on cardiomyocytes[J]. Exp Toxicol Pathol, 1999, 51 (3): 189-98.

[29] Yamazaki H, Hiramatsu N, Hayakawa K, et al. Activation of the Akt-NF-kappaB pathway by subtilase cytotoxin through the ATF6 branch of the unfolded protein response[J]. J Immunol, 2009, 183 (2): 1480-7.

[30] Kim JJ, Lee SB, Park JK, et al. TNF-alpha-induced ROS production triggering apoptosis is directly linked to Romo1 and Bcl-X (L)[J]. Cell Death Differ, 2010, 17 (9): 1420-34.

[31] Hasnain SZ, Lourie R, Das I, et al. The interplay between endoplasmic reticulum stress and inflammation[J]. Immunol Cell Biol. 2012, 90 (3): 260-70.

[32] Saini AS, Taliyan R, Sharma PL. Protective effect and mechanism of Ginkgo biloba extract-EGb 761 on STZ-induced diabetic cardiomyopathy in rats[J]. Pharmacogn Mag, 2014, 10 (38): 172-8.

[33] Chen CC, Chiang AN, Liu HN, et al. EGb-761 prevents ultraviolet B-induced photoaging via inactivation of mitogen-activated protein kinases and proinflammatory cytokine expression[J]. J Dermatol Sci, 2014, 75 (1): 55-62.

[34] Zhang Q, Wang GJ, A JY, et al. Application of GC/MS-based metabonomic profiling in studying the lipid-regulating effects of Ginkgo biloba extract on diet-induced hyperlipidemia in rats[J]. Acta Pharmacol Sin, 2009, 30 (12): 1674-87.

[35] Yao P, Song F, Li K, et al. Ginkgo biloba extract prevents ethanol induced dyslipidemia[J]. Am J Chin Med, 2007, 35 (4): 643-52.

First published: TIAN Jin-fan, LIU Yan-fei, LIU Yue, CHEN Ke-ji, LU Shu-zheng. Ginkgo biloba leaf extract protects against myocardial injury via attenuation of endoplasmic reticulum stress in streptozotocin-induced diabetic apoE$^{-/-}$ mice [J] . Oxid Med Cell Longev, 2018, 2018: 2370617.

A Novel Ca^{2+} Current Blocker Promotes Angiogenesis and Cardiac Healing after Experimental Myocardial Infarction in Mice

CUI Guo-zhen, XIN Qi-qi, TSENG Hisa Hui Ling, HOI Puiman, WANG Yan, YANG Bin-rui, CHOI In-leng, WANG Yu-qiang, YUAN Rong, CHEN Ke-ji, CONG Wei-hong, and LEE Simon Ming-yuen

Despite improvements in clinical care, more than 8 million acute myocardial infarctions (MI)occur worldwide annually and MI is the main cause of death worldwide in cardiovascular diseases (CVDs) [1]. Under physiological conditions, blood vessels deliver nutrients and oxygen to the whole body. MI is caused by necrosis of myocardium due to myocardial ischemia, an imbalance between coronary blood supply and myocardial demand. Hence, the main goal of MI medical therapy is to improve the blood flow and restore myocardium function [2]. The current main drugs for the treatment of patients with MI are vasodilators (including nitrodilators and calcium channel blockers), antiplatelet agents, anticoagulants, beta-blockers and angiotensin-converting enzyme inhibitors. Most of these drugs are effective therapeutically but may be associated with certain adverse effects in exposed patients [3].

Angiogenesis is a multi-step process including angiogenic endothelial cell proliferation, migration, and vessel formation. An imbalance of angiogenesis can lead to numerous disorders. For instance, insufficient angiogenesis causes tissue ischemia, impaired wound healing and preeclampsia and other disorders [4]. More importantly, it was reported that angiogenesis represents an important therapeutic goal in ischemic heart disease [5]. Although the mechanism of angiogenesis is complicated, involving a dynamic interaction among endothelial cells, vascular smooth muscle cells (VSMCs)and the corresponding extracellular environment, it was confirmed that the most important regulator is vascular endothelial growth factor (VEGF). The VEGF family consists of several members and VEGF (VEGF-A)is the main component that stimulates angiogenesis in healthy and disease states [6].

Accumulating preclinical and clinical evidence indicates that certain traditional herbs appear to significantly improve outcomes in patients with CVDs. For instance, the registered pharmaceutical product Danshen Dripping Pill is one of the most popular traditional Chinese herb medicines, with promising efficacy in treating coronary heart disease [7]. Herb medicines, as sources of novel drugs, have made contributions to commercial drugs including digitoxin from *Digitalis purpurea* to treat congestive heart failure, Lovastatin from Pu-erh tea for lowering cholesterol and the precursor to aspirin, salicin from *Salix alba* for inhibiting platelet aggregation to reduce the risk of CVDs. Our previous studies reported that a novel semi-synthetic small molecule named ADTM, produced by linking two natural compounds, Danshensu (DSS)and tetramethylpyrazine (TMP, also known as ligustrazine), displayed protective effects against oxidative stress-induced injury in cardiomyoblast H9c2 cells and myocardial ischemia in rats [8]. Further studies demonstrated that ADTM displayed versatile functions, including a relaxation action on rat coronary artery [9], inhibition of platelet aggregation both *in vitro* and *in vivo* [10], and protective effects against neurotoxin 6-hydroxydopamine-induced toxicity in neuronal PC12 cells and zebrafish [11,12]. Here, we reported a new angiogenic effect of ADTM that promoted revascularization and reduce cardiac infarction in an acute MI experimental mouse model.

MATERIALS AND METHODS

1 Chemical and Reagent

Compound ADTM was synthesized as described previously [13]. The natural products DSS and TMP were obtained from Xi`an Honson Biotechnology Co., Ltd. (Xi`an, China)and Shanghai Banghai Chemical Co., Ltd. (Shanghai, China), respectively. Perindopril was purchased from Servier Pharmaceytical Co., Ltd (Tianjin, China). The purity of all the compounds used in the present study was>95%. VEGF receptor (VEGFR) tyrosine kinase inhibitor II was obtained from Calbiochem Company (San Diego, CA, USA)and dissolved in DMSO. Kaighn's modification of Ham's F12 medium (F-12K), fetal bovine serum (FBS), penicillin-streptomycin (PS)and 0.25% (w/v)trypsin/1 mM EDTA were obtained from Invitrogen (Carlsbad, CA, USA). Dulbecco's modified Eagle's medium-high glucose (DMEM-HG), endothelial cell growth supplement (ECGS), gelatine and heparin were obtained from Sigma (St. Louis, MO, USA). MatrigelTM basement membrane matrix was purchased from BD Biosciences (Bedford, MA, USA). Antibodies used for immunofluorescence staining in this study were as follows: rabbit anti-differentiation 31 (CD31)and sheep anti-von Willebrand factor (vWF) antibodies were obtained from Abcam (Cambridge, UK). Alexa Fluor 555-conjugated donkey anti-rabbit antibodies and Alexa Fluor 488-conjugated donkey anti-sheep were from Molecular Probes (Carlsbad, CA, USA). All other chemicals were of analytical grade.

2 Maintenance of Zebrafish and Embryos

Transgenic zebrafish line *Tg* (*fli1*-EGFP), which expresses green fluorescent protein in endothelial cells, was kindly provided by ZFIN (Eugene, OR, USA)and maintained as described previously [14]. Ethical approval for the animal experiments was granted by the Animal Research Ethics Committee, University of Macau.

3 Embryo Collection and Drug Treatment

Zebrafish embryos were generated by natural pair-wise mating (6 months old)and cultured in embryo medium at 28.5oC. Zebrafish embryos at 24 hours post fertilization (hpf)were collected, distributed into a 12-well microplate with 15 fish in each well and pre-treated with 100 ng/mL VRI (VEGFR tyrosine kinase inhibitor II)for 3 h. VRI was then washed out and replaced with DSS (200 μM), TMP (200 μM), DSS (200 μM)+TMP (200 μM), and different concentrations (50-200 μM)of ADTM.

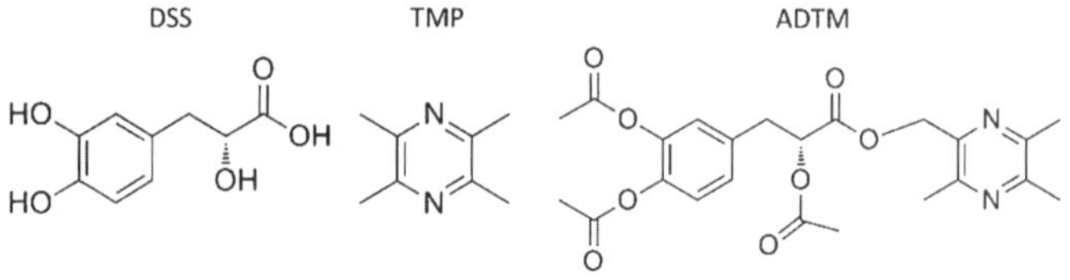

Figure 1 Chemical structures of DSS, TMP and ADTM

Embryos incubated with 0.1% DMSO served as a vehicle group. Embryos treated in the individual wells were then incubated at 28 ℃ for 48 h. Zebrafish were removed from microplates after drug treatment and observed for gross morphological changes under a fluorescence microscope as previously reported [15]. The number of intact intersegmental vessels (ISVs)in each zebrafish was counted as previously described [16].

4 Analysis of Gene Expression in ADTM-treated Zebrafish by Real-time PCR

Embryos were treated with ADTM according to the method described above. Total RNA of zebrafish was isolated at 72 hpf from each treatment group with the RNeasy Mini Kit (Qiagen, Valencia, CA, USA)according to the manufacturer's instructions. The RNA was converted to cDNA using the SuperScript III reverse transcriptase system with a mix of random hexamers and oligo (dT_{20})primers. The resulting cDNA was followed by real-time PCR with various primers (VEGFR, VEGFR1, VEGFR2, β-actin)as previously described (17). Housekeeping gene β-actin was used as a reference gene to normalize the expression ratios of VEGFR, VEGFR1 and VEGFR2.

5 Cell Culture

Human umbilical vein endothelial cells (HUVECs), rat thoracic VSMCs (A7r5)and H9c2 cardiomyoblast cells were purchased from the American Type Cell Culture Collection (ATCC; Rockville, MD, USA). HUVECs were maintained in F-12K medium with L-glutamine (2 mM), endothelial cell growth supplement (0.03 mg/mL), Hanks' balanced salt solution (5 ml), heparin (0.1 mg/mL), 10% FBS and 1% penicillin-streptomycin (100 U/mL). Cells were seeded on a 75 cm^2 tissue culture flask coated with 0.1% gelatine and incubated at 37 ℃ in a humidified 5% CO_2 atmosphere. HUVECs were used from passages 2 to 6. A7r5 and H9c2 cell lines were grown in Dulbecco's modified Eagle's medium (DMEM)supplemented with 10% FBS and 1% penicillin-streptomycin at 37 ℃ in a humidified 5% CO_2 atmosphere incubator.

6 Tube Formation Assay on HUVECs

BD MatrigelTM Basement Membrane Matrix was thawed at 4 ℃, quickly added to each well of a 24-well plate and allowed to solidify at 37 ℃ for 1 h. HUVECs were cultured on the top of the fixed matrix at a density of 1.2×10^6 cells per well in serum-free medium. After adhesion of cells for 1 h, ADTM was added at the indicated concentrations for 4 h and VEGF was used as a positive control. The formation of a capillary-like structure was examined under a microscope and images were taken by light microscopy.

7 HUVEC Proliferation by XTT Assay

The effects of ADTM on HUVEC viability were determined by XTT assay according to the manufacturer's instructions (Cell Proliferation Kit II; Roche Diagnostics GmbH, Mannheim, Germany). After confluence, HUVECs were digested with 0.25% trypsin and then cultured in 96-well plates pre-coated with 0.1% gelatine at 1×10^4 cells per in complete medium for 24 h. Then, the medium was removed and replaced by fresh medium containing 0.5% FBS with the indicated concentration of ADTM and further incubated for 48 h. Cells exposed to 20 ng/mL VEGF served as the positive control. Cell proliferation was determined by XTT assay. The XTT converted to formazan in active cells was determined by measuring absorbance at 450nm after subtracting the absorbance at 650 nm on a 96-well microplate reader. The reading of vehicle control was normalized to 100%, and readings from ADTM-treated cells were expressed as% of vehicle.

8 Mouse Model of MI And Drug Treatment

Male C57BL/6 mice (8-10 weeks old, 22 ± 2 g body weight)were purchased from Beijing Vital River Laboratory Animal Technology Co., Ltd. (Beijing, China). The mice were housed under conventional conditions (temperature of 22 ± 2 ℃, humidity $40 \pm 5\%$, under a 12 h light/dark cycle), and fed standard pellets and water *ad libitum*. Left ventricular acute MI was established in the mice via permanent ligation of the proximal aspect of the left anterior descending (LAD)coronary artery as previously described, with a slight modification [18]. Briefly, after animals were anesthetized with 4% chloral hydrate, the heart was exposed via a left-sided thoracotomy and the LAD was ligated with a single stitch via an 8-0 prolene suture to form an ischemia immediately. By closing the LAD, the remote area permitted no further blood flow; the color of infarcted myocardium became pale, indicating successful acute MI induction. The sham control group was subject to the above operations except for ligation. Acute MI mice were treated with vehicle, different dosages of ADTM (12 and 24 mg/kg, intraperitoneal injection) or perindopril (3 mg/kg, oral gavage)for 14 days by once daily before being sacrificed, respectively. Perindopril was served as positive control in this study. The serum from peripheral blood and heart were collected for further analysis. All protocols were performed in accordance with guidelines established by the Guide for the Care and Use of Laboratory Animals of China Academy of Chinese Medical Sciences.

9 Infarct Size Estimation with Masson's Trichrome Staining

Mice hearts were sliced into two segments from the ligation point (*n*=6-10). The left ventricle of the heart was removed and cut into halves along the ligated artery. The segment from the apex to the ligation point was fixed in 4% paraformaldehyde in phosphate-buffered saline solution for 48 h and processed for paraffin embedding and sectioning. The paraffin sections (5 μm)were cut from the ligation point and stained with Masson's trichrome staining. Quantification of fibrosis in infarcted mice hearts was carried out using ImageJ software (NIH, Bethesda, MD, USA).

10 Double Immunofluorescence Staining for CD31 and vWF of Heart Sections from Mice

Deparaffinized tissue sections were stained with antibodies against CD31/vWF (1: 200 dilution) and incubated at 4 ℃ overnight. Washed sections were incubated with appropriate Alexa Fluor 488 or 594-conjugated secondary antibodies (1: 300 dilution)at room temperature for 1 h before being mounted with DAPI-containing mountant (VectorLab, Burlingame, CA, USA). Histological vessel density was evaluated by morphometric examination. Five hot fields, with a high density of blood vessels at the theperi-infarct areas for each section, were selected and images were captured using an Olympus microscope and digital camera (Olympus DP71, Tokyo, Japan). Positive staining for both CD31 and vWF was confirmed in the vessel. Vessel density was analyzed by ImageJ. The mean vessel density in the five selected fields was expressed as vessel number per field. All morphometric studies were performed by examiners who were blinded to treatment.

11 Determination of VEGF Protein Level by ELISA

A7r5 cells were cultured in 96-well plates at 5×10^3 cells/well in DMEM with 10% FBS for 24 h. Cells were starved in low serum medium (0.2% FBS)for 12 h and then stimulated with ADTM at 25, 50, 100 and 200 μM for another 12 h. The medium with ADTM was then collected. VEGF levels in the medium and mice serum were measured by a VEGF ELISA (enzyme-linked immunosorbent assay)kit (R&D Systems, Minneapolis, MN, USA)according to the manufacturer's instructions.

12 Patch Clamp Experiments

Membrane currents were recorded by the whole-cell patch clamp method. H9c2 cells were superfused with the extracellular solution with the following compositions (mM): tetraethylammonium chloride (TEAC), 135; $CaCl_2$, 5.4; $MgCl_2$, 1; Tris, 5; and D-glucose, 10; pH was adjusted to 7.4 with HEPES. The pipettes (resistance 2-3 MΩ)were filled with intracellular pipette solution (mM): CsCl, 140; $MgCl_2$, 1; EGTA, 2; HEPES, 5; Mg-ATP, 5; pH 7.3. The recordings were made using an Axopatch-200B amplifier, Digidata-1321 interface, and pClamp10.0 software (Axon Instruments, Foster City, CA, USA). H9c2 cells were clamped at a holding potential of -50 mV, and the test potential was +10 mV, with pulses lasting 1000 ms.

13 Statistical Analysis

Data are presented as means ± SD and were analyzed using GraphPad Prism 6.0 software. Statistical significance was assessed by one-way ANOVA followed by Tukey's multiple comparison between each group. P values less than 0.05 were considered significant.

RESULTS

1 ADTM Restored Chemical-induced Blood Vessel Loss in Zebrafish

We evaluated the vascular regenerative activity of DSS, TMP, DSS+TMP and ADTM in a chemical-induced blood vessel loss model of zebrafish *in vivo*. We found that pretreatment with VEGF receptor tyrosine kinase inhibitor Ⅱ (VRI)at 100 ng/mL for 3 h reduced ISV and SIV (subintestinal vessel)branching and impaired DLAV (dorsal longitudinal anastomotic vessels)formation in the zebrafish embryos (Fig. 2B).

Exposure to ADTM rescued the VRI-induced blood vessel loss at SIV, ISV and DLAV in a concentration-dependent manner (Fig. 2F-H), and changes of ISV were quantified (Fig. 2I). In contrast, mild but insignificant restoration of an abnormal blood vessel phenotype by DSS or DSS+TMP was observed, while VRI or TMP alone group did not show any vascular regenerative activity (Fig. 2B-E). More importantly, 200μM ADTM could nearly restore all blood vessel loss induced by VRI in the zebrafish and exhibited a significantly vascular restoration effect compared with the other treatment groups.

2 ADTM Up-regulated Gene Expression of VEGFR1 and VEGFR2 in VRI- Induced Blood Vessel Loss in Zebrafish

In order to identify the molecular targets of the angiogenic effect of ADTM in zebrafish, mRNAs from different groups of whole zebrafish were isolated and reverse-transcribed to cDNA, and relative gene expression was measured using real-time PCR. Vascular endothelial growth factor (VEGF)is a key stimulator in physiological and pathological angiogenesis. Binding VEGF to two tyrosine kinase receptors, VEGFR1 and VEGFR2 allows coupling to downstream signal transduction pathway that regulates the proliferation, migration and differentiation of endothelial cells (19, 20). The bar charts in Fig. 3 showed that gene expression of VEGFR1 and VEGFR2 significantly decreased in the VRI group compared to the control group ($P < 0.05$). ADTM could reverse VRI-induced down-regulation of the expression of these genes in a dose-dependent manner. Therefore, the result suggested that ADTM triggered angiogenesis in zebrafish by up-regulation of VEGFR1 and VEGFR2 expression.

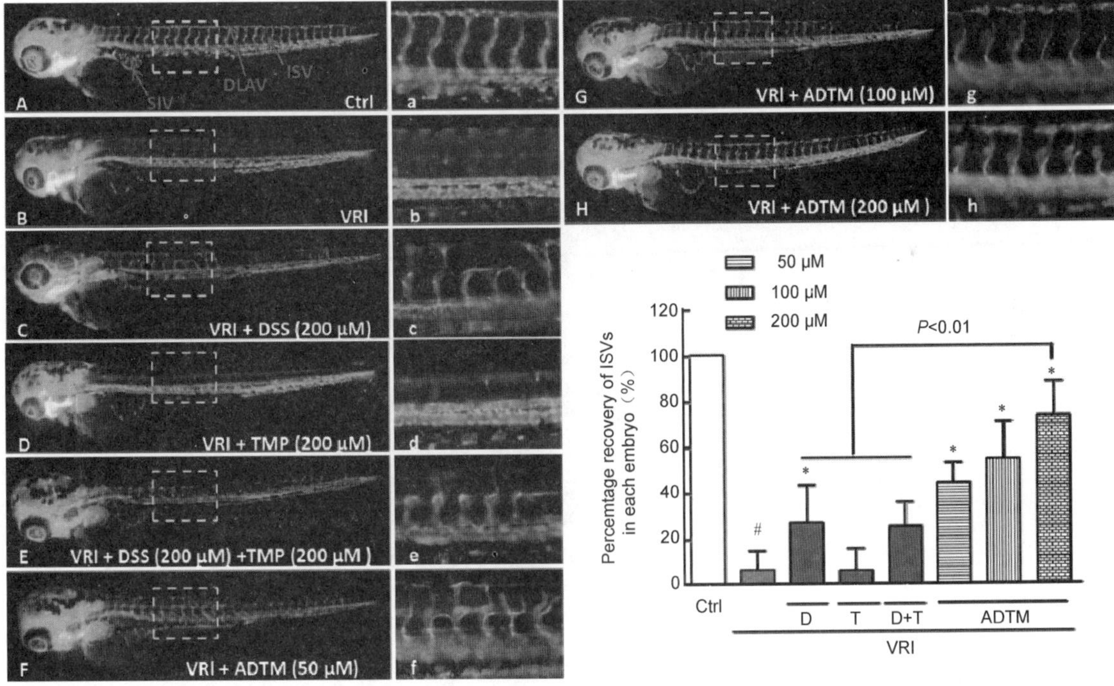

Figure 2 Effects of DSS, TMP and ADTM on VRI-induced Blood Vessel Loss in Zebrafish

Notes: (A)Embryos at 24 hpf were treated with 0.1% DMSO. The red arrow indicated SIV, DLAV and ISV of zebrafish. (B) VRI reduced blood vessel formation in ISV, SIV and DLAV; VRI pretreated zebrafish embryos, treated with 200μM DSS (C), 200μM TMP (D), 200μM DSS+TMP (E), 50μM, 100μM and 200μM ADTM (F, G and H). (I)The percentage recovery of ISVs was quantified by counting a minimum of eight zebrafish per group. Data are presented as means±SD of three independent experiments, $^{\#}P < 0.001$ versus ctrl group; $^{*}P < 0.01$ versus VRI treatment group. Ctrl, control; VRI, VEGFR tyrosine kinase inhibitor II; SIV, subintestinal vessel; DLAV, dorsal longitudinal anastomotic vessels; ISV, intersegmental vessels; DSS, Danshensu; TMP, tetramethylpyrazine; D, DSS; T, TMP. Scale bar (A-H): 250 μm; Scale bar (a-h): 50 μm.

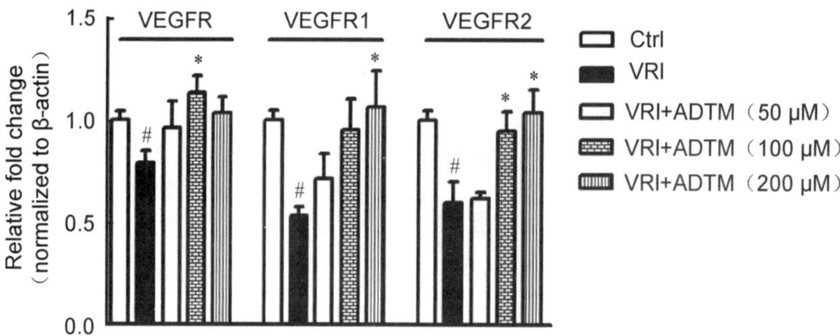

Figure 3　Effects of ADTM on VRI-induced Downregulation of VEGFR, VEGFR1 and VEGFR2 mRNA Expression

Notes: Zebrafish embryos at 24 hpf were pre-treated with VRI for 3 h and then washed out, followed by post-treatment with various concentrations of ADTM (50μM, 100μM, 200μM)for 48 h. Gene in whole zebrafish were determined by real-time PCR. ADTM reversed expression VRI-induced downregulation of VEGFR, VEGFR1 and VEGFR2 mRNA expression. Data are expressed as means ± SD from 3 independent experiments (n = 15 zebrafish in each group). $^{\#}P < 0.05$ versus control group; $^{*}P < 0.05$ versus VRI treatment group.

3 ADTM Did Not Stimulate Tube Formation on HUVECs

The process of angiogenesis is complex, typically consisted of cell proliferation and alignment to form tubular structures. In this study, we used an *in vitro* Matrigel model basement membrane to examine whether ADTM could induce HUVEC capillary tube formation. As expected, HUVECs formed tube-like structure on Matrigel under various treatments (Fig. 4A). As shown in Fig. 4B, the quantitative measurements of the tube

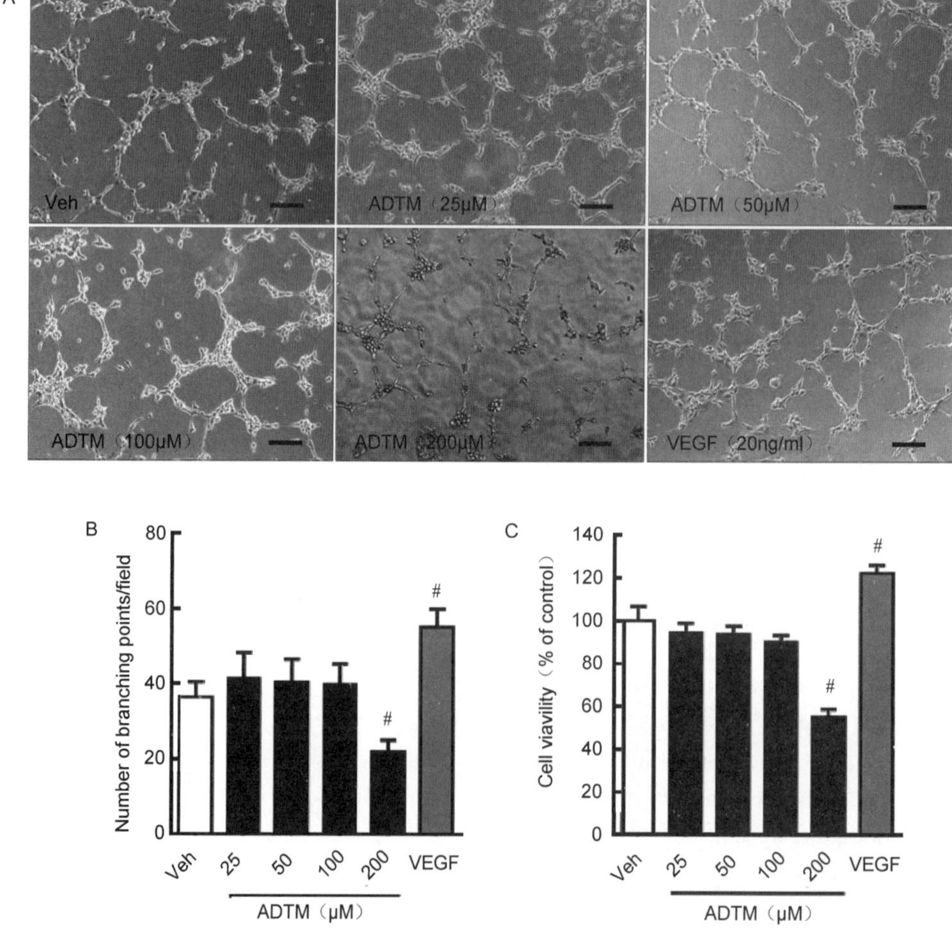

Figure 4　Tube Formation and Proliferation of ADTM-treated HUVECs

Notes: formation demonstrated that there was little tube formation when HUVECs were plated on Matrigel in medium supplemented with 0.5% FBS serum. Similarly, ADTM until 100 μM induced a slight increase in the number of branching points but there was no significant difference between two groups ($P>0.05$), while 200 μM demonstrated an obviously toxic effect ($P<0.05$), which was consistent with the result of XTT assay (Fig. 4C). In contrast, compared with the vehicle group, VEGF treatment significantly induced tube formation, quantified by measuring the number of branching points ($P<0.05$).

4 ADTM Did Not Induce HUVEC Proliferation

Endothelial cell proliferation is essential in the early stage of sprouting angiogenesis. The effect of ADTM on HUVEC proliferation was evaluated by XTT assay. As shown in Fig. 4C, ADTM could not promote HUVEC proliferation in a series of concentrations compared to vehicle control ($P>0.05$). A significant increase in cell proliferation was observed in VEGF-treated cells, which served as a positive control ($P<0.05$).

Various concentrations of ADTM (25μM, 50μM, 100μM, 200μM)were added for 4 h and VEGF was used as a positive control. The formation of a capillary-like structure was examined under a microscope and images were taken by light microscopy. (A)Microscopic view of tube formation of HUVECs. Scale bar: 200μm. (B) Quantitative analysis of the branching points in ADTM or VEGF-treated HUVECs. (C)Effect of ADTM on the proliferation of HUVECs compared with the vehicle group. VEGF was used as a positive control in the experiment. Data are expressed as means ± SD. $^{\#}P<0.05$ versus vehicle group. Veh: vehicle.

5 ADTM Attenuated Infarct Size After MI in Mice

To evaluate the infarct size after MI in mice, the animals were treated with vehicle, different dosages of ADTM (12 and 24 mg/kg)or perindopril once daily for 14 days, and heart sections were stained with masson's trichrome in the individual groups. In Fig. 5A, the blue colour shows collagen-rich fibrotic region (scar tissue)in the wall of the left ventricle and the red colour represents normal myocardium. The results of the quantitative analyses done with Image J software demonstrated that the fibrotic size (%)in the left ventricle cross-sectional area was significantly reduced in the ADTM treatment group (MI+12 mg/kg ADTM: 12.38% ± 1.6%; MI+24 mg/kg ADTM: 8.22% ± 2.3 %)and perindopril (7.22% ± 1.3%)compared with the vehicle-treated MI group (25.78% ± 2.9%; $P<0.05$). The therapeutic effects of ADTM (12-24 mg/kg)in myocardial infarct size were comparable to perindopril (3 mg/kg).

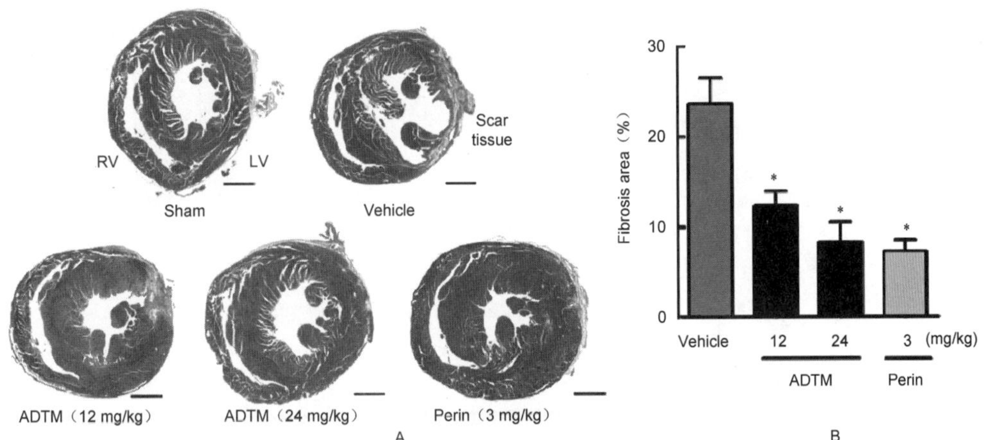

Figure 5 Histological Analysis of MI Sizes in Mice

Notes: Acute MI mice were treated with vehicle, different dosages of ADTM (12 and 24 mg/kg)or perindopril once daily for 14 days before being sacrificed. (A)Heart sections were stained with Masson's trichrome. Collagen-rich fibrotic region (scar tissue)in the wall of ventricles stained blue, and viable myocardium stained red. Scale bar: 1.0 mm. (B)Percentage of fibrotic area relative to that of the whole left ventricle. N=6-10 in each group. Data are presented as means ± SD. $^{\#}P<0.05$ versus vehicle-treated MI group. RV, right ventricle; LV, left ventricle; Perin, perindopril.

6 ADTM Increased the Vascular Density after MI in Mice

CD31 (green)and vWF (red)double-staining indicated the blood vessel density of mouse heart tissues. As shown in Fig. 6, compared with the sham group, LAD ligation induced mild but insignificantly increased blood vessel density in the infarct border of the left ventricular myocardium (147.56 ± 10.83 vs. 139.45 ± 11.22, $P>0.05$). This increase in blood vessel density resulted from increased angiogenesis, which acted as a compensatory mechanism for the salvage of damaged myocardium caused by infarction. Compared with the vehicle-treated MI group, treatment with ADTM at the doses of 12 mg/kg, 24 mg/kg and perindopril was associated with significant increases in blood vessel density (182.57 ± 18.26, 220.13 ± 18.21, and 227.59 ± 20.94, respectively, $P<0.05$). No significant difference was found among the ADTM 12 mg/kg, ADTM 24 mg/kg and perindopril treatment group ($P>0.05$).

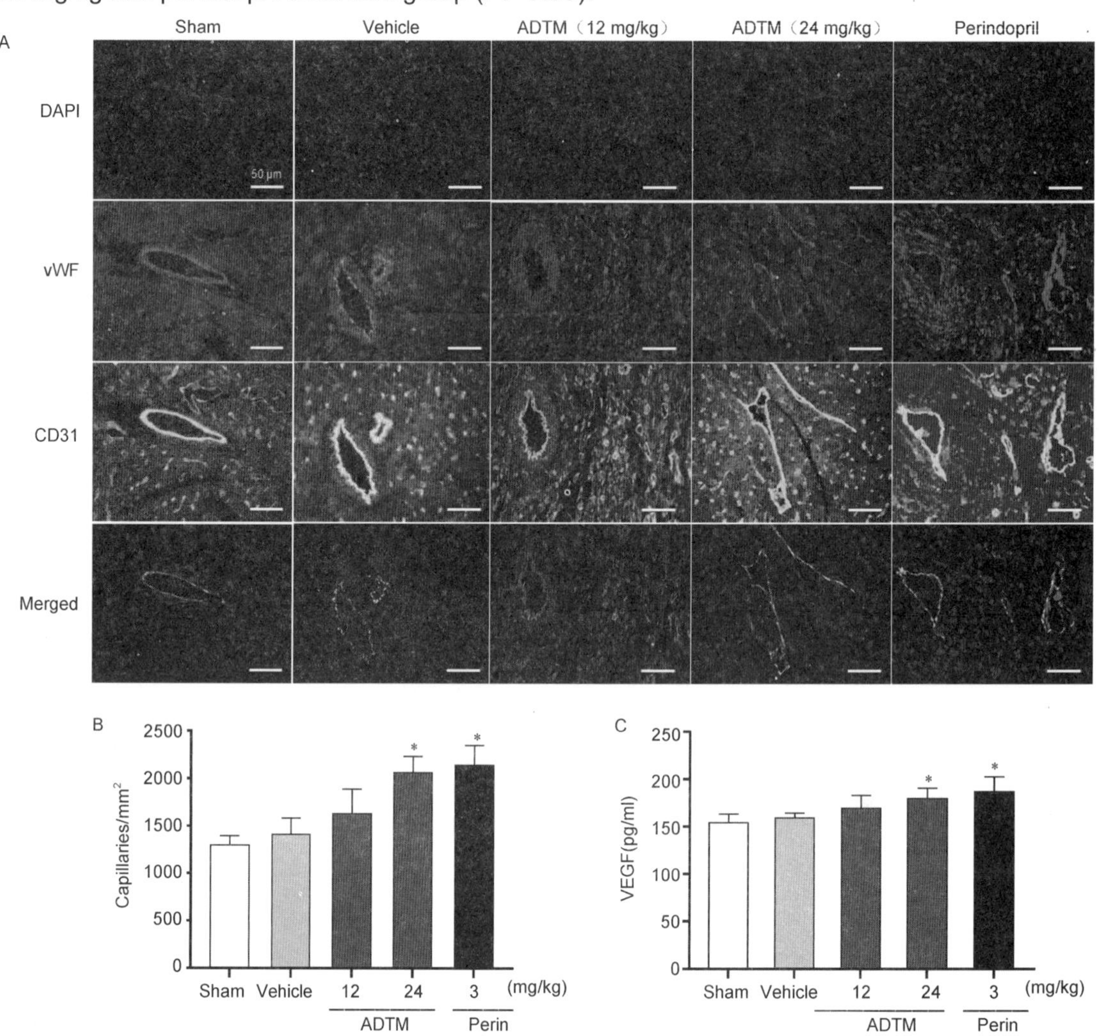

Figure 6 Effect of ADTM on Vessel Density and Serum VEGF Level in the Acute MI Mice

Notes: (A)Double immunofluorescence staining, for vWF (red)and CD31 (red), of heart sections from vehicle and ADTM (12 and 24 mg/kg)treatment groups. Cell nuclei were stained with DAPI (blue). Scale bar: 50 μm. (B)Quantitative measurement of vessel density in the peri-infarct area. Both vWF-and CD31-positive endothelial cell circles indicated vessels. The number of vessels per field was counted in each section. (C)The amount of VEGF protein in mouse serum. Data are presented as means±SD (n=6-8), $^*P<0.05$ versus vehicle-treated MI. Perin, perindopril.

7 ADTM Increased the Release of VEGF Protein into MI Mouse Serum and A7r5 Cell Medium

To unravel the mechanisms underlying the angiogenic effect of ADTM, ELISA analysis was performed to determine whether ADTM could regulate the secretion of VEGF both *in vivo and in vitro.* For *in vivo* study, the MI mice were treated without or with different concentrations of ADTM for 14 days before sacrifice. The serum from peripheral blood was collected. Compared with the sham group, MI has no significant effect on VEGF secretion in mouse serum. Treatment with ADTM (24 mg/kg)or perindopril (3 mg/kg)caused a significant increase in VEGF release compared with the vehicle-treated MI group ($P < 0.05$, Fig. 6C). For *in vitro* study, A7r5 cells were incubated with various concentrations of ADTM (12.5, 25, 50 and 100μM)for 24 h (n = 3-6 for each group). As shown in Fig. 7, ADTM (50 and 100 μM)significantly increased VEGF secretion in a concentration-dependent manner, with the maximal effect occurring at 100 μM.

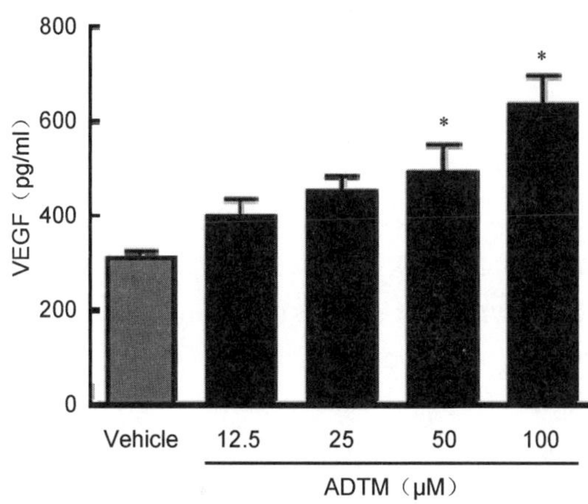

Figure 7　Effect of ADTM on the Release of VEGF Protein in A7r5 Cell Medium

A7r5 cells were exposed to either vehicle (0.1% DMSO)or various concentrations of ADTM for 24 h, and the medium was collected after centrifugation. The amount of VEGF protein in cell medium was assessed by ELISA. Data are expressed as means ± SD. $^{*}P < 0.01$ versus vehicle group.

8 ADTM Significantly Decreased I_{CaL} in H9c2 Cells

The L-type voltage-dependent Ca^{2+} channel is the primary route for Ca^{2+} entry into cardiac cells; they are known to be present in H9c2 cardiomyoblasts, which exhibit a rapidly activating voltage-dependent inward Ca^{2+} current (I_{CaL}) [21]. Therefore, we further examined the effect of ADTM on I_{CaL} in H9c2 by using whole cell

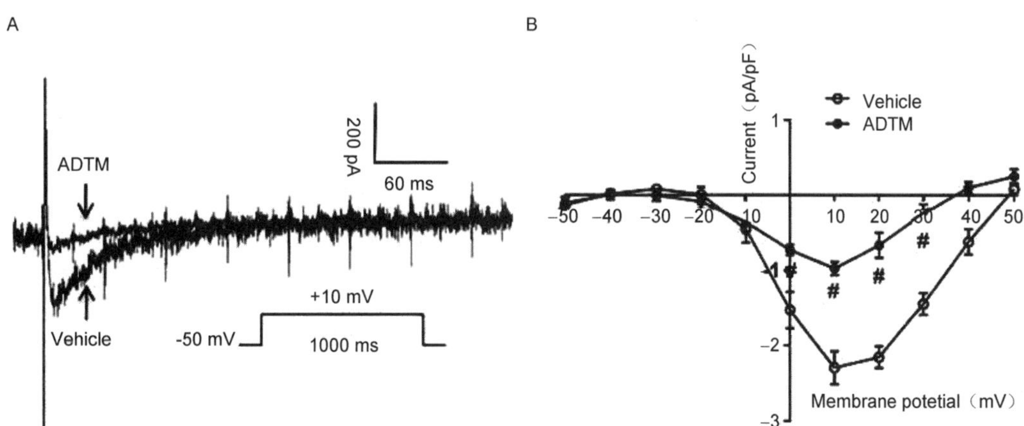

Figure 8　Effect of ADTM on Voltage-dependent Inward Ca^{2+} Currents (I_{CaL})in H9c2 Cells

Notes: H9c2 cells were superfused with vehicle or 200 ADTM (200μM)and whole cell currents at +10 mV were recorded with a depolarizing voltage pulse of 1, 000-ms duration. (A)Representative traces of Ca^{2+} currents at +10 mV in H9c2 recorded in the presence of ADTM (200 μM)or vehicle control (0.1% DMSO). (B)Current-voltage (I/V)graph for I_{CaL} in H9c2 cells in the presence of ADTM (200 μM)or vehicle control (0.1% DMSO). Data are presented shown as means±SD; $n = 6$; $^{\#}P < 0.01$ versus Vehicle.

patch clamp. H9c2 cells were superfused with ADTM and whole cell currents at +10 mV were recorded with a depolarizing voltage pulse of 1, 000-ms duration (Fig. 8A). It was observed that exposure to ADTM (200μM) inhibited the rapid inward movement of I_{CaL} in H9c2, which remained blocked for the rest of the stimulation period. Fig. 8B shows the current-voltage (I-V)relationship of I_{CaL} in H9c2. It was observed that ADTM (200μM) inhibited I_{CaL} at all depolarizing voltages, with＞50% inhibition at +10 mV. These results suggest that ADTM significantly inhibited I_{CaL} possibly by directly blocking the L-type Ca^{2+} channels present in H9c2.

DISCUSSION

We have previously reported a novel agent, named ADTM and originating from traditional Chinese medicine, which exhibited a number of pharmacological activities, such as antiplatelet activity [10], a relaxation effect on arteries [9], cytoprotection [8,12,22] and neuroprotection [11]. In the study described here, we demonstrated that twice daily treatment with ADTM for 14 days decreased the myocardial infarct size and increased the vessel density of the myocardial peri-infarct area in mice, the therapeutic efficacy of ADTM (24 mg/kg)was similar to that of perindopril, a well-known used drug to treat hypertension and congestive heart failure. These results suggest that more potential indications make ADTM to be a better option than perindopril. We also demonstrated that treatment with ADTM rescued the chemical-induced blood vessel loss in a zebrafish angiogenesis assay. However, ADTM did not directly promote the features of angiogenesis in HUVECs. Interesting, ADTM not only stimulated VEGF secretion into the serum of MI mice *in vivo,* but also culture medium of VSMCs *in vitro*. In addition, ADTM inhibited I_{CaL} at all depolarizing voltages, with＞50% inhibition at +10 mV. The current findings are important since they highlight the critical role of angiogenesis regulated by ADTM in the pathogenesis of acute MI, and suggest that stimulation of angiogenesis by small molecule-targeted VSMCs may offer a new strategy for the treatment of MI.

Angiogenesis is a complex and crucial step in the physiological process through which new vessels form preexisting vessels. In recent years, it was reported that some molecules, by stimulating myocardial angiogenesis to restore blood flow, opened an avenue for developing new and potentially effective therapeutic approaches for the treatment of acute MI (23,24). It has been demonstrated that growth factors such as VEGF play critical roles in triggering angiogenesis. VEGF is a specific growth factor for vascular endothelial cells. It was considered that VEGF administration alone may facilitate the formation of unstable capillaries. Due to the poor stability, rapid diffusion and short half-life *in vivo* of VEGF, several human clinical trials of VEGF in ischemic heart disease failed to find beneficial therapeutic effects in ischemic hearts [25,26]. In contrast, the results of the current study indicated that a novel small molecule, ADTM, could stimulate angiogenesis in zebrafish model by blocking VEGF signaling pathway-induced blood vessel loss and mouse acute MI model (Figs. 2&6). Interesting, ADTM treatment significantly attenuated infarct size after MI in mice (Fig. 5).

In our previous study, we reported a zebrafish angiogenesis assay, which was produced by blocking the VEGF signaling pathway; this was a more physiologically relevant assay for screening pro-angiogenic agents against various kinds of disease associated with angiogenesis deficiencies, especially ischemic heart disease [27]. In the current study, we found that ADTM displayed remarkably higher potency and efficacy than DSS and TMP, alone or in combination, for rescuing blood vessel loss in VRI-pretreated zebrafish embryos (Fig. 2). These data were consistent with our previous observations showing that ADTM exhibited much stronger protective effects than its parent compound, alone or in combination in models of oxidative stress-induced cardiomyoblast H9c2 cell injury, as well as neurotoxin-induced neuronal PC12 cell death [8,11]. Furthermore, similar results were observed with respect to the inhibitory effects of ADTM, shown by platelet aggregation and thrombus formation [10]. It was reported that the major metabolites of ADTM were 2-hydroxymethy-3, 5, 6-trimethylpyrazin (TMP-OH)and DSS in a rat model [28]. Previous studies demonstrated that TMP and DSS could inhibit voltage-dependent L-type Ca^{2+} channels [29-31]. The mechanism of action of ADTM on blocking calcium current may be contributed to the parent compounds TMP and DSS. However, the precise mechanism of the enhanced activity after chemical modification is still not fully known; further investigation is worthwhile to elucidate this mechanism because it may provide a promising and novel way to improve compound therapy efficacy by chemical modification.

The present study sought to evaluate the underlying angiogenic mechanism regulated by ADTM. However, the results of XTT and tube formation assays showed that ADTM conferred no angiogenic features in HUVECs (Fig. 4). Rat VSMCs are known to produce VEGF (32). Given the relative proximity of endothelial cells to smooth muscle in the vascular wall, we considered the possibility that angiogenic growth factors secreted by smooth muscle cells might mediate angiogenesis. Accordingly, we evaluated the effect of ADTM on VEGF levels in VSMCs by ELISA assay. Our findings indicated that ADTM promoted VEGF expression both in mice serum *in vivo* and A7r5 cells *in vitro* (Fig. 6C and 7). In addition, ADTM also increased the gene expression levels of VEGFR, VEGFR1 and VEGFR2 in response to ADTM in zebrafish (Fig. 3). These new findings demonstrated that ADTM treatment could enhance the VEGF level both in genes and protein. Therefore, it was anticipated that this phenomenon would potentiate the angiogenic effect of ADTM by targeting VSMCs, but not endothelial cells. Angiogenesis is also a critical step in the transition of tumors from benign state to malignant one, angiogenesis inhibitors are used to treat for various cancers, so it is logical to speculate that pro-angiogenesis agents such as ADTM, could promote tumor growth by promoting cancer expansion and aggressiveness on patients with cancer. Nonetheless, our previous pilot study demonstrated that ADTM did not show proliferation in breast cancer cells (33). These results indicate that ADTM could not exacerbate disease progress in patients with cancer. Besides the enhancement of angiogenesis, other molecular mechanisms, such as inhibition of the *I*CaL, responsible for the excitation-contraction coupling of cardiac cells, have been implicated in the therapeutic interventions against ischemic heart disease. The findings from the current study showed that ADTM significantly inhibited I_{CaL} (Fig. 8). Hence, the inhibition of I_{CaL} also appears to play a pivotal role in the therapeutic effects of ADTM in MI mice.

Drug screening is a complex process involving both *in vitro* and *in vivo* assays. It seems clear that *in vitro* drug screening assays usually require prior knowledge of the targets and are generally not amenable to identification of the active compound with a mode of action via multi-targets or metabolic product. Widely used *in vitro* assays of molecular-and cell-based methods cannot reflect the hidden effects of a compound, due to interaction with multiple molecular targets, cell types and metabolic tissue, subsequently leading to an overall beneficial effect in an organism. In contrast, zebrafish represent a small vertebrate model organism that possess the physiological complexity of mammalian animals, allowing for a more comprehensive analysis of a chemical's multi-target, off-target or metabolic effects in the context of the whole organism (34, 35). Our current study further shows the advantage of zebrafish over endothelial cells in angiogenesis assays, particularly when some compounds are only active in *in vivo* and not *in vitro*.

CONCLUSIONS

Taken together, this study provided new evidence that 14 days of treatment of acute MI mice with the novel cardioprotective agent ADTM could promote revascularization to reduce cardiac infraction, at least in part, through blocking of I_{CaL} and stimulating VEGF production in VSMCs, not endothelial cells. These findings indicate that ADTM could be a promising novel therapeutic agent for the rehabilitation of cardiovascular diseases, particularly ischemic heart disease.

REFERENCES

[1] Global Burden of Disease Study C. Global, regional, and national incidence, prevalence, and years lived with disability for 301 acute and chronic

diseases and injuries in 188 countries, 1990-2013: a systematic analysis for the Global Burden of Disease Study 2013[J]. Lancet. 2015； 386 (9995): 743-800.

[2] Shah AM, Mann DL. In search of new therapeutic targets and strategies for heart failure: recent advances in basic science[J]. Lancet. 2011； 378 (9792): 704-712.

[3] Ponikowski P, Voors AA, Anker SD, et al. 2016 ESC Guidelines for the diagnosis and treatment of acute and chronic heart failure: The Task Force for the diagnosis and treatment of acute and chronic heart failure of the European Society of Cardiology (ESC). Developed with the special contribution of the Heart Failure Association (HFA)of the ESC[J]. Eur J Heart Fail. 2016； 18 (8): 891-975.

[4] Carmeliet P. Angiogenesis in health and disease[J]. Nat Med. 2003； 9 (6): 653-660.

[5] Khan TA, Sellke FW, Laham RJ. Therapeutic Angiogenesis for Coronary Artery Disease[J]. Curr Treat Options Cardiovasc Med. 2002； 4 (1): 65-74.

[6] Nagy JA, Dvorak AM, Dvorak HF. VEGF-A and the induction of pathological angiogenesis[J]. Annu Rev Pathol. 2007； 2: 251-275.

[7] Jia Y, Huang F, Zhang S, et al. Is danshen (Salvia miltiorrhiza)dripping pill more effective than isosorbide dinitrate in treating angina pectoris? A systematic review of randomized controlled trials[J]. Int J Cardiol. 2012； 157 (3): 330-340.

[8] Cui G, Shan L, Hung M, et al. A novel Danshensu derivative confers cardioprotection via PI3K/Akt and Nrf2 pathways[J]. Int J Cardiol. 2013； 168 (2): 1349-1359.

[9] Li RW, Yang C, Shan L, et al. Relaxation effect of a novel Danshensu/tetramethylpyrazine derivative on rat mesenteric arteries. Eur J Pharmacol[J]. 2015； 761: 153-160.

[10] Cui G, Shan L, Guo L, et al. Novel anti-thrombotic agent for modulation of protein disulfide isomerase family member ERp57 for prophylactic therapy[J]. Sci Rep. 2015； 5: 10353.

[11] Cui G, Shan L, Chen Y, et al. A New Danshensu Derivative Protects Against 6-Hydroxydopamine-Induced Neurotoxicity In Vitro and In Vivo[J]. Am J Chin Med. 2016； 44 (7): 1349-1361.

[12] Cui G, Ho AW, Lee SM, et al. Development of the novel antiplatelet agent ADTM, originating from traditional Chinese medicine: a chemical proteomic analysis and in-vivo assessment of efficacy in an animal model[J]. Lancet. 2016； 388 Suppl 1: S37.

[13] Cui Q, Chen Y, Zhang M, et al. Design, synthesis, and preliminary cardioprotective effect evaluation of danshensu derivatives[J]. Chem Biol Drug Des. 2014； 84 (3): 282-291.

[14] Cui G, Chen H, Cui W, et al. FGF2 Prevents Sunitinib-Induced Cardiotoxicity in Zebrafish and Cardiomyoblast H9c2 Cells[J]. Cardiovasc Toxicol. 2016； 16 (1): 46-53.

[15] Tang JY, Li S, Li ZH, et al. Calycosin promotes angiogenesis involving estrogen receptor and mitogen-activated protein kinase (MAPK)signaling pathway in zebrafish and HUVEC[J]. Plos One. 2010； 5 (7): e11822.

[16] Yang BR, Hong SJ, Lee SM, et al. Pro-angiogenic activity of notoginsenoside R1 in human umbilical vein endothelial cells in vitro and in a chemical-induced blood vessel loss model of zebrafish in vivo[J]. Chin J Integr Med. 2016； 22 (6): 420-429.

[17] Tang JY, Li S, Li ZH, et al. Calycosin promotes angiogenesis involving estrogen receptor and mitogen-activated protein kinase (MAPK)signaling pathway in zebrafish and HUVEC[J]. PLoS One. 2010； 5 (7): e11822.

[18] Scherrer-Crosbie M, Ullrich R, Bloch KD, et al. Endothelial nitric oxide synthase limits left ventricular remodeling after myocardial infarction in mice[J]. Circulation. 2001； 104 (11): 1286-1291.

[19] Holmes K, Roberts OL, Thomas AM, et al. Vascular endothelial growth factor receptor-2: structure, function, intracellular signalling and therapeutic inhibition[J]. Cell Signal. 2007； 19 (10): 2003-2012.

[20] Moens S, Goveia J, Stapor PC, et al. The multifaceted activity of VEGF in angiogenesis -Implications for therapy responses[J]. Cytokine Growth Factor Rev. 2014； 25 (4): 473-482.

[21] Hescheler J, Meyer R, Plant S, et al. Morphological, biochemical, and electrophysiological characterization of a clonal cell (H9c2)line from rat heart[J]. Circ Res. 1991； 69 (6): 1476-1486.

[22] Cui G, Shan L, Chu IK, et al. Identification of disulfide isomerase ERp57 as a target for small molecule cardioprotective agents[J]. RSC Adv. 2015； 5 (91): 74605-74610.

[23] Awada HK, Johnson NR, Wang Y. Sequential delivery of angiogenic growth factors improves revascularization and heart function after myocardial infarction[J]. J Control Release. 2015； 207: 7-17.

[24] Cochain C, Channon KM, Silvestre JS. Angiogenesis in the infarcted myocardium[J]. Antioxid Redox Signal. 2013； 18 (9): 1100-1113.

[25] Hedman M, Hartikainen J, Syvanne M, et al. Safety and feasibility of catheter-based local intracoronary vascular endothelial growth factor gene transfer in the prevention of postangioplasty and in-stent restenosis and in the treatment of chronic myocardial ischemia: phase II results of the Kuopio Angiogenesis Trial (KAT)[J]. Circulation. 2003； 107 (21): 2677-2683.

[26] Henry TD, Annex BH, McKendall GR, et al. The VIVA trial: Vascular endothelial growth factor in Ischemia for Vascular Angiogenesis[J]. Circulation. 2003； 107 (10): 1359-1365.

[27] Li S, Dang YY, Che GOL, Kwan YW, Chan SW, Leung GPH, Lee SMY, Hoi MPM. VEGFR tyrosine kinase inhibitor II (VRI)induced vascular insufficiency in zebrafish as a model for studying vascular toxicity and vascular preservation[J]. Toxicol Appl Pharmacol. 2014； 280 (3): 408-420.

[28] Li S, Shan L, Zhang Z, et al. Pharmacokinetic and Metabolic Studies of ADTM: A Novel Danshensu Derivative Confers Cardioprotection by

HPLC-UV and LC-MS/MS[J]. J Chromatogr Sci. 2015; 53 (6): 872-878.

[29] Shan Au AL, Kwan YW, Kwok CC, et al. Mechanisms responsible for the in vitro relaxation of ligustrazine on porcine left anterior descending coronary artery[J]. Eur J Pharmacol. 2003; 468 (3): 199-207.

[30] Ren Z, Ma J, Zhang P, et al. The effect of ligustrazine on L-type calcium current, calcium transient and contractility in rabbit ventricular myocytes[J]. J Ethnopharmacol. 2012; 144 (3): 555-561.

[31] Lam FF, Yeung JH, Chan KM, et al. Relaxant effects of danshen aqueous extract and its constituent danshensu on rat coronary artery are mediated by inhibition of calcium channels[J]. Vascul Pharmacol. 2007; 46 (4): 271-277.

[32] Yamakawa K, Hosoi M, Koyama H, et al. Peroxisome proliferator-activated receptor-gamma agonists increase vascular endothelial growth factor expression in human vascular smooth muscle cells[J]. Biochem Biophys Res Commun. 2000; 271 (3): 571-574.

[33] Wang L, Zhang X, Cui G, et al. A novel agent exerts antitumor activity in breast cancer cells by targeting mitochondrial complex II[J]. Oncotarget. 2016; 7 (22): 32054-32064.

[34] Zon LI, Peterson RT. In vivo drug discovery in the zebrafish[J]. Nature Reviews Drug Discovery. 2005; 4 (1): 35-44.

[35] Seth A, Stemple DL, Barroso I. The emerging use of zebrafish to model metabolic disease[J]. Dis Model Mech. 2013; 6 (5): 1080-1088.

First published: CUI Guozhen, XIN Qiqi, TSENG Hisa Hui Ling, Hoi Maggie PuiMan, Wang Yan, YANG Bin-rui, CHOI InLeng, WANG Yu-qiang, YUAN Rong, CHEN Ke-ji, CONG Weihong, LEE Simon MingYuen. A novel Ca^{2+} current blocker promotes angiogenesis and cardiac healing after experimental myocardial infarction in mice[J]. Pharmacol. Res, 2018, 134: 109-117.

Tetramethylpyrazine and Paeoniflorin Inhibit Oxidized LDL-induced Angiogenesis in Human Umbilical Vein Endothelial Cells via VEGF and Notch Pathways

YUAN Rong, SHI Wei-li, XIN Qi-qi, YANG Bin-rui, HOI Puiman,
LEE Simon Ming-yuen, CONG Wei-hong, and CHEN Ke-ji

Acute coronary syndrome is often related to atherosclerotic plaque rupture and thrombosis, while angiogenesis is a key factor in plaque destabilization leading to rupture [1,2]. Angiogenesis is a complex process that involves cell proliferation, migration, basement membrane degradation and neovessel organization and maturation. Several studies suggest that angiogenesis contributes to the growth of atherosclerotic lesions and plaque destabilization by aggravating inflammation-related injury and causing intraplaque hemorrhage [3-5]. Oxidized low density lipoprotein (ox-LDL)is, at least in part, responsible for angiogenesis in atherosclerotic regions [6]. Previous studies have demonstrated that low concentrations of ox-LDL promote angiogenesis in human endothelial cells, thus leading to plaque vulnerability and intravascular thrombosis [7-10]. Therefore, the inhibition of angiogenesis has been considered as a potential therapeutic target in atherosclerosis [11].

Many leading researchers have advocated using combination approaches to pursue the optimum therapeutic efficacy and to improve the patient's health status [12]. *Ligusticum chuanxiong* Hort. and *Radix Paeoniae Rubra* have been used for many years in traditional Chinese medicine as an herb pair to treat atherosclerotic diseases and inflammatory problems, and the combination of these two drugs achieves optimum therapeutic efficacy. It is reported that the compound of active constituents of *Ligusticum chuanxiong* Hort. and *Radix Paeoniae Rubra* can stabilize plaques and inhibit angiogenesis in plaque lesions [13,14]. Tetramethylpyrazine (TMP)is the active ingredient of *Ligusticum chuanxiong* Hort., which could attenuate atherosclerosis development and protect endothelial cells [15]. Paeoniflorin (PF)is the active ingredient of *Radix Paeoniae Rubra*, which could inhibit cell proliferation and alleviate atherosclerosis [16,17]. However, the effect of TMP and PF on ox-LDL-induced angiogenesis has not been studied.

Combination therapy and synergistic analysis have been used to investigate herb pairs in Chinese medicine [18]. Therefore, we sought new strategies of combining TMP with PF to perform the synergistic analysis and then to observe whether they exhibit inhibitory effect on ox-LDL-induced angiogenic properties in human umbilical vein vascular endothelial cells (HUVECs). Moreover, the underlying mechanism of angiogenesis with combined treatment was also investigated.

Vascular endothelial growth factor (VEGF)is a key proangiogenic factor that promotes intraplaque angiogenesis. VEGF signaling is predominately mediated through the activation of VEGF receptor 2 (VEGFR2) on endothelial cells, which stimulates cell proliferation and migration and thus promotes the formation of new vessels; in turn, these events can induce plaque progression and eventual hemorrhage [19,20]. In addition, the Notch signaling pathway plays a significant role in angiogenesis. During Notch activation, the upregulation of Jagged1 signaling in endothelial cells promotes the nuclear translocation of the Notch1 intracellular domain, which is the biologically active signal transducer [21]. Jagged-dependent Notch signal activation promotes pathological angiogenesis [22]. However, little is known about whether these two pathways can be regulated by the individual or combined administration of TMP and PF.

In this study, we intend to determine the effect of TMP and PF on ox-LDL-induced angiogenesis and whether the VEGF and Notch pathways were regulated by TMP and PF in ox-LDL-induced HUVECs.

MATERIALS AND METHODS

1 Materials and Reagents

TMP hydrochloride and PF were purchased from Shanghai Yuanye Bio-Technology Co., Ltd. (Shanghai, China). Ox-LDL was purchased from Beijing Solarbio Science & Technology Co., Ltd. (Beijing, China). Endothelial Cell Medium (ECM)was purchased from Scien Cell Research Laboratories (CA, USA). ELISA kits for VEGF were purchased from Multi Sciences (Hangzhou, China). Primary antibodies against VEGFR2, Notch1, Jagged1 and Hes1 were purchased from Cell Signaling Technology (CA, USA). Primary antibodies against CD31 and vWF were purchased from Proteintech (Chicago, USA). Matrigel basement membrane matrix was purchased from Becton, Dickinson and Company (New Jersey, USA). L685458 was purchased from Med Chem Express (New Jersey, USA). Other reagents were of commercially available analytical grade.

2 Cell Culture and Induction

HUVECs were generated by extraction from human umbilical veins [23]. The cell line was cultured in ECM supplemented with 5% fetal bovine serum, 1% penicillin/streptomycin solution and 1% endothelial cell growth supplement at 37 ℃ in an atmosphere with 5% CO_2. HUVECs were then incubated with different concentrations (0, 1, 5, 10, 20, 40, or 80 μg/mL)of ox-LDL for 12 h and 24 h. Then a proper concentration was used in subsequent experiments. TMP, PF and L685458 (Notch inhibitor)were dissolved in DMSO to prepare stock solutions. Stock solutions were diluted further into cell culture medium immediately before use. The final concentration of DMSO was less than 0.2%.

3 Cell Proliferation

The ox-LDL-induced proliferation of HUVECs was measured using MTT assay [24]. Briefly, HUVECs were seeded in 96-well plates. After 24 h, cells were starved in low-serum medium (0.2%)for 12 h. Then, cells in the control group were treated with the vehicle (saline solution), whereas cells in the other groups were treated with ox-LDL for 24 h. Next, the control group and the ox-LDL-induced groups were treated with the vehicle, while the TMP and PF groups were treated with various concentrations of TMP (10, 1, 0.1, or 0.01 μmol/L)or PF (10, 1, 0.1, or 0.01 μmol/L), respectively. The combination groups were treated with TMP and PF at different concentration combinations. After drug stimulation for 24 h, the optical density (OD)was measured using a microplate reader (Epoch 2, BioTek Instruments, USA)after incubation with MTT solution for 4 h at 37 ℃ followed by incubation with DMSO for 5 min. Each condition included replicate wells with at least three independent repeats.

4 Drug Combination Analysis

The effects of the combination of TMP and PF were analyzed by CompuSyn software as previously described [25,26]. Effective rate data were acquired from the MTT assay, and the combination index (CI) values were generated for a range of fraction affected (Fa)levels from 0.05-0.9. The Fa-CI plot illustrates the numerical CI values at different levels. The CI value is a mathematical and quantitative representation of the pharmacological interplay of two drugs (CI＞1, antagonism; CI=1, additive; CI＜1, synergism).

5 Cell Migration

Cell migration was detected using a wound healing assay as described previously [27]. HUVECs were seeded in 48-well plates and incubated at 37 ℃ for 24 h. Subsequently, HUVECs were induced with ox-LDL and treated with TMP and PF, either alone or in combination, for 12 h. The tested concentrations of TMP and PF were selected based on synergistic analysis in cell proliferation. Confluent HUVECs were scratched with a pipette tip, and images were obtained before drug intervention and 12 h after drug intervention. Migration was quantified as the difference between the width of the wound area covered with cells and the width of the cell-free wound area. All assays were repeated three times independently.

6 Cell Tube Formation

Endothelial-like tube formation was examined as described previously [28]. A Matrigel basement membrane matrix was added to 96-well plates and incubated at 37 ℃ for 30 min to allow gel formation. Confluent HUVECs were harvested and diluted in 100 μL of low-serum medium containing ox-LDL and drugs; cells were then seeded in the Matrigel basement membrane matrix-coated 96-well plates and incubated at 37 ℃ for 8 h. Cells in the control group were treated with vehicle, whereas cells in the drug groups were treated with TMP and PF either alone or in combination. The network-like structures were examined under an inverted microscope. The number of branching points in 3 random fields per well was quantified by ImageJ software.

7 Immunofluorescence

The angiogenesis marker CD31 and vWF were examined as described previously [29]. HUVECs were seeded on coverslips in 12-well plates for 24 h and were then induced with ox-LDL for 24 h and subjected to drug intervention for 24 h. After drug stimulation, cells were fixed for 30 min with 4% formaldehyde, permeabilized with Triton X-100 for 5 min and blocked for 60 min. CD31 antibodies (1: 200)and vWF antibodies (1: 100)were added for overnight incubation (4 ℃). Subsequently, cells were washed with PBS and incubated with the appropriate secondary antibody (FITC-conjugated goat anti-rabbit IgG and Cy3-conjugated goat anti-mouse IgG)for 1 h. Nuclei were stained with DAPI for 5 min. Images were obtained at random using a fluorescence microscope, and the integral OD (IOD)was calculated. Each experiment was repeated on at least three occasions.

8 ELISA

HUVECs were seeded in 25 cm^2 culture flasks, induced with ox-LDL for 24 h and subjected to treatment with TMP and PF, either alone or in combination, for 24 h. The cell supernatant was harvested, and VEGF concentrations were detected with ELISA kits according to the manufacturer's instructions.

9 Western Blotting

Proteins were detected as previously described [30,31]. HUVECs were seeded in 25 cm^2 culture flasks, induced with ox-LDL for 24 h, and treated with TMP and PF, either alone or in combination, for 24 h. Proteins were extracted and protein concentrations were quantified with a BCA Protein Assay kit according to the instructions. Protein (20 μg)was separated by 8%-10% SDS-PAGE and then transferred to PVDF membranes. The membranes were blocked with 5% nonfat milk in TBST for 1 h at room temperature and were then probed with primary antibodies (dilution with 1: 1000)overnight at 4 ℃. Following incubation with the corresponding secondary antibody and three washes in TBST, the protein blots were visualized using a Chemi Doc XRS system with Image Lab software (Bio-Rad Laboratories, CA, USA).

10 Administration of the Notch Inhibitor L685458

L685458 is a potent inhibitor of amyloid β-protein precursor γ-secretase activity in the Notch signaling pathway. Cells were pre-treated with L685458 (10 μmol/L)for 30 min and then stimulated with ox-LDL for 24 h. Subsequently, western blotting was employed to evaluate the treatment effect, and the details of all treatments are indicated in the figure legends.

11 Statistical Analysis

One-way analysis of variance (ANOVA)was used to evaluate the statistical significance of data among the groups. $P \leqslant 0.05$ was considered statistically significant. All of the data were analyzed with SPSS 17.0

software and are presented as the means ± S.D.

RESULTS

1 TMP and PF Inhibit ox-LDL-induced HUVEC Proliferation with Synergistic Effect

In our results, 20 ug/ml ox-LDL enhanced HUVECs proliferation at 24 h when compared with control group ($P < 0.05$, Figure 1), and this concentration was used for the subsequent experiments. After 24-h treatment, TMP alone (10 μmol/L and 1 μmol/L)or PF alone (10 μmol/L, 1 μmol/L and 0.1 μmol/L)inhibited cell proliferation when compared with ox-LDL-induced group ($P < 0.05$, Figure 2). Then, HUVECs were treated with different effective concentrations of TMP and PF, either alone or in combination. All combinations of TMP and PF, except 10 μmol/L TMP + 10 μmol/L PF, 1 μmol/L TMP + 0.1 μmol/L PF and 10 μmol/L TMP + 1 μmol/L PF, exerted synergistic effects (CI < 1)and had a CI value of less than 1 at most Fa levels (Figures 3 (a)-3 (c)).

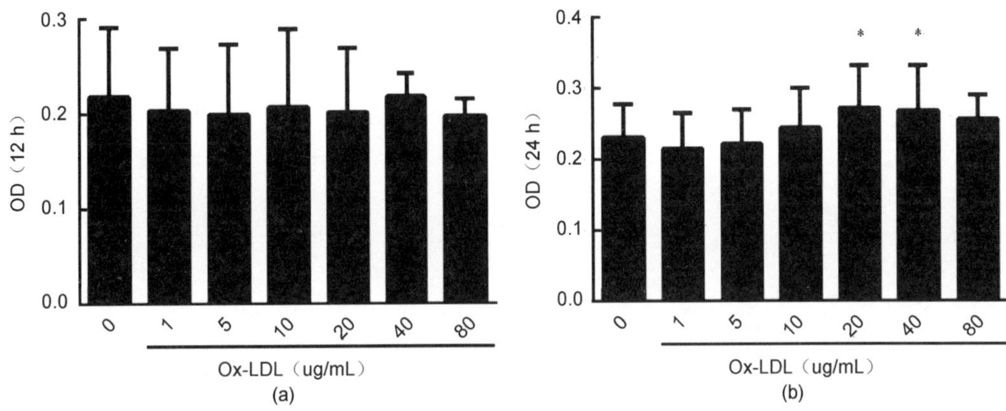

Figure 1 Ox-LDL Induced HUVEC Proliferation at (a)12 h and (b)24 h

Notes: Values are means±S.D. *$P < 0.05$ vs control group.

Specifically, TMP and PF (1: 10)displayed more effective synergistic activity at different dose and better dose-response relationship than did TMP and PF administered in the other ratios. Furthermore, the combination of 1 μmol/L TMP and 10 μmol/L PF, 1 μmol/L TMP and 1 μmol/L PF, 0.1 μmol/L TMP and 1 μmol/L PF significantly inhibited cell proliferation ($P < 0.05$), and the combination of 1 μmol/L TMP and 10 μmol/L PF showed the greatest inhibitory effect (Figure 3 (d)); thus, this concentration was used for the subsequent experiments.

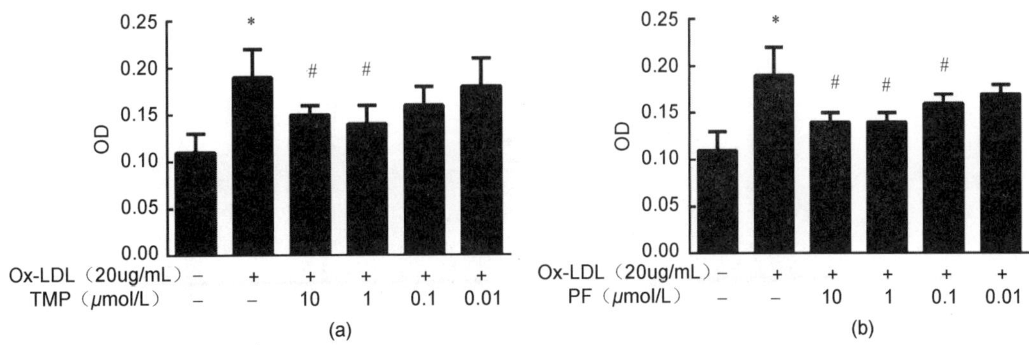

Figure 2 Effect of (a)TMP or (b)PF on ox-LDL-induced HUVEC Proliferation

Notes: Values are means±S.D. *$P < 0.05$ vs control group, #$P < 0.05$ vs ox-LDL-induced group.

2 TMP and PF Inhibit ox-LDL-induced HUVEC Migration

Ox-LDL intensively promoted the HUVEC migration when compared with control group ($P < 0.05$), while

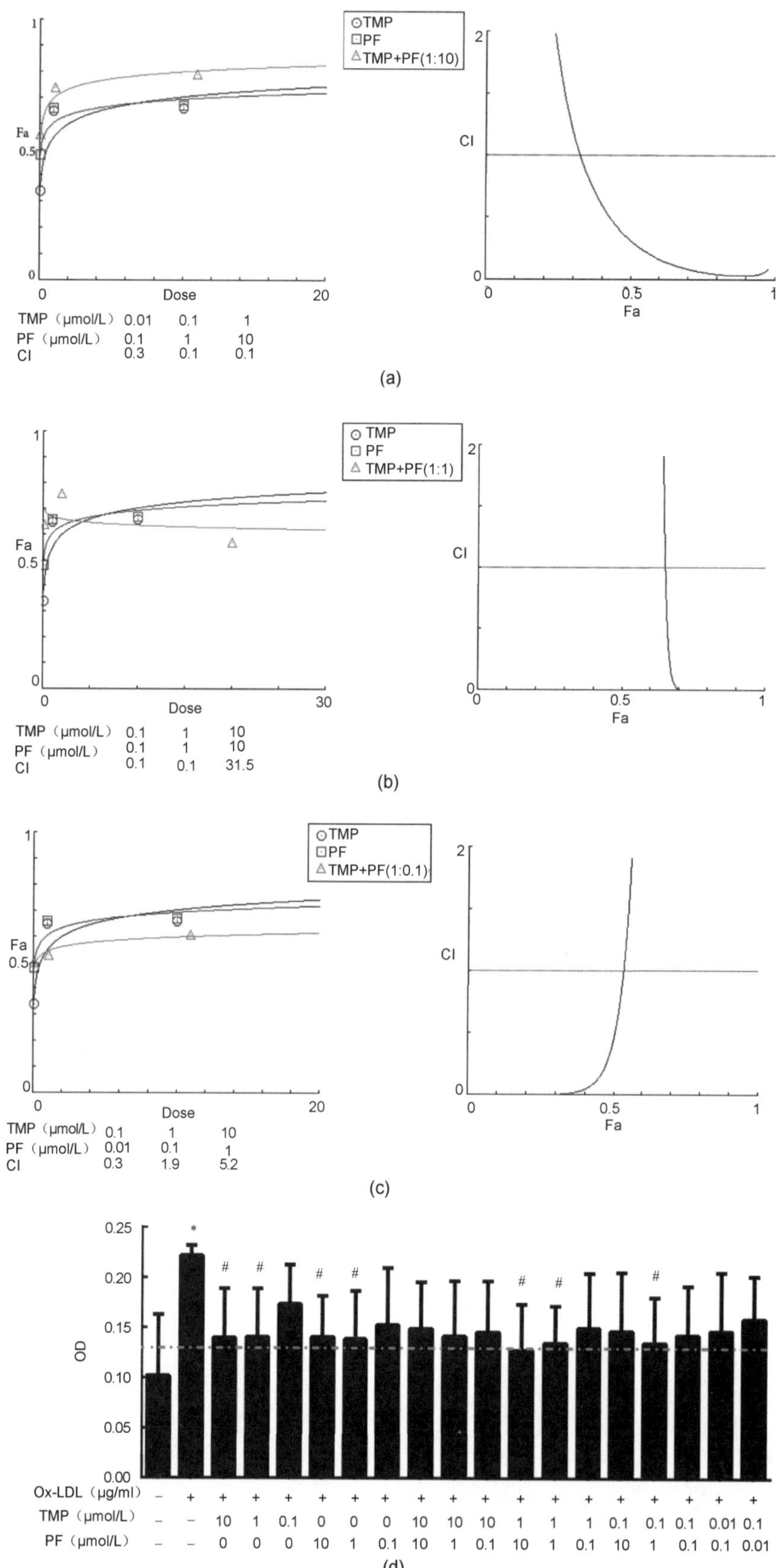

Figure 3　Combined Effects of TMP and PF on ox-LDL-induced HUVEC Proliferation

Notes: The Cl values and Fa-Cl plots generated using CompuSyn software for different concentration ratios of TMP and PF: (a)1: 10, (b)1: 1 and (c)1: 0.1. (d)Combined effects after treatment with 0, 0.01, 0.1, 1 or 10 μmol/L TMP in combination with either 0, 0.01, 0.1, 1, or 10 μmol/L PF for 24 h. Values are means±S. D, $^{*}P < 0.05$ vs control group, $^{\#}P < 0.05$ vs ox-LDL-induced group.

TMP and PF, either alone or in combination, suppressed the HUVEC migration when compared with ox-LDL-induced group ($P < 0.05$). Moreover, combination treatment with TMP and PF showed the strongest inhibitory effect (Figure 4). These results indicated that TMP and PF, either alone or in combination, exhibited inhibitory effects on ox-LDL-induced HUVEC migration.

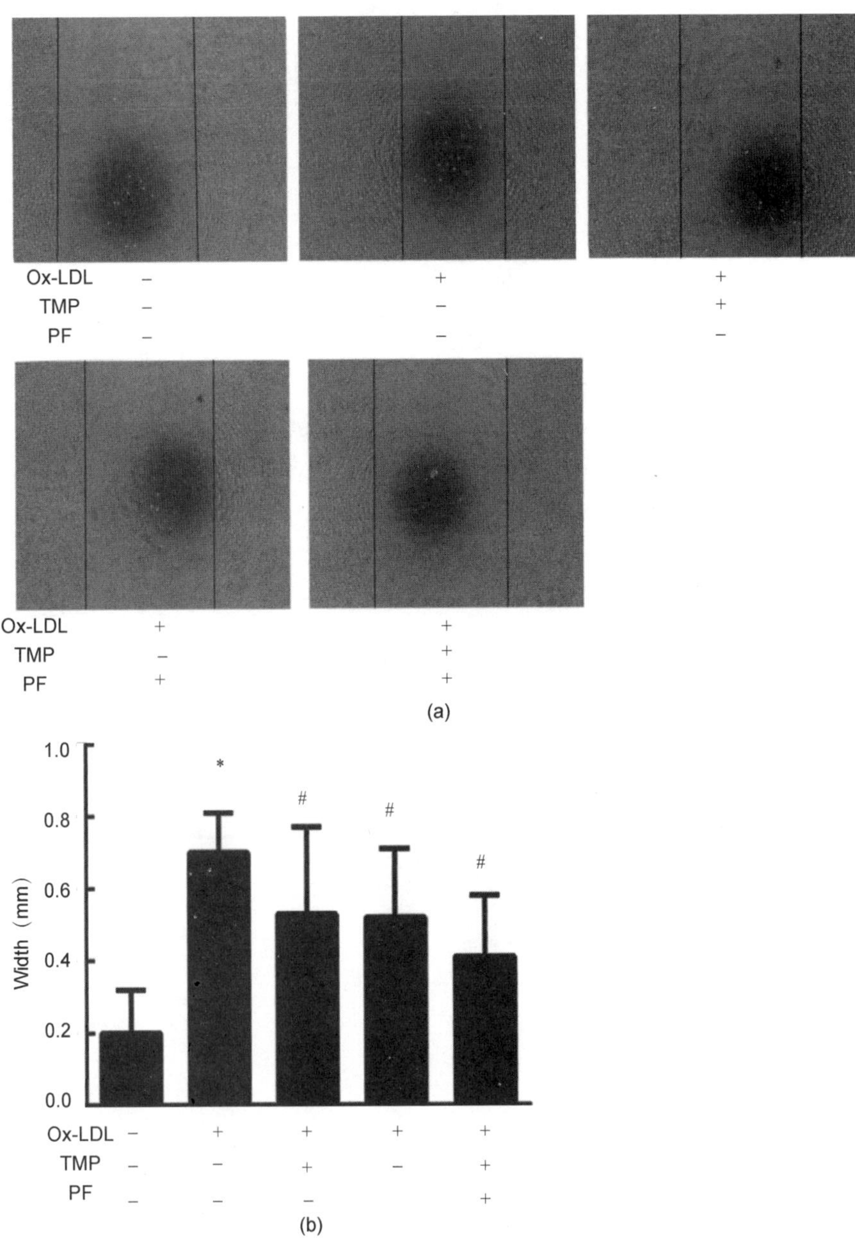

Figure 4 Effects of TMP and PF Alone or in Combination on ox-LDL-induced HUVEC Migration

Notes: (a)The scratches were examined under an inverted microscope after 12 h (10×). (b)Quantitative analysis of the migration width. Values are means±S.D. $^*P < 0.05$ vs control group, $^{\#}P < 0.05$ vs ox-LDL-induced group.

3 TMP and PF Inhibit ox-LDL-induced Tube Formation

Quantitative measurements showed that ox-LDL significantly increased the numbers of tube branch points ($P < 0.05$), while PF alone or in combination with TMP significantly decreased the number of tube branch points ($P < 0.05$) (Figure 5). These results indicated that PF alone or in combination with TMP exhibited inhibitory effects on ox-LDL-induced tube-forming ability of HUVECs.

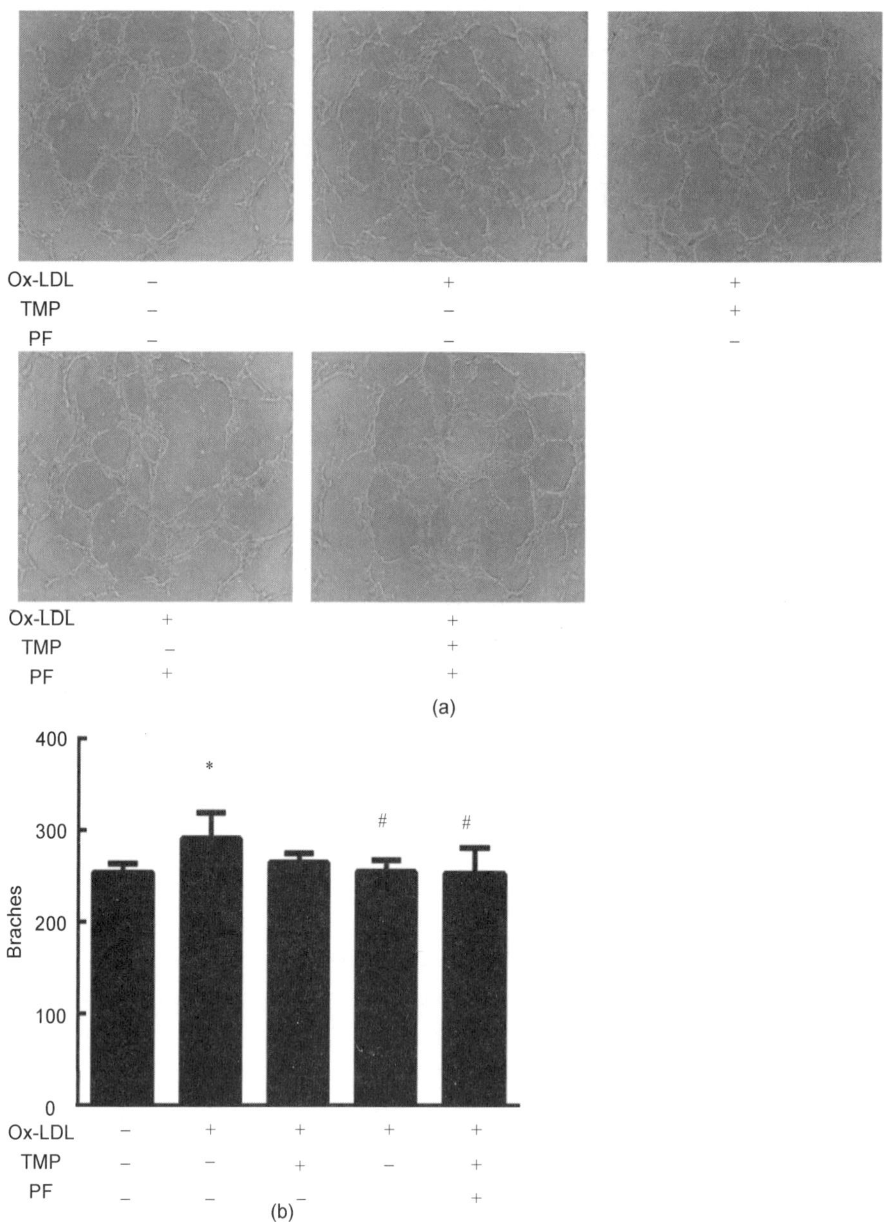

Figure 5　Effects of TMP and PF Alone or in Combination on Ox-LDL-induced Tube Formation

Notes: (a)The network-like structures were examined under an inverted microscope (20×). (b)Quantitative analysis of the number of branch points in ox-LDL-induced HUVECs. Values are means±S.D. $^{*}P<0.05$ vs control group, $^{\#}P<0.05$ vs ox-LDL-induced group.

4 Effect of TMP and PF on the ox-LDL-induced Expression of CD31 and vWF

We observed a higher level of CD31 fluorescence intensity in ox-LDL-induced cells than in control cells ($P<0.05$), which indicated that ox-LDL promoted neovascularization. PF alone or in combination with TMP was found to significantly decrease the CD31 fluorescence intensity ($P<0.05$)and thus inhibit ox-LDL-induced angiogenesis. However, TMP and PF alone or in combination failed to produce a detectable effect on the expression of vWF ($P>0.05$) (Figure 6), which is a marker of mature vessels.

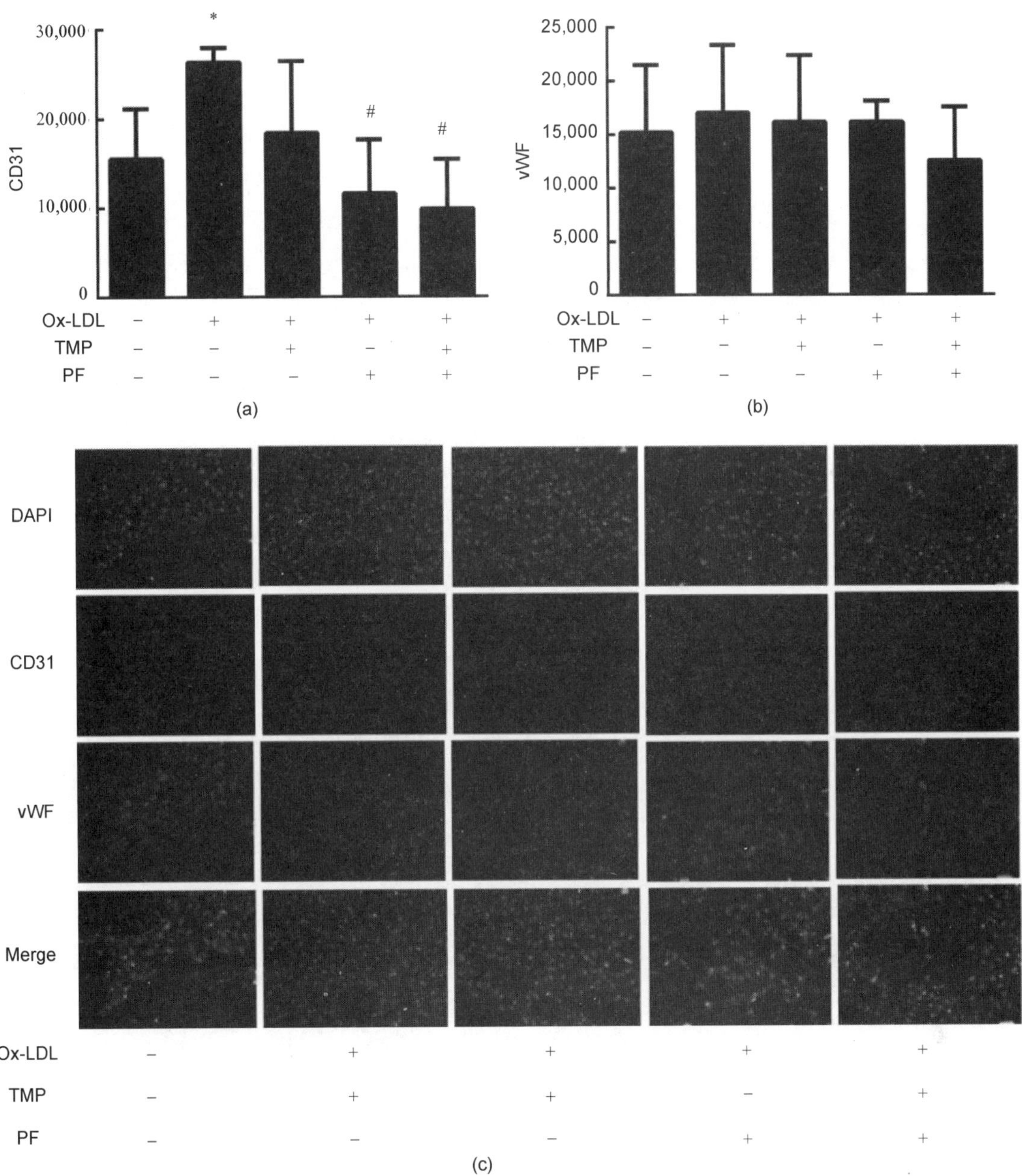

Figure 6 Effects of TMP and PF Alone or in Combination on CD31 and vWF Expression in Ox-LDL-induced HUVECs

Notes: Quantitative analysis of the IOD of (a)CD31 and (b)vWF. Values are means±S.D. $^*P < 0.05$ vs control group, $^\#P < 0.05$ vs ox-LDL-induced group. (c)The fluorescence intensity was examined under an inverted microscope (20×).

5 Effect of TMP and PF on the ox-LDL-induced Expression of Angiogenesis- Associated Protein

In our study, ox-LDL significantly increased the expression of VEGF, VEGFR2, Notch1, Jagged1 and Hes1 ($P < 0.05$), thus indicating that ox-LDL induced angiogenesis by activating the VEGF/VEGFR2 and Jagged1/Notch1 pathways. TMP downregulated VEGFR2 expression but did not regulate the expression of VEGF, Notch1, Jagged1 or Hes1; PF downregulated the expression of VEGF, VEGFR2 and Notch1 but did not regulate the expression of Jagged1 and Hes1. However, combination treatment not only decreased the expression of VEGF and VEGFR2 but also decreased the expression of Notch1, Jagged1 and Hes1 ($P < 0.05$), thus indicating that an antiangiogenic effect of the combination of TMP and PF is mediated through the VEGF/

VEGFR2 and Jagged1/Notch1 pathways. In addition, combination treatment with TMP and PF induced stronger inhibitory effects on the expression of Notch1 than did treatment with TMP alone ($P < 0.05$) (Figure 7).

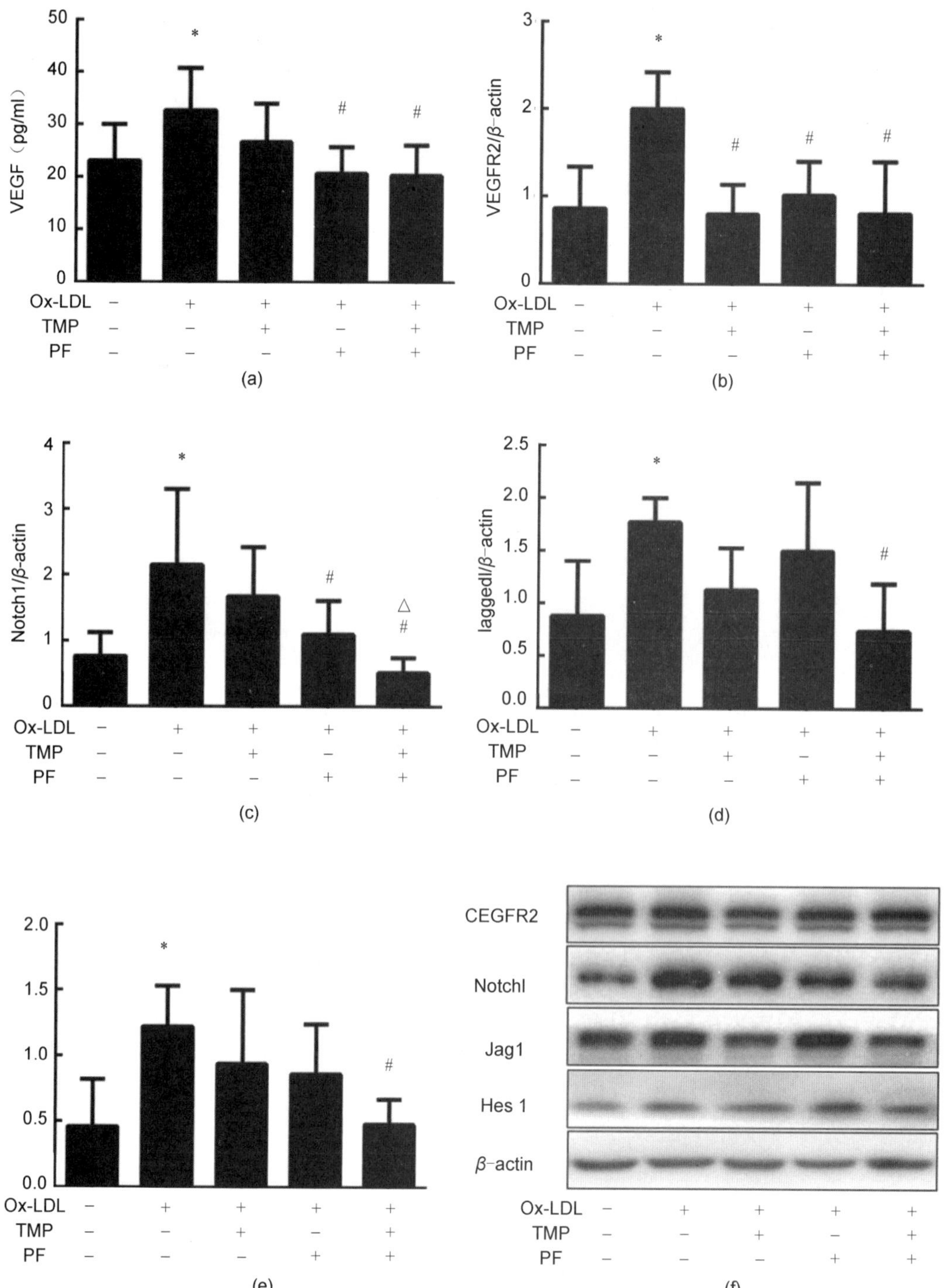

Figure 7 Analysis of Angiogenesis-associated Protein Expression

Notes: (a)Secreted VEGF protein level in the supernatant of ox-LDL-induced HUVECs was analyzed by an ELISA. Protein expression levels of (b)VEGFR2, (c)Notch1, (d)Jagged1 and (e)Hes1 were analyzed by western blot. Values are means±S. D. $^{*}P < 0.05$ vs control group, $^{\#}P < 0.05$ *vs* ox-LDL-induced group, $^{\triangle}P < 0.05$ *vs* TMP group. (F)Protein extracts were immunoblotted to determine the relative expression levels of VEGFR2, Notch1, Jagged1 and Hes1.

6 Inhibition by combination treatment and pathway inhibitor

To further examine the mechanisms by which changes in Notch1 and VEGFR2 expression alter angiogenesis upon combination treatment with TMP and PF, an inhibitor of the Notch signaling pathway was used. We found that Notch inhibitor not only inhibited the expression of Notch1, Jagged1 and Hes1, but also decreased the expression of VEGFR2 ($P < 0.05$). Additionally, the ox-LDL-induced expression of VEGFR2 was found to be reduced more by combination treatment than Notch inhibitor. Thus, we demonstrated that combination treatment with TMP and PF potentiated an antiangiogenic effect through the suppression of the Jagged1/Notch1 pathway and the further decrease in the expression of both Hes1 and VEGFR2, and not just through the suppression of the VEGF/VEGFR2 pathway (Figure 8).

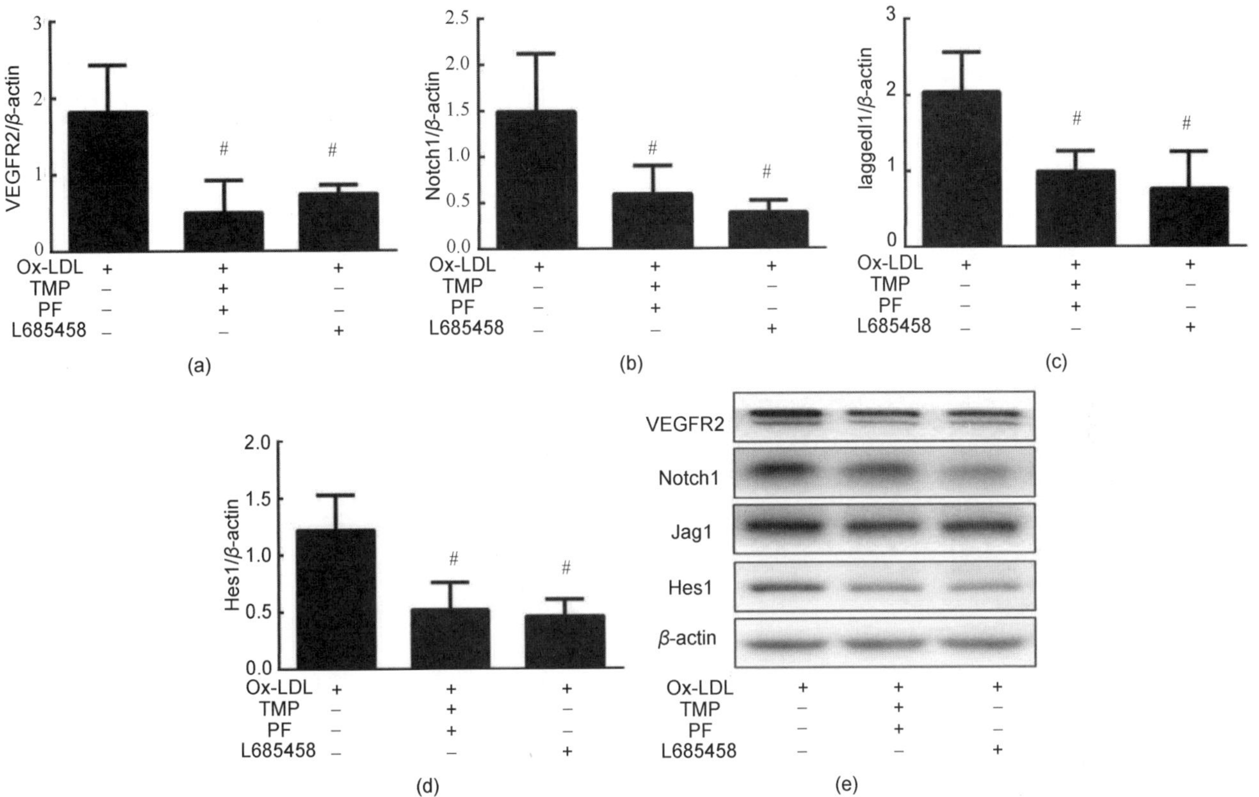

Figure 8 Analysis of the Effects of Combination Treatment and Notch Inhibitor Treatment on ox-LDL Induced-angiogenesis

Notes: Protein expression levels of (a)VEGFR2, (b)Notch1, (c)Jagged1 and (d)Hes1 were analyzed by western blot. Values are means±S.D. $^{\#}P < 0.05$ *vs* ox-LDL-induced group. (e)Protein extracts were immunoblotted to determine the relative expression levels of VEGFR2, Notch1, Jagged1 and Hes1.

DISCUSSION

Angiogenesis contributes to plaque instability in atherosclerosis, and the inhibition of ox-LDL-induced angiogenesis might stabilize plaques [4]. Our findings revealed that the combination of TMP and PF exhibited an antiangiogenic effect on ox-LDL-induced HUVECs, and the inhibitory effect was associated with its suppression of the VEGF/VEGFR2 and the Jagged1/Notch1 signaling pathways. These results indicated that combination treatment with TMP and PF inhibited ox-LDL-induced angiogenesis with advantages of multiple targets and multiple pathways, which might stabilize plaques (Figure 9).

Previous studies have shown that combination treatment with TMP and PF might be a promising therapeutic strategy for ischemic disease and optimal compatibility ratio is TMP 1 μmol/L and PF 10 μmol/L [32]. We evaluated synergistic effect in cell proliferation and found the optimal compatibility ratio 1: 10 for TMP and PF. These results suggest the potential of using lower TMP concentrations with higher PF concentrations to achieve an enhanced level of effectiveness. However, since the double-edged role of angiogenesis in myocardial ischemia and atherosclerosis [33], the effects of TMP and PF (1: 10)on coronary atherosclerotic heart disease require further investigation. Moreover, the other compatibility ratios of TMP and PF could also be investigated in the future to observe different interactions.

Recent evidence has demonstrated that combination therapy could provide greater therapeutic benefits to atherosclerosis, of which possesses complex pathophysiology and therefore is difficult to treat using single target approach [18]. Our study indicated that TMP inhibited cell proliferation and migration by decreasing the expression of VEGFR2; PF inhibited angiogenesis by mainly decreasing the expression of Notch1 and then decreasing the expression of VEGFR2; however, the combination of TMP and PF attenuated angiogenesis by inhibiting both the VEGF/VEGFR2 and Jagged1/Notch1 pathways. Therefore, combination treatment with TMP and PF exhibited an antiangiogenic effect through multiple targets and multiple pathways, which showed the advantages of combination therapy.

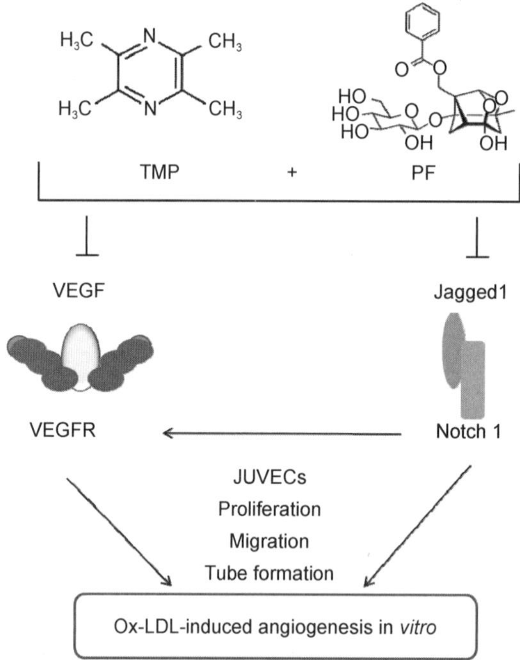

Figure 9 A Schematic Diagram of the Proposed Antiangiogenic Mechanisms of Combination Treatment with TMP and PF in ox-LDL-induced HUVECs

Notch1 selectively binds to Jagged1 under inflammatory conditions, and the Jagged1/Notch1 signaling pathway is then activated to promote angiogenesis in atherosclerosis [34,35]. In the present study, TMP had no effect on the Notch pathway and did not significantly inhibit tube formation; PF decreased the expression of Notch1 and inhibited angiogenesis; Combination treatment with TMP and PF significantly decreased the expression of Notch1 when compared with TMP treatment. These results indicated that Notch1may be one of the major regulatory factors in the antiangiogenic effect of combination treatment. Nevertheless, an in vivo study using ApoE-/-mice would be preferred in the future to examine the role of the Notch pathway in the antiangiogenic effect of combination treatment.

Herb pairs as the basic composition units of Chinese herbal formulae are of special clinical significance in traditional Chinese medicine, and their feature of simplicity can facilitate studies on mechanism investigation [36]. Previous reports have shown that compound of active constituents of *Ligusticum chuanxiong* Hort. and *Radix Paeoniae Rubra* has inhibitory effect on plaque angiogenesis *in vivo* [13,14]. Our study further examined the effect of TMP and PF on ox-LDL-induced angiogenesis *in vitro*, and partly elucidated the antiangiogenic mechanism of *Ligusticum chuanxiong* Hort. and *Radix Paeoniae Rubra* herb pair. Nowadays, endothelial to mesenchymal transition (EndMT)makes a major contribution to the vascular remodelling and neointimal formation, which correlates with the unstable plaques and promotes atherosclerosis progression [37]. Hence, the effects of TMP and PF on EndMT and the connection between angiogenesis and EndMT require further investigation. Moreover, it should be noted that further clinical research is required for verifying the efficiency of *Ligusticum chuanxiong* Hort. and *Radix Paeoniae Rubra* herb pair, and more research is needed for the standardization and safety evaluation.

CONCLUSION

Our results demonstrated that combination treatment with TMP and PF had an antiangiogenic effect on ox-LDL-induced HUVECs by inhibiting the VEGF/VEGFR2 and Jagged1/Notch1 signaling pathways, thus might stabilize plaques and decrease the incidence of cardiac and cerebrovascular events. Therefore, these results may provide a new direction for future drug treatment strategies in atherosclerosis.

REFERENCES

[1] Naito R, Miyauchi K, Daida H, et al. Impact of total risk management on coronary plaque regression in diabetic patients with acute coronary syndrome[J]. J Atheroscler Thromb, 2016, 23 (8): 922-931.

[2] van der Hoeven NW, Hollander MR, Yıldırım C, et al. The emerging role of galectins in cardiovascular disease[J]. Vascul Pharmacol, 2016, 81: 31-41.

[3] Eterafoskouei T, Allahyari S, Akbarzadehatashkhosrow A, et al. Methanolic extract of Ficus carica Linn. leaves exerts antiangiogenesis effects based on the rat air pouch model of inflammation[J]. Evid Based Complement Alternat Med, 2015, 2015: 760405.

[4] Liu MH, Tang ZH, Li GH, et al. Janus-like role of fibroblast growth factor 2 in arteriosclerotic coronary artery disease: atherogenesis and angiogenesis[J]. Atherosclerosis, 2013, 229 (1): 10-17.

[5] Camaré C, Pucelle M, Nègre-Salvayre A, et al. Angiogenesis in the atherosclerotic plaque[J]. Redox Biol, 2017, 12: 18-34.

[6] Dai Y, Zhang Z, Cao Y, et al. MiR-590-5p Inhibits oxidized-LDL induced angiogenesis by targeting LOX-1[J]. Sci Rep, 2016, 6: 22607-22610.

[7] Qiu J, Peng Q, Zheng Y, et al. OxLDL stimulates Id1 nucleocytoplasmic shuttling in endothelial cell angiogenesis via PI3K pathway[J]. Biochim Biophys Acta, 2012, 21 (10): 1361-1369.

[8] Wang L, Li G, Chen Q, et al. Octanoylated ghrelin attenuates angiogenesis induced by oxLDL in human coronary artery endothelial cells via the GHSR1a-mediated NF-κB pathway[J]. Metabolism, 2015, 64 (10): 1262-1271.

[9] Yu S, Wong SL, Lau CW, et al. Oxidized LDL at low concentration promotes in-vitro angiogenesis and activates nitric oxide synthase through PI3K/Akt/eNOS pathway in human coronary artery endothelial cells[J]. Biochem Biophys Res Commun, 2011, 407 (1): 44-48.

[10] Dandapat A, Hu C, Sun L, et al. Small concentrations of oxLDL induce capillary tube formation from endothelial cells via LOX-1-dependent redoxsensitive pathway[J]. Arterioscler Thromb Vasc Biol, 2007, 27 (11): 2435-2442.

[11] Wu W, Li X, Zuo G, et al. The Role of Angiogenesis in coronary artery disease: a double-edged sword: intraplaque angiogenesis in physiopathology and therapeutic angiogenesis for treatment[J]. Curr Pharm Des, 2018, 24 (4): 451-464.

[12] Yang Y, Zhang Z, Li S, et al. Synergy effects of herb extracts: Pharmacokinetics and pharmacodynamic basis[J]. Fitoterapia, 2014, 92 (2): 133-147.

[13] Xu H, Wen C, Chen KJ. Study on the effect of rhizoma Chuanxiong, *radix paeoniae rubra* and the compound of their active ingredients, Xiongshao Capsule, on stability of atherosclerotic plaque in ApoE (-/-)mice[J]. Zhongguo Zhong Xi Yi Jie He Za Zhi, 2007, 27 (6): 513-518.

[14] Zhang L, Jiang YR, Guo CY, et al. Effects of active components of red paeonia and rhizoma chuanxiong on angiogenesis in atherosclerosis plaque in rabbits[J]. Chin J Integr Med, 2009, 15 (5): 359-364.

[15] Zhang Y, Ren P, Kang Q, et al. Effect of tetramethylpyrazinc on atherosclerosis and SCAP/SREBP-1c signaling pathway in apoE-/-mice fed with a high-fat diet[J]. Evid Based Complement Alternat Med, 2017, 2017: 3121989.

[16] Li H, Jiao Y, Xie M. Paeoniflorin ameliorates atherosclerosis by suppressing TLR4-mediated NF-κB activation[J]. Inflammation, 2017, 40 (6): 2042-2051.

[17] Fan X, Wu J, Yang H, et al. Paeoniflorin blocks the proliferation of vascular smooth muscle cells induced by platelet-derived growth factor-BB through ROS mediated ERK1/2 and p38 signaling pathways[J]. Mol Med Rep, 2018, 17 (1): 1676-1682.

[18] Zhou X, Seto SW, Chang D, et al. Synergistic effects of Chinese herbal medicine: a comprehensive review of methodology and current research[J]. Front Pharmacol, 2016, 12 (7): 201-216.

[19] Yang Z, Wang H, Jiang Y, et al. VEGFA activates erythropoietin receptor and enhances VEGFR2-mediated pathological angiogenesis[J]. Am J Pathol, 2014, 184 (4): 1230-1239.

[20] Wang L, Chen Q, Ke D, et al. Ghrelin inhibits atherosclerotic plaque angiogenesis and promotes plaque stability in a rabbit atherosclerotic model[J]. Peptides, 2017, 90: 17-26.

[21] Nus M, Martínez-Poveda B, MacGrogan D, et al. Endothelial Jag1-RBPJ signalling promotes inflammatory leucocyte recruitment and atherosclerosis[J]. Cardiovasc Res, 2016, 112 (2): 568-580.

[22] Kangsamaksin T, Murtomaki A, Kofler NM, et al. NOTCH decoys that selectively block DLL/NOTCH or JAG/NOTCH disrupt angiogenesis by unique mechanisms to inhibit tumor growth[J]. Cancer Discov, 2015, 5 (2): 182-197.

[23] Jaffe EA, Hoyer LW, Nachman RL, et al. Synthesis of antihemophilic factor antigen by cultured human endothelial cells[J]. J Clin Invest, 1973, 52 (11): 2757-2760.

[24] Seibold S, Schürle D, Heinloth A, et al. Oxidized LDL induces proliferation and hypertrophy in human umbilical vein endothelial cells via regulation of p27Kip1 expression: role of RhoA[J]. J Am Soc Nephrol, 2004, 15 (12): 3026-3034.

[25] Chou TC. Preclinical versus clinical drug combination studies[J]. Leuk Lymphoma, 2008, 49 (11): 2059-2080.

[26] Chou TC, Talalay P. Quantitative analysis of dose-effect relationships: the combined effects of multiple drugs or enzyme inhibitors[J]. Adv Enzyme Regul, 1984, 22: 27-55.

[27] Xin QQ, Yang BR, Zhou HF, et al. Paeoniflorin promotes angiogenesis in a vascular insufficiency model of zebrafish *in vivo* and in human umbilical vein endothelial cells *in vitro*[J]. Chin J Integr Med, 2018, 24 (7): 494-501.

[28] Qin W, Xie W, Xia N, et al. Silencing of transient receptor potential channel 4 alleviates oxLDL-induced angiogenesis in human coronary artery endothelial cells by inhibition of VEGF and NF- κ B[J]. Med Sci Monit, 2016, 22: 930-936.

[29] Qin M, Guan X, Wang H, et al. An effective ex-vivo approach for inducing endothelial progenitor cells from umbilical cord blood CD34+ cells[J]. Stem Cell Res Ther, 2017, 8 (1): 25-27.

[30] Qiao H, Wang TY, Yan W, et al. Synergistic suppression of human breast cancer cells by combination of plumbagin and zoledronic acid *In vitro*[J]. Acta Pharmacol Sin, 2015, 36 (9): 1085-1098.

[31] Chen B, Wang HT, Yu B, et al. Carthamin yellow inhibits matrix degradation and inflammation induced by LPS in the intervertebral disc via suppression of MAPK pathway activation[J]. Exp Ther Med, 2017, 14 (2): 1614-1620.

[32] Wang Y, Guo G, Yang BR, et al. Synergistic effects of Chuanxiong-Chishao herb-pair on promoting angiogenesis at network pharmacological and pharmacodynamic levels[J]. Chin J Integr Med, 2017, 32 (9): 654-662.

[33] Yuan R, Shi WL, Xin QQ, et al. Holistic regulation of angiogenesis with Chinese herbal medicines as a new option for coronary artery disease[J]. Evid Based Complement Alternat Med, 2018, 2018: 3725962.

[34] Fu WB, Ding SF. Research progress of Notch signals and atherosclerosis[J]. Med Recapitul, 2014, 20 (1): 18-21.

[35] Yin Q, Wang W, Cui G, et al. Potential role of the Jagged1/Notch1 signaling pathway in the endothelial-myofibroblast transition during BLM-induced pulmonary fibrosis[J]. J Cell Physiol, 2018, 233 (3): 2451-2463.

[36] Wang S, Hu Y, Tan W, et al. Compatibility art of traditional Chinese medicine: from the perspective of herb pairs[J]. J Ethnopharmacol, 2012, 143 (2): 412-423.

[37] Evrard SM, Lecce L, Michelis KC, et al. Endothelial to mesenchymal transition is common in atherosclerotic lesions and is associated with plaque instability[J]. Nat Commun, 2016, 7: 11853.

First published: YUAN Rong, SHI Wei-li, XIN Qi-qi, YANG Bin-rui, HOI Maggie Puiman, LEE Simon Ming-yuen, CONG Wei-hong, CHEN Ke-ji. Tetramethylpyrazine and paeoniflorin inhibit oxidized LDL-induced angiogenesis in human umbilical vein Endothelial cells via VEGF and notch pathways[J]. Evid Based Complement Alternat Med, 2018, 2018: 3082507.

Sodium Tanshinone IIA Sulfate Adjunct Therapy Reduces High-sensitivity C-reactive Protein Level in Coronary Artery Disease Patients: A Randomized Controlled Trial

LI Si-ming, Jiao Yang, WANG Han-jay, SHANG Qing-hua, LU Fang, HUANG Li, LIU Jian-gang, XU Hao, and CHEN Ke-ji

Cardiovascular disease is the worldwide leading cause of death, and coronary artery disease (CAD) is responsible for the greatest mortality. Inflammation plays an important role both in the development of atherosclerosis and in triggering cardiovascular events[1]. As a robust marker of systematic inflammation, high-sensitivity C-reactive protein (hs-CRP)has been closely studied[2-5], and a meta-analysis showed that hs-CRP >3 mg/L is an independent risk factor for cardiovascular events[6]. Therefore, reducing the concentration of hs-CRP may further bene fits patients with CAD. In fact, the mortality reduction and cardiovascular benefits of statins, a cornerstone of evidence-based standard medical therapy for CAD, may partly attribute to its anti-inflammation effect.

Indeed, the JUPITER trial found that, among non-hyperlipidemic patients with elevated hs-CRP, statin therapy reduced hs-CRP levels by 37%, and led to a significantly lower rate of major adverse cardiovascular events after 1.9 years compared to placebo[7]. Nevertheless, despite intensive statin therapy, 22.4% of patients with acute coronary syndrome suffer a serious cardiovascular or cerebrovascular event within two years of initiating treatment[8], thus revealing the extent of residual cardiovascular risk, as well as the potential benefit of further dampening the inflammatory reaction of atherosclerosis.

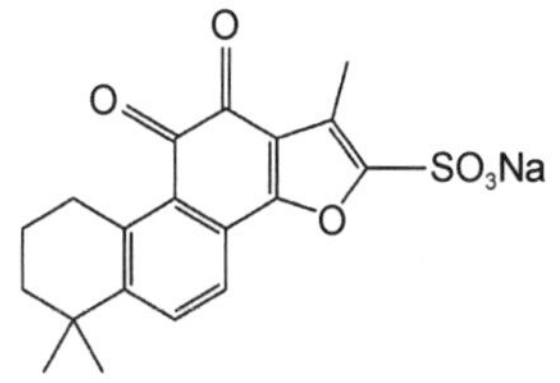

Figure 1 The Chemical Structure of Sodium Tanshinone IIA Sulfate

Tanshinone IIA, one of the most pharmacologically active components extracted from Radix Salviae miltiorrhizae, has been identified as a promising natural cardioprotective agent[9]. Most noteworthy is the ability of tanshinone IIA to decrease the levels of multiple inflammatory factors associated with the progression of atherosclerosis, such as CRP, interleukin-6 (IL-6), tumor necrosis factor alpha (TNF-α), vascular cell adhesion molecule-1 (VCAM-1), CD40, monocyte chemotactic protein-1 (MCP-1), and matrix metalloproteinase-9 (MMP-9)[10,11]. Because of the low oral bioavailability of tanshinone IIA[12], intravenous sodium tanshinone IIA sulfate (STS)has been developed (Fig. 1), and is the most widely used clinical formulation of tanshinone IIA in China for patients with CAD.

In this trial, we hypothesized that the addition of STS to standard statin-containing medical therapy for patients with CAD will: 1)further reduce the levels of serum hs-CRP and other circulating inflammatory markers after 14 days of treatment; 2)show a sustained effect on inflammatory marker levels at 30 days after treatment completion; 3)improve angina symptoms; and 4)be a safe treatment, compared to standard medical therapy alone.

METHODS

1 Ethics

The study protocol (2012XL022-2)was approved by the ethics review board of Xiyuan Hospital, China Academy of Chinese Medical Sciences (CACMS), and is available[23]. The study is registered at http: //www. iecrf. org (Chictr. org number: ChiCTR-TRC-12002361, registered on 07/22/2012). All aspects of our study were conducted with adherence to the current version of the Declaration of Helsinki, the guidelines established by the International Conference on Harmonization of Good Clinical Practice, and the laws of China. All participants signed informed consent forms before enrollment.

2 Trial Design and Settings

This trial was a parallel-group, prospective randomized open-label blinded-endpoint (PROBE)study conducted in China. The eligible participants were randomized 1: 1 into either the control group (standard medical therapy for CAD with uniformly-dosed atorvastatin)or the experimental group (control regimen plus 80 mg intravenous dose of STS daily). Because atorvastatin reduces hs-CRP to a greater extent than other statins[24], and is more popular in clinical practice, we treated participants with uniformly-dosed atorvastatin instead of simvastatin, as originally proposed in our published study protocol.

3 Participants

Hospitalized patients with unstable angina or non-ST-elevation myocardial infarction between 35 and 75 years of age were eligible if they were on statin therapies for at least 1 month, had increased hs-CRP level (between 3 mg/L and 15 mg/L)at enrollment, and with documented CAD (with at least 1 coronary artery stenosis ≥ 50% confirmed by previous coronary angiography, or with a documented history of myocardial infarction [coronary angiography not required]). The diagnosis of CAD was based on the standardized criteria established in "Nomenclature and criteria for diagnosis of ischemic heart disease," a joint report published by the International Society and Federation of Cardiology and the World Health Organization[25], and the ESC Guidelines for the management of acute coronary syndromes in patients presenting without persistent ST-segment elevation[26].

Exclusion criteria included severe heart failure (ejection fraction < 35%), reduced platelet count or other bleeding diatheses, cancer, sexually transmitted diseases, tuberculosis, rheumatoid arthritis or other autoimmune diseases, infection, fever, trauma, burn injury, surgery within one month prior to recruitment, or any history of serious pulmonary, hepatic, renal, neurological, psychiatric, or hematological diseases. Additional exclusion criteria included active use of any antibiotics or any traditional Chinese medicine with the function of clearing heat and removing toxins (e.g. Honeysuckle, Forsythiae Fructus, Taraxacum, Rheum officinale, Polygonum cuspidatum). Patients participating in other clinical trials were also excluded. Finally, patients must not have previously (within one month)undergone or currently be planning to undergo PCI or coronary artery bypass grafting, considering their effect on inflammatory factors.

Recruitment, intervention, and data collection took place at the inpatient department of Xiyuan Hospital, CACMS, and China-Japan Friendship Hospital in Beijing, China. Subjects were recruited from August 2012 to January 2014, and follow-up was completed by February 2014.

4 Interventions

Each patient in the control group received 20 mg atorvastatin orally once per evening, in addition to any other oral or intravenous medications (e.g. beta-blockers, ACEI/ARB, CCB, aspirin, clopidogrel, nitrates) deemed appropriate for a standard treatment of the patient's individual condition. Doses of ACEI/ARB or beta-blockers were titrated gradually to target levels whenever possible. These standard medications were prescribed by physicians who were not associated with the trial. Additionally, patients in the experiment group received intravenous STS (80 mg, once daily for 14 consecutive days, 10 mg per ampoule, Jiangsu Carefree Pharmaceutical Co., Ltd., national drug approval number: H31022558), diluted with 250 mL 0.9% sodium chloride solution.

All study participants received treatment as indicated above for 14 consecutive days. After 14 days, patients in both groups continued to receive guideline-based standard medical therapy for CAD.

5 Outcome Measures

Serum hs-CRP level was the primary outcome. Secondary outcomes included 1)the levels of other inflammatory mediators, including IL-6, TNF-α, VCAM-1, sCD40L, MCP-1, and MMP-9, as measured by enzyme-linked immunosorbent assay; 2)the extent of improvement in angina symptoms; and 3)treatment safety.

The extent of improvement in angina symptoms was evaluated by a scoring system (Supplementary Table S1)based on the frequency, duration, and intensity of angina episodes, as well as the dose of nitroglycerin utilized, according to "Cardiovascular Drug Clinical Research Guiding Principles" by the Ministry of Health, People's Republic of China, 1998. The total angina score ranges from a minimum 0 points (no angina)to a maximum 24 points, and higher score indicates more severe angina symptoms.

To assess treatment safety, patients were asked to report any side effects or changes in feelings that they had noticed. In addition, the results of routine blood, urine, and stool tests, liver and kidney function tests, coagulation tests, and electrocardiogram tests were also considered in the evaluation of safety. Finally, adverse events including death, adverse cardiovascular events (myocardial infarction, stroke, etc.)were closely monitored and recorded by the clinical researchers during the whole study period.

All outcomes were measured at baseline, immediately after completion of the 14-day treatment, and at 30 days after completion of treatment. No changes to the designated trial outcomes were made after the study commenced.

6 Sample Size Estimation

Because the data needed to perform an a priori sample size calculation for this pilot study was not available, we adopted the sample size of a comparable trial which involved 60 subjects randomized into two groups of 30 each[27]. For our study, planned to recruit 72 patients, assuming conservatively that 20% of the participants would be lost to follow-up. No interim analyses were undertaken.

7 Randomization and Blinding

A member of the Institute of Clinical Pharmacology (ICP)of Xiyuan Hospital who was independent of the study used SAS 9.3 software (SAS Institute, Cary, NC, USA)to perform a permuted-block randomization, generating a sequence of 72 random numbers. To maintain concealment, the group assignments were relayed by another member of the ICP using a central randomization strategy. Once a patient met all the criteria for enrollment in the trial, the group assignment was delivered by telephone to the clinical researchers. Given that the color of the STS solution is unique and challenging to emulate, unblinding was permitted at the physician and patient levels only after baseline data was collected. In order to minimize biases as much as possible, all other potential sources of information that may reveal treatment allocation to the patients were judiciously guarded. Additionally, the details of treatment allocation were not disclosed to any patient until the study had concluded, and all study participants were discouraged from discussing with one another their involvement in the trial. Finally, the clinical researchers strictly abided by the study's random design and interacted with the patients in each group with as few differences as possible. Blinding was maintained at the level of outcome assessment. The individuals performing laboratory blood analyses, data management, and statistical analysis were independent of the clinical component of the study, and were not provided with any information that may reveal treatment allocation details.

8 Statistical Analysis

Statistical analyses were performed with SAS9.3 software (SPSS, Inc., Chicago, IL, USA). Categorical data were reported as counts with the percentage of the total and continuous data as a mean with standard deviation, or as a median with 95% confidence interval (CI)or interquartile range (IQR). The χ^2 test or Fisher's exact test was used for comparisons of categorical data. Because serum levels of hs-CRP, IL-6, TNFα, VCAM-1, sCD40L, MCP-1, and MMP-9 were measurement data, an independent Student's t-test was used for the analysis of intergroup differences when the date meet the normal distribution; Wilcoxon rank-sum test was used when the distribution of levels of the data was non-normality. In addition, comparison of inflammatory markers levels within the group be conducted by paired t-test or paired Wilcoxon rank-sum test. Wilcoxon rank-sum test was used to the analysis of intergroup differences of total angina scores because the distribution of levels of the data was non-normality. All tests were two tailed and a statistical probability of $<$ 0.05 was considered significant.

RESULTS

1 Participant Characteristics

Study participants were recruited from August 2012 to January 2014, and final follow-up was completed by February 2014. A flow diagram illustrating the study design is shown in Fig. 2. A total of 280 inpatients were assessed for eligibility, and finally, 72 eligible participants were enrolled. Among which, 36 participants were randomly assigned to receive standard statin-containing medical therapy with uniformly-dosed atorvastatin 20 mg daily (control statin group)and 36 to standard medical therapy plus 80 mg intravenous STS daily (experimental statin+STS group). Two patients were subsequently excluded because of mis-inclusion: 1 patient in the statin group withdrew to receive percutaneous coronary intervention (PCI)during hospitalization, and 1 patient in the statin+STS group developed pneumonia. Ultimately, 70 participants (35 in each group) completed the 14-day treatment. During the 30-day follow-up period, 3 participants, 2 in the statin+STS group and 1 in the statin group, were lost to follow up. Among them, one declined to participate in the follow-up since she has left Beijing, two were unreachable for data collection. Intention-to-treat analysis was performed, involving all 70 patients who were successfully randomized, and the last-observation-carried-forward (LOCF) imputation method was used to account for missing data.

Of our 70 enrolled patients, 63 (90%)presented with unstable angina, and 7 (10%)presented with non-ST-elevation myocardial infarction (NSTEMI). CAD diagnosis was documented by previous coronary angiography performed any time prior to enrollment in 57 patients (81.4%), and via prior or present history of myocardial infarction in 13 patients (18.6%). The baseline characteristics of the participants are shown in Table 1, and the two groups were comparable in demographics, presenting diagnosis, cardiovascular risk factors, number of diseased vessels, thrombolysis in myocardial infarction (TIMI)risk score, and blood lipid concentrations. The use of other cardiovascular medications comprising standard medical therapy for CAD, including aspirin, clopidogrel, beta-blockers, angiotensin-converting enzyme inhibitors (ACEI), angiotensin receptor blockers (ARB), calcium channel blockers (CCBs), and agents for diabetes mellitus, was also similar between the groups.

2 Primary Endpoint

The levels of hs-CRP in the experimental statin+STS group and control statin group at baseline, immediately after 14 days of treatment, and at 30 days after completion of treatment are illustrated in Fig. 3. The data for comparisons in hs-CRP level between the statin+STS and statin groups are delineated in Table 2, while the data for comparisons within each group are presented in Table 3.

Baseline hs-CRP level was similar in the statin+STS and statin groups (5.35 vs 5.04 mg/L, respectively, $P = 0.3894$). After 14 days of treatment, however, hs-CRP level was significantly lower in the statin+STS group than in the statin group (1.72 vs 3.20 mg/L, $P = 0.0191$). Indeed, the magnitude of the absolute and relative reductions in hs-CRP level after 14 days of treatment were greater for the statin+STS group than for the statin group. Whereas a significant reduction in hs-CRP level was observed within the statin+STS group after 14 days of treatment compared to baseline (1.72 vs 5.35 mg/L, $P < 0.01$), the change in hs-CRP level within the statin group was not significant (3.20 mg/L after 14 days of treatment vs 5.04 mg/L at baseline, $P = 0.26$).

At 30 days after the completion of treatment, hs-CRP levels in the statin+STS and statin groups were not significantly different (1.80 vs 3.50 mg/L, respectively, $P = 0.2408$). The level of hs-CRP within the statin+STS group, however, remained significantly lower at 30 days after treatment completion than at baseline (1.80 vs 5.35 mg/L, $P < 0.01$). The level of hs-CRP within the statin group, too, was significantly lower at 30 days after treatment completion than at baseline (3.50 vs 5.04 mg/L, $P = 0.03$).

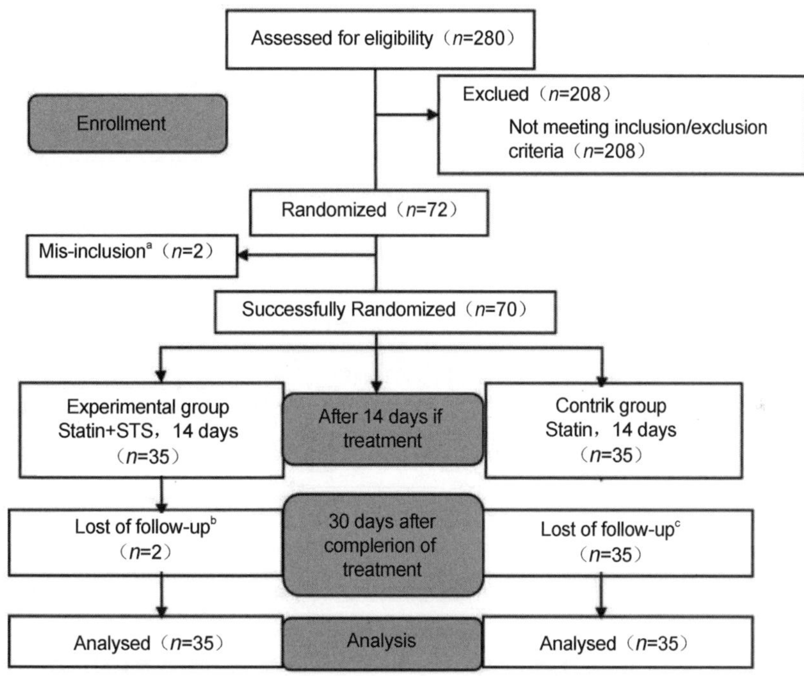

Figure 2 Flow Diagram of Study Design

Notes: [a]Two patients were excluded because of mis-inclusion: 1 patient in the control statin group elected to undergo percutaneous coronary intervention during hospitalization, and 1 patient in the experimental statin+STS group developed pneumonia. [b]Two patients were lost to follow up in the experimental statin+STS group, due to inability to contact the patients for data collection. [c]One patient was lost to follow up in the control statin group after the patient elected to withdraw from the study. STS, sodium tanshinone IIA sulfate.

In addition, the reduction of the experimental group was more significant than that of the control group (2.99 vs 1.54 mg/L, P=0.0485)after 14-day treatment, so as the percent change (71.75% vs 30%, P=0.0114) (Table 2).

3 Secondary Endpoints

Other circulating inflammatory marker levels. T e levels of IL-6, MCP-1, soluble CD40 ligand (sCD40L),

MMP-9, soluble VCAM-1 (sVCAM-1), and TNF-α in the experimental statin+STS group and control statin group at baseline, immediately after 14 days of treatment, and at 30 days after completion of treatment are illustrated in Fig. 4. The data for comparisons within each group are presented in Table 3.

For all the inflammatory markers above, baseline levels were similar between the 2 groups. After 14 days of treatment, the level of IL-6 in the statin+STS group was significantly less than that in the statin group (7.76 vs 9.55 pg/mL, *P* =0.0096), and the same was true of MCP-1 (301.65 vs 327.24 pg/mL, *P* =0.0014)and sCD40L (728.80 vs 848.90 pg/mL, *P* =0.0361). In addition, within both groups, all of the inflammatory markers were significantly decreased after 14 days of treatment compared to baseline.

At 30 days after the completion of treatment, the level of MCP-1 in the statin+STS group remained significantly less than that in the statin group (313.88 vs 337.91pg/mL, respectively, *P*=0.0078). Whereas levels of all the other inflammatory markers were similar between the 2 groups. Within the statin+STS group, the levels of all the inflammatory markers except sVCAM-1 remained significantly lower at 30 days after treatment completion than at baseline, and within the statin group, the same was true for all the inflammatory markers except sCD40L and sVCAM-1.

No significant differences in the levels of MMP-9, sVCAM-1, and TNF-α were observed between the 2 groups after 14 days of treatment, or at 30 days after the completion of treatment.

Angina. Total angina scores for the experimental statin+STS group and control statin group at each time point are presented in Table 4. T e median total angina score (no angina=0 points, maximum=24 points)was similar at baseline between the statin+STS and statin groups (10 *vs* 12 points, respectively, *P*=0.105). Median total angina score for the statin+STS group was significantly lower compared to that of the statin group both immediately after 14 days of treatment (0 vs 6 points, respectively, $P < 0.01$)and at 30 days after the completion of treatment (2 *vs* 8 points, $P < 0.01$).

Safety. No significant adverse side effects (e.g. bleeding events, abnormal liver or kidney function tests) or major adverse cardiovascular events (e.g. myocardial infarction, stroke, urgent coronary revascularization, death)were observed during the whole study period in all 72 participants. Two participants in the statin+STS group complained of mild dizziness (n=1)or headache (n=1)with initiation of treatment, which all fully disappeared the next day without special intervention. At 30 days after the completion of treatment, the survival in both groups was 100%.

Table 1 Baseline Characteristics.

Baseline Characteristics	Experimental group: Statin+STS (n=35)	Control group: Statin (n=35)
Demographics		
Male, N (%)	18 (51.4)	20 (57.1)
Age, mean ± SD	66 ± 7.28	67.47 ± 6.52
Diagnosis		
NSTEMI, N (%)	3 (8.6)	4 (11.4)
UA, N (%)	32 (91.4)	31 (88.6)
Number of diseased vessels, N (%)		
One	11 (31.4)	8 (22.9)
Two	6 (17.1)	6 (17.1)
three	4 (11.4)	8 (22.9)
Cardiovascular risk factors, N (%)		
Hypertension	27 (77.1)	33 (94.3)
Hyperlipidemia	26 (74.3)	30 (85.7)
Diabetes mellitus	17 (48.6)	13 (37.1)
Smoking history	9 (25.7)	8 (22.9)
BMI (mean ± SD, kg/m2)	24.47 ± 2.89	24.86 ± 3.72

Continued

Baseline Characteristics	Experimental group: Statin+STS (n=35)	Control group: Statin (n=35)
TIMI risk score, N (%)		
High risk (score 5-7)	2 (2.9)	3 (4.3)
Middle risk (score 3-4)	21 (30.0)	20 (28.6)
Low risk (score 0-2)	12 (17.1)	12 (17.1)
Medication, N (%)		
Beta-blocker	21 (60.0)	24 (68.6)
ACEI	9 (25.7)	12 (34.3)
ARB	10 (28.6)	10 (28.6)
CCB	17 (48.6)	19 (54.3)
Aspirin	34 (97.1)	29 (82.9)
Clopidogrel	17 (48.6)	24 (68.6)
Blood lipid (mean ± SD, mmol/L)		
TC	4.39 ± 1.28	4.22 ± 1.29
TG	1.71 ± 0.80	1.95 ± 0.92
LDL	2.73 ± 0.99	2.66 ± 0.85

All comparisons between the groups were not significantly different ($P>0.05$ for all). ACEI, angiotensin-converting enzyme inhibitor; ARB, angiotensin receptor blocker; BMI, body mass index; CCB, calcium channel blocker; IQR, interquartile range; LDL, low density lipoprotein; NSTEMI, non-ST segment elevation myocardial infarction; SD, standard deviation; TC, total cholesterol; TG, triglyceride; TIMI, Thrombolysis in Myocardial Infarction; UA, unstable angina.

DISCUSSION

Recent research has established a fundamental role for inflammation in atherosclerosis and CAD. Among the various systemic inflammatory markers, hs-CRP has the greatest predictive value for atherosclerotic plaque stability and acute cardiovascular events[5]. In the JUPITER trial, *de novo* initiation of rosuvastatin 20 mg daily reduced the incidence of major adverse cardiovascular events in apparently healthy persons without hyperlipidemia but with elevated hs-CRP level[7], thus suggesting the potential of hs-CRP to be a therapeutic target. A meta-analysis including 22 trials indicated that hs-CR$P>3$ mg/L was independently associated with risk of incident CAD events[6], while hs-CR$P>15$ mg/L may be more suggestive of infection. Therefore, hs-CRP was adopted as the primary outcome measure in this trial, but only patients with confirmed CAD and with elevated hs-CRP level between 3 mg/L and 15 mg/L were enrolled. Our results showed that 14 days of adjunctive STS therapy was more effective in reducing elevated hs-CRP level than standard medical therapy alone.

In addition to affecting hs-CRP, adjunctive STS therapy also reduced the levels of IL-6, MCP-1, and sCD40L further than did standard medical therapy alone. IL-6 is a potent pro-inflammatory cytokine that coordinates the release of CRP during the acute-phase response, and may have autocrine, paracrine, and endocrine mechanisms that all contribute to CAD pathogenesis[13]. Furthermore, MCP-1 plays an important role in atherosclerosis as a key chemokine regulating the migration and infiltration of mononuclear cells and macrophages[14], and CD40-mediated signaling has been implicated in the process of plaque destabilization[15]. Te upregulation of IL-6, MCP-1, and CD40L in the setting of CAD has each been associated with worse clinical outcomes[16-19], and as such, these important inflammatory factors represent additional targets for future anti-inflammatory CAD therapy. However, our study did not show a significant effect of adjunctive STS on levels of

TNF-α, MMP-9, and sVCAM-1, which differs from the results of previous experimental studies[10]. Nevertheless, STS represents a promising adjunctive therapy for mitigating residual cardiovascular risk secondary to inflammation in CAD patients. Indeed, Robertson et al. recently conducted a large-scale screening of anti-inflammatory compounds using zebrafish as an animal model, and identified tanshinone IIA as one of the most potent anti-inflammatory agents among thousands of compounds screened[20].

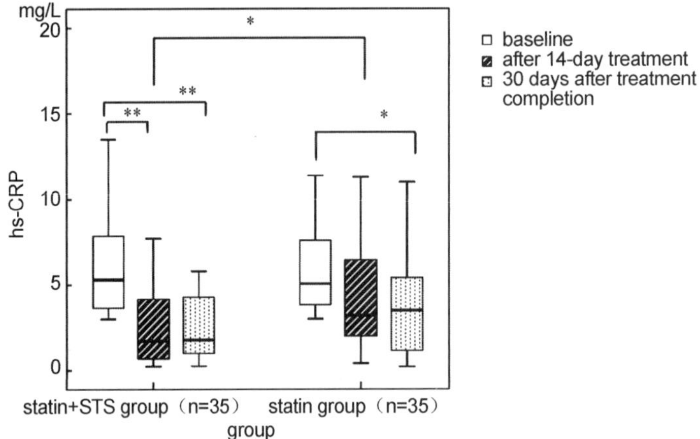

Figure 3　Comparison of hs-CRP Level Between Groups at Baseline, After 14-day Treatment, and at 30 days After Completion of treatment

Notes: *Statistically significant, $P < 0.05$. **Statistically signifcant, $P < 0.01$. hs-CRP, high-sensitivity C-reactive protein; STS, sodium tanshinone IIA sulfate.

Table 2　Comparison of hs–CRP between Groups at Baseline and After Treatment

Primary outcome: hs-CRP, median (IQR)	Experimental group: Statin+STS (*n*=35)	Control group: Statin (*n*=35)	*P* value
Baseline:			
hs-CRP, mg/L	5.35 (3.58, 8.00)	5.04 (3.81, 7.60)	0.3894
After 14-day treatment:			
hs-CRP, mg/L	1.72 (0.64, 4.24)	3.20 (1.99, 6.83)	0.0191
Absolute hs-CRP reduction, mg/L	2.90 (1.30, 6.05)	1.54 (-1.45, 3.51)	0.0485
Percent hs-CRP reduction, %	71.75 (24.07, 87.70)	30.00 (-22.14, 63.58)	0.0114
30 days after treatment completion:			
hs-CRP, mg/L	1.80 (0.90, 4.30)	3.50 (1.11, 5.60)	0.2408
Absolute hs-CRP reduction, mg/L	2.74 (0.86, 5.16)	1.38 (-0.25, 3.93)	0.1963
Percent hs-CRP reduction, %	69.14 (18.18, 84.44)	30.00 (-8.19, 77.98)	0.2309

Notes: hs-CRP, high-sensitivity C-reactive protein ; IQR, interquartile range ; STS, sodium tanshinone IIA sulfate. Inter-group comparison was analyzed using the Wilcoxon rank-sum test, due to non-normal distribution of the data.

Since STS is an intravenous preparation not suitable for long-term application, we investigated whether adjunctive STS therapy might yield sustained anti-inflammatory effects after discontinuation of treatment. Our results showed that the significant reduction in MCP-1 level following administration of integrative statin-STS therapy compared to standard medical therapy alone persisted to 30 days after the treatment was completed. Although there was no statistically significant difference in hs-CRP reduction between the groups at 30 days after the completion of treatment, we nevertheless observed a clear trend toward lower hs-CRP levels in the statin-STS group as compared to the control group. T is negative result might be due to the small sample size of this preliminary trial. Larger clinical trials with longer duration of follow-up are necessary to clarify whether there is a sustained, long-term effect of adjunctive STS on hs-CRP, and whether this promising anti-inflammatory effect might be translatable into clinical benefits.

In addition to anti-inflammatory effects, STS also possesses both anti-platelet and anticoagulant properties[21,22]. Considering the potential for drug interactions between STS and the various anti-thrombotic agents commonly used in conventional CAD treatment, increased hemorrhagic events associated with adjunctive STS therapy may be an issue of concern in clinical practice. In this short-term, small-sized clinical trial, we did not observe any bleeding events or any other serious adverse events associated with adjunctive STS therapy. Our results suggest that the addition of STS to standard medical therapy for CAD might not increase the risk of bleeding events or hepatorenal side effects, although the full safety profile of this integrative therapy should be further assessed in future larger scale clinical trials.

Table 3 Comparison of hs-CRP, IL-6, MCP-1, sCD40L, MMP-9, sVCAM-1, TNF-α Levels within Each Group at Baseline and After Treatment

Inflammatory Markers, Median (IQR)or Mean ± SD	Baseline	After 14-day treatment	30 days after treatment completion	△1	*P* value[1]	△2	*P* value[2]
hs-CRP, mg/L [b]							
Statin+STS group	5.35 (3.58, 8.00)	1.72 (0.64, 4.24)	1.80 (0.90, 4.30)	-2.83	0.00	-2.81	0.00
Statin group	5.04 (3.81, 7.60)	3.20 (1.99, 6.83)	3.50 (1.11, 5.60)	-1.01	0.26	-1.95	0.03
IL-6, pg/mL [b]							
Statin+STS group	14.58 (13.39, 18.45)	7.76 (5.98, 10.74)	9.30 (5.66, 13.11)	-6.30	0.00	-6.01	0.00
Statin group	15.18 (12.50, 18.15)	9.55 (8.35, 11.92)	8.81 (7.17, 11.33)	-3.67	0.00	-5.58	0.00
MCP-1, pg/mL [b]							
Statin+STS group	369.79 ± 36.24	301.65 ± 33.75	313.88 ± 37.91	-66.87	0.00	-53.06	0.00
Statin group	368.52 ± 37.18	327.24 ± 30.65	337.91 ± 27.62	-41.39	0.00	-30.71	0.00
sCD40L, pg/mL [a]							
Statin+STS group	934.48 ± 313.16	728.80 ± 196.68	853.19 ± 246.98	-215.71	0.00	-88.01	0.03
Statin group	941.03 ± 260.95	848.90 ± 267.89	878.73 ± 245.20	-93.88	0.02	-59.63	0.13
MMP-9, ng/mL [a]							
Statin+STS group	38.88 (23.73, 48.01)	17.61 (15.82, 20.11)	18.5 (14.17, 24.33)	-19.99	0.00	-19.43	0.00
Statin group	35.07 (23.73, 42.73)	19.22 (16.36, 24.92)	20.65 (16.25, 28.22)	-12.92	0.00	-13.46	0.00
sVCAM-1, ng/mL [a]							
Statin+STS group	807.25 ± 208.21	797.24 ± 242.28	753.27 ± 177.80	-74.39	0.01	-56.16	0.06
Statin group	731.76 ± 167.57	723.42 ± 216.73	745.08 ± 195.32	-68.24	0.02	-43.71	0.14
TNF-α, pg/mL [b]							
Statin+STS group	20.25 ± 7.99	14.26 (10.69, 19.05)	14.72 (10.24, 19.94)	-5.29	0.00	-4.20	0.00
Statin group	20.90 ± 10.03	13.99 (9.88, 30.15)	15.56 (10.97, 21.61)	-3.41	0.00	-4.43	0.00

Notes: hs-CRP, high-sensitivity C-reactive protein ; IL-6, interleukin-6 ; IQR, interquartile range ; MCP-1, monocyte chemotactic protein-1 ; MMP-9, matrix metalloproteinase-9 ; sCD40L, soluble CD40 ligand ; sVCAM-1, soluble vascular cell adhesion molecule-1 ; SD, standard deviation ; STS, sodium tanshinone IIA sulfate ; TNF-α, tumor necrosis factor alpha. △1 indicates the intra-group difference between baseline and immediately after 14-day treatment. △2 indicates the intra-group difference between baseline and at 30days after the completion of treatment. [1]p-value for intra-group comparisons between baseline and after 14-day treatment. [2]p-value for intra-group comparisons between baseline and at 30 days after the completion of treatment. [a]Intra-group comparison was analyzed using student's t-test, due to normal distribution of the data. [b]Intra-group comparison was analyzed using the Wilcoxon rank-sum test, due to non-normal distribution of the data.

Some limitations of this trial should be noted. First, the sample size was small, and thus the study may not have sufficient power to detect statistical differences between the 2 groups for each serum inflammatory marker. Second, the open-label design of our study introduces the potential for patients, physicians, or researchers to be influenced by their knowledge of a patient's treatment allocation. Nevertheless, blinded end-point assessment by outcome adjudicators, laboratory blood technicians, and data analysts minimized the potential biases. Third, the short 30-day follow-up period after the completion of treatment limits our ability to resolve the long-term effects of STS on serum inflammatory markers, and also hinders our ability to determine the potential benefit of STS in preventing recurrent cardiovascular events.

In conclusion, we demonstrate in this trial that an 80 mg intravenous dose of STS administered daily for 14 days, as an adjunct to standard medical therapy with uniformly-dosed atorvastatin, further reduced the levels of circulating inflammatory markers including hs-CRP, IL-6, MCP-1, and sCD40L in CAD patients compared to standard medical therapy alone. The apparent additive effect of STS in reducing the level of MCP-1 even persisted to 30 days after the completion of treatment. Our study also demonstrated a considerable improvement in angina symptoms, including the frequency and severity of angina pectoris, as compared with standard medical therapy alone. Given that no previous high-quality study has examined the effect of STS on hs-CRP and other inflammatory markers in CAD patients, our findings shed light on the benefit and safety of an integrative statin+STS regimen for CAD patients with enhanced inflammatory reaction, thereby offering potential implications for clinical practice. Whether the additional reduction of inflammatory factors in CAD patients will ultimately reduce future cardiovascular events and yield long-term prognostic benefit will be the focus of future clinical trials.

Table 4 Comparison of Angina Score between Groups at Baseline and After Treatment

Total Angina Score, median (IQR)	Experimental group: Statin+STS (*n*=35)	Control group: Statin (*n*=35)	*P* value
Baseline	10 (6, 12)	12 (8, 14)	0.105
After 14-day treatment	0 (0, 6)	6 (0, 10)	0.00
30 days after treatment completion	2 (0, 8)	8 (6, 10)	0.00

Notes: IQR, interquartile range ; STS, sodium tanshinone IIA sulfate.

Inter-group comparison was analyzed using the Wilcoxon rank-sum test, due to non-normal distribution of the data.

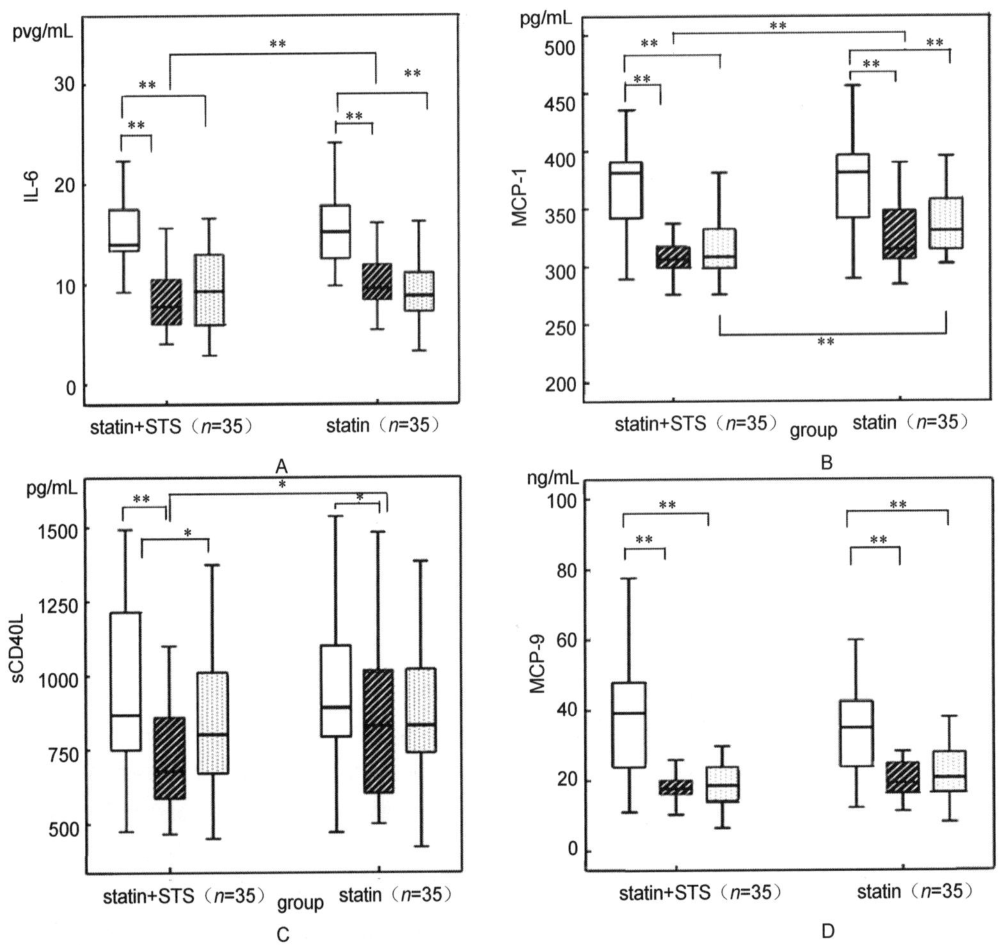

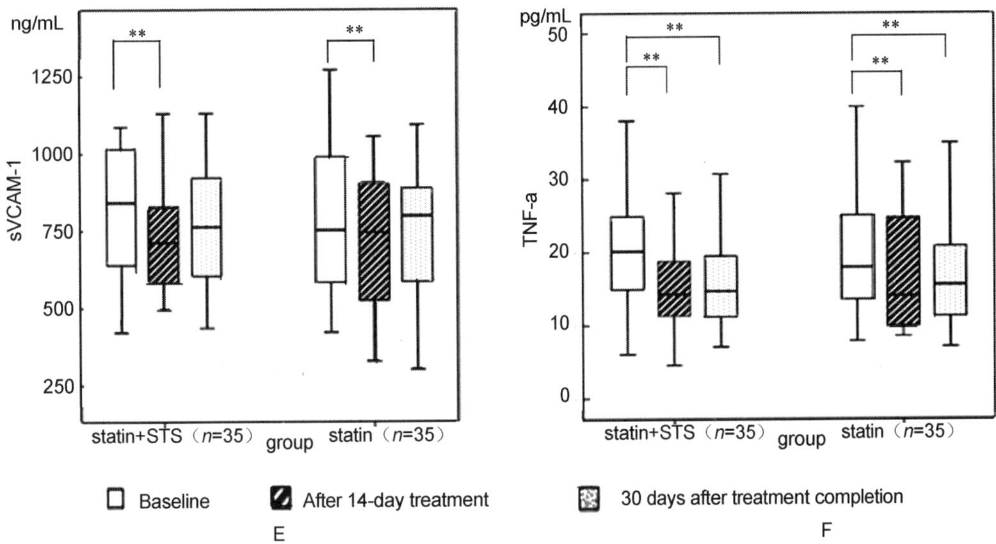

Figure 4 Comparison of IL-6, MCP-1, sCD40L, MMP-9, sVCAM-1, and TNF-α Levels between Groups at Baseline, after 14-day Treatment, and at 30 Days After Completion of Treatment

Notes: *Statistically significant, $P < 0.05$. **Statistically significant, $P < 0.01$. IL-6, interleukin-6; MCP-1, monocyte chemotactic protein-1; MMP-9, matrix metalloproteinase-9; sCD40L, soluble CD40 ligand; sVCAM-1, soluble vascular cell adhesion molecule-1; STS, sodium tanshinone IIA sulfate; TNF-α, tumor necrosis factor alpha.

REFERENCES

[1] Pepys MB, Hirschfield GM. C-reactive protein: a critical update[J]. J Clin Invest, 2003, 111: 1805-1812.

[2] Ridker PM. High-sensitivity C-reactive protein: potential adjunct for global risk assessment in the primary prevention of cardiovascular disease[J]. Circulation, 2001, 103: 1813-1818.

[3] Ridker PM., Hennekens, C. H., Buring, J. E. & Rifai, N. C-reactive protein and other markers of inflammation in the prediction of cardiovascular disease in women[J]. N Engl J Med, 2000, 342: 836-843.

[4] Danesh J. et al. Low grade inflammation and coronary heart disease: prospective study and updated meta-analyses[J]. BMJ, 2000, 321: 199-204.

[5] Koenig W. High-sensitivity C-reactive protein and atherosclerotic disease: from improved risk prediction to risk-guided therapy[J]. Int J Cardiol, 2013, 168: 5126-5134.

[6] Buckley DI, Fu R, Freeman M, et al. C-reactive protein as a risk factor for coronary heart disease: a systematic review and meta-analyses for the U. S. Preventive Services Task Force[J]. Ann Intern Med, 2009, 151: 483-495.

[7] Ridker PM, Danielson E, Fonseca FA, et al. Rosuvastatin to prevent vascular events in men and women with elevated C-reactive protein[J]. N Engl J Med, 2008, 359: 2195-2207.

[8] Auer J, Weber T, Eber B. Intensive versus moderate lipid lowering with statins after acute coronary syndromes[J]. N Engl J Med, 2004, 350: 1495-1504.

[9] Shang QH, Xu H, Huang L. Tanshinone IIA: a promising natural cardioprotective agent. Evid. Based Complement[J]. Alternat Med, 2012, 716459, https: //doi. org/10.1155/2012/716459.

[10] Gao S, Liu Z, Li H, et al. Cardiovascular actions and therapeutic potential of tanshinone IIA[J]. Atherosclerosis, 2012, 220: 3-10.

[11] Wang QL, Deng XJ, Li XQ, et al. Effect of sodium tanshinone injection on CRP and D-dimer level in patients with unstable angina[J]. J N Chin Med, 2007, 39: 16-17.

[12] Yu XY, Lin SG, Zhou ZW, et al. Role of P-glycoprotein in the intestinal absorption of tanshinone IIA, a major active ingredient in the root of Salvia miltiorrhiza Bunge[J]. Curr Drug Metab, 2007, 8: 325-40.

[13] Yudkin JS, Kumari M, Humphries SE, et al. Inflammation, obesity, stress and coronary heart disease: is interleukin-6 the link? [J]. Atherosclerosis, 2000, 148: 209-214.

[14] Namiki M, Kawashima S, Yamashita T, et al. Local overexpression of monocyte chemoattractant protein-1 at vessel wall induces infiltration of macrophages and formation of atherosclerotic lesion: synergism with hypercholesterolemia[J]. Arterioscler Thromb Vasc Biol, 2002, 122: 115-120.

[15] Schönbeck U, Mach F, Sukhova GK, et al. Regulation of matrix metalloproteinase expression in human vascular smooth muscle cells by T lymphocytes: a role for CD40 signaling in plaque rupture? [J]. Circ Res, 1997, 81 (3): 448-454.

[16] Biasucci LM, Vitelli A, Liuzzo G, et al. Elevated levels of interleukin-6 in unstable angina[J]. Circulation, 1996, 94 (5): 874-877.

[17] de Lemos JA, Morrow DA, Sabatine MS, et al. Association between plasma levels of monocyte chemoattractant protein-1 and long-term clinical outcomes in patients with acute coronary syndromes[J]. Circulation, 2003, 107 (5): 690-695.

[18] Pamukcu B1, Lip GY, Snezhitskiy V, et al. The CD40-CD40L system in cardiovascular disease[J]. Ann Med, 2011, 43 (5): 331-340.
[19] Zakynthinos E, Pappa N. Inflammatory biomarkers in coronary artery disease[J]. J Cardiol, 2009, 53: 317-333.
[20] Robertson AL, Holmes GR, Bojarczuk AN, et al. A zebrafish compound screen reveals modulation of neutrophil reverse migration as an anti-inflammatory mechanism[J]. Sci Transl Med, 2014, 6 (225): 225ra29.
[21] Li XJ, Zhou M, Li XH, et al. Effects of tanshinone IIa on cytokines and platelets in immune vasculitis and its mechanism[J]. J Exp Hematol, 2009, 17 (1): 188-192.
[22] Li CZ, Yang SC, Zhao FD. Effects of tanshinone II-A sulfonate on thrombus formation, platelet and blood coagulation in rats and mice[J]. Acta Pharmacol Sin, 1984, 5 (1): 39-42.
[23] Shang QH, Wang H, Li SM et al. The effect of sodium tanshinone IIA sulfate and simvastatin on elevated serum levels of inflammatory markers in patients with coronary heart disease: a study protocol for a randomized controlled trial[J]. Evid Based Complement Alternat Med, 2013: 756519, https: //doi. org/10.1155/2013/756519.
[24] Schaefer EJ, McNamara JR, Asztalos BF, et al. Effects of atorvastatin versus other statins on fasting and postprandial C-reactive protein and lipoproteinassociated phospholipase A2 in patients with coronary heart disease versus control subjects[J]. Am J Cardiol, 2005, 95 (9): 1025-1032.
[25] Nomenclature and criteria for diagnosis of ischemic heart disease: report of the Joint International Society and Federation of Cardiology/World Health Organization task force on standardization of clinical nomenclature[J]. Circulation, 1979, 59: 607-609.
[26] Hamm CW, Bassand JP, Agewall S, et al. ESC guidelines for the management of acute coronary syndromes in patients presenting without persistent ST-segment elevation: the Task Force for the management of acute coronary syndromes (ACS)in patients presenting without persistent ST-segment elevation of the European Society of Cardiology (ESC)[J]. Eur Heart J, 2011, 32 (23): 2999-3054.
[27] Chen H, Gao ZY, Xu H. Clinical study of unstable angina patients undergoing percutaneous coronary intervention treated with Chinese medicine for activating blood circulation and detoxification[J]. Chin J Integr Med Cardio/Cerebrovasc Dis, 2009, 7: 1135-1137.

First published: LI Si-ming, Jiao Yang, WANG Han-jay, SHANG Qing-hua, LU Fang, HUANG Li, LIU Jian-gang, XU Hao, CHEN Ke-ji. Sodium tanshinone IIA sulfate adjunct therapy reduces high-sensitivity C-reactive protein level in coronary artery disease patients: a randomized controlled trial[J]. Sci Rep, 2017, 7: 17451.

Roles and Mechanisms of Herbal Medicine for Diabetic Cardiomyopathy: Current Status and Perspective

TIAN Jin-fan, ZHAO Ying-ke, LIU Yan-fei, LIU Yue, CHEN Ke-ji, and LYU Shu-zheng

Diabetic cardiomyopathy (DCM)resulted from diabetes mellitus ultimately leads to heart failure, increasing the mortality in diabetic patients. There was a 2.4-fold increase in the risk of heart failure in the male diabetic subjects and flvefold in the female diabetic subjects[1]. DCM is characterized by left ventricular hypertrophy, myocardial flbrosis, and compromised left ventricular systolic/diastolic function[2]. Currently, there is still lack of feasible therapeutic approach for DCM. The Chinese traditional medicine has a long history in the treatment of glucose metabolism disorder and cardiovascular disease. Most recently, Li et al.[3] uncovered the antidiabetes effect of artemisinins, and this flnding has been published in the Journal of cell. Using herbs to treat many chronic diseases such as diabetes and its complication has been recognized by an increasing number of scientists and clinic physicians for their multitarget effect and comprehensive source. In this review, we discuss the molecular mechanisms for the pathogenesis of DCM and then the study progress of herbal medicines as potential therapeutic agents for DCM.

1 Pathophysiological Mechanisms of DCM

The function and structure of the heart are altered with the development of DCM. The left ventricular diastolic dysfunction is one of the pathological features of DCM, which occurs in isolation and precedes the development of systolic dysfunction [4]. The ventricular hypertrophy and myocardial flbrosis are the structural alteration of DCM. Hyperglycemia, insulin resistance, microcirculation dysfunction, and neurohormone activation are pathological triggers for DCM. The hyperglycemia and insulin resistance are responsible for altered substrate metabolisms including increased free fatty acid (FFA)oxidation, intra-myocardial triglyceride accumulation, and reduced glucose utilization. The altered substrate metabolisms contribute to morphological changes of cardiomyocytes. Moreover, oxidative stress, the dysfunction of mitochondrion, abnormalities in Ca^{2+} homeostasis, and cardiomyocyte apoptosis all promote DCM development (Figure 1).

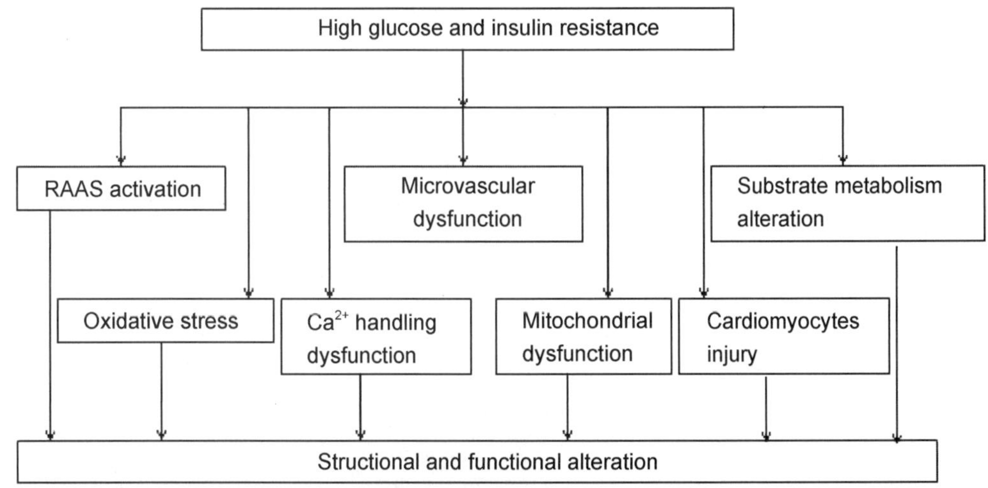

Figure 1 Pathophysiological Mechanisms for DCM

Notes: RASS: renin-angiotensin-aldosterone system; DCM: diabetic cardiomyopathy.

1.1 Neurohormone Activation and Microcirculation Dysfunction

Neurohormone activation is characterized by upregulation of sympathetic nervous system and renin-angiotensin-aldosterone system (RAAS). Circulating Ang II, the atrial natriuretic peptide (ANP), B-type natriuretic peptides (BNP), and catecholamines, as well as endothelin (ET-1)both in intramyocardium and circulating, are signiflcantly increased in the context of hyperglycemia. Activation of RAAS and elevated ET-1 contribute to the myocardial flbrosis. ET-1 is responsible for vasoconstriction and myocardial ischemia. Endothelia-derived NO, an endogenous vasodilator, is remarkably decreased in the diabetic status. Impaired microvascular blood flow, sustained hyperglycemia, and excess generation of reactive oxygen species (ROS) are contributors for endothelial dysfunction.

1.2 Altered Substrate Metabolism.

Substrate metabolism changes in diabetes are triggered by hyperglycemia and insulin resistance. In diabetes, the myocardial glucose utilization is signiflcantly reduced for the depletion of glucose transporter proteins 1 (GLUT-1)and GLUT-4, resulting in the diabetic rely almost exclusively on FA as an energy production source [5]. Elevated circulating and cellular FFAs are attributable for increased adipose tissue lipolysis and hydrolysis of accumulated myocardial triglyceride. FFAs can inhibit glucose oxidation by activating peroxisome proliferator-activator receptor-α (PPAR-α), which increases the expression of pyruvate dehydrogenase kinase 4 (PDK4)involved in regulating enhanced mitochondrial FA uptake and reducing glucose oxidation. Moreover, elevated circulating and cellular FFAs can enhance peripheral insulin resistance. In the long term, increased myocardial FA utilization leads to lipotoxicity to the cardiomyocytes, characterized by myocyte lipid accumulation, mitochondrial dysfunction, increased oxygen demand, and excessive generation of ROS[6,7]. Collectively, the enhanced peripheral insulin resistance, reduced cellular glucose utilization, and lipotoxicity are responsible for the cardiomyocyte injury and myocardial remodeling.

1.3 Oxidative Stress

In the physiological state, the ROS is eliminated by antioxidant system. However, in the diabetic settings, excessive production of ROS is responsible for oxidative stress and correlates with the development of DCM for its ability to damage proteins and DNA and lipid membranes. In the diabetic heart, ROS are derived from mitochondrial source, nicotinamide adenine dinucleotide phosphate (NADPH)oxidase, and uncoupled NO synthases (NOS). The role of NADPH oxidase is the most important of the three sources in the development of DCM. Tumor necrosis factor-α (TNF-α)could induce cardiomyocyte hypertrophy by triggering the activity of NADPH oxidase [8]. Moreover, ROS derived from NADPH oxidase promotes the myocardial interstitial flbrosis and the mechanism involving increased activation of matrix metalloproteinases (MMP), expression of proflbrotic genes, and activation of NF-κB[9]. As previously illustrated, mitochondrion is another major source for ROS production. The mitochondria themselves are susceptible to the ROS they produce, leading to local damage to mitochondrial DNA and membranes, generating more ROS as a result of a positive feedback mechanism [10].

1.4 Impaired Ca^{2+} Metabolism

Under the physiological state, Ca^{2+} influx induced by the activation of voltage-dependent L-type Ca^{2+} channels and then triggers the release of Ca^{2+} stored in the sarcoplasmic reticulum via ryanodine receptors (RyR)through a Ca^{2+}-induced Ca^{2+}-release mech-anism. Free Ca^{2+} binds to troponin C and results in cardiomyocyte contraction. [Ca^{2+}]is pumped out of cytosol and returns to a diastolic level mainly by the activation of the sarcolemmal Na^+/Ca^{2+} exchanger, the sarcoplasmic reticulum Ca^{2+}-ATPase2a (SERCA2a), and the sarcolemmal Ca^{2+}-ATPase[11]. In the diabetic state, the decreased activity of SERCA results from the interaction of advanced glycation end products (AGE)with SERCA and the overexpression of SERCA2a inhibitor phospholamban (PLB)and could be reversed by insulin treatment [11]. Suppression of SERCA2a ultimately leads to Ca^{2+} overload in the cytosol and diastolic dysfunction[12]. The activity and expression of Na^{+}/Ca^{2+} exchanger which contribute to the removal of[Ca^{2+}] is also decreased in the diabetic state. The abnormal function of RyR induced by AGE/RAGE and oxidative stress contributes to sarcoplasmic reticulum Ca^{2+} leak, decreased sarcoplasmic reticulum-stored Ca^{2+}, and systolic Ca^{2+} transient[13,14]. oreover, the decreased ATP synthesis rates which result from the reduced uptake of Ca^{2+} by mitochondria cause impaired contractility ability. Consequently, the disorder of Ca^{2+} handling contributes to diastolic/systolic dysfunction and left ventricular hypertrophy.

1.5 Cardiomyocyte Injury

Cardiomyocyte injury manners include apoptosis, necrosis, and autophagy. Apoptosis results from oxidative stress, mitochondrial dysfunction, and abnormalities in Ca^{2+} handling. Cardiomyocyte necrosis results in interstitial collagen deposition and ultimately leads to myocardial fibrosis [15]. Autophagy, a "housekeeping" subcellular process that maintains the cell nutrition homeostasis and self-renewal by degrading damaged proteins and organelles, is an alternate form of programmed cell death. Autophagy is also considered as a process that maintains cell survival in the condition of starvation and other cell stressors, for its regulation in the turnover of long-lived proteins, and protects cells. However, the dysregulated autophagy may result in excessive cell death. The role of autophagy in pathogenesis of DCM remains controversial. Xie et al. [16,17]reported that a low constitutive autophagy is essential for protecting cardiomyocytes from hyperglycemic damage, whereas, the defect autophagy in diabetes contributes to the development of DCM. Coincidence with this finding, Zhao et al. showed that enhanced autophagy prevents DCM induced by STZ administration [18]. However, Hou et al. showed that AGE impairs the cell viability of rat neonate cardiomyocytes in a dose-dependent manner by inducing autophagy [19]. Collectively, well-regulated autophagy is essential for DCM attenuation.

2 Molecules and Signaling Pathways

NF-κB is a key transcription factor that regulates inflammatory and cardiomyocyte injury processes. NF-κB consists of five members including p65 (RelA), RelB, c-Rel, NF-κB1 (p50 and its precursor p105), and NF-κB2 (p52 and its precursor p100). The most abundant form of the NF-κB family is the p65/p50 heterodimer. In resting cells, NF-κB is inactive by binding to IκBα in the cytoplasm. After high-glucose stimulation, the IκBα is phosphorylated by IκB kinase (IKK)complex, leading to the translocation of NF-κB to the nucleus and binding to NF-κB response element (RE)[20]. AMP-activated protein kinase (AMPK)suppresses NF-κB cascade through inhibition of IKK and decreased IκBα degradation. NF-κB cascade may be induced by phosphorylation of mitogen-activated protein kinase (MAPK). It has been also showed that signal transducer and activator of transcription (STAT)may contribute to activation of NF-κB and maintenance of NF-κB activity. PPAR has the ability to downregulate NF-κB activity by the interaction with the p65 subunit or inhibition of MAPK phosphorylation. Sirtuin 1 (SIRT1)inhibits NF-κB by inhibiting the APK or by increasing the interaction between PPAR and p65 subunit of NF-κB. SIRT1 activation leads to AMPK activation and deacetylation of PPAR-γ co-activator-1 (PGC1α). NF-κB decreases the activity of PGC-1α directly or indirectly by activating PKB/Akt. The activation of NF-κB leads to the increased proinflammatory cytokines, such as TNF-α, interleukin (IL)-6, and IL-1β, which contribute to the activation of profibrotic transforming growth factor beta (TGF-β)pathway. The NF-κB cascade is detailed in Figure 2. Herbs inhibit the activation of NF-κB by regulating AMPK, SIRT1, Akt, PPAR-γ, and MAPK cascades (Figure 2). Furthermore, herbs act on NFE2-related factor 2 (Nrf2), a master regulator of inflammation and oxidative status (Figure 3).

2.1 Mitogen-Activated Protein Kinase (MAPK)Cascade

Accumulated evidences have demonstrated that MAPK cascade including extracellular signal-regulated kinase 1/2 (ERK1/2), c-Jun N-terminal protein kinase (JNK), and p38 MAPK are involved in the diabetic complications[21]. p38 MAPK consists of four isoforms including p38α, p38β, p38γ, and p38δ. P38α is the major form expressed in a healthy heart, and p38β displays lower expression. p38 MAPK especially p38α MAPK contributes to the development of DCM owing to inflammation, oxidative stress, apoptosis, hypertrophy, metabolic abnormalities, and disordered Ca^{2+} handling. High glucose promotes the expression of protein kinase C (PKC)in the neonatal rat cardiomyocytes, leading to the upregulation of ROS, MAPK, and NF-κB[22]. ROS activates p38 MAPK, which in turn, promotes the production of ROS; alternatively, downregulation of p38 MAPK can inhibit ROS generation and oxidative stress [23]. p38α MAPK has been shown to promote the cardiomyocyte apoptosis by activating STAT1 and NF-κB and contribute to cardiomyocyte hypertrophy through activating the GATA4 transcription factor. MAPKPK-2 (MK2), a p38 MAPK downstream target, is responsible for downregulation of SERCA2a, FFA accumulation, and NF-κB activation in the development of DCM. On the contrary, the antiapoptotic function of p38β MAPK in DCM has been reported[21].

ERK1/2 signaling pathway is also known as the Ras-Raf-MEK-ERK cascade. ERK1/2 pathway is triggered by the activation of Ras at the myocyte membrane. The detrimental effects of ERK1/2 in a diabetic heart are manifested as oxidative stress, apoptosis, hypertrophy, and myocardial flbrosis. ERK1/2 activated by high glucose is associated with cardiac hypertrophy in DCM[24]. ROS and ET-1 stimulate the ERK1/2 cascade; hence, antioxidant agents block the ROS generation and ERK1/2 activation as well as cardiac hyper-trophy[25]. The hyperglycemia-induced increased TGF-β is suppressed by ERK1/2 inhibitor U0126, suggesting that ERK1/2 mediates upregulation of TGF-β, closely related to cardiomyocyte flbrosis[26]. Interestingly, Zhang et al. showed that flbroblast growth factor 21 (FGF21)protects the diabetic heart from cardiac apoptosis, remodeling, and dysfunction by activating ERK1/2, and this protection effect could be abolished by ERK1/2 inhibitor PD98059[27]. The antiapoptotic or proapoptotic effect of ERK1/2 is mainly dependent on the downstream effector activities. Taken together, ERK1/2 cascade is a two-edged sword in the development of DCM[28].

JNKs, members of the family of MAPKs, mediate inflammation and cell apoptosis. Tsai et al. [29]showed that hyperglycemia enhanced NADPH oxidase-derived superoxide generation, promoting activation of JNK and NF-κB activation as well as subsequent apoptosis of cardio-myocytes. JNK inhibitor and NF-κB siRNA abolished NF-κB-mediated inflammation and high-glucose-induced cardiomyocyte apoptosis.

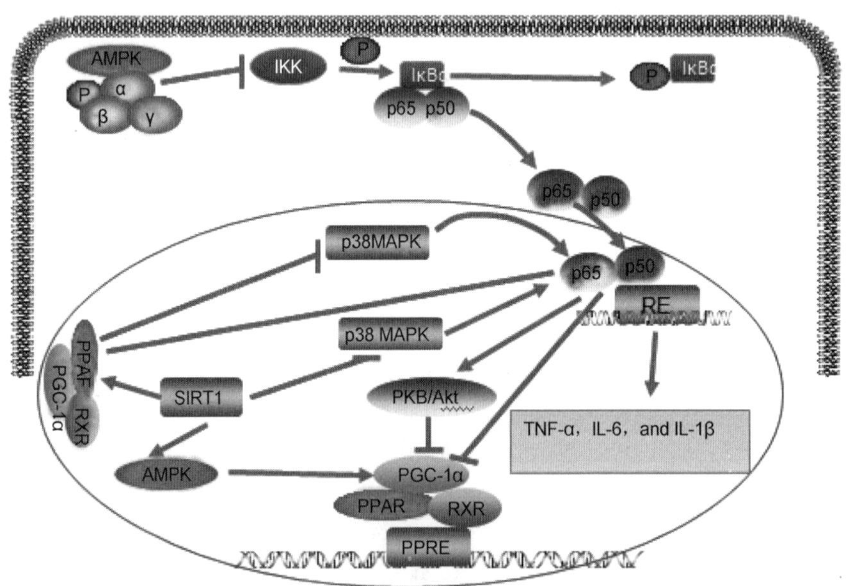

Figure 2　Inflammation Cascade in Pathogenesis of DCM

Notes: AMPK: AMP activated-protein kinase; MAPK: mitogen-activated protein kinase; SIRT1: sirtuin 1; IKK: IκB kinase; RE: response element; PPAR: peroxisome proliferator-activated receptor; PGC1α: PPAR-γ co-activator-1; RXR: retinoid X receptor; PPRE: PPAR response elements; TNF-α: tumor necrosis factor-α; IL: interleukin.

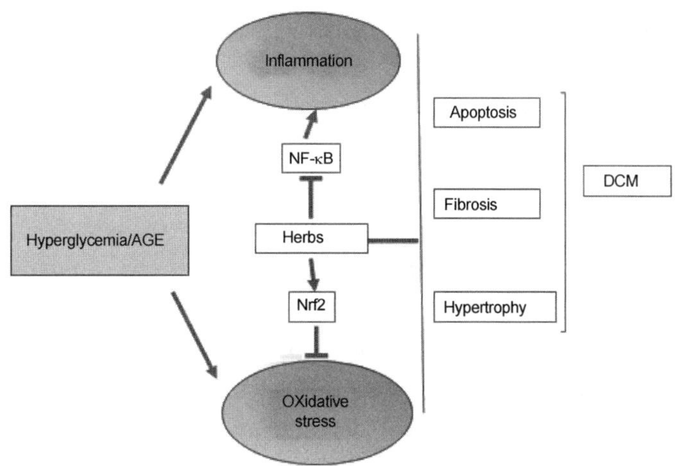

Figure 3 Potential Mechanisms of Herbal Medicine Protects Against Diabetic Cardiomyopathy

Notes: Nrf2: transcription factor NFE2-related factor 2.

2.2 AMPK Cascade

AMPK, consists of α, β, and γ subunits, is an important regulator of insulin signaling, cardiac energy homeostasis, and oxidative stress. The phosphorylation at T172 of the α subunit is well-known mechanisms for AMPK activation[30]. AMPK is upregulated in response to an enhanced AMP/ATP ratio in a stressed cellular state[31]. Both liver kinase B1 (LKB1)and Ca2+/calmodulin-dependent protein kinase kinase (CAMMKK) are responsible for phosphorylation at T172 of AMPK α subunit in the cardiomyocytes under the condition of energy depletion[32,33]. The activated AMPK facilitates the uptake of glucose by promoting myocardial GLUT-4 expression and translocation to the plasma membrane in a similar way to insulin[34]. Furthermore, AMPK increases FA uptake by cardiomyocytes via regulating the translocation of FA transporter (FAD/CD36) to the plasma membrane[35]. Carnitine palmitoyltransferase-1 (CPT-1)is responsible for the transportation of FAs into the mitochondria for β-oxidation. AMPK increases FA oxidation by inducing the phosphorylation-mediated inhibition of acetyl-COA carboxylase (ACC), leading to subsequent downregulation of malonyl-COA level, an inhibitor of CPT-1. Therefore, AMPK increases the energy production by increasing glucose uptake, FA oxidation, and glycolysis. However, AMPK inhibits lipolysis by inducing the phosphorylation of hormone-sensitive lipase[36]. The metabolic regulation by AMPK is illustrated in Figure 4.

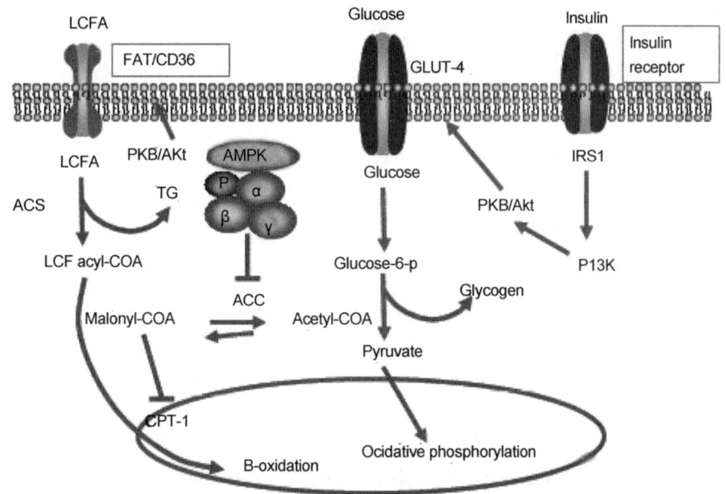

Figure 4 Metabolic Regulation for Normal Heart

Notes: LCFA: long-chain fatty acids; FAT/CD36: translocation of FA transporter; GLUT: glucose transporter proteins; ACC: acetyl-COA carboxylase; ACS: acyl-CoA synthetase; CPT1: carnitine palmitoyltransferase-1; PI3K: phosphatidylinositol 3-kinase; IRS-1: insulin receptor substrate 1.

AMPK exerts an antioxidant effect by regulating the activation of Nrf2, another transcription factor that protects cardiomyocyte against oxidative stress. AMPK inhibits the NF-κB cascade by inhibiting IKK activity and IκBα degra-dation, or by activating downstream targets such as SIRT1, Forkhead box O (FOXO), and cardiac-enriched PGC1α[37,38].

As previously illustrated, basic level of autophagy prevents against the apoptosis of cardiomyocytes. It has been demonstrated that AMPK directly activates ULK1, a homo-logue of yeast ATG1, through phosphorylation of Ser 317 and Ser 777 [39], or indirectly activates ULK1 by suppression of mammalian target of rapamycin complex 1 (mTORC1), resulting in enhanced autophagy[40]. Furthermore, AMPK regulates autophagy by activating FOXO, which upregulates expression of autophagy markers Bnip3, LC3, and ATG12 [30]. Recently, He et al.[41] reported that under starvation conditions, JNK1 activation leads to phosphorylation of BCL2 and dissociation of the Beclin1-BCL2 complex. However, diabetes inhibits the AMPK activity, suppresses its JNK1-BCL2 cascade, and promotes the interaction between Beclin1 and BCL2. Transfection of H9c2 cells with active JNK1 plasmid promotes BCL2 phosphorylation and disrupts the interaction between Beclin1 and BCL2, resulting in restoration of autophagy and reducing H9c2 cell apoptosis exposure to high glucose. Metformin, a well-known AMPK agonist, reduces apoptotic cell death and preserves the cardiac function by enhancing autophagy, and these effects were abolished by JNK1 inhibitor SP600125. These findings suggest that MAPK8/JNK1-BCL2 signaling is a new mechanism by which AMPK regulates autophagy[42].

2.3 PPAR Cascade

PPARs are responsible for the regulation of metabolism and inflammation. The subtypes of PPARs include PPAR α, PPAR β/δ, and PPAR-γ. Activation of PPARs is followed by the formation of heterodimers with the retinoid X receptor (RXR). Heterodimerization recruits PGC-1α and then binds to DNA-specific sequences called PPAR response elements (PPRE)and, consequently, allows the target gene transcription (CPT-1, FAT/CD36, PDK4, and GLUT-4 et al.). Of the three isoforms, PPAR α and PPAR β/δ express at high levels in the heart, while PPAR-γ enriched in adipose tissue shows a lower expression. According to Finck et al. [43] myocardial FA oxidation rates increased while glucose uptake and oxidation decreased in MHC-PPAR α mice, accompanied by the ventricular hypertrophy and systolic ventricular dysfunction. The MHC-PPAR α mice displayed metabolic phenotype and structure alteration similar to that of the diabetic heart. Burkart et al. [44] further showed that in contrast to MHC-PPAR α mice, MHC-PPAR β/δ mice did not develop cardiomyopathy, even in the context of a high-fat diet, owing to upregulation of GLUT-4 and enhanced rate of myocardial glucose uptake and utilization but without increased FA oxidation. Interestingly, in their study, both FAT/CD36 expression and GLUT-4 mRNA levels increased in MHC-PPAR-γ mice, suggesting that PPAR-γ shares the characteristic with both PPAR α and PPAR β/δ in regulation metabolism in diabetic hearts. Therefore, their findings provide the evidence that selective activation of PPAR β/δ is a promising therapeutic strategy for DCM. PGC-1α is the coactivator of PPARs enriched in the myocardium. PGC-1α regulates the mitochondrial biogenesis, FA oxidation, and glucose oxidative metabolism. PDK4 is a downstream molecule of PGC-1α. Selective overexpression of PDK4 in the heart of mice results in a remarkable decrease in glucose oxidation and an increase in FA oxidation. Overexpression of PGC-1α is associated with heart failure linked to increased FA oxidation. However, knockdown PGC-1α also leads to heart failure due to depletion of energy production in mitochondrion. According to Botta et al. [45]short-time exercise attenuated DCM in aged diabetic heart in db/db mice by activating PGC-1α. Wang et al. [46]showed that excise ameliorated DCM through activation of PGC-1α and Akt signaling.

All the three isoforms of PPARs exert anti-inflammation in the development of DCM for physical interaction with the p65 subunit of NF-κB and inhibit the activation of certain members of the MAPK signaling pathway[47–49]. Enhanced physical interaction between p65 and PGC-1α contributes to the decreased activation of PGC-1α.

2.4 Phosphatidylinositol 3-Kinase (PI3K)/PKB/Akt Cascade

PI3K takes a crucial role in insulin pathway and cardiac adaptation including protein synthesis, FA and glucose metabolisms, and cell survival regulation. Activation of PI3K subsequently targets to the upregulation of downstream effectors including PKB/Akt, glycogen synthase kinase (GSK)-3B, and mTOR. The activation of PKB/Akt increases the uptake of glucose by inducing the translocation of the GLUT-4 protein to the cell membrane (Figure 4). However, PI3K can induce the cardiac glycogen synthesis by inhibition of PKB/Akt downstream effector, GSK-3B. PI3K also has the ability to increase myocardial FA oxidation by promoting FAT/CD36 translocation to the sarcolemma in adult cardiomyocytes (Figure 4). PI3K stimulates autophagy by inhibiting mTORC1. NF-κB indirectly activates the PKB/Akt pathway, which phosphorylates PGC-1α and reduces its transcriptional activity.

2.5 SIRT1 Cascade

SIRT1, a class III (nicotinamide adeno-sine dinucleotide)NAD-dependent histone deacetylase, modulates AMPK activity by deacetylating LKB1 to induceits intracellular localization[50]. SIRT1 has the ability to promote the transcriptional activity of PGC-1α. SIRT1 inhibits NF-κB by enhancing the physical interaction between PPAR and p65 subunit or by inhibiting the phos-phorylation of p38 MAPK[51]. Furthermore, Sulaiman et al. showed that upregulation of SIRT1 restores the SER-CA2α gene expression in the context of hyperglycemia and improves the function left ventricular[52]. Taken together, SIRT1 prevents against the heart from diabetic injury by attenuating inflammation signaling cascade and improving Ca^{2+} handling[53].

2.6 Nrf2 Cascade

Under physiological conditions, Nrf2 locates in the cytoplasm and binds to its inhibitor kelch-like ECH-associated protein 1 (keap1). Under the condition of oxidative stress and high glucose, Nrf2 releases from keap1 and translocates into the nucleus to bind to antioxidant-responsive elements (AREs), leading to the expression of antioxidant enzymes such as NADPH quinone oxidore-ductase (NQO1), heme oxygenase-1 (HO-1), superoxide dismutase (SOD), and catalase (CAT). He et al. [54] investigated the protection role of Nrf2 in the development of DCM using Nrf2-KO mice. There was an increased level of ROS in the cardiomyocytes of Nrf2-KO mice, and high glucose further increased the ROS generation in concen-tration and time-dependent manners.

Zhao et al. [18]have demonstrated that HO-1 prevents cardiac dysfunction by promoting the phosphorylation of AMPK and increasing the autophagy marker LC3II and Beclin1 expression in the STZ-induced diabetic heart. Acti-vators target to Nrf2 are capable of protecting the heart from high-glucose injury.

2.7 MicroRNAs

miRNA is a class of conserved 19–25 nucleotide-noncoding RNAs that regulate gene expression posttranscriptionally. Recently, researchers have demon-strated that miRNAs play important roles in diabetes and related complications (Table 1). The miR-144 mimics enhance the generation of ROS and apoptosis in cardiomyocyte exposure to high glucose, which could be attenuated by an activator of Nrf2, Dh404. Inhibition of miR-144 results in suppressed ROS generation and cardiomyocyte apoptosis induced by high glucose, accompanied by the improved car-diac function in STZ-induced diabetic mice[55]. According to Jeyabal et al. [56], miR-9 expression was signiflcantly reduced in high-glucose cultured cardiomyocytes and human diabetic hearts. miR-9 mimics attenuated hyperglycemia-induced ELAV-like protein 1 (ELAVL1)and inhibited cardiomyocyte apoptosis. Inhibition of miR-9 increased ELAVL1 and caspase-1 expression [56]. Zheng et al. showed that miR-195 expression was increased, and its target protein SIRT1 was decreased in STZ-induced type 1 and db/db type 2 diabetic mouse hearts. Anti-miR-195 in the heart improved myocardial function in STZ-induced mice by upregulating the activity of SIRT1[57]. According to Liu et al., miR-21 promotes high-glucose-induced cardiac flbrosis though JAK/SAPK and p38 signaling pathway by suppression of dual speciflc phosphatase 8 (DUSP8)expression[58]. miR-200c expression is increased while its target molecule DUSP1 is decreased in DCM model and high-glucose-treated cardio-myocytes. Inhibition of miR-200c suppresses the expression of DUSP1, leading to decreased phosphorylation of ERK, p38, and JNK, as well as attenuating cardiomyocyte hypertrophy induced by high glucose[59]. Raut et al. showed that miR-30c overexpression attenuated high-glucose-induced cardiomyocyte hypertrophy by inhibiting the expression of cell division control protein 42 homolog (Cdc42)and p21-activated kinases (PAK1)[60]. Li et al. found that miR-30d promoted cardiomyocyte pyroptosis in DCM by direct repression of Foxo3a expression[61].

Table 1 miRNA functions in DCM

miR type	Experimental model	Mechanism	Target gene	Reference
miR-144	STZ-induced diabetic mice	Increased oxdative stress and cardiomyocyte apoptosis	Nrf2	[55]
miR-9	Human diabetic hearts, high-glucose cultured human	Prevented cardiomyocyte apoptosis	ELAVL1	[56]
miR-195	STZ-induced diabetic mice, db/db mice	Increased oxidative stress and apoptosis	SIRT1	[57]
miR-21	High-glucose cultured primary cardiac fibroblasts	Increased cardiac fibrosis	DUSP8	[58]
miR-200c	High-fat diet plus STZ-induced diabetic rat, high-glucose cultured cardiomyocytes	Decreased cardiomyocyte hypertrophy	DUSP1	[59]
miR-30c	STZ-induced diabetic rat, high-glucose cultured cardiomyocytes	Decreased cardiomyocyte hypertrophy	PAK1 and Cdc42	[60]
miR-30d	STZ-indcued diabetic rat	Increased cardiomyocyte pyroptosis	Foxo3a	[61]

Notes: Nrf2: factor-erythroid 2-related factor 2 ; ELAVL1: ELAV-like protein 1 ; SIRT1: sirtuin 1 ; DUSP: dual specific phosphatase ; PAK1: p21-activated kinases ; Cdc42: cell division control protein 42 homolog ; Foxo3a: Forkhead box O3.

Table 2 *In vitro* Studies of Herbs in the Application of DCM

Drug	Dosage	Experimental model	Reference
Triptolide	20 ng/ml	High-glucose cultured H9c2 rat cardiac cells	[64]
C66	2.5, 5, or 10 μmol/L	High-glucose cultured H9c2 cells	[69]
C66	2.5, 5, or 10 μmol/L	High-glucose cultured neonatal rat cardiomyocytes	[69]
Resveratrol	50 μM	High-glucose cultured neonatal rat cardiomyocytes	[79]
Astragalus polysaccharides	0.8 mg/mL	High-glucose cultured H9c2 cardiomyocytes	[85]
Myricitrin	25 μg/mL	AGE-induced H9c2 cells	[90]
Taxifolin	20, 40 μg/mL	High-glucose cultured H9c2 cells	[92]
Naringin	80 μM	High-glucose cultured H9c2 cells	[96]
Total saponins of Aralia taibaiensis	25, 50, and 75 μg/mL	G/GO cultured H9c2 cardiomyocytes	[109]

Notes: C66 ; Compound (2E, 6E)-2, 6-bis (2- (trifluoromethyl)benzylidene)cyclohexanone ; AGE: advanced glycation end products ; G/GO: 33 mM glucose + 15 mU glucose oxidase.

3 Herbal Medicines: Promising Therapeutic for DCM

Currently, a growing number of preclinical studies provide the evidences that herbal medicines are promising therapy for DCM (Tables 2 and 3). These herbs ameliorate cardiac injury of DCM owing to their antioxidant and anti-inflammation properties, via regulation of NF-κB and Nrf2 pathways (Figure 3).

3.1 Triptolide

Extracts of Tripterygium wilfordii Hook F are effective in traditional Chinese medicine for the treatment of immune inflammatory diseases including rheumatoid arthritis, systemic lupus erythematosus, and nephritis. Triptolide as the major active ingredient for Tripterygium wilfordii Hook F exerts immunosuppressive and anti-inflammatory functions[62] (Figure 5 (a)). Li et al.[63] showed that triptolide at 20 μg/kg/d and 100 μg/kg/d attenuated the myocardial fibrosis, cardiomyocyte hypertrophy, and restored the impaired cardiac function in the rat that underwent transverse aortic constriction, associated with decreased production of proflbrotic factors TNF-α and IL-1β. Wen et al. [64,65] showed that triptolide (100, 200, or 400 μg/kg/d p. o)administration for 6 weeks improved the left ventricular function of STZ-induced diabetic heart by inhibiting the expression of cardiac p38 MAPK in the upstream of NF-κB activation; triptolide with dose of 200 μg/kg/d displayed the best improvement. Furthermore, triptolide (20 ng/ml)atten-uated inflammation of H9c2 rat cardiac cell exposure to high glucose by inhibiting NF-κB activation. Guo et al.[66] showed that the left ventricle pathological structure and function of STZ-induced mice were signiflcantly improved by triptolide (50, 100 or 200 μg/kg/d p. o.) treatment for 8 weeks. The mechanism through which triptolide protects against DCM is involving inhibition of NF-κB/IL-1β and NF-κB/TNF-α cascades.

Table 3 *In vivo* Studies of Herbs in the Application of DCM

Drug	Dosage	Adminstration	Experimental model Model	Reference
Triptolide	100, 200 or 400 μg/kg/d	p. o. 6 weeks	STZ-induced diabetic rat	[64,65]
Triptolide	50, 100 or 200 μg/kg/d	p. o. 8 weeks	STZ-induced diabetic rat	[66]
Curcumin	100 mg/kg/d	p. o. 8 weeks	STZ-induced diabetic rat	[68]
C66	5 mg/kg/d	p. o. Every other day for 12 weeks.	STZ-induced diabetic mice	[69,70]
EGb761	100 mg/kg/d	p. o. 12 weeks	STZ-induced diabetic rat	[71,72]
EGb761	50 mg/kg/d	p. o. 3 weeks	STZ-induced diabetic rat	[75]
Resveratrol	2.5 mg/kg/d	p. o. 2 weeks	STZ-induced diabetic rat	[78]
Resveratrol	10 mg/kg/d	p. o. 4 weeks	STZ-induced diabetic rat	[80]
Resveratrol	Diet enrich with Resveratrol at 0.067%	p. o. 12 weeks	STZ-induced diabetic mice	[52]
Astragalus Polysaccharides	1-2 g/kg/d	p. o. 10 weeks	STZ-induced diabetic hamsters	[81-84]
Salvia miltiorrhiza	100 mg/kg/d	i. p. 4 weeks	STZ-induced diabetic rat	[86]
Cryptotanshinone	10 mg/kg/d	p. o. 28 days	STZ-induced diabetic rat	[87]
Myricitrin	300 mg/kg/d	p. o. 8 weeks	STZ-induced diabetic mice	[90]
Taxifolin	25, 50, 100 mg/kg/d	p. o. 4 weeks	STZ-induced diabetic mice	[92]
Troxerutin	150 mg/kg/d	p. o. 4 weeks	STZ-induced diabetic rat	[93]
Nobiletin	50 mg/kg/d	p. o. 11 weeks	STZ-induced diabetic mice	[95]
Liquirtin	8, 16 mg/kg	p. o. 10 weeks	High fructose-induced diabetic mice	[98]
Shengmaisan	4.5 g/kg/d	p. o. 24 weeks	db/db mice	[99]
Alcoholic ginseng root	200 mg/kg/d	p. o. 2or 4 months	STZ-induced diabetic mice and db/db mice	[101]
Dendrobium officinale kimura et Migo	75, 150, 300 mg/kg/d	p. o. 8 weeks	STZ-induced diabetic mice	[103]
Flos Puerariae Extract	100, 200 mg/kg/d	p. o. 10 weeks	STZ-induced diabetic mice	[104]
Mangiferin	20 mg/kg/d	p. o. 16 weeks	STZ and high-fat diet induced diabetic rat	[105]
TASAES	4.9, 9.8 and 19.6 mg/kg/d	p. o. 8 weeks	STZ-induced diabetic rat	[106]
Berberine	100 mg/kg/d	p. o, 16 weeks	High fat diet and STZ-induced diabetic rat	[109]

Notes: EGb761: *Ginkgo biloba* extract 761 ; TASAES: total aralosides of *Aralia elata* (Miq)seem.

3.2 Curcumin

Curcumin, a component of turmeric found in the *Curcuma longa* plant, has been used in treating inflammatory diseases for centuries due to its antioxidant property (Figure 5 (b)). Soetikno et al. [67] showed that curcumin exerts antiflbrotic effect in amelioration of diabetic nephropathy owing to inhibiting PKC-α and PKC-β2, as well as the downstream cascade ERK1/2. They also demonstrated that curcumin at dose of 100 mg/kg/d for an 8-week oral administration signiflcantly improved the left ventricular function and attenuated the progression of car-diac remodeling of STZ-induced diabetic rats by downregulating PKC-α and PKC-β2 and subsequently inactivating p38 MAPK, ERK1/2, and NF-κB. Moreover, the effect of improved blood glucose of diabetic rat partly explained the decreased oxidative stress [68]. Compound (2E, 6E)-2, 6-bis (2-(trifluoromethyl)benzylidene)cyclohexanone (C66)is a synthetic derivative of natural active curcumin. Pan et al. showed that pretreatment of H9c2 cells, and neonatal cardiomyocytes with C66, signiflcantly reduced the high-glucose-induced inflammation cytokine overexpression by inhibiting NF-κB. Treatment of STZ-induced diabetic mice with C66 at a dose of 5 mg/kg every other day for 12 weeks decreased the levels of plasma and cardiac TNF-α, endoplasmic reticulum stress, and cardiomyocyte apoptosis, as well as improved the cardiac dysfunction by inhibiting JNK phosphorylation [69,70].

3.3 Ginkgo biloba Extract (GBE).

Ginkgo biloba extract (GBE)contains terpenoids, flavonoids, alkylphenols, polyprenols, and organic acids. The standardized GBE, EGb761, is pharmacologically prepared containing ginkgo flavonoids (primarily quercetin, kaempferol, and isorhamnetin)com-prising 22%–24% of the GBE, 6% terpenoids (3.1% ginkgolides A, B, C, and J and 2.9% bilobalide), and < 5 ppm ginkgolic acid (Figures 5 (d), 5 (e), and 5 (f)). Fitzl et al. showed that 100 mg/kg/d EGb761 orally administered for 12 weeks signiflcantly reduced the increase of interstitial volume and collagen flbers in a diabetic rat heart[71,72]. Furthermore, EGb761 treatment improves the hypoxia tolerance of diabetic myocardium and myocardial microvessels[73,74]. Saini et al. [75]demonstrated that EGb761 at a dose of 50 mg/kg/d for 3 weeks signiflcantly attenuated the index of lipid peroxidation and oxidative stress in diabetic rats and inhibited the opening of mitochondrial permeability transition pore (mPTP), ultimately leading to improvement of cardiomyopathy.

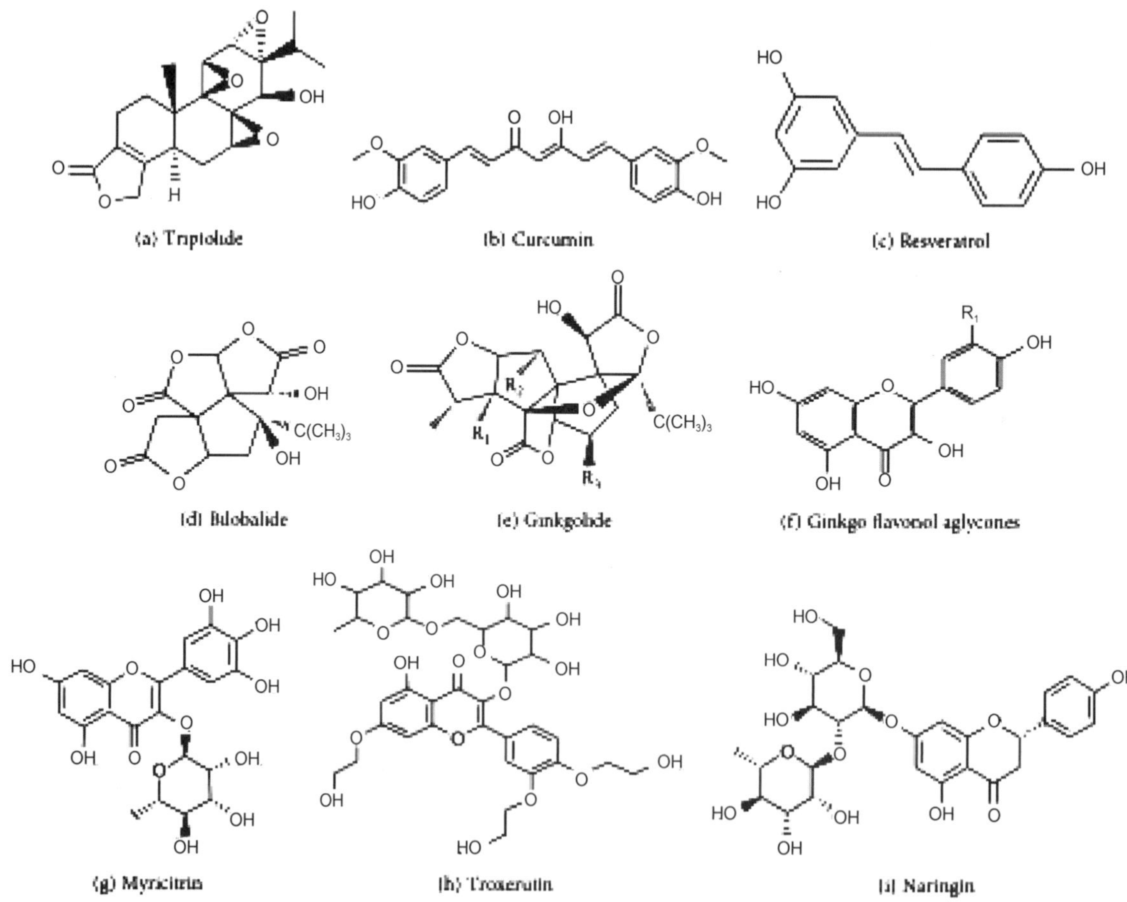

(a) Triptolide (b) Curcumin (c) Resveratrol

(d) Bilobalide (e) Ginkgolide (f) Ginkgo flavonol aglycones

(g) Myricitrin (h) Troxerutin (i) Naringin

Figure 5 Molecular Structure of the Compounds Described in This Review

3.4 Resveratrol

Resveratrol (3, 5, 4' -trihydroxylstilbene), a natural polyphenol present in red wine and grapes, is capable to reduce blood glucose level in STZ-induced diabetic rat[76,77] (Figure 5 (c)). GLUT-4 translocation and glucose uptake are increased in STZ-induced diabetic rat myocardium by orally administrated resveratrol at a dose of 2.5 mg/kg/d for 2 weeks, the mechanism involving activation of AMPK and AKt cascades by resveratrol[78]. Resveratrol prevents high-glucose cultured neonatal rat cardiomyocyte apoptosis by inhibiting NADPH-derived ROS production and by alleviating the reduction of cardiac antioxidant enzyme activities, possibly mediated by AMPK-related signaling pathway[79]. Yar et al. showed that 10 mg/kg/d resveratrol intraperitoneal injection for 4 weeks ameliorated diabetic heart failure by increasing the expression of SIRT1[80]. A special diet enriched with resveratrol at 0.067% (the consumption of resveratrol is estimated to be less than 100 mg/kg/d)for 12 weeks effectively restores SER-CA2α expression and cardiac function in diabetic mice, associated with STIR1 activation[52].

3.5 Astragalus Polysaccharides (APS)

APS is a main active extract from the traditional Chinese medicinal herb Astragalus membranaceus. Chen et al. demonstrated that APS improved cardiac function and myocardial collagen deposition by inhibiting the local chymase-Ang II system and Ang II-activated ERK1/2 in diabetic cardiomyopathy in hamsters[81–83]. They also showed that APS can ameliorate myocardial glucose metabolism disorders in diabetic hamster by promoting expression of myocardial GLUT-4 gene and inhibiting level of PPAR α[84]. Pretreatment of cells with 0.8 mg/ml APS could inhibit high-glucose-induced apoptosis of H9c2 cell by decreasing the expression of caspases and release of cytochrome C from mitochondria to cyto-plasm and by modulating the ratio of BCL-2 to Bax in mitochondria[85].

3.6 *Salvia Miltiorrhiza*

Salvia miltiorrhiza (Danshen), a traditional Chinese herbal medicine, is commonly used for the prevention and treatment of cardiovascular disease. According to Yu et al. [86]intraperitoneal injection Salviamiltiorrhiza 100 mg/kg/d for 4 weeks improved the heart function of diabetic rats and protected against cardiomyopa-thy by downregulating thrombospondin-1 (TSP-1)and TGF-β1 in myocardial tissue. Cryptotanshinone is an active principal ingredient isolated from *Salvia miltiorrhiza* (Danshen). Oral administration of 10 mg/kg/d cryptotan-shinone for 28 days attenuates the cardiac fibrosis in STZ-induced diabetic rats by inhibiting STAT3 pathway and MMP-9 expression [87].

3.7 Flavonoids

Chrysin, a PPAR-γ agonist, is a natural flavonoid present in honey, propolis, and various plant extracts. According to Rani et al. [88,89], chrysin attenuated isoproterenol-induced myocardial injury in diabetic rats by activating PPAR-γ and inhibiting AGE-RAGE-mediated inflammation and oxidative stress signaling pathway. Myricitrin (Figure 5 (g))is a flavone exact from the root bark of *Myrica cerifera*, Myrica esculenta, Ampelopsis grossedentata, and other plants. Zhang et al. [90]reported that pretreated AGE-cultured H9c2 cells with 25 μg/ml Myricitrin for 12 h significantly decreased the AGE-induced inflammation cytokines and cell apoptosis by activating Nrf2 and inhibiting NF-κB. Oral administration of Myricitrin 300 mg/kg/d for 8 weeks attenuated the cardiomyocyte apoptosis and inflammation of diabetic mice heart via regulation of AKt-and ERK-mediated Nrf2 pathways. Apigenin, a flavonoid derived in fruits and vegetables, has been shown to protect against isoproterenol-challenged diabetic myocardial injury by activation of PPAR-γ pathway [91]. Taxifolin is a flavo-noid abound in *Pseudotsuga taxifolia*, Dahurian larch, and syn Larix dahurica Turoz. According to Sun et al. [92], Taxifolin at concentration 20 and 40 μg/ml could decrease the apoptosis of high-glucose cultured H9c2 cells by inhibiting ROS generation. In vivo, Taxifolin attenuated the structure and function abnormalities by blocking NADPH oxidative activities. Troxerutin (Figure 5 (h)), a bioflavonoid, protects against DCM through suppression of NF-κB and JNK in a diabetic rat [93]. Hesperidin, a flavonoid isolated from citrus, has been shown to reduce oxidative stress and apoptosis and attenuate myocardial injury in isoproterenol-STZ rat via activation of PPAR-γ [94]. Nobiletin treatment (50 mg/kg/d p. o. 11 weeks)attenuates diabetic heart injury by suppression of oxidative stress, JNK, p38 MAPK, and NF-κB pathways [95]. 80 μM Naringin (4, 5, 7-trihydroxyflavonone-7-rhamno-glucoside, Figure 5 (i))pretreated for 2 hours protects H9c2 cells from high-glucose injury by ROS scavenging and MAPK cascade inhibiting [96]. Liquirtin, a major constitu-ent of Glycyrrhiza radix, exerts various pharmacological activities. Liquirtin prevents myocardial injury induced by high fructose feeding by inhibiting NF-κB and MAPK cascades [97,98].

3.8 Ginseng

Shengmaisan, a traditional Chinese recipe, consists of Radix Ginseng, Radix Ophiopogonis, and Fructus Schisandrae. According to Zhao et al. [99], cardiac dysfunction, hypertrophy, and fibrosis in diabetic mice are improved by 4.5 g/kg daily Shengmaisan treatment for 24 weeks through suppression of TGF-β pathway. Ni et al. [100] showed that Shengmai powder and Danshen decoction (consists of Radix Ginseng 9 g, Radix Ophiopogonis 9 g, Fructus Schisandrae 6 g, Radix Salviae Miltiorrhizae 30 g, Lignum Santali 6 g, and Fructus Amomi 6 g)inhibited the myocardial fibrosis in the diabetic rat through inhibiting TGF-β and TSP-1. Sen et al. [101]showed that alcoholic ginseng root (200 mg/kg/d, daily oral gavage)for 2 or 4 months is effective in the protection of cardiomyopathy in both type 1 and type 2 diabetic mice attributed to its antioxidative and antihyperglycemia properties. According to Gu et al.[102], total saponins of *Panax ginseng* 30 mg/kg/d by gavage for 12 weeks attenuated myocardial ultrastructural injury in diabetic rat and improved the lipid profile, blood glucose, and myocardial oxidative stress level as well. The mechanism involves regulation of citric acid cycle, fatty acid metabolism, and oxidative stress. Yu et al.[103] showed that Ginsenoside Rg1 dose dependently reduced serum levels of creatinine kinase MB and cardiac troponin I and attenuated diabetic rat myocardial ultrastructural disorder. Myocardial apoptosis was reduced by Ginsenoside Rg1 associated with reduced levels of caspase-3 and increased levels of B-cell lymphoma-extra-large (Bcl-xL)in the diabetic rat myocardium.

3.9 Others

Broccoli sprout extract at high dose (estimate an Nrf 2 activator-sulforaphane availability at 1.0 mg/kg) by gavage every other day for 3 months significantly prevents cardiac dysfunction of diabetic db/db mice by upregulating Nrf2 transcription[104]. Cardiac lipid accumulation and deposition of collagen are inhibited by 8-week oral treatment of Dendrobium offcinale Kimura et Migo at dose of 75, 150, and 300 mg/kg/d [105]. Dendrobium offcinale Kimura et Migo attenuates the diabetic heart injury by downregulating the NF-κB-mediated inflammation cascade[105]. Flos Puerariae extract at dose of 100 and 200 mg/kg/d for 10 weeks prevents myocardial apoptosis in STZ-induced diabetic heart through inhibiting oxidative stress, associated with suppres-sion of JNK and p38 MAPK activation [106]. Mangiferin (20 mg/kg/d p. o. 16 weeks)inhibits ROS accumulation, AGEs/RAGE production, and NF-κB nuclear translocation, attenuating cardiac injury induced by STZ and high-fat diet[107]. Total aralosides of *Aralia elata* (Miq)seem (TASAES)from Chinese traditional herb Longya *Aralia chinensis* L was found to prevent diabetes-induced cardiac dysfunction and pathological damage through upregulating L-type Ca^{2+} channel current in cardiac cells and decreasing connective tissue growth factor expression at dose of 4.9, 9.8 mg/kg, and 19.6 mg/kg/d by gavage, respectively, for 8 weeks[108]. Duan et al. [109] showed that the total saponins of Aralia taibaiensis exerted cytoprotective effects against oxidative stress induced by hyperglycemia through the Nrf2/ARE pathway. Chang et al. showed that berberine, a plant alkaloid, improves insulin resistance in H9c2 cardiomyocytes partly due to stimulation of AMPK activity[110]. They further found that berberine improved cardiac function and attenu-ated cardiac hypertrophy and fibrosis in a high-fat diet and STZ-induced diabetic rats through activation of AMPK and Akt[111]. According to Shen et al.[112], Shensong Yangxin Capsule inhibits diabetic myocardial fibrosis via suppressing TGF-β pathway.

4 Conclusion and Future Perspectives

DCM, featured by structure and function alteration, is a multifactorial disease. Extensive preclinical studies investigated the molecular targets for pathogenesis of DCM, and identified herbs that act on these targets are potential therapeutic approaches for DCM. However, at present, most clinical studies have small sample sizes and are not performed using a randomized design, and thus hamper the application of herbal medicines in patients with DCM. The combination of the herbs with Western medicine and joint application of herbal medicine on diabetic cardiomyopathy are superior to individual applications and are still under exploring. Hence, clinical trials in high-quality are needed in the future. Furthermore, exploring potential therapeutic target will contribute to detect new herbs for the treatment of DCM. The safety and drug interaction should be paid attention to ensure the wild and effective application of herbs in the DCM treatment.

REFERENCES

[1] Falcão-Pires I, Leite-Moreira AF. Diabetic cardiomyopathy: understanding the molecular and cellular basis to progress in diagnosis and treatment[J]. Heart Fail Rev, 2012, 17 (3): 325-44.

[2] Miki T, Yuda S, Kouzu H, et al. Diabetic cardiomyopathy: pathophysiology and clinical features[J]. Heart Fail Rev, 2013, 18 (2): 149-66.

[3] Li J, Casteels T, Frogne T, I et al. Artemisinins Target GABAA Receptor Signaling and Impair alpha Cell Identity[J]. Cell, 2017, 168 (1-2): 86-100. e15.

[4] Cosson S, Kevorkian JP. Left ventricular diastolic dysfunction: an early sign of diabetic cardiomyopathy? [J]. Diabetes Metab, 2003, 29 (5): 455-66.

[5] Amaral N, Okonko DO. Metabolic abnormalities of the heart in type II diabetes[J]. Diab Vasc Dis Res, 2015, 12 (4): 239-48.

[6] Taegtmeyer H, McNulty P, Young ME. Adaptation and maladaptation of the heart in diabetes: Part I: general concepts[J]. Circulation, 2002, 105 (14): 1727-33.

[7] Young ME, McNulty P, Taegtmeyer H. Adaptation and maladaptation of the heart in diabetes: Part II: potential mechanisms[J]. Circulation, 2002.105 (15): 1861-70.

[8] Zeng SY, Chen X, Chen SR, et al. Upregulation of Nox4 promotes angiotensin II-induced epidermal growth factor receptor activation and subsequent cardiac hypertrophy by increasing ADAM17 expression[J]. Can J Cardiol, 2013, 29 (10): 1310-9.

[9] Sirker A, Zhang M, Murdoch C, et al. Involvement of NADPH oxidases in cardiac remodelling and heart failure[J]. Am J Nephrol, 2007, 27 (6): 649-60.

[10] Duncan JG. Mitochondrial dysfunction in diabetic cardiomyopathy[J]. Biochim Biophys Acta, 2011, 1813 (7): 1351-9.

[11] Lebeche D, Davidoff AJ, Hajjar RJ. Interplay between impaired calcium regulation and insulin signaling abnormalities in diabetic cardiomyopathy[J]. Nat Clin Pract Cardiovasc Med, 2008, 5 (11): 715-24.

[12] Zhao XY, Hu SJ, Li J, et al. Decreased cardiac sarcoplasmic reticulum Ca2+ -ATPase activity contributes to cardiac dysfunction in streptozotocin-induced diabetic rats[J]. J Physiol Biochem, 2006, 62 (1): 1-8.

[13] Jiang X, Liu W, Deng J, et al. Polydatin protects cardiac function against burn injury by inhibiting sarcoplasmic reticulum Ca2+ leak by reducing oxidative modification of ryanodine receptors[J]. Free Radic Biol Med, 2013, 60: 292-9.

[14] Yan D, Luo X, Li Y, et al. Effects of advanced glycation end products on calcium handling in cardiomyocytes[J]. Cardiology, 2014, 129 (2): 75-83.

[15] Buja LM, Vela D. Cardiomyocyte death and renewal in the normal and diseased heart[J]. Cardiovasc Pathol, 2008, 17 (6): 349-74.

[16] Xie Z, He C, Zou MH. AMP-activated protein kinase modulates cardiac autophagy in diabetic cardiomyopathy[J]. Autophagy, 2011, 7 (10): 1254-5.

[17] Xie Z, Lau K, Eby B, et al. Improvement of cardiac functions by chronic metformin treatment is associated with enhanced cardiac autophagy in diabetic OVE26 mice[J]. Diabetes, 2011, 60 (6): 1770-8.

[18] Zhao Y, Zhang L, Qiao Y, et al. Heme oxygenase-1 prevents cardiac dysfunction in streptozotocin-diabetic mice by reducing inflammation, oxidative stress, apoptosis and enhancing autophagy[J]. PLoS One, 2013, 8 (9): e75927.

[19] Hou X, Hu Z, Xu H, et al. Advanced glycation endproducts trigger autophagy in cadiomyocyte via RAGE/PI3K/AKT/mTOR pathway[J]. Cardiovasc Diabetol, 2014, 13: 78.

[20] Palomer X, Salvadó L, Barroso E, et al. An overview of the crosstalk between inflammatory processes and metabolic dysregulation during diabetic cardiomyopathy[J]. Int J Cardiol, 2013, 168 (4): 3160-72.

[21] Wang S, Ding L, Ji H, et al. The Role of p38 MAPK in the Development of Diabetic Cardiomyopathy[J]. Int J Mol Sci, 2016.17 (7).

[22] Min W, Bin ZW, Quan ZB, et al. The signal transduction pathway of PKC/NF-kappa B/c-fos may be involved in the influence of high glucose on the cardiomyocytes of neonatal rats[J]. Cardiovasc Diabetol, 2009, 8: 8.

[23] Van Linthout S, Riad A, Dhayat N, et al. Anti-inflammatory effects of atorvastatin improve left ventricular function in experimental diabetic cardiomyopathy[J]. Diabetologia, 2007, 50 (9): 1977-86.

[24] Ko SY, Lin IH, Shieh TM, et al. Cell hypertrophy and MEK/ERK phosphorylation are regulated by glyceraldehyde-derived AGEs in cardiomyocyte H9c2 cells[J]. Cell Biochem Biophys, 2013, 66 (3): 537-44.

[25] Tanaka K, Honda M, Takabatake T. Redox regulation of MAPK pathways and cardiac hypertrophy in adult rat cardiac myocyte[J]. J Am Coll Cardiol, 2001, 37 (2): 676-85.

[26] Tang M, Zhang W, Lin H, et al. High glucose promotes the production of collagen types I and III by cardiac fibroblasts through a pathway dependent on extracellular-signal-regulated kinase 1/2[J]. Mol Cell Biochem, 2007, 301 (1-2): 109-14.

[27] Zhang C, Huang Z, Gu J, et al. Fibroblast growth factor 21 protects the heart from apoptosis in a diabetic mouse model via extracellular signal-regulated kinase 1/2-dependent signalling pathway[J]. Diabetologia, 2015, 58 (8): 1937-48.

[28] Xu Z, Sun J, Tong Q, et al. The Role of ERK1/2 in the Development of Diabetic Cardiomyopathy. Int J Mol Sci, 2016, 17 (12).

[29] Tsai KH, Wang WJ, Lin CW, et al. NADPH oxidase-derived superoxide anion-induced apoptosis is mediated via the JNK-dependent activation of NF-kappaB in cardiomyocytes exposed to high glucose[J]. J Cell Physiol, 2012, 227 (4): 1347-57.

[30] Jeon SM. Regulation and function of AMPK in physiology and diseases[J]. Exp Mol Med, 2016, 48 (7): e245.

[31] Cabarcas SM, Hurt EM, Farrar WL. Defining the molecular nexus of cancer, type 2 diabetes and cardiovascular disease[J]. Curr Mol Med, 2010, 10 (8): 744-55.

[32] Woods A, Johnstone SR, Dickerson K, et al. LKB1 is the upstream kinase in the AMP-activated protein kinase cascade[J]. Curr Biol, 2003, 13 (22): 2004-8.

[33] Woods A, Dickerson K, Heath R, et al. Ca^{2+}/calmodulin-dependent protein kinase kinase-beta acts upstream of AMP-activated protein kinase in mammalian cells[J]. Cell Metab, 2005, M 2 (1): 21-33.

[34] Holmes BF, Sparling DP, Olson AL, et al. Regulation of muscle GLUT4 enhancer factor and myocyte enhancer factor 2 by AMP-activated protein kinase[J]. Am J Physiol Endocrinol Metab, 2005, Dec；289 (6): E1071-6.

[35] Habets DD, Coumans WA, El Hasnaoui M, et al. Crucial role for LKB1 to AMPKalpha2 axis in the regulation of CD36-mediated long-chain fatty acid uptake into cardiomyocytes[J]. Biochim Biophys Acta, 2009, 1791 (3): 212-9.

[36] Garton AJ, Campbell DG, Carling D, et al. Phosphorylation of bovine hormone-sensitive lipase by the AMP-activated protein kinase. A possible antilipolytic mechanism[J]. Eur J Biochem, 1989, 179 (1): 249-54.

[37] Salminen A, Ojala J, Huuskonen J, et al. Interaction of aging-associated signaling cascades: inhibition of NF-kappaB signaling by longevity factors FoxOs and SIRT1[J]. Cell Mol Life Sci, 2008, 65 (7-8): 1049-58.

[38] Salminen A, Hyttinen JM, Kaarniranta K. AMP-activated protein kinase inhibits NF-kappaB signaling and inflammation: impact on healthspan and lifespan[J]. J Mol Med (Berl), 2011, 89 (7): 667-76.

[39] Egan D, Kim J, Shaw RJ, et al. The autophagy initiating kinase ULK1 is regulated via opposing phosphorylation by AMPK and mTOR[J]. Autophagy, 2011, 7 (6): 643-4.

[40] Shaw RJ. LKB1 and AMP-activated protein kinase control of mTOR signalling and growth[J]. Acta Physiol (Oxf), 2009, 196 (1): 65-80.

[41] He C, Zhu H, Li H, et al. Dissociation of Bcl-2-Beclin1 complex by activated AMPK enhances cardiac autophagy and protects against cardiomyocyte apoptosis in diabetes[J]. Diabetes, 2013, 62 (4): 1270-81.

[42] Zou MH, Xie Z. Regulation of interplay between autophagy and apoptosis in the diabetic heart: new role of AMPK[J]. Autophagy, 2013.9 (4): 624-5.

[43] Finck BN, Lehman JJ, Leone TC, et al. The cardiac phenotype induced by PPARalpha overexpression mimics that caused by diabetes mellitus[J]. J Clin Invest, 2002, 109 (1): 121-30.

[44] Burkart EM, Sambandam N, Han X, et al. Nuclear receptors PPARbeta/delta and PPARalpha direct distinct metabolic regulatory programs in the mouse heart[J]. J Clin Invest, 2007, 117 (12): 3930-9.

[45] Botta A, Laher I, Beam J, et al. Short term exercise induces PGC-1alpha, ameliorates inflammation and increases mitochondrial membrane proteins but fails to increase respiratory enzymes in aging diabetic hearts[J]. PLoS One, 2013, 8 (8): e70248.

[46] Wang H, Bei Y, Lu Y, et al. Exercise Prevents Cardiac Injury and Improves Mitochondrial Biogenesis in Advanced Diabetic Cardiomyopathy with PGC-1alpha and Akt Activation[J]. Cell Physiol Biochem, 2015, 35 (6): 2159-68.

[47] Buroker NE, Barboza J, Huang JY. The IkappaBalpha gene is a peroxisome proliferator-activated receptor cardiac target gene[J]. FEBS J, 2009, 276 (12): 3247-55.

[48] Planavila A, Rodríguez-Calvo R, Jové M, et al. Peroxisome proliferator-activated receptor beta/delta activation inhibits hypertrophy in neonatal rat cardiomyocytes[J]. Cardiovasc Res, 2005, 65 (4): 832-41.

[49] Asakawa M, Takano H, Nagai T, et al. Peroxisome proliferator-activated receptor gamma plays a critical role in inhibition of cardiac hypertrophy in vitro and in vivo[J]. Circulation, 2002, 105 (10): 1240-6.

[50] Lan F, Cacicedo JM, Ruderman N, et al. SIRT1 modulation of the acetylation status, cytosolic localization, and activity of LKB1. Possible role in

AMP-activated protein kinase activation[J]. J Biol Chem, 2008, 283 (41): 27628-35.

[51] Pan W, Yu H, Huang S, et al. Resveratrol Protects against TNF-alpha-Induced Injury in Human Umbilical Endothelial Cells through Promoting Sirtuin-1-Induced Repression of NF-KB and p38 MAPK[J]. PLoS One, 2016, 11 (1): e0147034.

[52] Sulaiman M, Matta MJ, Sunderesan NR, Gupta MP, Periasamy M, Gupta M. Resveratrol, an activator of SIRT1, upregulates sarcoplasmic calcium ATPase and improves cardiac function in diabetic cardiomyopathy[J]. Am J Physiol Heart Circ Physiol, 2010, 298 (3): H833-43.

[53] Karbasforooshan H, Karimi G. The role of SIRT1 in diabetic cardiomyopathy[J]. Biomed Pharmacother, 2017, 90: 386-392.

[54] He X, Kan H, Cai L, et al. Nrf2 is critical in defense against high glucose-induced oxidative damage in cardiomyocytes[J]. J Mol Cell Cardiol, 2009, 46 (1): 47-58.

[55] Yu M, Liu Y, Zhang B, et al. Inhibiting microRNA-144 abates oxidative stress and reduces apoptosis in hearts of streptozotocin-induced diabetic mice[J]. Cardiovasc Pathol, 2015, 24 (6): 375-81.

[56] Jeyabal P, Thandavarayan RA, Joladarashi D, et al. MicroRNA-9 inhibits hyperglycemia-induced pyroptosis in human ventricular cardiomyocytes by targeting ELAVL1[J]. Biochem Biophys Res Commun, 2016, 471 (4): 423-9.

[57] Zheng D, Ma J, Yu Y, et al. Silencing of miR-195 reduces diabetic cardiomyopathy in C57BL/6 mice[J]. Diabetologia, 2015, 58 (8): 1949-58.

[58] Liu S, Li W, Xu M, et al. Micro-RNA 21Targets dual specific phosphatase 8 to promote collagen synthesis in high glucose-treated primary cardiac fibroblasts[J]. Can J Cardiol, 2014, 30 (12): 1689-99.

[59] Singh GB, Raut SK, Khanna S, et al. MicroRNA-200c modulates DUSP-1 expression in diabetes-induced cardiac hypertrophy[J]. Mol Cell Biochem, 2017, 424 (1-2): 1-11.

[60] Raut SK, Kumar A, Singh GB, et al. miR-30c Mediates Upregulation of Cdc42 and Pak1 in Diabetic Cardiomyopathy[J]. Cardiovasc Ther, 2015, 33 (3): 89-97.

[61] Li X, Du N, Zhang Q, et al. MicroRNA-30d regulates cardiomyocyte pyroptosis by directly targeting foxo3a in diabetic cardiomyopathy[J]. Cell Death Dis, 2014, 5: e1479.

[62] Qiu D, Kao PN. Immunosuppressive and anti-inflammatory mechanisms of triptolide, the principal active diterpenoid from the Chinese medicinal herb Tripterygium wilfordii Hook. f[J]. Drugs R D, 2003, 4 (1): 1-18.

[63] Li R, Lu K, Wang Y, et al. Triptolide attenuates pressure overload-induced myocardial remodeling in mice via the inhibition of NLRP3 inflammasome expression[J]. Biochem Biophys Res Commun, 2017, 485 (1): 69-75.

[64] Wen HL, Liang ZS, Zhang R, et al. Anti-inflammatory effects of triptolide improve left ventricular function in a rat model of diabetic cardiomyopathy[J]. Cardiovasc Diabetol, 2013, 12: 50.

[65] Liang Z, Leo S, Wen H, et al. Triptolide improves systolic function and myocardial energy metabolism of diabetic cardiomyopathy in streptozotocin-induced diabetic rats[J]. BMC Cardiovasc Disord, 2015, 15: 42.

[66] Guo X, Xue M, Li CJ, et al. Protective effects of triptolide on TLR4 mediated autoimmune and inflammatory response induced myocardial fibrosis in diabetic cardiomyopathy[J]. J Ethnopharmacol, 2016, 193: 333-344.

[67] Soetikno V, Watanabe K, Sari FR, et al. Curcumin attenuates diabetic nephropathy by inhibiting PKC-alpha and PKC-beta1 activity in streptozotocin-induced type I diabetic rats[J]. Mol Nutr Food Res, 2011, 55 (11): 1655-65.

[68] Soetikno V, Sari FR, Sukumaran V, et al. Curcumin prevents diabetic cardiomyopathy in streptozotocin-induced diabetic rats: possible involvement of PKC-MAPK signaling pathway[J]. Eur J Pharm Sci, 2012, 47 (3): 604-14.

[69] Pan Y, Wang Y, Zhao Y, et al. Inhibition of JNK phosphorylation by a novel curcumin analog prevents high glucose-induced inflammation and apoptosis in cardiomyocytes and the development of diabetic cardiomyopathy[J]. Diabetes, 2014, 63 (10): 3497-511.

[70] Wang Y, Zhou S, Sun W, et al. Inhibition of JNK by novel curcumin analog C66 prevents diabetic cardiomyopathy with a preservation of cardiac metallothionein expression[J]. Am J Physiol Endocrinol Metab, 2014, 306 (11): E1239-47.

[71] Fitzl G, Martin R, Dettmer D, et al. Protective effects of Gingko biloba extract EGb 761 on myocardium of experimentally diabetic rats. I: ultrastructural and biochemical investigation on cardiomyocytes[J]. Exp Toxicol Pathol, 1999, 51 (3): 189-98.

[72] Welt K, Weiss J, Koch S, et al. Protective effects of Ginkgo biloba extract EGb 761 on the myocardium of experimentally diabetic rats. II. Ultrastructural and immunohistochemical investigation on microvessels and interstitium[J]. Exp Toxicol Pathol, 1999, 51 (3): 213-22.

[73] Fitzl G, Welt K, Martin R, et al. The influence of hypoxia on the myocardium of experimentally diabetic rats with and without protection by Ginkgo biloba extract. I. Ultrastructural and biochemical investigations on cardiomyocytes[J]. Exp Toxicol Pathol, 2000, 52 (5): 419-30.

[74] Welt K, Fitzl G, Schepper A. Experimental hypoxia of STZ-diabetic rat myocardium and protective effects of Ginkgo biloba extract. II. Ultrastructural investigation of microvascular endothelium[J]. Exp Toxicol Pathol, 2001, 52 (6): 503-12.

[75] Saini AS, Taliyan R, Sharma PL. Sharma, Protective effect and mechanism of Ginkgo biloba extract-EGb 761 on STZ-induced diabetic cardiomyopathy in rats[J]. Pharmacogn Mag, 2014, 10 (38): 172-8.

[76] Su HC, Hung LM, Chen JK. Resveratrol, a red wine antioxidant, possesses an insulin-like effect in streptozotocin-induced diabetic rats[J]. Am J Physiol Endocrinol Metab, 2006, 290 (6): E1339-46.

[77] Turan B, Tuncay E, Vassort G. Resveratrol and diabetic cardiac function: focus on recent in vitro and in vivo studies[J]. J Bioenerg Biomembr, 2012, 44 (2): 281-96.

[78] Penumathsa SV, Thirunavukkarasu M, Zhan L, et al. Resveratrol enhances GLUT-4 translocation to the caveolar lipid raft fractions through AMPK/Akt/eNOS signalling pathway in diabetic myocardium[J]. J Cell Mol Med, 2008, 12 (6A): 2350-61.

[79] Guo S, Yao Q, Ke Z, et al. Resveratrol attenuates high glucose-induced oxidative stress and cardiomyocyte apoptosis through AMPK[J]. Mol Cell Endocrinol, 2015, 412: 85-94.
[80] Yar AS, Menevse S, Alp E. The effects of resveratrol on cyclooxygenase-1 and -2, nuclear factor kappa beta, matrix metalloproteinase-9, and sirtuin 1 mRNA expression in hearts of streptozotocin-induced diabetic rats[J]. Genet Mol Res, 2011, 10 (4): 2962-75.
[81] Chen W, Li YM, Yu MH. Effects of Astragalus polysaccharides on chymase, angiotensin-converting enzyme and angiotensin II in diabetic cardiomyopathy in hamsters[J]. J Int Med Res, 2007, 35 (6): 873-877.
[82] Chen W, Yu MH, Li YM, et al. Beneficial effects of astragalus polysaccharides treatment on cardiac chymase activities and cardiomyopathy in diabetic hamsters[J]. Acta Diabetol, 2010, 47 Suppl 1: 35-46.
[83] Chen W, Li YM, Yu MH. Astragalus polysaccharides inhibited diabetic cardiomyopathy in hamsters depending on suppression of heart chymase activation[J]. J Diabetes Complications, 2010, 24 (3): 199-208.
[84] Chen W, Xia YP, Chen WJ, et al. Improvement of myocardial glycolipid metabolic disorder in diabetic hamster with Astragalus polysaccharides treatment[J]. Mol Biol Rep, 2012, 39 (7): 7609-15.
[85] Sun S, Yang S, Dai M, et al. The effect of Astragalus polysaccharides on attenuation of diabetic cardiomyopathy through inhibiting the extrinsic and intrinsic apoptotic pathways in high glucose -stimulated H9C2 cells[J]. BMC Complement Altern Med, 2017, 17 (1): 310.
[86] Yu J, Fei J, Azad J, et al. Myocardial protection by Salvia miltiorrhiza Injection in streptozotocin-induced diabetic rats through attenuation of expression of thrombospondin-1 and transforming growth factor-beta1[J]. J Int Med Res, 2012, 40 (3): 1016-24.
[87] Lo SH, Hsu CT, Niu HS, et al. Cryptotanshinone Inhibits STAT3 Signaling to Alleviate Cardiac Fibrosis in Type 1-like Diabetic Rats[J]. Phytother Res, 2017, 31 (4): 638-646.
[88] Rani N, Bharti S, Bhatia J, et al. Chrysin, a PPAR-gamma agonist improves myocardial injury in diabetic rats through inhibiting AGE-RAGE mediated oxidative stress and inflammation[J]. Chem Biol Interact, 2016, 250: 59-67.
[89] Rani N, Bharti S, Bhatia J, et al. Inhibition of TGF-beta by a novel PPAR-gamma agonist, chrysin, salvages beta-receptor stimulated myocardial injury in rats through MAPKs-dependent mechanism[J]. Nutr Metab (Lond), 2015, 12: 11.
[90] Zhang B, Shen Q, Chen Y, et al. Myricitrin Alleviates Oxidative Stress-induced Inflammation and Apoptosis and Protects Mice against Diabetic Cardiomyopathy[J]. Sci Rep, 2017, 7: 44239.
[91] Mahajan UB, Chandrayan G, Patil CR, et al. The Protective Effect of Apigenin on Myocardial Injury in Diabetic Rats mediating Activation of the PPAR-gamma Pathway[J]. Int J Mol Sci, 2017, 18 (4).
[92] Sun X, Chen RC, Yang ZH, et al. Taxifolin prevents diabetic cardiomyopathy in vivo and in vitro by inhibition of oxidative stress and cell apoptosis. [J]Food Chem Toxicol, 2014, 63: 221-32.
[93] Yu Y, Zheng G. Troxerutin protects against diabetic cardiomyopathy through NFkappaB/AKT/IRS1 in a rat model of type 2 diabetes[J]. Mol Med Rep, 2017, 15 (6): 3473-3478.
[94] Agrawal YO, Sharma PK, Shrivastava B, Arya DS, Goyal SN. Hesperidin blunts streptozotocin-isoprotemol induced myocardial toxicity in rats by altering of PPAR-gamma receptor[J]. Chem Biol Interact, 2014, 219: 211-20.
[95] Zhang N, Yang Z, Xiang SZ, et al. Nobiletin attenuates cardiac dysfunction, oxidative stress, and inflammatory in streptozotocin: induced diabetic cardiomyopathy[J]. Mol Cell Biochem, 2016, 417 (1-2): 87-96.
[96] Chen J, Guo R, Yan H, et al. Naringin inhibits ROS-activated MAPK pathway in high glucose-induced injuries in H9c2 cardiac cells[J]. Basic Clin Pharmacol Toxicol, 2014, 114 (4): 293-304.
[97] Zhang Y, Zhang L, Zhang Y, et al. The protective role of liquiritin in high fructose-induced myocardial fibrosis via inhibiting NF-kappaB and MAPK signaling pathway[J]. Biomed Pharmacother, 2016, 84: 1337-1349.
[98] Xie XW. Liquiritigenin attenuates cardiac injury induced by high fructose-feeding through fibrosis and inflammation suppression[J]. Biomed Pharmacother, 2017, 86: 694-704.
[99] Zhao J, Cao TT, Tian J, et al. Shengmai San Ameliorates Myocardial Dysfunction and Fibrosis in Diabetic db/db Mice[J]. Evid Based Complement Alternat Med, 2016, 2016: 4621235.
[100] Ni Q, Wang J, Li EQ, et al. Study on the protective effect of the Mixture of Shengmai Powder and Danshen Decoction on the myocardium of diabetic cardiomyopathy in the rat model[J]. Chin J Integr Med, 2011, 17 (2): 116-25.
[101] Sen S, Chen S, Wu Y, et al. Preventive effects of North American ginseng (Panax quinquefolius)on diabetic retinopathy and cardiomyopathy[J]. Phytother Res, 2013, 27 (2): 290-8.
[102] Gu JN, Niu J, Pi ZF, et al. Study on the mechanism of total saponins of panax ginseng in treatment of diabetic cardiomyopathy in rat assessed by urine metabonomics[J]. Chinese Journal of Analytical Chemistry, 2013, 41 (3): 371-376. [Article in Chinese]
[103] Yu HT, Zhen J, Pang B, et al. Ginsenoside Rg1 ameliorates oxidative stress and myocardial apoptosis in streptozotocin-induced diabetic rats[J]. Journal of Zhejiang University-SCIENCE B (Biomedicine & Biotechnology), 2015, 16 (5): 344-354.
[104] Xu Z, Wang S, Ji H, et al. Broccoli sprout extract prevents diabetic cardiomyopathy via Nrf2 activation in db/db T2DM mice[J]. Sci Rep, 2016, 6: 30252.
[105] Zhang Z, Zhang D, Dou M, et al. Dendrobium officinale Kimura et Migo attenuates diabetic cardiomyopathy through inhibiting oxidative stress, inflammation and fibrosis in streptozotocin-induced mice[J]. Biomed Pharmacother, 2016, 84: 1350-1358.
[106] Yu W, Zha W, Guo S, et al. Flos Puerariae extract prevents myocardial apoptosis via attenuation oxidative stress in streptozotocin-induced diabetic

mice[J]. PLoS One, 2014, 9 (5): e98044.

[107] Hou J, Zheng D, Fung G, et al. Mangiferin suppressed advanced glycation end products (AGEs)through NF-kappaB deactivation and displayed anti-inflammatory effects in streptozotocin and high fat diet-diabetic cardiomyopathy rats[J]. Can J Physiol Pharmacol, 2016, 94 (3): 332-40.

[108] Xi S, Zhou G, Zhang X, et al. Protective effect of total aralosides of Aralia elata (Miq)Seem (TASAES)against diabetic cardiomyopathy in rats during the early stage, and possible mechanisms[J]. Exp Mol Med, 2009, 41 (8): 538-47.

[109] Duan J, Wei G, Guo C, et al. Aralia taibaiensis Protects Cardiac Myocytes against High Glucose-Induced Oxidative Stress and Apoptosis[J]. Am J Chin Med, 2015, 43 (6): 1159-75.

[110] Chang W, Zhang M, Li J, et al. Berberine improves insulin resistance in cardiomyocytes via activation of 5'-adenosine monophosphate-activated protein kinase[J]. Metabolism, 2013, 62 (8): 1159-67

[111] Chang W, Zhang M, Meng Z, et al. Berberine treatment prevents cardiac dysfunction and remodeling through activation of 5'-adenosine monophosphate-activated protein kinase in type 2 diabetic rats and in palmitate-induced hypertrophic H9c2 cells[J]. Eur J Pharmacol, 2015, 769: 55-63.

[112] Shen N, Li X, Zhou Tet al. Shensong Yangxin Capsule prevents diabetic myocardial fibrosis by inhibiting TGF-beta1/Smad signaling[J]. J Ethnopharmacol, 2014, 157: 161-70.

First Published: TIAN Jin-fan, ZHAO Ying-ke, LIU Yan-fei, LIU Yue, CHEN Ke-ji, LU Shu-zheng. Roles and mechanisms of herbal medicine for diabetic cardiomyopathy: current status and perspective[J]. Oxid Med Cell Longev, 2017, 2017: 8214541.

Synergistic Effects of Chuanxiong-Chishao Herb-Pair on Promoting Angiogenesis at Network Pharmacological and Pharmacodynamic Levels

WANG Yan, GUO Gang, YANG Bin-rui, XIN Qi-qi, LIAO Qi-wen, LEE Simon Ming-yuen, HU Yuan-jia, CHEN Ke-ji, and CONG Wei-hong

Chinese medicine (CM)is a medical system characterized by the concept of organic wholeness as its principal theory and treatment based on syndrome differentiation as its diagnostic and therapeutic features. [1] CM has attracted considerable attention and acceptance in many countries due to its satisfactory therapeutic action. [2] Recent work involving CM has put forward the holistic philosophy of CM sharing much with the main ideas of emerging network pharmacology and network biology. [3] However, CM formula normally contains many active constituents which generally act upon multiple targets. [4] The complexity of the chemical constituents and the therapeutic targets pose big challenge to modern analytical chemistry and pharmacology methods. [5,6] The present work attempts to discover the candidate rule of CM from a systematic perspective at molecular level and pharmacodynamic level to interpret the abstract theory of CM through relatively simple two kinds of botanical drugs (Figure 1).

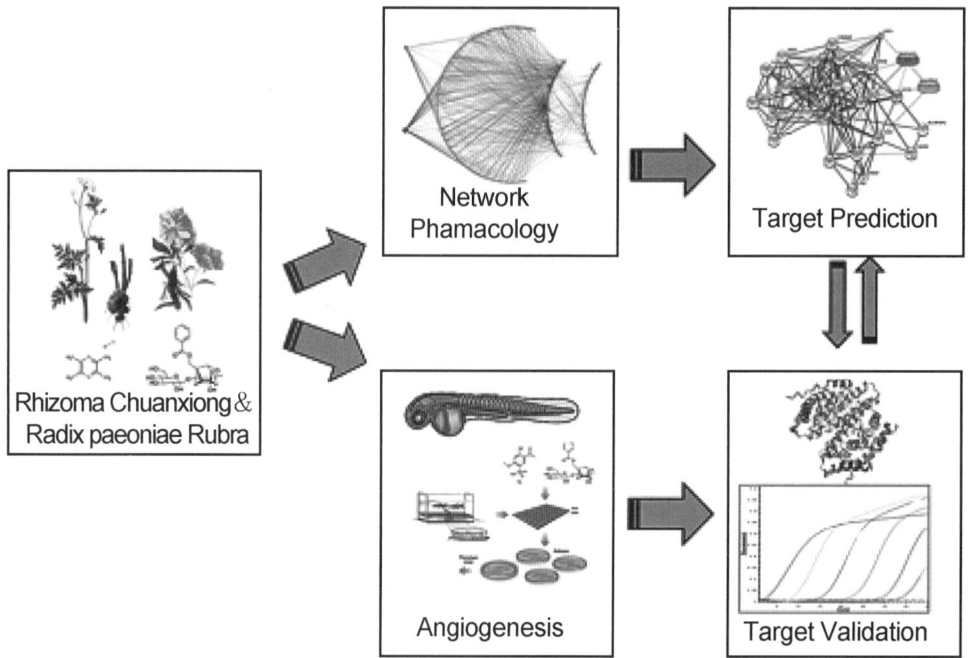

Figure 1　Schematic Diagram of Network Pharmacological and Pharmacodynamic Strategies

Chuanxiong (*Rhizoma Chuanxiong*)and Chishao (*Radix Paeoniae Rubra*)are two classical activating blood circulation herbs in China. Chuanxiong is one of the most popular herbal medicines in the World. [7] Ligustrazine (2, 3, 5, 6-tetramethylpyrazine, TMP, Figure 2A)and Paeoniflorin (PF, Figure 2B)are two representative bioactive compounds of the two herbs. TMP, a natural alkaloid and the predominant bioactive ingredient of Chuanxiong, had been demonstrated antioxidant, anti-platelet aggregation, anti-apoptosis, calcium-homeostasis and anti-inflammatory effect, which might contribute to protecting vascular diseases. [8] PF as a principle bioactive components of Chishao, had been widely studied as analgesic, antipyretic, anti-inflammatory, anti-oxidant, anti-hyperlipidemia, anti-hyperglycemia, anti-thrombotic and platelet-inhibitory agent. [9] In previous study, we had demonstrated that PF could promote angiogenesis in zebrafish in vivo and human umbilical vein endothelial cells (HUVECs)*in vitro* in a dose-dependent manner. [10]

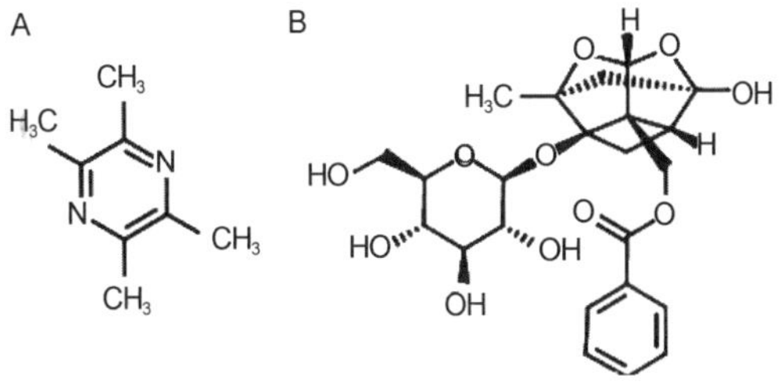

Figure 2 Chemical Structures of TMP (A)and PF (B)

Angiogenesis, an important natural process for healing and reproduction, refers to the establishment of a mature blood vessel network through expansion and remodeling of the pre-existing vascular primordium, [11] which had been continuously investigated as an innovative therapeutic approach for ischemic cardio-cerebrovascular diseases. [12]

Former experimental and clinical evidence had demonstrated the cardioprotective effects of TMP and PF. For example, TMP injection, which could prevent atherosclerosis as well as ischemia-reperfusion injury, had been extensively used in clinics in China for nearly 30 years; PF had been reported to protect against ischemic stroke with good permeation through the blood brain barrier[13] and exhibit pro-angiogenic action in zebraflsh *in vivo* and HUVECs *in vitro* model. However, further exploration is still needed, and limited information of TMP and PF had been exported from target prediction platform. In this study, we tried to use target prediction of these two ingredients to make a complementary understanding of Chuanxiong-Chishao herb-pair (CCHP).

METHODS

1 Data Collection

The data of chemical constituents, targets and diseases used for network pharmacological analysis in Chuangxiong and Chishao were collected from Traditional Chinese Medicine Systems Pharmacology Database (TCMSP). [14] In this platform, target information was obtained from DrugBank; [15] herb-target mappings were obtained from two sources: HIT[16] for experimentally validated herb-target pairs and the SysDT model[17] for compounds without validated targets. The disease information was obtained from TTD[18] and PharmGKB (https: // www. pharmgkb. org/). The knowledge about interactions between proteins and small molecules is essential for the understanding of molecular and cellular functions. We applied different database of known and predicted interactions between chemicals and proteins. To facilitate access to this data, Search Tool for Interactions of Chemicals (STITCH)database (http: //stitch. embl. de), SwissTargetPrediction (http: //www. swisstargetprediction. ch), Similarity Ensemble Approach (SEArch, http: //sea. bkslab. org/search/)and Chemmapper (http: //lilab. ecust. edu. cn/chemmapper/)were used to predict interact relations between TMP and PF, based on the concept that compounds sharing high 3D similarities may have relatively similar target association profile.

2 Establishment of Herb-Compound-Target-Cardiovascular Disease Network

To delineate the difference and similarity of chemicals between Chuanxiong and Chishao, we performed herbal compound comparison based on chemical constituents. Based on the Compound-Target-Disease Network of each herb, the cardiovascular disease system was selected manually and the related targets and compounds information of both herbs were extracted for further analysis. This extracted information was used to construct an Herb-Compound-Target-Cardiovascular Disease Network .

3 Analysis and Visualization of Network

The bipartite graphs were constructed by Cytoscape (version 3.4. 0 Boston, MA, USA). [19] In the network, the compounds, targets and diseases were represented by nodes, and each interaction between two nodes was represented by an edge. Since the therapeutic effectiveness of a CM formula was achieved through collectively modulating the molecular network by its active compounds, two crucial topological parameters, i. e., degree and betweenness centrality[20] were analyzed to specify the importance of each node in the network. The "degree" of a node was the number of edges connecting to the node, and the highly connected nodes (half of the maximum degree of nodes)were referred to as hubs. And the betweenness centrality of a node refers to its capacity located in the shortest communication paths between different pairs of nodes in the network. All the topological properties of these networks were analyzed using Network Analyzer of Cytoscape. [19]

4 Molecular Docking for Target Validation

To validate the compound-target associations, the molecular docking simulation was further performed on TMP and PF combined with their predicted targes by AutoDock software (version 4.2). AutoDock Tools-1.5. 6 was used to cluster the conformations. The program AutoGrid was used to generate the grid maps. The docking area of this grid was written by 60 × 60 × 60 with a 0.375 Å grid space. Lamarckian genetic algorithm (LGA)was employed in this simulation process. The binding free energy ($\triangle G_{bind}$) ≤ –5.0 kcal/mol indicated a high binding affinity of compound with their receptor. [21]

5 Chemicals and Reagents

Vascular endothelial growth factor (VEGF)receptor tyrosine kinase inhibitor Ⅱ (VRI)was obtained from Merck KGaA (Germany). Tetramethylpyrazine hydrochloride (TMP•HCl)were purchased from Chengdu Biopurify Phytochemicals Ltd. (Sichuan, China). PF was purchased from National Institute for Food and Drug Control (Beijing, China). Dimethyl sulfoxide (DMSO)was acquired from Sigma (St Louis, MO, USA). Stock solution of TMP•HCl (300 mmol/L in DMSO)and PF (300 mmol/L in DMSO)were prepared and appropriately diluted as required.

6 Maintenance of Zebrafish and Embryo Collection

The *Tg (fli-1a: EGFP)y1* zebrafish, in which endothelial cells (ECs)express enhanced green fluorescent protein (EGFP), were maintained as described in the Zebrafish Handbook. [22] Briefly, the zebrafish was maintained in standard conditions at the temperature of 28 ℃ with a 14 h: 10 h light/dark cycle. The zebrafish was fed twice daily with brine shrimp and also with general tropical fish food occasionally. Zebrafish embryos were generated by natural pairwise mating (3–12 months old)and were raised at 28.5 ℃ in E3 medium.

All animal experiments were conducted in accordance with the ethical guidelines of Institute of Chinese Medical Sciences, University of Macau and the protocol was approved by Institute of Chinese Medical Sciences-Animal Ethics Committee of the University of Macau.

7 Drug Treatment of TMP•HCl and PF

Healthy embryos were selected at 21 h postfertilization (hpf)and pretreated with 500 ng/mL VRI for 3 h. Afterwards, VRI was washed out and embryos were distributed into 24-well microplate (8 embryos in each well)containing 0.1% DMSO (v/v)or different concentrations of TMP•HCl (0.1–100 μmol/L), PF (0.1–100 μmol/L) and PF 10 μmol/L with different concentrations of TMP•HCl (0.1–10 μmol/L)for a treatment of 24 h at 28.5 ℃. Embryos receiving 0.1% DMSO (v/v)only served as vehicle control and were equivalent to no treatment. All experiments were repeated 3 times.

8 Morphological Observation of Zebrafish

At 48 hpf, Zebrafish embryos were removed from microplates and observed for viability and gross morphological changes under a fluorescence microscope (Olympus IX81 Motorized Inverted Microscope, Japan)equipped with a digital camera (DP controller, Soft Imaging System, Olympus). Images were analyzed with Adobe Photoshop 7.0.

9 Target Validation of TMP • HCl and PF in Zebrafish Using Real-Time Polymerase Chain Reaction

The 21 hpf healthy *Tg (fli-1a: EGFP)y1* zebrafish embryos were collected and distributed into 4 groups: vehicle control, VRI, TMP•HCl 1 μ mol/L and PF 10 μ mol/L, thereafter treated with 500 ng/mL VRI for 3 h apart from vehicle control group. Afterwards, VRI was washed out and embryos were exposed to 1 mL of E3 medium containing different drugs in 24-well plates (n=30). Total RNA was extracted from zebrafish embryos using RNeasy Mini Kit (Qiagen, USA)in accordance with the manufacturer's instructions, and converted into single-strand cDNA using SuperScript™ Ⅲ First-Strand Synthesis System followed by real-time polymerase chain reaction (RTPCR, Invitrogen™, USA)using the TaqMan® Universal PCR Master Mix (Branchburg, USA), corresponding probe from Universal Probe Library (Roche, Swiss). Then RT-PCR was performed in the ABI ViiA™ 7PCR System (Applied Biosystems)with the following amplification profile: hold at 50 ℃ for 2 min, hold at 95 ℃ for 10 min and 40 cycles at 95 ℃ for 15 s, 60 ℃ for 1 min. The expression of estrogen receptor α (ESRα)and hypoxia-inducible factor 1-α (HIF-1 α)mRNAs was normalized to the amount of β-actin, using the relative quantification method described by the manufacturer.

10 Statistical Analysis

All data were expressed as the mean ± standard deviations ($\bar{x} \pm s$). Data were analyzed with one-way ANOVA followed by Tukey's multiple comparison test with the following statistical criteria. *P* value less than 0.05 ($P < 0.05$)was considered significant. Chart was made with GraphPad Prism 6.0 software (San Diego, CA). Each experiment has been repeated at least 3 times independently.

RESULTS

1 Chuanxiong-Chishao-Compound-Target-Cardiovascular-Disease Network

Herb-Compound-Target-Disease interaction (Figure 3)was built by candidate compounds and their related targets, and the Target-Disease Network linking potential targets and diseases was constructed for exploring the protein interactions and the therapeutic targets for diseases.

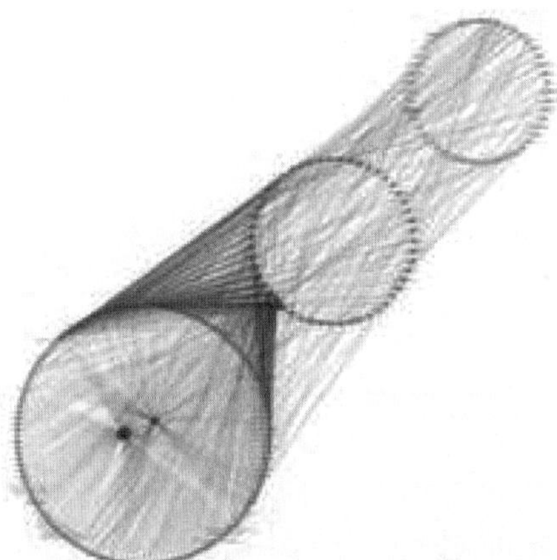

Figure 3 Cardiovascular Diseases Related Compound–Target–Disease Network of Chuanxiong–Chishao

Notes: The targets of Chuanxiong were concentrated in the whole cardiovascular system; Chishao placed emphasis on the anti-inflammatory effect and analgesics. Herb (hexagon, purple), compounds (ellipse, green), targets (triangle, red), cardiovascular diseases (round rectangle, yellow).

In this construction of network, 183 target proteinsof Chuanxiong were predicted, most of which were related to the above mentioned diseases, such as ESR related to myocardial infarction; [23] cell division protein kinase 2, nitric-oxide synthase endothelial and β 1 adrenergic receptor related to cardiovascular disease; [24,25] adenosine A2A receptor and mitogenactivated protein kinase 14 possibly involved in inflammation treatment. [26] Moreover, many compounds (i. e. Isobutyrophenone)have been predicted to target at α -1A adrenergic receptor; Chuanxiongol and (Z)-ligustilide have been predicted to target at adrenergic receptors, which are related to cardiovascular diseases.

The current work predicted 190 targets for Chishao, many of which showed relationships with inflammation and other diseases. For example, the main compounds, paeonin and baicalein, were highly connected with trypsin-1, which was involved in various pathological processes including inflammation, abnormal blood coagulation, tumor invasion, and atherosclerosis.

Among the targets, the protein with the highest degree was prostaglandin G/H synthase 2, followed by γ -aminobutyric acid receptor subunit α -1, prostaglandin G/H synthase 1, muscarinic acetylcholine receptor M2, muscarinic acetylcholine receptor M1, sodium-dependent noradrenaline transporter, etc.

2 Target Prediction of TMP and PF

A list of potential protein targets was ranked by the inference of chemical–protein association network whose edges weighed by the bioactivity of the similar compounds to the query. The biological annotations for each target, including name, species, function and involved pathway, were also displayed (Appendix 1, Figure 4).

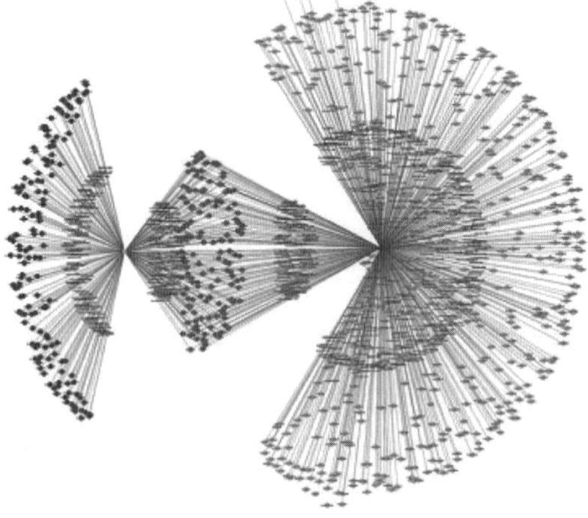

Figure 4 Target Prediction of TMP and PF

Notes: TMP (purple)and its targets (aqua), PF (yellow)and its targets (cobalt), mutual targets (magenta).

3 Target Validation

In docking analysis, TMP was able to bind ESR α (PDB code 3erd)and HIF-1 α (PDB code 5jwp), with the binding free energies were –5.67 and –6.94 kcal/mol, respectively. PF was also able to bind ESR α and HIF-1 α, with –6.94 and –5.59 kcal/mol, respectively (Figure 5).

4 Pro-angiogenic/Restorative Effect of TMP•HCl in Zebrafish Embryos

In vehicle control group, the intersegmental vessels (ISVs)sprouted and elongated from the dorsal aorta (DA)and posterior cardinal vein (PCV)to dorsal longitudinal anastomotic vessel (DLAV). [27] VRI displays anti-angiogenic properties and strongly inhibits the kinase activity of VEGF receptors. [28] VRI was demonstrated to induce significant blood vessel loss in ISVs, including a lack of physiological vessel formation and a loss of preexisting blood vessels in ISVs and DLAV in zebrafish embryos. After the treatment of TMP•HCl, several ISVs sprouted from DA or PCV, but did not reach DLAV to form intact ISVs. Moreover, VRI-induced vascular insufficiency in ISVs could be significantly rescued by TMP•HCl (10, 30 and 100 μ mol/L)post-treatment for 24 h in a dosedependent manner ($P < 0.01$). TMP•HCl at 100 μ mol/L restored ISVs sprouting close to normal level (Figure 6).

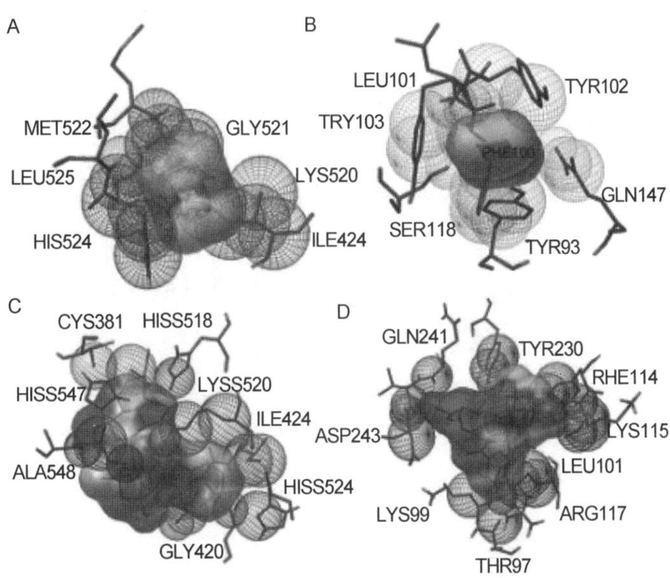

Figure 5 Ligands (TMP and PF)and Important Interactions in the Ligand-Binding Pocket of Receptors

Notes: A: TMP with ESR α; B: TMP with HIF-1α; C: PF with ESR α; D: PF with HIF-1α.

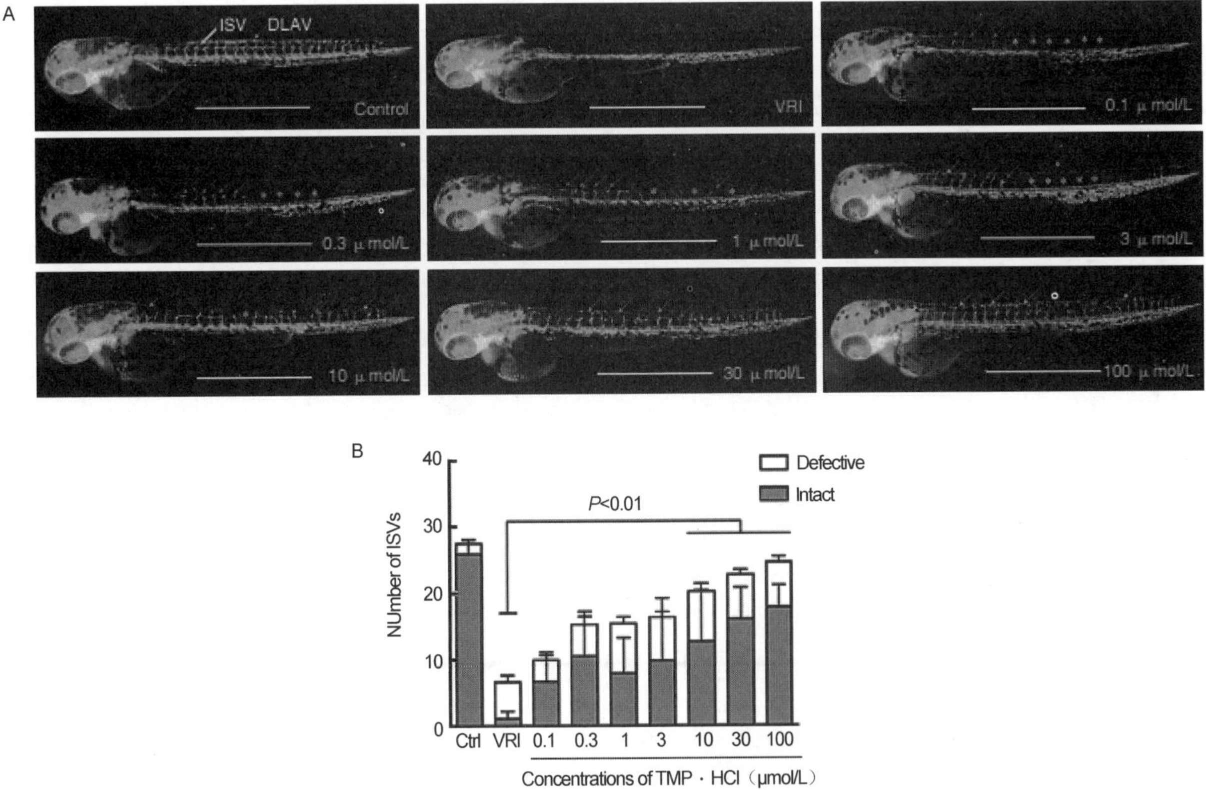

Figure 6 Pro-angiogenic Effect of TMP • HCl in Zebraflsh Embryos (n=3, $\bar{x} \pm s$)

Notes: A: VRI induced vascular insufficiency in zebrafish embryos. Yellow, blue and magenta arrows indicated normal ISVs, DLAV and abnormal ISVs, respectively. White asterisks indicated absent ISVs. B: Quantitative analysis showed the dose-dependent effect of TMP•HCl on the recovery of ISVs sprouting. Scale bar = 1.0 mm. Ctrl: control.

5 Pro-angiogenic/Restorative Effect of PF in Zebrafish Embryos

In vehicle control group, ISVs sprouted and elongated from DA and PCV to DLAV. After the treatment of PF (0.1–100 μ mol/L)for 24 h, ISVs at various concentrations sprouted from DA or PCV, but did not reach DLAV to form intact ISVs. VRI-induced vascular insufficiency in ISVs could be significantly rescued by PF at 30 μmol/L ($P < 0.01$, Figure 7).

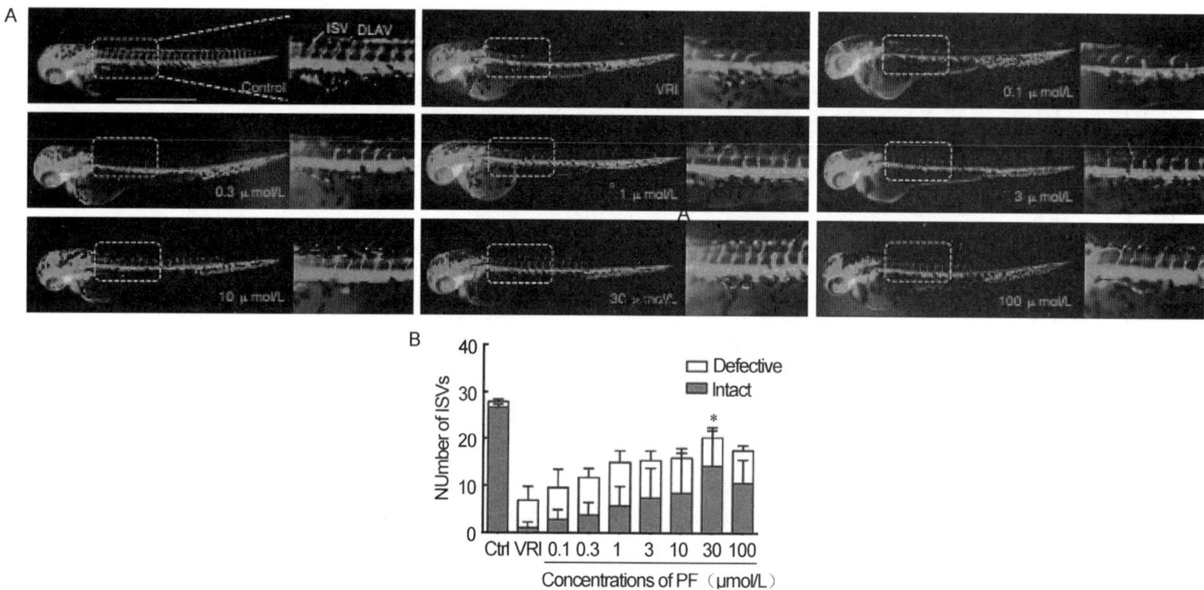

Figure 7 Pro-angiogenic Effect of PF in Zebraflsh Embryos (n=3, $\bar{x} \pm s$)

Note: A: VRI induced vascular insufficiency in zebraflsh embryos. Yellow, blue and magenta arrows indicated normal ISVs, DLAV and abnormal ISVs, respectively. White asterisks indicated absent ISVs. B: Quantitative analysis showed the dose-dependent effect of PF on the recovery of ISVs sprouting. $^*P < 0.01$, compared with the control group. Ctrl: control.

6 Synergistic Pro-angiogenic/Restorative Effect of Co-treatment of PF Paired with Different Concentrations of TMP•HCl in Zebrafish Embryos

The capacity of PF to protect against blood vessel loss in zebrafish embryos when treated at low dose (0.1–10 μ mol/L)was limited. However, this insufficiency of blood vessels could be significantly rescued by co-treatment of a lower concentration of PF (10 μ mol/L)paired with different concentrations of TMP•HCl (0.1–10 μ mol/L)for 24 h (Figure 8). The proangiogenic effect of cotreatmnet of PF 10 μ mol/L and TMP•HCl 1 μ mol/L was better than single use ($P < 0.05$). Quantitative analysis showed the PF 10 μ mol/L paired with TMP•HCl 1 μ mol/L co-treatment group might be of the optimal compatibility. TMP•HCl and PF post-treatment could promote angiogenic activity by activating ESR α (Figure 9).

DISCUSSION

In order to disclose the combination principle of CM, it is essential building the compound-target interaction profiles. [29] In this study, we applied Chuanxiong and Chishao, a representative herbpair of activating blood circulation, to analyze the network pharmacology. Subsequently, a set of CM network pharmacology methods were created to study the herbs in the context of targets and diseases networks, including predicting target profiles and pharmacological actions of main active compounds of Chuanxiong and Chishao, to prioritize disease-associated genes, and to reveal herb-gene-cardio-cerebrovascular disease co-module associations. The result showed that the targets of Chuanxiong were concentrated in the whole cardiovascular system, indicating that Chuanxiong might have antithrombotic, antihypertensive, antiarrhythmic, antiatherosclerotic effects, and be used for hypoxicischemic encephalopathy, ischemic stroke, myocardial infarction or heart failure. In addition, Chishao placed emphasis on the anti-inflammatory effect and analgesics. These data support the reasonability of the CM theory in construction of a formula (Appendix 2).

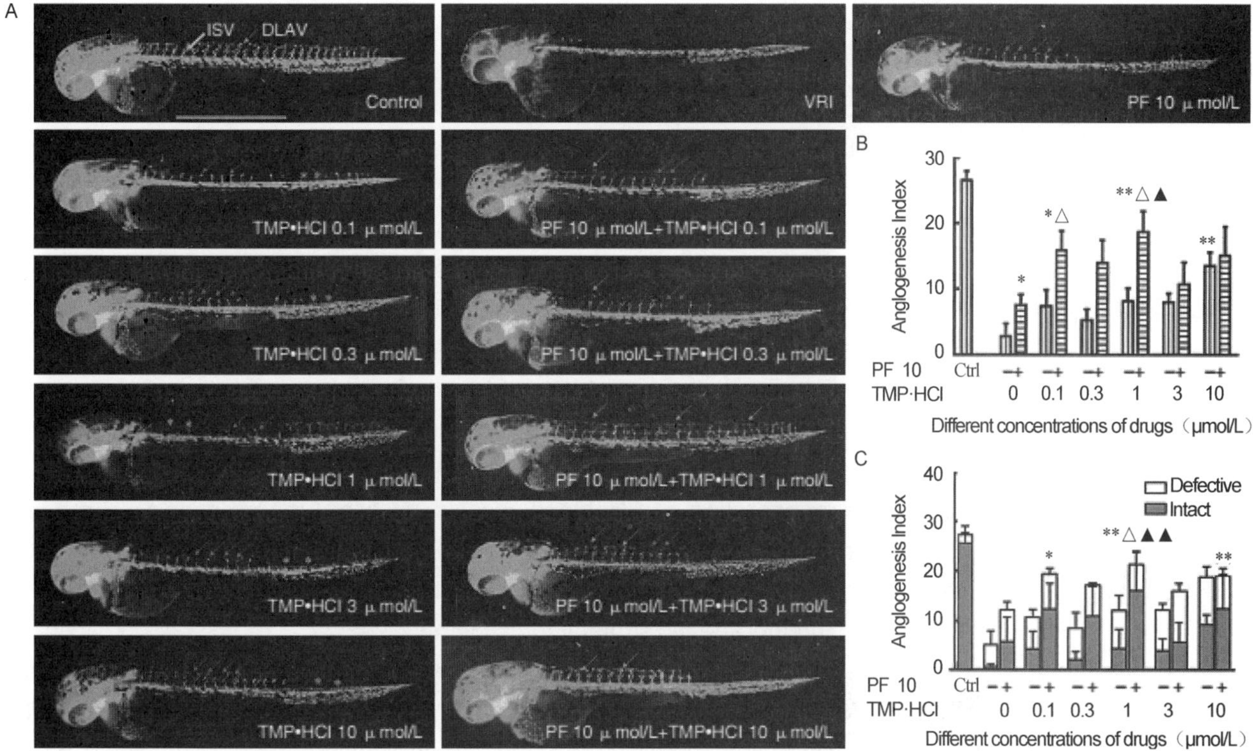

Figure 8 Pro-angiogenic Effect of Co-treatment of PF and TMP•HCl in Zebraflsh Embryos (n=3, $\bar{x} \pm s$)

Notes: A: Morphological observation of zebrafish embryos. B: After treatment of PF 10 μmol/L (with or without TMP•HCl), angiogenesis index (number of intact ISVs+0.5×number of defective ISVs)of ISVs sprouting was higher than without PF 10 μmol/L. PF 10 μmol/L paired with TMP•HCl 1 μmol/L co-treatment group showed signiflcant activity on rescuing the VRI-induced blood vessel loss in zebraflsh. $^{*}P < 0.05$, $^{**}P < 0.01$ compared with VRI group; $^{\triangle}P < 0.05$, compared with group treated with PF 10 μmol/L; $^{\blacktriangle}P < 0.05$, $^{\blacktriangle\blacktriangle}P < 0.01$ compared with corresponding group treated without PF 10 μmol/L. Ctrl: control. Yellow, blue and magenta arrows indicated normal ISVs, DLAV and abnormal ISVs, respectively. White asterisks indicated absent ISVs.

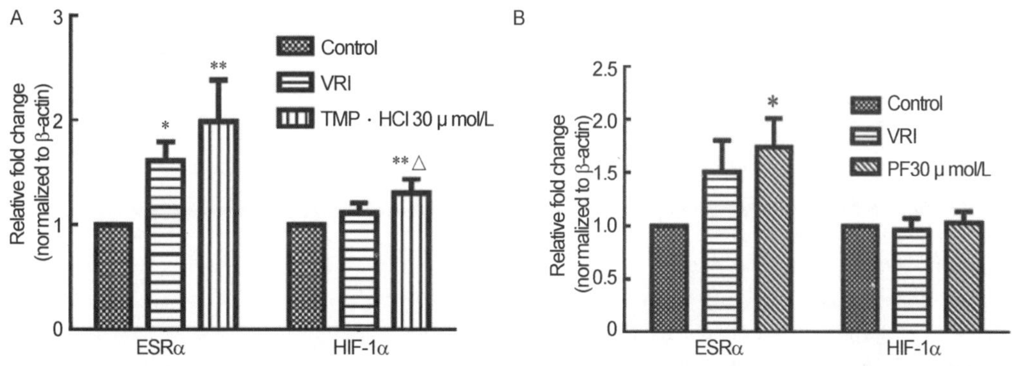

Figure 9 Effect of TMP•HCl and PF Post-treatment on ESR α Gene Expression

Notes: A and B: TMP•HCl and PF post-treatment could promote angiogenesis by activating ESR α in zebrafish embryos, respectively. $^{*}P < 0.05$, $^{**}P < 0.01$, compared with control group; $^{\triangle}P < 0.05$, compared with VRI group.

As an empirical system of multicomponent therapeutics, CM might have the potential of addressing a relationship between multicompound and drug synergistic effects, which is capable of systematically controlling various diseases such as the angiogenic disorders. [30,31] The application of network theory would be a very useful tool to visualize and analyze the interaction data among different components in the mixtures to capture the complexity in a simple, compact, and illustrative manner.

HIF-1 α is considered as the master transcriptional regulator of cellular and developmental response to decrease in available oxygen in the cellular environment, or hypoxia. [32,33] Recently, Nakada, et al [34] observed that exposure to hypoxaemia 7 days after myocardial infarction operation induced a robust regenerative response and highlighted the potential therapeutic role of hypoxia in regenerative medicine. Martínez-Lara, et al [35] demonstrated that HIF-1 α accumulation could lead to the expression of angiogenic proteins, which was ascribed to the upregulation of ESR α . There is evidence suggesting that ESR α is expressed in ECs, and that ESR α agonists, such as estrogen, could induce ECs proliferation, migration and vascular remodeling. [36,37] The molecular mechanisms of cardiovascular protection exerted by estrogens may be related a VEGF-A-delta-like ligand 4-notch1 axis signalling-mediated modulation of angiogenesis. [38] Previous study in our laboratory had demonstrated that ESR α -enhanced ROCK- Ⅱ signaling pathway activation was the critical mechanism of phytoestrogenic compounds in the promotion of angiogenesis. [39]

Previous studies had shown that TMP could inhibit neovascularization, fibrosis, thrombosis, and suppress angiogenesis and tumor growth of lung cancer. [40,41] On the contrary, the results of *in vivo* zebrafish experiment showed that VRI-pretreatment induced blood vessel loss in developing zebrafish; post-treatment of TMP · HCl and PF promoted the regeneration of new blood vessels involving up-regulating ESR α mRNA expression. The pharmacology results showed that co-treatment of TMP · HCl and PF could enhance the ISVs sprouting in VRI-induced vascular insufficiency zebrafish. Taken together, the compatibility treatment of TMP · HCl and PF might be a promising therapeutic strategy for ischemic disease.

The network pharmacological strategies combining drug target prediction and network analysis identified some putative targets of CCHP. Moreover, the transgenic zebrafish experiments demonstrated that the Chuanxiong-Chishao combination synergistically promoted angiogenic activity, probably involving ESR α signaling pathway. The discovered mechanisms of botanic drug pairs will be not only helpful to optimize the drug combinations in multi-component and multitargets therapeutics, but also critical for developing novel drug combinations that can lead to more efficient treatments of complex diseases.

REFERENCES

[1] Cheung F. TCM: made in China[J]. Nature, 2011, 480 (7378): S82-S83.

[2] Li SP, Zhao J, Yang B. Strategies for quality control of Chinese medicines[J]. J Pharm Biomed Anal, 2011, 55 (4): 802-809.

[3] Su SB, Jia W, Lu AP, et al. Evidence-based Zheng: a traditional Chinese medicine syndrome 2013[J]. Evid Based Complement Alternat Med, 2014, 2014: 1-2.

[4] Li P, Qi LW, Liu EH, et al. Analysis of Chinese herbal medicines with holistic approaches and integrated evaluation models[J]. Trends Analyt Chem, 2008, 27 (1): 66-77.

[5] Qiu J. Traditional medicine: a culture in the balance[J]. Nature, 2007, 448 (7150): 126-128.

[6] Tang F, Zhang QL, Nie Z, et al. Sample preparation for analyzing traditional Chinese medicines[J]. TrAC Trends Analytic Chem, 2009, 28 (11): 1253-1262.

[7] The State Pharmacopoeia Commission of the People's Republic of China. Chinese Pharmacopoeia[M]. Beijing: Chemical Industry Press, 2010, 1: 38.

[8] Guo M, Liu Y, Shi DZ. Cardiovascular actions and therapeutic potential of tetramethylpyrazine (active component isolated from Rhizoma Chuanxiong): roles and mechanisms[J]. Biomed Res Int, 2016, 2016: 1-9.

[9] Nizamutdinova IT, Jin YC, Kim JS, et al. Paeonol and paeoniflorin, the main active principles of Paeonia albiflora, protect the heart from myocardial ischemia/reperfusion injury in rats[J]. Planta Med, 2008, 74 (1): 14-18.

[10] Xin QQ, Yang BR, Zhou HF, et al. Paeoniflorin promotes angiogenesis in a vascular insufficiency model of zebrafish *in vivo* and in human umbilical vein endothelial cells *in vitro[J]*. Chin J Integr Med, 2016, 1-8.

[11] Franco CA, Liebner S, Gerhardt H . Vascular morphogenesis: a Wnt for every vessel? [J]. Curr Opin Genet Dev, 2009, 19 (5), 476-483.

[12] Ahn A, Frishman WH, Gutwein A, et al. Therapeutic angiogenesis: a new treatment approach for ischemic heart disease—part Ⅰ[J] . Cardiol Rev, 2008, 16 (4): 163-171.

[13] He XH, Xing DM, Ding Y, et al. Determination of paeoniflorin in rat hippocampus by high performance liquid chromatography after intravenous administration of Paeoniae Radix extract[J]. J Chromatogra B, 2004, 802 (2): 277-281.

[14] Ru JL, Li P, Wang JN, et al. TCMSP: a database of systems pharmacology for drug discovery from herbal medicines[J]. J Cheminformatics, 2014, 6 (1): 13.

[15] Knox C, Law CKV, Jewison T, et al. DrugBank 3.0: a comprehensive resource for 'omics' research on drugs[J]. Nucleic Acids Res, 2011, 39 suppl 1: 1035-1041.

[16] Ye H, Ye L, Kang H, et al. HIT: linking herbal active ingredients to targets[J]. Nucleic Acids Res, 2011, 39 suppl 1: 1055-1059.

[17] Yu H, Chen JX, Xu X, et al. A systematic prediction of multiple drug-target interactions from chemical, genomic, and pharmacological data[J]. PLoS One, 2012, 7: e37608.

[18] Zhu F, Shi Z, Qin C, et al. Therapeutic target database update 2012: a resource for facilitating target-oriented drug discovery[J]. Nucleic Acids Res, 2011, 40 (1): 1128-1136.

[19] Shannon P, Markiel A, Ozier O, et al. Cytoscape: a software environment for integrated models of biomolecular interaction networks[J]. Genome Res, 2003, 13 (11): 2498-2504.

[20] Azuaje FJ, Zhang L, Devaux Y, et al. Drug-target network in myocardial infarction reveals multiple side effects of unrelated drugs[J]. Sci Reports, 2011, 1: 52.

[21] Li XX, Xu X, Wang JN, et al. A system-level investigation into the mechanisms of Chinese traditional medicine: Compound Danshen Formula for cardiovascular disease treatment[J]. PLoS One, 2012, 7 (9): e43918.

[22] Westerfield M, ed. A guide for the laboratory usc of zebrafish (Danio rerio)[M]. The zebrafish book. 5th ed. Eugene: University of Oregon Press, 2007.

[23] Kabir ME, Singh H, Lu R, et al. G protein-coupled estrogen receptor 1 mediates acute estrogen-induced cardioprotection via MEK/ERK/GSK-3β pathway after ischemia/reperfusion[J]. PLoS One, 2015, 10: e0135988.

[24] Vecoli C. Endothelial nitric oxide synthase gene polymorphisms in cardiovascular disease[J]. Vitam Horm, 2014, 96: 387-406.

[25] Frishman WH. Beta-adrenergic receptor blockers in hypertension: alive and well[J]. Prog Cardiovasc Dis, 2016, 59: 247-252.

[26] Mohamed RA, Agha AM, Abdel-Rahman AA, et al. Role of adenosine A2A receptor in cerebral ischemia reperfusion injury: Signaling to phosphorylated extracellular signal-regulated protein kinase (pERK1/2)[J]. Neuroscience, 2016, 314: 145-159.

[27] Isogai S, Lawson ND, Torrealday S, et al. Angiogenic network formation in the developing vertebrate trunk[J]. Development, 2003, 130 (21): 5281-5290.

[28] Furet P, Bold G, Hofmann F, et al. Identification of a new chemical class of potent angiogenesis inhibitors based on conformational considerations and database searching[J]. Bioorg Med Chem Lett, 2003, 13 (18): 2967-2971.

[29] Rix U, Superti-Furga G. Target profiling of small molecules by chemical proteomics[J]. Nature Chem Biol, 2009, 5 (9): 616-624.

[30] Li XM, Brown L. Efficacy and mechanisms of action of traditional Chinese medicines for treating asthma and allergy[J]. J Allergy Clin Immunol, 2009, 123 (2): 297-306.

[31] Schmidt BM, Ribnicky DM, Lipsky PE, et al. Revisiting the ancient concept of botanical therapeutics[J]. Nature Chem Biol, 2007, 3 (7): 360-366.

[32] Wang GL, Jiang BH, Rue EA, et al. Hypoxiainducible factor 1 is a basic-helix-loop-helix-PAS heterodimer regulated by cellular O2 tension[J]. Proc Natl Acad Sci, 1995, 92: 5510-5514.

[33] Iyer NV, Kotch LE, Agani F, et al. Cellular and developmental control of O2 homeostasis by hypoxia-inducible factor 1 α[J] . Genes Dev, 1998, 92 (12): 149-162.

[34] Nakada YJ, Canseco DC, Thet SW, Abdisalaam S, Asaithamby A, Santos CX, et al. Hypoxia induces heart regeneration in adult mice[J]. Nature, 2017, 541: 222-227.

[35] Martínez-Lara E, Peña A, Calahorra J, et al. Hydroxytyrosol decreases the oxidative and nitrosative stress levels and promotes angiogenesis through HIF-1 independent mechanisms in renal hypoxic cells[J]. Food Function, 2016, 7: 540-548.

[36] Arnal JF, Fontaine C, Billon-Galés A, et al. Estrogen receptors and endothelium[J]. Arterioscl Thromb Vascul Biol, 2010, 30 (8): 1506-1512.

[37] Gopal S, Garibaldi S, Goglia L, et al. Estrogen regulates endothelial migration via plasminogen activator inhibitor (PAI-1)[J]. Mol Human Reprod, 2012, 18 (8): 410-416.

[38] Caliceti C, Aquila G, Pannella M, et al. 17β -Estradiol enhances signaling mediated by VEGF-A-delta-like ligand 4-notch1 axis in human endothelial cells[J]. PloS One, 2013, 8: e71440.

[39] Li S, Dang YY, Zhou XL, et al. Formononetin promotes angiogenesis through the estrogen receptor alpha-enhanced ROCK pathway[J]. Sci Reports, 2015, 5: 16815.

[40] Cai XX, Chen Z, Pan XK, et al. Inhibition of angiogenesis, fibrosis and thrombosis by tetramethylpyrazine: mechanisms contributing to the SDF-1/CXCR4 axis[J]. PLoS One, 2014, 9: e88176.

[41] Jia YC, Wang ZG, Zang AM, et al. Tetramethylpyrazine inhibits tumor growth of lung cancer through disrupting angiogenesis via BMP/Smad/Id-1 signaling[J]. Int J Oncol, 2016, 48 (5): 2079-2086.

First published: WANG Yan, GUO Gang, YANG Bin-Rui, XIN Qi-qi, LIAO Qi-wen, LEE Simon Ming-Yuen, HU Yuan-jia, CHEN Ke-ji, CONG Wei-hong. Synergistic effects of Chuanxiong-Chishao herb-pair on promoting angiogenesis at network pharmacological and pharmacodynamic levels[J] . Chin J Integr Med, 2017, 23: 654-662.

Zedoary Guaiane-Type Sesquiterpenes-Eluting Stents Accelerate Endothelial Healing without Neointimal Hyperplasia in a Porcine Coronary Artery Model

CUI Yuan-yuan, ZHAO Fu-hai, LIU Jian-gang, Wang Xin, DU Jian-peng, SHI Da-zhuo, and CHEN Ke-ji

Drug-eluting stents (DES)have effectively suppressed neointimal hyperplasia in patients undergoing percutaneous coronary interventions. [1] However, concern about DES-induced late stent thrombosis has raised. [2] Pathological studies have implicated incomplete reendothelialization induced by DES as a potential mechanism for late thrombotic events. [2,3] The antiproliferative drugs (sirolimus and paclitaxel)-associated antihealing effect plays a crucial role in deendothelialization. [4] Therefore, looking for a kind of drugs to facilitate endothelial healing along with inhibiting neointimal hyperplasia is encouraged in next generation stents.

Red arrow indicated naked struts, black arrow indicated platelets, and arrowhead indicated inflammatory cells. ZES: ZGS-eluting stents, SES: sirolimus-eluting stents, BMS: bare-metal stents.

Curcuma zedoaria, a Chinese medicinal herb, has been used to treat cancers for more than 100 years, including gastric cancer, [5] hepatoma, [6] and uterine cervical cancer, [7] while it has low toxicity on normal cells, such as human umbilical vein endothelial cells (HUVECs), [8] gastric epithelial cells, [9] and fibroblasts of human mucus lineage. [10] Moreover, Curcuma zedoaria has been demonstrated to prevent inflammation, [11,12] oxidant, [13] and hepatic injury activities. [14] Zedoary guaiane-type sesquiterpenoids (ZGS)are bioactive constituents of Curcuma zedoaria. Our previous study has demonstrated their effects on inhibiting neointimal hyperplasia in a porcine model. [15] However, the influence of ZGS on early reendothelialization *in vivo* and *in vitro* remains unclear. Therefore, the effects of ZGS on endothelial healing were examined in a porcine coronary artery model and detected by HUVECs.

METHODS

1 Stent Preparation

The stent platforms used were polymer-free 316L stainless metal with in situ nano/micropores on the surface. These nano/micropores ranged from 400 nm to 1 mm to release drugs steadily. The ZGS was kindly provide by Dalian Institute of Chemical Physics, Chinese Academy of Sciences, Dalian, China. The ZGS-eluting stents (ZES)were made by coating ZGS into the nano/micropores via freeze–drying technique. Sirolimus-eluting stents (SES; Lepu Medical Company, Beijing, China)and bare metal stents (BMS; Lepu Medical Company)with identical platforms were used as controls. All stents used in the experiments were 15 mm in length and 2.0 to 3.5 mm in diameter.

2 Stent Implantation

The process of experiment was conformed to the Guide for the Care and Use of Laboratory Animals published by the US National Institutes of Health (NIH Publication Number 85-23, revised 1996). The study protocol was approved by the Institutional Animal Care and Use Committee of Xiyuan Hospital.

Chinese minipigs (weight, 25-35 kg)were premedicated with aspirin (300 mg), clopidogrel (300 mg), and antibiotics (penicillin 1 g)orally 24 hours prior to stenting. Those animals were anesthetized with ketamine (20 mg/kg, intramuscularly [IM]), diazepam (0.4 mg/kg, IM), and 3% sodium pentobarbital via the marginal ear vein (25 mg/kg, intravenously). A 6F sheath was inserted into the right or left femoral artery under sterile conditions. Heparin (5000-10 000 U)was administered through the sheath to maintain an activated clotting time (250-300 seconds). Nitroglycerin was injected to avoid vasospasm. Coronary angiography was undertaken using Judkin-3.5 guiding catheter. The appropriate stent was delivered to the intended site with a stent to artery diameter ratio of 1.2: 1.0. Continuous hemodynamic and electrocardiographic monitoring was performed throughout the procedure. In each animal, the stents were randomly deployed into 3 coronary arteries. During the follow-up period, animals received oral aspirin (100 mg)and oral clopidogrel (50 mg)daily with a standard diet in the animal laboratory center.

3 Scanning Electron Microscopy Examination

Scanning electron microscopy (SEM)was carried out at 7, 14, and 28 days. The rate of reendothelialization was assessed by SEM (HITACHI S-3400N, Japan). Stented segments were opened longitudinally by fixing in 3% glutaraldehyde, then dried with liquid CO2, and coated with gold. The SEM photo-micrographs of each specimen were examined using a computer-assisted digital assessment system to determine the percentage of vascular coverage area compared to the total luminal surface area. Rate of endothelialization (%E)=(1-[nonendothelialized area/total stent area]) × 100[16].

4 Histomorphometry and Histopathology

Histological examination was performed at 7, 14, and 28 days. The hearts were harvested as described previously. [17] Stented segments were dehydrated in a graded series of ethanol, embedded in methylmethacrylate plastic, and stained with hematoxylin and eosin and elastic Van Gieson stains. Morphometric measurements were evaluated, including lumen area, stent area, neointimal area, and percentage of stenosis of each section, as described previously. [18]

For the pathological assessment, scores for reendothelialization, inflammation, and microthrombi of each stent were evaluated. Reendothelialization score with endothelial cells adhesion was assigned according to a semi-quantitative grading scale [18-20]: 0 for absent endothelium, 1 for present but＜25% of the lumen circumference, 2 for between 25% and 75% of the circumference, and 3 for complete endothelialization. Strut-associated inflammation was graded as follows: 0 for none, 1 for scattered inflammatory cells, 2 for moderate to dense cellular aggregate surrounding the strut noncircumferentially, and 3 for circumferential dense inflammatory cells infiltration of the strut. The microthrombi were assessed semi-quantitatively by the following scale21: values of 0 corresponding to absence; 1 for focal findings involving any portion of the artery but＜25% of the circumference of the artery; 2 for moderate accumulations involving＜25% of the circumference of the artery; and 3 for severe, involving＞25% of the circumference of the artery.

5 Cell Culture

The HUVECs were kindly provided by Women and Children's hospital of Haidian (Beijing, China). Cells were routinely cultured in endothelial cell medium (ECM; ScienCell, America)in a humidified atmosphere of 5% CO_2 at 37 ℃. Cells were subcultured once they reached 90% to 95% confluence. In all experiments, cells were used at passages 3 to 7.

6 Cell Viability Assay

The viability of cells was determined using the 3- (4, 5-dimethylthiazol-2yl)-2, 5-diphenyl-2H-tetrazoliumbromide (MTT)assay. The HUVECs were inoculated at a density of 5×10^4/mL in 96-well plates and treated with ECM containing different concentrations of ZGC (0, 10, 20, 40, 60, 80, 100, 200, 400, 600, 800, and 1000 mg/mL)for 24 and 72 hours. The original medium was removed, and 20 mL of 5% MTT was added to each well. Incubation of 4 hours required a humidified atmosphere containing 5% CO_2 and 95% air at 37 ℃ until MTT was taken up by active cells. Then, the medium was discarded, and the precipitated formazan was dissolved in 100 mL of dimethyl sulfoxide. The absorption value was measured at 490nm.

Table 1 Histological Results 7 Days After Implantation [a]

	ZES (*n* = 6)	SES (*n* = 6)	BMS (*n* = 6)
Neointimal area, mm^2	0.65 ± 0.27	0.79 ± 0.27	0.97 ± 0.26[b]
Lumen area, mm^2	3.32 ± 0.67	2.72 ± 0.25	2.64 ± 0.57
Stent area, mm^2	3.96 ± 0.36	3.50 ± 0.28	3.62 ± 0.49
Stenosis, %	22.52 ± 7.50	14.17 ± 2.64	22.84 ± 2.82
Naked strut, %	11.39 ± 5.58	51.82 ± 16.70[c]	47.79 ± 12.87[c]

Abbreviations: : BMS, bare metal stent ; SD, standard deviation ; SES, Sirolimus-eluting stent (SES) ; ZES zedoary guaiane-type sesquiterpenes-based eluting stent. [a]Data are presented as mean ± SD for each parameter. [b]$P < 0.05$ versus ZES. [c]$P < 0.01$ versus ZES.

Table 2 Histological Results 14 Days After Implantation [a]

	ZES (*n* =6)	SES (*n* = 6)	BMS (*n* =6)
Neointimal area, mm^2	0.78 ± 0.34	1.02 ± 0.39	1.56 ± 0.52[b]
Lumen area, mm^2	3.23 ± 0.21	2.88 ± 0.48	2.08 ± 0.71[b]
Stent area, mm^2	4.01 ± 0.45	3.91 ± 0.22	3.65 ± 0.32
Stenosis, %	18.90 ± 6.65	26.34 ± 10.44	38.60 ± 11.35[b]
Naked strut, %	9.47 ± 5.61	44.52 ± 24.98[c]	19.61 ± 3.55[c]

Abbreviations: BMS, bare metal stent ; SD, standard deviation ; SES, Sirolimus-eluting stent (SES) ; ZES zedoary guaiane-type sesquiterpenes-based eluting stent. [a]Data are presented as mean ± SD for each parameter. [b]$P < 0.01$ versus ZES. [c]$P < 0.05$ versus ZES.

Table 3 Histological Results 28 Days After Implantation [a]

	ZGS (*n*=9)	SES (*n*=9)	BMS (*n*=9)
Neointim area, mm^2	1.07 ± 0.48	0.94 ± 0.12	1.73 ± 0.69[b]
Lumen area, mm^2	2.77 ± 0.50	2.43 ± 0.80	2.12 ± 0.64[c]
Stent area, mm^2	3.84 ± 0.47	3.37 ± 0.86	3.92 ± 0.47
Stenosis, %	27.66 ± 12.20	28.87 ± 6.00	44.08 ± 15.03[b]
Naked strut/section, %	2.50 ± 3.75	22.10 ± 24.24c	13.99 ± 15.11

Abbreviations: BMS, bare metal stent ; SD, standard deviation ; SES, Sirolimus-eluting stent (SES) ; ZES zedoary guaiane-type sesquiterpenes-based eluting stent. [a] Data are presented as mean ± SD for each parameter. [b] $P < 0.01$ versus ZES. [c] $P < 0.05$ versus ZES.

7 Cell Cycle Assay

The cell cycle was analyzed by flow cytometry. The HUVECs were plated at a density of 1×10^5 cells/mL, treated with either ECM-containing sirolimus (1 g/mL)or different concentrations of ZGS (0, 600, 800, and 1000 mg/mL)for 24 hours. After harvesting, the cells were washed and fixed with ice-cold alcohol (75%)for more than 24 hours. Then, the cells were incubated with phosphate buffered saline (pH 7.4)containing RNaseA (5U)and propidium iodide (50 g/mL)for 15 minutes at 37 ℃. All samples were analyzed on a flow cytometry system. The percentage of cells in each phase of the cell cycle was estimated using the program of Cell FIT cell cycle analysis (Beckman Coulter, Germany).

8 Statistical Analysis

All results are expressed as mean ± standard deviation or standard error of the mean. Statistical comparisons were performed by 1-way analysis of variance with post hoc analysis for multiple comparisons. A P value of < . 05 was considered statistically significant. Statistical analyses were carried out using SPSS v16.0 software.

RESULTS

There were 21 Chinese minipigs implanted with 63 stents (ZES =21, SES=21, and BMS=21)in our experiment. All animals survived. One of the pigs in the BMS group had ventricular fibrillation while was saved by electrical defibrillation on time.

1 Scanning Electron Microscopy Findings

Seven days after implantation, 94.04% ± 5.01% of ZES was covered by neointima compared to either SES (47.59% ± 19.91%, $P < 0.01$)or BMS (59.58 ± 19.61, $P < 0.05$). At 14 days, the percentage of reendothelialization area was 96.37% ± 1.86% for ZES, 87.51% ± 8.58% for BMS, and 69.22% ± 16.44% for SES ($P < 0.05$ for ZES vs SES). At 28 days, the percentage of coverage area was 98.51% ± 1.86% for ZES, 86.18% ± 8.16% for SES ($P < 0.05$ for ZES vs SES), and 94.26% ± 5.58% for BMS, as shown in Figure 1.

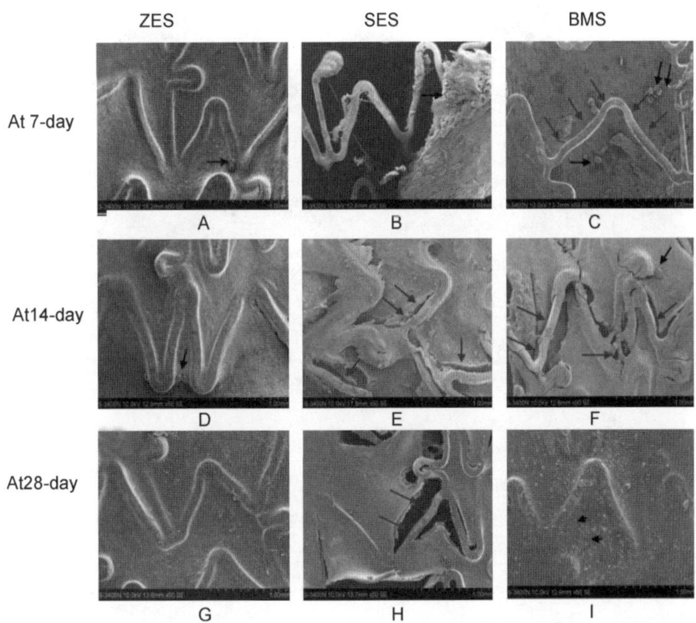

Figure 1 Scanning Electron Microscopy Showed re-endothelialization of Different Stents After Implantation (x50). (A), (D), and (G)Great endothelial coverage were observed in ZES. (B), (E), and (H)Uncovered struts were seen in SES. (C), (F), and (I) Different degree of endothelial coverage were showed in BMS. Although complete coverage was observed in BMS at 28 days, whereas mass of inflammatory cells were adhered.

2 Histomorphometric Analysis

Histomophometric analyses at different times are illustrated in Tables 1 to 3. Average injury score among the groups was of no difference ($P > 0.05$). At 7 days, there were no differences in the stent and lumen areas between ZES (3.96 ± 0.36 mm^2, 3.32 ± 0.67 mm^2), SES (3.50 ± 0.28 mm^2, 2.72 ± 0.25 mm^2), and BMS (3.62 ± 0.49 mm^2, 2.64 ± 0.57 mm^2, whereas percentage of naked struts was significantly less in ZES (11.39% ± 5.58%)when compared to SES (51.82% ± 16.70%, $P < 0.01$)or BMS (47.79% ± 12.87%, $P < 0.01$). At 14 days, nearly complete endothelial coverage was observed in ZES. Both SES and BMS showed naked struts. Moreover, SES exhibited stent thrombosis at 14 days. At 28 days, neointimal area, lumen area, and stent area were similar between ZES and SES, while percentages of naked struts per section were lower in ZES (2.50 % ± 3.75%)than SES (22.10% ± 24.24%, $P < 0.05$). Furthermore, neointimal area was much lower in ZES (1.07 ± 0.48 mm^2)than in BMS (1.73 ± 0.69 mm^2, $P < 0.01$), as shown in Figure 2.

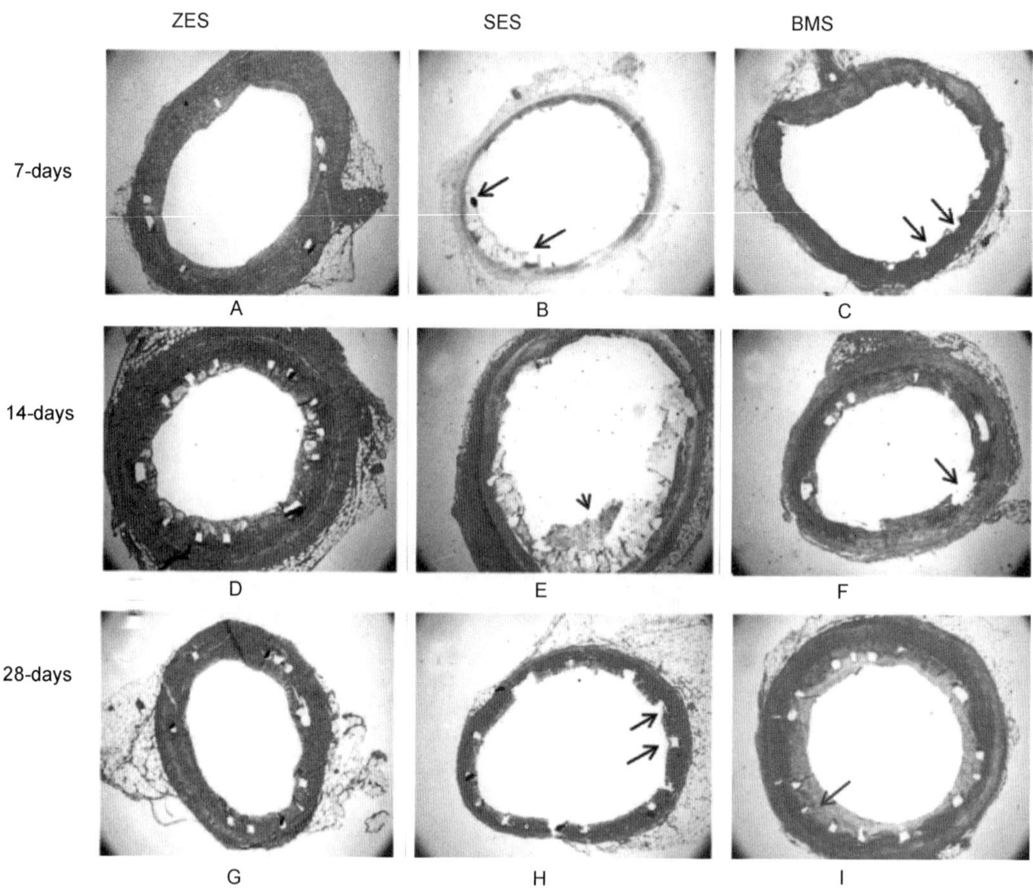

Figure 2　Histomorphology of Different Stents After Implantation (40)

Notes: (A), (D), and (G)Cross section of ZES showed complete endothe-lialium with thin neointimal thickness at 7, 14, and 28 days. (B), (E), and (H)uncovered struts were seen in SES at 7, 14, and 28 days. (C), (F), and (I)BMS showed nearly covered vessel surface, whereas neointimal hyperplasia was seen at 28 days. Black arrow indicated naked strut, arrowhead indicated stent-thrombus, and red arrow indicated neointimal hyperplasia.

3 Histopathological Analysis

The histopathological analyses were performed. At 28 days, reendothelialization score in ZES (2.83 ± 0.41)was higher than those in SES (1.43 ± 0.79, $P < 0.01$), while no difference was observed in BMS (2.17 ± 0.41, $P > 0.05$; Figure 3). Furthermore, the inflammation score was lower in ZES than either in SES or in BMS (both $P < 0.01$)at 28 days (Figure 4). And microthrombi were lower in ZES in compared with SES ($P < 0.05$)while was not different compared to BMS ($P > 0.05$). None of the stent thrombosis was observed in ZES during the experiment, whereas 2 cases in SES and 1 case in BMS occurred.

4 The Cell Viability Analysis and the Cell Cycle Analysis

The ZGS showed no harmful effect on HUVECs viability in comparison with the control group at 24 hours (data not shown). At 72 hours, increased viability was seen in ZGS, whereas sirolimus significantly reduced

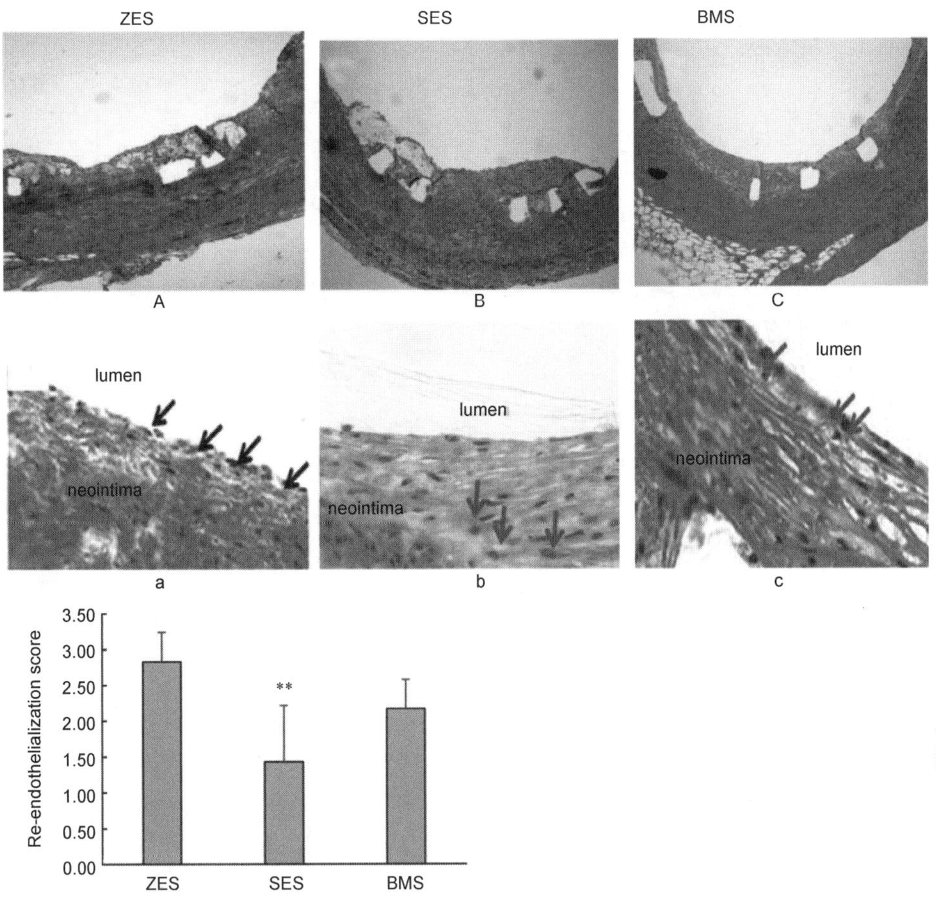

Figure 3 Re-endothelialization of Different Stents at 28 Days

Notes: (A), (B), and (C)Different stents exhibited the degree of re-endothelialization after implantation (100x). (a), (b)and (c) represented ports of (A), (B)and (C), respectively (400x). Black arrow indicated endothelial cells, and red arrow indicated inflammatory cells. Data stated mean+SD. $^{**}P < 0.01$, compared to ZMS.

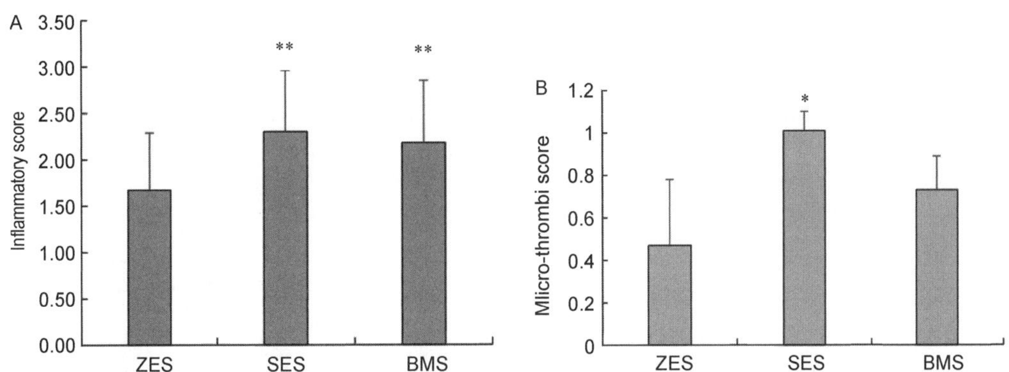

Figure 4 Inflammation and Micro-thrombi Scores for Stents at 28days

Notes: ZES indicated ZGS-eluting stents; SES, sirolimus-eluting stents; BMS, bare metal stents. Data are stated mean+SD (A) or mean +SE (B). $^{*}P < .05$, $^{**}P < .01$, compared to ZES.

HUVECs viability ($P < 0.01$)when compared to the control group (Figure 5).

Compared to the control group, ZGS (800 and 1000 mg/mL)and sirolimus suppressed HUVECs at G0/G1 phage. However, the concentrations of ZGS (600, 800, and 1000 mg/mL)showed reduced inhibition of cell cycle at G0/G1 phase (60.33% ± 3.00%, 63.64% ± 1.59%, 65.47% ± 8.26%)whencompared to sirolimus (73.88% ± 2.47%), as shown in Figure 6.

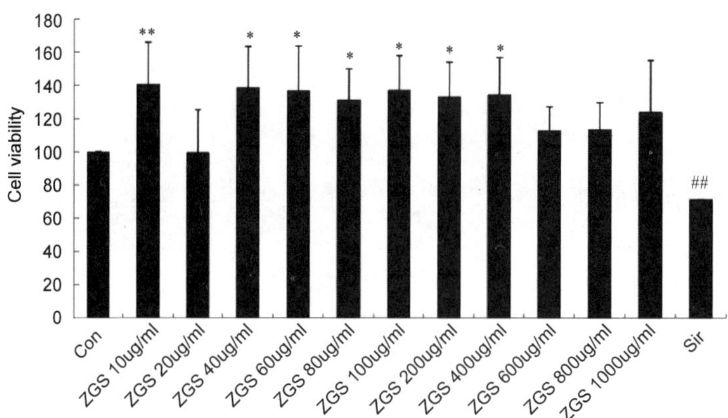

Figure 5　Improvement the Viability of HUVECs Treated with ZGS

Notes: HUVECs were incubated with ZGS (10*1000ug/ml)or sirolimus (1ug/ml)for 72 h. Values were mean + SE. Con indicated control group. Sir, sirolimus group. *$P < 0.05$, **$P < 0.01$ compared to Con; ##$P < 0.01$ compared to Con.

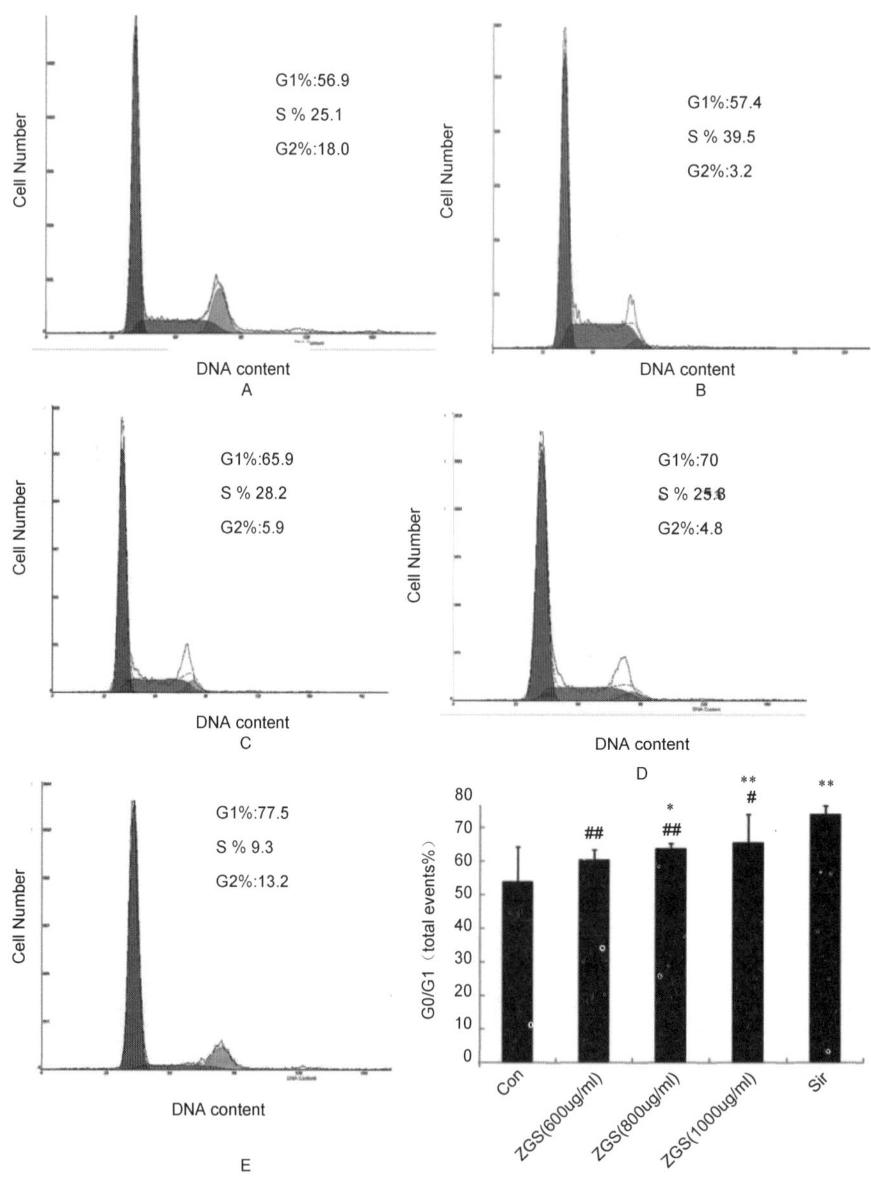

Figure 6　Effect of ZGS on the Cell Cycle of HUVECs

Notes: Cells were incubated with either increasing concentrations of ZGS (600*1 000 μg/mL)or sirolimus (1ug/ml)for 24 h. A*E indicated Con, ZGS (600 μg/mL), ZGS (800 μg/mL), ZGS (1 000 μg/mL), and siroliums (1ug/ml), respectively. Conindicated control group, Sir, sirolimus group. Values were means+SD, **$P < 0.01$, compared to control; #$P < 0.05$, ##$P < 0.01$, compared to the Sir.

DISCUSSION

The present study demonstrated that ZGS-based eluting stents nearly accomplished endothelial coverage 7 days after implantation and maintained thin neointima as effective as SES in a porcine coronary injury model at 28 days. Moreover, less inflammatory response was observed in ZES when compared to either SES or BMS. Microthrombi in ZES were significantly less than SES. In addition, ZGS also improved cell viability and reduced suppression of cell cycle at G0/G1 phase when compared to sirolimus.

Despite suppressing neointimal hyperplasia, sirolimus delays endothelial regrowth and function, therefore contributing to late thrombotic events to some extent. Looking for anti-proliferative drugs with less toxicity toward normal cells seems especially necessary. Previous studies demonstrated that Curcuma zedoaria, as an anticancer drug, has demonstrated to have less negative effects on normal cells, [8-10] showing that fibroblasts of human mucus lineage maintained stable cell viability from 0hours to 7 days, when treated with Curcuma zedoaria extract. In the present study, we found that ZGS, bioactive substances extracted from Curcuma zedoaria, increased the viability rates of HUVECs and significantly reduced the sup-pression of HUVECs cycle at the G0/G1 phase in comparison with sirolimus. Hence, ZGS had favorable endothelial viability and proliferation, indicating the advantages of its use in stents materials.

Using a stent implantation injury model, Rogers et al [22] demonstrated that despite a 60% loss in the endothelial cell monolayer within 1 hour after direct stent implantation, complete regeneration of the damaged endothelial cell layer occurred within 14 days. In the present study, ZES completed reendothelialization at 7 days. Although BMS completed reendothelialization at 14 days, neointimal hyperplasia was observed at 28 days. Part of SES struts were still naked during the experiment. Moreover, ZES suppressed neointimal hyperplasia as effective as SES. Histomorphology in our research showed that neointimal area and thickness, lumen area, and restenosis percentage were not different between ZES and SES, suggesting that ZES could promote reendothelialization effectively along with thin neointima.

Pathological studies demonstrated that Curcuma zedoaria inhibits growth of cancer cells at S/G (2)or induces cancer cell apoptosis by cleavage and activation of caspase-3, -8, and -9, polymerase cytochrome C translocation, or loss of mitochondrial membrane potential. [6, 23] Although the detailed mechanisms of suppression of smooth muscle cell (SMC)proliferation after treatment with ZGS was not investigated, it was obvious that reestablishment of an intact endothelium can inhibit SMC proliferation in our study and others. [24]

The layer of endothelial cells on the luminal surface of stents indicates restoration of an intact endothelium, serving as a natural "barrier" to regulate a variety of functions including inhibiting thrombosis and inflammation. [25,26] However, there was discrepancy among ZES, SES and BMS in neointimal components and the vascular responses. Hara et al [27] analyzed the neointimal tissue of stents in a rabbit study using intravascular near-infrared fluorescence molecular imaging, showing greater fibrin deposition and fibrin persistence in DES than in BMS at 7 and 28 days, respectively. Consistent with previous findings, [19] we also observed that less endothelial cells were adherent on neointimal surface of SES, hinting that neointima with less endothelial cells do not possess intimal functions, and endothelium of BMS may not be functional as reflected by inflammatory cells adhesion. In contrast, a layer of endothelialcells was adhesive onto the surface of ZES neointima, which could prevent against inflammation and thrombosis.

Persistent inflammatory cell infiltration largely induced by incomplete endothelium is a key factor to form late stent thrombosis. [28,29] In the present study, the relatively low level of inflammation in ZES was observed, whereas inflammation in both SES and BMS was increased, respectively, at 28 days. Accumulating researches have already identified the effects of sesquiterpenes of Curcuma zedoaria in preventinginflammatory responses. [12,30-32] Cho et al [33] demonstrated that zedoarondiol, a compound of ZGS, dose dependently inhibited lipopolysaccharide-stimulated tumor necrosis factor a, interleukin (IL)6, and IL-1b production in

RAW 264.7 macrophage and mouse peritoneal macrophage cells by sup-pressing the phosphorylation of Nuclear factor-kappB (IkappB)kinase (IKK)and Mitogen-activated protein kinases (MAPKs)and subsequently by inactivating the nuclear factor-kB pathway. This demonstrates that ZES prevents inflammation. In addition, research also showed that inflammation is closely associated with thrombosis. 34 There was no in-stent thrombosis in ZES, while these events occurred in both SES and BMS. The mechanism of antithrombosis in ZES required further investigation.

Although the animal studies demonstrated overall favorable outcomes using the ZGS-based eluting stents, it may be possible that the results will have disparity when applied to an atherosclerotic state. However, certain contents of Curcuma zedoaria have protective role against hypercholesterolemic and lipidemic conditions via modulation of PPAR-a, LXR-a, and associated genes involved in lipid metabolism and transport. [35,36] The effects of ZGS on cholesterol metabolism merit exportation in detail.

CONCLUSION

The present study suggested that ZGS-based eluting stents enhanced reendothelialization with suppression of neointimal hyperplasia in a porcine coronary artery model.

REFERENCES

[1] Pache J, Dibra A, Mehilli J, Dirschinger J, Scho ¨ mig A, Kastrati A. Drug-eluting stents compared with thin-strut bare stents for the reduction of restenosis: a prospective, randomized trial [J]. Eur Heart J, 2005, 26 (13): 1262-1268.

[2] Finn AV, Joner M, Nakazawa G, Kolodgie F, Newell J, John MC, Gold HK, Virmani R. Pathological correlates of late drug-eluting stent thrombosis: strut coverage as a marker of endothelialization [J]. Circulation, 2007, 115 (18): 2435-2441.

[3] Nakazawa G, Finn AV, Joner M, Ladich E, Kutys R, Mont EK, Gold HK, Burke AP, Kolodgie FD, Virmani R. Delayed arterial healing and increased late stent thrombosis at culprit sites after drug-eluting stent placement for acute myocardial infarction patients: an autopsy study [J]. Circulation, 2008, 118 (11): 1138-1145.

[4] Clever YP, Cremers B, Krauss B, Böhm M, Speck, U, Laufs U. Scheller B. Paclitaxel and sirolimus differentially affect growth and motility of endothelial progenitor cells and coronary artery smooth muscle cells. Eurointervention, 7 Suppl K (K), K32-42. . Paclitaxel and sirolimus differentially affect growth and motility of endothelial progenitor cells and coronary artery smooth muscle cells [J]. EuroIntervention, 2011, 7 (suppl K): K32-K42.

[5] Shi H, Tan B, Ji G, Lu L, Cao A, Shi S, Xie JQ. Zedoary oil (Ezhu You)inhibits proliferation of AGS cells[C]. Chin Med, 2013, 8: 13.

[6] Xiao Y, Yang FQ, Li SP, Hu G, Lee SM, Wang YT. Essential oil of Curcuma wenyujin induces apoptosis in human hepatoma cells [J]. World J Gastroenterol, 2008, 14 (27): 4309-4318.

[7] Sun XY, Zheng YP, Lin DH, Zhang H, Zhao F, Yuan CS. Potential anti-cancer activities of Furanodiene, a Sesquiterpene from Curcuma wenyujin [J]. Am J Chin Med, 2009, 37 (3): 589-596.

[8] Chen W, Lu Y, Gao M, Wu J, Wang A, Shi R. Anti-angiogenesis effect of essential oil from Curcuma zedoaria in vitro and in vivo [J]. J Ethnopharmacol, 2011, 133 (1): 220-226.

[9] Rouhollahi E, Moghadamtousi SZ, Hamdi OA, Fadaeinasab M, Hajrezaie M, Awang K, Looi CY, Abdulla MA, Mohamed Z. Evaluation of acute toxicity and gastroprotective activity of curcuma purpurascens BI. rhizome against ethanol-induced gastric mucosal injury in rats [J]. BMC Complement Altern Med, 2014, 14: 378.

[10] Fernandes JP, Mello-Moura AC, Marques MM, Nicoletti MA. Cytotoxicity evaluation of Curcuma zedoaria (Christm.)Roscoe fluid extract used in oral hygiene products [J]. Acta Odontol Scand, 2012, 70 (6): 610-614.

[11] Tohda C, Nakayama N, Hatanaka F, Komatsu K. Comparison of anti-inflammatory activities of six curcuma rhizomes: a possible curcuminoid-independent pathway mediated by curcuma phaeocaulis extract [J]. Evid Based Complement Alternat Med, 2006, 3 (2): 255-260.

[12] Makabe H, Maru N, Kuwabara A, Kamo T, Hirota M. Anti-inflammatory sesquiterpenes from Curcuma zedoaria [J]. Nat Prod Res, 2006, 20 (7): 680-685.

[13] Tao QF, Xu Y, Lam RY, Schneider B, Dou H, Leung P S, Shi SY, Zhou CX, Yang LX, Zhang RP, Xiao YC, Wu XM, Stockigt J, Zeng S, Cheng CH, Zhao Y. Diarylheptanoids and a monoterpenoid from the rhizomes of Zingiber officinale: antioxidant and cytoprotective properties [J]. J Nat Prod, 2008, 71 (1): 12-17.

[14] Matsuda H, Morikawa T, Ninomiya K, Yoshikawa M. Hepato protective constituents from Zedoariae rhizoma: absolute stereostructures of three new carabrane-type sesquiterpenes, curcumenolactones A, B, and C [J]. Bioorg Med Chem, 2001, 9 (4): 909-916.

[15] Zhao FH, Liu JG, Wang X, Zhang DW, Wang PL, Zhang L, Du JP, Li ZX, Ma YL, Shi Y, Shi DZ. Long-term effect of stent coating with zedoary essential components on neointimal formation in the porcine coronary artery [J]. Chin J Integr Med, 2013, 19 (10): 771-776.

[16] de Prado AP, Pérez-Mart′ınez C, Cuellas-Ramo′n C, Gonzalo-Orden J M, Regueiro-Purrinos M, Martinez B, Carcia-Iglesias MJ, Ajenjo JM, Altonaga JR, Diego-Nieto A, de Miguel A, Fernandez-Vazquez F. Time course of reendothelialization of stents in a normal coronary swine model: characterization and quantification [J]. Vet Pathol, 2011, 48 (6): 1109-1117.

[17] Waksman R, Pakala R, Baffour R, Hellinga D, Seabron R, Tio FO, Wittchow E , Tittelbach M , Diener T, Harder C, Virmani R, Jones R. Efficacy and safety of pimecrolimus-eluting stents in porcine coronary arteries [J]. Cardiovasc Revasc Med, 2007, 8 (4): 259-274.

[18] Cheneau E, John MC, Fournadjiev J, Chan RC, Waksman R. Time course of stent endothelialization after intravascular radiation therapy in rabbit iliac arteries [J]. Circulation, 2003, 107 (16): 2153-2158.

[19] Finn AV, Nakazawa G, Joner M, Kolodgie FD, Mont EK, Gold HK, Virmani R. Vascular responses to drug eluting stents: importance of delayed healing [J]. Arterioscler Thromb Vasc Biol, 2007, 27 (7): 1500-1510.

[20] Hong YJ, Jeong MH, Lee SR, Hong SN, Kim KH, Park HW, Kim JH, Kim W, Ahn Y, Cho JG, Park JC, Kang JC. Anti-inflammatory effect of abciximab-coated stent in a porcine coronary restenosis model [J]. J Korean Med Sci, 2007, 22 (5): 802-809.

[21] Shinke T, Geva S, Pendyala L, Jabara R, Li J, Chen JP, Venegoni A, Colley K, Klein R, Chronos NA, Robinson K, Hou D. Low-dose paclitaxel elution by novel bioerodible sol-gel coating on stents inhibits neointima with low toxicity in porcine coronary arteries [J]. Int J Cardiol, 2009, 135 (1): 93-101.

[22] Rogers C, Parikh S, Seifert P, Edelman ER. Endogenous cell seeding. Remnant endothelium after stenting enhances vascular repair [J]. Circulation, 1996, 94 (11): 2909-2914.

[23] Chen CC, Chen Y, Hsi YT, Chang CS, Ho CT, Way TD, Kao J. Chemical constituents and anticancer activity of Curcuma zedoaria roscoe essential oil against non-small cell lung carcinoma cells in vitro and in vivo [J]. J Agric Food Chem, 2013, 61 (47): 11418-11427.

[24] Sprague EA, Tio F, Ahmed SH, Granada JF, Bailey SR. Impact of parallel micro-engineered stent grooves on endothelial cell migration, proliferation, and function: an in vivo correlation study of the healing response in the coronary swine model [J]. Circ Cardiovasc Interv, 2012, 5 (4): 499-507.

[25] Otsuka F, Finn AV, Yazdani SK, Nakano M, Kolodgie FD, Virmani R. The importance of the endothelium in atherothrombosis and coronary stenting [J]. Nat Rev Cardiol, 2012, 9 (8): 439-453.

[26] Yang F, Feng B, Feng SC, Pang XJ, Li WX, Bi YH, Zhao Q, Zhang SX, Wang Y. Combination coating of chitosan and anti-CD34 antibody applied on sirolimus-eluting stents can promote endothelialization while reducing neointimal formation [J]. BMC Cardiovasc Disord, 2012, 12: 96.

[27] Hara T, Ughi GJ, McCarthy JR, Erdem SS, Mauskapf A, Lyon SC, Fard AM, Edelman E, Tearney G, Jaffer FA. Intravascular fibrin molecular imaging improves the detection of unhealed stents assessed by optical coherence tomography in vivo [J]. Eur Heart J, 2015, Pol: ehv677. [Epub ahead of print]

[28] Cook S, Ladich E, Nakazawa G, Eshtehardi P, Neidhart M, Vogel R, Togni M, Wenaweser P, Billinger M, Seiler C, Gay S, Meier B, Pichler WJ, Juni P, Virmani R. Correlation of intravascular ultrasound findings with histopathological analysis of thrombus aspirates in patients with very late drug-eluting stent thrombosis [J]. Circulation, 2009, 120 (5): 391-399.

[29] Nakazawa G, Otsuka F, Nakano M, Vorpahl M, Yazdani SK, Ladich E, Kolodgie FD, Finn AV, Virmani R. The pathology of neoatherosclerosis in human coronary implants bare-metal and drug-eluting stents [J]. J Am Coll Cardiol, 2011, 57 (11): 1314-1322.

[30] Jang MK, Sohn DH, Ryu JH. A curcuminoid and sesquiterpenes as inhibitors of macrophage TNF-alpha release from Curcuma zedoaria [J]. Planta Med, 2001, 67 (6): 550-552.

[31] Lou Y, Zhao F, He H, Peng KF, Zhou XH, Chen LX, Qiu F. Guaiane-type sesquiterpenes from Curcuma wenyujin and their inhibitory effects on nitric oxide production [J]. J Asian Nat Prod Res, 2009, 11 (8): 737-747.

[32] Ullah HM, Zaman S, Juhara F, Akter L, Tareq SM, Masum EH, Bhattacharjee R. Evaluation of antinocicep-tive, in-vivo & in-vitro anti-inflammatory activity of ethanolic extract of Curcuma zedoaria rhizome [J]. BMC Complement Altern Med, 2014, 14: 346.

[33] Cho W, Nam JW, Kang HJ, Windono T, Seo EK, Lee KT. Zedoarondiol isolated from the rhizoma of Curcuma heyneana is involved in the inhibition of iNOS, COX-2 and pro-inflammatory cytokines via the downregulation of NF-kappaB pathway in LPS-stimulated murine macrophages [J]. Int Immuno-pharmacol, 2009, 9 (9): 1049-1057.

[34] Wakefield TW, Strieter RM, Wilke CA, Kadell AM, Wrobleski SK, Burdick M, Schmidt R, Kunkel SL, Greenfield LJ. Venous thrombosis-associated inflammation and attenuation with neutralizing anti-bodies to cytokines and adhesion molecules [J]. Arterioscler Thromb Vasc Biol, 1995, 15 (2): 258-268.

[35] Tariq S, Imran M, Mushtaq Z, Asghar N. Phytopreventive anti-hypercholesterolmic and antilipidemic perspectives of zedoary (Curcuma Zedoaria Roscoe herbal tea [J]. Lipids Health Dis, 2016, 15: 39.

[36] Singh V, Jain M, Misra A, Khanna V, Rana M, Prakash P, Malasoni R, Dwivedi A, Dikshit M, Barthwal MK. Curcuma oil ameliorates hyperlipidaemia and associated deleterious effects in golden Syrian hamsters [J]. Br J Nutr, 2013, 110 (3): 437-446.

First published: CUI Yuan-yuan, ZHAO Fu-hai, LIU Jian-gang, WANG Xin, DU Jian-peng, SHI Da-zhuo, CHEN Ke-ji. Zedoary guaiane-type sesquiterpenes-eluting stents accelerate endothelial healing without neointimal hyperplasia in a porcine coronary artery model [J] . J Cardiovasc Pharmacol Ther, 2017, 22: 476-484.

miR-941 as A Promising Biomarker For Acute Coronary Syndrome

BAI Rui-na, YANG Qiao-ning, XI Rui-xi, LI LI-zhi, SHI Da-zhuo, and CHEN Ke-ji

Acute coronary syndrome (ACS)is a major cause of death and disability[1]. Rapid antiplatelet therapy and revascularization could prevent myocardial ischemia and reduce the incidence of cardiovascular events[2]. Thus, the early diagnosis of non-ST elevation ACS (NSTE-ACS)and ST-segment elevation myocardial infarction (STEMI)is essential for improved prognoses. Currently, the clinical diagnosis of ACS relies on assessment of symptoms, ischemia changes in electrocardiogram (ECG), and changes in troponin[2]. However, in elderly individuals and patients with diabetes, typical symptoms are not always observed. Moreover, changes in ECG can be easily influenced by left bundle branch blockage and chronic myocardial infarction. To a certain extent, unstable angina pectoris (UA), non-STEMI (NSTEMI), and STEMI reflect the pathological progress of ACS. Therefore, identification of novel biomarkers may facilitate the early diagnosis of ACS, particularly in patients with atypical symptoms of ACS.

MicroRNAs (miRNAs)are endogenous, small (22–24-nucleotide)noncoding RNA molecules that regulate the expression of mRNA by combining with the 3′ -untranslated region (3′ -UTR), subsequently triggering the degradation of mRNA or having negative effects on transcription[3]. miRNAs can regulate nearly 60% of coding genes to exert their biological functions[4,5]. Recently, many studies have shown that miRNAs can regulate endothelial dysfunction, inflammation, cell autophagy, platelet activation, and aggregation[6–9]. Moreover, miRNA expression can affect the stability of atherosclerotic plaques[10]. miRNAs possess tissue-specific expression and can be secreted into blood or urine. miRNAs of circulartory system can be used as bio-markers of diagnosis, treatment, and prevention of diseases, such as coronary heart disease [11–14]. However, it is still unclear whether miRNAs can be used as biomarkers of ACS and further evaluate the severity of ACS[15].

Therefore, in this study, we applied gene chip technology to analyze the expression of miRNAs in patients with stable angina (SA), NSTE-ACS, and STEMI. We then performed quantitative real-time reverse transcription polymerase chain reaction (qRT-PCR)to determine whether miRNAs could be used as biomarker for the diagnosis of ACS.

METHODS

1 Patients and Study Design

A total of 72 patients with chest pain who underwent diagnostic coronary angiography in Xiyuan Hospital, affiliated hospital of China Academy of Chinese Medical Sciences were enrolled from March 2015 to July 2015. The patients were divided into four groups as follows: 18 patients with STEMI, 18 patients NSTE-ACS, 20 patients with SA, and 16 patients without CAD. Patients in the control group did not have coronary stenosis as confirmed by coronary angiography, but had three or more risk factors for coronary heart disease (see schematic of the study in Fig. 1). Five cases were randomly selected from each group for analysis of gene expression profiles, using an Affymetrix GeneChip miRNA4.0. The differential expression of miRNAs between groups was analyzed according to the following criteria: fold-change (FC) $\geqslant 1.5$ and $P < 0.05$. qRT-PCR was applied to verify the differential expression of miRNAs (FC $\geqslant 2$ and $P < 0.05$). This study was registered in the Chinese Clinical Trial Registry (No. ChiCTR-IPR-15006336). The study was performed according to the guidelines of the Declaration of Helsinki and was approved by the Xiyuan Hospital Ethics Committee.

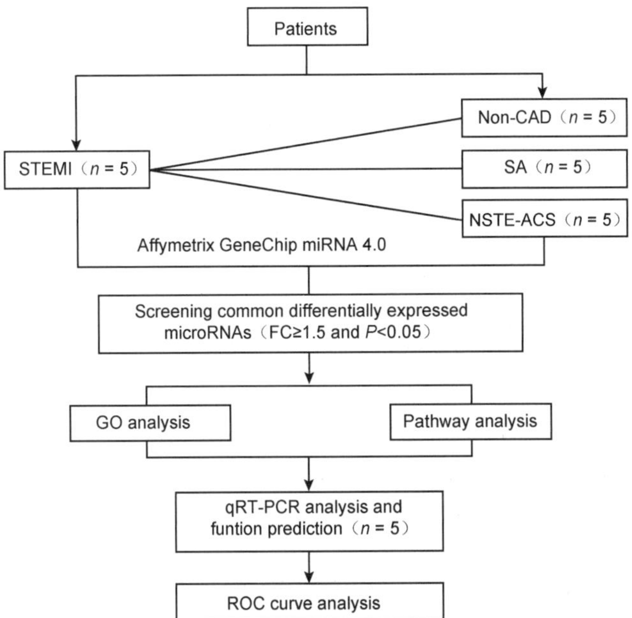

Fig. 1 Schematic of the Study Design

2 Diagnostic Criteria

In this study, patients with coronary heart disease were classified as having SA or ACS, including STEMI, NSTE-ACS, and UA. Diagnostic criteria was referred to the 2014 ACC/AHA/AATS/PCNA/SCAI/STS Focused Update of the Guideline for the Diagnosis and Management of Patients With Stable Ischemic Heart Disease [16], 2014 AHA/ACC Guideline for the Management of Patients with Non-ST-Elevation Acute Coronary Syndromes[2], and 2013 ACCF/AHA Guideline for the Management of ST-elevation Myocardial Infarction[17]. In addition, all patients presented stenosis (≥ 50% in at least one main coronary artery)as confirmed by coronary angiography[18].

3 Inclusion and Exclusion Criteria

The inclusion criteria were as follows: patients who met the diagnostic criteria, were 35–75 years old, and provided informed consent. The exclusion criteria were as follows: Patients with combined diseases, such as cardiomyopathy, valvular heart disease, severe arrhythmia, heart failure, and other accompanying diseases; patients encountered challenges with data collection, such as religious or language barriers; patients were pregnant or lactating and participating in other clinical studies.

4 Blood Collection and Storage

Venous blood samples were collected via antecubital venipuncture from each subject within 3–5 h of the onset of symptoms but before arteriography. Whole blood samples (2 mL)were collected directly into EDTA-containing tubes (BD, Franklin Lakes, NJ, USA), and three volumes of red blood cell lysis buffer (NH4CL2009; Haoyang, Tianjin, China)was added to obtain leukocytes, which were isolated within 2 h by centrifugation at 3000 rpm for 5 min at 4 ℃ to remove other blood elements. Next, 1 mL TRIzol (15596–026; Invitrogen Life Technologies)was added, and samples were then transferred to RNase/Dnase-free tubes and stored at –80 ℃.

5 RNA Isolation and Preparation

After collection of all samples, total RNA in leukocytes was isolated using a miRVana RNA Isolation Kit (p/n AM1556; Applied Biosystems, Foster City, CA, USA)according to the manufacturer's specifications.

Samples were then subjected to on-column DNase I treatment with RNase-free Dnase (#79254; Qiagen, Valencia, CA, USA). RNA quantity and quality were determined using a NanoDrop 2000 spectrophotometer (Thermo Scientific, USA)and an Agilent 2100 bioanalyzer. The RNA integrity was evaluated by agarose gel electrophoresis with ethidium bromide staining.

6 miRNA Array Analysis

Microarray analysis of gene expression was carried out using ELOSA QC Assays prior to array hybridization. Sample labeling, microarray hybridization, and washing were performed based on the manufacturer's standard protocols. Briefly, total RNA was modified with poly A tails and then labeled with biotin. Next, the labeled RNAs were hybridized onto the microarray. Slides were washed and stained, and the arrays were scanned using an Affymetrix Scanner 3000 (Affymetrix).

miRNA microarray analysis was performed to determine differential expression of blood-borne miRNAs among (i)non-CAD individuals and patients with STEMI (n=5), (ii)patients with SA and STEMI (n=5), and (iii)patients with NSTE-ACS and STEMI. Bioinformatic determination of downstream predicted targets for candidate miRNAs was performed as described previously by Selbach et al[19].

7 Reverse Transcription Quantitative Real-time Polymerase Chain Reaction (RT-qPCR) Analysis

Quantification was performed through two-step reaction process: reverse transcription (RT)and qPCR. Each RT re-action consisted of 1 μg RNA, 4 μL miScript HiSpec Buffer, 2 μL Nucleics Mix, and 2 μL miScript Reverse Transcriptase Mix (Qiagen, Germany), in a total volume of 20 μl. Reactions were performed in a GeneAmp PCR System 9700 (Applied Biosystems, USA)for 60 min at 37 ℃, followed by heat inactivation of the reverse transcriptase for 5 min at 95 ℃. The 20-μL reaction mix was then diluted 5-fold in nuclease-free water and stored at −20 ℃.

Real-time PCR was performed using a LightCycler 480II Real-time PCR Instrument (Roche, Switzerland) with 10 μL of the reaction mixture including 1 μL cDNA, 5 μL 2×LightCycler 480 SYBR Green I Master (Roche), 0.2 μL universal primers (Qiagen), 0.2 μL miRNA-specific primer, and 3.6 μL nuclease-free water. Reactions were incubated in a 384-well optical plate (Roche)at 95 ℃ for 10 min, followed by 40 cycles of 95 ℃ for 10 s and 60 ℃ for 30 s. Triplicates were averaged to calculate the expression value for each sample. At the end of the PCR cycling, melt curve analysis was performed to validate the specific generation of the expected PCR product. miRNA-specific primer sequences were designed in the laboratory and synthesized by Generay Biotech (Generay, PRC)based on the miRNA sequences obtained from the miRBase database (Release 20.0)as follows: *hsa-miR-182-5p*, UUUGG CAAUGGUAGAACUCACACU; *hsa-miR-363-3p*, AAU UGCACGGUAUCCAUCUGUA; and *hsa-miR-941*, CACCCGGCUGUGUGCACAUGUGC).

The expression levels of miRNAs were normalized to U6 and were calculated by the $2^{-\Delta\Delta Ct}$ method[20].

8 Statistical Analysis

Affymetrix GeneChip Command Console software (version4.0, Affymetrix)was used to analyze array images to obtain raw data, and RMA normalization was then carried out. Next, Genespring software (version 12.5, Agilent Technologies)was used for subsequent data analysis. Differentially expressed miRNAs were then identified through fold changes, and P-values were calculated using t-tests. The threshold set for up-and downregulated genes was a fold change of 1.5 or more and a P value of less than 0.05. Target genes of differentially expressed miRNAs were the intersection predicted with three databases (Targetscan, PITA, and microRNAorg). Gene ontology (GO) analysis and KEGG analysis were ap-plied to determine the roles of these target genes. Hierarchical clustering was performed to show distinguishable miRNA expression patterns among samples.

Paired and unpaired Student's t tests were performed to compare data as appropriate. Values are expressed as means ± standard deviations (SDs). *P* values of less than 0.05 (two-sided)were considered significant.

RESULTS

1 Patient Clinicopathological Information

Seventy-two patients (18 patients with STEMI, 18 patients with NSTE-ACS, 20 patients with SA, and 16 patients without CAD)were enrolled in this study. The clinicopathological characteristics of the patients are presented in Tables 1 and 2. There were no significant differences in clinical features among groups ($P>0.05$).

Table 1 Baseline Clinical Characteristics of Different Patient Groups Used in Microarray Analysis

Variable	CAD (*n* = 15)			Without CAD (*n* = 5)
	SA (*n* = 5)	NSTE-ACS (*n* = 5)	STEMI (*n* = 5)	
Age (years, mean ± SD)	55.8 ± 4.15	57.4 ± 11.19	52.8 ± 10.56	52.4 ± 13.23
Sex (male, n)	5	5	5	5
Risk factors (n)				
Hypertension	4	4	2	3
Dyslipidemia	5	3	4	3
Active smoker	4	3	5	1
Medications (n)				
Antiplatelet agents	5	5	5	0
β-Blockers	4	3	3	0
CCB	2	1	1	1
ACEI/ARB	4	4	4	2
Statins	5	5	5	1

Abbreviations: *SA* stable angina, *NSTE-ACS* non-ST elevation acute coronary syndrome, *STEMI* ST elevation myocardial infarction, *DM* diabetes mellitus, *CCB* calcium channel blocker, *ACEI* angiotensin-converting enzyme inhibitor, *ARB* angiotensin receptor blocker.

Table 2 Baseline Clinical Characteristics of Different Patient Groups Used in qRT–PCR Analysis

Variable	CAD (*n* = 56)			Without CAD (*n* = 16)
	SA (*n* = 20)	NSTE-ACS (*n* = 18)	STEMI (*n* = 18)	
Age (years, mean ± SD)	55.8 ± 9.15	56.4 ± 8.79	53.50 ± 10.56	52.5 ± 13.50
Sex (male, n)	12	15	16	9
Risk factors (n)				
Hypertension	14	15	13	11
Dyslipidemia	12	13	11	8
DM	9	10	9	7
Active smoker	12	15	14	8
Medications (n)				
Antiplatelet agents	12	16	18	0
β-Blockers	13	11	9	9
Statins	18	16	12	8

Abbreviations: *SA* stable angina, *NSTE-ACS* non-ST elevation acute coronary syndrome, *STEMI* ST elevation myocardial infarction, *DM* diabetes mellitus, *CCB* calcium channel blocker, *ACEI* angiotensin-converting enzyme inhibitor, *ARB* angiotensin receptor blocker.

2 miRNA Array Analysis

The differential expression of miRNAs among the patient groups was determined by gene chip analysis. The results showed that there exist 13 differentially expressed miRNAs in patients with STEMI comparing with those in patients without CAD and patients with SA and NSTE-ACS. After that, we chose *miR-941*, *miR-363-*

3p, and *miR-182-5p* (FC ≥ 2.0; $P < 0.05$)for further analysis by qRT-PCR (Table 3).

Table 3　Differentially Expressed miRNAs in Patients with ACS versus Patients without CAD and Patients with SA or NSTE-ACS in Microarray Analysis

miRNAs	STEMI versus without CAD			STEMI versus SA			STEMI versus NSTE-ACS		
	Fold change	*P* value	Regulation	Fold change	*P* value	Regulation	Fold change	*P* value	Regulation
miR-941	5.305	0.007	Up	4.544	0.003	Up	5.032	0.002	Up
miR-182-5p	2.331	0.013	Down	2.005	0.042	Down	2.121	0.024	Up
miR-363-3p	2.012	0.007	Down	2.016	0.018	Down	2.071	0.048	Up
hsa-mir-941-1	1.895	0.036	Up	2.051	0.001	Up	2.008	0.001	Up
hsa-mir-941-2	1.895	0.036	Up	2.051	0.001	Up	2.008	0.001	Up
hsa-mir-941-3	1.895	0.036	Up	2.051	0.001	Up	2.008	0.001	Up
hsa-mir-941-4	1.895	0.036	Up	2.051	0.001	Up	2.008	0.001	Up
hsa-miR-6798-5p	2.049	0.015	Up	1.866	0.019	Up	2.041	4.32E-04	Up
hsa-miR-4419a	1.737	0.013	Up	1.717	0.006	Up	1.851	9.32E-05	Up
hsa-miR-296-3p	1.811	0.031	Up	2.209	0.012	Up	1.726	0.109	Up
hsa-miR-1227-5p	1.549	0.013	Up	1.629	0.039	Up	1.653	0.147	Up
hsa-miR-4656	1.908	0.005	Up	1.617	0.025	Up	1.232	0.459	Up
hsa-miR-3064-3p	1.765	0.037	Down	1.529	0.001	Down	1.033	0.738	Down

Abbreviations: *SA* stable angina, *NSTE-ACS* non-ST segment elevation acute coronary syndrome, *STEMI* ST segment elevation acute myocardial infarction.

3 Gene Ontology (GO)Analysis

Differentially expressed miRNAs in patients without CAD and with SA or NSTE-ACS (compared with that in patients with STEMI)were found to be involved in inflammation, protein phosphorylation, RNA polymerase II-dependent transcription, cell adhesion, and other biological processes. Among these, inflammation, cell adhesion, T-cell proliferation, calcium transfer, and apoptosis were closely related to atherosclerosis (Fig. 2).

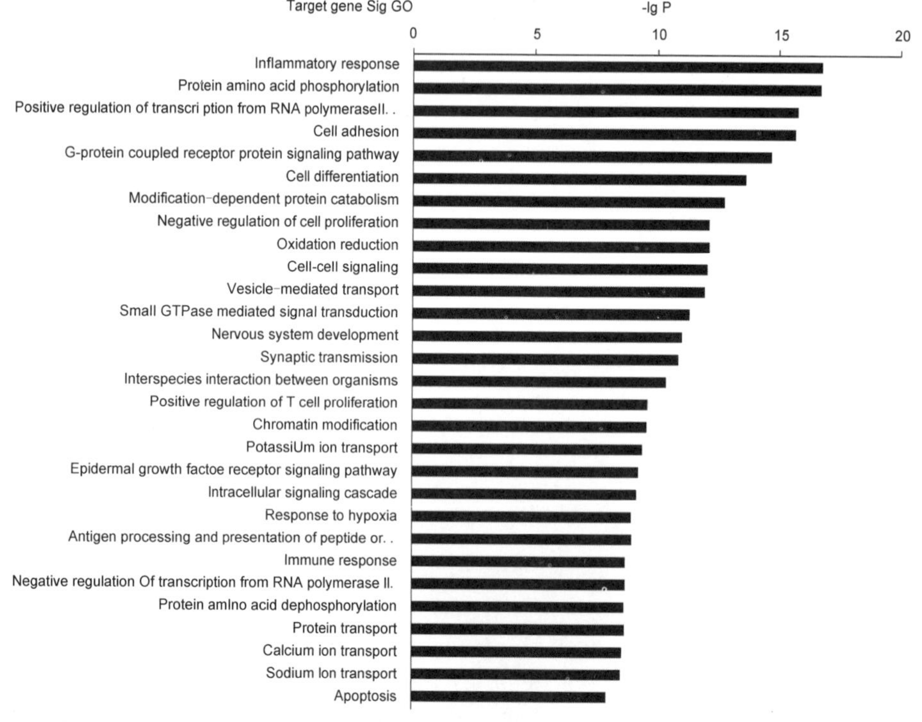

Fig. 2　Gene Ontology (GO)

4 Pathway Analysis

The KEGG database was used to analyze target genes of protein kinase (MAPK)signaling, tumorigenesis, and calcium ion signaling. Among the identified cell signaling pathways, we identified the following pathways involved in the pathological process of atherosclerosis: adhesion molecules, ErbB signaling, metabolism, Wnt signaling, insulin signaling, apoptosis, vascular endothelial growth factor signaling, and cell factor receptor interactions (Fig. 3).

miRNA-pathway network analysis showed that miR-941 can participate in regulation of T-cell receptor signaling, insulin signaling, and MAPK signaling. Additionally, *miR-182-5p* was related to vascular smooth muscle cell constriction and mammalian target of rapamycin (mTOR)signaling. *miR-363-3p* was involved in Toll-like receptor signaling and actin cytoskeleton regulation. Bioinformatics functional predictions showed that the differential expressed miRNAs could be related to the pathological process of cardiovascular disease (Fig. 4).

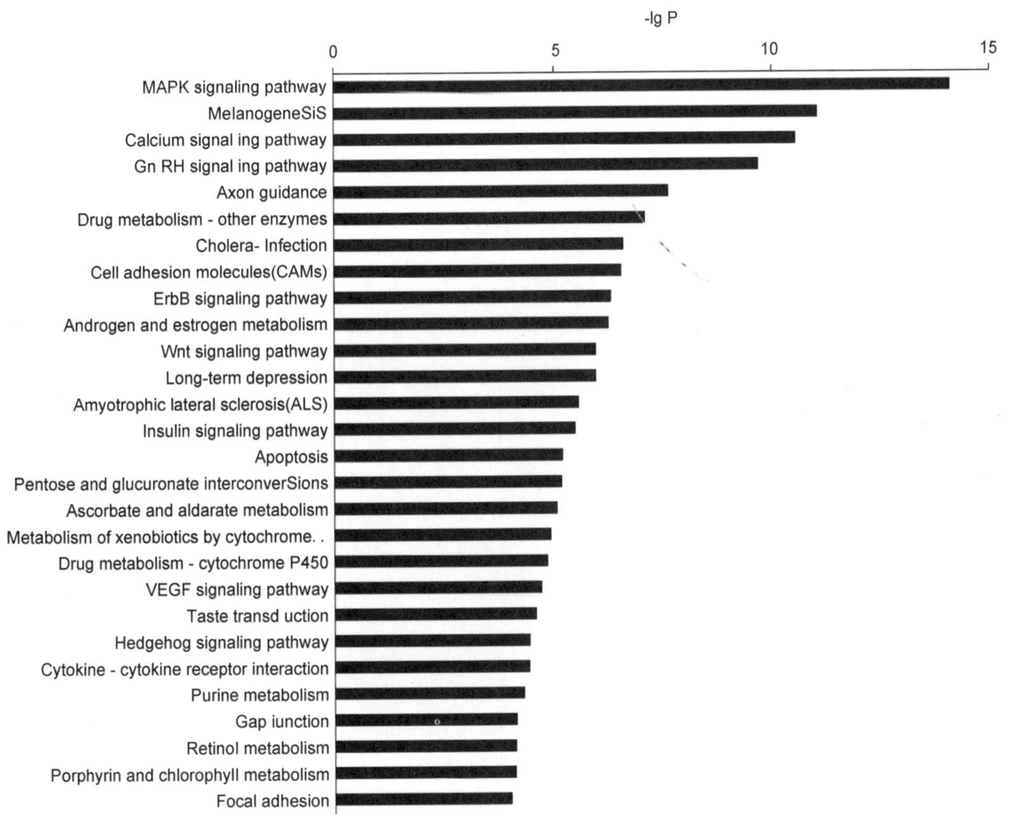

Fig. 3 Pathway Analysis

6 qRT-PCR

Next, we performed qRT-PCR to verify the different ex-pression of candidated gene like, *miR-941*, *miR-182-5p*, and *miR-363-3p*. The results showed that *miR-941* expression has no significant difference between the control patients (without CAD)and SA group. However, comparing with control patients, *miR-941* expression was significantly increased by 1.64-and 2.28-fold in patients with NSTE-ACS and STEMI, respectively, ($P < 0.05$; Fig. 5a).

There were no significant differences in *miR-182-5p* and *miR-363-3p* among groups ($P > 0.05$; Fig. 5b and c). Additionally, the expression of *miR-941* was increased by 1.66-fold in patients with STEMI compared with that in patients with SA ($P < 0.001$; Fig. 6a-1) and by 1.52-fold in patients with STEMI compared with that in patients with NSTE-ACS ($P < 0.05$; Fig. 6a-2). There were no significant differences in *miR-182-5p* and *miR-363-3p* ($P > 0.05$; Fig. 6b and c).

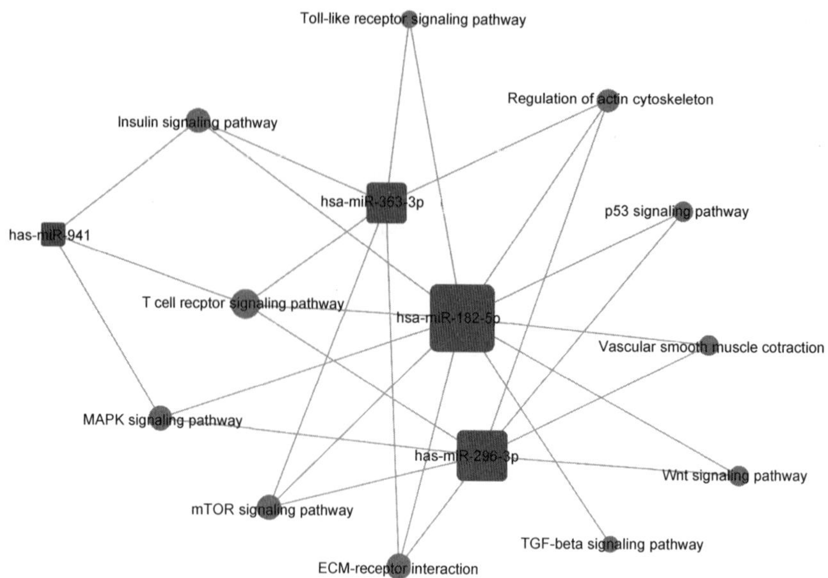

Fig. 4　Microarray Pathway Network

Notes: The red rectangles are miRNAs, the purple circle are pathways, and the green lines represented the regulatory connections between miRNAs and pathways.

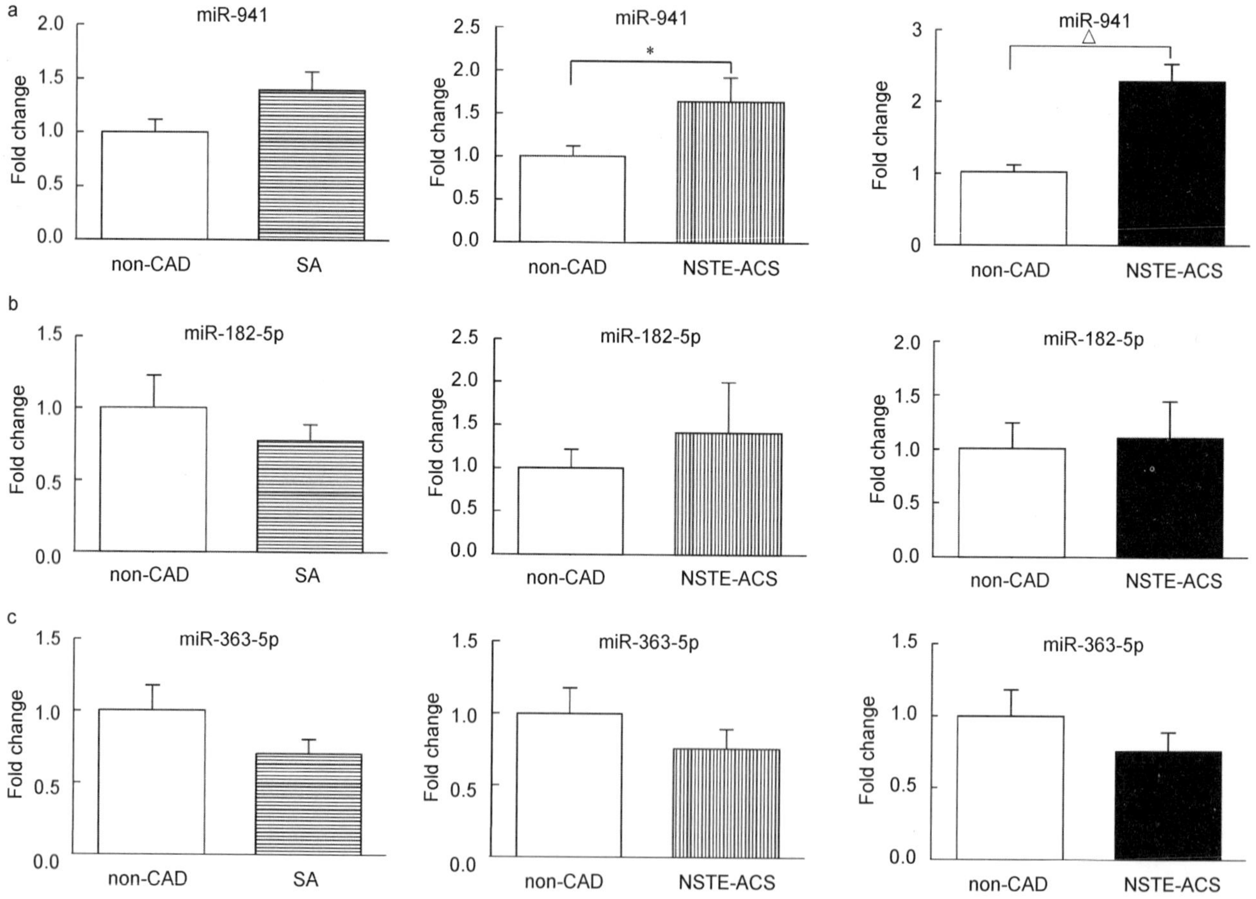

Fig. 5　Expression Profiles of Candidate miRNAs in Patients with and without CAD

Notes: The three candidate miRNAs were evaluated with qRT-PCR using 72 samples, including 16 non-CAD, 20 SA, 18 NSTE-ACS, and 18 STEMI samples. *miR-941* was significantly upregulated in the SA, NSTE-ACS, and STEMI groups compared with that in non-CAD patients (a). *miR-182-5p* (b)and *miR-363-3p* (c)were not significantly different in patients with CAD (SA, NSTE-ACS, and STEMI)compared with that in patients without CAD. Abbreviations: CAD: coronary artery disease, SA: stable angina, NSTE-ACS: non-ST elevation acute coronary syndromes, STEMI: ST elevation myocardial infarction. $^{*}P < 0.05$, $^{\Delta}P < 0.001$.

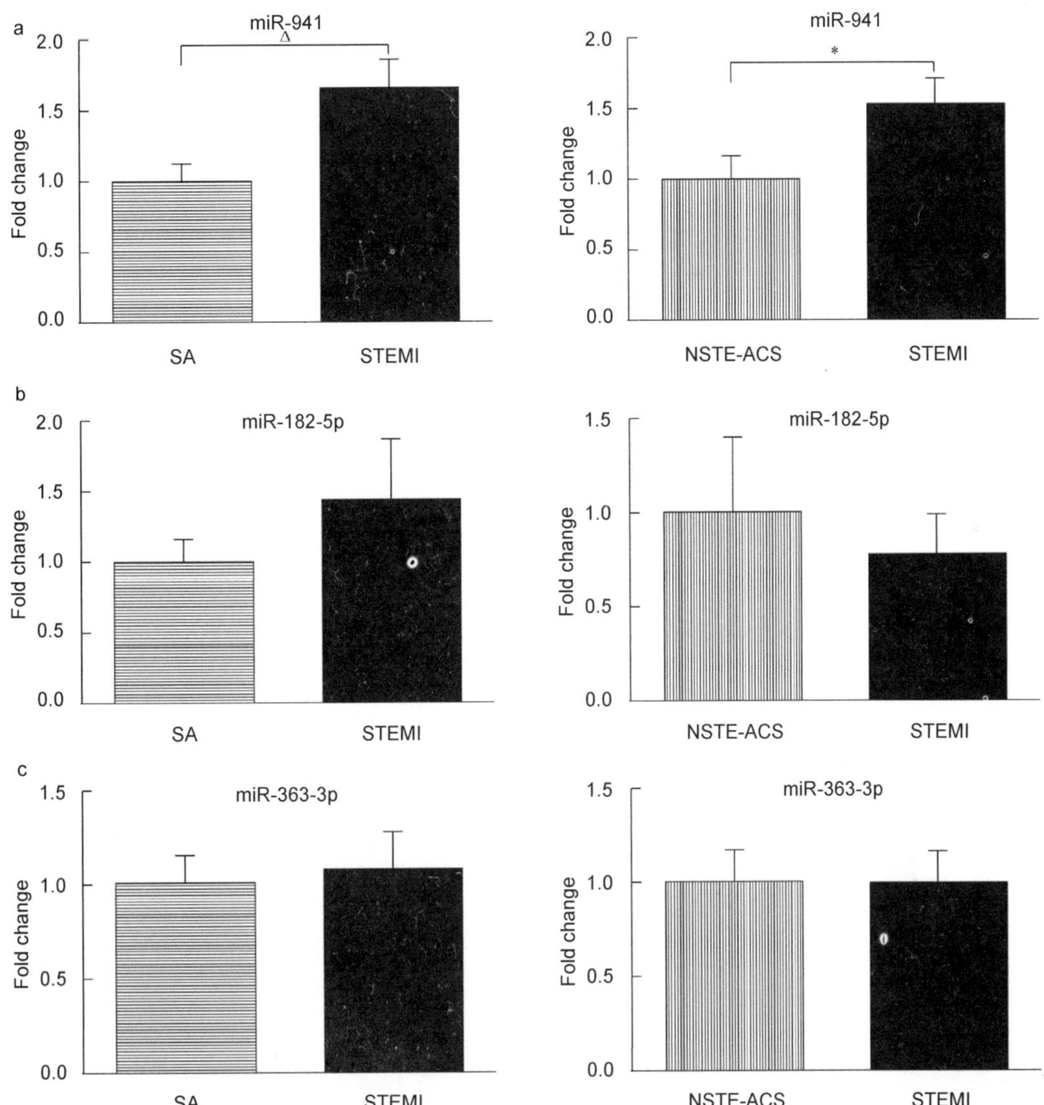

Fig. 6 Expression Profiles of Candidate miRNAs in Patients with SA, NSTE-ACS, and STEMI

Notes: The three candidate miRNAs were evaluated by qRT-PCR using 56 samples (20 cases of SA, 18 cases of NSTE-ACS, and 18 cases of STEMI). (a)*miR-941*, (b)*miR-182-5p*, and (c)*miR-363-3p* are shown. Abbreviations: CAD, coronary artery disease; SA, stable angina; NSTE-ACS, non-ST elevation acute coronary syndrome; STEMI, ST elevation myocardial infarction. $^{*}P < 0.05$, $^{\Delta}P < 0.001$.

Since there were no significant differences in *miR-941* expression between patients without CAD and patients with SA, we combined the two groups into the non-ACS group. Compared with that in the non-ACS group, the expression of *miR-941* was upregulated in the ACS group (FC: 1.62; $P < 0.01$; Fig. 7). NSTE-ACS and STEMI can reflect the degree of disease progression, and *miR-941* was significantly upregulated in patients with STEMI compared with that in patients in the non-ACS group (FC: 1.52; $P < 0.05$; Fig. 6a-2). The differential expression of *miR-941* in the two groups showed that the expression of *miR-941* was associated with the severity of ACS. Receiver operating characteristic (ROC)curve analysis Next, we performed ROC curve analysis to test the reliability of *miR-941* as a diagnostic biomarker of STEMI and ACS. Comparing with patients with STEMI, areas under the ROC curves were 0.896, 0.808, and 0.781 for patients in the control, SA, and NSTE-ACS groups, respectively; Comparing with patients in ACS group, the ROC curves of non-ACS group was 0.734 (Fig. 8). Thus, *miR-941* may act as a reliable biomarker of ACS, particularly STEMI. The area under the curve (AUC), 95% confidence intervals (CIs), and *p* values are summarized in Table 4.

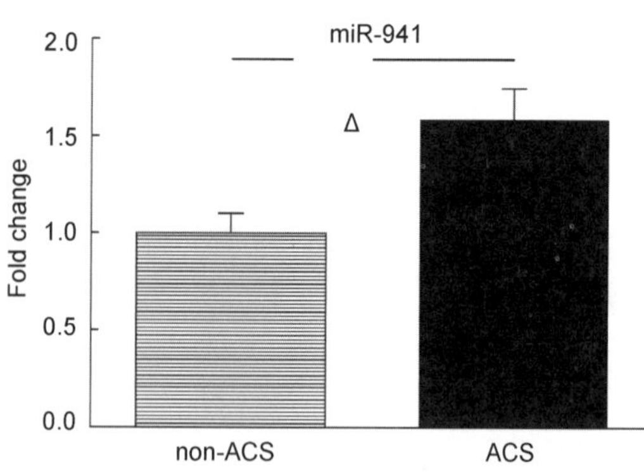

Fig. 7　Expression Profiles of *miR-941* in Patients with and without ACS.
Notes: *miR-941* expression was evaluated by qRT-PCR using 72 samples (36 patients without ACS and 36 patients with ACS). Abbreviations: ACS, acute coronary syndrome. $^{\Delta}P < 0.01$.

Table 4　ROC Curve Analysis of *miR-941* Expression in Patients with ACS and STEMI

miR-941	AUC	95% CI	*P* value
Non-ACS versus ACS	0.734	0.619–0.848	0.001
Without CAD versus STEMI	0.896	0.779–1.000	0.000
SA versus STEMI	0.808	0.670–0.947	0.001
NSTE-ACS versus STEMI	0.781	0.622–0.939	0.004

Abbreviations: *SA* stable angina, *ACS* acute coronary syndrome, *NSTE-ACS* non-ST segment elevation acute coronary syndrome, *STEMI* ST segment elevation acute myocardial infarction, *CAD* coronary artery disease, *ROC* receiver operating characteristic, *AUC* area under the curve.

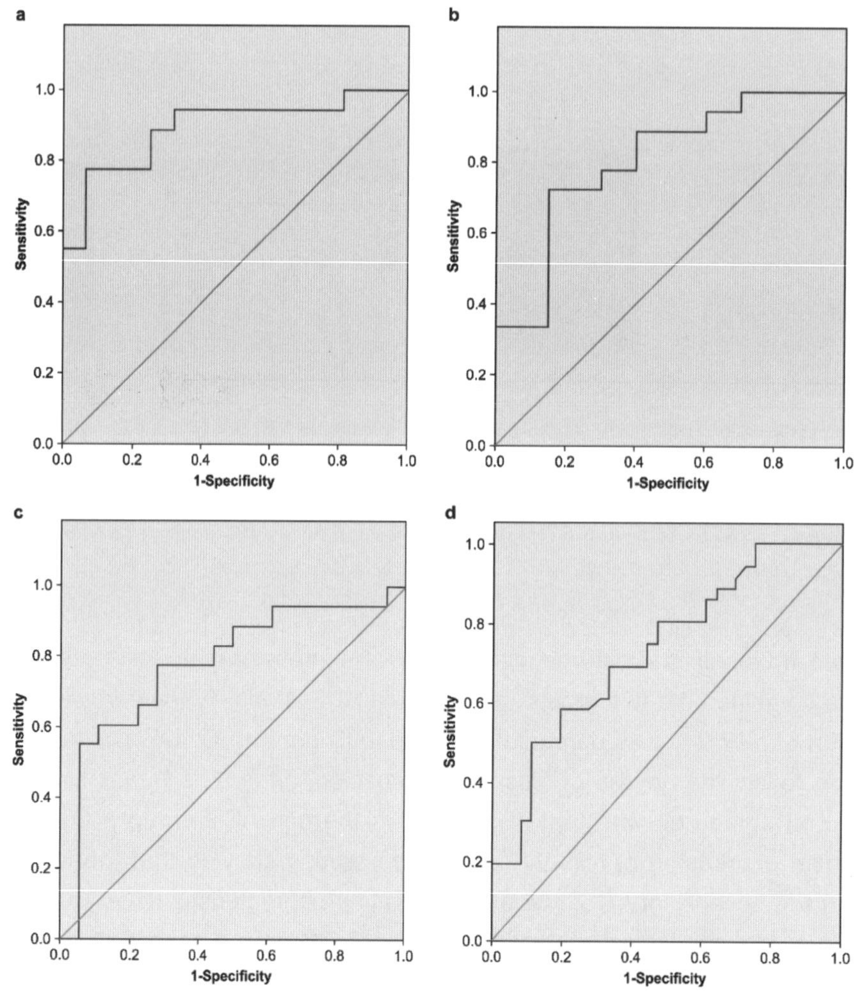

Fig. 8　ROC Curve Analysis
Notes: a. Expression profiles of *miR-941* in patients with STEMI and without CAD. b. Expression profiles of *miR-941* in patients with STEMI and SA. c. Expression profiles of *miR-941* in patients with STEMI and NSTE-ACS. d. Expression profiles of *miR-941* in patients with and without ACS.

DISCUSSION

Aberrant miRNA expression has been involved with a number of human diseases, including cardiovascular diseases[11, 21–23]. ACS has become a major public health problem owing to its high mortality and morbidity[24–26]. Thus, there is an urgent need to identify new diagnostic and therapeutic biomarkers of ACS; miRNAs may have such applications.

MiRNAs are involved in endothelial dysfunction, inflammation, apoptosis, angiogenesis, atherosclerosis, and other pathological processes involved in cardiovascular diseases[6,27,28], and miRNAs of circulartory system may be potential biomarkers of these diseases[7,29]. *miR-135a*, *miR-31*, *miR-378*, and *miR-147* are biological markers of stable coronary heart disease [30]; *miR-1*, *miR-126*, and *miR-133a* have potential value in the diagnosis of UA[31]; and *miR-208b*, *miR-499*, and *miR-1* play a key role in the diagnosis, progression, and prognosis of acute myocardial infarction (AMI)[15,32–34]. However, it is unclear whether miRNAs are differentially expressed with changes in the severity of coronary heart disease, including coronary stenosis and myocardial damage. Our findings suggested that *miR-363-3p*, *miR-941*, and *miR-182-5p* were differentially expressed among groups of patients with various types and degrees of coronary heart disease. Additionally, GO and KEGG pathway analysis showed that the differentially expressed miRNAs were involved in inflammatory responses, immune responses, MAPK signal, calcium pathway, ErbB signaling, and other cellular processes. In particular, MAPK signaling and immune responses are involved in the pathogenesis of atherosclerosis and affect the stability of plaques and the formation of blood clots. Furthermore, qRT-PCR analysis verified that *miR-941* was differentially expressed in plasma from patients with CADs (SA, NSTE-ACS, and STEMI) compared with that in patients without CAD. Thus, these data suggested that *miR-941* may have applications as a biomarker of CAD, with the ability to distinguish among ACS and non-ACS groups and to distinguish STEMI from SA and NSTE-ACS. Notably, *miR-941* was gradually upregulated as the degree of coronary artery stenosis and myocardial injury increased (SA < NSTE-ACS < STEMI); thus, *miR-941* was closely associated with the severity of ACS. Accordingly, we concluded that *miR-941* was a biomarker of ACS, particularly for STEMI, and could predict the severity and progression of coronary heart disease.

Recent bioinformatics analyses have shown that *miR-941* is involved in Wnt signaling, transforming growth factor (TGF)-β signaling, and insulin signaling[35,36]. However, no research has been reported the role of *miR-941* in atherosclerosis and coronary heart disease. In our study, we found that *miR-941* may be associated with metabolism, inflammation, cell proliferation, and other biological processes through regulation of components involved in insulin signaling, MAPK signaling, T-cell receptor signaling, and other related pathways. However, we were not able to confirm the direct relationship between *miR-941* and the pathogenesis of atherosclerosis. In vitro and in vivo experiments are needed to clarify the biological function of *miR-941* in the pathophysiology of atherosclerosis and to determine whether *miR-941* is involved in pathological processes of inflammation, immunity, metabolism, and platelet activation. Although we found that *miR-941* was differentially expressed between ACS and non-ACS groups, additional studies are needed to establish a rapid, inexpensive method for miRNA analysis. Additionally, greater sample sizes are needed to further confirm the potential applications of this miRNA as a promising diagnostic tool for diagnosis of ACS.

CONCLUSIONS

MiR-941 was relatively higher in patients with ACS and STEMI, and could predict the severity and progression of coronary heart disease. Thus, *miR-941* may be a potential biomarker of ACS or STEMI.

REFERENCES

[1] Go AS, Mozaffarian D, Roger VL, et al. Heart disease and stroke statistics—2014 update: a report from the American Heart Association[J]. Circulation, 2014, 129 (3): 399-401.

[2] Amsterdam EA, Wenger NK, Brindis RG, et al. 2014 AHA/ACC Guideline for the Management of Patients with Non-ST-Elevation Acute Coronary Syndromes: a report of the American College of Cardiology/American Heart Association Task Force on Practice Guidelines[J]. J Am Coll Cardiol, 2014, 64 (24): e139-e228.

[3] Diehl P, Fricke A, Sander L, et al. Microparticles: major transport vehicles for distinct microRNAs in circulation[J]. Cardiovasc Res, 2012, 93 (4): 633-644.

[4] Thomson DW, Bracken CP, Goodall GJ. Experimental strategies for microRNA target identification[J]. Nucleic Acids Res, 2011, 39 (16): 6845-6853.

[5] Noren Hooten N, Fitzpatrick M, Wood WH 3rd, et al. Age-related changes in microRNA levels in serum[J]. Aging, 2013, 5 (10): 725-740.

[6] Peng Y, Song L, Zhao M, et al. Critical roles of miRNA-mediated regulation of TGFβ signalling during mouse cardiogenesis[J]. Cardiovasc Res, 2014, 103 (2): 258-67.

[7] Small EM, Olson EN. Pervasive roles of microRNAs in cardiovascular biology[J]. Nature, 2011, 469 (7330): 336-342.

[8] Schroen B, Heymans S. Small but smart—microRNAs in the centre of inflammatory processes during cardiovascular diseases, the metabolic syndrome, and ageing[J]. Cardiovasc Res, 2012, 93 (4): 605-613.

[9] Edelstein LC, Bray PF. MicroRNAs in platelet production and activation[J]. Blood, 2011, 117: 5289-5296.

[10] Menghini R, Stohr R, Federici M. MicroRNAs in vascular aging and atherosclerosis[J]. Ageing Res Rev, 2014, 17 (2): 68-78.

[11] Small EM, Frost RJ, Olson EN. MicroRNAs add a new dimension to cardiovascular disease[J]. Circulation. 2010, 121 (8), 1022-1032.

[12] Kataoka M, Wang DZ. Non-coding RNAs including miRNAs and lncRNAs in cardio-vascular biology and disease[J]. Cell, 2014, 3 (3): 883-898.

[13] Creemers EE, Tijsen AJ, Pinto YM. Circulating microRNAs: novel biomarkers and extracellular communicators in cardiovascular disease? [J]. Circ Res, 2012, 110 (3): 483-495.

[14] van Rooij E. The art of microRNA research[J]. Circ Res, 2011, 108: 219-234.

[15] Li C, Pei F, Zhu X, et al. Circulating microRNAs as novel and sensitive biomarkers of acute myocardial infarction[J]. Clin Biochem, 2012, 45 (10-11): 727-732.

[16] Fihn SD, Blankenship JC, Alexander KP, et al. 2014 ACC/AHA/AATS/PCNA/SCAI/STS focused update of the guideline for the diagnosis and management of patients with stable ischemic heart disease: a report of the American College of Cardiology/American Heart Association Task Force on Practice Guidelines, and the American Association for Thoracic Surgery, Preventive Cardiovascular Nurses Association, Society for Cardiovascular Angiography and Interventions, and Society of Thoracic Surgeons[J]. J Am Coll Cardiol, 2014, 64 (3): 1929-1949.

[17] American College of Emergency Physicians, Society for Cardiovascular Angiography and Interventions, O'Gara PT, et al. 2013 ACCF/AHA guideline for the management of ST-elevation myocardial infarction: a report of the American College of Cardiology Foundation/American Heart Association Task Force on Practice Guidelines[J]. J Am Coll Cardiol, 2013, 61 (1): e78-e140.

[18] Libby P, Theroux P. Pathophysiology of coronary artery disease[J]. Circulation, 2005, 111: 3481-3488.

[19] Selbach M, Schwanhäusser B, Thierfelder N, et al. Widespread changes in protein synthesis induced by microRNAs[J]. Nature, 2008, 455 (7209): 58-63.

[20] Livak KJ, Schmittgen TD. Analysis of relative gene expression data using real-time quantitative PCR and the 2 (-Delata Delta C (T))method[J]. Methods, 2001, 25 (4): 402-408.

[21] Lagos-Quintana M, Rauhut R, Lendeckel W, et al. Identification of novel genes coding for small expressed RNAs[J]. Science, 2001, 294 (5543): 853-858.

[22] Gomes da Silva AM, Silbiger VN. miRNAs as biomarkers of atrial fibrillation[J]. Biomarkers, 2014, 19: 631-636.

[23] Zeller T, Keller T, Ojeda F, et al. Assessment of microRNAs in patients with unstable angina pectoris[J]. Eur Heart J, 2014, 35 (31): 2106-2114.

[24] McManus DD, Lin H, Tanriverdi K, et al. Relations between circulating microRNAs and atrial fibrillation: data from the Framingham Offspring Study[J]. Heart Rhythm, 2014, 11 (4): 663-669.

[25] Pagidipati NJ, Gaziano TA. Estimating deaths from cardiovascular disease: a review of global methodologies of mortality measurement[J]. Circulation, 2013, 127 (6): 749-756.

[26] Arbab-Zadeh A, Nakano M, Virmani R, et al. Acute coronary events[J]. Circulation, 2012, 125: 1147-1156.

[27] Dangwal S, Bang C, Thum T. Novel techniques and targets in cardiovascular microRNA research[J]. Cardiovasc Res, 2012, 93 (4): 545-554.

[28] Fichtlscherer S, Zeiher AM, Dimmeler S. Circulating microRNAs: biomarkers or mediators of cardiovascular diseases? [J]. Arterioscler Thromb Vasc Biol, 2011, 31 (11): 2383-2390.

[29] Sayed AS, Xia K, Salma U, et al. Diagnosis, prognosis and therapeutic role of circulating miRNAs in cardiovascular diseases[J]. Heart Lung Circ, 2014, 23 (6): 503-510.

[30] D'Alessandra Y, Carena MC, Spazzafumo L, et al. Diagnostic potential of plasmatic MicroRNA signatures in stable and unstable angina[J]. PLoS One, 2013, 8 (11): e80345.

[31] Long G, Wang F, Duan Q, et al. Human circulating microRNA-1 and microRNA-126 as potential novel indicators for acute myocardial

infarction[J]. Int J Biol Sci, 2012, 8 (6): 811-818.

[32] Sayed AS, Xia K, Yang TL, Peng J. Circulating microRNAs: a potential role in diagnosis and prognosis of acute myocardial infarction[J]. Dis Markers, 2013, 35 (5): 561-566.

[33] Liu P, Qiu C, Li B, et al. Clinical impact of circulating miR-133, miR-1291 and miR-663b in plasma of patients with acute myocardial infarction[J]. Diagn Pathol, 2014, 1 (9): 89.

[34] Liebetrau C, Mollmann H, Dorr O, et al. Release kinetics of circulating muscle-enriched microRNAs in patients undergoing transcoronary ablation of septal hypertrophy[J]. J Am Coll Cardiol, 2013, 62 (11): 992-998.

[35] Zhang PP, Wang XL, Zhao W, et al. DNA methylation-mediated repression of miR-941 enhances lysine (K)-specific demethylase 6B expression in hepatoma cells[J]. J Biol Chem, 2014, 289 (35): 24724-24735.

[36] Hu HY, He L, Fominykh K, et al. Evolution of the human-specific microRNA miR-941[J]. Nat Commun, 2012, 3: 1145.

First Published: BAI Rui-na, YANG Qiao-ning, XI Rui-xi, LI Lizhi, SHI Da-zhuo, CHEN Ke-ji. miR-941 as a promising biomarker for acute coronary syndrome[J] . BMC Cardiovasc Disord, 2017, 17: 227.

Efficacy of Danlou Tablet (丹蒌片) in Patients with Non-ST Elevation Acute Coronary Syndrome Undergoing Percutaneous Coronary Intervention: Results from a Multicentre, Placebo-Controlled, Randomized Trial

WANG Lei, ZHAO Xu-jie, MAO Shuai, LIU Shao-nan, GUO Xin-feng, GUO Li-heng, DU Ting-hai, YANG Hai-yu, ZHAO Fu-hai, WU Keng, Cong Hong-liang, WU Keng, YANG Phillip C, CHEN Ke-ji, and ZHANG Min-zhou

Over the past several decades, percutaneous coronary intervention (PCI)has emerged as the predominant therapeutic administration for ischemic heart disease. However, the high incidence of periprocedural myocardial infarction (PMI)following PCI severely impaired the benefits of coronary revascularization. It has been demonstrated that approximately 30% of patients undergoing PCI therapy developed PMI, which is significantly associated with bad long-term prognosis [1,2].

Clinical trials have revealed the efficacy of high-dose statin treatment in significantly reducing the incidence of PMI among patients after coronary revascularization [3–5]. However, high-dose statin administration has been asso-ciated with severe side effects, including increased risk of new-onset diabetes, liver damage, rhabdomyolysis, and intracerebral haemorrhage [6–8]. Therefore, recent studies endeavored to discover alternative natural agents that could reduce the incidence of myocardial necrosis after coronary intervention with low risk of side effects[9,10].

Over the past several years, there has been a surge of interest in the use of Chinese medicine for alleviating cardiovascular diseases, including angina pectoris, myocardial infarction, and chronic heart failure[11–13]. According to the theory of Traditional Chinese Medicine (TCM), the primary cause of coronary heart disease is intermingled phlegm and blood stasis. The Danlou Tablet, a patented Chinese medicine, has been approved by China Food and Drug Administration for patients with coronary heart disease and angina pectoris in 2005. The Danlou Tablet has been demonstrated to significantly alleviate phlegm and stasis mutual obstruction, decrease the serum level of inflammation molecular, and improve the quality of life in patients with unstable angina pectoris[14]. Furthermore, basic research has shown that it could decrease the area of myocardial ischemia and increase ion transport channel-related enzyme activities for the arrhythmia model rats induced by transient myocardial ischemia/reperfusion [15]. Ultraperformance liquid chromatography-tandem mass spectrometer (UPLC-MS/MS)was also used to analyse 15 quality-control markers of Danlou Tablet, and good consistency of the active markers was found among 12 different batches (Figure 1).

In the current study, we evaluated the hypothesis that Danlou Tablet treatment in patients with non-st-segment elevation acute coronary syndromes (NSTE-ACS)undergoing PCI would decrease the incidence of PMI and improve the clinical outcome by a multicentre, randomized, prospective, double-blind, placebo-controlled trial.

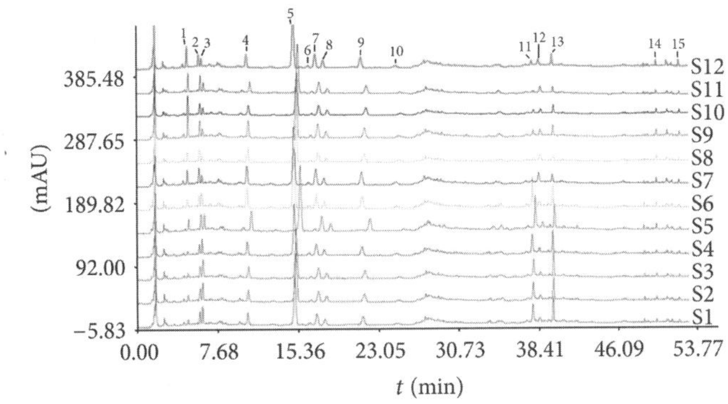

Figure 1 UPLC fingerprints of 15 batches of Danlou Tablets. 2: 5-hydroxymethyl furfural; 3: danshensu; 5: puerarin; 9: daidzin; 11: SalB; 13: Sal A; and 15: tanshinone II A

METHODS

1 Study Design

The protocol of this clinical trial has been revealed in detail previously[16]. Briefly, the study followed the Declaration of Helsinki and was approved by Institutional Ethics Committee of Guangdong Provincial Hospital of Traditional Chinese Medicine and participating hospitals (Acknowledgments Section). Statin-naive patients aged ≥ 18 years with non-ST-segment elevation ACS including unstable angina or non-ST-segment elevation myocardial infarction (NSTEMI)with selective coronary angioplasty to be under-taken within 72 h of admission were screened. Patients with acute ST-segment elevation myocardial infarction (STEMI), fraction < 30%), or hepatic dysfunction with elevated alanine aminotransferase and aspartate aminotransferase serum levels for any reason were excluded from this study. Written informed consent was obtained from each participating patient.

2 Interventions

Eligible patients were randomized to either the experimental group or the control group. Patients in the experimental group received the treatment of Danlou Tablet (4.5 g per day for 48 hours before PCI and a further 4.5 g per day for 90 days after PCI). Patients in the control group received the administration of placebo. All enrolled patients received standard management care in accordance with the uidelines for the Management of Patients with Unstable Angina/NSTEMI [17], including anti-platelet agents, anticoagulation agents, lipid-lowering agents, antiventricular remodeling, or antihypertensive therapy depending on the conditions of patients, irrespective of the randomization assignment. In particular, atorvastatin served as the unique lipid-lowering agent in the study, administrated with the moderate-intensity dose of 10 mg/day before and after PCI without any loading doses for the purpose of minimizing the effect of statin on the results.

Enrolled patients were assessed at 48 h before PCI, 8 h and 24 h after PCI, and 30 days and 90 days after PCI. Assessments included physical examination, vital signs, quality-of-life measurement, electrocardiogram (ECG), and echocardiography. Furthermore, blood samples were collected for laboratory tests, including cardiac biomarkers (troponin I and creatine kinase-myocardial band [CK-MB]), lipids, biochemistry, haematology, C-reactive protein (CRP), and urinalysis.

3 Randomization and Blinding

Participants were randomly assigned into two groups. Randomization was stratified by centre with permuted block size. The randomized sequence was generated by computer with SAS 9.2 software (SAS institute Inc., Cary, USA)and saved in China-Australia International Research Centre for Chinese Medicine (CAIRC-CM), Guangdong Academy of Chinese Medical Sciences. Allocation of treatments was distributed by sealed, opaque, and numbered envelopes. Practitioners and participants were unaware of their assignment. One statistician who generated the blinding code was aware of the drug allocation. Participants, physicians, outcome assessors, and other statisticians and practitioners, however, remained blind to treatment assignments before the results were revealed. The placebo was prepared and packed by a pharmaceutical company (Jilin Connell Pharmaceutical Co. Ltd., China). The placebo was designed similarly to Danlou Tablet in shape, size, and taste. Each participant was provided with a bottle of water labelled with their unique number according to randomization.

4 Outcomes

The primary endpoints of this trial were the incidence of death, nonfatal myocardial infarction, target vessel revascularization (bypass surgery or repeat PCI), and rehospitalization due to acute cardiovascular events (severe angina or heart failure)within 30 days of the procedure. Secondary endpoints included the incidence of major adverse cardiovascular events (MACEs)within 90 days of PCI, the proportion of patients with elevated biomarkers of myocardial injury (troponin I)at 8 h and 24 h after PCI, and the proportion of patients with elevated CRP level at these time points. Nonfatal myocardial infarctions included spontaneous myocardial infarction, PMI, and myocardial infarctions related to stent thrombosis. PMI was defined as a postprocedural increase of cardiac troponin I (cTn I)values more than 5 × 99th percentile of the upper reference limit (URL)or a rise of cTn I values if baseline values were elevated. Spontaneous myocardial infarctions were considered to be related to ischemia due to plaque erosion and/or rupture, fissuring, or dissection [18].

Furthermore, the safety and tolerability of experimental drugs were evaluated by the incidence, severity, and relation-ship to treatment of adverse events (AEs), including clinically significant changes in vital signs, physical examination findings, and laboratory measurements.

5 Sample Size Estimation

The sample size was calculated based on the reduction of incidence of MACE by a two-sided test with level size of 5% and a power of 80% chance of detecting a difference. A previous trial revealed the incidence of MACE as 17% in patients treated with low-dose statin therapy within 30 days after PCI [3]. Assuming a MACE incidence of 5% in the experimental group, it was calculated that a minimum of 99 patients would be required for each group. Additionally, we estimated that up to 10% of initial participants may withdraw from the trial (PASS 11.0 software, NCSS, Utah, USA). We thus determined that 232 eligible cases would be required.

6 Statistical Analysis

The trial database was blindly reviewed before the data were locked and unblended by the independent data collection centre, China-Australia International Research Centre for Chinese Medicine. Data from all participants who underwent randomization were analyzed based on the intention-to-treat (ITT)principle. A per-protocol (PP) analysis was performed to test the robust-ness of the trial results. Baseline clinical and demographic characteristics were expressed as mean ± SD, median, or interquartile range (IQR). For comparisons, two samples were compared by t-test for normally distributed values; otherwise the Mann–Whitney U test was used. Proportions were analyzed using the Chi-square test or the exact test method. Kaplan-Meier plots of cumulative incidence freedom of overall MACEs were constructed from the 30-day and (two-tailed)was considered statistically significant. All calculations were conducted using SPSS software version 18.0 (IBM Inc., New York, USA).

RESULTS

1 Patient Population

Between November 25, 2012, and March 23, 2014, 340 patients were screened: among them, 60 were excluded because of previous or current treatment with statins; 35 were excluded because they required an emergency PCI approach; 21 were excluded because of severe heart failure with ejection fraction < 30%, and 5were excluded because of contraindications to statin treatment (e.g., hepatic dysfunction or serious adverse reaction) (Figure 2). Eligible patients (*n*= 219)received the study assignment drug (Danlou Tablet or placebo)before PCI. Procedural success was obtained in all patients; 4 patients (2 in each group)had no-reflow or slow-flow phenomenon, which was significantly alleviated following intracoronary administration of platelet glycoprotein IIb/IIIa inhibitors (tirofiban). The last subject completed follow-up in June, 2014. Data entry was completed by November, 2014.

Demographic and clinical features of patients in the Danlou Tablet group and placebo group are indicated in Table 1. Patient characteristics were not significantly different in age, gender, cardiovascular risk factors, concomitant diseases, clinical presentation, cardiac function, blood creatinine levels, and medical therapy at the time of intervention. In comparing the main procedural features treatments in both the Danlou Tablet and placebo groups, there were statistically significant differences in the stent length (indicated in Table 2), but there were no statistically significant differences in coronary anatomy, multivessel lesion type, procedural characteristics of intervention, number of stents per patient, or the diameter of implanted stents ($P>0.05$).

2 Cardiovascular Events

The primary endpoint was assessed at 30 days after coronary revascularization (Table 3). There was no statistically significant difference in the incidence of MACE in the Danlou Tablet group (22.0% . of patients[24 of 109])in the Danlou Tablet group compared to the placebo group (33.6% of patients [37 of 110]) (P= 0.06). At 90 days after PCI, however, the incidence of MACE in the Danlou Tablet group was significantly lower than in the placebo group (23.9% versus 37.3%, P= 0.03, Table 4).

Furthermore, Kaplan-Meier curves showed that MACE-free survival rates at the 90-day follow-up were significantly greater in Danlou Tablet group than in the placebo group (n = 0.04, Figure 3). The lower rate of MACE at 90 days in the Danlou Tablet group was mostly driven by a reduced incidence of nonfatal myocardial infarction (22% versus 34.5%, P= 0.04). The vast majority of nonfatal myocardial infarction cases occurred within 24 hours after PCI and were defined as PMIs (Figure 4). One patient (0.9%)in the placebo group died due to probable stent thrombosis complicated with cardiac shock. In two patients (1.8%)in the Danlou Tablet group and five patients (4.5%)in the placebo group, instent restenosis occurred, and coronary revascularization had to be repeated. There was no statistically significant difference in the incidences of target vessel revascularization between the treated and placebo groups (P= 0.45).

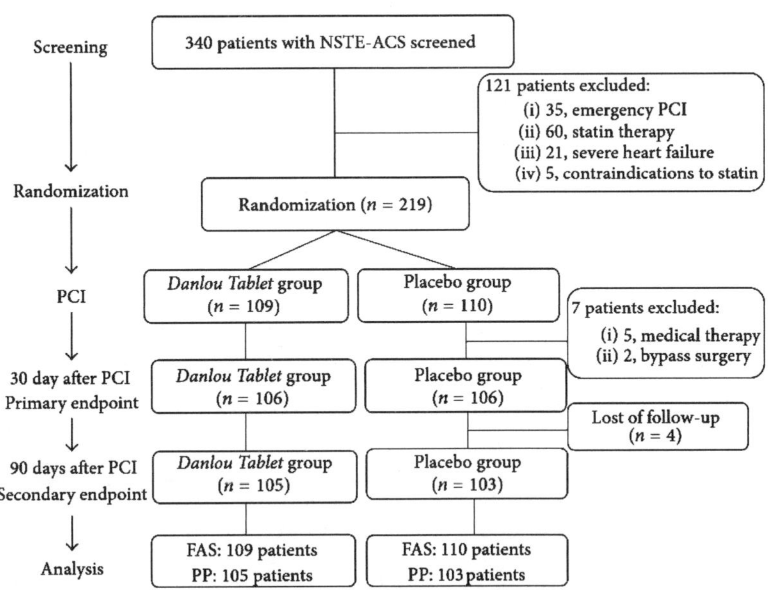

Figure 2 Flow diagram of Danlou Tablet for patients with ACS undergoing PCI.

Notes: FAS, full-analysis set; NSTE-ACS, non-ST-segment elevation acute coronary syndrome; PCI, percutaneous coronary intervention; and PP, per protocol.

Table 1 Main Demographic and Clinical Features of the Two Groups

Variable	Danlou Tablet group (n = 109)	Placebo group (n = 110)	χ^2 (Z)	P value
Age, yr	62.89 ± 9.23	63.89 ± 10.03	0.04	0.44
Men, number (%)	72 (66.1)	74 (67.3)	0.04	0.85
Body weight, kg	66.91 ± 10.14	66.65 ± 9.54	-0.6	0.55
Height, cm	166.41 ± 6.85	166.00 ± 8.17	-0.23	0.82
Family history of coronary disease, number (%)	18 (16.5)	10 (9.1)	2.71	0.10
Concomitant diseases, number (%)				
Previous coronary heart disease	41 (37.6)	47 (42.7)	0.60	0.44
Previous coronary intervention	9 (8.3)	17 (15.5)	2.71	0.10
Systemic hypertension	51 (46.8)	63 (57.3)	2.41	0.12
Diabetes mellitus	21 (19.3)	19 (17.3)	0.15	0.70
Dyslipidemia	38 (34.9)	38 (34.5)	0.002	0.96
Heart failure	1 (0.9)	4 (3.6)		0.37*
Arrhythmia	4 (3.7)	10 (9.1)	2.69	0.10
Stroke	7 (6.4)	8 (7.3)	0.06	0.80
Current smoker, number (%)	47 (43.1)	44 (40.0)	0.22	0.64
Cardiac Marker Elevation, number (%)	30 (27.5%)	33 (30.0%)	0.16	0.69
Clinical pattern, number (%)				
Unstable angina	88 (80.7)	87 (79.1)	0.09	0.76
NSTEMI	21 (19.3)	23 (20.9)		
Cardiac function, number (%)				
Level I	41 (37.6)	41 (37.3)		
Level II	53 (48.6)	53 (48.2)	0.03	0.99
Level III	15 (13.8)	16 (14.5)		

Notes: Values are given as number of patients (%)or mean ± SD. NSTEMI, non-ST-segment elevation myocardial infarction; PCI, percutaneous coronary intervention; ACE, angiotensin-converting enzyme; and ARB, angiotensin II receptor blocker. * P value is from Fisher's exact test.

Table 2 Angiographic and Procedural Features of the Two Groups

Variable	Danlou Tablet group (n= 109)	Placebo group (n= 110)	χ^2 (Z)	P value
Multivessel coronary artery disease, number (%)	62 (56.9)	63 (57.3)	0.00	0.95
Vessel treated, number (%)				
Left main	2 (1.8)	2 (1.8)		1.00*
Left anterior descending	73 (67.0)	65 (59.1)	1.46	0.23
Left circumflex	26 (23.9)	34 (30.9)	1.37	0.24
Right coronary artery	35 (32.1)	30 (27.3)	0.61	0.43
Restenotic lesions, number (%)	1 (0.9)	1 (0.9)		1.00
Multivessel intervention, number (%)	24 (22.0)	18 (16.4)	1.13	0.29
Type of intervention, number (%)				
Balloon only	1 (0.9)	1 (0.9)		1.00*
Stent	108 (99.1)	109 (99.1)		1.00*
Number of stents per patient	1.49 ± 0.70	1.41 ± 0.67	-0.89	0.37
Stent diameter, mm	2.94 ± 0.43	2.92 ± 0.43	-0.87	0.39
Total stent length, mm	20.52 ± 7.01	22.37 ± 7.46	-2.34	0.02

Notes: Values are given as number of patients (%)or mean ± SD. *P value is from Fisher's exact test.

Table 3 MACE at 30 Days after PCI in the Danlou Tablet and Placebo Groups

	Incidence		Treatment difference (%)	
	Danlou Tablet group	Placebo group	Difference[a] of incidence (95% CI)	*P* value
Full-analysis set	*N* = 109	*N* = 110		
Total MACE, *n* (%)	24 (22.0)	37 (33.6)	1.8 (1.0, 3.3)	0.06[c]
Cardiac death, *n* (%)	0	0		
Nonfatal MI, *n* (%)	24 (22.0)	37 (33.6)	1.8 (1.0, 3.3)	0.06[c]
Target vessel revascularization, *n* (%)	0	1 (0.9)		1.0[d]
Rehospitalization due to CVE[b], *n* (%)	0	0		
Per-protocol analysis set	*N* = 107	*N* = 109		
Total MACE, *n* (%)	24 (22.4)	36 (33.0)	1.7 (0.9, 3.1)	0.08[c]
Cardiac death, *n* (%)	0 (0)	0 (0)		
Nonfatal myocardial infarction, *n* (%)	24 (22.4)	36 (33.0)	1.7 (0.9, 3.1)	0.08[c]
Target vessel revascularization, *n* (%)	0	1 (0.9)		
Rehospitalization due to CVE[b], *n* (%)	0	0		

Notes: CI, confidence interval ; CVE, cardiovascular events ; MACE, major adverse cardiac event ; and MI, myocardial infarction. [a]Difference of incidence = Danlou Tablet - placebo. [b]Cardiovascular events included severe angina or heart failure (NYHF ⩾ IV). [c]*P* value is from the continuity-adjusted Chi-square test. [d]*P* value is from Fisher's exact test.

3 Biomarker Results

Before the procedure, there were no significant differences in the percentage of patients with abnormal cTn I elevation between two group (27.5% versus 30.0%, *P* = 0.69, Table 1). After the procedure, 8 and 24 hr post-PCI cTn I>3×99th percentile of URL occurred more frequently in the placebo arm than in the Danlou Tablet group (25.7% versus 40.9%, *P*= 0.02, and 30.3% versus 41.8%, *P*= 0.08) (Figure 5 (a)). Moreover, the proportion of patients with elevated levels of cTn I>5×99th percentile of URL was significantly lower in the Danlou Tablet group at 8 h (22.0% versus 35.4%, *P*= 0.04)and 24 h after PCI (23.9% versus 38.2%, *P*= 0.02) (Figure 5 (b)). Analyses on the population with elevated CRP levels showed no statistically significant differences between the Danlou Tablet group and the placebo group at 8 h (37.1% versus 32.0%, *P*= 0.44) and 24 h (47.6% versus 42.7%, *P*= 0.48)after PCI.

4 Safety Analysis

Only two patients in Danlou Tablet group had minor gastrointestinal adverse events (nausea and diarrhea), which were relieved after two days of suspension in the management of the experimental drug. Meanwhile, therewere no significant ECG or physical examination findings or changes in laboratory parameters potentially associated with experimental drugs.

Table 4 MACE at 90 Days after PCI in the Danlou Tablet and Placebo Groups

	Incidence		Treatment difference (%)	
	Danlou Tablet group	Placebo group	Difference[a] of incidence (95% CI)	*P* value
Full-analysis set	*N* = 109	*N* = 110		
Total MACE, *n* (%)	26 (23.9)	41 (37.3)	1.9 (1.1, 3.4)	0.03[c]
Cardiac death, *n* (%)	0	1 (0.9)		1.00[d]
Nonfatal MI, *n* (%)	24 (22.0)	38 (34.5)	1.9 (1.0, 3.4)	0.04[c]
Target vessel revascularization, *n* (%)	2 (1.8)	5 (4.5)	2.5 (0.5, 13.4)	0.45[d]
Rehospitalization due to CVE[b], *n* (%)	0	0		
Per-protocol analysis set	*N* = 105	*N* = 103		

Continued

	Incidence		Treatment difference (%)	
	Danlou Tablet group	Placebo group	Difference[a] of incidence (95% CI)	*P* value
Total MACE, *n* (%)	25 (23.8)	35 (34.0)		
Cardiac death, *n* (%)	0	1 (1.0)	1.6 (0.9, 3.0)	0.11[c]
Nonfatal myocardial infarction, *n* (%)	23 (21.9)	32 (31.1)	1.6 (0.9, 3.0)	0.50[d]
Target vessel revascularization, *n* (%)	2 (1.9)	5 (4.9)	2.6 (0.5, 13.9)	0.13[c]
Rehospitalization due to CVE[b], *n* (%)	0	0		0.28[d]

CI, confidence interval ; CVE, cardiovascular events ; MACE, major adverse cardiac event ; and MI, myocardial infarction. [a]Difference of incidence = Danlou Tablet-placebo. [b]Cardiovascular events included severe angina or heart failure (NYHF ≥ IV). [c]*P* value is from the continuity-adjusted Chi-square test. [d]*P* value is from Fisher's exact test.

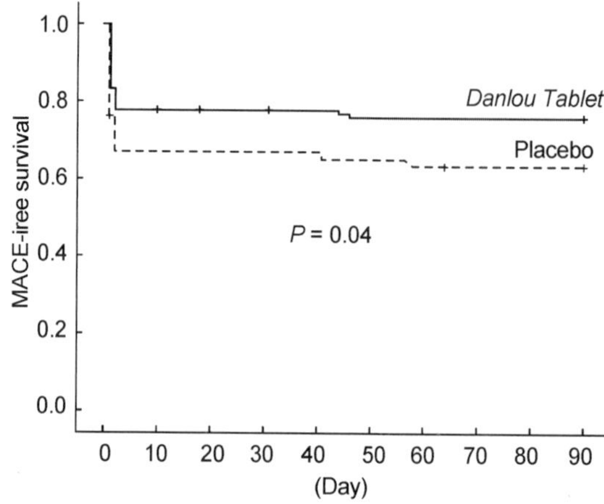

Figure 3　Survival Curves

Notes: Kaplan-Meier curves of 90-day major adverse cardiac event- (MACE-)free survival in the 2 arms. MACE, major adverse cardiac event (death, nonfatal myocardial infarction, target vessel revascularisation, and rehospitalization due to acute cardiovascular events).

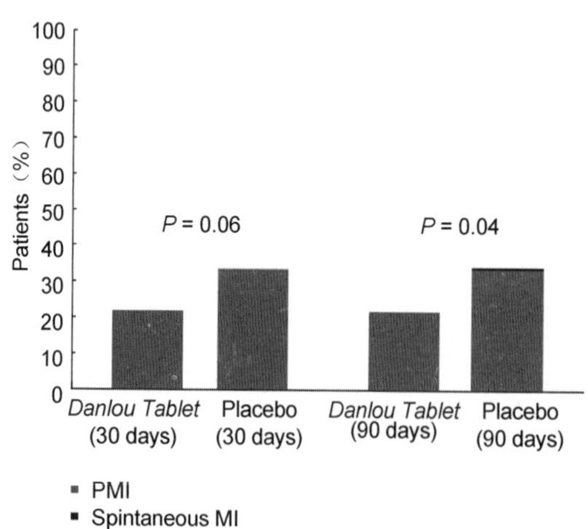

Figure 4　Non-fatal MI

Notes: *PMI: periprocedure myocardial infarction.

DISCUSSION

It has been reported that a large number of patients under-going PCI might suffer from myocardial injuries arising from the procedure itself, which is significant enough to serve as a negative prognostic factor [19]. Although previous studies have shown that pretreatment with high-dose statin is associated with reduced incidence of PMI in patients with acute coronary events[3,4], still more studies did not demonstrate similar results[20,21]. Particularly, a trial in which statin-naive Korean and Chinese patients with NSTE-ACS received additional loading high-dose atorvastatin before PCI showed that there were no benefits compared with usual post-PCI atorvastatin treatment[21]. Moreover, recent trials revealed that there were no expected benefits of high-intensity statin treatments in East Asian patients compared with moderate-or low-intensity statin treatments [22,23]. The reason why there were the different benefits of high-dose statin between Asian and Caucasians population could be attributed to the race difference of statin pharmacokinetics. Therefore, strong evidence-based natural agents to improve East Asian patient management and reduce the incidence of PMI are critical to address this challenge.

The present study was a multicentre, randomized controlled trial conducted in a statin-naive Chinese ACS population undergoing selective PCI. Herein, we compare a group in which Danlou Tablet was administered for 2 days before elective PCI following a further treatment with the control group who received placebo based on usual care including moderate-intensity statin treatment (atorvastatin, 10 mg/day). Our study demonstrated that the proportion of patients with elevated levels of troponin I was significantly lower in the Danlou Tablet group at 8 h and 24 h, suggesting that Danlou Tablet pretreatment was associated with a significantly lower occurrence of PMI (Figure 5 (b)). There was a tendency towards a lower occurrence of major cardiac events 30 days after PCI in patients with ACS undergoing selective interventional therapy (22.0% versus 33.6%, P = 0.06). The MACE-free Kaplan-Meier curves showed a significantly better event-free survival at 90 days in the Danlou Tablet arm. This change may be attributed to a significant reduction of nonfatal myocardial infarctions. The incidence of PMI in our trial was higher than that in the ARMYDAR-ACS[4] or ROMA trials[5]. The different diagnostic criteria of PMI may have led to this result; in the latter trials, PMI was diagnosed by the increase of creatine kinase-MB instead of cTn I.

The predominant mechanisms of PMI are complicated, including vulnerable plaque disruption[24], ischemia/reperfusion injury[25], oxidative stress, platelet activation[26], and inflammatory cytokines activation [27] induced by balloon pressure inflation or stent implantation during the procedure. The Danlou Tablet is a potent herbal compound mainly consisting of Salvia, *Ligusticum chuanxiong* Hort, Trichosanthes kirilowii, and Alliummacrostemon. Chen et al. [28] report that Danlou Tablet may accelerate blood circulation and eliminate intravascular phlegm, which have critical roles in managing the ischemic disease based on the Traditional

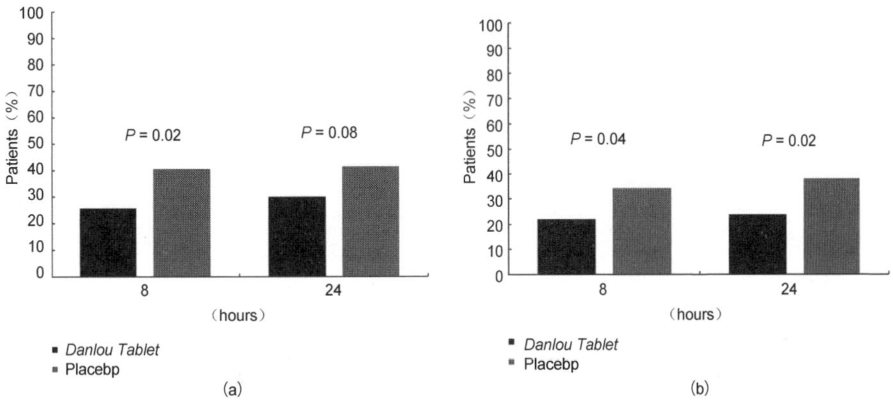

Figure 5 Cardiac Marker Elevations

Notes: (a)TnI > 3 × 99th percentile of the upper reference limit (URL)at 8 and 24 hours after PCI in the Danlou Tablet group and in the placebo group. (b)TnI > 5 × 99th percentile of the URL at 8 and 24 hours after PCI in the Danlou Tablet group and in the placebo group.

Chinese Medicine (TCM)theory. An increasing number of studies have been conducted to elucidate the cardioprotective effects of Danlou Tablet. Liu et al. investigated the efficacy of Danlou Tablet in improving cardiac function in miniature swine with experimental coronary disease and found that the Danlou Tablet treatment significantly improved cardiac function and histopathology and downregulated malondialdehyde (MDA)and superoxide dismutase (SOD)serum levels [29]. Guo et al. examined the effects of Danlou Tablet on arrhythmia model rats induced by transient myocardial ischemia/reperfusion (I/R)and revealed that Danlou Tablet inhibited the incidence of fatal and nonfatal ventricular fibrillation. The reduced frequency and duration of ventricular tachycardia might be related to lowering the degree of myocardial ischemia and increasing ion transport channel related enzyme activities (Na^+-K^+ ATPase and CaATPase)[15]. Similarly, our recent studies also suggested that administration of Danlou Tablet could alleviate the severity of risk region myocardial ischemia and reperfusion arrhythmia in vivo [30]. Moreover, recent studies revealed that puerarin, the main component of Danlou Tablet by UPLC-MS/MS analysis (Figure 1), could significantly protect cardiomyocytes from anoxia/reoxygenation injury in vitro[31,32].

In addition, endothelial injury induced by balloon or stent inflating is another key contributor for PMI [33]. Yang et al. found that the original superfine Danlou Tablet improved endothelial function in rats with arterial endothelial injury by downregulating the cardiac chymase signal pathway and chymase-mediated angiotensin II production [34]. Hong's study suggested that Danlou Tablet may protect vascular endothelium and improve formation of new capillaries on the edges of the ischemic myocardial zones, thereby contributing to the ultimate reduction of the infarct size and subsequent alleviation of the progressive heart failure[35]. Furthermore, another possible mechanism underlying the beneficial effects of Danlou Tablet may involve the alleviation of inflammatory reactions at the atherosclerotic plaque [28]. A clinical trial by Wang et al. showed the treatment of Danlou Tablet could alleviate inflammatory activation by reducing the serum level of hs-CRP, soluble CD40, and interleukin-6 [14]. However, our study demonstrated that there was no significant difference in the serum level of hs-CRP between two arms. Consequently, the anti-inflammation effects of this patented Chinese herbneed to be further explored by more studies in vitro and in vivo.

Therefore, the benefits of Danlou Tablet in reducing PMI could be explained by the reported multiple mechanisms by which the treatment or its components inhibit ischemia reperfusion injury, decrease oxidative stress responses, and improve endothelial dysfunction and microvessel coronary circulation. Pre-PCI treatment of Danlou Tablet in NSTE-ACS patients may consequently translate into clinical positive outcomes.

LIMITATIONS

This study has some limitations. Firstly, the figures we used to estimate the sample size were not consistent with the actual results, which led to relatively lower power than expected. Secondly, biochemical measurements (e.g., CRP and cTnI)were not performed in the laboratory, which may have decreased the reliability of results. Furthermore, this trial was undertaken in China; whether the effects of the trial drugs would be similar in other ethnic groups is unknown.

CONCLUSION

In conclusion, the present trial implied that treatment with Danlou Tablet based on the low-dose of statin could reduce the incidence and magnitude of PMI and subsequently improve clinical outcomes in patients receiving elective revascularization with unstable angina and non-ST-segment elevation acute coronary syndromes. If confirmed by larger additional randomized studies, these findings may support the indication of "upstream" administration of this alternative natural agent in patients with acute coronary syndromes treated with an early invasive strategy.

REFERENCES

[1] Ganesha Babu G, Malcolm Walker J, Yellon D M, and Hausenloy D J. Peri-procedural myocardial injury during percutaneous coronary intervention: an important target for cardioprotection[J]. European Heart Journal, 2011, 32 (1): 23-31.

[2] Nettleman M D, Banitt L, Barry W, Awan I, and Gordon E E. Predictors of Survival and the Role of Gender in Postoperative Myocardial Infarction[J]. American Journal of Medicine, 1997, 103 (5): 357-362.

[3] Pasceri V, Patti G, Nusca A, Pristipino C, Richichi G, and Di Sciascio G. Randomized trial of atorvastatin for reduction of myocardial damage during coronary intervention: Results from the ARMYDA (Atorvastatin for Reduction of Myocardial Damage during Angioplasty)study[J]. Acc Current Journal Review, 2004, 13 (11): 53-53.

[4] Patti G, Pasceri V, Colonna G, et al. Atorvastatin Pretreatment Improves Outcomes in Patients With Acute Coronary Syndromes Undergoing Early Percutaneous Coronary Intervention: Results of the ARMYDA-ACS Randomized Trial[J]. Journal of the American College of Cardiology, 2007, 49 (12): 1272-1278.

[5] Sardella G, Conti G, Donahue M, et al. Rosuvastatin pretreatment in patients undergoing elective PCI to reduce the incidence of myocardial periprocedural necrosis: The ROMA trial[J]. Catheterization & Cardiovascular Interventions Official Journal of the Society for Cardiac Angiography & Interventions, 2013, 81 (1): E36-E43.

[6] Preiss D Seshasai S R K, Welsh P, et al. Risk of Incident Diabetes With Intensive-Dose Compared With Moderate-Dose Statin Therapy: A Meta-analysis[J]. The Journal of the American Medical Association, 2011, 305 (24): 2556-2564.

[7] Armitage J. The safety of statins in clinical practice[J]. The Lancet, 2007, 370 (9601): 1781-1790.

[8] Pandit A K, Kumar P, Kumar A, et al. High-dose statin therapy and risk of intracerebral hemorrhage: a meta-analysis[J]. Acta Neurologica Scandinavica, 2016, 134 (1): 22-28.

[9] Li Guang-Ping, Zheng Xin-Tian, Wang Huai-Zhen, et al. Multicenter investigation of compound danshen dripping pills on short-term clinical events in patient with ST elevation myocardial infarction undergoing primary PCI (MICD-STEMI PCI)[J]. Chinese Journal of Interventional Cardiology, 2011, 19 (1): 24-28.

[10] Mao S, Wang L, Zhao X, et al. Sodium tanshinone IIA sulfonate for reduction of periprocedural myocardial injury during percutaneous coronary intervention (STAMP trial): Rationale and design[J]. International Journal of Cardiology, 2015, 182: 329-333.

[11] Shang H, Zhang J, Yao C, et al. Qi-Shen-Yi-Qi Dripping Pills for the Secondary Prevention of Myocardial Infarction: A Randomised Clinical Trial[J]. Evidence-Based Complementary and Alternative Medicine, 2013, 2013: 1-9.

[12] Wang L, Guo L, Zhang M, et al. Clinical pathways based on integrative medicine in chinese hospitals improve treatment outcomes for patients with acute myocardial infarction: A multicentre, nonrandomized historically controlled trial[J]. Evidence-Based Complementary and Alternative Medicine, 2012, 2012 Article ID 821641.

[13] Li X, Zhang J, Huang J, et al. A Multicenter, Randomized, Double-Blind, Parallel-Group, Placebo-Controlled Study of the Effects of Qili Qiangxin Capsules in Patients With Chronic Heart Failure[J]. Journal of the American College of Cardiology, 2013, 62 (12): 1065-1072.

[14] Shi-Han W, Jie W, Ji Li. Efficacy Assessment of Treating Patients with Coronary Heart Disease Angina of Phlegm and Stasis Mutual Obstruction Syndrome by Danlou Tablet[J]. Chinese Journal of Integrated Traditional and Western Medicine, 2012, 32 (8): 1051-1055.

[15] Guo L L, Wang J, Lin F, et al. Effect of danlou tablet on arrhythmia model rats induced by transient myocardial ischemia/reperfusion[J]. Chinese Journal of Integrated Traditional & Western Medicine, 2014, 34 (9): 1125-1129.

[16] Effect of Danlou Tablet (丹蒌片)on peri-procedural myocardial injury among patients undergoing percutaneous coronary intervention for non-ST elevation acute coronary syndrome: a study protocol of a multicenter, randomized, controlled trial[J]. Chinese Journal of Integrative Medicine, 2015, 21 (9): 662-666.

[17] Wright R S, Anderson J L, Adams C D, et al. 2011 ACCF/AHA Focused Update Incorporated Into the ACC/AHA 2007 Guidelines for the Management of Patients With Unstable Angina/Non-ST-Elevation Myocardial Infarction: A Report of the American College of Cardiology Foundation/American Heart Association Task Force on Practice Guidelines[J]. Journal of the American College of Cardiology, 2011, 57 (19): e215-e367.

[18] Thygesen K, Alpert J S, Jaffe A S, Simoons M L, Chaitman B R, and White H D. Third universal definition of myocardial infarction[J]. Journal of the American College of Cardiology, 2012, 60 (16): 1581-1598.

[19] Nienhuis M B, Ottervanger J P, Bilo H J G, et al. Prognostic value of troponin after elective percutaneous coronary intervention: A meta-analysis[J]. Catheterization and Cardiovascular Interventions, 2008, 71 (3): 318-324.

[20] Veselka J, David Zemánek, Petr Hájek, et al. Effect of Two-Day Atorvastatin Pretreatment on the Incidence of Periprocedural Myocardial Infarction Following Elective Percutaneous Coronary Intervention: A Single-Center, Prospective, and Randomized Study[J]. American Journal of Cardiology, 2009, 104 (5): 630-633.

[21] Jang Y, Zhu J, Ge J, et al. Preloading with atorvastatin before percutaneous coronary intervention in statin-naive Asian patients with non-ST elevation acute coronary syndromes: A randomized study[J]. Journal of Cardiology, 2014, 63 (5): 335-343.

[22] Li Y F, Feng Q Z, Gao W Q, Zhang X J, Huang Y and Chen Y D. The difference between Asian and Western in the effect of LDL-C lowering therapy on coronary atherosclerotic plaque: a meta-analysis report[J]. BMC Cardiovascular Disorders, 2015, 15 (1): article 6.

[23] Zhao S P, Yu B L, Peng D Q, et al. The effect of moderate-dose versus double-dose statins on patients with acute coronary syndrome in China:

Results of the CHILLAS trial[J]. Atherosclerosis, 2014, 233 (2): 707-712.

[24] Kawamoto T, Okura H, Koyama Y, et al. The Relationship Between Coronary Plaque Characteristics and Small Embolic Particles During Coronary Stent Implantation[J]. Journal of the American College of Cardiology, 2007, 50 (17): 1635-1640.

[25] Sinha, M. K. Ischemia Modified Albumin Is a Sensitive Marker of Myocardial Ischemia After Percutaneous Coronary Intervention[J]. Circulation, 2003, 107 (19): 2403-2405.

[26] Cuisset T, Frere C, Quizlike J, et al. High post-treatment platelet reactivity is associated with a high incidence of myonecrosis after stenting for non-ST elevation acute coronary syndromes. [J]. Thromb Haemost, 2007, 97 (02): 282-287.

[27] Saleh N, Svane B, Jensen J, et al. Stent implantation, but not pathogen burden, is associated with plasma C-reactive protein and interleukin-6 levels after percutaneous coronary intervention in patients with stable angina pectoris[J]. American Heart Journal, 2005, 149 (5): 876-882.

[28] Chen J, Cai H W, Miao J, et al. Danlou Tablet Fought against Inflammatory Reaction in Atherosclerosis Rats with Intermingled Phlegm and Blood Stasis Syndrome and Its Mechanism Study[J]. Zhongguo Zhong xi yi jie he za zhi Zhongguo Zhongxiyi jiehe zazhi = Chinese journal of integrated traditional and Western medicine, 2016, 36 (6): 703-708.

[29] Jian-Xun L, Cheng-Ren L, Jian-Xun R, et al. Protective effect of formula of removing both phlegm and blood stasis on myocardial tissues of Chinese mini-swine with coronary heart disease of phlegm-stasis cementation syndrome[J]. China Journal of Chinese Materia Medica, 2014, 39 (4): 726-732.

[30] Qi J Y, Wang L, Gu D S, et al. Protect effects of Danlou Tablet (丹蒌片)against murine myocardial ischemia and reperfusion injury in vivo[J]. Chinese Journal of Integrative Medicine, 2016.

[31] Ma Y, Gai Y, Yan J, et al. Puerarin Attenuates Anoxia/Reoxygenation Injury Through Enhancing Bcl-2 Associated Athanogene 3 Expression, a Modulator of Apoptosis and Autophagy[J]. Medical science monitor: international medical journal of experimental and clinical research, 2016, 22: 977-983.

[32] Tang L, Liu D, Yi X, et al. The protective effects of puerarin in cardiomyocytes from anoxia/reoxygenation injury are mediated by PKC ε [J]. Cell Biochemistry and Function, 2014, 32 (4): 378-386.

[33] Jaffe R, Charron T, Puley G, et al. Microvascular obstruction and the no-reflow phenomenon after percutaneous coronary intervention[J]. Circulation, 2008, 117 (24): 3152-3156.

[34] Zhen Y, Tie H, Yu-Mei L. Protection of Danlou Tablets on Hyperlipidemia and Vascular Endothelial Injury in Rats[J]. World Journal of Integrated Traditional and Western Medicine, 2010, 5 (6): 491-494.

[35] Mei H. Effects of Danlon Tablet on Myocardial Infarct Size and Ventricular Remodeling in Rats[J]. Chinese Journal of Experimental Traditional Medical Formulae, 2011, 17 (10): 208-211.

First published: WANG Lei, ZHAO Xu-jie, MAO Shuai, LIU Shao-nan, GUO Xin-feng, GUO Li-heng, Du Ting-hai, YANG Hai-yu, ZHAO Fu-hai, WU Keng, Cong-Hongliang, WU Keng, YANG Phillip C, CHEN Ke-ji, ZHANG Min-zhou. Efficacy of Danlou Tab letin patients with Non-ST elevation acute coronary syndrome undergoing percutaneous coronary intervention: results from a multicentre, placebo-controlled, randomized trial[J] . Evid Based Complement Alternat Med, 2016, 2016: 7960503.

Neoatherosclerosis after Drug-Eluting Stent Implantation: Roles and Mechanisms

CUI Yuan-yuan, LIU Yue, ZHAO Fu-hai, SHI Da-zhuo, and CHEN Ke-ji

The emergence of first-generation drug-eluting stents (DES)has greatly minimized the limitations of bare metal stents (BMS); however, concern about in-stent neoatherosclerosis (NA)has attracted much attention owing to its close association with late complications such as revascularization and late stent thrombosis[1–3]. NA is characterized by accumulation of yellow-lipid-laden foamy macrophages within neointima with or without necrotic core and/or calcification after stent implantation [4]. Pathological studies have revealed that advanced NA with neointimal rupture and thrombosis is the most common mechanism of definite vary late stent thrombosis and is also associated with a high frequency of ST-segment elevation myocardial infarction[5,6].

Theoretically, accomplishing endothelial coverage after stenting is considered to be safe to prevent against vascular pathological changes, including thrombosis and inflammation. Nevertheless, "neointima" of DES seems not effective as normal because recent studies have reported that patients with first-and second-generation DES have a high frequency of NA, which was less seen in bare metal stents (BMS)[7,8]. DES-induced endothelial dysfunction plays a critical role in NA formation[9,10]. Here, we try to describe the detailed pathological and cellular mechanisms for DES-induced NA.

1 Clinical Evidence of Neoatherosclerosis

Traditionally, promoting stent coverage after stenting is considered as an important index to evaluate efficacy and safety of current or advanced stents. However, neointimal function after stenting seems anxious for the emergency of NA. Data from the CVPath (Gaithersburg, Maryland)stent registry, including 209 first-generation DES (103 sirolimus-DES [SES] and 106 paclitaxel-DES [PES])and 197 BMS with implant duration of>30 days, showed that the incidence of NA was greater in DES (30%)than in BMS (16%; $P<0.001$)[1]. Furthermore, Ali et al. [7] analyzed 65 symptomatic patients with in-stent restenosis (ISR)33 months of follow-up, finding that optical coherence tomography- (OCT-)verified NA was greater in first-generation DES than with BMS (68% versus 36%, $P = 0.02$). These results suggest that NA is more prevalent in first-generation DES when compared with BMS.

The advent of second-generation DES, including everolimus-eluting stents (EES)and zotarolimus-eluting stents (ZES), has been improved with more biocompatible polymers and thinner strut stent backbones than those with first-generation DES [11]. Neointimal growths developed within those second-generation DES have been documented. Kim et al. [12] reported that second-generation DES (ZES; Endeavor)facilitated strut coverage and reduced rate of malapposed strut compared with first-generation DES. In contrast, results from another multicenter OCT analysis, including 212 patients with first-or second-generation DES (second-generation DES: 40 zotarolimus, 36 everolimus, and 35 biolimus; first-generation DES: 65 sirolimus and 36 paclitaxel), showed that the second-generation DES was not more protective against NA than the first-generation DES [13]. Even second-generation cobalt-chromium EES (CoCr-EES), possessing greater strut coverage with lower incidence of late/very late stent thrombosis than SES and PES in human autopsy analysis, findings showed that the frequency of NA in CoCr-EES was not statistically different when compared with first-generation devices [14]. "neointima" of DES is not functional as normal vessels, and further examination of the neointimal components of DES is needed.

2 Pathological Characteristics of Neointima

Neointima of DES has several features distinguishing from these of BMS, including its components, developing time, progression, and prognosis. Pathological studies, including coronary angioscopy, intravascular ultrasonography (IVUS), histological analysis, and OCT researches, have been performed to investigate the features of neointima in both DES and BMS-associated segments, as shown in Table 1.

Table 1 Different Characteristics of NA between BMS and DES

	Neointima of BMS	Neointima of DES
Tissue components	Smooth muscle cells and proteoglycans-rich extracellular matrix	Fibrin deposition；larger necrotic；calcified components；and less smooth muscle cells
lipid-laden plaque	Small	Large
Inflammatory cell infiltration	Less Inflammatory cell infiltration	Many kind of inflammatory cells: macrophages, multinucleated giant cells, lymphocytes, and granulocytes
Developing time	Slow (>1 year after stenting)	Rapid (< 1year after stenting)
Type of NA	Less of thin-cap NA	Thin-cap NA
Progression	Slow or disappeared	Growing
Prognosis	Relatively stable	High frequency of late stent failure

Early histopathologic studies revealed that neointimal components of DES lesion were similar to those in BMS where the neointima was mainly composed of proliferative smooth muscle cells with proteoglycans-rich extracellular matrix. However, emerging evidence suggests that neointimal components of DES are of obvious difference compared to BMS. Hara et al. [15] conducted a rabbit study by using intravascular near-infrared fluorescence (NIRF)molecular imaging (high-resolution imaging of fibrin)in combination with simultaneous OCT, showing greater fibrin deposition and fibrin persistence in DES than in BMS at 7 and 28 days, respectively. Moreover, neointimal tissue of DES (n = 34)and BMS (n = 27), identified in 61 lesions by using iMap IVUS which allows identifying neointimal tissue components in vivo, showed that the neointima in DES placement showed smaller fibrotic component (67% versus 78%, $P < 0.0001$), larger necrotic (14% versus 9%, $P < 0.0001$), and calcified (15% versus 7%, $P < 0.0001$)components compared to BMS[16]. These results suggest that fibrin deposition rather than endothelial cells is a major surface component for DES-neo-intima [17], indicating that neointima with less endothelial cells in DES does not possess its native functions.

Lipid deposition within neointima of DES is one of the most characteristics which differs from BMS, where the latter is mainly composed of smooth muscle cells. Nakano et al. [18] examined the neointimal characteristics of both DES and BMS and demonstrated that neointimal compositions of DES restenosis showed greater proteoglycan deposition and less smooth muscle cellularity over time, whereas BMS showed greater cell density and collagen deposition. Furthermore, Ali et al. [7] reported the findings using OCT and NIFS with IVUS for patients with ISR, finding the total lipid core burden index and the density of lipid core burden index (34 versus 9, $P < 0.001$；144 versus 26, $P < 0.001$, resp.)to be higher in DES than in BMS. Similarly, Yonetsu et al. [19] revealed a greater incidence of lipid-laden plaque (37% versus 8%, P = 0.02)and a higher percentage of lipid-rich plaque (12.9% versus1.2%, P = 0.01)that were found in DES compared to BMS within 9 months. Interestingly, a significant difference in the regression of NA is notable in DES and BMS. Awata et al. [20] reported a serial hagioscopic evidence of neointima after SES and BMS up to 2-year follow-up, revealing that yellow plaques were exposed in 71% of SES at the first follow-up (3.6 ± 1.1 months)and remained exposed until the third follow-up (21.1 ± 2.2 months), whereas yellow plaque in BMS has disappeared by the time of the second follow-up (10.5 ± 1.6 months). Of note, to assess neointimal hyperplasia after DES placement, data from a clinical study including 37 angina patients undergoing repeated percutaneous coronary intervention showed that the late phase (mean follow-up, 40 ± 23.9 months)had a greater percentage of lipid components and relative larger necrotic volume compared to the early phase (< 1 year), suggesting that lipid plaque of DES grew persistently and rapidly with time [21]. Lipid deposition within neointima in DES segments seems to increase risks of adverse events. On the one hand, the prevalence of thrombus was significantly higher on the yellow than on the white neointimal area [22]. On the other hand, patients with yellow plaque after stenting showed great frequency of late stent failure, including cardiac death, acute myocardial infarction or unstable angina, or need for revascularization associated with stent site, compared to those without yellow plaque (8.1%)[23].

Clinical reports and pathological findings from patients with DES postulate a hypersensitivity inflammation as an important factor in nonatherosclerotic development[23,24]. Potential culprits responsible for hypersensitivity include arachidonic acid metabolites, proteolytic enzymes, and inflammatory cells such as macrophages, T-lymphocytes, mast cells, and eosinophils [25]. Pfoch et al. [24] reported that patients with a polymer-based PES (Taxus, Boston Scientific)presented with characteristics of hypersensitivity: disseminated wheals, pruritus, bronchial asthma, and synovitis and were cured by initial intravenous injection followed by oral antihistamine treatment for 1 month until paclitaxel was eluted totally. Moreover, in noninjured coronary arteries of domestic swine (n = 58), overlapping stents (SES, PES, and BMS)were implanted to detect circumferential granulomatous inflammation, defined as inflammation consisting of macrophages, multinucleated giant cells, lymphocytes, and granulocytes, including many eosinophils in stented segments. Results showed that circumferential granulomatous inflammation was more prevalent in SES (9 of 23, 39%)compared with BMS (0 of 44)in the combined 90-and 180-day cohort. Recently, Niccoli et al. [26] considered that mammalian target of rapamycin- (mTOR-)inhibited DES stent type is associated with an increase of eosinophil cationic protein in serum levels of patients undergoing stent implantation, possibly triggered by permanent polymer. However, Fu et al. [27] analyzed neointimal coverage of polymer-free sirolimus-DES in coronary arteries of 8 normal swine; lymphocyte infiltration of peristrut was more frequently seen in heterogeneous sections than in homogeneous sections. And Cook et al. [28] reported histology findings in 54 patients with DES (28 patients with very late DES stent thrombosis and 26 controls), suggesting that very late DES thrombosis was associated with histopathological signs of inflammation, and eosinophilic infiltrates were more common in thrombi harvested from very late DES thrombosis. These results suggested that antiproliferative drugs-mediated DES may play a role in hypersensitivity, partly contributory to promote progression of NA.

NA is classified as I (thin-cap NA), II (thick-cap NA), and III (peristrut NA)types, topographically. The types of NA between DES and BMS are discrepant. Ali et al. [7] detected the cap neointima of both DES (n = 51)and BMS (n = 14)in 65 patients with in-stent restenosis (ISR)at 33-month follow-up and suggested that the type 1 thin-cap neoatheroma was greater in DES than BMS (20% versus 3%, P = 0.01). Similarly, Ando et al. [29] also found this phenomenon in patients with ISR after SES (n = 20)or BMS (n = 34)implantation, finding that a smaller fibrous tissue percentage in neointimal tissue by integrated backscatter IVUS was observed in SES than in BMS (72.6% versus 82.0%, P = 0.011). Moreover, Kang et al. [30] analyzed 50 patients (30 stable, 20 unstable angina)with 50 DES-ISR with 32.2-month follow-up, revealing that 52% of lesions had at least 1 OCT-defined in-stent thin-cap fibroatheroma- (TCFA-)containing neointima, and patients presenting with unstable angina showed a thinner fibrous cap (0.55 mm)and higher incidence of OCT-defined TCFA-containing neointima compared to stable patients. Like vulnerable plaque characterized by a thin cap of lesions (< 0.65 mm), these results suggest that NA of DES is responsible for late complications for its favor of rupturing over time.

3 Cellular Mechanisms of Neoatherosclerosis

Many pathological factors have been elucidated as indicators of NA, such as delayed arterial healing[12], hypersensitivity [26], stent types, stent age, and patient characteristics[31,32], including current smoking and chronic kidney disease. Antiproliferative drugs-induced incomplete reendothelialization plays a key role in neoatherosclerotic development. Nakazawa et al. [33] analyzed 44 New Zealand White rabbits with induced atheroma by bilateral iliac artery stents to evaluate endothelial coverage between DES (SES, ZES, and EES) and BMS. Findings showed a significant lower level of endothelial nitric oxide synthase (eNOS)expression in DES than BMS, although endothelial coverage was comparable between DES and BMS, suggesting that regenerated endothelium was dysfunctional in DES. Therefore, antiproliferative drugs such as sirolimus and paclitaxel inhibit endothelial cells proliferation and induce endothelial dysfunction which contributes to NA.

3.1 Reactive Oxygen Species (ROS)Production Induced by Antiproliferative Drugs

Jabs et al. [8] analyzed the effect of sirolimus in vascular dysfunction using Wistar rats undergoing infusion (5 mg/kg/day)for 7 days for mimicking the continuous sirolimus exposure of a stent vessel. Results showed that sirolimus caused a marked endothelial dysfunction and a desensitization of the vasculature to the endothelium- independent vasodilator nitroglycerin； moreover, upregulated superoxide production was observed, in part by nicotinamide adenine dinucleotide phosphate (NADPH)oxidase via stimulating of p67phox/rac1 expression and increased rac1 membrane association. Similarly, paclitaxel also increases ROS production via activation of NADPH oxidase, including p47 (phox)mRNA and gp91 (phox)mRNA in arteries and human coronary artery endothelial cells, while the level of nitric oxide (NO)is reduced [34]. In view of the ROS production, evidence suggests that ROS may mediate endothelial caveolae-mediated transcytosis [35] and paracellular pathway [36] which are potentially associated with neoatherosclerosis development. Detailed explanations will be discussed in the following sections.

Transcytosis of vascular endothelial cells is a basic process for maintaining vascular homeostasis [6]. Caveolae-mediated transcytosis is a major conduit for transporting macro-molecules (＞3nm of molecular radius), including albumin, insulin, and LDL, from one side of a cell to the other via membrane-bounded caveolae [37–39]. Known that many excellent articles about caveolae structure and functions have been introduced in detail[40,41], our focus is on the effects of ROS on nonatherosclerotic development via caveolae-mediated transcytosis pathway.

3.2 ROS Promote Lipid Uptake via Caveolae-Mediated Tran-scytosis

Impairment of endothelial barrier function is implicated in many vascular disorders. One prevalent mechanism of endothelial dysfunction is an increase in ROS under oxidative stress. As mentioned in pathological studies, both sirolimus and paclitaxel-eluting stents are associated with increased vascular level of ROS, consequently altering endothelial function in the treated artery [42]. Although there is no direct evidence to demonstrate the effects of DES in increasing lipid uptake, ROS-associated lipid deposition in vessels is widely described. By exposing an aortic endothelial smooth muscle cell bilayer to a free-radical generating system to detect the influence of superoxides in lipid permeability and uptake, increased level of 125I-LDL uptake was observed via transcellular pathway [43]. Moreover, transcytosis of FITC-labelled LDL simulated by C-reactive protein (CRP)was examined in human umbilical vein endothelial cells and ApoE (-/-)mice, pointing out that CPR-stimulated LDL uptake within in vitro and in vivo was increased closely associating with increased ROS production. This action was blocked by an NADPH oxidase inhibitor (inhibition of ROS production)[44]. Therefore, these results indicate that ROS production stimulate lipoprotein uptake in endothelial cells.

ABC transporters (such as ABCA1 and ABCG1)play an important role in cholesterol homeostasis, especially in liver. In contrast to smooth muscle cells and macrophages that form the atherosclerotic plaque, neither ABC transporters nor scavenger receptor B-I is required for vascular endothelial cholesterol efflux, indicating that other pathways may be involved in the lipid transport for endothelial cells [45]. Caveolae-related transcytosis and their generated channels are the main cellular instruments for trafficking cargoes in endothelial cells. Endothelial-specific cav-1 expression is essential for the progression of atherosclerosis [46]. cav-1, as a primary structural protein of caveolae, greatly regulates caveolae formation and caveolae-mediated endocytosis and transcytosis in microvascular endothelial cells [47]. Many studies have already investigated the relationship between ROS and cav-1-mediated caveolae pathway [48,49].

Evidence showed that ROS upregulate cav-1 protein expression via increasing binding of Sp1 to the cav-1 promoter region containing the two GC-rich boxes [49]. Overexpression of cav-1 inhibits thioredoxin reductase-1 (TrxR1), an important antioxidant enzyme that controls cellular redox homeostasis. Lack of TrxR1, which fails to localize to caveolae and binds to cav-1, constitutively induces oxidative stress-mediated endothelial dysfunction [50]. Some key signaling pathways, including activation of Src kinase family members and extracellular signal-regulation kinases (ERK1/2), have been specifically incriminated in ROS-mediated barrier disruption. Src signaling has been demonstrated to be a crucial "switch" in the regulation of caveolae-mediated transcellular transport via phosphorylation of cav-1 at tyrosine 14, followed by phosphorylation of dynamin-2 to fission of caveolae. P90 ribosomal S6 (p90RSK)is a potentially important downstream effector of Src and ERK1/2. H_2O_2 activates p90RSK by ROS via Fyn and Ras to activate several transcription factors [51]. The nuclear erythroid 2 p45-related factor-2 (Nrf2), a transcription factor that mediated cytoprotective response against stress, is inhibited by expression of cav-1 [52], leading to alteration of endothelial barrier.

ROS not only induce cav-1 upregulation, but also cause phosphorylation of cav-1 via activation of c-Abl, an upstream kinase of cav-1[53,54], to promote the growth of microscopic voids (caveolae formation)within the cellular bilayer [55]. Prdx1 is one of the antioxidant enzymes that plays a protective role in cells against oxidative stress. In cytoplasm, Prdx1 exists as a protein complex with c-Abl-SH domain and protects c-Abl from phosphorylation. Under oxidative stress, oxidant dissociates Prdx1 and c-Abl complex and then induces c-Abl phosphorylation [56], therefore leading to caveolae formation. In addition, Jin and Michel found [57] that actin-binding protein myristoylated alanine-rich C-kinase substrate (MARCKS), an important mediator of the oxidative stress (H_2O_2), could induce endothelial permeability change by regulating cytoskeletal reorganization in endothelial cells via a signaling cascade from Rac1 to Ab1, phospholipase Cg1, and PKCd, eliciting altered endothelial permeability.

Fission of caveolae is an important progress in migration of caveolae to the basal membrane for endothelial cells. The GTPase dynamin on oligomerization plays a crucial role in transcytosis for triggering fission by constriction of caveolae necks. Dynamin-2 is mainly involved in the scission of newly formed caveolae from the membrane by self-assembles to form spiral structures on the neck of invaginated pits during endocytosis by stimulating its GTPase activity. Activated Src kinase increases dynamin-2 phosphorylation, promotes association with cav-1, and localizes dynamin to caveolae, hence increasing macromolecule transports [58]. Oxidative stress-induced ROS cause recruitment of dynamin 2 and c-Abl to caveolin-enriched microdomains [59]; c-Abl tyrosine-phosphorylated dynamin 2 enhances p47phox/dynamin 2 association, therefore increasing the number and fission of caveolae formation and leading to increased lipid uptake and retention within vessels [59], as shown in Figure 1.

3.3 Paracellular Transport Pathway

Under physiological conditions, endothelial cell-cell contacts and vascular endothelial barrier integrity are mediated by tight junctions, adherens junctions, and gap junctions to regulate physiological process, especially inhibiting inflammatory cell transendothelial migration (TEM). Opening of interendothelial cell-cell junctions or disruption of endothelial-matrix contacts within the vasculature after DES placement has a pivotal role in inducing inflammatory cell infiltration, including macrophages, eosinophils, multinuclear giant cells, and lymphocytes [60,61]. Antiproliferative drugs, potent mTOR inhibitor, may be important in disrupting cell-cell conjunctions [62].

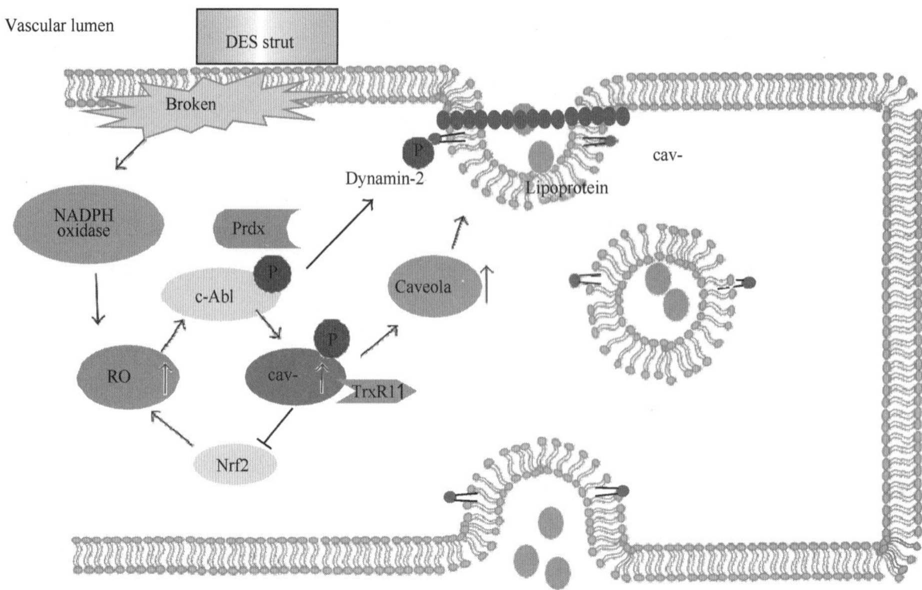

Figure 1 Caveolae-associated Transcytosis

Notes: Dysfunctional endothelial cells increase lipoprotein uptake by increased cav-1 expression and phosphorylation induced by DES-mediated ROS production.

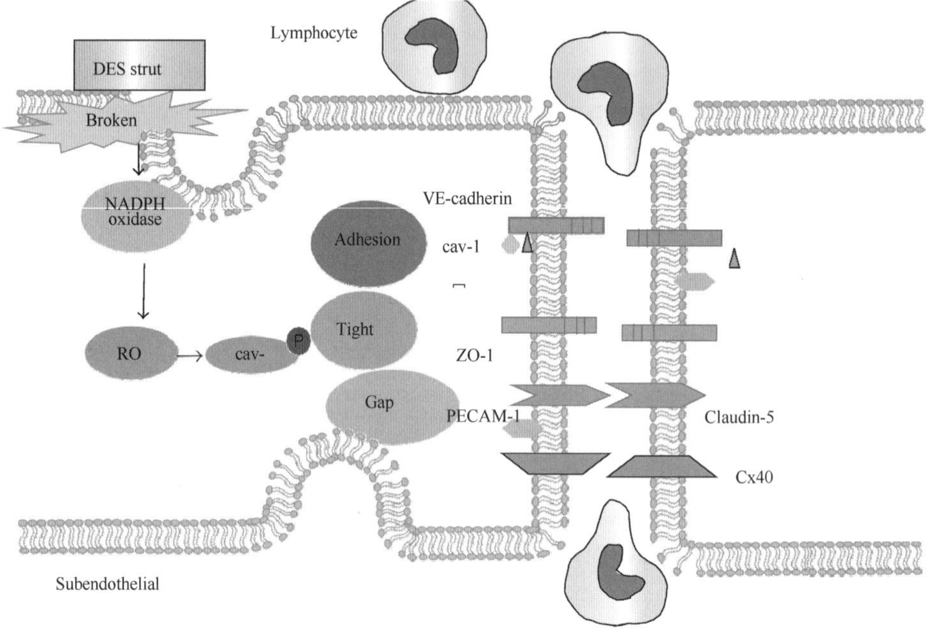

Figure 2 Paracellular-associated Pathway

Notes: DES-induced dysfunctional endothelial cells show broken cell-cell junctions, further eliciting inflammatory cell migration.

Vascular endothelial- (VE-)cadherin and its associated catenins are important to form adherens junction complexes for controlling endothelial cell-cell adhesion. Data from mTORC2 deficient mice showed that a blocking mTOR or the upstream kinase phosphoinositide 3-kinase (PI3K)dose-dependently decreased VE-cadherin mRNA and protein expression[63]. Furthermore, prolonged rapamycin treatment significantly decreased cytoskeletal adaptor protein Nck by reducing the expression of total mTOR, rictor expression, and mTORC2 formation, finally leading to high permeability [64]. This concept has been confirmed by Walid et al. [65] who clarified that rapamycin, a specific mTOR inhibitor, damaged cell junctions and subsequent tubule formation, facilitating inflammatory cell TEM.

Oxidative stress-induced endothelial cell filamin translocation (from the membrane to the cytosol), cytoskeletal rearrangement, and intercellular gap formation are related to increased monolayer permeability, which contribute to destabilization of junctions[66]. As mentioned above, sirolimus-and paclitaxel-DES induced increase in ROS production may be associated with disruption of endothelial integrity, as shown in Figure 2.

VE-cadherin plays a key role in maintaining cell-cell integrity. The VE-cadherin cytoplasmic tail is highly homologous to other cadherins and binds b-catenin or g-catenin. b-or g-catenin binds a-catenin to stabilize the adherens junction anchorage to the actin cytoskeleton. In addition, confocal images and coimmunoprecipitation technology show significant colocalization of cav-1 and b-catenin at cell-cell borders in a nonphosphorylated state [36]. Disruption of binding between b-catenin and VE-cadherin interferes with the association of adherens junctions with the actin cytoskeleton, therefore resulting in decreased cell adhesion strength and subsequent barrier disruption [67]. H_2O_2 induces the disassociation between cav-1 and b-catenin at the endothelial cells borders in cav-1 phosphorylated state. b-catenin is tyrosine phosphorylation by ROS via redox-sensitive proline-rich tyrosine kinase 2 [68]. Then, the assciation of VE-cadherin and b-catenin is reduced upon H_2O_2 stimulation [69], and b-catenin translocates into cytosolic compartment, resulting in endothelial barrier disruption. These results suggest that loss of cell-cell conjunctions is partly induced by disruption of b-catenin/VE-cadherin complexes via oxidant-induced paracellular pathway. In the bEnd3 monolayer of mouse endothelial cells, elevated level of cellular ROS led to VE-cadherin and zona occludens-1 (ZO-1)disruption, whereas antioxidant (N-acetylcysteine and tempol)treatment significantly lowered the permeability induced by ROS[70].

In addition to decreasing assembly of adherens junctions, ROS also affect the formation of endothelial tight junctions. Under pathological conditions, ROS significantly contribute to blood-brain barrier dysfunction and inflammation in the brain by enhancing cellular migration, paralleling with cytoskeleton rearrangements and redistribution of disappearance of tight junctions proteins claudin-5 and occludin [71]. Production of ROS induced by HIV-transactivator of transcription/cocaine activates Ras/Raf/ERK1/2 pathway contributing to disruption of tight junction protein [72]. Hence, opening of tight junctions after endothelium damage facilitates inflammatory cell migration. Conversely, the NADPH oxidase inhibitor DPI reversed the events, including impaired tight proteins ZO-1 and claudin-5, decreased transendothelial electrical resistance, and significantly increased cytosolic ROS in brain endothelial cells, indicating that ROS play a key role in this process [73].

Immunofluorescent staining for the tight junctional protein occludin and ZO-1 demonstrated that oxidant challenge caused a loss of endothelial tight junction organization. Protein phosphatase 2A (PP2A)interacts with epithelial tight junctions and negatively regulates the integrity of the tight junctions. PP2A-calpha protein and PP2A activity were coimmunoprecipitated with occludin, and this coimmunoprecipitation was rapidly increased by H_2O_2. H_2O_2-induced dephosphorylation of occludin on threonine residues and redistribution of occludin and ZO-1 from the intercellular junctions is caused by a Src kinase-dependent mechanism [74]. Rhodamine phalloidin staining of the actin cytoskeleton showed that H_2O_2 stimulated increased stress fiber formation with concomitant gap formation between adjacent endothelial cells [75]. In addition, ROS could activate myosin light chain kinase, followed by decreased tight junction complex, while providing antioxidant prevented brain endothelial injury[76].

Connexins (Cx)are recognized as structural constituents of gap-junctional intercellular communication (GJIC). Downregulated Cx43 expression and damaged GJIC function in HUVECs along with intracellular ROS production were observed by asymmetric dimethylarginine (ADMA), whereas these events could be attenuated by NADPH oxidase inhibitor [77]. Adhesion molecules that localize at endothelial cells junctions or cell-cell contracts regions are essential to the process of TEM. Activated endothelial cells presented with cell-surface adhesion molecules expressions[78] cause monocytes fixed adhesion on the endothelium, facilitating TEM via paracellular pathway. These molecules include platelet/EC adhesion molecule-1 (PECAM-1), CD99, junctional adhesion molecules A and C (JAM-A and JAM-C), and JAM-like protein (JAML)[79]. Among these adhesion molecules, PECAM-1 acts as a sensor of oxidative stress during the process of TEM. PECAM-1-mediated TEM is dependent on its tyrosine phosphorylation. An inducer of oxidative stress (t-BuooH) in HUVECs caused two fold increase in the TEM of monocyte like HL-60 cells and a fivefold increase in PECAM-1 phosphorylation [80]. H_2O_2 supports PECAM-1/SHP-2 complex formation via an "oxidative burst" and sufficiently high concentrations of H_2O_2 for a sufficiently long period of time[81], a process that is similar to DES implantation. Conversely, antioxidant enzyme and superoxide dismutase conjugated with antibodies to PECAM-1 quench the corresponding ROS and alleviate vascular oxidative stress and inflammation.

ROS disassemble the endothelial cell actin dense peripheral band, followed by an increase in the number and diameter of intercellular gaps. Millimolar concentrations of reactive oxygen metabolites lead to nonspecific endothelial cell injury, and micromolar concentrations activate inflammatory second messenger cascades which produce distributional changes in endothelial cell cytoskeletal proteins, causing translocation of filamin, attributed to rearrangement of the dense peripheral band of F-actin [82].

4 Biodegradable Polymer Stents and Drug-Eluting Absorbable Stents

The slow and often incomplete endothelial regrowth after injury is the primary cause of serious short- and long-term complications, including thrombosis and neoatherosclerosis. Rapid endothelium restoration has the potential to prevent these sequelae [83]. The emergence of biodegradable polymer stents seems attractive because its polymer degrades and eliminates itself from the body leaving the permanent metallic stent without polymer, which would facilitate reendothelialization. Karjalainen et al. [84] performed a clinical study enrolling 44 patients with acute coronary syndrome receiving either a biodegradable polymer-based SES (BP-SES)or durable polymer-based ZES (DP-ZES). Results showed that BP-SES provided better stent strut coverage at 3 months compared with the DP-ZES group, although neither was fully covered. However, a 5-year follow-up research, in which 30 patients with 33 stents (10 with 12 biodegradable polymer biolimus-eluting stents [BES], 10 with 11 SES, and 10 with 10 BMS)showed that lipid-laden neointima with BES had no statistical discrepancy when compared with those with SES or BMS, respectively [85]. Therefore, the safety of biodegradable stents should still be further developed.

Several prospective, multicenter, clinical trials have been performed to directly investigate the effect of bioabsorbable stents on neointimal function. Mattesini et al. [86] designed a clinical study in which 100 complex coronary lesions were treated with a bioabsorbable vascular scaffold (BVS)or second-generation DES. The findings showed that the BVS group had a higher tissue prolapsed area and greater incidence of incomplete strut apposition at the proximal edge compared to the DES group. Furthermore, Christiansen et al. [87] published the results of the SORT OUT V trial in which 2468 patients received either BVS or SES, showing that significantly more patients in the BVS group had definite thrombosis at 12 months than those in the SES group (risk difference. 0.6%；P = 0.034), suggesting that the effects of biodegradable stents on vascular reendothelialization merit further validation.

Endothelial dysfunction or damage by oxidants is associated with an enhanced risk of platelet activation and subsequent atherothrombotic complications [88]. To investigate the biocompatibility of biodegradable polymers, cultured monocytes differentiated into functional macrophages were incubated with various polymers including poly-L-lactide, polycaprolactone, or poly-D, L-lactide-co-glycolide for up to 5 days and showed that biodegradable polymers were associated with macrophage adhesion, NADPH oxidase-induced generation of ROS, and excess apoptosis [89]. Furthermore, Hietala et al. [90] examined the possible differences between biodegradable polylactide (PLA)and stainless steel (SS)stents in platelet attachment and morphology after whole blood perfusion. Results revealed that more platelets deposited on PLA stents than on SS stents under all study ($P < 0.03$), while among all biodegradable stents, the braided PLA stent coated with PCL-PLA-heparin accumulated the fewest platelets ($P < 0.02$), indicating that materials, design, and coating techniques of biodegradable stents must be further developed.

ROS could activate platelets, increasing their adhesion to the vascular wall. Evidence showed that platelet recruitment (PR)inhibited by rosuvastatin was associated with downregulation of platelet release of the prothrombotic molecule CD40L, lower production of platelet ROS and is isoprostane, and activation of the glycoprotein IIb/IIIa. Detailed mechanisms revealed that platelet isoprostane formation, platelet CD40L, and sNOX2-dp mainly depend on NADPH oxidase, and inhibition of NOX2-derived oxidative stress could impair platelet activation [91]. Moreover, the soluble CD40L (sCD40L)/CD40 axis is a thromboinflammmatory mediator that affects platelet and endothelial functions. Khzam et al. [92] found that pretreatment of early outgrowth cells (EOCs)with sCD40 reduced their inhibitory effect on platelet aggregation. In contrast, blockade of ROS reversed the effects of sCD40-treated EOCs on platelet aggregation. Similar results were observed in disease of anoxia-reoxygenation, where platelets undergoing anoxia-reoxygenation simultaneously increase ROS, thromboxane (Tx)B_2, and isoprostanes. These events were associated with NOX2 activation and could be inhibited by NOX2-blocking peptide, vitamin C, and the inhibitor of phospholipase A [93]. Therefore, production of ROS is an important factor in platelet recruitment and thrombotic events, and strategies to decrease oxidative stress can encourage reendothelialization and reduce the incidence of NA.

5 Effects of Antioxidants on Reendothelialization after Vascular Injury

Targeting of endothelial function by antioxidants may be promising to promote endothelial healing and to prevent against NA formation after stent implantation. Early trial of probucol (an antioxidant)administration in animal models of stent implantation showed antirestenosis and antithrombotic properties, which are related to promoting in-stent reendothelialization [94]. Moreover, in another study, animals of expanded polytetrafluoroethylene grafts in the abdominal aorta were treated with probucol, showing increased endothelial cell coverage and decreased intimal hyperplasia, suggesting that reducing oxidative stress promotes healing of prosthetic grafts [95]. The mechanisms involved beneficial effects on oxidative stress and improvement of endothelial functional activities and reduced LDL oxidative state [96].

Hanratty et al. [97] found that low flow resulted in greater lumen loss in segments form the same vessel subject to balloon injury, by greater enhancement, whereas the antioxidant pyrrolidine dithiocarbamate effectively reduced intima formation and inward remodeling after balloon-injured vessels. Cicero et al. [98] performed a crossover, double-blind, placebo-controlled randomized clinical trial to detect if a short-term treatment with monacolins combined with antioxidant, red yeast rice, improves lipid pattern and endothelial function in a small cohort-moderately hyper-cholesterolemic subjuncts. Results showed that monacolin treatment with red yeast rice appeared to safely reduce cholesterolemia, hs-CRP, and improve endothelial function. The detailed mechanisms for improvement of endothelial function are via inhibiting of oxidative stress, downregulating cav-1, upregulating eNOS expression, and decreasing whole blood viscosity [99]. These data suggest that strategies that promote functional healing of vascular endothelium may be cardinal methods, consequently decreasing the risks of late complications [100].

6 Conclusion and Perspectives

In summary, it is already demonstrated that reendothelialization with complete function is essential to maintain safety and performance of coronary stents. ROS are released following PCI and are closely associated with neoatherosclerosis formation, which is one of the main mechanisms for late thrombosis. The use of antioxidants may inhibit such complications, by encouraging endothelial coverage, improving endothelial function via mediating lipid uptake and inflammation. Although the current DES and advanced biodegradable stents have tried their best to reduce the rates of adverse cardiac events, including nonfatal myocardial infarction, stroke, repeat target vessel revascularization, or death, inadequate endothelial healing in stented segments plays a key role in the dilemma. It is likely that stents which conquer the overwhelming influence of ROS on the arterial healing process will gain a delighted achievement.

REFERENCES

[1] Nakazawa G, Otsuka F, Nakano M, et al. The pathology of neoatherosclerosis in human coronary implants: bare-metal and drug-eluting stents [J]. Journal of the American College of Cardiology, 2011, 57 (11): 1314-1322.

[2] Sang S J, Mintz GS, Akasaka T, et al. Optical coherence tomographic analysis of in-stent neoatherosclerosis after drug-eluting stent implantation [J]. Circulation, 2011, 123 (25): 2954-2963, .

[3] Karanasos A, Ligthart J M, Regar E. Regar. In-stent neo-atherosclerosis: a cause of late stent thrombosis in a patient with 'full metal jacket' 15 years after implantation: insights from optical coherence tomography [J]. JACC: Cardiovascular Interventions, 2012, 5 (7): 799-800.

[4] Otsuka F, Byrne, RA, Yahagi K, et al. Neoatherosclerosis: overview of histopathologic findings and implications for intravascular imaging assessment [J]. European Heart Journal, 2015, 36 (32): 2147-2159.

[5] Kang SJ, Lee CW, Song H, et al. OCT analysis in patients with very late stent thrombosis [J]. JACC: Cardiovascular Imaging, 2013, 6 (6): 695-703.

[6] Nakazawa G, Finn AV, Vorpahl M, et al. Coronary responses and differential mechanisms of late stent thrombosis attributed to first-genera-tion sirolimus-and paclitaxel-eluting stents[J]. Journal of the American College of Cardiology, 2011, 57 (4): 390-398.

[7] Ali ZA, Roleder T, Narula J, et al. Increased thin-cap neoatheroma and periprocedural myocardial infarction in drug-eluting stent restenosis multimodality intravascular imaging of drug-eluting and bare-metal stents [J]. Circulation, 2013, 6 (5): 507-517.

[8] Jabs A, GOBel S, Wenzel P, et al. Sirolimus-induced vascular dysfunction: increased mitochondrial and nicotinamide adenosine dinucleotide phosphate oxidase-dependent superoxide production and decreased vascular nitric oxide formation[J]. Journal of the American College of Cardiology, 2008, 51 (22): 2130-2138.

[9] Joner M, Finn A V, Farb A, et al. Pathology of drug-eluting stents in humans: delayed healing and late thrombotic risk [J]. Journal of the American College of Cardiology, 2006, 48 (1): 193-202.

[10] Van d HM, Sorop O, van Beusekom HM, et al. Endothelial dysfunction after drug eluting stent implantation [J]. Minerva Cardioangiologica, 2009, 57 (5): 629-643.

[11] Whitbeck MG, Applegate RJ. Applegate. Second generation drug-eluting stents: a review of the everolimus-eluting platform [J]. Clinical Medicine Insights: Cardiology, 2013, 7: 115-126.

[12] Kim JS, Jang IK, Kim TH, et al. Optical coherence tomography evaluation of zotarolimus-eluting stents at 9-month follow-up: comparison with sirolimus-eluting stents [J]. Heart, 2009, 95 (23): 1907-1912.

[13] Lee SY, Hur SH, Lee SG, et al. Optical coherence tomographic observation of in-stent neoatherosclerosis in lesions with more than 50% neointimal area stenosis after second-generation drug-eluting stent implantation [J]. Circulation: Cardiovascular Interventions, 2015, 8 (2): Article ID e001878.

[14] Otsuka F, Vorpahl M, Nakano M, et al. Pathology of second-generation everolimus-eluting stents versus first-generation sirolimus-and paclitaxel-eluting stents in humans [J]. Circulation, 2014, 129 (2): 211-223.

[15] Hara T, Ughi GJ, Mccarthy JR, et al. Intravascular fibrin molecular imaging improves the detection of unhealed stents assessed by optical coherence tomography in vivo [J]. European Heart Journal, 2015.

[16] Tsujita K, Takaoka N, Kaikita K, et al. Neointimal tissue component assessed by tissue characterization with 40 MHz intravascular ultrasound imaging: comparison of drug-eluting stents and bare-metal stents[J]. Catheterization and Cardiovascular Interventions, 2013, 82 (7): 1068-1074.

[17] Finn A V, Nakazawa G, Joner M, et al. Vascular responses to drug eluting stents: importance of delayed healing [J]. Arteriosclerosis, Thrombosis, and Vascular Biology, 2007, 27 (7): 1500-1510.

[18] Nakano M, Otsuka F, Yahagi K, et al. Human autopsy study of drug-eluting stents restenosis: histomorphological predictors and neointimal characteristics [J]. European Heart Journal, 2013, 34 (42): 3304-3313.

[19] Yonetsu T, Kim JS, Kato K, et al. Comparison of incidence and time course of neoatherosclerosis between bare metal stents and drug-eluting stents using optical coherence tomography [J]. American Journal of Cardiology, 2012, 110 (7): 933-939.

[20] Awata M, Kotani JI, Uematsu M, et al. Serial angioscopic evidence of incomplete neointimal coverage after sirolimus-eluting stent implantation: comparison with bare-metal stents [J]. Circulation, 2007, 116 (8): 910-916.

[21] Araki T, Nakamura M, Sugi K. Characterization of in-stent neointimal tissue components following drug-eluting stent implantation according to the phase of restenosis using a 40-MHz intravascular ultrasound imaging system[J]. Journal of Cardiology, 2014, 64 (6): 423-429.

[22] HigoT, Ueda Y, Oyabu J, et al. Atherosclerotic and thrombo-genic neointima formed over sirolimus drug-eluting stent: an angioscopic study [J]. JACC: Cardiovascular Imaging, 2009, 2 (5): 616-624.

[23] Ueda Y, Matsuo K, Nishimoto Y, et al. In-stent yellow plaque at 1 year after implantation is associated with future event of very late stent failure: the DESNOTE study (detect the event of very late stent failure from the drug-eluting stent not well covered by neointima determined by angioscopy)[J]. JACC: Cardiovascular Interventions, 2015, 8 (6): 814-821.

[24] Pfoch L, Mahler V, Sticherling M. Sticherling. Drug-eluting coronary stents: hypersensitivity reactions to paclitaxel [J]. Dermatology, 2009, 218 (1): 52-55.

[25] Chen JP, Hou D, Pendyala L, et al. Drug-eluting stent thrombosis. The kounis hyper-sensitivity-associated acute coronary syndrome revisited [J]. Journal of the American College of Cardiology: Cardiovascular Inter-ventions, 2009, 2 (7)583-593.

[26] Niccoli G, Calvieri C, Minelli S, et al. Permanent polymer of drug eluting stents increases eosinophil cationic protein levels following

percutaneous coronary intervention independently of C-reactive protein [J]. Atherosclerosis, 2014, 237 (2): 816- 820.

[27] Fu Q, Hu H, Chen W, et al. Histological validation of frequency domain optical coherence tomography for the evaluation of neointimal formation after a novel polymer-free sirolimus-eluting stent implantation[J]. International Journal of Clinical and Experimental Pathology, 2015, 8 (9): 11068-11075.

[28] Cook S, Ladich E, Nakazawa G, et al. Correlation of intravascular ultrasound findings with histopathological analysis of thrombus aspirates in patients with very late drug-eluting stent thrombosis [J]. Circulation, 2009, 120 (5)391-399.

[29] Ando H, Amano T, Takashima H, et al, Murohara T. Differences in tissue characterization of restenoticneointima between sirolimus-eluting stent and baremetal stent: Integrated backscatter intravascular ultrasound analysis for in-stent restenosis[J]. European Heart Journal Cardiovascular Imaging, 2013, 14 (10): 996-1001.

[30] Kang S J, Mintz GS, Akasaka T, et al. Optical coherence tomographic analysis of in-stent neoatherosclerosis after drug-eluting stent implantation[J]. Circulation, 2011, 123 (25): 2954-2963.

[31] Yonetsu T, Kato K, Kim SJ, et al. Predictors for neoathero-sclerosis: a retrospective observational study from the optical coherence tomography registry [J]. Circulation: Cardiovascular Imaging, 2012, 5 (5): 660-666.

[32] Kim C, Kim BK, Lee SY, et al. Incidence, clinical presen-tation, and predictors of early neoatherosclerosis after drug-eluting stent implantation [J]. American Heart Journal, 2015, 170 (3): 591-597.

[33] kazawa, G, Nakano M, Otsuka F, et al. Evaluation of polymer-based comparat or drug-eluting stents using a rabbit model of iliac artery atherosclerosis [J]. Circulation: Cardiovascular Interventions, 2011, 4 (1): 38-46.

[34] Serizawa KI, Yogo K, Aizawa K, et al. Paclitaxel-induced endothelial dysfunction in living rats is prevented by nicorandil via reduction of oxidative stress [J]. Journal of Pharmacological Sciences, 2012, 119 (4): 349-358.

[35] Layne J, Majkova Z, Smart EJ, et al. Caveolae: a regulatory platform for nutritional modulation of inflammatory diseases [J]. Journal of Nutritional Biochemistry, 2011, 22 (9): 807-811.

[36] Sun Y, Hu G, Zhang X, et al. Phosphorylation of caveolin-1 regulates oxidant-induced pulmonary vascular permeability via paracellular and transcellular pathways [J]. Circulation Research, 2009, 105 (7): 676-685.

[37] Frank P G, Lisanti M P. Role of caveolin-1 in the regulation of the vascular shear stress response [J]. The Journal of Clinical Investigation, 2006, 116 (5): 1222-1225.

[38] Hansen CG, Nichols BJ. Exploring the caves: cavins, caveolins and caveolae [J]. Trends in Cell Biology, 2010, 20 (4): 177-186.

[39] Tuma P, Hubbard A L. Transcytosis: crossing cellular barriers [J]. Physiological Reviews, 2003, 83 (3): 871-932.

[40] Parton RG, Del Pozo MA. Caveolae as plasma membrane sensors, protectors and organizers [J]. Nature Reviews Molecular Cell Biology, 2013, 14 (2): 98-112.

[41] Del Pozo MA, Balasubramanian N, Alderson NB, et al. Phospho-caveolin-1 mediates integrin-regulated membrane domain internalization[J]. Nature Cell Biology, 2005, 7 (9): 901-908.

[42] Juni RP, Duckers HJ, Vanhoutte PM, et al. Oxidative stress and pathological changes after coronary artery interventions [J]. Journal of the American College of Cardiology, 2013, 61 (14): 1471-1481.

[43] Alexander JJ, Graham DJ, Miguel R. Oxygen radicals alter LDL permeability and uptake by an endothelial-smooth muscle cell bilayer [J] Journal of Surgical Research, 1991, 51 (5): 361-367.

[44] Bian F, Yang X, Zhou F, et al. C-reactive protein promotes atherosclerosis by increasing LDL transcytosis across endothelial cells [J]. British Journal of Pharmacology, 2014, 171 (10): 2671-2684.

[45] O "Connell B, Denis M, Genest J. Cellular physiology of cholesterol efflux in vascular endothelial cells [J]. Circulation, 2004, 110 (18): 2881-2888.

[46] Fernández-Hernando C, Yu J, Suárez Y, et al. Genetic evidence supporting a critical role of endothelial caveolin-1 during the progression of atherosclerosis [J]. Cell Metabolism, 2009, 10 (1): 48-54.

[47] Rothberg KG, Heuser JE, Donzell WC, et al. Caveolin, a protein component of caveolae membrane coats [J]. Cell, 1992, 68 (4): 673- 682.

[48] Zhang M, Lee SJ, An C, et al. Caveolin-1 mediates Fas-BID signaling in hyperoxia-induced apoptosis [J]. Free Radical Biology and Medicine, 2011, 50 (10): 1252-1262.

[49] Bartholomew JN, Galbiati F. Mapping of oxidative stress response elements of the caveolin-1 promoter [J]. Methods in Molecular Biology, 2010, 594: 409-423.

[50] Volonte D, Galbiati F. Inhibition of thioredoxin reductase 1 by caveolin 1 promotes stress-induced premature senescence [J]. EMBO Reports, 2009, 10 (12): 1334-1340.

[51] Abe J, Okuda M, Huang Q, et al, Berk BC. Reactive oxygen species activate p90 ribosomal S6 kinase via Fyn and Ras [J]. The Journal of Biological Chemistry, 2000, 275 (3): 1739-1748.

[52] Li W, Liu H, Zhou JS, et al. Caveolin-1 inhibits expression of antioxidant enzymes through direct interaction with nuclear erythroid 2 p45-related factor-2 (Nrf2)[J]. Journal of Biological Chemistry, 2012, 287 (25): 20922-20930.

[53] Sanguinetti A R, Mastick CC. c-Abl is required for oxida-tive stress-induced phosphorylation of caveolin-1 on tyrosine 14[J]. Cell Signaling, 2003, 15 (3): 289-298.

[54] Sun X, Majumder P, Shioya H, et al. Activation of the cytoplasmic c-Abl tyrosine kinase by reactive oxygen species [J]. The Journal of Biological

Chemistry, 2000, 275 (23): 17237-17240.

[55] Howland MC, Parikh AN. Model studies of membrane disruption by photogenerated oxidative assault [J]. Journal of Physical Chemistry B, 2010, 114 (19): 6377-6385.

[56] Takeuchi K, Morizane Y, Kamami-Levy C, et al. AMP-dependent kinase inhibits oxidative stress-induced caveolin-1 phosphorylation and endocytosis by suppressing the dissociation between c-Abl and Prdx1 proteins in endothelial cells[J]. The Journal of Biological Chemistry, 2013, 288 (28)20581-20591.

[57] Jin BJ, Michel T. MARCKS protein mediates hydrogen peroxide regulation of endothelial permeability [J]. Proceedings of the National Academy of Sciences of the United States of America, 2012, 109 (37): 14864-14869.

[58] Shajahan AN, Timblin BK, Sandoval R, et al. Role of Src-induced dynamin-2 phosphorylation in caveolae-mediated endocytosis in endothelial cells [J]. The Journal of Biological Chemistry, 2004, 279 (19): 20392-20400.

[59] Singleton PA, Pendyala S, Gorshkova I A, et al. Dynamin 2 and c-Abl are novel regulators of hyperoxia-mediated NADPH oxidase activation and reactive oxygen species production in caveolin-enriched microdomains of the endothelium [J]. Journal of Biological Chemistry 2009, 284 (50): 34964-34975, .

[60] Palabrica T, Lobb R, Furie BC, et al. Leukocyte accumulation promoting fibrin deposition is mediated in vivo by P-selectin on adherent platelets [J]. Nature, 1992, 359 (6398): 848-851.

[61] Nakazawa G, Granada JF, Alviar C L, et al. Anti-CD34 antibodies immobilized on the surface of sirolimus-eluting stents enhance stent endothelialization [J]. JACC: Cardiovascular Interventions, 2010, 3 (1): 68-75.

[62] Vollenbröker B, George B, Wolfgart M, et al. mTOR regulates expression of slit diaphragm proteins and cytoskeleton structure in podocytes[J]. American Journal of Physiology Renal Physiology, 2009, 296 (2): F418-F426.

[63] Bieri M, Oroszlan M, Zuppinger C, et al. Bio-synthesis and expression of VE-cadherin is regulated by the PI3K/mTOR signaling pathway [J]. Molecular Immunology, 2009, 46, (5)866-872.

[64] Vollenbröker B, George B, Wolfgart M, et al. mTOR regulates expression of slit diaphragm proteins and cytoskeleton structure in podocytes [J]. American Journal of Physiology—Renal Physiology, 2009, 296 (2): F418-F426.

[65] Walid S, Eisen R, Ratcliffe D R, Dai K, Ojakian G K. The PI 3-kinase and mTOR signaling pathways are important modulators of epithelial tubule formation[J]. Journal of Cellular Physiology, 2008, 216 (2): 469-479.

[66] Zhang YW, Yao XS, Murota S, et al. Inhibitory effects of eicosapentaenoic acid (EPA)on the hypoxia/re-oxygenation-induced tyrosine kinase activation in cultured human umbilical vein endothelial cells [J]. Prostaglandins Leuko-trienes and Essential Fatty Acids, 2002, 67 (4): 253-261.

[67] Wang L, Dudek SM. Regulation of vascular permeability by sphingosine 1-phosphate [J]. Microvascular Research, 2009, 77 (1): 39-45.

[68] Van Buul J D, Anthony E C, Fernandez-Borja M, Burridge K, Hordijk P L. Proline-rich tyrosine kinase 2 (Pyk2)mediates vascular endothelial-cadherin-based cell-cell adhesion by regulating-catenin tyrosine phosphorylation [J]. The Journal of Biological Chemistry, 2005, 280 (22): 21129-21136.

[69] Haidari M, Zhang W, Wakame KD. Disruption of endothelial adherens junction by invasive breast cancer cells is mediated by reactive oxygen species and is attenuated by AHCC [J]. Life Sciences, 2013, 93 (25-26): 994-1003.

[70] Bao L, Shi H. Arsenite induces endothelial cell permeability increase through a reactive oxygen species-vascular endothelial growth factor pathway [J]. Chemical Research in Toxicology, 2010, 23 (11): 1726-1734.

[71] Schreibelt G, Kooij G, Reijerkerk A, et al. Reactive oxygen species alter brain endothelial tight junction dynamics via RhoA, PI3 kinase, and PKB signaling[J]. FASEB Journal, 2007, 21 (13): 3666-3676.

[72] Dalvi P, Wang K, Mermis J, et al. HIV-1/Cocaine induced oxidative stress disrupts tight junction protein-1 in human pulmonary microvascular endothelial cells: role of RAS/ERK1/2 pathway [J]. PLoS ONE, 2014, 9 (1), Article ID e85246.

[73] Usatyuk PV, Parinandi NL, et al. Redox regulation of 4-hydroxy-2-nonenal-mediated endothelial barrier dysfunction by focal adhesion, adherens, and tight junction proteins [J]. Journal of Biological Chemistry, 2006, 281 (46): 35554-35566.

[74] Sheth P, Samak G, Shull JA, et al. Protein phosphatase 2A plays a role in hydrogen peroxide-induced disruption of tight junctions in Caco-2 cell monolayers [J]. Bio-chemical Journal, 2009, 421 (1): 59-70.

[75] Kevil CG, Oshima T, Alexander JS. The role of p38 MAP kinase in hydrogen peroxide mediated endothelial solute permeability [J]. Endothelium, 2001, 8 (2): 107-116.

[76] Ramirez SH, Rotula R, Fan S, et al. Methamphetamine disrupts blood-brain barrier function by induction of oxidative stress in brain endothelial cells[J]. Journal of Cerebral Blood Flow and Metabolism, 2009, 29 (12): 1933-1945.

[77] Jia SJ, Zhou Z, Zhang BK, et al. Asymmetric dimethylarginine damages connexin43-mediated endothelial gap junction intercellular communication [J]. Biochemistry & Cell Biology, 2009, 87 (6): 867-874.

[78] Liao JK. Linking endothelial dysfunction with endothelial cell activation [J]. Journal of Clinical Investigation, 2013, 123 (2): 540-541.

[79] Guo YL, Bai R, Chen XJ, et al. Role of junctional adhesion molecule-like protein in mediating monocyte transendothelial migration [J]. Arteriosclerosis, Thrombosis, and Vascular Biology, 2009, 29 (1): 75-83.

[80] Rattan V, Sultana C, Shen Y, et al. Oxidant stress-induced transendothelial migration of monocytes is linked to phosphorylation of PECAM-1[J]. American Journal of Physiology Endocrinology and Metabolism, 1997, 273 (3): E453-E461.

[81] Maas M, Wang R, Paddock C, et al. Reactive oxygen species induce reversible PECAM-1 tyrosine phosphorylation and SHP-2 binding [J].

American Journal of Physiology Heart and Circulatory Physiology, 2003, 285 (6): H2336-H2344.

[82] Hastie LE, Patton WF, Hechtman HB, et al. Filamin redistribution in an endothelial cell reoxygenation injury model [J]. Free Radical Biology and Medicine, 1997, 22 (6): 955-966.

[83] Adamo RF, Fishbein I, Zhang K, et al. Magnetically enhanced cell delivery for accelerating recovery of the endothelium in injured arteries [J]. Journal of Controlled Release, 2016, 222: 169-175.

[84] Karjalainen PP, Varho V, Nammas W, et al. Early neointimal coverage and vasodilator response following biodegradable polymer sirolimus-eluting vs. Durable polymer zotarolimus-eluting stents in patients with acute coronary syndrome-HATTRICK-OCT trial [J]. Circulation Journal, 2015, 79 (2): 360-367.

[85] Kuramitsu S, Sonoda S, Yokoi H, et al, Long-term coronary arterial response to biodegradable polymer biolimus-eluting stents in comparison with durable polymer sirolimus-eluting stents and bare-metal stents: five-year follow-up optical coherence tomography study [J]. Atherosclerosis, 2014, 237 (1): 23- 29.

[86] Mattesini A, Secco GG, Dall"Ara G, et al. ABSORB bio-degradable stents versus second-generation metal stents: a comparison study of 100 complex lesions treated under OCT guidance [J]. JACC: Cardiovascular Interventions, 2014, 7 (7): 741-750.

[87] Christiansen EH, Jensen LO, Thayssen P, et al. Biolimus-eluting biodegradable polymer-coated stent versus durable polymer-coated sirolimus-eluting stent in unselected patients receiving percutaneous coronary intervention (SORT OUT V): a randomised non-inferiority trial [J]. The Lancet, 2013, 381 (9867): 661-669.

[88] Bonnefont-Rousselot D. Glucose and reactive oxygen species [J]. Current Opinion in Clinical Nutrition and Metabolic Care, 2002, 5 (5): 561-568.

[89] Potnis PA, Tesfamariam B, Wood SC. Induction of nicotinamide-adenine dinucleotide phosphate oxidase and apoptosis by biodegradable polymers in macrophages: implications for stents [J]. Journal of Cardiovascular Pharmacology, 2011, 57 (6): 712-720.

[90] Hietala EM, Maasilta P, Juuti H, et al. Platelet deposition on stainless steel, spiral, and braided polylactide stents. A comparative study [J]. Thrombosis and Haemostasis, 2004, 92 (6): 1394-1401.

[91] Pignatelli P, Carnevale R, Santo SD, et al, Violi F. Rosuvastatin reduces platelet recruitment by inhibiting NADPH oxidase activation [J]. Biochemical Pharmacology, 2012, 84 (12): 1635-1642.

[92] Khzam LB, Hachem A, Zaid Y, et al. Soluble CD40 ligand impairs the anti-platelet function of peripheral blood angiogenic outgrowth cells via increased production of reactive oxygen species [J]. Thrombosis and Haemostasis, 2013, 109 (5): 940-947.

[93] Basili S, Pignatelli P, Tanzilli G, et al. Anoxia-reoxygenation enhances platelet thromboxane A2 production via reactive oxygen species-generated NOX2: effect in patients undergoing elective percutaneous coronary intervention [J]. Arteriosclerosis, Thrombosis, and Vascular Biology, 2011, 31 (8): 1766-1771.

[94] Kleinedler JJ, Foley JD, Alexander JS, et al. Synergistic effect of resveratrol and quercetin released from drug-eluting polymer coatings for endovascular devices [J]. Journal of Biomedical Materials Research-PartB Applied Biomaterials, 2011, 99 (2): 266-275.

[95] Rosenbaum MA, Miyazaki K, Colles SM, et al. Graham. Antioxidant therapy reverses impaired graft healing in hypercholesterolemic rabbits [J]. Journal of Vascular Surgery, 2010, 51 (1): 184-193.

[96] Aviram M, Fuhrman B. LDL oxidation by arterial wall macrophages depends on the oxidative status in the lipoprotein and in the cells: role of prooxidants vs. antioxidants [J]. Molecular and Cellular Biochemistry, 1998, 188 (1-2): 149-159.

[97] Hanratty C G, Murrell M, Khachigian L M, et al. Low flow promotes instent intimal hyperplasia: comparison with lumen loss in balloon-injured and uninjured vessels and the effects of the antioxidant pyrrolidine dithiocarbamate [J]. Atherosclerosis, 2004, 177 (2): 269-274.

[98] Cicero AF, Morbini M, Parini A, Urso R, Rosticci M, Grandi E, Borghi C. Effect of red yeast rice combined with antioxidants on lipid pattern, hs-CRP level, and endothelial function in moderately hypercholesterolemic subjects [J]. Therapeutics & Clinical Risk Management, 2016, (12): 281-286.

[99] Zhu XY, Li P, Yang YB, Liu ML. Xuezhikang, extract of red yeast rice, improved abnormal hemorheology, suppressed caveolin-1 and increased eNOS expression in atherosclerotic rats [J]. PLoS ONE, 2013, 8 (5): article e62731.

[100] Douglas G, Van Kampen E, Hale A B, Mcneill E, Patel J, Crabtree MJ, Ali Z, Hoerr RA, Alp NJ, Channon KM. Endothelial cell repopulation after stenting determines in-stent neointima formation: effects of bare-metal vs. drug-eluting stents and genetic endothelial cell modification [J]. European Heart Journal, 2013, 34 (43): 3378-3388.

First published: Cui Yuan-yuan, LIU Yue, ZHAO Fu-hai, SHI DAžhuo, and CHEN Ke-ji: Neoatherosclerosis after Drug-εlutirg Stert Implantation: roles and mechanisms [J]. Oxid Med Cell Longev, 2016, 2016: 592423.

Mechanisms and Clinical Application of Tetramethylpyrazine (an Interesting Natural Compound Isolated from *Ligusticum Wallichii*): Current Status and Perspective

ZHAO Ying-ke, LIU Yue, and CHEN Ke-ji

Tetramethylpyrazine (ligustrazine, TMP)is a natural compound isolated from Chinese herbal medicine Ligusticum wallichii (chuanxiong), which has been extensively used for medicinal purpose for more than 2000 years. TMP was firstly isolated in 1957 and has been increasingly studied for its action on myocardial and cerebral infarction since 1970s [1]. In the past decades, researchers explored other pharmacological capabilities of TMP in various diseases, such as coronary heart disease, diabetes, cancers and liver injury. Accordingly, laboratory study verified that the regulation ability of this agent in multiple molecular targets, such as anti-inflammation, antioxidant, antiplatelet, antiapoptosis. The pharmacology of TMP has been well reviewed in the past [2-4]. This paper will briefly summarize the pharmacological mechanisms and its clinical application status, moreover research about TMP derivatives, also a highly popular topic due to its inherent low bioavailability, will then be discussed [5]. (see Figure 1)

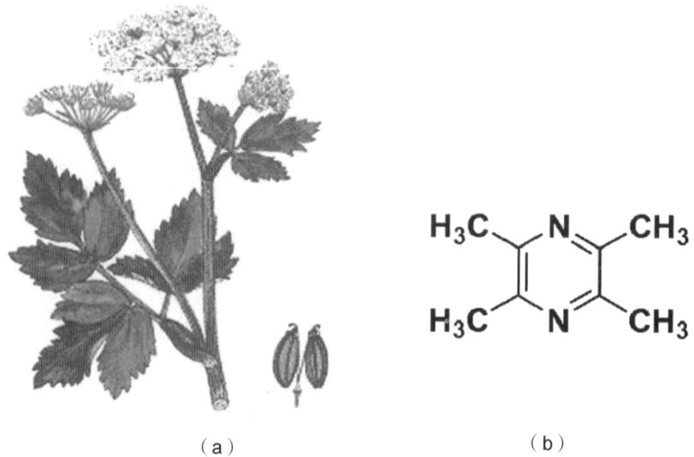

Figure 1 Illustration of *Ligusticum wallichii* (*Chuan Xiong*)Plant
Notes: (a)and chemical structure of ligustrazine (b).

1 Medicinal Use of TMP

1.1 Cardiovascular System

The cardiovascular pharmacological effects of TMP aroused widespread interest among researchers in recent years [2,4]. There are considerable documents supporting the view that this monomer can be a promising botanical remedy for cardiovascular diseases. The possible mechanism of its action might include modulating ion channels, stimulating the release of NO production, inhibiting vascular smooth muscle cell proliferation and migration, scavenging ROS, regulating inflammation and apoptosis, and preventing platelet aggregation (see Figure 2).

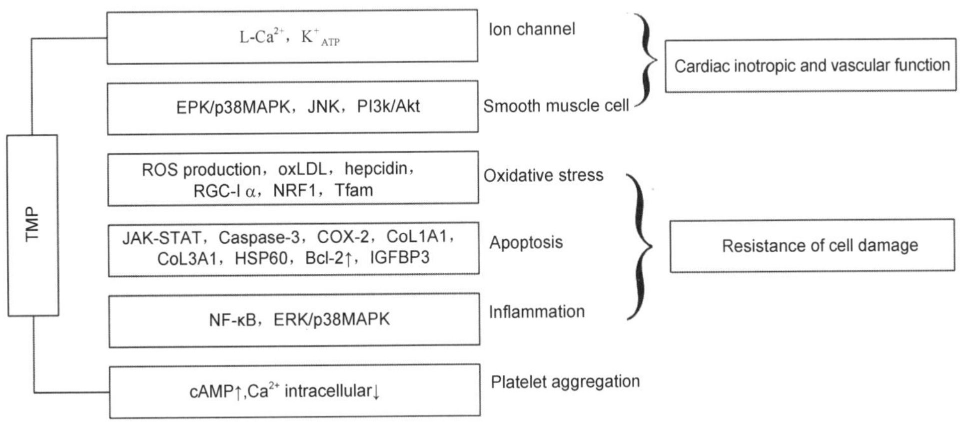

Figure 2 Putative Mechanisms Underlying Cardiovascular Protective Effects of TMP

1.1. 1 Regulation of Cardiac Inotropic and Vascular Functions

(1)Ion Channels. TMP was described as "calcium antagonist" [6] and produce a vasodilation effect via inhibiting Ca^{2+} influx and the release of intracellular Ca^{2+} at first [7]. Tsai et al. [8] introduced the cultured vascular smooth muscle (A7r5)to prove that TMP can affect the calcium influx, at least partly, by mediating the opening of potassium channel. Moreover, Kim et al. [9] verified that TMP-induced vasorelaxation in isolated rat aortic rings was determined by ATP-dependent potassium channels. TMP was also reported to have a direct effect on L-type Calcium current (I_{Ca-L}), since it can reduce calcium transient in a dose-dependent manner when applied to rabbit ventricular myocyte [10]. The combination of tetramethylpyrazine phosphate (TMPP) and Ginsenoside-Rb1 (Rb1)in $cTnT^{R141W}$ mouse model also obtained some benefit; the downregulated level of calmodulin 1 and calcium/calmodulin-dependent protein kinase Ⅱβ (Camk2b)indicated that TMP might regulate Ca^{2+}/CaM/CaMKⅡ [11]. However, current evidence is quite preliminary; the specific link between TMP and ion channel still needs to be thoroughly investigated. Despite the potentially involved ions which has been listed in the publications, the corresponding pathways, genes or cytokines that might responsible for the activation of ion channels are barely understood.

(2)Nitric Oxide Pathway. TMP can stimulate NO production in pulmonary arteries of rat [12], Lv et al. [13] demonstrated that Akt and the endothelial isoform of nitric oxide synthase (eNOS)phosphorylation were significantly up-regulated after TMP pretreatment *in vivo*, this effect could be blocked by NO synthase (NOS) inhibitor consequently. PI3K/Akt pathway might play a pivotal role in activating eNOS and increasing NO production. Numerous researches verified the result of TMP on NO production; they believed that there are certain kinds of relationship between TMP and Akt, while the result remains controversial. Some reported TMP exerts an inhibition role in phosphorylation of Akt in N9 microglial cells [14], although others claimed that TMP can activate Akt in vascular endothelial cells [15]. Despite different cell phenotypes involved in these experiments, the relationship between TMP and Akt pathway requires further exploration. Besides, there is no clear and standard therapeutic dosages of TMP, which makes the antioxidative effect of TMP not as evident as proposed.

(3)Smooth Muscle Cell Proliferation and Migration. TMP can suppress the proliferation of VSMC in rabbit aortic vascular [16]. Additionally, there is a study which intended to investigate the effect of TMP on the airway smooth muscle; their data indicate that TMP might suppress the airway smooth cells proliferation via ERK1/2 signaling pathway, as the level of PDGF and p-ERK 1/2 proteins has decreased significantly in the TMP group [17]. Recently, another researcher [18] pointed out that TMP can inhibited PDGF-BB induced proliferation of VSMC, and results expressed that differentiated VSMC can be reversed by TMP and ERK and p38 MAPK might be involved in this process. Interestingly, most studies emphasized inhibitory effect on proliferation when TMP administered before proliferation occurs, although few related mechanism or targets have been identified.

1.1. 2 Resistance of Cell Damage

(1)Oxidative Stress. Clinical and laboratory studies on herbal medicine paid special attention to ROS-pathway-mediated injury in CVDs [19]. The scavenging ROS function of TMP on hypoxia induced pulmonary vascular leakage had been explored [20], and H_2O_2-induced human umbilical vein endothelial cells (HUVECs) were also employed to evaluate protective effect of TMP on oxidative stress, as well as its antiapoptotic properties [21]. By testing its effect on C2C12 myotube, Gao and his coworkers [22] reported that TMP can restrain mitochondrial ROS generation and upregulate the expression of PGC1, NRF1 and Tfam, which reflects mitochondrial biogenesis. TMP also exerts an endothelium protective property via downregulating the expression of ICAM-1 and HSP60 [23]. Considering the precise mechanism is still not quite clearly clarified, further studies focusing on the specific roles of TMP should be emphasized.

(2)Apoptosis. TMP can decrease the ANP mRNA expression in cardiomyocyte hypertrophy rat model and suppress the level of pJAK2, pJAK1 or pSTAT3, demonstrated that TMP can inhibit JAK-STAT signal transduction [24]. Researchers evaluated the effect of tetramethylpyrazine phosphate (TMPP)on the dilated cardiomyopathy (DCM)and reported that TMPP can prevent the progressive LV dilation and systolic dysfunction, as well as the collagen deposition and gene expression reduction of procollagens COL1A1 and COL3A1 [25]. Moreover, the upregulated level of Bcl-2 and the reduction of Caspase-3 also had been observed in apoptosis myocyte after TMP intervention [26]. TMP can exert anti-apoptosis ability by inhibiting macrophage COX-2 [27]. Recently, a piece of work [28] successfully tested the protective effect of TMP in H9c2 cardiomyoblasts; the result is consistent with previous report from Zheng et al. [29].

(3)Inflammation. TMP can restrain LPS-induced IL-8 overexpression in HUVECs at both the protein and mRNA levels, which is possibly due to blocking the activation of the NF- κ B-dependent pathway, the activation of ERK and p38 MAPK signaling pathway has also been observed [30]. Hepcidin has emerged as a positive regulator of atherosclerotic plaque destabilization since 2007 by Sullivan [31]; its expression can be regulated by TMP [32]. SD rats with high-fat diet for 8 weeks were employed in the study; TMP group was injected with TMP at 40 mg/ (kg · d), while hepcidin group was injected with heparin at 5 mg/ (kg · d). After treatment, relevant markers such as blood lipid, hepcidin, ET-1, ROS, MDA, and SOD were detected. The results supported that the protective effect of TMP on endothelium might be related to inhibiting overexpressed level of hepcidin. However, direct pathways involved in regulating hepcidin need to be investigated in the future.

1.1. 3 Antiplatelet

Platelet aggregation plays a key role in the pathogenesis of atherothrombosis, and a variety of Chinese herbals have been examined for their antiplatelet property [33]. TMP has been commonly reported on its effect of antiplatelet since the 1980s [34]; stimulating cAMP production and inhibiting of intracellular calcium mobilization were assumed to be the potential mechanism [35]. There is plenty of evidence for the suppression of platelet aggregation, although few publications were related to the platelet release reaction. A piece of research was conducted on patients who were diagnosed with acute coronary syndrome and received percutaneous coronary intervention. After TMP treatment, the level of CD63, an indicator of platelet activation, decreased significantly [36]. TMP might have an effect on inhibition of platelet release, although no experimental study is conducted to verify the role of TMP in platelet release reaction.

1.2 Protection on cerebra and spinal cord injury

The application of TMP in the treatment of ischemic stroke has been well documented for ages [37]. Tsai and Liang [38] directly evaluated its ability to penetrate blood brain barrier by using microdialysis technique that provide evidence for the following studies on central action of TMP. Its neuroprotective property is partly due to modulating thioredoxin transcription [39] and down-regulating the expression of neuronal isoform of NO synthase (nNOS)[40]. TMP also could attenuate the inflammation associated with ischemia by regulating the expression of NF-E2-related factor 2 (Nrf2)and heme oxygenase-1 (HO-1), which plays a role against ischemic reperfusion brain injury [40,41]. Researchers also claimed that TMP can protect mitochondrial function and enzymatic antioxidants [42]; nevertheless, sufficient evidence is needed. Recently, there is evidence about the effects of TMP on functional recovery and dendritic plasticity after ischemia [43]. The neuroprotective effects of TMP have also been tested on spinal cord injury [44,45]. Moreover, other researchers [46] explored anti-inflammatory properties of TMP in Alzheimer's disease. Considering there is limited publications currently in this field, rigorous experiments can be warranted.

1.3 Cancer

Liu et al[47]firstly investigated the effect of TMP on lymphocytes proliferation response. Later on, it has been tested on various cancers, such as leukemia [48,49], lung cancer[50,51], ovarian carcinoma[52], liver cancer [53], glioma [54], osteosarcoma [55], chemotherapy-resistant breast cancer [56] and prostate cancer [57]; the probable mechanism includes anti-inflammatory and promoting apoptosis. Studies intended to examine the effect of TMP derivatives like tetramethylpyrazine hydrochloride (TMPH)had yielded a similar conclusion. Large quantities of agents are currently reported as an anticarcinogen via numerous pathways, as determined in experimental environments, while few display the same effects in clinic. How to apply the laboratory finding in the clinical practice is a critical issue that remains to be settled.

1.4 Diabetes

As there is abundant evidence for the vascular protective action of TMP, Lee and his colleagues hypothesized to investigate this characteristic on the diabetic model at the outset. Streptozotocin-induced diabetic mice model was adopted to test lipid peroxidation level, which is one of marked pathological changes in diabetes, and the result indicated that TMP can effectively alleviate glucose and blood urea nitrogen concentration (BUN)[58]. Later on, researchers also attempt to conduct similar experiments on streptozotocin-induced diabetic nephropathy rat model; their result was consistent with the previous one on the mice model. Moreover, they demonstrated that the level of insulin, angiotensin II and P-selectin also decreased [58,59]. Additionally, there is a piece of study reporting protective role of TMP regarding this disorder [60].

1.5 Liver injury

Liu et al[61]detected hepatoprotective effect of TMP on acute econazole-induced liver injury. The probable explanation for this action includes inhibition of membrane lipid peroxidation [62] and oxidative stress [63]. Likewise, recent evidence indicated that TMP exerts a protective property on sepsis-induced acute liver injury mainly by ameliorating the aquaporin 8 expression [64]. Besides, there are also publications related to its inhibitory effect on hepatic fibrosis, PI3/AKT and ERK pathways, NLRP3 inflammasome pathway might be engaged [65,66].

1.6 Renal Injury

TMP can attenuate the Cisplatin-induced nephrotoxity in rats, antioxidative stress might be one of the proposed mechanisms [67,68]. Similar effects had also been tested in rat renal tubular cells [69]. Its therapeutic effect on hepatic/renal ischemia-reperfusion injury in rats [70], as well as the fibrosis of renal interstitial, had been verified [71,72]. Moreover, TMP can protect rat renal tubular cells from adriamycin-induced apoptosis [73,74]; this action, to some extent, is due to the inhibition of p38 MAPK and FoxO1 pathways [75].

1.7 Others

Since TMP was reported to possess a broad spectrum of pharmacological effects, such as antioxidant, anti-inflammatory, antifibrosis effects, diseases, such as asthma and colitis, suffered from such pathological changes and had been further investigated [76-80]. However, the precise mechanism still needs to be further explored.

2 Current Status of Therapeutic Uses of TMP

The injection solution of TMP has been broadly used especially in China to treat ischemic stroke [81], coronary heart disease [36], diabetic nephropathy [82], knee osteoarthritis [83]. Large amount of research is about the efficacy of TMP injection. For example, in a systematic review, they evaluated the efficacy of 22 Chinese patent medicines for stroke, there are 11 randomized controlled trials with 1652 patients related to TMP injection [84]. Although, it seems that lots of evidence have been stated the efficacy, the reliability of these trials is doubtful. Few of the studies report the adverse events [82,85,86]; the poor methodology of the design makes the problem even worse. Even for the treatment of the same disease, the dosage of TMP injection is quite different. Similar problem was confronted when talking about the treatment course. What is more, there are lots of combination use of other herbal injections during the treatment, which might be difficult to figure out the interactions. Due to the low quality of clinical trials in this field, the safety concerns about the herbal injection have long been a major dispute [87].

3 Approaches to Improve the Bioavailability of TMP

3.1 Problems Associated with Drug Delivery

Early pharmacokinetic research has determined the metabolism rate of TMP and verified its in vivo short half-life of $T_{1/2}$=2.89 h. Besides, the accumulated toxicity is another potential threat to the patients for keeping an effective concentration via frequently administration [88,89]. Considering the drug delivery deficiency of TMP [90], enormous experiments were conducted to improve its pharmacological activity since 1990s. There are two primary approaches which can improve the biological activity.

3.2 Improvement of Dosage Form

The conventional TMP dosage forms include injection, oral tablet and capsule. Conventionally, the oral administration, is the most preferable route for chronic diseases. However, this form might not be suitable, considering that hepatic first-pass metabolism can probably result in a lower bioavailability [5]. However, the intravenous injection does not help; drug concentration of injection form was peaked within 20 min but undetected after 120 min [38]. A great deal of formulation has been proposed in order to solve the deficiency during drug delivery, such as porosity osmotic pump, microemulsions, ethosomes, transdermal patch. The administration route has changed accordingly, transdermal, intranasal, intraperitoneal injection, and ocular delivery were introduced [5,91,92]. It is of importance to quantify the drug concentration in different sites (such as brain, liver and skin). Research related to *in vitro* drug release, *in vivo* distribution, and the optimum dosage is urgently needed. Another unsatisfactory situation is that most of the newly designed forms were conducted at laboratory level, and extensively clinical evidence needs to be layed out to validate the clinical effect accordingly.

3.3 Structural Modification of TMP

The structural formula of TMP shows that pyrazine largely determined its pharmacodynamics, while the side chain might be mainly responsible for its pharmacokinetics. Given its inherent characteristics, the structure modification to improve the bioavailability has been broadly investigated, which opened new perspective for drug discovery. During the past decades, over 300 novel TMP derivatives has been designed and synthesized [93]. In general, most of the modifications were derived from 4 primary intermediates of TMP. They are 2-bromomethyl-3, 5, 6-trimethylpyrazine (TMP-Br), 3, 5, 6-trimethylpyrazin-2-yl (TMP-OH), 3, 5, 6-trimethylpyrazine-2-carboxylic acid (TMP-COOH), and 2, 5-dimethylol-3, 6-dimethyl pyrazine (OH-

TMP-OH) (Figure 3). The first step of the structural modification is the synthesis of these four fundamental compounds. With the obtained intermediates, we can easily link other reactive groups with TMP. Not only small chemical groups be used for structural modification, but considerable herbal compounds were also introduced into synthesis process. For example, TMP-ferulic acid derivatives that combined TMP and ferulic acid, another active ingredient of Ligusticum wallichii, as precursors. Both TMP and ferulic acid had been extensively reported because of their anti-platelet aggregation effects [94]. Given the structural properties, calcium antagonists also could be combined to pyrazine to form new derivatives. Further study should be conducted, enabling a better understanding of the pharmacokinetics of these derivatives. After modification, further experiment is needed to demonstrate the biological activities and pharmacological characteristics of original derivatives. After 21 new derivatives had been developed, Li and his coworkers conducted experiment to evaluate the protective effect of newly designed derivatives on the HUVECs. The data proved that some of the newly compounds had better protective effect compared with the reference drug TMP [95]. Most of the results seems very preferable, which reported a better effect over TMP. Although the interaction and toxicity of new derivatives have not been studied comprehensively, the active parts of the new drugs, as well as their metabolism parameters, signal transmission might be different from TMP, which also needs to be further confirmed.

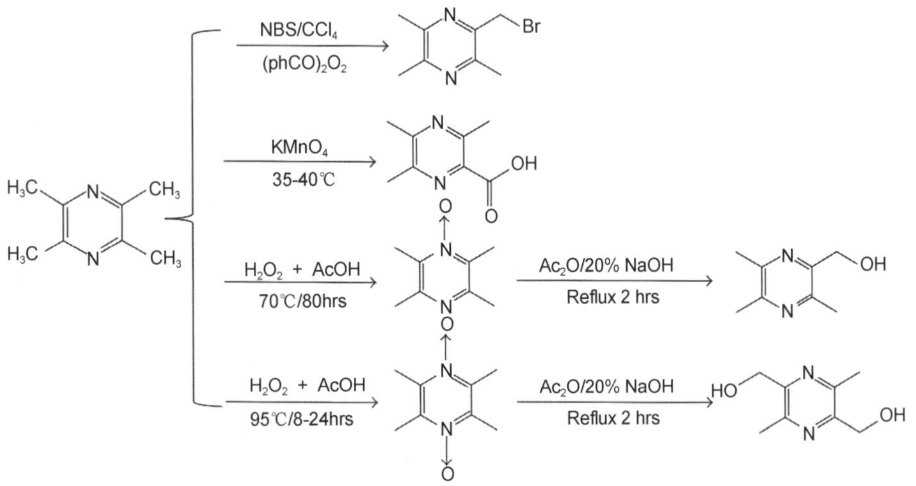

Figure 3 Primary Intermediates of TMP

4 Conclusion

As an effective and multi-target product, TMP is promising and worth of further investigation. Large amount of trials has been conducted to assess it clinical efficacy; their results seem too good to be true. So far, there is no clear evidence that give us the standard dosage, treatment course, as well as the reporting of adverse events which is necessary for clinical trials. It would be more helpful if standardized usage of TMP was established. In that case, the results of clinical trials would be more persuasive, providing reliable evidence for decision making in practice. Despite enormous interests in the clinical uses, there is still a great deal of challenge facing the academics, such as the effectiveness, pharmacological effect, and toxicity. Nowadays, the action and mechanisms of TMP have been investigated in multi-systems and multi-diseases, and the involved pathways and targets seem quite complex. With advances in the technique of laboratory, such as genomic, proteomic data, as well as spectrometric analysis, our understanding of herbal compounds like TMP will be more systematic. As our knowledge about its mechanism as well as disease pathophysiology has been expanded, TMP can be used more extensively and more targeted. In the future, more preclinical studies to determine its mechanisms and potential toxic effects and to answer questions related to absorption and metabolism are needed. After this preclinical work has been completed, well-designed and clinical studies can be conducted. In summary, multifunction and the structural advantage make TMP a promising candidate for further study to achieve maximum therapeutic efficacy and minimum toxicity.

REFERENCE

[1] Guo SK, Chen KJ, Qian ZH, et al. Tetramethylpyrazine in the treatment of cardiovascular and cerebrovascular diseases Planta Medica[J]. 1983, 47 (2): 89.

[2] Guo M, Liu Y, Shi D. Cardiovascular actions and therapeutic potential of tetramethylpyrazine (active component isolated from Rhizoma Chuanxiong): roles and mechanisms[J]. BioMed Research International, 2016 (5): 243.

[3] Gao HJ, Liu PF. Ligustrazine monomer against cerebral ischemia/ reperfusion injury[J]. Neural Regeneration Research, 2015, 10, (5): 832-840.

[4] Qian W, Xiong X, Fang Z, et al. Protective effect of tetramethylpyrazine on myocardial ischemia-reperfusion injury[J]. Evidence-Based Complementary and Alternative Medicine, 2014: 9.

[5] Mei D, Mao S, Sun W, et al. Effect of chitosan structure properties and molecular weight on the intranasal absorption of tetramethylpyrazine phosphate in rats[J]. European Journal of Pharmaceutics and Biopharmaceutics, 2008, 70 (3): 874-881.

[6] Zhou XB, L. Salganicoff, and R. Sevy, The pharmacological effect of ligustrazine on human platelets[J]. Acta Pharmaceutica Sinica, 1985, 2 (5): 334-339.

[7] C. Y. Kwan, E. E. Daniel, et al. Inhibition of vasoconstriction by tetramethylpyrazine: does it act by blocking the voltage-dependent Ca channel? [J]. Journal of Cardiovascular Pharmacology, 1990, 15 (1): 157-162.

[8] C C Tsai, Lai TY, Huang WC, et al. Tetramethylpyrazine as potassium channel opener to lower calcium influx into cultured aortic smooth muscle cells[J]. Planta Medica, 2003, 69 (6): 557-558.

[9] E Y Kim, J H Kim, and M R Rhyu. Endothelium-independent vasorelaxation by ligusticum wallichii in isolated rat aorta: comparison of a butanolic fraction and tetramethylpyrazine, the main active component of ligusticum wallichii [J]. Biological and Pharmaceutical Bulletin, 2010, 33, (8): 1360-1363, .

[10] Ren Z, Ma J, P, et al. The effect of ligustrazine on L-type calcium current, calcium transient and contractility in rabbit ventricular myocytes[J]. Journal of Ethnopharmacology, 2012, 144 (3): 555-561.

[11] Lu D, Shao HT, Ge WP, et al. Ginsenoside-RB1 and tetramethylpyrazine phosphate act synergistically to prevent dilated cardiomyopathy in cTnTR141W transgenic mice[J]. Journal of Cardiovascular Pharmacology, 2012, 59 (5): 426-433.

[12] Peng W, D Hucks, R M Priest, et al. Ligustrazine-induced endothelium-dependent relaxation in pulmonary arteries via an NO-mediated and exogenous L-arginine-dependent mechanism[J]. British Journal of Pharmacology, 1996, 119 (5): 1063-1071.

[13] Lv L, Jiang SS, Xu J, et al. Protective effect of ligustrazine against myocardial ischaemia reperfusion in rats: the role of endothelial nitric oxide synthase[J]. Clinical and Experimental Pharmacology and Physiology, 2012, 39 (1): 20-27.

[14] Liu HT, Du YG, He JL, et al. Tetramethylpyrazine inhibits production of nitric oxide and inducible nitric oxide synthase in lipopolysaccharide-induced N9 microglial cells through blockade of MAPK and PI3K/Akt signaling pathways, and suppression of intracellular reactive oxygen species[J]. Journal of Ethnopharmacology, 2010, 129 (3): 335-343.

[15] Kang Y, Hu M, Zhu Y, et al. Antioxidative effect of the herbal remedy Qin Huo Yi Hao and its active component tetramethylpyrazine on high glucose-treated endothelial cells[J]. Life Sciences, 2009, 84 (13): 428-436.

[16] Li S, Wang JH, and Chen SL. Inhibitory effect of ligustrazine on proliferation of rabbit vascular smooth muscle cells after arterial injury[J]. Acta Pharmacologica Sinica, 1999, 20 (10): 917-922.

[17] Qu YJ, Bai HB, Wang CZ, et al. Inhibition of tetramethylpyrazine on the proliferation of rat airway smooth muscle cells[J]. Chinese Pharmacological Bulletin, 2010, 26 (6): 814-818.

[18] Yu L, Huang X, Huang K, et al. Ligustrazine attenuates the platelet-derived growth factor-BB-induced proliferation and migration of vascular smooth muscle cells by interrupting extracellular signal-regulated kinase and P38 mitogen-activated protein kinase pathways[J]. Molecular Medicine Reports, 2015, 12 (1): 705-711.

[19] Li L, Zhou X, Li N, et al. Herbal drugs against cardiovascular disease: traditional medicine and modern development[J]. Drug Discovery Today, 2015, 20 (9): 1074-1086.

[20] Zhang L, Deng M, and Zhou S. Tetramethylpyrazine inhibits hypoxia-induced pulmonary vascular leakage in rats via the ROS-HIF-VEGF pathway[J]. Pharmacology, 2011, 87 (5-6): 265-273.

[21] Li WM, Liu HT, Li XY, et al. The effect of tetramethylpyrazine on hydrogen peroxide-induced oxidative damage in human umbilical vein endothelial cells[J]. Basic and Clinical Pharmacology and Toxicology, 2010, 106 (1): 45-52.

[22] Gao X, Zhao XL, Zhu YH, et al. Tetramethylpyrazine protects palmitate-induced oxidative damage and mitochondrial dysfunction in C2C12 myotubes[J]. Life Sciences, 2011, 88 (17-18): 803-809.

[23] H J, Hao WJ, Wang SQ, et al. Protective effects of ligustrazine on TNF--induced endothelial dysfunction[J]. European Journal of Pharmacology, 2012, 674 (2): 365-369.

[24] Gao MH, Zhang L, Li B, et al. Effect of tetramethylpyrazine on JAK-STAT signal transduction in cardiomyocyte hypertrophy[J]. Chinese Journal of Cellular and Molecular Immunology, 2011, 27 (5): 519-524.

[25] Zhao HP, Lu D, Zhang W, et al. Protective action of tetramethylpyrazine phosphate against dilated cardiomyopathy in cTnTR141W transgenic mice[J]. Acta Pharmacologica Sinica, 2010, 31 (3): 281-288.

[26] Yang Y, Li ZH, Liu H, et al. Inhibitory effect of tetramethylpyrazine preconditioning on overload training-induced myocardial apoptosis in rats[J]. Chinese Journal of Integrative Medicine, 2014, 21 (6): 423-430.

[27] Wan JY, Ye DY, Wu P, et al. Effect of tetramethylpyrazine on lipopolysaccharides induced macrophage cyclo-oxidase-2 expression and apoptosis of cardiac myocytes[J]. Chinese Journal of Integrated Traditional and Western Medicine, 2004, 24 (10): 906-911.

[28] Lin KH, Kuo WW, Jiang AZ, et al. Tetramethylpyrazine ameliorated hypoxia-induced myocardial cell apoptosis via HIF-1α/JNK/p38 and IGFBP3/BNIP3 inhibition to upregulate PI3K/Akt survival signaling[J]. Cellular Physiology and Biochemistry, 2015, 36 (1): 334-344.

[29] Zheng H, Wang S, Zhou P, et al. Effects of Ligustrazine on DNA damage and apoptosis induced by irradiation[J]. Environmental Toxicology and Pharmacology, 2013, 6 (3): 1197-1206.

[30] Li XY, He JL, Liu HT, et al. Tetramethylpyrazine suppresses interleukin-8 expression in LPS-stimulated human umbilical vein endothelial cell by blocking ERK, p38 and nuclear factor- κ B signaling pathways[J]. Journal of Ethnopharmacology, 2009, 125 (1): 83-89.

[31] J. L. Sullivan. Macrophage iron, hepcidin, and atherosclerotic plaque stability[J]. Experimental Biology and Medicine, 2007, 232 (8): 1014-1020.

[32] Sun MY, Guo CY, Wang JS, et al. Correlation between high expression of hepcidin and vascular endothelial damage as well as intervention of tetramethylpyrazine[J]. Chinese Traditional and Herbal Drugs, 2015, 46 (15): 2265-2269.

[33] Liu Y, Yin HJ, Shi DZ, et al. Chinese herb and formulas for promoting blood circulation and removing blood stasis and antiplatelet therapies[J]. Evidence-Based Complementary and Alternative Medicine, 2012: 8.

[34] Zeng GY, Zhou YP, Zhang LY, et al. Effects of tetramethylpyrazine on cardiac haemodynamics in dogs[J]. Acta Pharmaceutica Sinica, 1982, 17 (3): 182-186.

[35] Liu SY and D. M. Sylvester, Antithrombotic/antiplatelet activity of tetramethylpyrazine[J]. Thrombosis Research, 1990, 58 (2): 129-140.

[36] Chen ZQ, Hong L, Wang H, Effect of tetramethylpyrazine on platelet activation and vascular endothelial function in patients with acute coronary syndrome undergoing percutaneous coronary intervention[J]. Chinese Journal of Inte-grated Traditional and Western Medicine, 2007, 27 (12): 1078-1081.

[37] Chen KJ and Chen K, Ischemic stroke treated with Ligusticum chuanxiong[J]. Chinese Medical Journal, 1992, 105 (10): 870-873.

[38] T. -H. Tsai, C. -C. Liang. Pharmacokinetics of tetramethylpyrazine in rat blood and brain using microdialysis[J]. International Journal of Pharmaceutics, 2001, 216 (1-2): 61-66.

[39] Jia J, Zhang X, Hu YS et al. Protective effect of tetraethyl pyrazine against focal cerebral ischemia/reperfusion injury in rats: therapeutic time window and its mechanism[J]. Thrombosis Research, 2009, 123 (5)727-730.

[40] Xiao X, Liu Y, Qi C, et al. Neuroprotection and enhanced neurogenesis by tetramethylpyrazine in adult rat brain after focal ischemia[J]. Neurological Research, 2010, 32 (5): 547-555.

[41] Li M, Zhang X, Cui L, et al. The neuroprotection of oxymatrine in cerebral ischemia/reperfusion is related to nuclear factor erythroid 2-related factor 2 (Nrf2)-mediated antioxidant response: role of Nrf2 and hemeoxygenase-1 expression[J]. Biological and Pharmaceutical Bulletin, 2011, 34 (5): 595-601.

[42] Li SY, Jia YH, Sun WG, et al. Stabilization of mitochondrial function by tetramethylpyrazine protects against kainate-induced oxidative lesions in the rat hippocampus[J]. Free Radical Biology and Medicine, 2010, 48 (4): 597-608.

[43] Lin JB, Zheng CJ, Zhang X, et al. Effects of tetramethylpyrazine on functional recovery and neuronal dendritic plasticity after experimental stroke[J]. Evidence-based Complementary and Alternative Medicine, 2015: 10.

[44] Xiao Z, Hu J, Lu H, et al. Effect of tetramethylpyrazine on the expression of macrophage migration inhibitory factor in acute spinal cord injury in rats[J]. Journal of Central South University (Medical Sciences), 2012, 37 (10): 1031-1036.

[45] J. -W. Shin, J. -Y. Moon, J. -W. Seong et al. Effects of tetramethylpyrazine on microglia activation in spinal cord compression injury of mice[J]. The American Journal of Chinese Medicine, 2013, 41 (6): 1361-1376.

[46] M. Kim, S. -O. Kim, M. Lee et al. Tetramethylpyrazine, a natural alkaloid, attenuates pro-inflammatory mediators induced by amyloid and interferon-in rat brain microglia[J]. European Journal of Pharmacology, 2014, 740: 504-511.

[47] Liu J, Qiang W, Ye S. Effect of tetramethylpyrazine on lymphocytes proliferation response of murine splenocytes[J]. Journal of West China University of Medical Sciences, 1995, 26 (2): 177-179.

[48] Li N, Jia XH, Wang JY. Effects of tetramethylpyrazine on apoptosis of human leukemia cells and the expressions of apoptotic-relevant proteins[J]. Tumor, 2014, 34 (10): 919-923.

[49] Wang XJ, Xu YH, Yang GC, et al. Tetramethylpyrazine inhibits the proliferation of acute lymphocytic leukemia cell lines via decrease in GSK-3β[J]. Oncology Reports, 2015, 33 (5): 2368-2374.

[50] Xu XY, Yan PK, Chen G, et al. Inhibition of tetramethylpyrazine on Lewis lung carcinomas, microvessel growth and VEGF expression in mice[J]. Chinese Pharmacological Bulletin, 2004, 20 (2): 151-154.

[51] Zheng CY, Xiao W, Zhu MX, et al. Inhibition of cyclooxygenase-2 by tetramethylpyrazine and its effects on A549 cell invasion and metastasis[J]. International Journal of Oncology, 2012, 40 (6): 2029-2037.

[52] Yin J, Yu C, Yang Z et al. Tetramethylpyrazine inhibits migration of SKOV3 human ovarian carcinoma cells and decreases the expression of interleukin-8 via the ERK1/2, p38 and AP-1 signaling pathways[J]. Oncology Reports, 2011, 26 (3): 671-679.

[53] Cao J, Miao Q, Miao S, et al. Tetramethylpyrazine (TMP)exerts antitumor effects by inducing apoptosis and autophagy in hepatocellular carcinoma[J]. International Immunopharm acology, 2015, 26 (1): 212-220.

[54] Chen Z, Pan X, A. G. Georgakilas et al. Tetramethylpyrazine (TMP)protects cerebral neurocytes and inhibits glioma by down regulating chemokine receptor CXCR4 expression[J]. Cancer Letters, 2013, 336 (2): 281-289.

[55] Wang Y, Fu Q, and Zhao W. Tetramethylpyrazine inhibits osteosarcoma cell proliferation via downregulation of NF- κ B in vitro and in vivo[J]. Molecular Medicine Reports, 2013, 8 (4): 984-988.

[56] Zhang Y, Liu X, Zuo T, et al. Tetramethylpyrazine reverses multidrug resistance in breast cancer cells through regulating the expression and function of Pglycoprotein[J]. Medical Oncology, 2012, 29 (2): 534-538.

[57] Han J, Song J, Li X et al. Ligustrazine suppresses the growth of HRPC Cells through the inhibition of cap-dependent translation via both the mTOR and the MEK/ERK pathways[J]. Anti-Cancer Agents in Medicinal Chemistry, 2015, 15 (6): 764-772.

[58] L. M. Lee, Liu CF, Yang PP. Effect of tetramethylpyrazine on lipid peroxidation in streptozotocin-induced diabetic mice[J]. The American Journal of Chinese Medicine, 2002, 30 (4): 601-608.

[59] Fu YJ, Zhou Y, Pan JQ, et al. The therapeutic effects and mechanisms of tetramethylpyrazine on streptozocin-induced-nephropathy in type 2 diabetic rats[J]. Chinese Pharmaceutical Journal, 2012, 47 (22): 1807-1812.

[60] Yang QH, Liang Y, Xu Q, et al. Protective effect of tetramethylpyrazine isolated from Ligusticum chuanxiong on nephropathy in rats with streptozotocin-induced diabetes[J]. Phytomedicine, 2011, 18 (13): 1148-1152.

[61] Liu CF, Lin CC, L. -T. Ng, et al. Hepatoprotective and therapeutic effects of tetramethylpyrazine on acute econazole-induced liver injury[J]. Planta Medica, 2002, 68 (6): 510-514.

[62] E. C. So, K. -L. Wong, Huang TC, et al. Tetramethylpyrazine protects mice against thioacetamide-induced acute hepatotoxicity[J]. Journal of Biomedical Science, 2002, 9 (5): 410-414.

[63] Lu C, Jiang Y, Zhang F, et al. Tetramethylpyrazine prevents ethanol-induced hepatocyte injury via activation of nuclear factor erythroid 2-related factor 2[J]. Life Sciences, 2015, 141: 119-127.

[64] Wang JQ, Zhang L, Tao XG, et al. Tetramethylpyrazine upregulates the aquaporin 8 expression of hepatocellular mitochondria in septic rats[J]. Journal of Surgical Research, 2013, 185 (1): 286-293.

[65] Zhang F, Zhang Z, Kong D et al. Tetramethylpyrazine reduces glucose and insulin-induced activation of hepatic stellate cells by inhibiting insulin receptor-mediated PI3K/AKT and ERK pathways[J]. Molecular and Cellular Endocrinology, 2014, 382 (1): 197-204.

[66] Wu X, Zhang F, Xiong X, et al. Tetramethylpyrazine reduces inflammation in liver fibrosis and inhibits inflammatory cytokine expression in hepatic stellate cells by modulating NLRP3 inflammasome pathway[J]. IUBMB Life, 2015, 67 (4): 312-321.

[67] B. H. Ali, M. Al-Moundhri, M. T. Eldin, et al. Amelioration of cisplatin-induced nephrotoxicity in rats by tetramethylpyrazine, a major constituent of the chinese herb ligusticum wallichi[J]. Experimental Biology and Medicine, 2008, 233 (7): 891-896.

[68] Lan Z, Bi KS, Chen XH. Ligustrazine attenuates elevated levels of indoxyl sulfate, kidney injury molecule-1 and clusterin in rats exposed to cadmium[J]. Food and Chemical Toxicology, 2014, 63: 62-68.

[69] Y. -M. Sue, Cheng CF, Chang CC, et al. Antioxidation and anti-inflammation by haemoxygenase-1 contribute to protection by tetramethylpyrazine against gentamicin-induced apoptosis in murine renal tubular cells[J]. Nephrology Dialysis Transplantation, 2009, 24 (3): 769-777.

[70] Chen JL, Zhou T, Chen WX, et al. Effect of tetramethylpyrazine on P-selectin and hepatic/renal ischemia and reperfusion injury in rats[J]. World Journal of Gastroenterology, 2003, 9 (7): 1563-1566.

[71] Yuan XP, Liu LS, Fu Q, et al. Effects of ligustrazine on ureteral obstruction-induced renal tubulointerstitial fibrosis[J]. Phytotherapy Research, 2012, 26 (5): 697-703.

[72] Li J, Yu J, Liu Y, et al. Expression of the matrix metalloproteinases and the tissue inhibitor of metalloproteinase factors are affected by tetramethylpyrazine treatment in a renal interstitial fibrosis rat model[J]. Journal of Hard Tissue Biology, 2014, 23 (3): 309-316.

[73] Cheng CY, Y. -M. Sue, Chen CH, et al. Tetramethylpyrazine attenuates adriamycin-induced apoptotic injury in rat renal tubular cells NRK-52E[J]. Planta Medica, 2006, 72 (10): 888-893.

[74] Juan SH, Chen CH, Y. -H. Hsu et al. Tetramethylpyrazine protects rat renal tubular cell apoptosis induced by gentamicin[J]. Nephrology Dialysis Transplantation, 2007, 22 (3): 732-739.

[75] Gong X, Wang Q, Tang X, et al. Tetramethylpyrazine prevents contrast-induced nephropathy by inhibiting p38 MAPK and FoxO1 signaling pathways[J]. American Journal of Nephrology, 2013, 37 (3): 199-207.

[76] Che XW, Zhang Y, Wang H, et al. Effect of ligustrazine injection on levels of interleukin-4 and interferon- γ in patients with bronchial asthma[J]. Chinese Journal of Integrative Medicine, 2008, 14 (3): 217-220.

[77] Ji NF, Xie YC, Zhang MS, et al. Ligustrazine corrects Th1/Th2 and Treg/Th17 imbalance in a mouse asthma model[J]. International Immunopharmacology, 2014, 21 (1): 76-81.

[78] Xu XY, Ye L, Chen G, et al. Effect of tetramethylpyrazine on expression of vascular cell adhesion molecule-1 in mice with ulcerative colitis[J]. China Journal of Chinese Materia Medica, 2006, 31 (19): 1608-1611.

[79] He X, Zheng Z, Yang X, et al. Tetramethylpyrazine attenuates PPAR- γ antagonist-deteriorated oxazolone-induced colitis in mice[J]. Molecular Medicine Reports, 2012, 5 (3): 645-650.

[80] Lu Y, Zhu M, Chen W, et al. Tetramethylpyrazine improves oxazolone-induced colitis by Inhibiting the NF- κ B pathway[J]. Clinical &

Investigative Medicine, 2014, 37 (1): E1-E9.

[81] Ni X, Liu S, Guo X. Medium and long-term efficacy of ligustrazine plus conventional medication on ischemic stroke: a systematic review and meta-analysis[J]. Journal of Traditional Chinese Medicine, 2013, 33 (6): 715-720.

[82] Wang B, Ni Q, Wang X, et al. Meta-analysis of the clinical effect of ligustrazine on diabetic nephropathy[J]. The American Journal of Chinese Medicine, 2012, 40 (1): 25-37.

[83] Hu JZ, Luo CY, Kang M, et al. Therapeutic effects of intraarticular injection of ligustrazine on knee osteoarthritis[J]. Journal of Central South University, 2006, 31 (4): 591-594.

[84] Wu B, Liu M, Liu H, et al. Meta-analysis of traditional Chinese patent medicine for ischemic stroke[J]. Stroke, 2007, 38 (6): 1973-1979.

[85] Shao H, Zhao L, Chen F, et al. Efficacy of ligustrazine injection as adjunctive therapy for angina pectoris: a systematic review and meta-analysis[J]. Medical Science Monitor, 2015, 21: 3704-3715.

[86] Li JS, Wang HF, Bai YP, et al. Ligustrazine injection for chronic pulmonary heart disease: a systematic review and meta-analysis[J]. Evince-Based Complementary and Alternative Medicine, 2012: 8.

[87] S. A. Jordan, D. G. Cunningham, and R. J. Marles. Assessment of herbal medicinal products: challenges, and opportunities to increase the knowledge base for safety assessment[J]. Toxicology and Applied Pharmacology, 2010, 243 (2): 198-216.

[88] Xu R, Li Y, and Huang X. Pharmacokinetic developments in ligustrazine[J]. Journal of Anhui Traditional Chinese Medicine College, 2002, 21: 58-61.

[89] C. Ligong, Y. Yili, and N. Shanqiu. Research on the mechanism of the action of tetramethylpyrazine on mesenteric capillary of rabbits[J]. Journal of Chinese Microcirculation, 1998, 1: 5.

[90] Cai W, Dong SN, Lou YQ. HPLC determination of tetramethylpyrazine in human serum and its pharmacokinetic parameters. Acta Pharmaceutica Sinica, 1989, 24 (12): 881-886.

[91] Wei L, N. Marasini, Li G, et al. Development of ligustrazine-loaded lipid emulsion: formulation optimization, characterization and biodistribution[J]. International Journal of Pharmaceutics, 2012, 437 (1-2): 203-212.

[92] Tang Z, Wang Q, Xu H, et al. Microdialysis sampling for investigations of tetramethylpyrazine following trans-dermal and intraperitoneal administration[J]. European Journal of Pharmaceutical Sciences, 2013, 50 (3-4): 454-458.

[93] Xu K, Wang P, Xu X, et al. An overview on structural modifications of ligustrazine and biological evaluation of its synthetic derivatives[J]. Research on Chemical Intermediates, 2015, 41 (3): 1385-1411.

[94] Ran X, Ma L, Peng C, et al. *Ligusticum chuanxiong* Hort: a review of chemistry and pharmacology[J]. Pharmaceutical Biology, 2011, 49 (11): 1180-1189.

[95] Li Z, Yu F, Cui L, et al. Ligustrazine derivatives. Part 8: design, synthesis, and preliminary biological evaluation of novel ligustrazinyl amides as cardiovascular agents[J]. Medicinal Chemistry, 2014, 10 (1): 81-89.

First published: ZHAO Ying-ke, LIU Yue, CHEN Ke-ji. Mechanisms and Clinical application of tetramethylpyrazine (an interesting natural compound isolated from *ligusticum wallichii*): current status and perspective[J] . Oxid Med Cell Longev, 2016, 2016: 2124638.

Expecting the Holistic Regulation from Traditional Chinese Medicine Based on the"Solar System"Hypothesis of Ischemic Heart Disease

LUO Jing, WANG An-lu, XU Hao, SHI Da-zhuo, and CHEN Ke-ji

By definition, ischemic heart disease (IHD)is caused by a mismatch between blood supply to, and demand by the heart. [1] However, it is generally accepted that coronary artery stenosis is an absolute requirement for IHD. As a result, "coronary heart disease" (CHD)has been used as a synonym for IHD.

In 1977, Andreas Grüntzig successfully performed the first percutaneous transluminal coronary angioplasty in a patient with stenosis of the left anterior descending coronary artery. [2] The strategy of revascularization has witnessed rapid evolvement, [3] and has substantially improved clinical outcomes of patients with IHD. [4] Coronary revascularization, exemplified by percutaneous coronary intervention (PCI)and coronary artery bypass grafting (CABG), has now become the mainstay in the treatment of IHD. [5]

Despite its huge success, significant challenges remain, including but not limited to myocardial reperfusion injury and 'no-reflow' phenomenon. [6,7] The most troublesome problem is restenosis: patients presenting with drug-eluting stent in-stent restenosis nearly had 19% binary restenosis rate. [8] To complicate issues further, patients with myocardial ischemia do not always have visible coronary artery stenosis (≥50%)on angiography, whereas many patients with severe coronary artery stenosis have neither angina nor evidence of myocardial ischemia. [9]

1 The"solar system"Hypothesis of IHD

The diagnosis and treatment of IHD have focused on coronary artery stenosis over the previous decades. [10] Such an emphasis is reflected by the fact that IHD is often referred to as CHD. CHD and IHD are clearly not the same identities: many studies have failed to demonstrate that all patients with coronary artery stenosis have IHD, and *vice versa*. [11,12] Moreover, many large clinical trials, such as COURAGE (Clinical Outcomes Utilizing Revascularization and Aggressive Drug Evaluation)trial (n=2, 287), FAME (Fractional Flow Reserve versus Angiography for Multivessel Evaluation)study (n=1, 005), and STICH (Surgical Treatment for Ischemic Heart Failure)trial (n=1, 212), showed that removing stenosis does not necessarily result in improvement of IHD. [13-15] The distinction between IHD and CHD was emphasized by Marzilli et al., who put forward a "solar system" hypothesis to argue that coronary artery stenosis is only one of the contributors to myocardial ischemia and treatment focusing exclusively on coronary artery stenosis is not appropriate. [16]

In Marzilli's "solar system" hypothesis, myocardial ischemia is the central issue that is in turn affected by six pathological underpinnings: coronary artery stenosis, inflammation, endothelial dysfunction, platelet dysfunction/thrombosis, microvascular dysfunction, and vasospasm. Marzilli and colleagues summarized ample evidence by showing that, despite the critical importance of coronary artery stenosis, all six pathologic features participate in the initiation and evolvement of myocardial ischemia. They argue that, when considered in isolation in the diagnosis and treatment of IHD, coronary artery stenosis does not capture the whole scenario.

2 Evidence from Traditional Chinese Medicine

On the basis of a holistic regulation and individualized medicine, traditional Chinese medicine (TCM) has been used in the real-world setting to manage a variety of diseases, including IHD, for more than two thousand years. Many clinical studies[17-20] have revealed beneficial effects of TCM in patients with IHD, including reduction of mortality, major adverse cardiac events (MACEs), and the rate of restenosis. A systematic review including 65 randomized controlled trials (RCTs)containing 12, 022 patients with myocardial infarction (MI)indicated that compared with Western medicine treatment alone, adding Chinese herbal medicine to Western medicine could further reduce all-cause mortality (relative risk reduction (RRR)0.37, 95 % confidence interval (CI)0.28 to 0.45)and cardiac mortality (RRR 0.39, 95% CI 0.22 to 0.52). A multicenter prospective observational study[18] registering 5, 284 hospitalized patients with coronary artery disease found that treatment with TCM plus Western medicine is independently associated with reduced in-hospital mortality and MACEs within 1 year (e.g., death, acute MI, PCI and CABG) (odds ratio (OR)0.69, 95% CI 0.49 to 0.97).

A Cochrane review[19] including four RCTs involving 694 patients after PCI showed that *Xiongshao* capsule (a TCM recipe)plus Western medicine produced more robust reduction in restenosis either to placebo plus Western medicine (risk ratio (RR)0.52, 95% CI 0.33 to 0.80)or Western medicine treatment alone (RR 0.41, 95% CI 0.22 to 0.75). An open-label multicenter RCT[20] including 808 patients with acute coronary syndrome after PCI showed that Chinese proprietary medicines (*Xinyue* capsule and *Fufang Chuanxiong* capsule)added to conventional treatment could further reduce the incidence of composite endpoints containing cardiac death, nonfatal recurrent MI and ischemia-driven revascularization during one year follow up (2.7% versus 6.2%, (hazard ratio (HR)0.43, 95% CI 0.21 to 0.87, P=0.015).

3 The Holistic Regulation from Traditional Chinese Medicine

A number of preclinical studies have been conducted to explore the potential mechanisms of TCM on the treatment of IHD. The following is a brief summary of the potential mechanisms, which shows the holistic regulation of TCM based on the “solar system” hypothesis of IHD.

3.1 Anti-inflammation

Inflammation is a central feature in the formation and pathologic progression of atherosclerotic plaques. [21] Zhang *et al.* [22] investigated the effect of *Tongxinluo* capsule on vascular inflammatory response and neointimal hyperplasia using a mouse carotid artery ligation model. They found that treatment with *Tongxinluo* capsule for 3 weeks dose-dependently inhibited vascular inflammation and neointimal hyperplasia. A mechanistic study[23] using miR-155$^{-/-}$mice suggested that the action is mediated by suppressing the expression of miR-155, a key player in promoting vascular inflammation and atherosclerosis, and blocking the feedback loop between miR-155 and tumor necrosis factor-α (TNF-α). A study[24] using cultured human umbilical vein endothelial cells showed that *Salvia miltiorrhiza* (a Chinese herb)inhibited TNF-α induced expression and release of vascular cell adhesion molecule (VCAM)-1 and intercellular adhesion molecule (ICAM)-1, in addition to reducing the levels of interleukin (IL)-6, IL-8 and monocyte chemoattractant protein (MCP)-1. Using a rat atherosclerotic model, Xue *et al.* [25] found that sub-chronic treatment with *Shenshao* decoction attenuated the progression of aortal atherosclerosis by inhibiting the expression of IL-1β, IL-17A, and IL-23.

3.2 Improving Endothelial Function

Endothelial cells modulate the vasomotor tone by releasing a number of vaso-active substances, such as nitric oxide (NO)and prostacyclin (PGI_2). [26] *Danhong* injection is a Chinese proprietary medicine consisting of extracts from *Salvia miltiorrhiza* and *Flos Carthami*. Wang *et al.* [27] showed that *Danhong* injection promoted endothelial-dependent dilatation of rat aorta both *in vivo* and *in vitro*, by increasing prostacyclin production (e.g., PGI_2). Fan *et al.* [28] demonstrated that Tanshinone IIA, an active lipophilic ingredient of *Salvia miltiorrhiza*, enhanced the expression of endothelial NO synthase (eNOS)and NO production, thus leading to vasodilatation. A metabonomics study[29] based on liquid chromatography-mass spectrometry analysis of urine samples found that abnormal metabolism occurred in the pathways of adenine, phenylalanine, tryptophan, porphyrin, and riboflavin in rats with endothelial dysfunction, while *Tongxinluo* capsule prevented endothelial dysfunction by restoring the above multiple metabolic pathways to their normal state.

3.3 Improving Microvascular Function

Coronary microvascular dysfunction, which may be triggered by dysfunction of endothelial cells, smooth muscle cells and the autonomic nervous system, can lead to symptoms of myocardial ischemia and affect ventricular remodeling through altering the supply of blood to the myocardium. [30] Coronary microvascular reflow is crucial for myocardial survival during ischemia and reperfusion of ischemic myocardium. In this case, coronary microvascular dysfunction often gives rise to myocardial perfusion abnormalities, which may influence the outcome of reperfusion therapies. In a study using porcine closed-chest models, Han *et al.* showed that intravenous salvianolate (exact of *salvia miltiorrhiza*)improved myocardial microvascular reflow and reduced myocardial apoptosis. [31] A study of rats with anterior descending branch of coronary artery ligated found that Tanshinone IIA had protective function on myocardial ischemia reperfusion injury through inhibiting inflammation and the increase of reactive oxygen species. [32]

3.4 Inhibiting Platelet Aggregation and Thrombosis

Both *in vitro* and *in vivo* studies[33] showed that salvianolic acids (extract of *Salvia miltiorrhiza*)and notoginsengnosides (extract of *Panax notoginseng*)inhibited platelet aggregation. Maione *et al.* [34] found that Tanshinone IIA inhibited platelet aggregation induced by reversible adenosine diphosphate stimuli in mice. A study by Lee et al. [35] assessed the effects of morusinol (extract of *Morus alba*)on the formation of thromboxane B2 and platelet aggregation *in vitro* as well as on thrombus formation using an *in vivo* thrombosis model. The results showed that morusinol inhibited arterial thrombosis by suppressing platelet aggregation and thromboxane B2 formation.

3.5 Relieving Vasospasm

Using isolated rat aortas, Koon *et al.* [36] showed that *Erigerontis herba* (a Chinese herb)caused a concentration-dependent vasorelaxation by decreasing the influx of calcium and increasing the influx of potassium. Lam *et al.* [37,38] found that both dihydrotanshinone and cryptotanshinone (active components of *Salvia miltiorrhiza*)produced vasorelaxant effect on rat coronary artery by inhibiting Ca^{2+} influx in vascular smooth muscle cells. A study by Chang et al. [39] showed that magnesium lithospermate B (extract of *Salvia miltiorrhiza)*reduced vasospasm in a rat model of subarachnoid hemorrhage through enhancing expression of eNOS and decreasing endothelin-1 level.

3.6 Improving Anoxia-tolerance and Self-healing Ability

Rhodiolarosea is a perennial flowering plant growing at high altitudes in the Arctic and mountainous regions throughout Asia and Europe. It is known for its ability to reduce fatigue, enhance work performance, and prevent high altitude sickness. [40] A recent systematic review[41] including 13 RCTs containing 1672 patients with IHD showed that *Rhodiolarosea* alone, or in combination with Western medicine, produced beneficial effects on angina symptoms and electrocardiogram. Mechanistic studies have revealed the following mechanisms underlying the cardio-protective effects of *Rhodiolarosea*: reducing hypoxia/ischemia-induced myocardial apoptosis, [42,43] decreasing ischemia-reperfusion injury, [44] and promoting angiogenesis in ischemic or anoxic myocardium. [45] Such findings suggest that *Rhodiolarosea* could enhance the tolerance of the myocardium to ischemia and promote self-healing capability.

4 Implications and Future Challenges

Revascularization is a breakthrough in the management of IHD. However, other aspects of the underlying pathophysiology have been increasingly noted in modern medicine. As a matter of fact, current practice has shifted towards a broader framework that also includes the use of pharmacotherapies to inhibit platelet aggregation and to relieve coronary spasm. Such a shift in the general attitude is reflected in both diagnosis and management of IHD.

TCM emphasizes holism. [46] Under the principles of TCM, the human being is viewed as an organic and dynamic integration of the spirit, physical body, and environment. In clinical practice, specific pathologic changes are noted, but within a larger context. Pattern identification is a critical step in the diagnosis. Individuals with identical disease (s)often present with distinct patterns, with vastly different and sometimes opposing treatment strategies. [47] Such a strategy is equivalent to individualized medicine in Western medicine. For IHD specifically, we believe that: 1)in addition to revascularization, physicians need to consider strategies of anti-inflammation, improving endothelial function and microvascular function, inhibiting platelet aggregation and thrombosis, relieving vasospasm, enhancing anoxia-tolerance and self-healing ability, 2)physicians need to evaluate the relative contribution of the above-mentioned aspects in a given patient, and tailor the treatment accordingly.

Despite increasing evidence for the benefit of TCM in prevention and treatment of IHD, we still face two major challenges. From a practical viewpoint, the level of evidence for TCM efficacy is low. Towards this end, we have made some efforts in establishing data registries to evaluate the real-world effectiveness of TCM treatments. In addition, the number of clinical trials that conform to the CONSORT statement has been increasing. At the conceptual level, the mechanisms of TCM are largely unclear.

To summarize, we believe that the "solar system" hypothesis has been increasingly implemented in the management of IHD in modern medicine despite the general lack of formal recognition. In our opinion, the "solar system" hypothesis is a metaphor of the holistic view of TCM, and a comprehensive approach should be established to treat IHD. At the theoretical level, the central features of this approach include a holistic view of disease and human subjects, as well as individualized medicine. At the practical level, this approach emphasizes anoxia-tolerance and self-healing. TCM is a complementary but promising treatment for IHD patients. There is a strong need for the two "worlds" to come together: Western medicine could tap into TCM for a more theoretical interpretation of IHD, TCM could benefit from Western medicine in clarifying specific mechanistic view of IHD as well as more solid methodologies of research.

REFERENCES

[1] Nomenclature and Criteria for Diagnosis of Ischemic Heart Disease. Report of the joint International Society and Federation of Cardiology/World Health Organization task force on standardization of clinical nomenclature[J]. Circulation, 1979, 59 (3): 607-609.

[2] Meier B, Bachmann D, Lüscher T. 25 years of coronary angioplasty: almost a fairy tal[J]. Lancet, 2003, 361 (9356): 527.

[3] Lopes RD, Leonardi S, Neely B, et al. Spontaneous MI After Non-ST-Segment Elevation Acute Coronary Syndrome Managed Without Revascularization: The TRILOGY ACS Trial[J]. J Am Coll Cardiol, 2016, 67 (11): 1289-1297.

[4] Lee PH, Lee SW, Park HS, et al. Successful Recanalization of Native Coronary Chronic Total Occlusion Is Not Associated With Improved Long-Term Survival[J]. JACC Cardiovasc Interv, 2016, 28 (9): 530-538.

[5] Osnabrugge RL, Magnuson EA, Serruys PW, et al. Cost-effectiveness of percutaneous coronary intervention versus bypass surgery from a Dutch perspective[J]. Heart, 2015, 101 (24): 1980-1988.

[6] Yellon DM and Hausenloy DJ. Myocardial reperfusion injury[J]. N Engl J Med, 2007, 357 (1): 1121-1135.

[7] Celık T, Balta S, Demır M, et al. Predictive value of admission red cell distribution width-platelet ratio for no-reflow phenomenon in acute ST segment elevation myocardial infarction undergoing primary percutaneous coronary intervention[J]. Cardiol J, 2016, 23 (1): 84-92.

[8] Alfonso F, Pérez-Vizcayno MJ, Cárdenas A, et al. A Prospective Randomized Trial of Drug-Eluting Balloons Versus Everolimus-Eluting Stents in Patients With In-Stent Restenosis of Drug-Eluting Stents: The RIBS IV Randomized Clinical Trial[J]. J Am Coll Cardiol, 2015, 66 (1): 23-33.

[9] Patel MR, Peterson ED, Dai D, et al. Low diagnostic yield of elective coronary angiography[J]. N Engl J Med, 2010, 362 (1): 886-895.

[10] Wright RS, Anderson JL, Adams CD, et al. 2011 ACCF/AHA focused update incorporated into the ACC/AHA 2007 Guidelines for the Management of Patients with Unstable Angina/Non-ST-Elevation Myocardial Infarction: a report of the American College of Cardiology Foundation/American Heart Association Task Force on Practice Guidelines developed in collaboration with the American Academy of Family Physicians, Society for Cardiovascular Angiography and Interventions, and the Society of Thoracic Surgeons[J]. J Am Coll Cardiol, 2011, 57

(19): e215-e367.

[11] Lin F, Shaw LJ, Berman DS, et al. Multidetector computed tomography coronary artery plaque predictors of stress-induced myocardial ischemia by SPECT[J]. Atherosclerosis, 2008, 197 (2): 700-709.

[12] Akasaka T. What can we expect in PCI in patients with chronic coronary artery disease. -Indication of PCI for angiographically significant coronary artery stenosis without objective evidence of myocardial ischemia (Con)[J]. Circ J, 2011, 75 (1): 211-217.

[13] Boden WE, O'Rourke RA, Teo KK, et al. Optimal medical therapy with or without PCI for stable coronary disease[J]. N Engl J Med, 2007, 356 (15): 1503-1516.

[14] Pijls NH, Fear Optimal medical therapy with or without PCI for stable coronary disease on WF, Tonino PA, et al. Fractional flow reserve versus angiography for guiding percutaneous coronary intervention in patients with multivessel coronary artery disease: 2-year follow-up of the FAME (Fractional Flow Reserve Versus Angiography for Multivessel Evaluation)study[J]. J Am Coll Cardiol, 2010, 56: 177-184.

[15] Velazquez EJ, Lee KL, Deja MA, et al. Coronary-artery bypass surgery in patients with left ventricular dysfunction[J]. N Engl J Med, 2011, 364: 1607-1616.

[16] Marzilli M, Merz CN, Boden WE, et al. Obstructive coronary atherosclerosis and ischemic heart disease: an elusive link![J]. J Am Coll Cardiol, 2012, 60 (11): 951-956.

[17] Chung VC, Chen M, Ying Q, et al. Add-on effect of chinese herbal medicine on mortality in myocardial infarction: systematic review and meta-analysis of randomized controlled trials[J]. Evid Based Complement Alternat Med, 2013, 2013: 675906.

[18] Gao ZY, Xu H, Shi DZ, et al. Analysis on outcome of 5284 patients with coronary artery disease: the role of integrative medicine[J]. J Ethnopharmacol, 2012；141 (2): 578-83.

[19] Zheng GH, Liu JP, Chu JF, et al. Xiongshao for restenosis after percutaneous coronary intervention in patients with coronary heart disease[J]. Cochrane Database Syst Rev, 2013, 31 (5): CD009581.

[20] Wang SL, Wang CL, Wang PL, et al. Combination of Chinese Herbal Medicines and Conventional Treatment versus Conventional Treatment Alone in Patients with Acute Coronary Syndrome after Percutaneous Coronary Intervention (5C Trial): An Open-Label Randomized Controlled, Multicenter Study[J]. Evid Based Complement Alternat Med, 2013, 2013: 741518.

[21] Ross R. Atherosclerosis--an inflammatory disease[J]. N Engl J Med, 1999, 340: 115-126.

[22] Zhang RN, Zheng B, Li LM, et al. Tongxinluo inhibits vascular inflammation and neointimal hyperplasia through blocking positive feedback loop between miR-155 and TNF-α[J]. Am J Physiol Heart Circ Physiol, 2014, 307: H552-H562.

[23] Nazari-Jahantigh M, Wei Y, Noels H, et al. MicroRNA-155 promotes atherosclerosis by repressing Bcl6 in macrophages[J]. J Clin Invest, 2012, 122 (1): 4190-4202.

[24] Stumpf C, Fan Q, Hintermann C, et al. Anti-inflammatory effects of danshen on human vascular endothelial cells in culture[J]. Am J Chin Med, 2013, 41 (5): 1065-1077.

[25] Xue ZW, Shang XM, Lv SH, et al. Effects of Shenshao Decoction on the inflammatory response in the aorta of a rat atherosclerotic model[J]. Chin J Integr Med, 2013, 19 (5): 347-352.

[26] Csányi G, Gajda M, Franczyk-Zarow M, et al. Functional alterations in endothelial NO, PGI and EDHF pathways in aorta in ApoE/LDLR-/- mice[J]. Prostaglandins Other Lipid Mediat, 2012, 98 (3-4): 107-115.

[27] Wang D, Fan G, Wang Y, et al. Vascular reactivity screen of Chinese medicine danhong injection identifies Danshensu as a NO-independent but PGI2-mediated relaxation factor[J]. J Cardiovasc Pharmacol, 2013, 62 (5): 457-465.

[28] Fan G, Zhu Y, Guo H, et al. Direct vasorelaxation by a novel phytoestrogen tanshinone IIA is mediated by nongenomic action of estrogen receptor through endothelial nitric oxide synthase activation and calcium mobilization[J]. J Cardiovasc Pharmacol, 2011, 57 (3): 340-347.

[29] Dai W, Wei C, Kong H, et al. Effect of the traditional Chinese medicine tongxinluo on endothelial dysfunction rats studied by using urinary metabonomics based on liquid chromatography-mass spectrometry[J]. J Pharm Biomed Anal, 2011, 56 (1): 86-92.

[30] Herrmann J, Kaski JC, Lerman A. Coronary microvascular dysfunction in the clinical setting: from mystery to reality[J]. Eur Heart J 2012, 33 (22): 2771-2782b.

[31] Han B, Zhang X, Zhang Q, et al. Protective effects of salvianolate on microvascular flow in a porcine model of myocardial ischaemia and reperfusion[J]. Arch Cardiovasc Dis, 2011, 104 (5): 313-324.

[32] Hu H, Zhai C, Qian G, et al. Protective effects of tanshinone IIA on myocardial ischemia reperfusion injury by reducing oxidative stress, HMGB1 expression, and inflammatory reaction[J]. Pharm Biol, 2015, 53: 1752-1758.

[33] Yao Y, Wu WY, Liu AH, et al. Interaction of salvianolic acids and notoginsengnosides in inhibition of ADP-induced platelet aggregation[J]. Am J Chin Med, 2008, 36 (2): 313-328.

[34] Maione F, De Feo V, Caiazzo E, et al. Tanshinone IIA, a major component of Salvia milthorriza Bunge, inhibits platelet activation via Erk-2 signaling pathway[J]. J Ethnopharmacol, 2014, 155 (2): 1236-1242.

[35] Lee JJ, Yang H, Yoo YM, et al. Morusinol extracted from Morusalba inhibits arterial thrombosis and modulates platelet activation for the treatment of cardiovascular disease[J]. J AtherosclerThromb, 2012, 19: 516-522.

[36] Koon CM, Fong S, Wat E, et al. Mechanisms of the dilator action of the ErigerontisHerba on rat aorta[J]. J Ethnopharmacol, 2014, 155 (3): 1561-1567.

[37] Lam FF, Yeung JH, Chan KM, et al. Mechanisms of the dilator action of cryptotanshinone on rat coronary artery[J]. Eur J Pharmacol 2008, 578

(2-3): 253-260.

[38] Lam FF, Yeung JH, Chan KM, et al. Dihydrotanshinone, a lipophilic component of Salvia miltiorrhiza (danshen), relaxes rat coronary artery by inhibition of calcium channels[J]. J Ethnopharmacol, 2008, 119 (2): 318-321.

[39] Chang CZ, Wu SC, Kwan AL, et al. Magnesium lithospermate B alleviates the production of endothelin-1 through an NO-dependent mechanism and reduces experimental vasospasm in rats[J]. Acta Neurochir (Wien), 2011, 153 (11): 2211-2217.

[40] Kelly GS. Rhodiolarosea: a possible plant adaptogen[J]. Altern Med Rev, 2001, 6: 293-302.

[41] Yu L, Qin Y, Wang Q, et al. The efficacy and safety of Chinese herbal medicine, Rhodiola formulation in treating ischemic heart disease: A systematic review and meta-analysis of randomized controlled trials[J]. Complement Ther Med, 2014, 22 (4): 814-825.

[42] Zhong H, Xin H, Wu LX, et al. Salidroside attenuates apoptosis in ischemic cardiomyocytes: a mechanism through a mitochondria-dependent pathway[J]. J Pharmacol Sci, 2010, 114 (4): 399-408.

[43] Zhang J, Liu A, Hou R, et al. Salidroside protects cardiomyocyte against hypoxia-induced death: a HIF-1alpha-activated and VEGF-mediated pathway[J]. Eur J Pharmacol, 2009, 607 (1-3): 6-14.

[44] Wu T, Zhou H, Jin Z, et al. Cardioprotection of salidroside from ischemia/reperfusion injury by increasing N-acetylglucosamine linkage to cellular proteins[J]. Eur J Pharmacol, 2009, 613 (1-3): 93-99.

[45] Gao XF, Shi HM, Sun T, et al. Effects of Radix et RhizomaRhodiolaeKirilowii on expressions of von Willebrand factor, hypoxia-inducible factor 1 and vascular endothelial growth factor in myocardium of rats with acute myocardial infarction[J]. Journal of Chinese Integrative Medicine, 2009, 7 (5): 434-440.

[46] Wang P, Wang Q, Yang B, et al. The Progress of Metabolomics Study in Traditional Chinese Medicine Research[J]. Am J Chin Med, 2015, 43 (7): 1281-1310.

[47] Ferreira AS, Lopes AJ. Chinese medicine pattern differentiation and its implications for clinical practice[J]. Chin J Integr Med, 2011, 17 (11): 818-823.

First published: LUO Jing, WANG An-Lu, XU Hao, SHI Da-zhuo, CHEN Ke-ji. Expecting the holistic regulation from Chinese medicine based on the "solar system" hypothesis of ischemic heart disease[J] . Chin J Integr Med, 2016, 22 (11): 805-810.

Effect of Danlou Tablet (丹蒌片)on Peri-procedural Myocardial Injury among Patients undergoing Percutaneous Coronary Intervention for Non-ST Elevation Acute Coronary Syndrome: A Study Protocol of A Multicenter, Randomized, Controlled Trial

WANG Lei, MAO Shuai, QI Jian-yong, REN Yi, GUO Xin-feng, CHEN Ke-ji, and ZHANG Min-zhou

Over the past few years, a high incidence of adverse cardiovascular events following percutaneous coronary intervention (PCI), including peri-procedural myocardial injury, received a great deal of attention in spite of major improvements in this therapy. [1]As estimated, 75, 000 to 450, 000 patients with coronary artery disease have sustained a peri-procedural myocardial injury, in which the incidence is similar to the annual rate of spontaneous myocardial infarction. Peri-procedural myocardial injury, also known as myocardial necrosis was assessed by cardiac biomarker elevation. As many retrospective observational studies found that the extent of cardiac biomarkers increase is related to subsequently adverse cardiovascular events and mortality rate. [2] Despite many strategies have been proposed to address this issue, procedural ischemic myocardial injury remains the primary complication after coronary angioplasty. [3]

Recently, many clinical trials demonstrated the efficacy of 3-hydroxy-3-methylglutaryl coenzyme-A reductase inhibitors (statins)in significant reduction of peri-procedural myocardial infarction in patients with acute coronary syndromes following coronary intervention. [4]For instance, the ARMYDA (Atorvastatin for Reduction of Myocardial Damage During Angioplasty)trial revealed that treatment with atorvastatin in statin-naive patients undergoing selective PCI for chronic stable angina was associated with a considerable decrease in the occurrence of peri-procedural myocardial injury. [5]This myocardial protection was confirmed by the ARMYDA-ACS (Atorvastatin for Reduction of Myocardial Damage During Angioplasty–Acute Coronary Syndromes)trial, in which a pre-treatment with high-dose atorvastatin 12-h prior to procedure of coronary revascularization in statin-naive patients with acute coronary syndromes undergoing early invasive strategy improved outcomes during a period of 30-day follow-up. [6]Furthermore, the ROMA (Rosuvastatin Pretreatment in Patients Undergoing Elective PCI to Reduce the Incidence of Myocardial Periprocedural Necrosis)trial established that a single, high loading dose of rosuvastatin (40 mg)within 24 h before elective PCI in patients with stable coronary artery disease could decrease the rate of post-procedural elevation of cardiac biomarkers compared with the standard treatment. [7] Nevertheless, high-dose or even super-high-dose statin pretreatment and maintenance might increase the risk of liver damage or rhabdomyolysis. [8]Therefore, numerous studies, including that presented in this paper, aim at elucidating whether such myocardial injury could be averted after administration of some natural herbs or agent that reduce the incidence of peri-procedural myocardial necrosis after non-emergency coronary angioplasty. [3]

Chinese medicine (CM)has been practiced for thousands of years and a series of studies have suggested that it bring multiple benefits to people with coronary heart disease (CHD)due to the discovery of their effectiveness in alleviating symptoms of myocardial infarction, angina pectoris, arrhythmia, hypertension and other cardiovascular conditions. [9]In particular, Danlou Tablet (丹蒌片), a Chinese patent medicine, has been successfully utilized by many cardiologists and internists for its induction of promoting blood circulation and eliminating phlegm. It consists of the following ingredients: Salvia, miltiorrhiza Bunge, Ligusticum chuanxiong

Hort, Trichosanthes kirilowii Maxim and Allium macrostemon Bunge, etc.

Moreover, recent experimental research has indicated that Danlou Tablet may reduce blood lipid level of rats with hyperlipidemia and improve vascular endothelial function in rats with arterial endothelial injury. [10] In addition, it could reduce myocardial necrosis area and promote infarct healing, prevention and treatment of early left ventricular remodeling in rats exposed to myocardial ischemia-reperfusion injury. [11]Importantly, a multicenter trial demonstrated that administration of Danlou Tablet improved clinical symptoms, inhibited the inflammation reaction of patients with CHD and decreased the frequency of major atherogenetic complications (plaque rupture and thrombosis). [12]Thus, we hypothesized that administration of Danlou Tablet may provide benefits for myocardial necrosis in patients with acute coronary syndrome (ACS)undergoing invasive surgery, which is similar to statins.

METHODS

1 Aim of the Study

The primary objective is to evaluate the major adverse cardiac clinical events (MACE)in terms of cardiac death, peri-procedural myocardial infarction (MI), spontaneous MI and target vessel revascularization (TVR). According to the literature, the peri-procedural MI was defined as a creatine kinase-MB (CK-MB)elevation＞3 upper limit of normal (ULN)value alone or associated with chest pain in patients undergoing PCI.

The secondary objective is to evaluate the efficacy of the sequential peri-PCI Danlou Tablet treatment strategy, which means pre-PCI loading doses of Danlou Tablet and post-PCI Danlou Tablet treatment for 30 days, in reducing 30-day primary cardiovascular endpoints in patients undergoing PCI with non-ST elevation acute coronary syndrome, and the rate of peri-procedural rise of myocardial biomarkers (troponin I and CK-MB and hyper sensitive C-reactive protein (hs-CRP)greater than the normal value within 8 and 24 h after PCI. In addition, the effect of Danlou Tablet treatment on the serum level of triglycerides and cholesterol, and the efficacy of peri-procedural CM therapy on clinical outcomes including quality of life and CM syndromes 3 months following surgery will also be investigated.

2 Study Design

This is a multicenter, randomized, prospective, double-blind, placebo-controlled, parallel-group study performed in 9 institutions (Guangdong Provincial Hospital of Chinese Medicine；Xiyuan Hospital of China Academy of Chinese Medical Sciences；Yueyang Hospital of Integrated Medicine of Shanghai University of Chinese Medicine；Dongfang Hospital of Beijing University of Chinese Medicine；First Affiliated Hospital of Zhejiang University of Chinese Medicine；China-Japan Friendship Hospital of Ministry of Health；Affiliated Hospital of Guangdong Medical College；First Affiliated Hospital of Henan College of Chinese Medicine；Tianjin Chest Hospital；Wuyi Hospital of Chinese Medicine of Jiangmen City). This study has been reviewed and approved by the Institutional Ethics Committee at Guangdong Provincial Hospital of Chinese Medicine (B2011-41-01)and is currently enrolled in the Chinese Clinical Trail Registry (ChiCTR- RC-12001929).All patients have to personally sign and date an informed consent document before randomization.

3 Study Population

The inclusion criteria included: patients' age greater than 18 and less that 80 years old, selective coronary angiography due to non-ST-segment elevation ACS, unstable angina or non-ST elevation (NSTE) acute myocardial infarction. Eligible patients also suffer from the Chinese medicine syndrome of intermingled phlegm and blood stasis (IPBS)based on its own theory.

According to the protocol, clinical exclusion criteria included ST-segment elevation acute myocardial infarction (STEMI); NSTE-ACS with a high risk for emergency coronary angiography; previous myocardial infarction within 30 days, cardiac shock or left ventricular ejection fraction < 30%; a history of taking any dose of statin (such as simvastatin, pravastatin, fluvastatin or rosuvastatin)during the past 2 weeks; hepatic dysfunction, active hepatic disease, or elevated of alanine aminotransferase and aspartate aminotransferase serum levels; severe renal dysfunction (serum creatinine concentration > 3 mg/dL or 264 μmol/L); myopathy or elevated creatine kinase; serious adverse reaction to Danlou Tablet or statins; malignant disease or other diseases with life expectancy < 6 months; participate in other interventional clinical trials using drugs or devices; pregnancy or lactation; the increased risk of adverse event or abnormal laboratory finding.

4 Interventions and Comparisons

Enrolled patients will be randomly allocated to indicated study group according to a computer-generated site-stratified, block randomization schedule. Eligible patients were randomized to receive placebo or Danlou Tablet (4.5 g/day for 2 consecutive days before coronary angiography, with a further 4.5 g/day for 90 days after the procedure). Simultaneously, all patients after intervention were received standard ischemic and antihypertensive therapy according to patients' conditions, such as aspirin, clopidogrel, angiotensin-converting enzyme inhibitors or β-blockers, irrespective of the initial randomization assignment. Physicians will prescribe these medicines according to the clinical guidelines. In particular, atorvastatin was unified administrated so that patients from both groups do not receive any dose of statins before the coronary angiography whereas receive atorvastatin 10 mg/day for 90 days after the procedure. Three-month clinical follow-up was scheduled in all study patients by investigators at 30 days and 3 months after the procedure. Physicians performing the procedure and the follow-up assessment were not aware of the randomization assignment.

Blood samples were collected and baseline standard biomarkers, including CK-MB and troponin I, were determined at admission time. Following the procedure, levels of CK-MB and troponin-I were assessed at 8-, 12-, and 24-h post-PCI. Levels of C-reactive protein (CRP)were also measured before PCI and at 8, 12 and 24 h after intervention. The ULN was defined as the 99th percentile of normal population with a total imprecision of 10%, according to Joint European Society of Cardiology/American College of Cardiology guidelines. CK-MB and troponin-I values were considered abnormal if > 3 ULN (0.01 ng/mL). Pre-procedural and post-procedural electrocardiograms were performed. Peri-procedural values of total and low-density lipoprotein (LDL)cholesterol were measured.

5 End Points

The primary end point of this trial was 30-day incidence of MACE: cardiac death, MI, documented unstable angina requiring revascularization (bypass surgery or repeat PCI), rehospitalization due to severe angina and heart failure for a 30-day period after randomization.

Peri-procedural myocardial infarction was defined as a post-procedural increase of CK-MB > 5 ULN, which is consistent with the consensus statement of the Joint European Society of Cardiology/American College of Cardiology Committee for the Redefinition of Myocardial Infarction for clinical trials on coronary intervention.

Secondary end points of the study were:

(1)any post-procedural changes of myocardial biomarkers (CK-MB and troponin-I)occurring within 24 h of the procedure; (2)post-procedural variations from baseline of CRP levels at 8 and 24 h after the procedure; (3)serum levels of triglycerides and cholesterol before treatment and 90 days after PCI; and (4)quality of life by Seattle Angina Scale and CM syndromes scale during 3-month follow-up; (5)proportion of patients who take a reduced dose of atorvastatin, withdraw from the study treatment, or withdraw from the study due to adverse events over 3-month follow-up. Study design is shown in Figure 1.

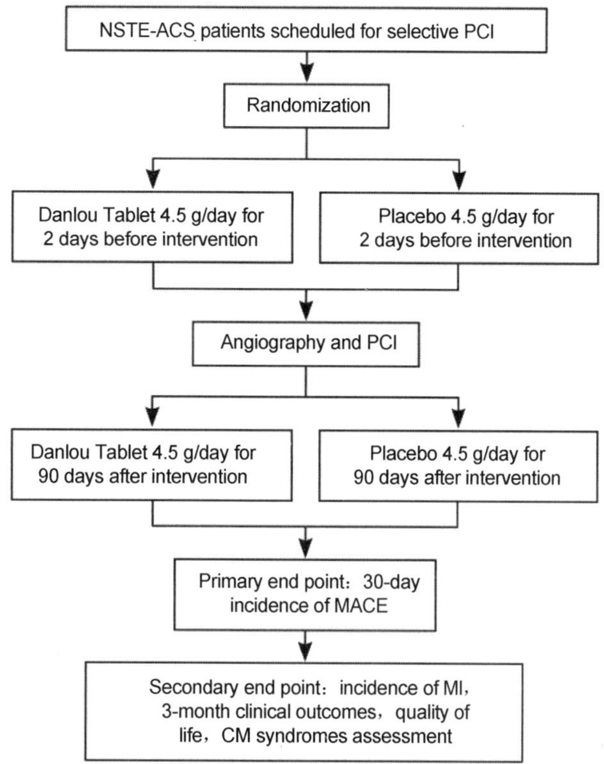

Figure 1 Study Design of Danlou Tablet for Patients with ACS undergoing PCI

Notes: CK-MB: creatine kinase-MB; hs-CRP: high sensitive C-reactive protein; MI: myocardial infarction; NSTE-ACS: non-ST-segment elevation acute coronary syndrome; PCI: percutaneous coronary intervention; TVR: target vessel revascularization.

6 Sample Size Estimation

The objective of the statistical test on the primary response is to detect a difference in the incidence of primary endpoint events between the experiment and the control groups within 30 days after PCI. In the ARMYDA-ACS trial, [6]the morbidity of MACEs in the control group without intervention of statin was around 17%. With the protocol presented in this study, it is expected that MACEs in the experiment and the control groups will be 5% and 17%, respectively. On the basis of a two-sided test size of a level of 5% and a power of 80%, it has been calculated that a minimum of 99 patients would be required for each group (total 198 patients). Allowing for 10% of patients who may withdraw from the study within 3 months after PCI, 232 eligible cases will be required.

DISCUSSION

Some impressive trials showed clinical benefit of treatment with statins in patients undergoing PCI for ACS, such as ARMYDA (Atorvastatin for Reduction of MYocardial Damage During Angioplasty, 81% risk reduction of periprocedural myocardial infarction), MIRACL (Myocardial Ischemia Reduction with Aggressive Cholesterol Lowering; 16% risk reduction), [13]A to Z (Aggrastat to Zocor; 25% risk reduction), ARMYDA-ACS (88% risk reduction)or PROVE-IT (Pravastatin or Atorvastatin Evaluation and Infection Therapy; 28% risk reduction).

However, the possible mechanisms underlying these cardio-protective effects of statin are indistinguishable Because of a longer duration of medication, this could not be attributable to cholesterol-lowering effects. [14]Experimental evidence indicates various lipid-independent and pleiotropic effects of statin treatment for instance improvement of endothelial function, [15]vasodilation of coronary microvessels, [16]and direct antithrombotic effect. Furthermore, experimental studies have demonstrated that Chinese herbs, in particular Danlou Table, have cardio-protective effects, similar to statin, in the animal model of hyperlipidemia, arterial endothelial injury and acute ischemia. [10-11,17] Despite these advances, the incidence of side-effect in treatment with statins, like rhabdomyolysis or liver damage, should not be ignored. Therefore, this study protocol has been designed to assess whether Danlou Tablet may improve clinical outcomes in patients with ACS (unstable angina or non-ST-segment elevation myocardial infarction)undergoing PCI.

Inflammation, reflected by the level of hs-CRP, contributes to the pathogenesis of coronary artery disease. [18] Myocardial necrosis is associated with an increase in inflammatory biomarkers. [19]Elevation of both pre-procedural and/or post-procedural hs-CRP is an independent predictor of a higher incidence of MACE. [20] The anti-inflammatory effects of Danlou Tablet are demonstrated in a previous clinical study, [12]suggesting that Danlou Tablet may play an important role in improving outcomes in patients with hs-CRP. Thus the assessment of hs-CRP in the current study protocol is necessary.

Furthermore, the unified statin management included in the current study protocol, i. e., neither groups receive any dose of statin before PCI and receive a usual dose of statin post PCI, was enforced in order to eliminate the confounding factor coming from statin pretreatment on the background of complying with the ethical principles. The results of this study will provide important evidence on the efficacy and safety of peri-procedural serial CM pre-treatment in patients with ACS syndrome undergoing selective PCI. Besides the 30-day primary outcomes, this study is going to evaluate the incidence of 3-month MACEs and find out whether short-term Danlou Tablet therapy could yield long-term benefit for patients undergoing PCI.

REFERENCES

[1] Nomoto K, Watanabe I, Oba T, Nagao K, Kushiro T, Hirayama A. Safety and efficacy of sirolimus-eluting stent in patients with acute coronary syndrome undergoing emergency procedure[J]. Circ J, 2008, 72: 1054-1058.

[2] Ellis SG, Chew D, Chan A, Whitlow PL, Schneider JP, Topol EJ. Death following creatine kinase-MB elevation after coronary intervention: identification of an early risk period: Importance of creatine kinase-MB level, completeness of revascularization, ventricular function, and probable benefit of statin therapy[J]. Circulation, 2002, 106: 1205-1210.

[3] Nallamothu BK, Bates ER. Periprocedural myocardial infarction and mortality: causality versus association[J]. J Am Coll Cardiol, 2003, 42: 1412-1414.

[4] Patti G, Cannon CP, Murphy SA, Mega S, Pasceri V, Briguori C, et al. Clinical benefit of statin pretreatment in patients undergoing percutaneous coronary intervention. A collaborative patient-level meta-analysis of 13 randomized study[J]. Circulation, 2011, 123: 1622-1632.

[5] Pasceri V, Patti G, Nusca A, ARMYDA Investigators. Randomized trial of atorvastatin for reduction of myocardial damage during coronary intervention: results from the ARMYDA (Atorvastatin for Reduction of Myocardial Damage During Angioplasty)study[J]. Circulation, 2004, 110: 674-678.

[6] Giuseppe P, Vincenzo P, Giuseppe C, Miglionico M, Fischetti D, Sardella G, et al. A torvastatin pretreatment improves outcomes in patients with acute coronary syndromes undergoing early percutaneous coronary intervention: results of the ARMYDA-ACS randomized trial[J]. J Am Coll Cardiol, 2007, 49: 1272-1278.

[7] Sardella G, Conti G, Donahue M, Mancone M, Canali E, De Carlo C, et al. Rosuvastatin pretreatment in patients undergoing elective PCI to reduce the incidence of myocardial periprocedural necrosis: The ROMA trial[J]. Catheter Cardiovasc Interv, 2013, 86: E36-E43.

[8] Jane A. The safety of statins in clinical practice[J]. Lancet, 2007, 370: 1781-1790.

[9] Wang L, Zhang MZ, Guo LH, Qi JY, Luo HM, He HK, et al. Clinical pathways based on integrative medicine in Chinese hospitals improve treatment outcomes for patients with acute myocardial infarction: A multi-centre, non-randomized historically controlled trial[J]. Evid Based Complement Alternat Med, 2012: ID821641.

[10] Yang Z, Hong T, Liu YM. Protection of Danlou Tablet on hyperlipidemia and vascular endothelial injury in rats[J]. World J Integr Tradit West Med (Chin), 2010, 5: 491-494.

[11] Hong M. Effects of Danlou Tablet on myocardial infarction size and ventricular remodeling in rats[J]. Chin J Exp Tradit Med Formul (Chin), 2011, 17: 208-211.

[12] Wang SH, Wang J, Li J. Efficacy assessment of treating patients with coronary heart disease angina of phlegm and stasis mutual obstruction syndrome by Danlou Tablet[J]. Chin J Integr Tradit West Med (Chin), 2012, 32: 1051-1055.

[13] Di Sciascio G, Patti G, Pasceri V, Gaspardone, A, colonna G, Montinaro A. Efficacy of atorvastatin reload in patients on chronic statin therapy

undergoing percutaneous coronary intervention: results of the ARMYDA-RECAPTURE (Atorvastatin for Reduction of Myocardial Damage During Angioplasty)Randomized Trial[J]. J Am Coll Cardiol, 2009, 54: 558-565.

[14] Ray KK, Cannon CP. Early time to benefit with intensive statin treatment: could it be the pleiotropic effects[J]. Am J Cardiol, 2005, 96: 54F-60F.

[15] Wassmann S, Faul A, Hennen B, Scheller B, Böhm M, Nickenig G. Rapid effect of 3-hydroxy-3-methylglutaryl coenzyme A reductase inhibition on coronary endothelial function[J]. Circ Res, 2003, 93: e98-e103.

[16] Hinoi T, Matsuo S, Tadehara F, Tsujiyama S, Yamakido M. Acute effect of atorvastatin on coronary circulation measured by transthoracic Doppler echocardiography in patients without coronary artery disease by angiography[J]. Am J Cardiol, 2005, 96: 89-91.

[17] Fu J, Hong M, Leng JY, Huang HL, Huang YP. The protective effects of Danlou Tablet on the rat model of acute ischemia induced by isoproterenol[J]. Chin J Gerontol (Chin), 2011, 31: 1204-1207.

[18] Hansson GK. Mechanisms of disease: Inflammation, atherosclerosis, and coronary artery disease[J]. N Engl J Med, 2005, 352: 1685-1695.

[19] Versaci F, Gaspardone A, Tomai F, Crea F, Chiariello L, Gioffrè PA. Predictive value of C-reactive protein in patients with unstable angina pectoris undergoing coronary artery stent implantation[J]. Am J Cardiol, 2000, 85: 92-95.

[20] Delhaye C, Sudre A, Lemesle G, Maréchaux S, Broucqsault D, Hennache B, et al. Preprocedural high-sensitivity C-reactive protein predicts death or myocardial infarction but not target vessel revascularization or stent thrombosis after percutaneous coronary intervention[J]. Cardiovasc Revasc Med, 2009, 10: 144-150.

First published: WANG Lei, MAO Shuai, QI Jian-yong, REN Yi, GUO Xin-feng, CHEN Ke-ji, ZHANG Min-zhou. Effect of Danlou Tablet on peri-procedural myocardial injury among patients undergoing percutaneous coronary intervention for non-ST elevation acute coronary syndrome: a study protocol of a multicenter, randomized, controlled trial[J]. Chin J Integr Med, 2015, 21 (9): 662-666.

The Effect of Xuefuzhuyu Oral Liquid on Aspirin Resistance and its Association with rs5911, rs5787 and rs3842788 Gene Polymorphisms

XUE Mei, YANG Lin, KOU Na, MIAO Yu, WANG Ming-ming, ZHAO Quan-li, REN Jun-hua, ZHANG Shao-yan, SHI Da-zhuo, and CHEN Ke-ji

Platelet activation and aggregation have a pivotal role in the thrombotic complications that occur in patients undergoing percutaneous coronary intervention (PCI)[1]. Aspirin and clopidogrel (dual)anti-platelet therapy is recommended by the guidelines for the prevention of ischemic complications after PCI [2,3]. However, bleeding events limit their clinical application. It is also recommended in the guidelines that if the risk of morbidity from bleeding outweighs the anti-platelet benefit of a recommended duration of P2Y12 inhibitor therapy after stent implantation, earlier discontinuation ($<$ 12 months)of P2Y12 inhibitor therapy is reasonable [4]. After PCI, aspirin administration should be continued indefinitely at a low dose. However, some patients still experience cardiovascular events despite its regular intake, a phenomenon which is known as aspirin resistance (AR)[5].

Gene polymorphisms can affect individual drug response. Detecting genetic variation may help to predict a patient's response to drugs and could be used as a tool to optimize therapy strategy, tailor dosage regimens, and improve clinical outcomes [6]. A number of studies have examined the association of AR with single nucleotide polymorphisms (SNPs)in the genes for COX-1 and for several receptors on the surface of platelets [7-9]. Maree reported COX-1 haplotypes [A-842G, C22T (R8W), G128A (Q41Q), C644A (G213G)and C714A (L237M)] were significantly associated with aspirin response determined by AA-induced platelet aggregation (P = 0.004； 4 d. f.) in patients (n = 144)with stable coronary heart disease (CHD)from Ireland [7]. Platelet glycoprotein (GP)IIb/IIIa receptors play an inevitable role in platelet aggregation[10]. Pamukcu reported that GP IIIa (PlA)polymorphism is related to aspirin resistance in Turkish patients with intracoronary stent restenosis, while our previous study has shown that there are only PlA1, A1 alleles of GP IIIa in 212 CHD patients and 39 healthy volunteers in the Chinese Han population [11,12]. Therefore, it is important to find specific genetic markers for different ethnic groups.

Traditional Chinese medicines exhibiting good anti-platelet effects are the most commonly used drugs for patients after interventional therapy for activating blood circulation to remove blood stasis [13]. Xuefuzhuyu oral liquid, derived from the classic recipe Xuefuzhuyu decoction, can effectively inhibit platelet activation and reduce platelet aggregation and showed good effects in the clinical treatment of CHD [12]. But it still remains unknown whether Xuefuzhuyu oral liquid could relieve AR in patients after interventional therapy, and if there are some specific gene polymorphisms related to the drug response. Therefore a control randomized study was designed to investigate the effects of Xuefuzhuyu oral liquid on AR in patients with chronic stable angina after PCI and the possible associated genetic markers for the drug response.

MATERIALS AND METHODS

1 Patients

Patients were recruited from Xiyuan hospital, China Academy of Chinese Medical Sciences from March 2012 to November 2014. The protocol was approved by the institutional Ethics Committee of China Academy of Chinese Medical Sciences, and all patients gave written informed consent. Trial registration number: Chinese Clinical Trial Register: ChiCTR-TRC-12002416.

2 Diagnostic Criteria

Chronic stable angina patients with coronary angiography showed stenosis ≥ 50% in at least one coronary artery or previous myocardial infarction[14]. Classification of CHD syndrome referred to the "Criterion of Syndrome Differentiation for CHD" by Cardiovascular Specialty Committee, China Association of Integrative Medicine [15]. Stasis syndrome differentiation and scores were made according to the "diagnostic criteria of blood stasis syndrome (BSS)" [17].

3 Inclusion and Exclusion Criteria

Inclusion criteria included (1)stable angina patients after post-revascularization or myocardial infarction, (2)35 years old ≤ age ≤ 75 years old, (3)taking aspirin for more than 7 days, and (4)aspirin resistance: ①platelet aggregation rate ≥ 70% when diphosphate adenosine (ADP, 10 μM)induced; ②platelet aggregation rate ≥ 20% when arachidonic acid (AA, 0.5 mg/ml)induced, complied with one of them is defined as aspirin semi-resistance. Exclusion criteria included (1)family or personal history of bleeding disorders, (2)platelet count $< 100 \times 10^9$/L, or $> 450 \times 10^9$/L, (3)hemoglobin < 90 g/L, (4)taking other anti-platelet, anticoagulant drugs or non-steroidal anti-inflammatory drugs, (5)taking other herbs besides Xuefuzhuyu oral liquid which are activating blood circulation to remove blood stasis within the latest two weeks, (6)history of trauma or surgery in the latest two weeks, (7)severe primary diseases like renal insufficiency, liver dysfunction, hematopoietic system diseases, mental disorder or malignant tumor, and (8)female in pregnancy or lactation period.

4 Clinical Design and Treatment Procedure

The enrolled aspirin resistance or semi-resistance patients were randomly divided into control and treatment groups using a randomized block design. Conventional western medicine treatment and aspirin (75 mg)once daily were used in the control group, while Xuefuzhuyu oral liquid (10 ml, three times per day) was added in the treatment group for four consecutive weeks. The enrolled patients should not take anti-platelet, anticoagulant drugs, non-steroidal anti-inflammatory drugs, and any other herbs activating blood circulation to remove blood stasis besides Xuefuzhuyu oral liquid during the research period. Biochemical indicators of liver and kidney function, platelet aggregation rate and BSS scores were detected before and after treatment. Xuefuzhuyu oral liquid (national medicine permit No. Z10950063, batch No. 1211010)was kindly provided by Jilin Aodong Yanbian Pharmaceutical Co., Ltd (Jilin, China).

5 Platelet Aggregation Studies

Platelet aggregation rate was determined among different patients groups using turbidimetry (Platelet Aggregation Instrument, LBYNJ2, Beijing Lipusheng Co., China). The inducer of platelet aggregation was ADP (10 μM, Chrono-log Co., Havertown, USA)and AA (0.5 mg/ml, Chrono-log Co., Havertown, USA).

6 DNA Preparation and Genotyping

Genomic DNA was isolated from whole blood using a Wizard® Genomic DNA Purification Kit (Promega Co., USA)in accordance with the manufacturer's instructions as previously described [17]. Patients were genotyped for three single nucleotide polymorphisms in COX-1 (rs5787, rs3842788)and GPIIb (rs5911) (Table 1). Genotyping was performed using Taqman probe technique (rs5787 and rs5911)and gene sequencing technology (rs3842788)on an ABI PRISM 7900 HT Fast Real-time instrument (Applied Biosystems, Foster City, CA)and an ABI PRISM 3730 DNA Sequencer (Applied Biosystems, Foster City, CA, USA)respectively as has previously been described [12,17].

Table 1 COX–1 and GPIIb single nucleotide polymorphisms

	Region	Contig position	mRNA position	dbSNP rs# cluster id	RefSNP allele	Protein residue	Codon position	Amino acid position
COX-1	exon_4	32462028	458	rs5787	G	Arg [R]	2	108
					A	Gln [Q]	2	108
	exon_3	32461411	258	rs3842788	A	Gln [Q]	3	41
					G	Gln [Q]	3	41
GPIIb	exon_26	1106870	2653	rs5911	A	Ile [I]	2	874
					C	Ser [S]	2	874

Notes: dbSNP: single nucleotide polymorphism database, RefSNP: reference single nucleotide polymorphism.

7 Statistical Analysis

Continuous variables were expressed as means ± standard deviation (SD). One-way analysis of variance (ANOVA)was carried out for the comparison of means. Categorical data were described by frequency tables, percentage, or constituent ratio and analyzed by Chi-square test. All statistical analysis was performed with SPSS version 13.0, and *P* value of less than 0.05 was considered statistically significant.

RESULTS

1 General Clinical Characteristics

43 patients diagnosed as having aspirin resistance or semi- resistance were randomly divided into control and treatment groups after screening 207 stable CHD patients, and there were no significant adverse reactions occurring before and after treatment. There was no statistical difference between the two groups in age, sex and body mass index ($P>0.05$). The risk factors (myocardial infarction, hypertension, dyslipidemia and diabetes history)and statins medication history was comparable between the two groups ($P>0.05$) (Table 2). All the patients enrolled carried only the G/G allele in both rs5787 and rs3842788 gene polymorphisms. The C haplotype of rs5911 was carried by 76.2% and 72.7% of patients in the two groups respectively without significant difference ($P>0.05$).

Table 2 Baseline Characteristics of Study Participants

	Control group (*n* = 21)	Treatment group (*n* = 22)
Age, y	62.8 ± 6.3	67.0 ± 8.1
Male sex, *n* (%)	6 (28.6)	10 (45.5)
Body mass index, kg/m^2	24.7 ± 2.9	26.9 ± 6.1
Statins, *n* (%)	15 (71.4)	15 (68.2)
Myocardial infarction history, *n* (%)	3 (14.3)	5 (22.7)
Hypertension, *n* (%)	14 (66.7)	18 (81.8)
Dyslipidemia, *n* (%)	16 (76.2)	16 (72.2)
Diabetes, *n* (%)	10 (47.6)	11 (50)
rs5787 GG, *n* (%)	21 (100)	22 (100)
rs5911 AA/ (AC+CC)	5/16	6/16
rs3842788 GG, *n* (%)	21 (100)	22 (100)

2 Improvement of Aspirin Resistance Before and After Treatment

90.5% of patients retained aspirin resistance or aspirin semi-resistance in the control group after conventional western medicine treatment, while only 18.2% retained resistance in the treatment group after combination therapy with Xuefuzhuyu oral liquid ($P < 0.01$) (Table 3).

Table 3 Improvement of Aspirin Resistance Before and After Treatment

	aspirin resistance/aspirin semi-resistance	
	Before Treatment *n* (%)	After Treatment *n* (%)
Control group	21 (100)	19 (90.5)
Treatment group	22 (100)	4 (18.2)$^{**\wedge\wedge}$

Notes: $^{**}P < 0.01$, compared with the control group ; $^{\wedge\wedge}P < 0.01$, compared with before treatment.

3 Comparison of BSS Patients and BSS Scores between Groups

There were 12 patients (57.1%)and 18 patients (81.8%)with BSS respectively in the control and treatment groups with no statistical difference ($P > 0.05$) (Table 4). The BSS scores in the treatment group were reduced significantly after combination therapy with Xuefuzhuyu oral liquid compared to the control group, which indicated that Xuefuzhuyu oral liquid could reduce the degree of blood stasis in patients.

Table 4 Comparison of BSS Patients and BSS Scores between Groups

	BSS Patientsn (%)	Non-BSS Patientsn (%)	BSS Scores	
			Before Treatment	After Treatment
Control group	12 (57.1)	9 (42.9)	20.25 ± 5.59	19.92 ± 4.81
Treatment group	18 (81.8)	4 (18.2)	21.11 ± 3.38	13.5 ± 3.36$^{*\wedge}$

Notes: $^{*}P < 0.05$, compared with the control group ; $^{\wedge}P < 0.05$, compared with before treatment.

4 Correlation between Gene Polymorphism and the Effects of Xuefuzhuyu Oral Liquid on AR

ADP-induced platelet aggregation was significantly lower ($P < 0.05$, $P < 0.01$)after treatment in combination with Xuefuzhuyu oral liquid, no matter what kind of genotypes (A/A or A/C+C/C)the patients had, while AA-induced platelet aggregation provoked no significant change (Table 5), which indicated that Xuefuzhuyu oral liquid improves aspirin resistance by inhibiting ADP-induced platelet aggregation.

Table 5 Effect of rs5911 Genotyping on the Effects of Xuefuzhuyu Oral Liquid

rs5911 Genotyping	Group	*n*	ADP-induced Platelet Aggregation Rate	AA-induced Platelet Aggregation Rate
A/A	Before Treatment	6	77.06 ± 6.48	12.21 ± 7.17
	After Treatment	6	63.65 ± 4.27**	11.48 ± 4.73
A/C+C/C	Before Treatment	16	72.09 ± 14.20	16.38 ± 7.18
	After Treatment	16	60.88 ± 13.37*	14.03 ± 3.32

Notes: $^{*}P < 0.05$, $^{**}P < 0.01$, compared with before treatment.

5 Comparison of BSS Scores in Patients with Different Genotypes Before and After Treatment

After treatment in combination with Xuefuzhuyu oral liquid, BSS scores decreased significantly in patients with A/C or C/C genotype, which illustrated that patients carrying the C allele were more responsive to the improvement of blood stasis symptoms and more sensitive to the treatment of Xuefuzhuyu oral liquid.

Table 6 Comparison of BSS Scores in Patients with Different Genotypes Before and After Treatment

rs5911 Genotyping	Group	*n*	BSS Scores
A/A	Before Treatment	8	19.88 ± 3.23
	After Treatment	8	15.75 ± 3.65
A/C+ C/C	Before Treatment	22	21.09 ± 4.69
	After Treatment	22	16.18 ± 5.56**

Notes: * $P < 0.05$, ** $P < 0.01$, compared with before treatment.

DISCUSSION

An aspirin maintenance dose should be continued indefinitely in patients after interventional therapy, and it was reported that aspirin could reduce serious vascular events by 25% in patients with high risk conditions [18]. However, its effectiveness is limited because 10% to 40% of patients with arterial thrombosis who are treated with aspirin have recurrent vascular events during long-term follow-up [19]. Eikelboom reported that AR patients, defined as failure of suppression of thromboxane generation, had a 2-times-higher risk of myocardial infarction and a 3.5-times-higher risk of cardiovascular death than those with low expression of thromboxane[20]. It has been suggested that higher doses of aspirin or dual antiplatelet therapy may be required in AR patients to achieve the optimal antithrombotic effect[21]. However, bleeding and upper gastrointestinal damage have been serious complications of this therapeutic strategy with high morbidity and mortality[22,23]. Therefore, it is urgent to find novel effective and safe antiplatelet agents, which provides a great opportunity for traditional Chinese medicine with multi-target effects.

Xuefuzhuyu oral liquid, derived from the classic recipe Xuefuzhuyu decoction, has been well documented to inhibit platelet aggregation and to improve hemorheology [13]. In the present study, 43 enrolled patients with chronic stable angina after PCI exhibing aspirin resistance or semi-resistance were randomly divided into control and treatment groups using a randomized block design. Only 18.2% of patients retained AR or ASR in the treatment group after combination therapy with Xuefuzhuyu oral liquid, while 90.5% retained resistance in the control group, which illustrated that Xuefuzhuyu oral liquid could effectively improve AR in patients with chronic stable angina after PCI. The BSS scores in the treatment group were reduced significantly after combination therapy with Xuefuzhuyu oral liquid compared to the control group, which indicated that Xuefuzhuyu oral liquid could reduce the degree of blood stasis in patients. Aspirin exerts its major antithrombotic effect by irreversibly acetylating platelet cyclo-oxygenase-1 (COX-1). One of the possible explanations for AR is that platelets can be activated by pathways that are not blocked by aspirin [20]. ADP-induced platelet aggregation was significantly lower after treatment in combination with Xuefuzhuyu oral liquid, while AA-induced platelet aggregation provoked no significant change, which demonstrated that Xuefuzhuyu oral liquid improves AR by inhibiting ADP-induced platelet aggregation.

Many researches are currently focusing on identifying variants of genes that affect drug response. Because aspirin exhibited anti-platelet aggregation effects by irreversible inhibition of COX-1, polymorphisms of the COX-1 gene are in the focus of many researches, but the role of COX-1 SNPs in the mechanism of AR have not been fully elucidated. Rs3842788 has been shown to be significantly associated with aspirin response determined by AA-induced platelet aggregation and serum TXB2 generation in Irish patients with cardiovascular disease, while Xu ZH et al. reported that the mutation of rs3842788 (4.44% mutant)was not related to AR in patients accepting aspirin treatment in China [7,24]. An in vitro study proved rs5787 variants exerts the largest functional effects on decreasing the antiplatelet effectiveness of aspirin among four SNPs, with evidence for impaired interactions with a COX substrate and inhibitors[25]. In our present study, no variants of rs5787 and rs3842788 were detected among 207 stable CHD patients enrolled, and because the mutations of rs5787 and rs3842788 were very uncommon, they were not suitable as representative gene polymorphisms for AR in the Chinese population. The GPIIb/IIIa receptor is critical in the process of thrombus formation since it serves as the final common pathway for platelet aggregation[26]. Several polymorphisms of the GP IIb/IIIa receptor have been identified in the general population. As compared to rs5911 C/C homozygotes, individuals with the rs5911 A/C genotype showed significantly increased inhibition of platelet aggregation in healthy Chinese male volunteers. In the present study, BSS scores decreased significantly in patients with A/C or C/C genotype after treatment with Xuefuzhuyu oral liquid, which showed that patients carrying the C allele were more responsive to the improvement of blood stasis symptoms and more sensitive to the treatment of Xuefuzhuyu oral liquid.

Therefore, Xuefuzhuyu oral liquid therapy in addition to aspirin administration for the treatment of chronic stable angina patients after PCI leads to greater protection from AR, and the patients with the rs5911 variants of GPIIb exhibited better drug response upon treatment with Xuefuzhuyu oral liquid. More rigorous randomized controlled trials are necessary to provide clinicians with evidence regarding the use of Xuefuzhuyu oral liquid in the treatment of AR.

REFERENCES

[1] Sweeny JM, Gorog DA, Fuster V, et al. Antiplatelet drug ‘resistance’ . Part 1: mechanisms and clinical measurements[J]. Nat Rev Cardiol, 2009, 6 (4): 273-282, 2009.

[2] Yusuf S, Zhao F, Mehta SR, et al. Effects of clopidogrel in addition to aspirin in patients with acute coronary syndromes without ST-segment elevation[J]. N Engl J Med, 2001, 345 (7): 494-502.

[3] Steinhubl SR, Berger PB, 3rd Mann IT, et al. Early and sustained dual oral antiplatelet therapy following percutaneous coronary intervention: a randomized controlled trial[J]. JAMA, 2001, 288 (19): 2411-2420.

[4] Amsterdam EA, WengerNK, Brindis RG, et al. 2014 AHA/ACC guideline for the management of patients with non-ST-elevation acute coronary syndromes: executive summary: a report of the American College of Cardiology/American Heart Association Task Force on Practice Guidelines[J]. Circulation, 2014, 130 (25): 2354-2394.

[5] Szczeklik A, Musiał J, Undas A, et al. Aspirin resistance[J]. J Thromb Haemost, 2005, 3 (8): 1655-1662.

[6] Cambria-Kiely JA, Gandhi PJ. Aspirin resistance and genetic polymorphisms[J]. J Thromb Thrombolysis, 2002, 14 (1): 51-58.

[7] Maree AO, Curtin RJ, Chubb A, et al. Cyclooxygenase-1 haplotype modulates platelet response to aspirin[J]. J Thromb Haemost, 2005, 3 (10): 2340-2345.

[8] Xu ZH, Jiao JR, Yang R, et al. Aspirin resistance: clinical significance and genetic polymorphism[J]. J Int Med Res, 2012, 40 (1): 282-292.

[9] Li XL, Cao J, Fan L, et al. Genetic polymorphisms of HO-1 and COX-1 are associated with aspirin resistance defined by light transmittance aggregation in Chinese Han patients[J]. Clin Appl Thromb Hemost, 2013, 19 (5): 513-521.

[10] Papp E, Havasi V, Bene J, et al. Glycoprotein IIIA gene (PlA)polymorphism and aspirin resistance: is there any correlation? ” Ann Pharmacother, 2015, 39 (6): 1013-1018.

[11] Pamukcu B, Oflaz H, Nisanci Y. The role of platelet glycoprotein IIIa polymorphism in the high prevalence of in vitro aspirin resistance in patients with intracoronary stent restenosis[J]. Am Heart J, 2005, 149 (4): 675-680.

[12] Xue M, Chen KJ, Yin HJ. Relationship between polymorphism of platelet membrane glycoprotein IIIa and coronary heart disease with blood-stasis syndrome in Chinese Han population[J]. Zhong Xi Yi Jie He Xue Bao, 2009, 7 (4): 325-329.

[13] Liao F. Herbs of activating blood circulation to remove blood stasis[J]. Clin Hemorheol Microcirc, 2000, 23 (2-4): 127-131.

[14] Chinese Society of Cardiology. Guidelines for the diagnosis and management of patients with chronic stable angina[J]. Chin J Cardiol, 2007, 35 (3): 159-206.

[15] Cardiovascular Specialty Committee and China Association of Integrative Medicine. Criterion of syndrome differentiation for CHD[J]. Zhong Guo Zhong Xi Yi Jie He Za Zhi, 1991, (11): 257.

[16] Wang J. Study on diagnostic criteria of blood stasis syndrome[J]. Beijing: United Publishing House of Beijing Medical University and Chinese Union Medical University, 1993.

[17] Xue M, Chen KJ, Yin HJ. Association between platelet membrane glycoprotein IIb polymorphism and coronary heart disease in Han people[J]. Zhong Guo Bing Li Sheng Li Za Zhi, 2009, 25 (10): 1898-1902.

[18] Antithrombotic Trialists' Collaboration. Collaborative meta-analysis of randomised trials of antiplatelet therapy for prevention of death, myocardial infarction, and stroke in high risk patients[J]. BMJ, 2002, 324 (7329): 71-86.

[19] Patrono C, Coller B, Dalen JE, et al. Platelet-active drugs: the relationships among dose, effectiveness, and side effects[J]. Chest, 2001, 119 (1 Suppl): 39S-63S.

[20] Eikelboom JW, Hirsh J, Weitz JI, et al. Aspirin resistant thromboxane biosythesis and the risk of myocardial infarction, stroke, or cardiovascular

death in patients at high risk for cardiovascular events[J]. Circulation, 2002, 105 (14): 1650-1655.

[21] Petreñas Cañivano L, Yubero García C. Resistance to aspirin: prevalence, mechanisms of action and association with thromboembolic events. A narrative review[J]. Farm Hosp, 2010, 34 (1): 32-43.

[22] Hennekens CH, Sechenova O, Hollar D, et al. Dose of aspirin in the treatment and prevention of cardiovascular disease: current and future directions[J]. J Cardiovasc Pharmacol Ther, 2006, 11 (3): 170-176.

[23] Mehran R, Baber U, Steg PG, et al. Cessation of dual antiplatelet treatment and cardiac events after percutaneous coronary intervention (PARIS): 2 year results from a prospective observational study[J]. Lancet, 2013, 382 (9906): 1714-1722.

[24] Xu ZH, Jiao JR, Yang R, et al. Aspirin resistance: clinical significance and genetic polymorphism[J]. J Int Med Res, 2012, 40 (1): 282-292.

[25] Liu W, Poole EM, Ulrich CM, et al. Decreased cyclooxygenase inhibition by aspirin in polymorphic variants of human prostaglandin H synthase-1[J]. Pharmacogenet Genomics, 2012, 22 (7): 525-537.

[26] Vita De M, Coluccia V, Burzotta F, et al. Intracoronary use of GP IIb/IIIa inhibitors in percutaneous coronary interventions[J]. Curr Vasc Pharmacol, 2012, 10 (4): 448-453.

[27] Li MP, Xiong Y, Xu A, et al. Association of platelet ITGA2B and ITGB3 polymorphisms with ex vivo antiplatelet effect of ticagrelor in healthy Chinese male subjects[J]. Int J Hematol, 2014, 99 (3): 263-271.

First published: YANG Lin, KOU Na, MIAO Yu, WANG Ming-ming, ZHAO Quan-li, REN Jun-hua, ZHANG Shao-yan, SHI Da-zhuo, and CHEN Ke-ji. The Effect of Xuefuzhuyu Oral Liquid on aspirin resistance and its association with rs5911, rs5787, and rs3842788 gene polymorphisms [J]. Evid Based Complement Alternat Med, 2015, 2015: 507349.

Oral Chinese Proprietary Medicine for Angina Pectoris: an Overview of Systematic Reviews/Meta-analyses

LUO Jing, XU Hao, YANG Guo-yan, QIU Yu, LIU Jian-ping, and CHEN Ke-ji

In the hierarchy of evidence-based medicine, systematic reviews/meta-analyses of high quality randomized controlled trials (RCTs)are considered as golden standard for health care intervention evidence, which can help clinicians, patients, and policy/guideline makers to make rational decisions about health care [1,2]. With the introduction of evidence-based medicine in the field of traditional Chinese medicine (TCM), the number of TCM systematic reviews/meta-analyses grows dramatically [3].

Angina pectoris, defining as cardiac-induced pain, is triggered by decreased myocardial oxygen supply or increased myocardial oxygen demand, and is a common type of coronary heart disease (CHD)[4]. It occurs when coronary arteries are narrowed or blocked by hardening of the arteries (atherosclerosis), by spasm, or by a blood clot. In 2009, approximately 94.9 of every 100 thousand urban residents died of CHD in China [5], and nearly one of every six deaths was attributable to CHD in the United States [6]. Individuals with angina pectoris may have an increased risk of subsequent acute fatal cardiovascular events. Recently, an estimated 10.2 million Americans experience angina pectoris, with approximately 500, 000 new cases occurring each year.

Chinese proprietary medicine (CPM), also known as Chinese patent medicine, is a common type of drugs in TCM nowadays. There have been 520 kinds of CPM (one CPM may involves more than one kind of preparation but based on the same Chinese medicine formula)approved in China since 2012 [7]. Moreover, many kinds of oral CPM such as Compound Danshen dropping pill and Tong Xin Luo capsule have been widely used for angina in China so far. A systematic review published in International Journal of Cardiology in 2012 [8] indicated that Compound Danshen dropping pill was more effective than isosorbide dinitrate in treating angina. Similar effectiveness of another oral CPM (Xin Xue Kang capsule)was found by a recent meta-analysis [9]. However, a previous systematic review [10] showed that herbal medicinal products were associated with cardiovascular adverse effects. What's more, two literature reviews[3,11] reported that most TCM systematic reviews published in Chinese journals had serious methodological and reporting flaws, which limited the quality of evidence. Although use of oral CPM is popular for the treatment of angina and many relevant systematic reviews/meta-analyses are available, evidence from these reviews haven't been summarized and evaluated before recommendation and application. This overview aims to investigate the general characteristics, methodological quality and reporting characteristics of systematic reviews/meta-analyses on oral CPM in treating angina pectoris.

MATERIALS AND METHODS

The protocol of this overview was documented in PROSPERO International Prospective Register of Systematic Reviews (ID=CRD42013004468)[12].

1 Source of Literature and Search Strategy

We searched the following databases from their inception until March 2013: The Cochrane Library, Pubmed, Embase, Chinese Biomedical Database (CBM), Chinese VIP Information (VIP), China National Knowledge Infrastructure (CNKI) (including academic journals, dissertation and conference proceedings), and

Wanfang Database (including academic journals, dissertation and conference proceedings). Search strategies used in English electronic databases were listed in Appendix 1, and were adapted for Chinese electronic databases with appropriate Chinese terms.

In addition, we screened the reference lists of retrieved review articles to identify missing systematic reviews/meta-analyses.

2 Inclusion and Exclusion Criteria

We included systematic reviews and meta-analyses reporting oral CPM as intervention for the treatment of any kind of angina pectoris, irrespective of language and publishing status. The CPM was limited to orally taken. If systematic reviews or meta-analyses assessed oral CPM and other preparations of the same Chinese medicine (s), they were also included. All types of control were considered. CPM was identified by *Clinical Guide of the Chinese Pharmacopeia: Traditional Chinese Medicine* [13], *Pharmacopoeia of the People's Republic of China 2010* [14], and the China Food and Drug Administration website data query system [7].

Articles were excluded if they were published as abstracts or protocols, or if the interventions focused on a broad concept of TCM (e.g., different Chinese medications or TCM treatment methods/principles), of which the objectives were irrelevant to oral CPM).

3 Data Collection And analysis

3.1 Study Selection

Two authors (Luo J and Yang GY)independently screened the titles and abstracts of citations for potentially relevant systematic reviews/meta-analyses. Full texts of potentially eligible articles were retrieved for further assessment according to the inclusion and exclusion criteria. Any disagreement was resolved by discussion or by consulting a third author (Liu JP).

3.2 Data Extraction and Management

Two authors (Luo J and Xu H)independently extracted data from each included review in accordance with a self-developed data extraction form using Excel (version Microsoft Excel 2007), and data were validated by a third author (Liu JP). Disagreements were resolved by consensus. Extracted data items included study design included, the number of trials included, types of comparisons, outcomes, author's conclusions, etc.

According to the "Outcomes Research in Cardiovascular Disease Report" of National Heart, Lung, and Blood Institute (NHLBI)Working Group[15], we categorized the outcomes into the following types: 1)endpoints: including all-cause mortality, cardiac mortality, and acute cardiovascular events such as nonfatal myocardial infarction and coronary revascularization; 2)quality of life (QOL): including health-related and generic QOL; 3) symptoms: improvement of symptoms including reduction of angina frequency and/or persistence time, decrease of consumption of nitroglycerine, etc. ; 4)surrogate outcomes: changes in clinical risk, such as improvement of electrocardiogram (ECG)and serum markers; 5)adverse events; and 6)economic evaluations.

For author's conclusion describing the overall effectiveness of the interventions, we categorized them into the following types: (A)the oral CPM was effective; (B)reliable conclusions could not be drawn due to limited methodological quality of evidence; (C)reliable conclusions could not be drawn due to insufficient evidence; (D) the oral CPM was ineffective or harmful, considering both the statements of author (s)and the quality of evidence.

3.3 Assessment of Methodological Quality and Reporting Characteristics

3.3.1 Methodological Quality of Included Reviews

Two authors (Luo J and Xu H)independently appraised the methodological quality of each included review using the Assessment of Multiple Systematic Reviews (AMSTAR)scale [16] containing 11 items. We judged each item as "yes" when the criterion was explicitly met, "no" when the criterion was explicitly not met, "can't answer" when the item was relevant but not described adequately or not reported at all, and "not applicable" when the item was not relevant. For literature search (item 3), we judged it as "yes" when authors searched two of the following English electronic databases: the Cochrane Library, Pubmed/medline and Embase, and two of the following Chinese electronic databases: CBM, CNKI, VIP and Wanfang databases.

We also calculated the quality scores according to other previous studies [17],[18] used AMSTAR: it was given 1 point if the item was judged as "yes", otherwise it was given 0. In addition, based on the rating system used by the Canadian Agency for Drugs and Technologies in Health (CADTH)[19], we graded the methodology quality of each review on the overall score and reported it as "low" (range 0 to 4), "moderate" (range 5 to 8), or "high" (range 9 to 11). Disagreements were resolved by discussion or consultation from a third author (Liu JP).

3.3.2 Reporting Assessment of Included Reviews

Two authors (Luo J and Xu H)independently assessed the reporting characteristics of each review according to the Preferred Reporting Items for Systematic Reviews and Meta-analyses (PRISMA)statement [20] composing of 27 items. For each item, a "yes" indicated that the item was reported adequately; a "no" showed that none content of the item was reported; otherwise, if an item was reported inadequately, we judged it as "partially reported". Disagreements were resolved by consensus.

3.4 Data Analysis

We used SPSS (version 17.0)for data analyses. All of the analyses were descriptive. Continuous variables were reported as means with standard deviations (SDs) (normally distributed)or medians with inter-quartile ranges (IQRs) (non-normally distributed). Categorical variables were presented as frequencies with percentages.

RESULTS

1 Study Identification

According to the search strategy, we identified 391 records, of which 212 were excluded for duplicates among databases. After screening titles and abstracts, we excluded 136 articles. A total of 81 records were retrieved for further identification, of which 45 were excluded because they did not meet the pre-specified eligibility criteria described in the methods. Finally, 36 systematic reviews/meta-analyses [8,9,21-54] were included in this overview (Fig 1).

2 Characteristics of Included Reviews.

The characteristics of the included 36 systematic reviews/meta-analyses are summarized in Table 1. Publication year of the 36 reviews ranged from 2004 to 2013, and the number of reviews published in 2011 and 2012 contributed to more than half of these reviews (19/36, 52.7%). Of the 36 reviews, eight (8/36, 22.2%) were published in English [8,9,21-26] and 28 (28/36, 77.8%)were in Chinese. The reviews included a median of 4.1 authors (IQR: 3.0-4.8)while three (3/36, 8.3%)of them were single authored [34,42,51]. No review reported as an update of their previous reviews although two Cochrane reviews [21,22] required updating every two years from published date.

Most (27/36, 75.0%)of the reviews included only RCTs, four reviews (4/36, 11.1%)included RCTs and quasi-RCTs, and five (5/36, 13.9%)contained RCTs and controlled clinical trials. One review [49] containing 35 trials did not report any data about the number of participants. The remaining reviews (35/36, 97.2%) included a median of 18 trials (IQR: 14.0-27.0), involving a median of 2, 152.0 participants (IQR: 1, 062.0-3, 153.0)per review, and the total number of participants in these reviews was 82, 105. A total of 13 kinds of oral CPM were assessed in the 36 reviews (Table 2), of which Compound Danshen dropping pill was the most

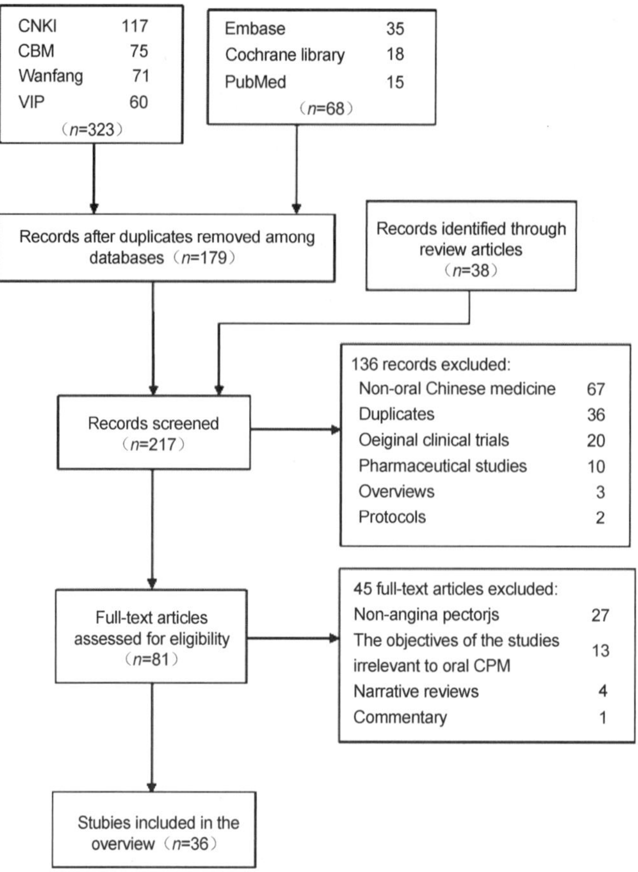

Figure 1 Flow Chart of Reviews Search and Identiflcation

popular one evaluated in 14 reviews (14/36, 38.9%). The majority (29/36, 80.6%)of the reviews assessed single oral CPM, while others evaluated oral CPM and other different preparations of the same medicine (s). There were a variety of comparisons in the reviews including oral CPM vs conventional medicine, oral CPM plus conventional therapy vs conventional therapy, oral CPM plus conventional therapy vs placebo plus conventional therapy, and other comparisons (e.g., oral CPM (a)vs oral CPM (b)). More than one third of the reviews (14/36, 38.9%)assessed single comparison, of which nearly half (6/14, 42.9%)focused on oral CPM vs conventional medicine. One review [52] used indirect comparison, a comparison of oral CPM (a)and oral CPM (b)by comparing them with a common intervention (c), respectively.

For outcomes (Fig 2), most of the reviews assessed surrogate outcomes (34/36, 94.4%), adverse events (31/36, 86.1%), and symptoms (30/36, 83.3%). Eight reviews reported two other outcomes: one [44] reported the improvement of TCM syndrome (1/36, 2.8%), and seven reported composite outcomes referring to total effective rate (7/36, 19.4%). Few reviews assessed endpoints (2/36, 5.6%)and QOL (1/36, 2.8%). No review considered economic evaluations.

Notes: Others included composite outcomes (seven reviews)and TCM syndrome (one review).

Six (6/36, 16.7%)of the reviews drew definitely positive conclusions in favour of a certain oral CPM, while the others (30/36, 83.3%)suggested that there might be some benefits, but the findings should be interpreted with caution due to the poor quality of trials. It should be noted that the (potential)benefits of oral CPM for angina included few adverse events in addition to the improvements of symptoms and surrogate outcomes such as ECG. Only one review [21] drew a conclusion of the potential benefit on endpoints, and no conclusion of the reviews related to QOL. After considering the author's findings and limited quality of evidence, we assigned all of the author's conclusions into category B.

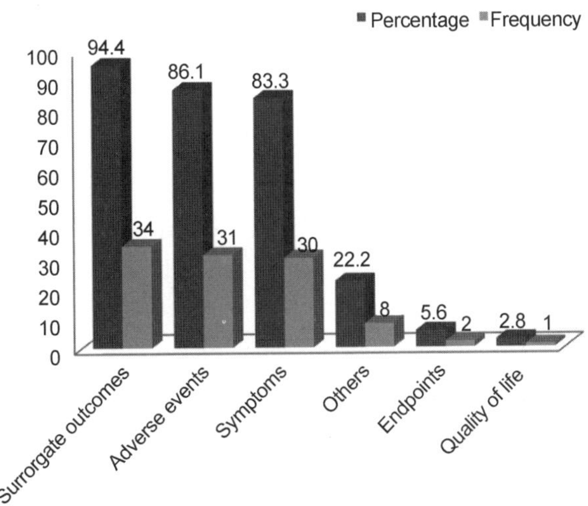

Figure 2 Outcomes Reported in Included Reviews (n = 36)

3 Methodological Quality and Reporting Characteristics of Included Reviews

3.1 Methodological Quality

The compliance with AMSTAR checklist items ranged from 5.6% to 94.4% (Table 3). Of the 36 reviews, three (3/36, 8.3%)provided a registered protocol, 14 reviews (14/36, 38.9%)conducted study selection and data extraction respectively by two reviewers independently. Nearly half of the reviews (16/36, 44.4%) adequately described the characteristics of the included trials, while only two Cochrane reviews provided a list of included and excluded studies. 23 reviews (23/36, 63.9%)synthesized the data of trials appropriately. Reasons of inappropriate data synthesis included that results of trials were pooled despite the trials had different control treatments (11/36, 30.6%), and fixed effect model was used in meta-analyses when there was a large heterogeneity ($I^2 \geqslant 75\%$; 2/36, 5.6%). Almost all of the reviews (34/36, 94.4%)assessed and documented the methodological quality of the included trials, and 32 reviews (32/36, 88.9%)assessed publication bias using funnel plots. Furthermore, most of the reviews (31/36, 86.1%)appropriately used the methodological quality of the included trials in formulating conclusions. Less than one third of reviews (10/36, 27.8%)stated the conflict of interest.

For literature search, over half of the reviews performed a comprehensive literature search (22/36, 61.1%). The mean number of electronic databases searched in the reviews was 5.7 (SD 2.5, range 1 to 12). Most of the reviews searched the following databases: Pubmed (24/36, 66.7%), the Cochrane Library (23/36, 63.9%), Embase (16/36, 44.4%), and Chinese databases (CNKI (30/36, 83.3%), CBM (21/36, 58.3%), VIP (17/36, 47.2%) and Wanfang (16/36, 44.4%)). Six reviews (6/36, 16.7%)applied language restriction to English and Chinese literature, and seven other reviews (7/36, 19.4%)only searched Chinese databases. 15 reviews (15/36, 41.7%) performed hand-searches and 15 reviews conducted additional searches considering the reference lists of relevant articles. Nearly half of the reviews considered grey literatures (19/36, 52.8%)while only one review [26] included an unpublished trial. In addition, five reviews (5/36, 13.9%)searched ongoing trials but none had available data.

The overall scores on AMSTAR ranged from 2 to 10 (maximum score: 11)with a mean score of 6.3 (SD 2.1). Finally, 20 reviews (20/36, 55.5%)were categorized as of "moderate" quality for their overall scores ranging from 5 to 8.10 reviews (10/36, 27.8%)were categorized as of "low" quality and only six reviews including two Cochrane reviews[21,22] (6/36, 16.7%)were categorized as of "high" quality.

3.2 Reporting Characteristics

The overall compliance on each checklist item of PRISMA ranged from 8.3% to 100% (Appendix 2). Almost all of the reviews (35/36, 97.2%)used the term "systematic review" or "meta-analysis" in the title. However, only nine reviews (9/36, 25%)provided a structured summary. 13 reviews (13/36, 36.1%)described the rationale adequately. 25 reviews (25/36, 69.4%)provided explicit objectives in the introduction section.

For methods section, three reviews (3/36, 8.3%)reported their protocols, while most reviews (34/36, 94.4%)stated the principal summary measures, such as risk ratio. More than half of the reviews reported each of the following items adequately: information sources, the process for study selection, the method of data extraction, the methods used for assessing risk of bias of individual studies, the methods of handling data and pooling data of studies, any assessment of risk of bias across studies, and the methods of additional analyses. In addition, 17 reviews (17/36, 47.2%)specified eligibility criteria, six reviews (6/36, 16.7%)presented full electronic search strategy for at least one database, and 12 reviews (12/36, 33.3%)listed and defined data items.

For results section, all reviews presented results of each meta-analysis. Most reviews were adequately compliant with the following items: presented data on risk of bias of each study (28/36, 77.8%), presented results of any assessment of risk of bias across studies (27/36, 75%), reported results of individual studies (25/36, 69.4%), and gave results of additional analyses (22/36, 61.1%). However, less than half of the reviews reported study selection (15/36, 41.7%)as well as study characteristics (14/36, 38.9%)adequately. Six reviews (6/36, 16.7%)reported the flow chart, while one review [49] stated no information about the review process, and the remaining reviews (29/36, 80.6%)just reported inadequate information of the reasons for excluding trials.

For discussion and funding sections, most of the reviews (30/36, 83.3%)provided a summary of results and a conclusion. Ten reviews (10/36, 27.8%)discussed limitations at study, outcome and review level, and most of the other reviews did not discuss limitations at review level. Nine reviews (9/36, 25%)described sources of funding.

DISCUSSION

This overview described the general characteristics, methodological quality as well as reporting quality of 36 systematic reviews/meta-analyses on oral CPM for the treatment of angina. Most of the reviews indicated a potential benefit, while the others concluded a certain oral CPM was definitely effective in treating angina mainly on the improvements of symptoms and ECG, with less adverse events. The overall methodological quality of the reviews was "moderate" or "low", and the reporting quality was limited, with many serious flaws.

Outcomes assessed in trials and systematic reviews should be selected carefully based on their importance for decision making. For angina pectoris, endpoint outcomes such as mortality should be addressed. Surrogate outcomes and symptoms often have limited clinical value. Nevertheless, most of the included reviews assessed surrogate outcomes, adverse events and symptoms, few reviews assessed endpoints and QOL. Due to the short duration of treatment in trials, long term data (e.g., mortality and nonfatal myocardial infarction)which are important for patients with angina were often missed. Considering patients with angina may have an increased risk of acute cardiovascular events and have poor QOL, we recommend that future clinical trials on the effectiveness of oral CPM for angina should have long term follow-up to evaluate endpoint outcomes such as death, or cardiovascular events, as well as QOL and other patient reported outcomes. A previous study [55] and a literature review [56] have identified that selective outcome reporting bias might occur in systematic reviews because few reviews addressed primary outcomes. Our overview indicated a similar finding. Therefore, selective outcome reporting bias might exist in systematic reviews.

For the conclusions, it is worth to mention that some included reviews drew positive conclusions taking no account of the methodological quality of included trials. Despite all included reviews suggesting positive effectiveness (potential or definite benefits)of oral CPM in treating angina, we still can not draw a confirmative conclusion on the beneficial effect of oral CPMs for angina due to the poor methodological quality of evidence. It is well known that trials with positive findings are likely to be published, thus reporting bias and publication bias might exist in trial level and review level. Our results found no negative conclusion in the included reviews on oral CPM for angina. Thus, stakeholders should take critical thinking about the positive conclusions. We recommend that researchers should incorporate the findings with methodological quality of included trials to make a reasonable conclusion. Moreover, high-quality evidence from rigorous clinical trials and relevant systematic reviews are bases to support the clinical recommendation for oral CPM for the treatment of angina.

It is difficult to evaluate the methodological quality of a systematic review due to the insufficient reporting. In this overview, majority of the included systematic reviews had serious methodological and reporting flaws. First, most of the reviews didn't provided registration information or accessible protocol, which is consistent to a previous literature review [3]. Cochrane reviews publish their protocols in the Cochrane Library. For non-Cochrane reviews, PROSPERO [57] is an optional international database for prospective registering systematic review information in health and social care. Protocols can help researchers to conduct reviews transparently. Without protocols, selection bias and reporting bias might occur at review stage. Second, majority of the reviews didn't report whether they conducted study selection as well as data extraction by two reviewers independently. Therefore, selection bias might exist in these reviews. Third, over half of the reviews reported unspecified eligibility criteria, such as the details of outcomes and control treatment. Therefore, the findings could not be interpreted properly to represent clinical generalizaton of the review findings. In addition, incomprehensive literature search, and inappropriate data synthesis were also identified in some of the reviews. All these flaws might influence the reliability of conclusions in the reviews. It is worth mentioning that two included Cochrane reviews were of high methodological and reporting quality, which were the most promising and were worth prioritizing the CPM intervention for independent reproduction in future researches because of the rigorous design, performance and reporting. Future researches should refer to the approach of Cochrane reviews, appropriately design and conduct their systematic reviews according to AMSTAR scale, and transparently report information in keeping with PRISMA statement, so to improve the quality of systematic reviews.

There are also a number of limitations in this overview. First, we might miss some relevant reviews, since for grey literature we tried to search unpublished reviews from dissertation and conference in CNKI and Wanfang databases, and we didn't conduct hand-search or search for ongoing reviews. Second, we could not assess the possible publication bias for our findings due to the lack of relevant strategies. Thus, publication bias might exist in our results. Third, our overview was performed on the basis of reviews' report. If the reviews did not report certain important details adequately, it is difficult for us to judge whether the reviews designed and conducted appropriately.

CONCLUSIONS

Many systematic reviews/meta-analyses suggested oral CPM had potential benefits in treating angina mainly on the improvements of symptoms and ECG, and adverse events. However, the overall methodological and reporting quality of the reviews was limited, with many serious flaws. Thus, the findings should be interpreted cautiously. We recommend further systematic reviews should perform and report according to AMSTAR and PRISMA. Further high quality evidence from relevant systematic reviews would form the basis for support or refute the use of oral CPM for angina pectoris.

REFERENCES

[1] Young D. Policymakers. experts review evidence-based medicine[J]. Am J Health Syst Pharm, 2005, 62 (04): 342-343.

[2] The Medical Research Library of Brooklyn. The Evidence Pyramid. January 2004. Available from: http: //library. downstate. edu/EBM2/2100. htm. [Accessed 12th April 2013].

[3] Ma B, Guo J, Qi G, et al. Epidemiology, quality and reporting characteristics of systematic reviews of traditional Chinese medicine interventions published in Chinese journals[J]. PLoS One, 2011, 6 (05): e20185.

[4] Tobin KJ. Stable angina pectoris: what does the current clinical evidence tell us? [J]. J Am Osteopath Assoc, 2010, 110 (07): 364-370.

[5] National Center for Cardiovascular Diseases, CHINA (NCCD). Report on cardiovascular diseases in China (2011)[J]. Beijing, China: Encyclopedia of China Publishing House, 2012: 7-12.

[6] Go AS, Mozaffarian D, Roger VL, et al. Heart disease and stroke statistics-2013 update: a report from the American Heart Association[J]. Circulation, 2013, 127 (01): e6-e245.

[7] State food and drug administration. The China Food and Drug Administration (SFDA)website data query system. Available from: http: //app2. sfda. gov. cn/datasearchp/gzcxSearch. do? formRender=cx. [Accessed 13th May 2013].

[8] Jia YL, Huang F, Zhang S, et al. Is danshen (Salvia miltiorrhiza)dripping pill more effective than isosorbide dinitrate in treating angina pectoris? A systematic review of randomized controlled trials[J]. Int J Cardiol, 2012, 157 (03): 330-340.

[9] Jia YL, Chen C, Ng CS, et al. Meta-analysis of randomized controlled trials on the efficacy of Di'ao Xinxuekang Capsule and isosorbide dinitrate in treating angina pectoris[J]. Evid Based Complement Alternat Med, 2012, 2012. [Article ID 904147].

[10] Ernst E. Cardiovascular adverse effects of herbal medicines: a systematic review of the recent literature[J]. Can J Cardiol, 2003, 19 (7): 818-827.

[11] Zhang JH, Shang HC, Gao XM, et al. Methodology and reporting quality of systematic review/meta-analysis of traditional Chinese medicine[J]. J Altern Complement Me, 2007, 13 (08): 797-805.

[12] Luo J, Xu H, Yang GY, et al. Oral Chinese proprietary medicine for angina pectoris: an overview of systematic reviews/meta-analyses. PROSPERO 2013: CRD42013004468. Available from http: //www. crd. york. ac. uk/PROSPERO_REBRANDING/display_record. asp? ID=CRD42013004468

[13] Chinese Pharmacopoeia Commission. Clinical guide of the Chinese pharmacopeia: traditional Chinese medicine (2005 edition). Beijing, China: People's Medical Publishing House, 2005.

[14] Chinese Pharmacopoeia Commission. Pharmacopoeia of the People's Republic of China 2010 (Vol Ⅰ). Beijing, China: China Medical Science Press, 2010.

[15] National Heart, Lung, and Blood Institute Working Group. Outcomes Research in Cardiovascular Disease Report of the NHLBI Working Group. January, 2004. Available from: http: //www. nhlbi. nih. gov/meetings/workshops/cvdoutcomes. htm. [Accessed 12th April 2013].

[16] Shea BJ, Grimshaw JM, Wells GA, et al. Development of AMSTAR: a measurement tool to assess the methodological quality of systematic reviews[J]. BMC Med Res Methodol, 2007, 7: 10. [PubMed: 17302989]

[17] Sequeira-Byron P, Fedorowicz Z, Jagannath VA, et al. An AMSTAR assessment of the methodological quality of systematic reviews of oral healthcare interventions published in the Journal of Applied Oral Science (JAOS)[J]. J Appl Oral Sci, 2011, 19 (05): 440-447.

[18] Shea BJ, Bouter LM, Peterson J, et al. External validation of a measurement tool to assess systematic reviews (AMSTAR)[J]. PLoS One, 2007, 2 (12): e1350.

[19] Canadian Agency for Drugs and Technologies in Health (CADTH). Interventions Directed to Consumers. Available from: http: //www. cadth. ca/en/resources/rx-for-change/interventions-consumers. [Accessed 13th April 2013].

[20] Moher D, Liberati A, Tetzlaff J, et al. Preferred reporting items for systematic reviews and meta-analyses: the PRISMA statement[J]. Ann Intern Med, 2009, 151 (4): 264-269.

[21] Wu T, Harrison RA, Chen X, et al. Tongxinluo (Tong xin luo or Tong-xin-luo)capsule for unstable angina pectoris[J]. Cochrane Database Syst Rev, 2006, (4): 1-41.

[22] Duan X, Zhou L, Wu T, et al. Chinese herbal medicine suxiao jiuxin wan for angina pectoris[J]. Cochrane Database Syst Rev, 2008, (1): 1-28.

[23] Zhang JH, Shang HC, Gao XM, et al. Compound Salvia droplet pill, a traditional Chinese medicine, for the treatment of unstable angina pectoris: a systematic review[J]. Med Sci Monit, 2008, 14 (1): RA1-7.

[24] Wang G, Wang L, Xiong ZY, et al. Compound salvia pellet, a traditional Chinese medicine, for the treatment of chronic stable angina pectoris compared with nitrates: a meta-analysis[J]. Med Sci Monit, 2006, 12 (1): SR1-7.

[25] Li YF, Wang YL, Qi Y, et al. Compound Danshen dripping pills for stable angina: meta-analysis of randomized controlled trials[J]. J Med Plant Res, 2011, 5 (11): 2245-2251.

[26] Jia YL, Bao FF, Huang FY, et al. Is tongxinluo more effective than isosorbide dinitrate in treating angina pectoris? A systematic review and meta-analysis of randomized controlled trials[J]. Journal of Alternative and Complementary Medicine, 2011, 17 (12): 1109-1117.

[27] Chen W, Qin LM, Liu ZH, et al. Systematic assessment on randomized controlled trials for treatment of stable angina pectoris by Compound Danshen dripping pill[J]. Journal of Shandong University of Traditional Chinese Medicine, 2012, 36 (04): 287-291.

[28] Wang L, Xiong ZY, Wang G, et al. Systematic assessment on randomized controlled trials for treatment of stable angina pectoris by compound salvia pellet[J]. Chinese Journal of Integrated Traditional and Western Medicine, 2004, 24 (06): 500-504.

[29] Zhang JH, Shang HC, Gao XM, et al. Systemic evaluation of compound preparation of Salvia Miltiorrhiza in treating stable angina in a randomized controlled trial[J]. Tianjin Journal of Traditional Chinese Medicine, 2007, 24 (03): 195-200.

[30] Wang Y, Kuang YX. Meta-analysis of effect of Tong Xin Luo capsule on coronary heart disease angina[J]. Modern Journal of Integrated Traditional Chinese and Western Medicine, 2012, 21 (08): 801-803.

[31] Liu JX, Liang H, Sun X, et al. A meta-analysis on curative effect of Nao Xin Tong capsules in treatment of unstable angina[J]. Chinese Journal of

Evidence-Based Cardiovascular Medicine, 2012, 4 (02): 97-100.

[32] Zheng GH, Chen HY, Chu JF, et al. Systematic review of randomize controlled trials on Xuefu Zhuyu capsule for angina pectoris in patients with coronary heart disease[J]. Journal of Traditional Chinese Medicine, 2012, 53 (02): 117-121.

[33] Ye TS, Zhang YW, Hu HK. Systematic evaluation of efficacy and safety of Compound Salvia droplet pills for angina pectoris[J]. Herald of Medicine, 2013, 32 (1): 100-105.

[34] Li KJ. Preparation of Salvia Miltiorrhiza in treating stable angina: a systematic review of randomized controlled trial[J]. Herald of Medicine, 2007, 26 (04): 383-386.

[35] Wang XJ, Xu BN. Meta-analysis on of Chinese herbal medicine Suxiao Jiuxin wan on the treatment of angina pectoris[J]. Shaanxi Journal of Traditional Chinese Medicine, 2008, 29 (09): 1249-1251.

[36] Zhou XG, Wang HW, Yu GB. Meta-analysis on of Chinese herbal medicine Shexiang Baoxin wan on the treatment of angina pectoris[J]. Chinese Traditional Patent Medicine, 2004, 26 (S1): 1-6.

[37] Hao CH, Zhang JY. Meta-analysis of Tong Xin Luo capsule for coronary heart disease angina[J]. China Modern Doctor, 2010, 48 (14): 6-9.

[38] Guo MG, Zhao TT, Li JT. Meta-analysis of randomized controlled trials on Compound Danshen dropping pills compared with other three common drugs in treatment of acute angina[J]. Medical Journal of West China, 2012, 24 (03): 486-490.

[39] Zhang MZ, Wang L, Chen BJ, et al. Meta-analysis of document on Compound Danshen dropping pills (DSP)in treatment of patients with stable angina[J]. Chinese Journal of Integrative Medicine on Cardio/Cerebrovascular Disease, 2004, 2 (06): 311-314.

[40] Xu CX, Zhao YQ, Hu Y, et al. Shexiang Baoxin pills for coronary disease angina pectoris: a systematic review[J]. China Pharmacy, 2011, 22 (44): 4196-4200.

[41] Jiang SY, Tong JC, Sun RY, et al. Meta-analysis of Compound Danshen dropping pills (DSP)in treating coronary heart disease angina[J]. Practical Pharmacy and Clinical Remedies, 2007, 10 (06): 334-337.

[42] Li KJ. Preparation of Salvia Miltiorrhiza in treating unstable angina: a systematic review of randomized controlled trial[J]. Guangming Journal of Chinese Medicine, 2007, 22 (02): 37-40.

[43] Zhao W, Xiang JS, Ye K. Systematic review on randomized controlled trials for treatment of UAP by Ginkgo extract[J]. Journal of Liaoning University of Traditional Chinese Medicine, 2010, 12 (11): 216-220.

[44] Wang X, Zhu YY, Hu LS. A systematic review of Rhodiola L. for treating angina[J]. Progress in Modern Biomedicine, 2006, 6 (02): 42-45.

[45] Chen XT, Guo SS, Guo Y. Meta-analysis of Chinese herbal medicine Xin Ke Shu for angina pectoris[J]. Journal of Changchun University of Traditional Chinese Medicine, 2010, 26 (03): 357-359.

[46] Xu YY, Xu KK. Systematic review of Ginkgo Leaves tablet for angina[J]. Chinese Journal of Experimental Traditional Medical Formulae, 2011, 17 (16): 288-293.

[47] Jiang GF, Jiang YD, Zhan T. A systematic review and meta-analysis of Shexiang Baoxin pill for the treatment of unstable angina pectoris[J]. Practical Journal of Cardiac Cerebral Pneumal and Vascular Disease, 2011, 19 (12): 2030-2033.

[48] Cui HJ, He HY, Xing ZH. System evaluation and meta analysis of Xuefu Zhuyu decoction on unstable angina pectoris[J]. Journal of Emergency in Traditional Chinese Medicine, 2011, 20 (07): 1071-1074.

[49] Yang Y, Zeng LX. Meta-analysis of efficacy and safety of Nao Xin Tong capsule for treatment of angina pectoris of coronary heart disease[J]. Chinese Journal of Integrative Medicine on Cardio-/Cerebrovascular Disease, 2012, 10 (07): 769-772.

[50] Xu GL, Lin SH, Qin L. Systematic review of Tong Xin Luo capsule on effectiveness and safety of elderly patients with unstable angina[J]. Journal of Emergency in Traditional Chinese Medicine, 2012, 21 (03): 409-410.

[51] Liu JG. Efficacy and safety evaluation on the treatment of coronary artery disease with Shexiang-baoxin pill and complex Danshen drop pill[J]. International Journal of Traditional Chinese Medicine, 2012, 34 (9): 779-781.

[52] Jia YL, Zhang SK, Bao FF, et al. Indirect comparison of Tongxinluo Capsule and Danshen dripping pill for angina pectoris: a systematic review[J]. Chinese Journal of Evidence-Based Medicine, 2011, 11 (08): 919-931.

[53] Ng CS, Wang SP, Cheong JL, et al. Systematic review and meta-analysis of randomized controlled trials comparing Chinese patent medicines Compound Danshen dripping pills and Di'ao Xin Xue Kang in treating angina pectoris[J]. Journal of Chinese Integrative Medicine, 2012, 10 (01): 25-34.

[54] Xu GL, Wu HD, Du B, et al. A systemic review of the efficacy and safety on comparison Tong Xin Luo capsule with Danshen tablet in the treatment of angina pectoris[J]. Chinese Journal of Difficult and Complicated Cases, 2012, 11 (01): 2-5.

[55] Silagy CA, Middleton P, Hopewell S. Publishing protocols of systematic reviews: Comparing what was done to what was planned[J]. JAMA, 2002, 287 (21): 2831–2834.

[56] Moher D, Tetzlaff J, Tricco AC, et al. Epidemiology and reporting characteristics of systematic reviews. PLoS Med, 2007, 4 (3): e78.

[57] Http: //www. crd. york. ac. uk/PROSPERO/

First publishe: LUO Jing, XU Hao, YANG Guo-yan, QIU Yu, LIU Jian-ping, and CHEN Ke-ji. Oral Chinese proprietary medicine for angina pectoris: An overview of systematic reviews/meta-analyses[J]. Complementary Therapies in Medicine, 2014, 22 (4): 787-800.

Potential Benefits of Chinese Herbal Medicine for Elderly Patients with Cardiovascular Diseases

LUO Jing, XU Hao, and CHEN Ke-ji

China and some other developing countries are experiencing an increasing prevalence of Cardiovascular diseases (CVDs)which is now still the leading cause of death[1,2]. Data from The Global Burden of Disease Study 2010 (GBD 2010)shows that one in four deaths was attributable to heart disease or stroke, and ischemic heart disease was the first cause of global disability-adjusted life years (DALYs)in 2010. Moreover, a greater proportion of deaths are taking place among elderly people (older than 70 years)in 2010, compared with 1990[3,4]. With aging of population, CVDs will have a higher prevalence and place a huge financial and social burden on human development. Despite improvement of clinical outcomes with percutaneous coronary intervention (PCI)and conventional Western medicine, elderly patients with CVDs remain at certain risk of recurrent acute cardiovascular events, complications as well as unfavorable quality of life.

Traditional Chinese medicine (TCM), the amazing part of traditional Chinese culture, with a history of several thousand years, has both unique theories and rich experience. For lacking of objective and quantitative evaluation criteria, TCM is currently considered as a complementary or alternative medicine (CAM)in most Western countries. In China, however, it is reported that more than 71.2% patients who had experienced western medicine, TCM, and integrative medicine (IM), preferred IM therapeutic method, and 18.7% took TCM therapeutic method as their favorite[5]. Moreover, CAM, including TCM is increasingly welcomed in many developed countries such as Australia and the United States[6]. Recently, as more clinicians successfully applied TCM in CVDs prevention and treatment based on conventional therapy, the effects of TCM for CVDs especially in elderly patients with CVDs have drawn greater attention[7,8]. In this paper, we briefly commented the potential benefits of Chinese herbal medicine (CHM), the most common form of TCM, for CVDs in the elderly.

1 Characteristics of CVDs in the Elderly

Most of patients with CVDs are elderly. The characteristics of these patients have to be taken into account before treatment. (1)The organs are in age-related declines, which may be a key factor of frailty. In this case, individuals may have the problem of impaired immunity[9]. What's more, with hepatic and renal function in declines, the application of many drugs will be affected, which will increase the risk of adverse effects[10,11]. (2)Usage of multiple drugs due to multiple diseases. Elderly patients with CVDs always have one or more comorbidities such as diabetes, hyperlipidemia, or hypertension. They often need receiving several prescribed drugs daily, even more than 10 medications, which place them at a high risk for adverse effects, including drug interactions[12]. (3)Elderly patients with CVDs usually have hepatic and/or renal insufficiency. Thus, many drugs need a dose adjustment, and some drugs should be limited or avoided. For example, with hepatic dysfunction, statins should be limited or avoided. Similarly, with renal dysfunction, digoxin and most angiotensin converting enzyme inhibitor (ACEIs), which are renally eliminated, should be started at lower doses. However, elderly patients receiving 'target' (high)dose ACEI therapy might have better cardiac outcomes with an insignificant increase in adverse effects[13,14]. These usually put clinicians in a dilemma. (4)Pharmacokinetic and pharmacodynamic changes in older patients[15]. Aging significantly affects drug distribution and elimination triggered by the age-related changes in hepatic and renal function, muscle mass, and plasma proteins. In addition, some comorbidities such as diabetes can lead to renal dysfunction, which also result in pharmacokinetic and pharmacodynamic changes.

2 Present Treatment of CVDs in the Elderly

Western medicine, TCM, and IM are current three major models of health care in China, with Western medicine considered as the mainstream medicine. The evolution of Western medicine has substantially reduced mortality and morbidity associated with CVDs[16,17]. At present, most patients with CVDs can receive more effective treatments such as antithrombotic therapy combined with timely reperfusion therapy, PCI or coronary artery bypass grafting (CABG). However, particularly to the elderly patients, potentially serious adverse effects associated with Western therapy such as bleeding[18], orthostatic hypotension, bradycardia, and congestive heart failure are still key challenges. In addition, unfavorable quality of life resulting from drug-related gastrointestinal reactions, depression, dizziness, and cognitive impairment also bring clinicians into perplexity.

3 CHM for CVDs

Many experimental studies indicated that some Chinese herbs (e.g., "*Ren Shen*" (*Radix Ginseng*), "*Chuan Xiong*" (*Rhizoma Canxiong*)and "*Dan Shen*" (*Radix Salviae Miltiorrhizae*))have potential benefits for CVDs[19-22]. Recent clinical trials and systematic reviews[23-28] showed that CHM (e.g., Xiongshao capsule, Tong Xin Luo capsule and Danshen dripping pill)can improve health-related quality of life, lower the restenosis rate after PCI, reduce cardiovascular events, improve electrocardiogram (ECG)and serum myocardial injury biomarkers, decrease consumption of some chemicals, etc. Furthermore, only few mild side effects with spontaneous remission such as abdominal distention from common CHM in elderly patients with CVDs can be found clinically. In fact, natural products with fewer side effects are what often come to mind while TCM once mentioned. Nevertheless, it is too early to draw a conclusion of the safety of CHM for elderly patients with CVDs yet due to the insufficient evidence. Rigorously designed clinical trials with detailed description of adverse events are warrant to further demonstrate the safety of CHM for CVDs.

It is worthy to mention that CHM will be a good choice for elderly patients with CVDs combined with other diseases such as tumor, autoimmune disease, and metabolic disease. CHM can improve quality of life, reduce drug-resistance and toxic effects of chemicals, and assist in the decrease or withdrawal of glucocorticoids[29-31]. Nowadays, with an ever-growing number of people adopting CHM for the clinical effectiveness and safety[5-8,32], CHM is playing an important role in the treatment of elderly patients with CVDs in China.

4 Features and Advantages of CHM

4.1 Holistic Regulation

TCM is characterized by "holistic regulation". As a basic theory of TCM, holism is a concept of the organism as a whole, which refers to the integral unity of the human body and its close relationship with the outer world. In TCM theory, either excessiveness or insufficiency is illness, getting equilibrium of human being is considered as the therapeutic objective. Under these guidelines, practitioners pay more attention to the diseased patients rather than the suffered diseases in the clinical practice of TCM. They often treat patients by reinforcing the body's immunity, eliminating pathogenic factors, and improving the ability of body's self-healing capacity.

4.2 Syndrome Differentiation Based Treatment

As another feature of TCM, "syndrome differentiation based treatment (SDT)" refers to diagnosis and treatment based on an overall analysis of the illness and the patient's unbalanced condition. What's more, practitioners timely modify formulae in accordance with the patients' varying syndromes and clinical manifestations. As a basis of holistic regulation, a correct SDT always makes great contribution to the improvement of outcomes. On the other hand, SDT is an individualized treatment for different patients with same disease.

4.3 Complex Interventions

The 2008 Medical Research Council Guide described complex interventions as interventions that contain several interacting components, which may be to do with the range of possible outcomes, or their variability in the target population, rather than with the number of elements in the intervention package itself[33]. As a typical kind of complex interventions, the complexity of TCM is mainly reflected in SDT and the composition of a formula. A single herb contains interacting components, which play crucial roles in the comprehensive effects of CHM. Furthermore, TCM formulae exert comprehensive effects by containing several herbs served as "king-minister-assistant-envoy". In fact, many researches on pharmacology and chemistry[34-37] have indicated that both single herbs and formulae have features of multi-level regulation and multi-targets. These features may be the inherent foundation of complex interventions. In the theory of TCM, complex interventions are seen as a basis of holistic regulation. CHM handles the relationship between mind and body, disease and medicine in the view of holism, dynamic and dialectic. Finally, SDT, holistic regulation, and complex interventions, help the unbalanced body return to a harmony state.

4.4 Homology of Medicine and Food

As a distinguished feature of TCM, "Homology of Medicine and Food" means that CHM and foods originate from the same source. Traditionally, Chinese people prefer foods to drugs for health care, and certain kinds of herbs are regarded as both medicines and foods[38]. For example, "*Shan Zha*" (hawthorn fruit)is also a medicine for its effects on dyspepsia and dyslipidemia. This to some extent, reflects why CHM have few side effects.

5 Comparison between CHM and Western Medicine

With the development of modern medical technology and biomedicine, Western medicine has made great contributions to the elderly patients with CVDs. However, there are still some challenges as stated above, which are associated with both elderly patients themselves and Western medicine. Focusing on a specific physiological target, Western medicine often has a strong effect on a disease. For example, statins can reduce the level of low-density lipoprotein cholesterol (LDL-C)dramatically. It is widely accepted that particular Western medicines usually work against specific pathological process rather than a patient. Due to the strong pertinence, Western medicine will inevitably cause adverse effects. Compared with Western medicine, CHM mainly has the following advantages: complex interventions, holistic regulation, individualized treatment and fewer side effects.

In fact, both CHM and Western medicine have their own advantages and disadvantages. They can complement each other to give full play to their advantages in clinical practice[8] e.g., by IM. Recently, a multicenter randomized double-blind placebo-controlled trial indicated that administration of Xiongshao capsule in addition to standardized Western medication was effective and safe in reducing post-PCI restenosis and recurrent angina in elderly patients with coronary heart disease[25]

6 Potential Benefits of CHM for Elderly Patients with CVDs

In recent decades, more and more clinicians have accepted and used CHM. CHM has made and continues to make great contributions to the health of CVDs patients. Due to the foregoing characteristics: frailty, polypharmacy, potential hepatic and renal insufficiency, and changes in drug distribution and elimination, elderly CVDs patients are often at an increased risk of adverse effects. To this special population, cardiovascular therapy requires more frequent monitoring, and individualized intervention with minimum adverse effects would be a good choice.

The various factors including characteristics of elderly patients with CVDs, features of CHM, and relevant clinical evidences, discussed before, demonstrate the potential benefits of CHM for elderly patients with CVDs. The potential benefits may embody in individualized treatment, fewer side effects, improvement of health-related quality of life, lowering the restenosis rate after PCI, reducing cardiovascular events, decreasing consumption of some chemicals, etc.

In a word, although the efficacy of CHM is not as strong as chemicals on a pathological process of CVDs, CHM is indeed an alternative and complementary choice for elderly patients with CVDs due to its holistic regulation, individualized and complex intervention as well as fewer side effects. What's more, with mutual complementary, Western medicine and TCM together shall benefit the elderly patients with CVDs. We expect more evidence from high quality trials to support the extensive clinical use of CHM for elderly patients with CVDs.

REFERENCES

[1] National Center for Cardiovascular Diseases, CHINA (NCCD). Report on cardiovascular diseases in China (2011)[M]. Beijing: Encyclopedia of China Publishing House, 2012, 7-12.

[2] Go AS, Mozaffarian D, Roger VL, et al. Heart disease and stroke statistics-2013 update: a report from the American Heart Association[J]. Circulation, 2013, 127 (1): e6-e245.

[3] Horton R. GBD 2010: understanding disease, injury, and risk. The Lancet 2012, 380 (9859): 2053-2054.

[4] Murray CJ, Vos T, Lozano R, et al. Disability-adjusted life years (DALYs)for 291 diseases and injuries in 21 regions, 1990-2010: a systematic analysis for the Global Burden of Disease Study 2010[J]. The Lancet, 2012, 380 (9859): 2197-2223.

[5] Chen KJ and Lv AP. Situation of Integrative Medicine in China: Results from a National Survey in 2004[J]. Chinese Journal of Integrative Medicine, 2006, 12 (3): 161-165.

[6] World Health Organization. Traditional medicine strategy 2002-2005, 2002. Available from: http: //whqlibdoc. who. int/hq/2002/WHO_EDM_TRM_2002.1. pdf. [Accessed 8th June 2013].

[7] Ferreira AS and Lopes AJ. Chinese medicine pattern differentiation and its im-plications for clinical practice[J]. Chinese Journal of Integrative Medicine, 2011, 17 (11): 818-823.

[8] Xu H and Chen KJ. Integrating Traditional Medicine with Biomedicine Towards a Patient-Centered Healthcare System[J]. Chinese Journal of Integrative Medicine, 201117 (2): 83-84.

[9] Lambert ND, Ovsyannikova IG, Pankratz VS, et al. Understanding the immune response to seasonal influenza vaccination in older adults: a systems biology approach[J]. Expert Rev Vaccines, 2012, 11 (8): 985-994.

[10] Schmucker DL. Liver function and phase I drug metabolism in the elderly: a pa-radox[J]. Drugs Aging, 2001, 18 (11): 837-851.

[11] Lindeman RD. Changes in renal function with aging. Implications for treatment[J]. Drugs Aging, 1992, 2 (5): 423-431.

[12] Lesage J. Polypharmacy in geriatric patients[J]. Nurs Clin North Am, 1991, 26 (2): 273-290.

[13] Chen YT, Wang Y, Radford MJ, et al. Angiotensin-converting enzyme inhibitor dosages in elderly patients with heart failure[J]. Am Heart J, 2001, 141 (3): 410-417.

[14] Gattis WA, Larsen RL, Hasselblad V, et al. Is optimal angiotensin-converting enzyme inhibitor dosing neglected in elderly patients with heart failure? [J]. Am Heart J, 1998, 136 (1): 43-48.

[15] Howland RH. Effects of aging on pharmacokinetic and pharmacodynamic drug processes[J]. J Psychosoc Nurs Ment Health Serv, 2009, 47 (10): 15-18.

[16] White HD and Chew DP. Acute myocardial infarction[J]. The Lancet, 2008, 372 (9638): 570-584.

[17] Eugene B. The treatment of acute myocardial infarction: the Past, the Present, and the Future[J]. European Heart Journal: Acute Cardiovascular Care, 2012, 1 (1): 9-12.

[18] Manoukian SV, Feit F, Mehran R, et al. Impact of major bleeding on 30-day mortality and clinical outcomes in patients with acute coronary syndromes: an analysis from the ACUITY Trial[J]. J Am Coll Cardiol, 2007, 49 (12): 1362-1368.

[19] Wang JR, Zhou H, Yi XQ, et al. Total ginsenosides of Radix Ginseng modulates tricarboxylic acid cycle protein expression to enhance cardiac energy metabolism in ischemic rat heart tissues[J]. Molecules, 2012, 17 (11): 12746-12757.

[20] Li HX, Han SY, Ma X, et al. The saponin of red ginseng protects the cardiac myocytes against ischemic injury in vitro and in vivo[J]. Phytomedicine, 2012, 19 (6): 477-483.

[21] Zhou W, Ruigrok TJ. Protective effect of danshen during myocardial ischemia and reperfusion: an isolated rat heart study[J]. Am J Chin Med, 1990, 18 (1-2): 19-24.

[22] Liu Y, Yin HJ, Jiang YR, et al. Correlation between Platelet Gelsolin and Platelet Activation Level in Acute Myocardial Infarction Rats and Intervention Effect of Effective Components of Chuanxiong Rhizome and Red Peony Root[J]. Evid Based Complement Alternat Med, 2013.

[23] Chen KJ, Shi DZ, Xu H, et al. XS0601 reduces the incidence of restenosis: a prospective study of 335 patients undergoing percutaneous coronary intervention in China[J]. Chin Med J (Engl), 2006, 119 (1): 6-13.

[24] Xu H, Gao ZY, Chen KJ. A prospective study on the diagnostic and therapeutic status and prognosis of 1864 elderly patients with coronary heart disease[J]. Chinese Journal of Geriatrics, 2008, 27 (8): 617-622.

[25] Shang QH, Xu H, Lu XY, et al. A multi-center randomized double-blind placebo-controlled trial of Xiongshao Capsule in preventing restenosis after percutaneous coronary intervention: a subgroup analysis of elderly patients[J]. Chinese Journal of Integrative Medicine, 2011, 17 (9): 669-674.

[26] Du BM, Lu ZL, Wu YF, et al. China coronary secondary prevention study: conclusion in aged coronary heart disease patients with or without hypertension[J]. Chinese Journal of geriatric cardiovascular and cerebrovascular diseases, 2006, 8 (2): 82-86.

[27] Wu T, Harrison RA, Chen X, et al. Tongxinluo (Tong xin luo or Tong-xin-luo)capsule for unstable angina pectoris[J]. Cochrane Database of Systematic Reviews, 2006, 18 (4): 1-40.

[28] Jia YL, Huang F, Zhang S, et al. Is danshen (Salvia miltiorrhiza)dripping pill more effective than isosorbide dinitrate in treating angina pectoris? A systematic review of randomized controlled trials[J]. Int J Cardiol. 2012, 157 (3): 330-340.

[29] Hu XM, Liu F, Zheng CM, et al. Effect and prognostic analysis of treatment for acute myeloid leukemia using Chinese drugs combined with chemotherapy[J]. Chinese Journal of Integrative Medicine, 2009, 15 (3): 193-197.

[30] Song XR and Hou SX. Research progress in the reversion of traditional Chinese medicine on multidrug resistance of tumor[J]. Chin J Chin Mater Medica, 2005, 30 (16): 1300-1304.

[31] Wu GL, Fan YS, Han YM, Yu GY. Effect of Yangyin jiedu Huoxue Recipe on hormone withdrawal and disease activity in patients with systemic lupus erythematosus[J]. Chin J Integr Tradit West Med, 2009, 29 (9): 780-782.

[32] LV AP, Ding XR, Chen KJ. Current Situation and Progress in Integrative Medicine in China[J]. Chinese Journal of Integrative Medicine, 2008, 14 (3): 234-240.

[33] Craig P, Dieppe P, Macintyre S, Michie S, Nazareth I, Petticrew M, Medical Research Council Guidance. Developing and evaluating complex interventions: the new Medical Research Council guidance[J]. British Medical Journal, 2008, 337: a1655.

[34] Zhao J, Jiang P, Zhang W. Molecular networks for the study of TCM pharma-cology[J]. Brief Bioinform, 2012, 11 (4): 417-430.

[35] Terstappen GC, Reggiani A. In silico research in drug discovery[J]. Trends Pharmacol. Sci, 2001, 22 (1): 23-26.

[36] Ma XH, Zheng CJ, Han LY, et al. Synergistic therapeutic actions of herbal in-gredients and their mechanisms from molecular interaction and network perspectives[J]. Drug Discov Today, 2009, 14 (11-12): 579-588.

[37] Hou JY. Pharmacology of Traditional Chinese Medicine[M]. Beijing: China Press of traditional Chinese Medicine, 2002: 21.

[38] Wang L. Guidelines for the Selection of Therapeutic Food[M]. Beijing: China Light Industry Press, 2000.

First published: LUO Jing, XU Hao, and CHEN Ke-ji. Potential benefits of Chinese Herbal Medicine for elderly patients with cardiovascular diseases[J]. J Geriatr Cardiol, 2013, 10: 305-309.

Oral *Panax notoginseng* Preparation for Coronary Heart Disease: A Systematic Review of Randomized Controlled Trials

SHANG Qing-hua, XU Hao, LIU Zhao-lan, CHEN Ke-ji, and LIU Jian-ping

Coronary heart disease (CHD)is one of the most leading causes of morbidity and mortality in many countries with large economic and human burdens, and it accounts for 20% of overall mortality in the United State[1]. It is reported that Ischaemic heart disease is the second leading cause for males and the third leading cause of global burden of disease for females, accounting for 6.8% and 5.3% respectively[2]. Although the benefit of some conventional drugs, such as aspirin and statin, have been demonstrated in reducing CHD mortality, annually 17.3 million people die from cardiovascular disease (CVD)worldwide (WHO 2008), and over 80% of CVD deaths take place in low and middle income countries, it is reported that by 2030 more than 23 million people will die annually from CVDs [3].

In recent years, traditional medicines have been playing more and more important roles in the maintenance of health, the prevention and treatment of diseases, and plant-based drug discovery[4–8]. Chinese herbal medicine or its products have been administered widely for treating CHD in China. There are more than one hundred kinds of patent herbal medicine for CHD available at present. Puerarin injection[9], Danshen preparations[10], Tongxinluo[11], compound salvia pellet[12], Suxiao jiuxin wan[13] or traditional Chinese herbal products[14] have been shown as potential benefits recently by systematic reviews. Sanqi is one of the most widely used herbal medicines in China, with function of invigorating the blood circulation according to TCM theory. *Panax notoginseng* was the active and effective component purified from sanqi. Oral *Panax notoginseng* products included xuesaitong capsule, xuesaitong dripping pills, xuesaitong pill, xuesaitong effervescent tablet, xuesaitong granule, xuesaitong dispersible tablet, sanqishutong capsule, *Panax notoginseng* saponins (PNS)tablet and PNS capsule. The content of *Panax notoginseng* varies in different agents. All of the agents have been used in clinic for patients with CHD for decades of years. Recent researches found its antioxidative[15], antiatherogenic, lipid-lowering and anti-inflammatory[16] effects and angiogenic effect[17]. A Cochrane systematic review indicated that *Panax notoginseng* was effective in preventing stroke[18]. Some recent clinical trials also proved that it could benefit CHD patients[19,20]. Therefore, this systematic review aims to evaluate the safety and effectiveness of oral *Panax notoginseng* preparations for CHD patients.

METHOD

1 Inclusion Criteria

We included randomized controlled trials (RCTs)or cross-over trials in English and Chinese regardless of publication type in this review. Quasirandomized trials were excluded and the first stage of data was used if it was cross-over trial. Any adult participant with CHD meeting with at least one of the current or past definitions or guidelines of CHD (including acute coronary syndrome (ACS)and X syndrome)was considered. Those who did not introduce diagnostic criteria in the text but stated patients with definite CHD were also included. The trial was included if oral *Panax notoginseng* preparation was in intervention group regardless of dosage, treatment course, and agents; trials should be excluded if there were other Chinese herbal medicines in intervention group; trials also should be excluded if there was a combination of *Panax notoginseng* preparation and a kind of western medicine on the basis of control group. Chinese herbal injection should be excluded in this review. Placebo, no intervention, or nitrate was considered in control group, Chinese herbal medicine in control group should be excluded. Oral *Panax notoginseng* preparations versus conventional therapy (except for nitroglycerin)were excluded for limited extension.

Outcome measures include primary outcomes: all cause mortality, cardiovascular events (e.g., CHD mortality, incidence of myocardial infarction (MI), revascularization, andrehospitalization for unstable angina); secondary outcomes: quality of life, attack of angina pectoris (measuring by recurrence of angina pectoris, frequency of angina pectoris, duration of angina pectoris, dosage of nitroglycerin, decrement of nitroglycerin, efficacy of angina pectoris, and others), electrocardiogram (ECG), and adverse events. We defined the efficacy of angina pectoris as improvement was more than 50%; the efficacy of ECG as elevation of ST segment was more than 0.05 mv.

2 Search Strategy

Two review authors (Qinghua Shang, Hao Xu)searched the following databases up to January 2013 independently for the identifications of trials (publication or nonpublication): the Cochrane Library, Pubmed, Chinese Biomedical database (CBM), China National Knowledge Infrastructure (CNKI), Chinese VIP Information (VIP), and Wanfang databases. We used the terms as follows: coronary heart disease, CHD, coronary artery disease, angina pectoris, myocardial infarction, acute coronary syndrome, cardi, sanqi, sanchi, jinbuhuan, tiansanqi, tianqi, panlongqi, tongpitiegu, xueshancao, liuyuelin, xuesaitong, xueshuantong, notoginseng, pseudoginseng, *Panax notoginseng*, ginsenosides *Panax*, sanchinoside, and so forth. Because of different characteristics of various databases, MeSH terms and free text terms were used regardless of the report types in full text, title, keyword, subject terms, or abstract.

3 Data Extraction and Quality Assessment

Data Extraction and Quality Assessment. Two review authors (Qinghua Shang, Hao Xu)independently extracted data according to a data extraction form made by the authors. Disagreements were resolved by consensus or consultation from a third reviewer (Jianping Liu or Zhaolan Liu). The methodological quality of trials was assessed independently using criteria from the Cochrane Handbook for Systematic Review of Interventions, Version 5.0. 1 (Qinghua Shang, HaoXu)[15]. The items included random sequence generation (selection bias), allocation concealment (selection bias), blinding of participants and personnel (performance bias), blinding of outcome assessment (detection bias), incomplete outcome data (attrition bias), selective reporting (reporting bias), and other biases. We judged each item from three levels ("Yes" for a low of bias, "No" for a high risk of bias, and "Unclear" otherwise), and then we assessed the trials and categorized them into three levels: low risk of bias (all the items were in low risk of bias), high risk of bias (at least one item was in high risk of bias), and unclear risk of bias (otherwise).

4 Data Synthesis

We used Revman 5.1 software provided by the Cochrane Collaboration for data analyses. Studies were stratified by the types of comparisons. We will express dichotomous data as risk ratio (RR)and its 95% confidence intervals (CI). Continuous outcome will be presented as mean difference (MD)and its 95% CI. Heterogeneity was recognized significant when $I^2 \geqslant 50\%$. Fixed effects model was used if there is no significant heterogeneity of the data; random effects model was used if significant heterogeneity existed ($50\% < I^2 < 85\%$). Sensitive analysis would be used if there was any heterogeneity (including differences of clinical characteristics among trials and the statistical heterogeneity); subgroup analysis would be used in patients prescribed Xuesaitong softy capsule. Publication bias was explored using a funnel plot.

RESULTS

1 Description of Included Trials

17 RCTs (17 papers)[19,21–36] were included. All of the papers were published in Chinese and 2 were in postgraduate dissertations (unpublished study)[23,24]. The whole process of trials selection was demonstrated in Figure 1. The characteristics of included trials were listed in Table 1.

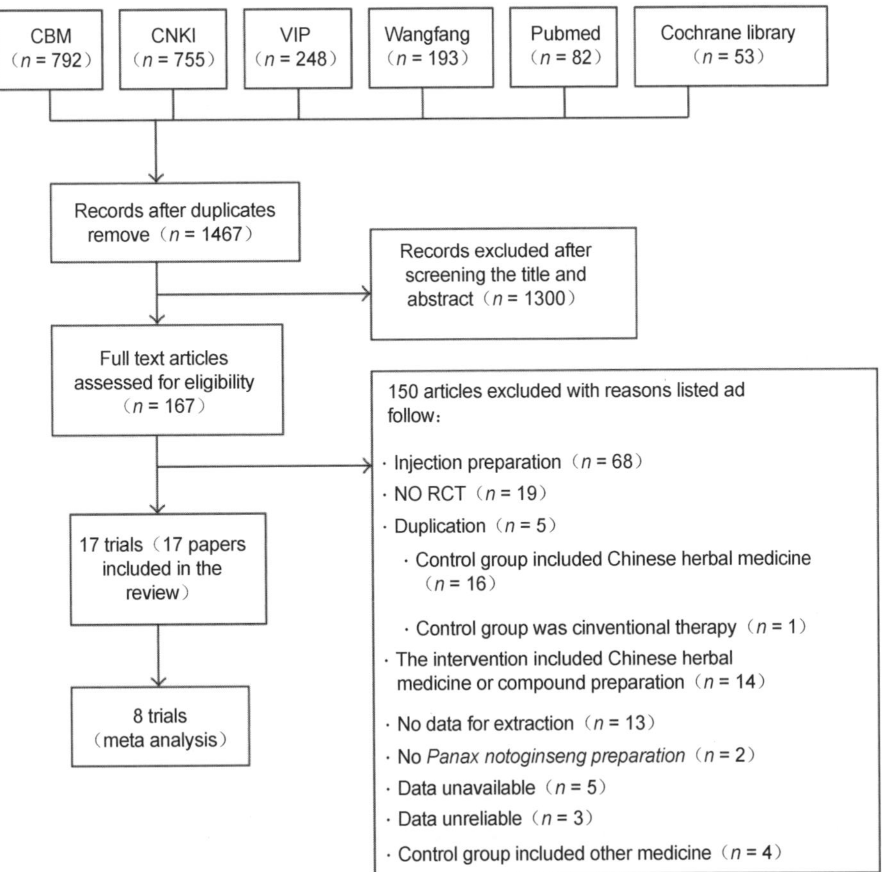

Figure 1 The Process of Included and Excluded Studies

1747 Participants were included (864 in the intervention group and 883 in the control group). 906 males and 581 females were included in 17 trials (two of the trials did not report the number in each gender group). A total of 7 criteria of CHD (including ACS)were involved. 5 trials[21,27,30,33,36] did not introduce criteria of CHD but mentioned that "patients with CHD were eligible to be included." One trial[23] included patients who need to take percutaneous coronary intervention (PCI)the next day; 8 trials[19,21,22,24,27,28,31,33] included patients with unstable angina; 2 trials[34,35] included patients with stable angina pectoris; 1 trial[25] included patients with either stable angina or unstable angina; the other 5 trials[26,29,30,32,36] did not introduce the types of CHD, but two of them recruited hospitalized patients[29,32].

Patients in 11 trials[19,21-23,26-29,31,33,36] were prescribed Xuesaitong softy capsule 2 tablet (120 mg, 60 mg *Panax notoginseng* Saponins [PNS] in each capsule)BID (regulation was conducted for the course); patients in 2 trials[32,35] were prescribed Xuesaitong softy capsule 2 tablet (120 mg, 60 mg PNS in each capsule)TID; patients in 1 trial[34] were prescribed Sanqi guanxinning pills 2–4 pills (100 mg PNS in each pill)TID; 1 trial[25] prescribed PNS tablets 2–4 pill (50 mg PNS in each pill)TID, oral administration or sublingual administration, 2 trials[26,30] used sanqi power (the purity is unclear)in the treatment group. The treatment course of treatment ranged from 7 days to 6 months.

There were 2 comparisons in the review according to various control groups: (1)*Panax notoginseng* preparations and conventional therapy versus conventional therapy (15 trials)[19,21–24,26–29,31–36]; (2)*Panax notoginseng* preparations and conventional therapy versus nitrates and conventional therapy (2 trials)[25,30]. Two trials[24,28] were designed as three groups and four groups, respectively. Wang et al. [28] designed three groups with 2 comparisons: *Panax notoginseng* preparations and conventional therapy versus conventional therapy; *Panax notoginseng* preparations and trimethazine and conventional therapy versus conventional therapy; however, we extracted the data of first comparison for inclusion criteria. Ji and Zhang[24] designed four groups with 3 comparisons: *Panax notoginseng* coarse power and conventional therapy versus conventional therapy; *Panax notoginseng* semi-micron power and conventional therapy versus conventional therapy; *Panax notoginseng* micron power and conventional therapy versus conventional therapy; however, we summed up the three groups included *Panax notoginseng* as intervention group and conventional therapy as control group for data analysis.

2 Methodological Quality of Included Trials

According to the criteria introduced above, no trial was evaluated as low risk of bias. Only one trial of the 17 trials reported the method to generate the allocation sequence (random number table)[23]. Two trials were assessed as having adequate concealment (concealed letter cover)[19,23]. No trial reported blinding method. One trial[31] reported the result of follow up. No trial reported information on withdrawal/dropout. All of trials provided baseline data for the comparability among groups. The results of the assessment of risk of bias are presented in a "risk of bias summary" figure produced by Revman 5.1 automatically (Figure 2).

3 (Tables 2 and 3)

3.1 Cardiovascular Mortality

There was only1 trial[31] that reported the cardiovascular mortality in the comparisons *Panax notoginseng* preparations (Xuesaitong softy capsule)and conventional therapy versus conventional therapy with no significant difference between the two groups [RR 0.50; 95% CI 0.05 to 5.34; 1 trial, n=100]. In the followup of 4 months, 2 patients died of heart failure in the conventional therapy group and 1 patient died of arrhythmia in the combined therapy group.

3.2 Incidence of Myocardial Infarction (MI)

There were 2 studies[28,31] reporting MI incidence in one comparison. Compared with no intervention on the basis of conventional therapy, *Panax notoginseng* preparations (Xuesaitong softy capsule)showed no significant reduction of incidence of MI (RR 0.17; 95% CI 0.02 to 1.37; 2 trials)[28,31].

3.3 Incidence of Intractable Angina Pectoris

One trial[28] reported the intractable angina pectoris in 2 different comparisons. In the comparisons of *Panax notoginseng* prepa-ration (Xuesaitong softy capsule)and conventional therapy versus conventional therapy, *Panax notoginseng* preparation (Xuesaitong softy capsule)showed no significant difference in controlling intractable angina pectoris.

3.4 Rehospitalization for Unstable Angina

There was 1 trial[23] reporting rehospitalization. Compared with no treatment on the basis of conventional therapy, *Panax notoginseng* preparation (Xuesaitong softy capsule)showed no significant difference in the number of rehospitalization (RR 0.33; 95% CI 0.04 to 3.03; 1 trial).

3.5 Recurrence of Angina Pectoris

One trial[23] reported recurrence of angina pectoris. Compared with no treatment on the basis of conventional therapy, *Panax notoginseng* preparation (Xuesaitong softy capsule)showed significant difference in reducing recurrence of angina pectoris (RR 0.38； 95% CI 0.16 to 0.94； 1 trial).

3.6 Reduction of Nitroglycerin

The definition of successful nitroglycerin reduction was that the patients in the trial stopped using nitroglycerin or the dosage of nitroglycerin was cut off more than 50% after the trial. Two trials[24,30] reported the condition of nitroglycerin. The results showed no significant improvement of *Panax notoginseng* preparation comparing with no treatment on the basis of conventional therapy (RR 1.41； 95% CI 0.89 to 2.24； 2 trials, n=250).

3.7 Angina Pectoris Alleviation

We defined the efficacy of angina pectoris as alleviation of more than 50%. There were 7 studies[22,24,27,29,31–33] reporting angina pectoris alleviation. The results showed significant improvement of *Panax notoginseng* preparations as compared with no treatment on the basis of conventional therapy (RR 1.20； 95% CI 1.12 to 1.28； 7 trials, n=791). Subgroup analysis showed that Xuesaitong softy capsule in 6 trials[17,23,25,27–29] was more effective than no treatment in the basis of conventional therapy (RR 1.19； 95% CI 1.11 to 1.27； 6 trials, n=641).

3.8 Electrocardiogram Improvement

We defined the efficacy of ECG as elevation of depressed ST segment of more than 0.05 mv. There were 9 trials[19,22,24–27,31,32,35] reporting the electrocardiogram improvement. The results in 8 trials[19,22,24,26,27,31,32,35] showed significant improvement of *Panax notoginseng* preparation comparing with no treatment on the basis of conventional therapy (RR 1.35； 95% CI 1.19 to 1.53； 8 trials, n=727). 1 trial[25] showed that notoginsenoside pill had no immediate effect on improving ECG compared with isosorbide dinitrate (RR 0.79； 95% CI 0.41 to 1.52； 1 trial, n=80). Subgroup analysis showed that Xuesaitong softy capsule[19,22,26,27,31,32,35] was superior to no treatment on the basis of conventional treatment in improving ECG (RR 1.39； 95% CI 1.21 to 1.59； 7 trials, n=612).

3.9 Angina Pectoris Immediate Effect

There was only one trial[25] which reported the angina pectoris immediate effect. 2 notoginsenoside pills were prescribed in this trial when angina pectoris happened. The criterion was defined as remarkably effective (angina was alleviated in 3 minutes)； effective (angina was alleviated in 3–5 minutes)； no effect (angina was alleviated in more than 5 minutes or need to add other medicines). The result indicated that notoginsenoside pill had similar effect compared with isosorbide dinitrate (RR 0.96； 95% CI 0.81 to 1.15； 1 trial, n=80).

3.10 Angina Pectoris Frequency

There were 4 studies[21,26,29,33] reporting frequency of angina pectoris in the unit of times/week. Compared with no intervention on the basis of conventional therapy, *Panax notoginseng* preparation (Xuesaitong softy capsule)showed a reduction in angina pectoris frequency (MD -2.16； 95% CI -3.02 to -1.30； 4trials, n=572). Sensitivity analysis also indicated that *Panax notoginseng* preparation was effective in reducing angina pectoris frequency (MD -2.34； 95% CI -2.53 to -2.16； 2 trials, n=292)[21,29]. There was 1 trial[33] which reported the frequency of angina pectoris in the unit of times/day. The result indicated that *Panax notoginseng* (Xuesaitong softycapsule)could reduce angina pectoris frequency compared with no treatment on the basis of conventional therapy (MD-2.76； 95% CI -3.87 to -1.65； 1 trial, n=28).

3.11 Angina Pectoris Duration

There was 3 trials[21,29,33] reporting the duration of angina pectoris. The result showed that *Panax notoginseng* preparation (Xuesaitong softy capsule)significantly reduced angina pectoris duration comparing with no treatment on the basis of conventional therapy (MD -2.10； 95% CI -2.58 to -1.62； 3 trials, *n* =472). However, there was significant statistical heterogeneity among these three trials (I^2=91%). Further sensitivity analysis also indicated the benefit of *Panax notoginseng* preparation (Xuesaitong softy capsule)in reducing angina pectoris frequency in hospitalized patients (MD -1.88； 95% CI -2.08 to -1.69； 2 trials, n=292)[21,29].

3.12 Dosage of Nitroglycerol

There were 2 studies[21,26] reporting dosage of nitroglycerol in the unit of mg/week. Compared with no intervention on the basis of conventional therapy, oral *Panax notoginseng* preparation (Xuesaitong softy capsule)showed a reduction of nitroglycerol dosage (MD -1.13； 95% CI -1.70 to -0.56； 2 trials, *n*=212). There was 1 study[36] reporting dosage of nitroglycerol in the unit of mg/day, which showed *Panax notoginseng* preparation (Xuesaitong softy capsule)also reduced the nitroglycerol dosage significantly (MD -4.10； 95% CI -5.58 to -2.62； 1 trial, *n*=28).

4 Publication Bias

A funnel plot analysis of the 7 trials in comparison of *Panax notoginseng* preparation and conventional therapy versus conventional therapy on angina pectoris improvement was conducted and shown in Figure 3； there might be a publication bias in this review for small sample, negative report, and low quality of the included trials.

5 Adverse Events

There were 9 trials[21-25,29-31,33] reporting adverse events (Ads) (Table 4). 6 trials[21–24,29,33] indicated no Ads in the duration of treatment. 1 trial[25] reported reduction of blood pressure and increasement of heart rate (RR 0.03； 95% CI 0.00 to 0.543； 1 trial, *n*=80)； 1 trial[30] reported nausea (RR 3.0； 95% CI 0.13 to 70.16； 1 trialn=48)； 1 trial[30] reported dizziness (RR 0.33； 95% CI 0.01 to 7.80； 1 trial, n=48)； 1 trial[30] reported vomit (RR 0.33； 95% CI 0.01 to 7.80； 1 trial, *n*=48)； 1 trial[31] reported erythra (RR 3.00； 95% CI 0.13 to 71.92； 1 trial, *n*=100). All Ads were not significantly different between the intervention group and the control group (Table 4).

DISCUSSION

This systematic review included 17 RCTs and a total of 1747 participants. The review showed that, (1) comparing with no intervention on the basis of conventional therapy, oral *Panax notoginseng* showed no significant improvement for reducing the cardiovascular events, but it could relieve angina pectoris and related symptoms (including reducing the recurrence of angina pectoris, duration and frequency of angina pectoris, and dosage of nitroglycerol, as well as ECG changes)； (2)oral *Panax notoginseng* showed similar immediate effect on angina pectoris compared with nitrate, but we could not make a significant conclusion from this equivalence due to small sample and low methodological quality trial； (3)The results also showed that oral *Panax notoginseng* was safe for CHD patients according to the information in hand, but it was too limited to make a conclusion for high risk bias and small sample in these trials. Oral *Panax notoginseng* preparations have been used widely for treating CHD in China. Most of the researchers paid more attention to their pharmacological mechanism. Yang et al. comprehensively collected the pharmacological action of *Panax notoginseng* and concluded that it could provide protective effects against cardiovascular diseases through

Table 1 Characteristics of trials.

Study ID	Type of CHD and syndrome	Members (I/C)	Age	Gender (M/F)	Interventions group	Control group	Product	Outcome evaluation
Du and Chen 2009 [21]	UA	56/56	58.8 ± 9.2	62/50	C + Xuesaitong softy capsule, 2 capsules, BID, 4 weeks	Conventional therapy (aspirin, *β* blocker agent, nitroglycerin, CCB, low molecular heparin 5–7 days, antihypertensive drugs and medicine used to treat 2 diabetes)	Xuesaitong softy capsule* (Shenghuo Pharmaceutical Holdings Yunnan kunming, China, Z19990022, containing PNS 60 mg/capsule)	Angina pectoris (extension, frequency, duration), dosage of nitroglycerin, Ads.
Ge and Zhao 2010 [22]	UA	48/48	I: 56; C: 54 (in average)	I: 22/26 V: 25/23	C + Xuesaitong softy capsule, 2 capsules, BID, 4 weeks	Conventional therapy (aspirin, *β* blocker agent, nitroglycerin, CCB, low molecular heparin 5–7 days, antihypertensive drugs and medicine used to treat 2 diabetes)	Xuesaitong softy capsule* (Shenghuo Pharmaceutical Holdings Yunnan kunming China, Z19990022, containing PNS 60 mg/capsule)	Angina pectoris relievement, ECG, Ads.
Han and Chen 2008 [23]	PCI patients	30/30	I: (64.1 ± 10.8); C: (63.7 ± 11.7)	I: 23/7; C: 21/9	C + Xuesaitong softy capsule, 2 capsules, BID in the first 2 weeks, then 1 capsule, TID, 12 weeks	Conventional therapy (anticoagulant agent, antiplatelet agent, medicine for modifying blood lipid, antihypertensive drug and medicine used to treat 2 diabetes)	Xuesaitong softy capsule* (Shenghuo Pharmaceutical Holdings Yunnan kunming, China, Z19990022, containing PNS 60 mg/capsule)	Angina pectoris, rehospitalization
Ji and Zhang 2003 [24]	UA	30/90	I1: (69.0 ± 7.5); I2: (69.2 ± 6.0); I3: (68.5 ± 5.4); C: (68.7 ± 7.3)	I1: 20/10; I2: 18/12; I3: 21/9; C: 17/13	I1: C + coarse power 1 g, TID; I2: C + semi-micron power 1 g, TID; I3: C + micron power 1 g, TID	Isosorbide Mononitrate 20 mg BID; Aspirin 75 mg, QD; Metoprolol 25 mg BID; DTZ 30 mg, TID or QID; Plendil 5 mg QD or BID or Acertil 4 mg, QD for hypertension; Nitroglycerol 0.5 mg subligual administration or nitroglycerol injection 10 mg, iv.	*Panax notoginseng* coarse power: WF-2000 pulverizer; *Panax notoginseng* micron power: BFM-6 pulverizer; *Panax notoginseng* semi-micron power: BFM-6 pulverizer and starch.	Efficacy of Angina pectoris, ECG, symptoms, Ads
Liu et al. 2008 [19]	UA and BSS	30/30	I: (64.6 ± 5.4); C: (63.6 ± 4.5)	Unclear	C + Xuesaitong softy capsule, 2 capsules, BID, 4 weeks	Conventional therapy (no detail)	Xuesaitong softy capsule (Yunnan weihe Pharmaceutical company, containing PNS 60 mg/capsule)	Syndrome, pulse, heart rate, heart rhythm, blood pressure, angina pectoris, ECG
Meng 2003 [25]	UA and SA	60/20	I: (61–78); C: (61–78)	I: 44/16 C: 16/4	PNS pill, 2 tablets, sublingual when angina pectoris attacked	Isosorbide dinitrate when angina pectoris attacked (5 mg/tables)	PNS pill, 2 tablet**, Sublingual	Duration of angina pectoris relievement, blood pressure, heart rate, and ECG after 2 hours of prescription.
Song et al. 2005 [26]	Unclear	50/50	I: (36–77), (61.21 ± 5.73); C: (38–74), (60.77 ± 5.61) in average	I: 31/19 C: 33/17	C + Xuesaitong softy capsule, 2 capsules, BID, 4 weeks	Conventional therapy (aspirin, *β* blocker agent, nitroglycerin, CCB, low molecular heparin 5–7 days, antihypertensive drugs and medicine used to treat diabetes)	Xuesaitong softy capsule* (Shenghuo Pharmaceutical Holdings Yunnan kunming, China)	Efficacy of angina pectoris, ECG, dosage of nitroglycerin
Wan 2011 [27]	UA	26/26	I: 65.7 in average; C: No report	I: 15/11 C: 13/13	C + Xuesaitong softy capsule, 2 capsules, BID, 4 weeks	Conventional therapy (aspirin, *β* blocker agent and et al.)	Xuesaitong softy capsule* (Shenghuo Pharmaceutical Holdings Yunnan kunming, China)	Efficacy of angina pectoris, ECG
Wang et al. 2009 [28]	UA	100/100	36–75	Unclear	**T1:C1** + Xuesaitong softy capsule, 2 capsules, BID, 30 days; **T2:C2** + trimetazidine + Xuesaitong softy capsule, 2 capsules, BID, 30 days;	C1: conventional therapy (ant platelet, Nitrates, CCB, *β* blocker agent, statin, trimetazidine); C2: Conventional therapy (ant platelet, Nitrates, CCB, *β* blocker agent, astatine)	Xuesaitong softy capsule	Efficacy of angina pectoris and cardiovascular events in 30 d followup.
Wei 2010 [29]	Unclear	90/90	60.4 ± 3.5	113/67	C + Xuesaitong softy capsule, 2 capsules, BID, 4 weeks	Conventional therapy (Nitrate, *β* blocker agent, CCB, low molecular heparin)	Xuesaitong softy capsule* (Shenghuo Pharmaceutical Holdings Yunnan kunming, China)	Angina pectoris, Ads, ECG
Yan 2005 [30]	Unclear	24/24	I: (48–67), 60 in average; C: (47–69), 62 in average	I: 13/11 C: 14/10	Isosorbide mononitrat 5 mg TID + *Panax notoginseng* power 6 g BID, 7 days	Isosorbide Mononitrate, 10 mg, TID	*Panax notoginseng* power 6 g BID	Efficacy of angina pectoris, ECG, ADs
Yu 2010 [31]	UA	50/50	I: (64.18 ± 12.13); C: (62.8 ± 10.8)	I: 29/21 C: 28/22	C + Xuesaitong softy capsule, 2 capsules, BID, 4 weeks	Conventional therapy (aspirin, *β* blocker agent, nitroglycerin, CCB and et al.)	Xuesaitong softy capsule* (Shenghuo Pharmaceutical Holdings Yunnan kunming, China)	Efficacy of angina pectoris, ECG, ADs, cardiovascular events
Zhou and Bai 2009 [32]	Unclear	43/43	65 ± 6	I: 32/11 C: 34/9	C + Xuesaitong softy capsule, 2 capsules, TID, 4 weeks	Conventional therapy (nitrate, Metoprolol, aspirin, Nitroglycerin if necessary)	Xuesaitong softy capsule$^{\Delta}$ (Luotai, Kunming Pharmaceutical incorporated corporation)	Efficacy of angina pectoris, ECG

BSS: blood stasis syndrome ; PNS: *panax notoginseng* saponins ; I: intervention group ; C: control group ; DTZ: dilthiazem ; ECG: electrocardiogram ; Ads: adverse event. *Xuesaitong softy capsule produced by Shenghuo Pharmaceutical Holdings, Yunnan kunming, China (Z19990022)contains PNS 60 mg/capsule. **There was no purity of PNS pill in this trial. According to the internet, PNS pill produced by Yunnan Weihe Pharmaceutical company contains PNS 50 mg/pill. $^{\Delta}$Xuesaitong softy capsule$^{\Delta}$ (Luotai, Kunming Pharmaceutical incorporated corporation, China)contains PNS 100 mg/capsule. $^{\Delta}$Sanqi guanxinning tablets (Z53020028), there is no introduction in the paper about the composition and the purity. According to the internet, Sanqi guanxinning producted by Yunnan JinBuHuan (group)Co., ltd. pharmaceutical branch, containing 100 mg PNS/tablet.

Continued

Study ID	Type of CHD and syndrome	Members (I/C)	Age	Gender (M/F)	Interventions group	Control group	Product	Outcome evaluation
Kuang et al. 2011 [33]	UA	90/90	I: (56.3 ± 6.9); C: (57.1 ± 7.2)	I: 47/43 C: 46/44	C + Xuesaitong softy capsule, 2 capsules, BID, 4 weeks	Conventional therapy (aspirin, β blocker agent, nitroglycerin, CCB, low molecular dextran, and others)	Xuesaitong softy capsule* (Shenghuo Pharmaceutical Holdings Yunnan kunming, China, containing PNS 60 mg/capsule)	Efficacy of angina pectoris, ECG, ADs
Bao 2011 [34]	SA, BSS	63/64	I: (52.3 in average); C: (51.6 in average)	I: 35/28 C: 37/27	C + Sanqi guanxinning tablets (Z53020028), 2–4 tables, TID, 6 weeks	Conventional therapy (nitroglycerin, β blocker agent, and others)	Sanqi guanxinning tablets$^{\Delta\Delta}$ (Z53020028)	Efficacy of angina pectoris
Zhao and Li 2012 [35]	SA	60/58	I: (57.4 ± 9.9, 42–70); C: (59.6 ± 9.7, 41–68)	I: 38/22 C: 40/18	C + Xuesaitong softy capsule, 2 capsules, TID, 4 weeks	Conventional therapy (aspirin, J20080078, 100 mg) Qd, isosorbide mononitrate (H20030418, 60 mg Qd), β blocker (H32025391)	Xuesaitong softy capsule* (Shenghuo Pharmaceutical Holdings Yunnan kunming, China, Z19990022)	Efficacy of ECG
Yang 2012 [36]	Unclear	14/14	(67.3 ± 1.1), 51–78	19/9	C + Xuesaitong softy capsule, 2 capsules BID in the first two weeks, 1 capsule BID in the later weeks	Conventional therapy (aspirin, β blocker agent, nitroglycerin, CCB, and others)	Xuesaitong softy capsule* (Shenghuo Pharmaceutical Holdings Yunnan kunming, China, containing PNS 60 mg/capsule)	Frequency of angina pectoris, dosage of nitroglycerin, frequency of premature ventricular contraction

many pharmacological mechanisms including improving myocardial microcirculation, reducing arrhythmia, regulating blood lipid, preventing atherosclerosis, lower-ing blood pressure, and antishock[37]. Du et al. summarized the experiments on *Panax notoginseng* for MI and concluded that *Panax notoginseng* could inhibit the inflammatory reaction and improve ischemia reperfusion injury in patients with MI[38]. Chan et al. concluded

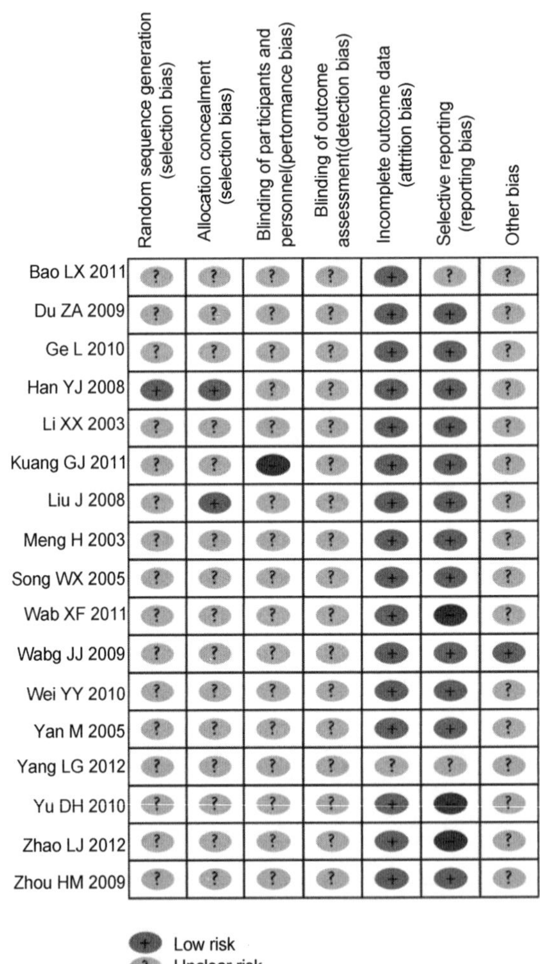

Figure 2　Risk of Bias Summary

that Trilinolein purified from *Panax notoginseng* could provide protective effects against cardiovascular disease including reducing thrombogenicity and arrhythmia and increase erythrocyte deformability. It was also an antioxidant which could counteract free radical damage associated with atherogenesis and myocardial damage[39]. All these experiments provided us laboratory evidence on protective effect of *Panax notoginseng*

Table 2 Analysis of Cardiovascular Events and Angina Pectoris

Outcomes (comparisons)	Treatment group (n/N)	Control group (n/N)	RR	95% CI
(1) Cardiovascular mortality				
Panax notoginseng preparation and conventional therapy versus conventional therapy				
Yu 2010 [31]	1/50	2/50	0.50	[0.05, 5.34]
(2) Myocardial infarction incidence				
Panax notoginseng preparation and conventional therapy versus conventional therapy				
Wang et al. 2009 [28]	0/100	3/100	0.14	[0.01, 2.73]
Yu 2010 [31]	0/50	2/50	0.20	[0.01, 4.06]
	Overall all (FEM, I^2 = 0%)		0.17	[0.02, 1.37]
(3) Incidence of intractable angina pectoris				
Panax notoginseng preparation and conventional therapy versus conventional therapy				
Wang et al. 2009 [28]	6/100	11/100	0.55	[0.21, 1.42]
(4) Rehospitalization incidence for unstable angina				
Panax notoginseng preparation and conventional therapy versus conventional therapy				
Han and Chen 2008 [23]	1/30	3/30	0.33	[0.04, 3.03]
(5) Recurrence of angina pectoris				
Panax notoginseng preparation and conventional therapy versus conventional therapy				
Han and Chen 2008 [23]	5/30	13/30	0.38	[0.16, 0.94]
(6) Nitroglycerol decreasement				
Panax notoginseng preparation and conventional therapy versus conventional therapy				
Ji and Zhang 2003 [24]	19/30	65/120	1.17	[0.85, 1.61]
Song et al. 2005 [26]	26/50	14/50	1.86	[1.11, 3.12]
	Overall all (REM, I^2 = 59%)		1.41	[0.89, 2.24]
(7) Angina pectoris relievement				
Panax notoginseng preparation and conventional therapy versus conventional therapy				
Ge and Zhao 2010 [22]	44/48	36/48	1.22	[1.02, 1.47]
Ji and Zhang 2003 [24]	24/30	77/120	1.25	[1.00, 1.56]
Wan 2011 [27]	24/26	19/26	1.26	[0.98, 1.64]
Wei 2010 [29]	84/90	75/90	1.12	[1.01, 1.25]
Yu 2010 [31]	48/50	43/50	1.12	[0.98, 1.27]
Zhou and Bai 2009 [32]	37/43	30/43	1.23	[0.98, 1.55]
Bao 2011 [34]	57/63	45/64	1.29	[1.08, 1.54]
	Overall all (FEM, I^2 = 0%, N = 791)		1.20	[1.12, 1.28]
Subgroup analysis (excluded Ji and Zhang [24])	Overall (FEM, I^2 = 0%, N = 641)		1.19	[1.11, 1.27]
(8) Electrocardiogram improvement				
15.1 *Panax notoginseng* preparation and conventional therapy versus conventional therapy				
Ge and Zhao 2010 [22]	42/48	36/48	1.17	[0.96, 1.42]
Ji and Zhang 2003 [24]	67/86	19/29	1.19	[0.89, 1.58]
Liu et al. 2008 [19]	12/30	8/30	1.50	[0.72, 3.14]
Song et al. 2005 [26]	36/50	27/50	1.33	[0.98, 1.82]
Wan 2011 [27]	19/26	12/26	1.58	[0.98, 2.55]
Yu 2010 [31]	28/50	19/50	1.47	[0.96, 2.27]
Zhou and Bai 2009 [32]	35/43	27/43	1.30	[0.99, 1.70]
Zhao and Li 2012 [35]	24/60	12/58	1.93	[1.07, 3.49]
	Overall all (FEM, I^2 = 0%, N = 727)		1.35	[1.19, 1.53]
Subgroup analysis (excluded Ji and Zhang [24])	Overall (FEM, I^2 = 0%, N = 612)		1.39	[1.21, 1.59]
15.2 *Panax notoginseng* preparation and conventional therapy versus isosorbide dinitrate and conventional therapy				
Meng 2003 [25]	19/60	8/20	0.79	[0.41, 1.52]
(9) Angina pectoris immediate effect				
Panax notoginseng preparation and conventional therapy versus isosorbide dinitrate and conventional therapy				
Meng 2003 [25]	52/60	18/20	0.96	[0.81, 1.15]

FEM: fixed effects model；REM: random effects model；RR: relative risk；CI: credibility interval.

Table 3 Analysis of Efficacy of Angina Pectoris

Angina pectoris (comparison)	Intervention group Mean	Intervention group SD	Control group Mean	Control group SD	Weight (%)	MD	95% CI
(1) Angina pectoris frequency							
Panax notoginseng preparation and conventional therapy versus conventional therapy (times/week)							
Du and Chen 2009 [21]	3.24	0.61	5.63	0.92	33.6	−2.39	[−2.68, −2.10]
Kuang et al. 2011 [33]	3.53	0.61	6.83	1.92	14.1	−3.30	[−3.72, −2.88]
Song et al. 2005 [26]	0.75	0.79	1.36	1.31	32.4	−0.61	[−1.03, −0.19]
Wei 2010 [29]	4.27	0.87	6.58	0.75	34.0	−2.31	[−2.55, −2.07]
	Overall (REM, I^2 = 96%, N = 572)				**100**	**−2.16**	**[−3.02, −1.30]**
Sensitive analysis (excluded Song et al. 2005 [26] Kuang et al. [33])	Overall (FEM, I^2 = 0%, N = 292)					**−2.34**	**[−2.53, −2.16]**
Panax notoginseng preparation and conventional therapy versus conventional therapy (times/day)							
Yang 2012 [36]	1.22	0.97	3.98	1.89	28	−2.76	[−3.87, −1.65]
(2) Angina pectoris duration (minute/time)							
Panax notoginseng preparation and conventional therapy versus conventional therapy							
Du and Chen 2009 [21]	2.86	0.72	4.82	0.63	60.7	−1.96	[−2.21, −1.71]
Kuang et al. 2011 [33]	2.23	0.62	4.78	0.83	45.4	−2.55	[−2.76, −2.34]
Wei 2010 [29]	4.56	1.08	6.32	1.05	39.3	−1.76	[−2.07, −1.45]
	Overall (REM, I^2 = 91%, N = 472)				100	−2.10	[−2.58, −1.62]
Sensitive analysis (excluded Kuang et al., [33])	Overall (FEM, I^2 = 0%, N = 292)					**−1.88**	**[−2.08, −1.69]**
(3) Dosage of nitroglycerol							
Panax notoginseng preparation and conventional therapy versus conventional therapy (mg/week)							
Du and Chen 2009 [21]	2.94	2.26	4.26	1.94	53.0	−1.32	[−2.10, −0.54]
Song et al. 2005 [26]	2.95	2.25	3.87	1.97	47.0	−0.92	[−1.75, −0.09]
	Overall (FEM, I^2 = 0%, N = 212)				100	−1.13	[−1.70, −0.56]
Panax notoginseng preparation and conventional therapy versus conventional therapy (mg/day)							
Yang 2012 [36]	1.3	0.4	5.4	2.8	100	−4.10	[−5.58, −2.62]

FEM: fixed effects model；REM: random effects model；MD: mean difference；CI: credibility interval.

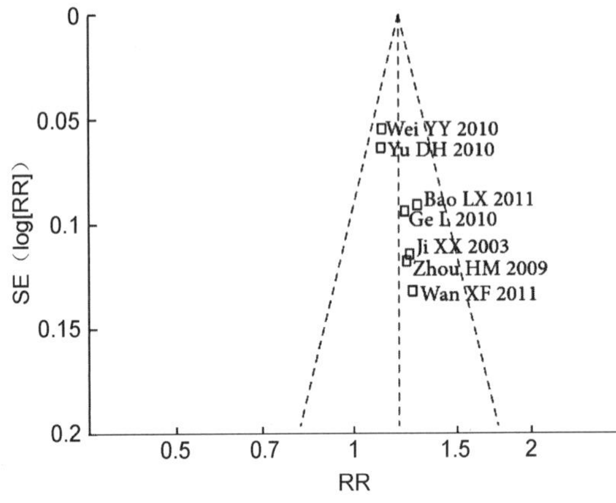

Figure 3 Funnel Plot of Comparison: Conventional Therapy and *Panax notoginseng* preparation versus Conventional Therapy, outcome: 3.3. 7 Angina Pectoris Alleviation

Table 4 Adverse Events

Study ID	ADs
Du and Chen 2009 [21]	No abnormal changes appeared and no Ads was reported in the trial.
Ge and Zhao 2010 [22]	Blood regular test, urine regular test, and blood biochemistry test had no changes compared with the previous.
Han and Chen 2008 [23]	No serious Ads were reported in the trial; blood, urine, and stool routine tests, blood biochemistry test had no changes comparing with the previous.
Ji and Zhang 2003 [24]	Blood, urine, and stool routine tests, and blood biochemistry test had no changes compared with the previous. No Ads was reported in the trial.
Meng 2003 [25]	Reduction of blood pressure and increasement of heart rate: intervention group: 0/60; control group: 5/20. RR: 0.03. 95% CI: [0.00, 0.54].
Wei 2010 [29]	Blood, urine, and stool routine tests, and blood biochemistry test had no changes compared with the previous. No Ads was reported in the trial.
Yan 2005 [30]	Nausea: intervention group (1/24), control group (0/24), RR: 3.0, 95% CI: [0.13, 70.16]. Dizziness: intervention group (0/24), control group (1/24), RR: 0.33, 95% CI: [0.01, 7.80]. Vomit: intervention group (0/24), control group (1/24), RR: 0.33, 95% CI: [0.01, 7.80].
Yu 2010 [31]	Erythra: intervention group (1/50), control group: (0/50). RR: 3.00; 95% CI: [0.13, 71.92].
Kuang et al. 2011 [33]	No abnormal changes appeared and no Ads was reported in the trial.

for CHD. Although many clinical trials were conducted on effect of oral *Panax notoginseng* preparations for CHD, there was no critical appraisal for these up to now. There was still no enough evidence for clinicians to prescribe oral *Panax notoginseng* preparations in CHD patients.

The impact of this review was to take a light on oral *Panax notoginseng* for CHD. Although it failed to prove the protective effect of *Panax notoginseng* on major cardiovascular events (cardiovascular mortality, MI incidence, and rehospitalization), it demonstrated that *Panax notoginseng* preparation might be recommended for improving symptoms of angina pectoris.

However, before translating the conclusion of this review to clinical practitioners, we have to consider the following weaknesses in this review. (1)Firstly, the "randomization" was not clear in most of the trials for insucient reporting of generation methods of the allocation sequence, allocation concealment. Most trials stated only that patients were randomly assigned. (2)Secondly, no trial used placebo in control group, most of trials did not introduce double blind in this review, and one trial introduced blinding of outcome assessment. Therefore, in nonplacebo-controlled and nondouble blind trials, placebo effects may add to the complexity of interpreting the conclusion. (3)Thirdly, most of the trials did not introduce the study plan, and attrition bias and selective reporting bias might exist in this conclusion. (4)Fourthly, funnel plot indicated that publication bias would exist in this review. The reasons we considered were as follows: we only selected trials published in Chinese and English trials published in other languages or originated from other countries might be omitted; we only identified unpublished studies from conference paper or academic thesis, and negative trials might not be reported and induce publication bias.

Although this review suggested some benefit of *Panax notoginseng* preparation for CHD, the recommendation should be discreet due to poor quality and high risk bias of these trials, further rigorously designed, and well reported RCTs are still needed to prove the effectiveness and safety of Panax notoginseng preparation for CHD.

CONCLUSION

In this systematic review, oral *Panax notoginseng* preparation did not show benefit on reducing major cardiovascular events and relapse (including cardiovascular death, MI incidence, incidence of intractable angina pectoris, and rehospitalization), although it was effective in alleviating angina pectoris (including the recurrence, frequency, and duration of angina pectoris, ECG presentation, and dosage of nitroglycerin) with low adverse reaction. However, the small sample size and potential bias of most trials influence the convincingness of this conclusion. Before recommending oral *Panax notoginseng* preparation as an alternative herbal medicine in CHD patients, more rigorous trials with high quality are needed to prove the benefit of oral *Panax notoginseng* preparation and provide high level of evidence.

REFERENCES

[1] American Heart Association. Heart disease and stroke statistics—2007 update. 2007, http: //www. americanheart. org/ statistics.

[2] World Heart Organization. The World Health Report 2003— Shaping the Future. 2003, http: //www. who. int/whr/2003/en/.

[3] http: //www. who. int/cardiovascular diseases/en/, http: //www. who. int/cardiovascular diseases/resources/atlas/en/.

[4] Xu H, Chen KJ. Integrative medicine: the experience from China[J]. Journal of Alternative and Complementary Medicine, 2008, 14 (1): 3-7.

[5] Robinson N, Integrative medicine—traditional Chinese medicine, a model? [J] Chinese Journal of Integrative Medicine, 2011, 17 (1): 21-25.

[6] Xu H, Chen KJ. Integrating traditional medicine with biomedicine towards a patient-centered healthcare system[J]. Chinese Journal of Integrative Medicine, 2011, 17 (2): 83-84.

[7] Dobos G, Tao I. The model of western integrative medicine the role of chinese medicine[J]. Chinese Journal of Integrative Medicine, 2011, 17 (1): 11-20.

[8] Balasubramani S. P, Venkatasubramanian P, Kukkupuni S. K, et al. Plant-based Rasayana drugs from Ayurveda[J]. Chinese Journal of Integrative Medicine, 2011, 17 (2): 88-94.

[9] Wang Q, Wu TX, Chen XY et al. Puerarin injection for unstable angina pectoris[J]. Cochrane Library, 2009.

[10] Wu TX, Ni J, Wei JF. Danshen (Chinese medicinal herb)preparations for acute myocardial infarction[J]. Cochrane Library, 2009.

[11] Wu TX, Harrison R. A, Chen XY, et al. Tongxinluo (tong xin luo or tong-xin-luo)capsule for unstable angina pectoris[J]. Cochrane Library, 2009.

[12] Wang G, Wang L, Xiong ZY, et al. Compound salvia pellet, a traditional Chinese medicine, for the treatment of chronic stable angina pectoris compared with nitrates: a meta-analysis[J]. Medical Science Monitor, 2006, 12 (1): SR1-SR7.

[13] Duan X, Zhou L, Wu T, et al. Chinese herbal medicine suxiao jiuxin wan for angina pectoris[J]. Cochrane Database of Systematic Reviews, 2008 (1), Article ID CD004473.

[14] Zhuo Q, Yuan Z, Chen H, and T. Wu et al. Traditional Chinese herbal products for stable angina[J]. Cochrane Database of Systematic Reviews, 2010 (5), Article ID CD004468.

[15] Guo JW, Li LM, Qiu GQ, et al. Effects of Panax notoginseng saponins on ACE2 and TNF-alpha in rats with post-myocardial infarction-ventricular remodeling[J]. Zhong Yao Cai, 2010.33 (1): 89-92.

[16] Wan JB, Lee S. M. Y, Wang JD, et al. Panax notogin-seng reduces atherosclerotic lesions in ApoE-deficient mice expression and monocyte adhesion[J]. Journal of Agricultural and Food Chemistry, 2009.57 (15): 6692-6697.

[17] Zhang ZR, Li X, Wang YH, et al. Angiogenic effect of total saponins extracted from root and flower of panax notoginseng in zebrafish model[J]. Universitatis Traditionis Medicalis Sinensis Pharmacologiaeque Shanghai, 2013, 27 (1): 45-49.

[18] Chen XY, Zhou MK, Li QF, et al. Sanchi for acute ischaemic stroke[J]. Cochrane Library, 2008.

[19] Liu X, Li J, Yang G, et al. Study on effect of promoting blood circulation drugs components in treating unstable angina in patients with blood stasis inflammatory levels[J]. Zhongguo Zhongyao Zazhi, 2008, 33 (24): 2950-2953.

[20] Higgins J. P. T, Green S. Cochrane handbook for systematic reviews of interventions, version 5.0. 2 [updated september 2009]. The Cochrane Collaboration, 2011, http: //www. cochrane-handbook. org/.

[21] Du Z, Chen GL. Effect of Xuesaitong softy capsule for angina pectoris on endothelin and C reaction protein[J] . Chinese Journal of Modern Drug Application, 2009, 3 (4): 140-141.

[22] Ge L, Zhao SZ. Effect of Xuesaitong softy capsule for ustable angina pectoris[J]. Hebei Journal of Traditional Chinese Medicine, 2010, 32 (8): 1223-1224.

[23] Han YJ, Chen QX. Clinical study on intervention of Xuesaitong soft capsule on coronary heart disease patients after PCI [M. S. thesis]. Guangzhou University of Chinese Medicine, 2008.

[24] Ji XX, Zhang WG. Clinical and experimental study of micro-powder of panax notoginseng on both treating unstable angina and protecting in isoproterenol induced myocardial necrosis in rats [M. S. thesis]. Shandong University of Chinese Medicine, 2003.

[25] Meng H. Analysis of Panax Notoginseng Saponins tablets for 60 patients with angina pectoris[J]. Academic Journal of Traditional Chinese Medicine, 2003, 21 (6): 1007.

[26] WX, Wang ZT, Zeng SY. Clinical observation of Xuesaitong soft capsule for angina pectoris[J]. Journal of Emergency in Traditional Chinese Medicine, 2005, 14 (8): 707-708.

[27] Wan XF. Effect observation of Xuesaitong soft capsule for unstable angina pectoris[J]. Practical Journal of Cardiac Cerebral Pneumal and Vascular Disease, 2011, 19 (10): 1768.

[28] Wang JJ, Zhang SL, Liu QY, et al. Clinical effect of Xuesaitong soft capsule and trimetazidine for unstable angina pectoris[J]. Shandong Medical Journal, 2009, 49 (37): 92-93.

[29] Wei YY. Effect of Xuesaitong soft capsule for 90 patients with angina pectoris[J]. Chinese Journal of Modern Drug Application, 2010, 4 (23): 20-21.

[30] Yan M. Report of isosorbide 5-mononitrate and panax noto-ginseng for angina pectoris[J]. Gansu Journal of Traditional Chinese Medicine, 2005, 18 (1): 28.

[31] Yu DH. Clinical effect analysis of Xuezhikang soft capsule for unstable angina pectoris[J]. Proceeding of Clinical Medicine, 2010, 19 (1): 38-39.

[32] Zhou HM, Bai J. Effect of Xuesaitong soft capsule for angina pectoris and influence on serum endothelin and nitric oxide[J]. Chinese Journal of Practical Meicine, 2009, 36 (14): 82.

[33] Kuang GJ, Huang ZJ, Bai CW et al. Effect of Xuesaitong soft capsule for unstable angina pectorisand inhibits TNF-induced endothelial adhesion moleculeand influence on Electrocardiogram QT dispersion degree[J]. Lingnan Journal of Emergency Medicine, 2011, 16 (6): 455-456.

[34] Bao LX. Clinical trial of Sanqi Guanxinning for stable angina pectoris[J]. Journal of Chinese Medicine, 2011, 26 (162): 1371-1372.

[35] Zhao LJ, Li FE. Clinical observation of Xuesaitong softy capsule for 60 patients with stable angina pectoris[J]. Hebei Journal of Traditional Chinese Medicine, 2012, 34 (7): 1049- 1050.

[36] Yang LG. Clinical effect of xuesaitong for coronary heart disease[J]. Contemporary Medicine, 2012, 18 (35): 79-80.

[37] Yang ZG, Chen AQ, Yu SD. Research Progress of pharmacological actions of Panax notoginseng[J]. Shanghai Journal of Traditional Chinese Medicine, 2005, 39 (4): 59-62.

[38] Du WS, Xiao XF, Zhu MD, et al. Inflammatory response, damage, repairing in necrotic area and effect of Panax notogin-seng for patient with myocardial infarction[J]. Lishizhen Medicine and Materia Medica Research, 2010.21 (10): 2560-2562.

[39] Chan P, Thomas G. N, Tomlinson B. Protective effects of trilinolein extracted from Panax notoginseng against cardiovascular disease[J]. Acta Pharmacologica Sinica, 2002, 23 (12): 1157-1162.

First published: Shang QH, Xu H, Liu ZL, Chen KJ, Liu JP. Oral Panax notoginseng preparation for coronary heart disease: a systematic review of randomized controlled trials. [J]. Evidence-Based Complementray and Alternative Medicine, 2013, 2013 (1): 940125.

Effect of Qingxuan Granule (清眩颗粒)on Blood Pressure Variability of Hypertensive Patients with and without Obstructive Sleep Apnea

CHEN Yi-yu, CHEN Jing, ZHANG Jing-chun, and CHEN Ke-ji

Hypertension is closely related to obstructive sleep apnea (OSA). In 1984, Lavie, et al[1] found out that there were 11 hypertensive patients suffered from OSA in total 16 hypertensive patients. In 2000, Peppard, et al[2] found out that OSA patients had a growing risk of hypertension along with the increasing index of apnea and hyponea in the 4-year and 8-year follow-up visit. It is proved that OSA is an independent risk factor of hypertension. About 30% primary hypertension is combined with OSA, and 50% of OSA is associated with hypertension. [3] In 2003, the seventh report of the Joint National Committee on prevention, detection, evaluation, and treatment of high blood pressure had clearly included OSA as an etiological factor of hypertension. [4]

The research of the medicine intervention on hypertensive patients with OSA is significant for target organ protection and cardiovascular diseases prevention. The improvement of blood pressure variability (BPV)and OSA needed to take into account when choosing different hypotensors. In this study Qingxuan Granule (清眩颗粒)was given to the hypertensive patients with or without OSA, and the change of BPV was observed.

METHODS

1 Diagnostic Criteria

1.1 Hypertension Diagnostic Criteria

According to World Health Organization (WHO)/ International Society of Hypertension (ISH)statement on management of hypertension, [5] Guidelines for Prevention and Treatment of Hypertension in China (2005), [6] and Guiding Principle of Clinical Researches on New Drugs of Traditional Chinese Medicine, [7] mild and moderate primary hypertensive patients [systolic blood pressure (SBP)from 140–179 mm Hg, or diastolic blood pressure (DBP)from 90–109 mm Hg] with yin deficiency and yang hyperactivity syndrome were selected. Ambulatory blood pressure monitoring (ABPM)[9027-ABP, SP (a)celabs Medical, USA] was applied before and after treatment for measuring blood pressure.

1.2 OSA Diagnostic Criteria

With the Guideline for Diagnosis and Treatment for Obstructive Sleep Apnea Hypopnea Syndrome in 2002[8] and the Experts Consensus on Obstructive Sleep Apnea and cardio-vascular diseases, [9] the OSA diagnosis criteria include: (1)snoring and irregular breath at night, somnolence during daytime; (2) polysomnography indicated that the OSA and hypopnea would occur more than 30 times during 7 h at night, or the apnea hypopnea index (AHI)is more than 5 times per hour. In this study the portable sleep monitor which was widely accepted in clinical research trials was used before and after treatment for diagnosis of OSA. [10,11]

2 Inclusion Criteria

Hypertensive patients untreated or met the diagnostic criteria after 2-week washout period, aged from 18–75 years old, and signed the informed consent were included.

3 Exclusion Criteria

Those who did not meet the hypertensive inclusion criteria were excluded. Those who snored due to central nervous system diseases or maxillofacial deformity or otolaryngology diseases were excluded.

4 Withdrawal Criteria

The patients who violated the protocol, had poor compliance, needed continuous positive airway pressure (CPAP)or operation immediately were withdrawal from the study.

5 Trial Design

This study adopted the method of stratified, double-blind, and placebo-controlled. Hypertensive patients were assigned to two subgroups, one with OSA group (group A), one without OSA group (group B). Then the patients in group A were randomly assigned to the treatment group (group A1)and the control group (group A2), and the patients in group B were randomly assigned to treatment group (group B1)and control group (group B2). Both treatment groups (groups A1 and B1)received Amlodipine Besylate (5 mg, once daily), and Qingxuan Granule (10.3 g, twice daily); while both control groups (groups A2 and B2)received placebo (10.3 g, twice daily); and Amlodipine Besylate (5 mg, once daily).

The random number table was performed by SAS 9.2, and saved in a sealed envelope in the Medical Statistics Office of Xiyuan Hospital. The patients and investigator were blind in the trial. Each envelop was prepared. Investigation could uncover the emergency envelop with monitor if a serious adverse event happened.

6 Patients Selection

Hypertensive patients from Xiyuan Hospital of China Academy of Chinese Medical Sciences were selected from January 2010 to December 2010 (Figure 1).

7 Drugs and Interventions

The treatment groups (groups A1 and B1)received Amlodipine Besylate (5 mg, once daily)which was provided by Pfizer Pharmaceuticals Ltd., USA and Qingxuan Granule (10.3 g, extracted from the following crude drugs: Cortex Eucommiae 15 g, Ramulus Uncariae cum Uncis 15 g, Rhizoma Gastrodiae 15 g, Radix Scutellariae 7.5 g and Folium Ilicis Latifoliae 7.5 g, twice daily)which was provided by New Green

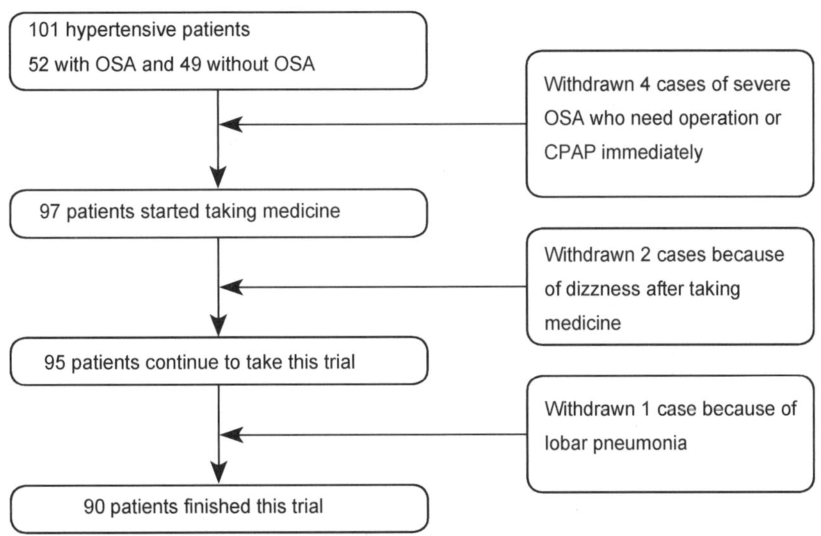

Figure 1 Flow Diagram of Clinical Trial

Pharmaceutical Co., Ltd., Sichuan, China (batch No. 100718206)for successive 2 months. The control group (groups A2 and B2)received Amlodipine Besylate (5 mg, once daily)and placebo (10.3 g, twice daily) for successive 2 months. The placebo was consistent with Qingxuan Granule on appearance, packaging, color, and smell, which was designed and produced by the above mentioned manufacture (New Green Pharmaceutical Co., Ltd., Sichuan, China)and packed by those not participating in the trial.

8 Indicators of Observation

8.1 Mean Value of Blood Pressure (MBP)

The 24-h SBP, DBP, day-time SBP and DBP, and night-time SBP and DBP were detected. The standard of antihypertensive effective rate was as follows: markedly effective: (1)the decrease of DBP was more than 10 mm Hg and reached the normal level, or (2)decrease of DBP was more than 20 mm Hg though above the normal level; effective: (1)the decrease of DBP was less than 10 mm Hg and reached the normal level, or (2) decrease of DBP was between 10–19 mm Hg though above the normal level, or (3)the decrease of SBP was more than 30 mm Hg; ineffective: none of the above standard was achieved.

8.2 Blood Pressure Variability

Blood pressure standard deviation (SD)and coefficient of variation (CV)were applied in this study as blood pressure variability (BPV)indicator. [12,13]

8.3 OSA Indicator

Portable sleep monitor was applied in this study (SW-SM2000CB, Kaidi Thai Company, USA). Apnea index (AI), hypopnea index (HI), AHI, lowest SaO2%, and oxygen desaturation index (ODI)were included in this study.

8.4 Medical Ethics

This study was approved by Ethics Committees of Xiyuan Hospital, China Academy of Chinese Medical Sciences (No. 2010XL016). All patients had signed the information consents before entering the trial, comprehensively understanding the purpose, procedures and possible risks and benefits on participation in this study.

9 Drug Safety Evaluation

The adverse events incidence according to patients' spontaneous report or doctors' direct observation or non-revulsant inquisition; laboratory detection including blood, urine, biochemical indices, and electrocardiogram (ECG).

10 Statistical Analysis

The statistical analysis was performed by SAS 9.2. The measurement data was described as mean ± standard deviation. P-values less than 0.05 were accepted as statistical difference. Independent sample t-test was used for comparison between different groups, and paired sample t-test was applied for comparison before and after treatment in the same group.

In this study the increase or decrease of all indices after treatment were measured by difference (D)-value (D-value = pre-treatment level-post-treatment level)which was accepted as dependent variable Y. D-value was influenced by three independent variables, namely treatment method (considered as factor a), the base level of all indicators before treatment (considered as factor b), and OSA condition (considered as factor c), so covariance analysis of generalized linear models was also applied in this trial: (1)if $Pa > 0.05$, $Pb > 0.05$, indicated there was no difference in the D-value of the treatment groups (groups A1+B1)and the control groups (groups A2+B2), and OSA did not affect this result; (2)if $Pa < 0.05$, $Pb > 0.05$, indicated the D-value in treatments (groups A1+B1)and control groups (groups A2+B2)were statistically different and OSA did not affect this result; (3)if $Pb < 0.05$, indicated that OSA would affect the D-value of all indices, therefore the patients were divided into two subgroups, patients with OSA (group A)and patients without OSA (group B), and further analysis between group A1 and A2, group B1 and B2 were performed. If a value of $P < 0.05$, indicated the D-value of group A1 (or group B1)were different from group A2 (or group B2). The base level of all indicators before treatment was considered as factor c to calibrate its effect on D-value. Moreover, D-value in the following tables were the original difference before and after treatment which could not used for comparison directly, and in order to exclude the influences of independent variables, D-value was transformed to adjusted mean D', namely least squares means (LS means)for comparison.

RESULTS

1 General Information

A total of 90hypertensive patients with yin deficiency and yang hyperactivity were included in this study, 46 (51.11%)patients with OSA, 44 (48.89%)patients without OSA; the age was 55.11 ± 10.07 years old; mean waistline was 93.43 ± 10.24 cm, mean hipline was 105.09 ± 7.89 cm, the ratio of waistline to hipline was 0.88 ± 0.06, the mean neck circumference was 8.75 ± 2.16 cm, and the mean body mass index (BMI)was 26.34 ± 3.36 kg/m^2. The groupings of patients were shown in Figure 2.

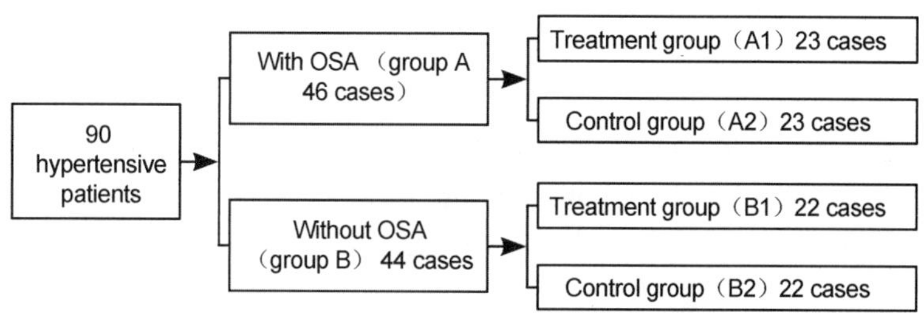

Figure 2　Diagram of Stratified Randomized Trial

2 Change of Blood Pressure after Treatment

2.1 Comparison of Antihypertensive Effective Rate

According to the Office Blood Pressure Measure (OBPM), the total antihypertensive effective rates in groups A1, A2, B1, and B2 were 78.26%, 5.21%, 90.90%, and 81.81%, respectively, without statistical difference (Table 1, χ^2=3.15, P=0.075).

Table 1　Comparison of Antihypertensive Effect [Case (%)]

Group	Case	Markedly effective	Effective	Ineffective	Total effective
A1	23	6 (26.08)	12 (52.17)	5 (21.73)	18 (78.26)
A2	23	4 (17.39)	11 (47.82)	8 (34.78)	15 (65.21)
B1	22	13 (59.09)	7 (31.81)	2 (9.09)	20 (90.90)
B2	22	8 (36.36)	10 (45.45)	4 (18.18)	18 (81.81)

2.2 Comparison of OBPM before and after Treatment

Compared with the same group before treatment, the SBP and DBP in all groups decreased after treatment ($P < 0.05$). However, compared with the control group (group A2, or B2, or A2+B2)after treatment, there was no significant difference of SBP or DBP in the treatment group (group A1, or B1, or A1+B1, respectively, $P > 0.05$). Also, there was no significant difference of D-value of SBP in the treatment groups (groups A1+B1)and control groups (groups A2+B2, Pa=0.10), neither did D-value of DBP (Pa=0.12). OSA did not affect the D-value of SBP or DBP (Pb=0.16, Pb=0.10, respectively, Table 2).

Table 2　Comparison of OBPM before and after Treatment (mmHg, $\bar{x} \pm s$)

Index	Time	Subgroup				Total group	
		With OSA (Group A)		Without OSA (Group B)		With or without OSA (Groups A+B)	
		Group A1	Group A2	Group B1	Group B2	Groups A1+B1	Groups A1+B1
SBP	Pre-treat.	150.65 ± 9.82	149.00 ± 9.84	143.72 ± 4.99	143.90 ± 4.12	147.28 ± 8.50	146.93 ± 8.09
	Post-treat.	131.95 ± 9.32*	134.56 ± 14.64*	125.59 ± 6.47*	129.86 ± 10.34*	128.84 ± 8.59*	132.26 ± 12.80*
	D-value	18.69 ± 11.51	14.72 ± 12.65	18.18 ± 9.28	14.05 ± 12.12	18.44 ± 10.36	14.66 ± 12.26
DBP	Pre-treat.	92.73 ± 8.49	92.60 ± 9.72	87.81 ± 7.36	87.50 ± 5.89	90.33 ± 8.25	90.11 ± 8.39
	Post-treat.	83.60 ± 9.15*	85.00 ± 9.20*	76.20 ± 10.34*	80.00 ± 10.07*	80.02 ± 10.33*	82.55 ± 9.88*
	D-value	8.69 ± 8.39	7.72 ± 3.67	11.54 ± 8.40	7.5 ± 12.29	10.31 ± 8.55	7.55 ± 8.87

Notes: *$P < 0.01$, compared with pre-treatment in the same group；D-values in the table were the original difference before and after treatment which could not be used for comparison directly；the same in the following tables.

2.3 Comparison of MBP before and after Treatment

Compared with the same group before treatment, the SBP and DBP of 24-h, day-time and night-time in all groups declined after treatment ($P < 0.05$). However, compared with the control group (group A2, or B2, or A2+B2)after treatment, there was no significant difference of 24-h, day-time, night-time SBP or DBP in the treatment groups (group A1, or B1, or A1+ B1, respectively)was found ($P > 0.05$).

The D-value of MBP in the treatment groups (groups A1+B1)did not differ from those of control groups (groups A2+B2, Pa＞0.05)；OSA could affect the D-value of night-time SBP (Pb=0.024), D-value of night-time SBP in OSA patients (3.72 mm Hg)was smaller than that of those without OSA patients (10.37 mm Hg, $P < 0.05$)；in all subgroups, there was no significant difference of D-value of MBP between the treatment and the control groups ($P > 0.05$, Table 3).

Table 3　Comparison of MBP before and after Treatment ($\bar{x} \pm s$, mmHg)

Item	Time	Subgroup				Total group	
		With OSA (Group A)		Without OS	A (Group B)	With or without OSA (Groups A+B)	
		Group A1 (23 cases)	Group A2 (23 cases)	Group B1 (22 cases)	Group B2 (22 cases)	Groups A1+B1 (45 cases)	Groups A2+B2 (45 cases)
SBP							
	Pre-treat.	142.60 ± 14.80	143.30 ± 11.84	126.72 ± 7.06	130.72 ± 6.86	136.93 ± 12.49	135.06 ± 13.25
24-h	Post-treat.	133.52 ± 10.65*	135.91 ± 16.03*	123.27 ± 6.80*	126.04 ± 8.33*	129.22 ± 9.71	130.37 ± 14.16
	D-value	9.08 ± 15.18	6.40 ± 16.32	3.45 ± 6.78	4.68 ± 8.96	6.33 ± 12.05	6.06 ± 13.36
	Pre-treat.	145.13 ± 12.45	148.48 ± 10.96	130.73 ± 5.81	132.91 ± 6.42	147.75 ± 9.03	146.46 ± 7.43
Day-time	Post-treat.	136.17 ± 11.59**	139.52 ± 17.09*	125.59 ± 6.47*	129.86 ± 10.34*	132.44 ± 10.55**	133.35 ± 15.24*
	D-value	8.95 ± 14.89	7.90 ± 15.63	5.13 ± 6.23	3.04 ± 9.78	16.28 ± 11.40	12.13 ± 14.39
	Pre-treat.	133.13 ± 14.78	136.87 ± 12.31	119.36 ± 8.39	120.00 ± 7.73	127.66 ± 14.59	127.60 ± 12.41
Night-time	Post-treat.	129.21 ± 13.10**	131.08 ± 9.85*	115.09 ± 9.67*	115.05 ± 8.73*	122.93 ± 12.91	122.40 ± 13.01
	D-value	8.13 ± 12.25	8.90 ± 19.98	4.27 ± 8.02	5.90 ± 12.13	6.24 ± 10.46	7.71 ± 16.34
DBP							
	Pre-Treat.	84.60 ± 11.38	89.13 ± 10.9	81.31 ± 5.07	81.31 ± 6.46	84.22 ± 9.89	84.08 ± 8.92
24-h	Post-treat.	79.86 ± 8.54**	82.82 ± 12.76**	75.09 ± 9.64*	76.86 ± 10.39*	77.60 ± 10.55	79.84 ± 10.85
	D-value	4.73 ± 6.06	5.90 ± 9.45	6.22 ± 7.48	4.45 ± 8.56	5.46 ± 6.76	5.40 ± 8.96
	Pre-treat.	87.39 ± 11.33	91.17 ± 11.00	83.81 ± 4.92	83.22 ± 6.68	86.48 ± 9.83	86.44 ± 9.04
Day-time	Post-treat.	81.95 ± 9.64**	85.39 ± 13.56*	76.63 ± 9.64**	79.00 ± 10.38*	79.75 ± 11.12	81.86 ± 11.40
	D-value	5.43 ± 7.15	5.36 ± 10.21	7.18 ± 9.34	4.22 ± 8.94	6.28 ± 8.28	5.02 ± 9.52

Continued

Item	Time	Subgroup				Total group	
		With OSA (Group A)		Without OS	A (Group B)	With or without OSA (Groups A+B)	
		Group A1 (23 cases)	Group A2 (23 cases)	Group B1 (22 cases)	Group B2 (22 cases)	Groups A1+B1 (45 cases)	Groups A2+B2 (45 cases)
	Pre-treat.	78.30 ± 10.91	81.56 ± 11.90	75.40 ± 6.09	75.36 ± 9.73	78.04 ± 10.70	77.37 ± 9.58
Night-time	Post-treat.	73.08 ± 7.94**	74.82 ± 11.92*	70.40 ± 10.13*	69.31 ± 10.02*	71.13 ± 10.53	72.82 ± 9.93
	D-value	5.21 ± 7.22	6.36 ± 10.81	5.00 ± 8.76	5.95 ± 10.47	5.11 ± 7.92	6.35 ± 10.48

Notes: $^{*}P < 0.05$, $^{**}P < 0.01$, compared with pre-treatment in the same group.

2.4 Comparison of BPV before and after Treatment

Compared with the same group before treatment, SD (day-time and night-time SBP; 24-h, daytime, night-time DBP), and heart rate decreased in all groups after treatment ($P < 0.05$), and CV (24-h and night-time DBP)in the treatment groups (group A1, B1 or A1+B1)decreased after treatment. Compared with the control groups (group A2, or B2, or A2+B2)after treatment, there was significant difference in SD (night-time SBP; 24-h, day-time and night-time DBP), and CV (24-h DBP)in the treatment groups (group A1, or B1, or A1+B1, respectively, $P < 0.05$). The night-time DBP and SBP decreasing rate increased in the patients without OSA ($P < 0.05$, Table 4).

The D-values of SD (24-h, day-time, night-time SBP and DBP), CV (24-h, night-time DBP)decreased in the treatment groups (groups A1+B1)compared with those in the control groups (groups A2+B2. Pa < 0.05, Tables 4 and 5). There was no significant difference between the treatment groups and the control groups in the following D-values: day-time SBP CV (Pa=0.62), day-time DBP CV (P a=0.83)night SBP and DBP decreasing rate (Pa=0.57 and 0.55, respectively). OSA could affect the D-values of the following indicators: 24-h SBP SD, day-time SBP SD, night-time SBP SD, 24-h DBP SD, 24-h DBP CV, day-time DBP SD, night-time DBP SD and CV, heart rate, and the night-time SBP DBP decreasing rate (Tables 4 and 6, Pb < 0.05). OSA did not affect the D-values of the following indicators: day-time DBP CV (Pb=0.15)and night-time DBP CV (Pb=0.054).

Table 4 Comparison of BPV before and after Treatment ($\bar{x} \pm s$, mmHg)

Item	Time	Subgroup				Total group	
		With OSA (Group A)		Without OS A (Group B)		With or without OSA (Groups A+B)	
Item	Time	Group A1 (23 cases)	Group A2 (23 cases)	Group B1 (22 cases)	Group B2 (22 cases)	Group A1+B1 (45 cases)	Group A2+B2 (45 cases)
SBP BPV							
Pre-treat.		17.52 ± 3.57	17.36 ± 4.08	13.76 ± 2.19	13.37 ± 2.46	15.68 ± 3.50	15.41 ± 3.91
24-h SD	Post-treat.	12.72 ± 1.53$^{**\triangle}$	14.47 ± 3.58	10.92 ± 1.90$^{**\triangle}$	12.09 ± 1.69**	11.84 ± 1.93$^{**\triangle}$	13.31 ± 3.03**
D-value		4.79 ± 4.48°	2.43 ± 3.70	2.83 ± 2.95°	1.28 ± 2.34	3.83 ± 3.90°	2.10 ± 3.48
Pre-treat.		12.41 ± 2.77	11.72 ± 2.49	10.90 ± 1.90	10.27 ± 2.05	11.43 ± 2.93	11.02 ± 2.38
24-h CV (%)	Post-treat.	10.16 ± 2.24**	10.36 ± 2.64*	10.53 ± 2.22	9.99 ± 1.87	10.34 ± 2.19	10.18 ± 2.28
D-value		2.25 ± 2.92	1.16 ± 2.68	0.36 ± 2.30	0.28 ± 2.65	1.09 ± 3.17	0.83 ± 2.74
Pre-treat.		14.52 ± 3.39	15.21 ± 3.66	11.77 ± 2.18	12.09 ± 2.86	13.17 ± 3.15	13.68 ± 3.62
Day-time SD	Post-treat.	10.87 ± 1.74**	12.65 ± 3.01*	9.04 ± 2.55$^{**\triangle}$	10.45 ± 1.92*	9.97 ± 2.34$^{**\triangle}$	11.57 ± 2.74*
	D-value	3.65 ± 3.65°	2.36 ± 5.12	2.72 ± 3.67°	1.63 ± 3.44	3.20 ± 3.65°	2.11 ± 4.34
	Pre-treat.	10.04 ± 2.49	10.33 ± 2.87	9.00 ± 1.61	9.11 ± 2.15	8.92 ± 1.96	9.33 ± 2.57
Day-time CV (%)	Post-treat.	8.53 ± 1.94**	9.11 ± 3.94	6.72 ± 2.82**	6.46 ± 3.09**	7.65 ± 2.55*	7.19 ± 3.69**
	D-value	1.51 ± 2.56	2.11 ± 4.98	2.27 ± 2.90	2.64 ± 3.57	1.27 ± 2.57	2.14 ± 4.41

Continued

		Subgroup				Total group	
		With OSA (Group A)		Without OS A (Group B)		With or without OSA (Groups A+B)	
Item	Time	Group A1 (23 cases)	Group A2 (23 cases)	Group B1 (22 cases)	Group B2 (22 cases)	Group A1+B1 (45 cases)	Group A2+B2 (45 cases)
	Pre-treat.	13.30 ± 3.67	14.26 ± 5.15	10.00 ± 3.23	10.5 ± 3.12	11.68 ± 3.81	12.42 ± 4.64
Night-time SD	Post-treat.	9.17 ± 2.57$^{**\triangle}$	11.69 ± 4.9*	7.22 ± 1.84$^{**\triangle}$	8.72 ± 2.89*	8.22 ± 2.42$^{*\triangle}$	10.24 ± 4.27*
	D-value	4.13 ± 4.20°	1.95 ± 4.44	2.77 ± 3.87	1.77 ± 3.67	3.46 ± 4.05°	2.17 ± 4.50
	Pre-treat.	10.01 ± 3.20	9.57 ± 4.76	7.78 ± 3.36	7.97 ± 3.71	8.92 ± 3.43	9.03 ± 4.02
Night-time CV (%)	Post-treat.	7.67 ± 2.41**	8.46 ± 5.07	5.91 ± 2.53*	6.67 ± 3.61	6.81 ± 2.60*	7.59 ± 4.46*
	D-value	2.34 ± 3.62	1.15 ± 4.66	1.53 ± 3.34	0.81 ± 2.77	2.11 ± 3.54	1.44 ± 4.07
	Pre-treat.	5.58 ± 7.41	4.86 ± 7.56	11.20 ± 3.80	9.88 ± 6.09	8.33 ± 6.52	7.32 ± 7.29
Night-time decreasing rate (%)	Post-treat.	7.96 ± 8.27	8.47 ± 6.52	15.19 ± 3.41$^{**\triangle}$	12.52 ± 5.13*	11.49 ± 7.29*	10.45 ± 6.16*
D-value		−2.38 ± 7.86	−3.92 ± 9.45	−3.98 ± 3.46	−2.64 ± 5.84	−3.16 ± 6.10	−3.13 ± 7.77
DBP BPV							
Pre-treat.		11.42 ± 1.26	12.34 ± 3.07	9.61 ± 1.72	10.15 ± 2.41	10.53 ± 1.74	11.26 ± 2.95
24-h SD	Post-treat.	9.27 ± 1.45$^{**\triangle}$	10.64 ± 1.63**	7.72 ± 1.22$^{**\triangle}$	8.87 ± 1.22*	8.51 ± 1.54$^{**\triangle}$	9.77 ± 1.69**
D-value		2.14 ± 1.88°	1.49 ± 2.80	1.89 ± 1.76	1.27 ± 2.77	2.02 ± 1.81°	1.49 ± 2.82
Pre-treat.		13.67 ± 1.99	13.88 ± 3.09	11.85 ± 2.17	12.48 ± 2.66	12.78 ± 2.25	13.20 ± 2.94
24-h CV (%)	Post-treat.	11.72 ± 2.19$^{\triangle}$	13.08 ± 2.53	10.38 ± 1.78$^{\triangle}$	11.68 ± 1.78	11.06 ± 2.09$^{\triangle}$	12.39 ± 2.28
D-value		1.95 ± 2.22	0.65 ± 3.14	1.47 ± 2.39°	0.8 ± 2.57	1.71 ± 2.29°	0.80 ± 2.85
Pre-treat.		9.95 ± 2.24	10.43 ± 3.23	7.68 ± 1.93	8.18 ± 1.89	8.84 ± 2.37	9.33 ± 2.86
Day-time SD	Post-treat.	7.26 ± 1.28$^{**\triangle}$	8.21 ± 1.59**	6.04 ± 1.55$^{**\triangle}$	7.13 ± 1.78*	6.66 ± 1.53$^{**\triangle}$	7.68 ± 1.75**
	D-value	2.36 ± 2.63°	1.95 ± 3.27	1.63 ± 2.27	1.04 ± 2.29	2.17 ± 2.49°	1.64 ± 2.96
	Pre-treat.	11.47 ± 2.72	11.35 ± 3.48	9.17 ± 2.25	9.88 ± 2.39	10.35 ± 2.76	10.63 ± 3.05
Day-time CV (%)	Post-treat.	8.95 ± 1.75**	8.85 ± 3.28*	7.75 ± 3.55*	7.76 ± 3.74*	8.36 ± 2.83**	8.25 ± 3.58**
	D-value	2.52 ± 2.90	1.89 ± 3.99	1.42 ± 4.37	2.27 ± 3.81	1.98 ± 3.69	2.38 ± 4.32
	Pre-treat.	10.65 ± 2.83	11.04 ± 3.79	7.18 ± 2.19	8.22 ± 2.40	8.95 ± 3.06	9.66 ± 3.46
Night-time SD	Post-treat.	7.47 ± 1.92$^{**\triangle}$	9.34 ± 3.60*	5.63 ± 1.29$^{**\triangle}$	6.81 ± 2.13*	6.57 ± 1.87$^{**\triangle}$	8.11 ± 3.20*
	D-value	3.17 ± 3.96**	1.54 ± 3.81	1.54 ± 1.87	1.40 ± 2.88	2.37 ± 3.19°	1.55 ± 3.34
	Pre-treat.	13.74 ± 3.99	12.61 ± 5.57	8.84 ± 3.94	9.27 ± 4.92	11.35 ± 4.64	10.98 ± 5.47
Night-time CV (%)	Post-treat.	10.40 ± 2.99**	11.45 ± 5.78	7.42 ± 3.14*	8.79 ± 4.75	8.94 ± 3.39**	10.15 ± 5.41
	D-value	3.34 ± 5.52	0.68 ± 6.43	1.16 ± 2.93	0.04 ± 4.70	2.40 ± 4.39	0.82 ± 0.50
	Pre-treat.	13.74 ± 3.99	12.61 ± 5.57	8.84 ± 3.94	9.27 ± 4.92	11.35 ± 4.64	10.98 ± 5.47
Night-time CV (%)	Post-treat.	10.40 ± 2.99	11.45 ± 5.78	7.42 ± 3.14	8.79 ± 4.75	8.94 ± 3.39	10.15 ± 5.41
	D-value	3.34 ± 5.52	0.68 ± 6.43	1.16 ± 2.93	0.04 ± 4.70	2.40 ± 4.39	0.82 ± 0.50
	Pre-treat.	7.35 ± 6.05	9.77 ± 7.07	11.97 ± 6.08	12.26 ± 5.75	9.61 ± 6.44	10.80 ± 7.02
Night-time CV (%)	Post-treat.	10.33 ± 9.01	11.90 ± 8.28	14.85 ± 4.24*	15.45 ± 6.54	12.54 ± 7.37	13.64 ± 7.61
	D-value	−2.98 ± 10.64	-2.46 ± 11.30	−2.87 ± 5.79	−3.18 ± 7.66	−2.93 ± 8.52	−2.83 ± 9.44
	Pre-treat.	77.43 ± 11.35	75.37 ± 8.15	73.19 ± 7.67	70.13 ± 8.76	75.36 ± 9.85	72.81 ± 8.76
Night-time CV (%)	Post-treat.	72.59 ± 9.90**	72.01 ± 7.44	64.00 ± 3.24**	67.46 ± 6.90*	68.39 ± 8.54**	69.79 ± 7.46*
	D-value	4.83 ± 7.08	2.90 ± 6.84	9.19 ± 8.09°	2.67 ± 5.76	6.96 ± 7.82°	3.02 ± 6.38

Notes: $^{*}P < 0.05$, $^{**}P < 0.01$, compared with pre-treatment in the same group；$^{\triangle}P < 0.05$, compared with the control group after treatment；$^{\circ}P < 0.05$, D-value in the treatment groups compared with those in the control groups, and the adjusted D'-value which were statistically different between the two groups were shown in Tables 5–8.

Table 5 Comparison of D'-Value in Treatment Groups and Control Groups

BPV		Time	D'-value of BPV indices		
			Groups A1+B1	Groups A2+B2	Pa-value
SD	SBP	24-h	3.73	2.2	0.0028
		Day-time	3.43	1.87	0.0016
		Night-time	3.71	1.93	0.0069
	DBP	24-h	2.29	1.21	0.0001
		Day-time	2.38	1.43	0.0036
		Night-time	2.61	1.31	0.0064
CV	DBP	24-h	1.85	0.29	0.0047
		Night-time	0.021	0.0038	0.029
Heart rate			6.42	3.56	0.026

Table 6 Comparison of D'-Value in OSA and non-OSA Patients

BPV		Time	D'-value		
			OSA	non-OSA	P -value
SD	SBP	24-h	2.16	3.81	0.032
		Day-time	1.62	3.73	0.002
		Night-time	2.08	3.59	0.032
	DBP	24-h	1.10	2.43	< 0.0001
		Day-time	1.45	2.38	0.0082
		Night-time	1.26	2.70	0.0078
CV	SBP	Day-time	0.99	2.45	0.014
	DBP	24-h	0.85	1.68	0.047
Heart Rate			2.93	7.14	0.0013
Night-time SBP Decreasing rate			-1.34	-5.04	0.0057
Night-time DBP Decreasing rate			-1.21	-4.63	0.03

Notes: the D-value in the above content was transformed to adjusted mean D', namely least squares means (LS means)for comparison.

Table 7 The Comparison of D'-Value in Treatment and Control Group in OSA Patients

BPV		Time	D'-value of BPV indices	
			Group A1	Group A2
SD	SBP	24-h	4.72	2.95*
		Day-time	4.01	2.20*
		Night-time	4.45	2.23*
	DBP	24-h	2.52	1.31*
		Day-time	2.92	1.98*
		Night-time	3.33	1.53*

Note: *$P < 0.05$, compared with group A1.

Table 8 The Comparison of D'–Value in Treatment and Control group in non–OSA Changhua Christian Hospital Patients

BPV			D'-value of BPV indices	
			Group B1	Group B2
SD	SBP	24-h	2.67	1.44*
		Day-time	2.90	1.46*
	DBP	Day-time	1.70	0.56*
		Night-time	8.20	3.66*
CV	DBP	24-h	1.70	0.56*

Note: *$P < 0.05$, compared with group B1.

2.5 Comparison of OSA Indices before and after Treatment

In OSA patients, HI decreased in the treatment group compared with that in the control group ($P < 0.05$), other indicators had improving tendency after treatment without statistical difference ($P > 0.05$, Table 9).

Table 9 Comparison of OSA Indicators before and after Treatment ($\bar{x} \pm s$)

Item	Time	Group A1	Group A2
AHI (Time/h)	Pre-treat	14.59 ± 10.60	16.61 ± 14.40
	Post-treat.	13.87 ± 9.88	16.07 ± 14.06
HI (Time/h)	Pre-treat	8.94 ± 6.25	8.88 ± 6.46
	Post-treat.	7.27 ± 6.62*	8.69 ± 6.04
AI (Time/h)	Pre-treat	5.70 ± 6.24	7.66 ± 10.99
	Post-treat.	6.60 ± 5.67	7.33 ± 10.91
Lowest SaO2 (%)	Pre-treat	83.43 ± 5.25	82.73 ± 7.61
	Post-treat.	85.08 ± 4.91	82.91 ± 7.11
ODI (Time/h)	Pre-treat	14.31 ± 13.97	17.48 ± 15.77
	Post-treat.	13.29 ± 12.73	17.75 ± 16.00

Notes: *$P < 0.05$, compared with pre-treatment in the same group.

2.6 Safety Analysis

There was no obvious change in results of blood, urine, biochemical indices, and ECG before and after treatment.

DISCUSSION

The increase of BPV is closely related to the target organ damage in hypertension patients. The research showed that the decrease of BPV could improve the baroreflex sensitivity, and protect the target organ. [14] BPV is more important than MBP in aspect of target organ protection. The result of the Anglo-Scandinavian Cardiac Outcomes Trial Blood Pressure Lowering Arm (ASCOT-BPLA)showed that BPV has stronger predictive value in cerebral apoplexy and cardiovascular diseases, especially in mild and moderate hypertensive patients. [15]

According to Chinese medicine (CM)theory, the hypertension is caused by the imbalance of Liver (Gan), Kidney (Shen), and Heart (Xin), and the main syndrome is yin deficiency and yang hyperactivity, hypertension with OSA would cause pathological fire, wind and phlegm. There are few researches on hypertensive patients with OSA treating with CM. In this trial the clinical hypertensive patients were selected, and divided into OSA and non-OSA subgroups according to portable sleep monitoring examination, then the patients were randomly assigned to treatment group and control group in each subgroup. The antihypertensive effect was observed in this trial.

After treatment, we could conclude that Amlodipine Besylate was effective to decline the MBP as a fundamental hypotensor. Compared with the placebo, the MBP treated by Qingxuan Granule had a down tendency without statistical difference ($P > 0.05$). To exclude the interference of OSA and base level of blood pressure, we analyzed the D-value of blood pressure before and after treatment by covariance analysis of generalized linear models, and there was no difference of MBP between D-values of treatment and control groups.

Compared with BPV of the control group after treatment, Qingxuan Granule could decrease BPV in these patients ($P < 0.05$). To exclude the interference of OSA and base BP level we analyzed the D-value of BPV, the results showed that the D-value of treatment group was more than that of the control group ($P < 0.05$)which indicated that Qingxuan Granule could improve the BPV in these patients, and this effect could weakened by OSA ($P < 0.05$).

Also, the results suggest that OSA patients' night-time BPV did not improve which was due to the airway obstruction during night, and oral medicine could not effectively solve this problem. While for those patients without OSA, Qingxuan Granule could improve the night-time BPV and modulate the circadian rhythm obviously.

The decrease of BPV is the effective measurement to prevent cardiovascular diseases, so it is important to pay attention to BPV besides MBP. A meta-analysis revealed that calcium antagonists could effectively reduce BPV than angiotensin Ⅱ receptor blocker (ARB)or angiotensin-converting enzyme inhibitors (ACEI). [16] Rothwell PM, [15] et al found that calcium antagonists could reduce the risk of apoplexy through reducing the BPV, while β-blocker had opposite effect on BPV. From these researches we could conclude that the improving of BPV would be an important aim to prevent cardiovascular diseases besides the control of MBP. For hypertension patients with OSA, the treatment of CPAP, oral appliance or operation could promote the airway obstruction obviously to eliminate or reduce the hypoxia and respiratory effort-related arousals, which would improve the baroreflex sensitivity, and BPV. From this trial, we could conclude that Amlodipine Besylate would not aggravate OSA, and Qingxuan Granule could improve the hypopnea in OSA patients. More researches about different hypotensors are needed to explore the effect of these medicine on hypertension patients with OSA.

In this research Qingxuan Granule was taken as treatment method. Granular preparation was a new CM form including the process of extraction, concentration, granulation, and packaging. It is more convenient for patients to take granule than traditional decoction, [17] and this would improve the globalization of CM.

REFERENCES

[1] Lavie P, Ben Yousef R, Rubin AE. Prevalence of sleep apnea syndrome among patients with essential hypertension[J]. Am Heart J 1984; 108: 373-376.

[2] Peppard PE, Young T, Palta M, Skatrud J. Prospective study of the association between sleep-disordered breathing and hypertension[J]. N Engl J Med 2000; 342: 1378-1384.

[3] Somers VK, White DP, Amin R, Abraham WT, Costa F, Culebras A, et al. Sleep apnea and cardiovascular disease: an American Heart Association/American College of Cardiology Foundation Scientific Statement from the American Heart Association Council for High Blood Pressure Research Professional Education Committee, Council on Clinical Cardiology, Stroke Council, and Council on Cardiovascular Nursing[J]. J Am Coll Cardiol 2008; 52: 686-717.

[4] Chobanian AV, Bakris GL, Black HR, Cushman WC, Green LA, Izzo JL, et al. Seventh report of the Joint National Committee on prevention, detection, evaluation, and treatment of high blood pressure[J]. Hypertension 2003; 42: 1206-1252.

[5] Whitworth JA. World Health Organization, International Society of Hypertension Writing Group. 2003 World Health Organization (WHO)/ International Society of Hypertension (ISH)statement on management of hypertension (guidelines and recommendations)[J]. J Hypertens 2003; 21: 1983-1992.

[6] Ministry of Health of the People's Republic of China. Guidelines for prevention and treatment of hypertension in China (2005). 2005.

[7] Zheng XY, ed. Guiding principle of clinical research on new drugs of traditional Chinese medicine[M]. Beijing: China Medical Science Press;

2002: 73-77.

[8] Sleep Breathing Disorder Group, Branch of Respiratory Disease, Chinese Medical Association. Guidlines of diagnosis and treatment for obstructive sleep apnea hypopnea syndrome (draft)[J]. Chin J Tubercul Resp Dis (Chin)2002；25: 195-198.

[9] Experts Consensus on OSA. The expert consensus on obstructive sleep apnea and cardiovascular diseases[J]. Chin J Intern Med (Chin)2009；48: 1059-1067.

[10] Chan AS, Phillips CL, Cistulli PA. Obstructive sleep apnoea—an update[J]. Intern Med J 2010；40: 102-106.

[11] Zou D, Grote L, Peker Y, Lindblad U, Hedner J. Validation a portable monitoring device for sleep apnea diagnosis in a population based cohort using synchronized home polysomnography[J]. Sleep 2006；29: 367-374.

[12] Mancia G, Grassi G. Mechanisms and clinical implications of blood pressure variability[J]. J Cardiovasc Pharmacol 2000；35 (Suppl 4): 15-19.

[13] Kikuya M, Hozawa A, Ohokubo T, Tsuji I, Michimata M, Matsubara M, et al. Prognostic significance of blood pressure and heart rate variabilities: the Ohasama study[J]. Hypertension 2000；36: 901-906.

[14] Su DF. The relationship of blood pressure variability, baroreflex sensitivity and target organ in spontaneously hypertensive rats when treated with different kinds of antihypertensive drugs[J]. Chin J Hypertens (Chin)2007；15: 38.

[15] Rothwell PM, Howard SC, Dolan E, O'Brien E, Dobson JE, Dahlöf B, et al. Effects of β blockers and calcium-channel blockers on within-individual variability in blood pressure and risk of stroke[J]. Lancet Neurol 2010；9: 469-480.

[16] Webb AJ, Fischer U, Mehta Z, Rothwell PM. Effects of antihypertensive-drug class on interindividual variation in blood pressure and risk of stroke: a systematic review and meta-analysis[J]. Lancet 2010；375: 906-915.

[17] He L, Yao R. The current research situation and prospect of Chinese medicine granular form[J]. Chin Modern Med (Chin)2010；17 (9): 82-83.

First published: CHEN Yi-yu, CHEN Jing, ZHANG Jing-chun, and CHEN Ke-ji. Effect of Qingxuan Granule (清眩颗粒)on blood pressure variability of hypertensive patients with and without obstructive sleep apnea[J]. Chin J Integr Med, 2013: 1-9.

The Expression of CD14⁺CD16⁺ Monocyte Subpopulation in Coronary Heart Disease Patients with Blood Stasis Syndrome

HUANG Ye, WANG Jing-shang, YIN Hui-jun, and CHEN Ke-ji

The way of disease-syndrome combination is an important style to diagnose and treat disease in traditional Chinese medicine (TCM)clinical practice today. Study on the blood stasis syndrome (BSS)is the most active field of integration of traditional and western medicine research in China [1]. To normalize and standardize the BSS, the way of disease-syndrome combination is used to explore the essence of BSS, which will be the inevitable tendency in the future. Study on CHD with BSS initiated by research team of CHEN Ke-ji is the model of the way of disease syndrome combination. In our previous study, we found that Fc receptor III A of immunoglobulin G (Fc γ RIIIA, also called $CD14^{+}CD16^{+}$ monocyte subpopulation)is one of the differentially expressed genes related to coronary heart disease (CHD)patients using the oligonucleotide microarray technique[2], and high level of Fc γ RIIIA in CHD patients observed previously was verified by both mRNA level and its protein content[3]. Our recent study suggested an important role of Fc γ RIIIA in the atherosclerotic formation by elevating the adhesive efficiency of monocytes to HUVECs in vitro, by increasing expression of inflammatory cytokines and also by kindling the atherosclerotic plaque destabilization in $ApoE^{-/-}$ mouse[4]. Additionally, we also investigated that traditional Chinese medicine of activation of blood and dissolving stasis, effective components of Chuanxiong Rhizome and Red Peony Root, could stabilize the atherosclerotic plaque by suppressing inflammation, and its target was relative with Fc γ RIIIA[5]. However, whether or not the deregulation of the expression of CD14+CD16+ monocyte subpopulation is implicated in the pathogenesis of CHD patients with BSS has not yet been elucidated.

METHODS

1 Patients and Healthy Control

All patients with coronary heart disease were the inpatients of Beijing Anzhen Hospital, from May 2010 to December 2010, diagnosed by a diameter stenosis of at least 50% from standard selective coronary angiography [6,7]. These CHD patients were selected into blood stasis syndrome (BSS)group and non-BSS group based on the standard diagnostic criteria established by the Special Committee of Promoting Blood Circulation and Removing Blood Stasis, Chinese Association of Integrative Medicine[8]. Patients with severe valvulopathy, serious primary diseases such as liver or kidney dysfunction, malignant tumors, medication history of antiplatelet therapy, and women in pregnancy or lactation stage were excluded from enrollment. Forty age-and sex-matched healthy individuals from the physical examination center of Xiyuan Hospital were selected as a control group. These individuals were without any history of chest pain or evidence of cardiac or other systemic disease verified by history examination, chest film, electrocardiogram, and blood routine examination, and none was taking any medication. Our study was in accordance with the Helsinki Declaration, with ethical approval granted by the Ethics Committee at Xiyuan Hospital, China Academy of Chinese Medical Sciences, and a written informed consent was obtained from all study participants. The clinical characteristics of the participants are shown in Table 1.

Table 1 Characteristics of the CHD Patients with BSS/non-BSS and Healthy Individuals Participated in the Study

	CHD patients			
	BSS patients (*n*=50)	Non-BSS patients (*n*=50)	Healthy control (*n*=40)	P value
Age (year)	53.00 ± 6.43	52.92 ± 6.03	49.50 ± 8.71	0.507
Sex (male/female)	36/14	33/17	28/12	0.804
BMI (kg/m^2)	25.50 ± 2.77	25.10 ± 2.57	24.29 ± 1.57	0.509
SAP (n)	12	13	-	-
ACS (n)	38	37	-	-
UAP (n)	31	31	-	-
AMI (n)	7	6	-	-
Hypercholesterolemia (>230 mg/dL) (yes/no)	7/43	5/45	-	-
Hypertension (yes/no)	31/19	30/20	-	-
Diabetes (n)	20/30	20/30	-	-
Monocyte count (mmol/L)	0.38 ± 0.11	0.37 ± 0.20	0.36 ± 0.11	0.891

BMI: body mass index ; SAP: stable angina pectoris ; ACS: acute coronary syndrome ; UAP: unstable angina ; AMI: acute myocardial infarction. Data are expressed as mean SD.

2 Blood Samples

Peripheral blood was collected from the CHD patients with BSS/non-BSS and healthy subjects under standardized conditions. Blood from CHD patients was drawn before coronary angiography was performed. For the analyses of cytometry or mRNA expression or flow cytometry, 2 mL ethylenediaminetetraacetate-(EDTA-)anticoagulated blood was taken and immediately analyzed. For the detection of inflammatory cytokines by ELISA assay, blood was centrifuged at 3, 000 rpm for 20 min, and serum was frozen at −80 ℃ until analysis.

3 RT-PCR

Fcγ RIIIA mRNA expression was investigated by the quantitative real-time polymerase chain reaction (PCR)assay. Total RNA samples were extracted from leukocytes using Trizol reagent (Invitrogen, USA) according to the manufacturer's protocol. The purity and integrity of RNA were determined on a UV spectrophotometer (Eppendorf, Germany)by 260–280nm absorbance ratio and agarose gel electrophoresis (1.5%)and ethidium bromide staining, respectively. cDNA preparations were performed at 42 ℃ for 1 h, with reverse transcriptase, 2 μL RNase, 2 μL of an oligo (dT)primer, and 10 mM of each dNTP in a total volume of 50 μL of 1x first strand cDNA synthesis buffer, incubated at 70 ℃ for 10 min. PCR assays were carried out in a PCR (ABI 7500, USA). 1.5 μL of cDNA mixture was subjected to amplification in a 20 μL mixture. The following primer sequences with the predicted size were used for amplification: Fcγ RIIIA: forward, 5'-TGTTCAAGGAGGAAGACCCT-3, reverse, 5 GAAGTAGGAGCCGCTGTCTT-3'; GAPDH: forward, 5'-GGGTGTGAACCATGAGAAGT-3', reverse, 5'-GGCATGGACTGTGGTCATGA-3'. PCR conditions were as follows: initial denaturation at 94 ℃ for 15 min followed by 40 cycles of denaturation for 15 s at 94 ℃, annealing at 60 ℃ for 34 sec, extending at 72 ℃ for 15 sec, and a final extension at 72 ℃ for 10 min. Glyceraldehydes-3-phosphate dehydrogenase (GAPDH)was used as an internal control in all PCR reactions. The PCR products were subjected to 2% agarose gel electrophoresis. The relative mRNA expression level of the target gene in each individual was calculated using the comparative cycle time (Ct)method [9].

4 Flow Cytometry

Fcγ RIIIA protein level was assessed by flow cytometry. Ethylenediaminetetraacetic-Acid- (EDTA-) anticoagulated peripheral blood (PB)samples were collected from all patients and healthy controls for flow cytometric analysis performed previously described [10]. Briefly, PB samples were stained with saturating concentrations of fluorescein-isothiocyanate- (FITC-)conjugated anti-CD14 monoclonal antibody (mAb) (BD Biosciences, Lot: 74003)and phycoerythrin- (PE-)conjugated anti-CD16 mAb (BD Biosciences, Lot: 73903) or isotype-matched control mAb for 20 min at room temperature in the dark. After erythrocytes were lysed by incubation with lysing solution for 8 min, PB mononuclear cells were resuspended in PBS with 1% fetal calf serum. The surface expression of CD14 and CD16 on PB monocytes was performed by a fluorescence-activated cell sorter (FACS)cytometer (Becton Dickinson). The test data were obtained by FS versus SS gate and analyzed by Expo32 special software. Monocytes were identified by gating CD14+ events, and all additional analyses were performed on this population. Fcγ RIIIA protein content defined by the percentage of CD16 on the monocyte population ($CD14^+/CD16^+$%)was measured.

5 Enzyme-Linked Immunosorbent Assay (ELISA)

Concentrations of TNF-α (R&D, USA, Lot: 1007143), IL-1 (R&D, USA, Lot: 1007155), and soluble CD14 (sCD14) (R&D, USA, Lot: 1010179)in sera were determined by double-antibody sandwich avidin-biotin peroxidase complex enzyme-linked immunosorbent assay (ABC-ELISA), according to manufacturer's instructions.

6 Statistical Analysis

All data are expressed as mean ± SD. The SPSS Statistics 15.0 package was utilized to analyze the data. Differences among groups were analyzed using the one-way analysis of variance (ANOVA), followed by multiple comparisons by LSD test. Difference was considered significant at $P < 0.05$.

RESULTS AND DISCUSSION

BSS is a pathological state, which is the outward manifestation of some certain pathological stage of various diseases. Due to lack of objective diagnosis criteria, the essence of BSS is studied into the bottleneck stage. Recently, based on the way of disease-syndrome combination, much effective exploration of the essence of BSS was the foundation of BSS objective diagnosis criteria construction. During the past 50 years, we found a correlation between CHD with BSS and inflammatory, hemodynamics, platelet, and microcirculation[11].

Atherosclerosis, a chronic inflammatory immune state, is chiefly responsible for the development of CHD. Various leukocytes have been shown to influence atherogenesis. Monocytes and their descendant macrophages are central protagonists in the development of atherosclerosis [12]. Monocyte migration to the vessel wall is an initial event in the growth of atherosclerotic lesions [13]. Once monocytes are activated, adhesion to endothelial cells was induced by the transform of phenotype, which led to myocardium injury, inducing the proinflammatory cytokines such as TNF-α and IL-1 synthesis to initiate the inflammatory cascade reaction and oxidative stress injury, producing matrix metalloproteinase (MMP)and releasing many media to induce plaque instability and even fracture [14,15]. Therefore, monocytes played the key role in the chronic inflammation immunoreaction of the arterial vessels. In our study, we investigated that there was no significant difference of monocyte count based on CBC count among CHD patients with BSS, non-BSS, and healthy control (Table 1). However, the level of sCD14 which is the indicator of activated monocyte [16] was obviously increased in CHD patients with BSS, compared to non-BSS and healthy control (Figure 1). The increased level of sCD14 in sera in CHD patients with BSS indicated monocytes activation. To demonstrate the correlation between deregulated expression of $CD14^+CD16^+$monocyte subpopulation and pathogenesis of CHD with BSS, its mRNA expression at the leukocyte level was assessed. As shown in Figure 2, relative expression level of $CD14^+CD16^+$ monocyte subpopulation in both CHD patients with BSS and non-BBS was largely increased by 99% and 77%, respectively, compared to the healthy control ($P < 0.01$). However, there was no significant difference of this relative expression level between CHD patients with BSS and non-BSS (Figure 2).

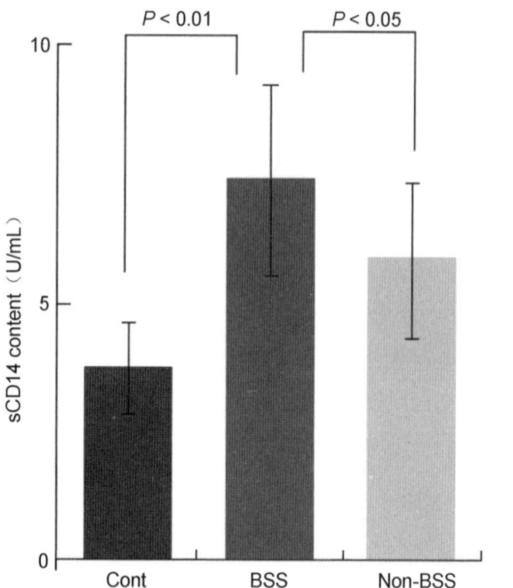

Figure 1　The Significant Level of Soluble CD14 in Sera in CHD Patients with BSS by ELSIA Assay

Notes: Results were presented as mean ± SD.

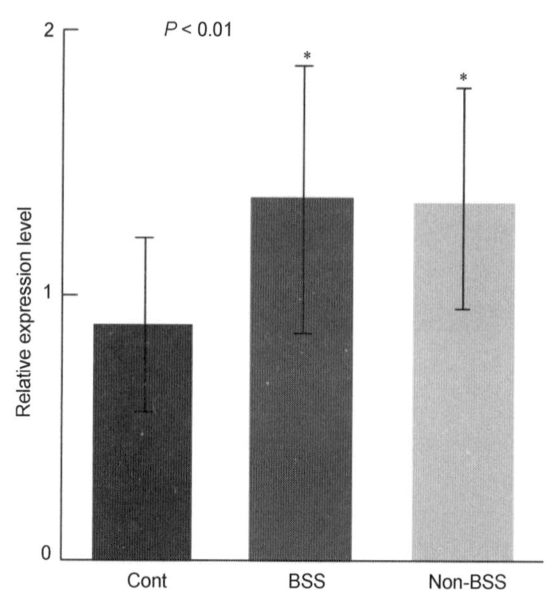

Figure 2　The mRNA Level of CD14$^+$CD16$^+$ Monocyte Subpopulation in Leukocytes in CHD Patients with BSS by qRT-PCR

Notes: $^*P < 0.01$ compared to the control group. Results were presented as mean±SD.

The expression of biological traits was controlled by gene, and the biological traits were reflected by protein. To investigate whether or not the expression change of CD14$^+$CD16$^+$ monocyte subpopulation in both CHD patients with BSS and non-BSS at its protein level, therefore, we further analyzed the protein level of CD14$^+$CD16$^+$ on monocyte member using 2-color immunofluorescent staining (Figure 3 (a)). The FACS results showed that the protein level of CD14$^+$CD16$^+$ on monocyte member was significantly increased in the CHD patients with BSS, when compared to the CHD patients with non-BSS and the healthy control ($P < 0.01$ or $P < 0.05$, Figure 3 (b)).

TNF-α is one of the cytokines with various biological activation, and one previous study confirms that increased level of TNF-α was existed in the monocyte/macrophage, smooth muscle cells, and endothelial cells in the atherosclerotic plaque, and this high level was correlated to the severity of atherosclerosis [17]. IL-1 was released by active monocyte/macrophage, which induced the releasing of many cytokines and growth factors by monocyte/macrophage and the expression of adhesion molecules such as ICAM-1. Additionally, IL-1 could stimulate vascular endothelium to produce many inflammatory factors such as TNF-α, aggravated local inflammatory reaction, and promote the development of atherosclerosis [18,19]. Additionally, previous studies indicated that the circulation of CD14$^+$CD16$^+$ monocytes could spontaneously produce TNF and IL-1[20], which could provoke cell proliferation and migration of smooth muscle cells and macrophages in the atherosclerotic plaque[21].

Therefore, protein level of TNF-α and IL-1 in sera was also assessed in our study by ELISA. The significant increased serum of TNF-α and IL-1 level was observed in CHD patients with BSS and non-BSS compared to the healthy control ($P < 0.01$, Figure 4), and the level of TNF-α and IL-1 in CHD patients with BSS was much higher than that in CHD patients with non-BSS ($P < 0.05$, Figure 4).

In the current study, we investigated that there were monocyte activation and an increased CD14$^+$CD16$^+$ monocyte subpopulation at protein level and its downstream inflammatory cytokines such as TNF-α and IL-1

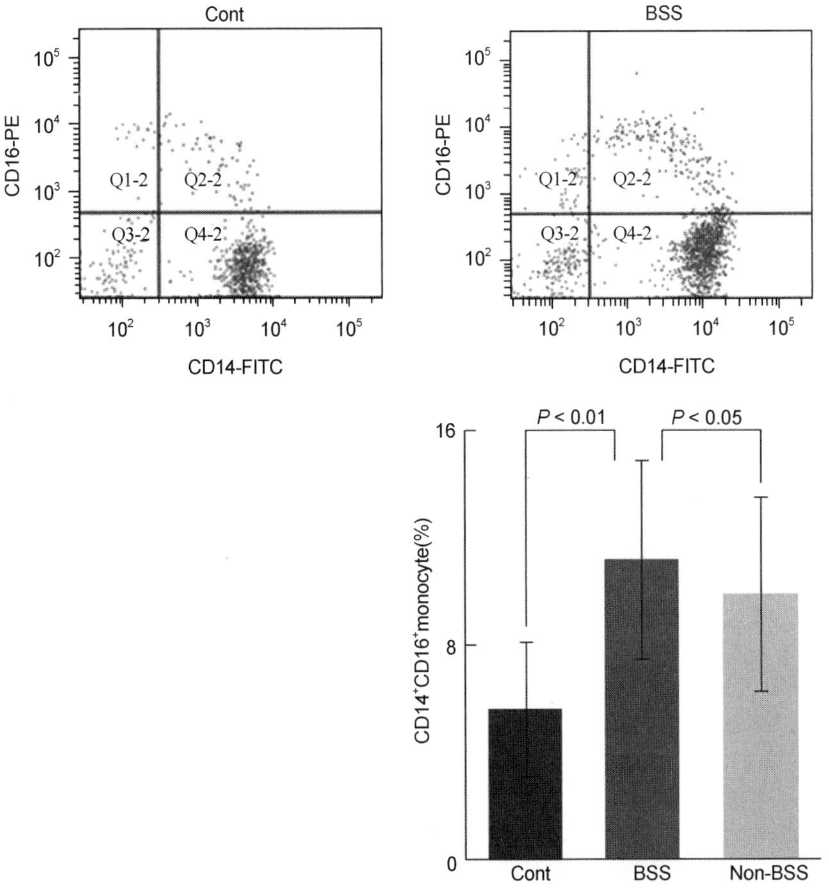

Figure 3 The Protein Level of CD14^{+}CD16^{+} Monocyte Subpopulation in CHD Patients with BSS by FACS Analysis

in sera in CHD patients with BSS. Herein, we presumed that monocyte activation in the CHD patient with BSS induced the phenotype of monocyte member transforming to CD14^{+}CD16^{+}monocyte subpopulation which was involved in the pathogenesis of CHD with BSS.

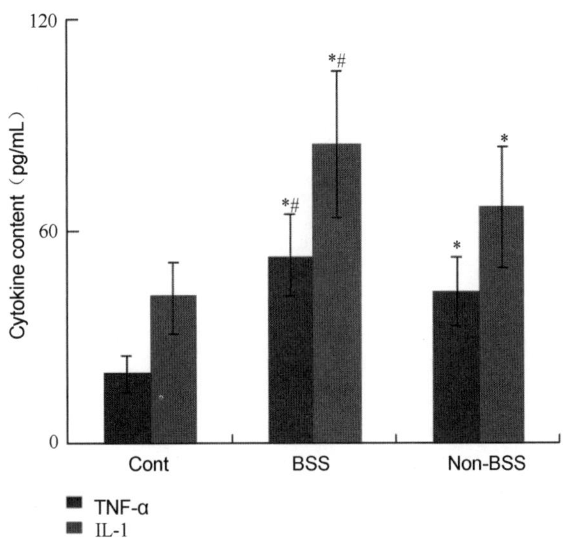

Figure 4 The Changes of Inflammatory Cytokines of TNF-α and IL-1 in Sera in CHD Patients with BSS

Notes: $^{*}P < 0.01$ compared to the control group. $^{\#}P < 0.05$ compared to the CHD patients with non-BSS. Results were presented as mean±SD.

CONCLUSION

Overall, the present work confirmed the correlation between increased $CD14^+CD16^+$ monocyte subpopulation at protein level and CHD patients with based on the way of disease syndrome combination. Thus, the increased $CD14^+CD16^+$ monocyte subpopulation and its downstream inflammatory cytokines in CHD patient with BSS indicated that $CD14^+CD16^+$ monocyte subpopulation was one of the sensitive markers in the pathogenesis of CHD with BSS.

REFERENCES

[1] Liu Y, Yin HZ, Shi DZ, et al. Chinese herb and formulas for promoting blood circulation and removing blood stasis and antiplatelet therapies[J]. Evidence-Based Complementary and Alternative Medicine, 2012, Article ID 184503.

[2] Ma XJ, Yin HJ, Chen KJ. Differential gene expression profiles in coronary heart disease patients of blood stasis syndrome in traditional Chinese medicine and clinical role of target gene[J]. Chinese Journal of Integrative Medicine, 2009, 15 (2): 101–106.

[3] Huang Y, Yin HJ, Wang JS, et al. The significant increase of Fc γ RIIIA (CD16), a sensitive marker, in patients with coronary heart disease[J]. Gene, 2012, 504 (2): 284–287.

[4] Huang Y, Yin HJ, Wang JS, et al. Aberrant expression of Fc γ RIIIA (CD16)contributes to the development of atherosclerosis[J]. Gene, 2012, 498 (1): 91–95.

[5] Huang Y, Yin HJ, Ma XJ et al. Correlation between Fc γ RIII a and aortic atherosclerotic plaque destabilization in ApoE knockout mice and intervention effects of effective components of Chuanxiong Rhizome and Red Peony Root[J]. Chinese Journal of Integrative Medicine, 2011, 17 (5): 355–360.

[6] Braunwald E, Antman EM, Beasley JW, et al. ACC/AHA 2002 guideline update for the management of patients with unstable angina and non-ST-segment elevation myocardial infarction—summary article: a report of the American College of Cardiology/American Heart Association Task Force on Practice Guidelines (committee on the management of patients with unstable angina)[J]. Journal of the American College of Cardiology, 2002, 40 (7): 1366–1374.

[7] Gibbons RJ, Chatterjee K, Daley J, et al. ACC/AHA/ACPASIM guidelines for the management of patients with chronic stable angina: executive summary and recommendations. A report of the American College of Cardiology/American Heart Association task force on practice guidelines (committee on management of patients with chronic stable angina)[J]. Circulation, 1999, 99 (21): 2829–2848.

[8] Society of Cardiology, Chinese Association of the Integrative Medicine, The diagnostic criteria of Chinese medicine in coronary heart disease[J]. Chinese Journal of Integrated Traditional and Western Medicine, 1991 11: 257.

[9] Meijerink JPP, Mandigers C, Van De Locht, E, et al. Anovel method to compensate for different amplification efficiencies between patient DNA samples in quantitative real-time PCR[J]. Journal of Molecular Diagnostics, 2001, 3 (2): 55–61.

[10] Gremmel T, Kopp CW, Seidinger D, et al. Te formation of monocyte-platelet aggregates is independent of on-treatment residual agonists'-inducible platelet reactivity[J]. Atherosclerosis, 2009, 207 (2): 608–613.

[11] Chen KJ. Exploration on the possibility of reducing cardiovascular risk by treatment with Chinese medicine recipes for promoting blood-circulation and relieving blood-stasis[J]. Zhong Guo Zhong Xi Yi Jie He Za Zhi, 2008, 28 (5): 389.

[12] Pittet MJ, Swirski FK. Monocytes link atherosclerosis and cancer[J]. European Journal of Immunology, 2011, 41 (9): 2519–2522.

[13] Woollard KJ, Geissmann F. Monocytes in atherosclerosis: subsets and functions[J]. Nature Reviews Cardiology, 2010, 7 (2): 77–86.

[14] Pamukcu B, Lip JYH, Devitt A. Te role of monocytes in atherosclerotic coronary artery disease[J]. Annals of Medicine, 2010, 42 (6): 394–403.

[15] Saha P, Modarai B, Humphries J, et al. Te monocyte/macrophage as a therapeutic target in atherosclerosis[J]. Current Opinion in Pharmacology, 2009, 9 (2): 109–118.

[16] Kruger C, Schutt C, Obertacke U, et al. Serum CD14 levels in polytraumatized and severely burned patients[J]. Clinical and Experimental Immunology, 1991, 85 (2): 297–301.

[17] Barath P, Fishbein MC, Cao J, , et al. Detection and localization of tumor necrosis factor in human atheroma[J]. American Journal of Cardiology, 1990, 65 (5): 297–302.

[18] Merhi-Soussi F, Kwak BR, Magne D, et al. Interleukin-1 plays a major role in vascular inflammation and atherosclerosis in male apolipoprotein E-knockout mice[J]. Cardiovascular Research, 2005, 66 (3): 583–593.

[19] Isoda K, Sawada S, Ishigami N, et al. Lack of interleukin-1 receptor antagonist modulates plaque composition in apolipoprotein E-defcient mice[J]. Arteriosclerosis, Trombosis, and Vascular Biology, 2004, 24 (6): 1068–1073.

[20] Frankenberger M, Sternsdorf T, Pechumer H, et al. Differential cytokine expression in human blood monocyte subpopulations: a polymerase chain reaction analysis[J]. Blood, 1996, 87 (1): 373–377.

[21] de Bont N, Netea MG, Rovers C, et al. LPS-induced release of IL-1, IL-1Ra, IL-6, and TNF-αin whole blood from patient with familial hypercholesterolemia: no effect of cholesterol-lowering treatmen, Journal of Interferon and Cytokine Research, 2006, 26 (2): 101-107.

First published: HUANG Ye, WANG Jing-shang, YIN Hui-jun, CHEN Ke-ji. The Expression of $CD14^+CD16^+$ monocyte subpopulation in coronary heart disease patients with blood stasis syndrome[J]. Evid Based Complement Alternat Med, 2013, 2013: 416932.

Effect of Chinese Drugs for Activating Blood Circulation and Detoxifying on Indices of Thrombosis, Inflammatory Reaction, and Tissue Damage in a Rabbit Model of Toxin-Heat and Blood Stasis Syndrome

XUE Mei, YIN Hui-jun, WU Cai-feng, MA Xiao-juan, GUO Chun-yu
HUANG Ye, SHI Da-zhuo, and CHEN Ke-ji

Blood stasis is considered as a major contributing factor for the pathogenesis of chronic cardiovascular and cerebrovascular diseases. The pathophysiological basis of blood stasis involves platelet adhesion, aggregation, activation, coagulation, and thrombosis. However, inflammation reaction, oxidative stress injury, tissue necrosis, and other pathological changes during the process of diseases may not be fully explained by blood stasis syndrome. Based on the interpretation of pathogenic roles of toxins in Chinese medicine, it has been believed that "stasis" and "toxin" act together to contribute to the disease etiology. Researches that attempt to elucidate of "toxin" and detoxification have been carried out using modern biology research tools.[1-3] However, the casual relationship and the interaction of "toxin" and "toxin" during pathogenesis are not well understood. Further, there have not been well-established indicators or indices that can be used as sensitive measures for exploring the therapeutic benefit of treatments that are aimed at antagonizing "stasis" and "toxin".

In the current study, utilizing a rabbit compound model of hyperlipidemia, immune injury, and endotoxininduced endothelial injury, we intended to systematically analyze the pathophysiological changes, including tissue damage, inflammation reaction, and thrombosis. At the same time, we planned to evaluate and compare the effect of Chinese medicines with activating blood circulation (ABC)activity and those with activating blood circulation and detoxifying (ABCD)activities on these pathophysiological changes. It was anticipated that the findings in the study would also provide a molecular basis for understanding the interplay of "stasis" and "toxin" in disease pathogenesis.

METHODS

1 Animals and Forage

Fifty-four male purebred New Zealand rabbits, weighting 2.0–2.5 kg, were purchased from Beijing Vital River Experimental Animals Technical Ltd. Co., with a certificate serial number SCXK (Beijing)2005-0002. Hypercholesterol forage (ordinary forage with 2% cholesterol and 5% lard)was purchased from the Experimental Animal Center of Academy of Military Medical Sciences, China.

2 Reagents and Apparatus

Percoll was purchased from Pharmacia (P8370). Rabbit antihuman factor Ⅷ related antigen (CAT: bs-0434R, LOT: 080417)and fluorescein isothiocyanate (FITC)-conjugated polyvalent goat antirabbit IgG (CAT: bsF-0295G, LOT: 080301)were purchased from Beijing Biosynthesis Biotechnology Ltd., Co., China. Bovine serum albumin (A738328)and endotoxin (L2880)were purchased from Roche and Sigma, USA respectively. Enzyme-linked immunoassay (ELISA)kits, which included matrix metalloproteinase-9 (MMP-9) (CAT: E0553Rb, LOT: 090113), tissue inhibitors tometalloproteinase (TIMP-1, CAT: E0128Rb, LOT: 090108), granule membrane protein-140 (GMP-140, CAT: E00602Rb, LOT: 090114), plasminogen activator inhibitor-1 (PAI-1, CAT: E0532Rb, LOT: 090114), highsensitivity C-reactive protein (hs-CRP, CAT: E0821Rb, LOT: 090116), interleukin-6 (IL-6, CAT:

E0079Rb, LOT: 090119), and tumor necrosis factor-α (TNF-α, CAT: E0133Rb, LOT: 090114), were all purchased from USCNLIFE Company, China, and a microplate reader (Thermo Multiskan 3, China)was used for the assay.

3 Drugs

Simvastatin was purchased from Hangzhou Merck Sharp & Dohme Pharmaceutical Ltd., Co., 40 mg/tablet, batch No. 07432. Simvastatin was grinded into powder form and dissolved in double-distilled water to have a suspension. Xiongshao Capsule (芎芍胶囊, XSC, composed of Rhizoma Chuanxiong and *Radix Paeoniae rubra*, 0.25 g/capsule, content of drug markers: paeoniflorin 28 mg, ferulic acid 3.5 mg, and gallic acid 34 mg each capsule)was purchased from Dalian Institute of Chemical Physics, China, batch No. 070929. Huanglian Capsule (黄连胶囊), 0.25 g/pill, with ingredient of chinensis Franch, was purchased from Hubei Xianglian Pharmaceutical Ltd., Co., China, with a national medicine permit No. Z19983042. XSC with the ABC activity would be compared with XSC+Huanglian Capsule that possesses ABCD activity.

4 Grouping and Model Establishment

After 7 days of acclimation, 10 of 54 rabbits were randomly taken to form the normal control group, which were fed with normal diets. The other 44 rabbits were injected with bovine serum albumin (0.5 g each)and fed with high-fat diet for 6 weeks. They were then randomly assigned into 1 of 4 treatment groups, namely, the model group (no treatment), simvastatin group, activating blood circulation (ABC)group, and activating blood circulation and detoxifying (ABCD)group, with 11 animals per group. Rabbits with high-fat diet received ear vein injection of endotoxin (1 μg/kg)on the 28th day of highfat diet, and the normal control group received normal saline. The rabbits on high-fat diet continued with the same diet plus treatment of simvastatin[4] (0.93 mg/kg per day), XSC (0.07 g/kg per day), or XSC (0.07 g/kg per day)and Huanglian Capsule (0.14 g/kg per day)administered to the simvastatin group, ABC group, and ABCD group, respectively, for an additional 2 weeks. At the end of the treatment, blood (12 mL)samples from all rabbits were taken from the abdominal aorta. The first 6 mL of the blood was collected into a sodium citrate tube and centrifuged for 15 min at 3 000r/min. The resulting plasma was stored in a −20 ℃ refrigerator to determine levels of specific serum proteins. The next 3 mL of blood was collected in a siliconized glass tube with 3.8% sodium citrate (0.33 mL)for quantification of circulating endothelial cells. [5,6] The last 3 mL of blood was collected to determine blood lipids.

5 Determination of Blood Lipids

Total cholesterol (TC), triglyceride (TG), and low-density and high-density lipoprotein cholesterol (LDL-C and HDL-C)were measured with an automatic biochemical analyzer (Hitachi 7600-020, JAPAN).

6 Determination and Quantification of Circulating Endothelial Cells

Circulating endothelia cells (CECs)were separated by Percoll density gradient. Two Percoll suspensions with a specific gravity of 1.060 g/mL and 1.045 g/mL were used. The specific gravity of 1.060 g/mL (100 mL) was obtained by mixing 42.9 mL of stock Percoll suspension, 10 mL of pooled human serum, 37.1 mL of Earle's medium, and 10 mL of 3.8% sodium citrate. The specific gravity of 1.045 g/mL (100 mL)was obtained by mixing 30.3 mL of stock Percoll suspension, 10 mL of pooled human serum, 49.7 mL Earle's medium, and 10 mL of 3.8% sodium citrate. The 3-mL of each Percoll suspension was mixed in a centrifuge tube. Anticoagulant blood diluted 1: 1 with Hanks was layered over the mixed Percoll suspension and centrifuged for 20 min at 1 800r/min at room temperature. The interface containing cells were collected using a capillary pipette and transferred to another a centrifuge tube.

Cells were precipitated by centrifugation and resuspended in 0.5 mL of saline. Cell viability was determined by 0.5% trypan blue staining (viability of>95% was required). Total cell count was obtained under a light microscope. Indirect immunofluorescence assay was performed to identify the CECs. Cell suspension was spread on a glass slide and fixed with acetone for 30 s at 4 ℃. Slides were washed with PBS (0.1 mol/L)3 times, incubated with rabbit anti-human factor Ⅷ related antigen (20 μL)for 30 min at 37 ℃, washed 3 times with PBS, stained with FITC-conjugated polyvalent goat anti-rabbit IgG (20 μL)30 min at 37 ℃, washed 3 times with PBS, and embedded in 87% glycerol in PBS (9: 1). CECs were enumerated under a fluorescent microscope (Olympus BX51, JAPAN). Negative controls were processed similarly except the rabbit antihuman factor Ⅶ related antigen was replaced with PBS.

7 Pathological Examination of the Atherosclerotic Plaque

At the end of the 2-week treatment, all rabbits were sacrificed and a 1.5-cm-long aortic arch segment was obtained from each rabbit. Samples were rinsed with normal saline, and the section with the most prominent atherosclerotic plaque was dissected. The identical section of the aortic arch was also obtained from the normal control group. Samples were then fixed with 10% formalin, embedded in paraffin, and sliced into 2-μm thickness slices. After HE staining, plaques were examined under the light microscope for foam cells, lipid storage, and cholesterol crystals.

8 Determination of Indices of Tissue Damage, Thrombosis and Inflammation Reaction

The indices of tissue damage (serum MMP-9 and TIMP-1), the indices of thrombosis (serum GMP-140 and PAI-1), and the indices of inflammation reaction (serum hs-CRP, IL-6, and TNF-α)were detected by ELISA.

9 Statistical Analysis

Statistical analysis was performed with SPSS 11.5 software, and the values of $P < 0.05$ were considered statistically significant. For enumeration data, Chi-square test was used; while for quantitative data, t test was used for comparisons between groups, and one-way ANOVA was applied for significance test in multiple-group comparisons.

RESULTS

1 General Observations

After infection of endotoxin, 5 rabbits in the model group, 2 rabbits in Simvastatin group, 5 rabbits in ABC group, and 4 rabbits in ABCD group died of infective fever. Data presented below were taken from the remaining 38 rabbits.

2 Comparison of the Level of Blood Lipids

Compared with the normal control group, the levels of TC, TG, and LDL-C increased in the model group ($P < 0.01$), but there was no change in the level of HDL-C ($P > 0.05$). Compared with the model group, the levels of TC and TG in the simvastatin group and the level of TG in the ABCD group reduced significantly ($P < 0.05$, Table 1).

Table 1 Comparison of the Levels of Blood Lipids (mmol/L, $\bar{x} \pm s$)

Group	n	TC	TG	HDL-C	LDL-C
Normal control	10	1.00 ± 0.34	0.72 ± 0.22	1.07 ± 0.43	0.43 ± 0.23
Model	6	29.93 ± 3.10*	4.61 ± 1.29*	0.94 ± 0.29	13.38 ± 3.34*
Simvastatin	9	23.89 ± 3.26△	2.24 ± 0.73*△	1.07 ± 0.33	12.21 ± 3.66
ABC	6	28.77 ± 2.86	3.58 ± 1.02	1.17 ± 0.65	13.07 ± 2.74
ABCD	7	27.92 ± 4.38	2.29 ± 0.62△	0.95 ± 0.29	12.31 ± 2.61

Notes: *$P < 0.01$, compared with the normal control group; △$P < 0.05$, compared with the model group.

3 Pathological Changes in Aortic Arch in Rabbits

Figure 1 shows the HE staining of the aortic arch tissue sections from all groups. There were no foam cells and lipid storage in the aortic media and intima in the normal control group under normal diets. In the model group fed with high-fat diet, the aortic intima was significantly thickened in comparison to the normal control group and contained numerous foam cells. There was a small amount of cholesterol crystals under the endothelium. Compared with the model group, the overall pathological changes in the all drug intervention groups appeared less severe, including thickening of the aortic intima, swelling and degeneration of endothelial cells, and the quantities of foam cells and cholesterol crystals.

4 Determination and Quantification of CECs

Endothelial cells after immunofluorescence staining appeared as cells with yellow-green fluorescence under the fluorescence microscope, and none of the cells from the negative control showed any fluorescence, confirming that the fluorescent cells were CECs. Table 2 listed the CECs counts in all groups. Compared with the normal control group, the number of CECs was significantly increased in the model group ($P < 0.01$). In contrast, the number of CECs was significantly reduced after treatment with simvastatin, ABC, or ABCD when compared with the model group ($P < 0.01$). There was no significant difference among the drug intervention groups ($P > 0.05$).

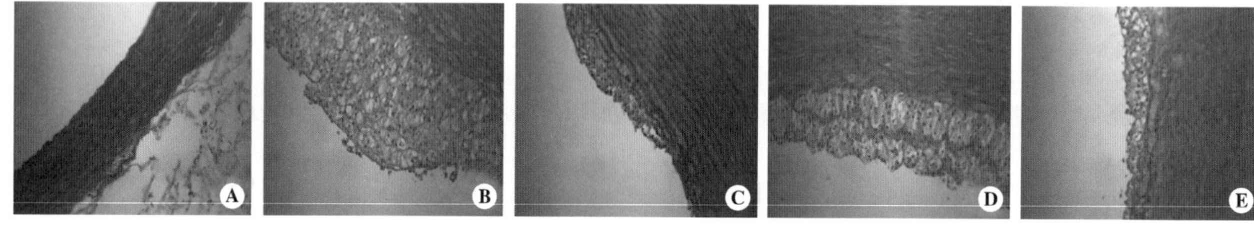

Figure 1　Histomorphologic Changes of Atherosclerosis Plaque in the Aortic Arch (HE staining, ×200)
Notes: A: normal control group, B: model group, C: simvastatin group, D: ABC group, E: ABCD group.

Table 2　Comparison of the Number of CECs in Rabbits among Groups (0.9 μg, $\bar{x} \pm s$)

Group	n	the number of CECs
Normal control	10	2.00 ± 1.25
Model	6	7.83 ± 1.72*
Simvastatin	9	3.67 ± 1.00△
ABC	6	4.00 ± 0.63△
ABCD	7	4.00 ± 1.41△

Notes: *$P < 0.01$, compared with the normal group；△$P < 0.01$, compared with the model group.

5 Comparison of Indices of Thrombosis

Compared with the normal control group, serum GMP-140 and PAI-1 were increased significantly in the model group ($P < 0.01$). Compared with the model group, serum GMP-140 and PAI-1 were decreased significantly in the simvastatin group and ABCD group ($P < 0.05$). A decrease in both GMP-140 and PAI-1 was also observed in the ABC group when compared with the model group, but the difference was not statistically significant ($P > 0.05$, Table 3).

Table 3 Comparison of the Levels of GMP-140 and PAI-1 (ng/mL, $\bar{x} \pm s$)

Group	n	GMP-140	PAI-1
Normal control	10	0.53 ± 0.12	3.83 ± 0.98
Model	6	$1.08 \pm 0.31^{*}$	$7.28 \pm 2.01^{*}$
Simvastatin	9	$0.78 \pm 0.33^{\triangle}$	$5.37 \pm 2.26^{\triangle}$
ABC	6	0.92 ± 0.20	5.92 ± 1.57
ABCD	7	$0.79 \pm 0.20^{\triangle}$	$5.23 \pm 1.39^{\triangle}$

Notes: $^{*}P < 0.01$, compared with the normal group ; $^{\triangle}P < 0.05$, compared with the model group.

6 Comparison of Indices of Inflammation Reaction

Compared with the normal control group, serum hs-CRP, IL-6, and TNF-α all increased in the model group ($P < 0.01$). Compared with the model group, reductions in levels of all three molecules were evident in all drug intervention groups; however, only reductions in hs-CRP observed in the simvastatin group and IL-6 in the ABCD group were statistically significant ($P < 0.05$, Table 4).

Table 4 Changes of the Level of Serum hs-CRP、IL-6 and TNF-α ($\bar{x} \pm s$)

Group	n	hs-CRP (ng/mL)	IL-6 (pg/mL)	TNF-α (pg/mL)
Normal control	10	5.76 ± 1.61	33.65 ± 7.31	15.24 ± 4.16
Model	6	$11.82 \pm 3.52^{*}$	$54.44 \pm 13.56^{*}$	$31.58 \pm 8.39^{*}$
Simvastatin	9	$8.54 \pm 3.76^{\triangle}$	44.34 ± 11.32	23.69 ± 9.71
ABC	6	9.53 ± 2.97	44.56 ± 12.26	25.87 ± 7.66
ABCD	7	9.02 ± 2.75	$40.64 \pm 10.11^{\triangle}$	24.14 ± 6.72

Notes: $^{*}P < 0.01$, compared with the normal group ; $^{\triangle}P < 0.05$, compared with the model group.

7 Comparison of Indices of Tissue Damage

Compared with the normal control group, serum MMP-9 was increased in the model group ($P < 0.01$) and serum TIMP-1 was reduced ($P < 0.05$). Compared with the model group, a reduction in MMP-9 and an increase in TIMP-1 were observed for all drug intervention groups, but only the reduction in MMP-9 in the simvastatin group reached statistical significance ($P < 0.05$, Table 5).

Table 5 Comparison of the Levels of Serum MMP-9 and TIMP-1 ($\bar{x} \pm s$)

Group	n	MMP-9 (ng/mL)	TIMP-1 (pg/mL)
Normal control	10	0.39 ± 0.11	329.21 ± 91.79
Model	6	$0.81 \pm 0.24^{**}$	$195.38 \pm 97.34^{*}$
Simvastatin	9	$0.58 \pm 0.26^{\triangle}$	239.39 ± 119.18
ABC	6	0.66 ± 0.22	241.66 ± 79.15
ABCD	7	0.63 ± 0.21	290.79 ± 103.89

Notes: $^{*}P < 0.05$, $^{**}P < 0.01$, compared with the normal group ; $^{\triangle}P < 0.05$, compared with the model group.

DISCUSSION

With high-fat diets and bovine serum albumin injection, lipid disorders and persistent chronic inflammatory reaction are the main underlying mechanism for plaque formation in the rabbit model of atherosclerosis. [7] Intravenous injection of endotoxin induces systemic inflammatory response, which accelerates the atherogenic process. [8]In the current study, rabbits in the model group, when compared with the normal control group, showed a significant increase in the levels of TC, TG, and LDL-C, atherosclerotic changes in the aortic arch, an increase in CECs, a rapid elevation of serum GMP-140, PAI-1, hs-CRP, IL-6, TNF-α, and MMP-9, and a reduction in TIMP-1. The protein molecules affected in the disease model have been shown in other studies to be markers or play a role in disease pathogenesis. GMP-140 is a known marker of the later stage platelet activation, which is one of the microcosmic dialectical indices of blood stasis；[9] PAI-1 promotes the development of atherosclerosis and thrombosis；[10] Hs-CRP, IL-6, and TNF-α are typical inflammatory markers and have a variety of biological effects in body response to infection and tissue damage. [11] The balance between MMP and TIMP plays an important role in the inflammatory response and tissue repair. [12]

In the rabbit model, a series of physiological responses and pathological changes occurred, including dyslipidemia, vascular endothelial cells damage, inflammation reaction, platelet activation, thrombosis and tissue damage. Pathological changes, including platelet activation and thrombosis, are always attributed to "blood stasis". Chinese medicine considers "toxin": the etiology of diseases as well as causative agent for pathological changes. Based on this concept, pathological changes, such as tissue necrosis and inflammation reaction, observed in the rabbit model could be attributed to the action of "toxin", the etiologic and pathogenic agent. The overall findings in the model could be attributed to the joint action of "toxin" and "toxin". In this model, injection of bovine serum albumin and endotoxin induced immune damage and fever. These initial responses resemble the diseases caused by pathogenic toxin in humans that are characterized by sudden onset, rapid deterioration, and muscle damage. It appears that the rabbit model used in the current study was established as a result of initial "toxin-heat" attack and subsequent "blood stasis", and both contributed to the eventual changes described above.

Huanglian Capsule is effective in detoxification and heat reduction. XSC was extracted from the traditional activating blood circulation prescription, Xuefu Zhuyu Decoction (血府逐瘀汤), and has been shown to be an effective prescription for the treatment of coronary heart disease. In this study, we used XSC (ABC)and XSC with Huanglian Capsule (ABCD)as two different treatments to assess and compare the effect of the ABC and ABCD activities in the rabbit model of toxic-heat and blood stasis syndrome. Our study results show that the rabbits treated with simvastatin had a decrease in the level of serum TC and TG, a reduction in CECs, and a decrease in the levels of serum GMP-140, PAI-1, hs-CRP, and MMP-9, compared with the rabbits in the model group that received no treatment. The results demonstrated that simvastatin had an anti-inflammatory effect in addition to its lipid lowering function. The results also showed that simvastatin had an anti-atherosclerosis effect as demonstrated by its inhibition in the expression of platelet-activating factor GMP-140, fibrinolytic system PAI-1, and tissue damage factor MMP-9 and by reduction of endothelial injury. Our observation was consistent with the previous findings. [13-16]A similar trend of improvement was also observed in the rabbits treated with the ABCD drug, and this was reflected by the improvement in the serum TG level and in the pathological changes in the aortic arch and a reduction in the number of CECs and in the levels of serum GMP-140, PAI-1, and IL-6.

In contrast, although the rabbits treated with the ABC drug had, to a lesser extent, mprovement in the pathological changes in the aortic arch and a reduction in CECs, there was no significant difference in the levels of serum GMP-140, PAI-1, hs-CRP, IL-6, TNF-α, MMP-9, and TIMP-1 when compared with the rabbits in the model group. Previous studies confirmed that some activating blood circulation and detoxifying prescription (extract of Rhizoma Polygoni Cuspidati with XSC)and an effective component of activating blood circulation and detoxifying prescription (extrac of Rhizoma Polygoni Cuspidati and the alcoholic extract of Rhubarb) could reduce the expression of hs-CRP, TNF-α, and MMP-9 in apolipoprotein E gene knockout mice. [1-3]The discrepancy of the findings might be associated with different models utilized and different indices selected in each individual studies.

In our rabbit model of toxin-heat and blood stasis symdrome, a rapid and dramatic rise in the indices selected to represent thrombosis (GMP-140 and PAI-1), inflammation reaction (hs-CRP, IL-6, and TNF-α), and tissue damage (MMP-9 and TIMP-1)was observed in comparison to the normal control group, indicating that these measurements could be used as molecular biomarkers in the diagnosis of toxin-induced stasis and both toxin-and stasis-induced diseases. Further, based on the principle of syndrome differentiation through formula effect assessment, the superior therapeutic benefit of the ABCD drug compared with the ABC drug provided an alternative validation to the rabbit model of toxin-heat and blood stasis. Our study also indicated that serum GMP-140, PAI-1, and IL-6 were sensitive molecular indices for determining the therapeutic effect of drugs with activating blood circulation and detoxifying activities.

REFERENCES

[1] Zhang JC, Chen KJ, Zheng GJ, et al. Regulatory effect of Chinese herbal compound for detoxifying and activating blood circulation on expression of NF- κ B and MMP-9 in aorta of apolipoprotein E gene knocked-out mice[J]. Chin J Integr Tradit West Med (Chin), 2007, 27 (1): 40-44.

[2] Zhang JC, Chen KJ, Liu JG, et al. Effect of assorted use of Chinese drugs for detoxifying and activating blood circulation on serum high sensitive C-reactive protein in apolipoprotein E gene knock-out mice[J]. Chin J Integr Tradit West Med (Chin), 2008, 28 (4): 330-333.

[3] Zhou MX, Xu H, Chen KJ, et al. Effects of some active ingredients of Chinese drugs for activating blood circulation and detoxicating on blood lipids and atherosclerotic plaque inflammatory reaction in ApoE-gene knockout mice[J]. Chin J Integr Tradit West Med (Chin), 2008, 28 (2): 126-130.

[4] Chen Q. Methodological Study of Chinese Herbs pharmacology[M]. People's Medical Publishing House. 1996, 8, 1103-1105.

[5] Gan WJ, Liu JT, Lin R. The protective effect of quercetin on the vascular endothelial cells injured by homocysteine in rabbits[J]. Chin Pharmacol Bull (Chin), 2004, 20 (6): 647-651.

[6] R Sbarbati, M de Boer, M Marzilli, et al. Immunologic detection of endothelial cells in human whole blood[J]. Blood, 1991, 77 (4): 764-769.

[7] Ding J, Chen HY, Kong J, et al. Effect of Rosiglitazone on cardiovascular ultrastructure of atherosclerosis in rabbits[J]. Chin J Gerontology (Chin), 2008, 28 (4): 342-344.

[8] Wang KF, Lu FE, Xu LJ, et al. Study on the dynamic changes of body temperature and plasma endotoxin levels in rabbits after infusion with endotoxin[J]. Acta Universitatis Medictnae Tangji (Chin), 2001, 30 (2): 129-133.

[9] Chen KJ, Xue M, Yin HJ. The Relationship between Platelet Activation and Coronary Heart Disease and Blood-stasis Syndrome[J]. Journal of Capital Medical University (Chin), 2008, 29 (3): 266-269.

[10] Chen LH, Lu GP, Wu CF, et al. Effect of pravastatin on arterial gene expression of plasminogen activator inhibitor type 1 in atherosclerotic rabbits[J]. Chinese Journal of Cardiology (Chin), 2001, 29 (2): 115-117.

[11] Ma XJ, Yin HJ, Chen KJ. Research progress of correlation between blood-stasis syndrome and inflammation[J]. Chin J Integr Med (Chin), 2007, 27 (7): 669-672.

[12] Bruno G, Todor R, Lewis I, et al. Vascular extracellular matrix remodeling in cerebral aneurysms[J]. J Neurosurg, 1998, 89: 431-440.

[13] Ji Y, Zhang RY, Lu G, et al. Effect of simvastatin on the expressions of P-selectin and ICAM-1 in atherosclerotic iliac artery of rabbits[J]. Chin J Geriatrics (Chin), 2003, 22 (3): 165-168.

[14] Qin L, Zhu Y, Huang KX. Study on expression of plasminogen activator inhibitor type-1 and its correlation with cholesterolemia in the atherosclerotic rabbits[J]. J Clin Cardiology (Chin), 2006, 22 (9): 538-540.

[15] Zhang L, Jiang YR, Xue M, et al. of simvastatin on the atherosclerotic plaque stability and the angiogenesis in atherosclerotic plaque of rabbits[J]. Chinese Sci Bull (Chin), 2009, 54 (15): 2228-2232.

[16] Yip HK, Sun CK, Chang LT, et al. Strong suppression of high-sensitivity C-reactive protein level and its mediated pro-atherosclerotic effects with simvastatin: in vivo and in vitro studies[J]. Int J Cardiol, 2007, 121 (3): 253-60.

First published: XUE Mei, YIN Hui-jun, WU Cai-feng, MA Xiao-juan, GUO Chun-yu, HUANG Ye, SHI Da-zhuo, CHEN Ke-ji. Effect of Chinese drugs for activating blood circulation and detoxifying on indices of thrombosis, inflammatory reaction, and tissue damage in a rabbit model of toxin-heat and blood stasis syndrome[J] . Chin J Integr Med, 2013, 19 (1): 42-47.

Correlation between Platelet Gelsolin and Platelet Activation Level in Acute Myocardial Infarction Rats and Intervention Effect of Effective Components of Chuanxiong Rhizome and Red Peony Root

LIU Yue, YIN Hui-jun, JIANG Yue-rong, XUE Mei, GUO Chun-yu, SHI Da-zhuo, and CHEN Ke-ji

Despite recent medical advances, cardiovascular diseases remain the predominant cause of morbidity and mortality all over the world[1,2]. Rupture of atherosclerotic plaque and the ensuing thrombotic changes are the triggers for acute coronary event. Platelet activation and aggregation play crucial roles in this process of atherothrombosis. The emergence of antiplatelet drug is the milestone of prevention and therapy of cardiovascular disease and provides the primary therapeutic strategy to combat cardiovascular diseases. The proper application of antiplatelet drug in reducing the mortality and morbidity of acute myocardial infarction successfully has been verified by a large number of large-scale clinical trials[3]. Antiplatelet drug, such as aspirin, now is recommended for the secondary prevention of cardiovascular disease (CVD)in patients with CVD because it decreases the risk of CVD events and mortality in clinical trials of men and women with CVD[4]. But many clinical problems arose along with the wide range of application of antiplatelet drugs (such as aspirin and clopidogrel, etc.) during the past 10 years[5,6]. Despite their proven benefits, recurrent cardiovascular events still occur in those taking antiplatelet drugs. This has led to the concept of "antiplatelet drug resistance," most commonly aspirin or clopidogrel resistance. The latest research shows that aspirin prophylaxis in people without prior CVD does not lead to reductions in cardiovascular death, for the benefits are further offset by clinically important bleeding events[7], which limit the clinical practice of antiplatelet drugs widely. These phenomena suggest that other pathways capable of stimulating platelet activation may exist and provide an impetus for developing new antiplatelet drugs which possess higher efficacy and fewer adverse effects.

Proteomics technology has been successfully applied to platelet research during the past 5 years, contributing to the emerging field of platelet proteomics which led tothe identification of a considerable amount of novel platelet proteins, many of which have been further studied at their functional level[8]. Our previous work[9] indicated that platelet gelsolin is the main platelet differential functional protein between patients of coronary heart disease and healthy people by platelet proteomics. Studies have also shown that platelet gelsolin is highly expressed in patients with acute coronary syndrome (ACS)and the blood-stasis syndrome (BSS)of traditional Chinese medicine (TCM)[10,11]. Gelsolin is known to have one of the key roles in extra-myocardial infarction (AMI)is unclear. On the prevention of cellular actin-scavenger system (EASS)[12], but the biology-atherosclerosis or vulnerable plaque, Chinese medicine and Western medicine agree on stabling plaque and promoting blood circulation. Based on the agreed thoughts of the Eastern and Western worlds, the application of Chinese herbs for activating blood circulation (ABC herbs)has valuable significance in the exploration of reducing the risk of cardiovascular event[13,14]. Chuanxiong rhizome and Red peony root are the two classical ABC herbs in China and have been used for thousands of years in the prevention and treatment of CVD. Xiongshao capsule (XSC)is a patent drug in China and is composed of effective components of Chuanxiong rhizome and Red peony root. Our previous studies have showed that paeoniflorin, ferulic acid and total phenolic acid are the major active principles of the water extract from Xiongshao capsule[15,16]. Clinical studies indicated that XSC can effectively prevent restenosis after percutaneous coronary intervention (PCI)[17], but the antiplatelet target of XSC is not defined.

In the present study, we used AMI as a disease model to investigate the correlation between platelet gelsolin and platelet activation level in rat model of AMI and the prophylaxis mechanism of XSC *in vivo*.

MATERIALS AND METHODS

1 Drug and Reagents

Xiongshao Capsule (XSC), which contained paeoniflorin (more than or equal to 28 mg each capsule), ferulate (more than or equal to 3.5 mg each capsule), and total phenolic acid (more than or equal to 34 mg each capsule), 0.25 g per capsule, were provided by Beijing International Institute of Biological Products (batch no. 200091, Beijing, China); aspirin, 0.1 g per capsule, was purchased from Bayer HealthCare Manufacturing (batch no. BJ01653, Beijing, China); verapamil, 0.04 g per tablet, was purchased from the Central Pharmaceutical Co., Ltd (batch no. 100402, Tianjing, China). All the drugs were dissolved in pure water before use. Fluo-3AM was purchased from Sigma (St Louis, MO, USA); rabbit anti-gelsolin polyclonal antibody was purchased-actin monoclonal antibody was purchased from Sigma (St Louis, MO, USA); FITC-Phalloidin was purchased from Sigma (St Louis, MO, USA); enzyme-linked immunosorbent assay (ELISA) kit of P-selectin, gelsolin, F-actin, vitamin D binding protein (VDBP), CK-MB, cTnI, TXB, and COX-1 were purchased from Huamei Biological Technology Company (Wuhan, Hubei province, China).

2 Animal Grouping and Treatment

Sprague Dawley (SD)rats (male, weight 220–250 g, *n*=90)were obtained from Beijing University Laboratory Animal Center (the animal certificate No: SCXK (Jing)2006–0009). The rats were housed in humidity-controlled (55 ± 5)% rooms at (22 ± 2)℃ with a 12 h on/12 h off light cycle. The animals were maintained with free access to standard diet and tap water.

After one week of adaptive feeding, we randomly allocated the SD rats into six groups of 15 rats each as fol-lows: Model group, Sham group, Aspirin group, Xscd group (the high dose group), Xscx group (the low doses group), and Verapamil group. Aspirin 40 mg/kg/day, verapamil 4 mg · $kg^{-1}d^{-1}$, and XSC 390 mg/kg/day, 195 mg/kg/day per gavage for 3 consecutive weeks were administrated to the aspirin, verapamil, Xscd and Xscx groups respectively. Rats in the Sham and Model groups received the same volume of distilled water, per gavage for 3 weeks. After 3 weeks, myocardial infarction (MI)model was created in rats by ligating the left anterior descending coronary artery (LAD)as described before[18]. The Animal Care and Use Committee of Xiyuan hospital approved the experimental protocol.

3 Sample Preparation

After 3 hours of ligation, all the rats were killed after anesthesia by intraperitoneal injection of 20% urethane (0.5 mL/100 g). Fresh blood (10 mL)was drawn from the abdominal aorta and collected into vacutainer tubes containing acid citrate dextrose (ACD)9% v/v (trisodium citrate 22.0 g/L, citric acid 8.0 g/L, dextrose 24.5 g/L)as anti-coagulant. The initial 2 mL of blood was discarded to avoid spontaneous platelet activation. The blood was centrifuged for 10 min at 150 × g at room temperature to obtain platelet-rich plasma (PRP)and the remaining blood centrifuged for 20 min at 800 × g to obtain platelet poor plasma (PPP). Ischemic heart tissue was taken after blood collection and preserved at 80 ℃ for detection of gelsolin expression by western blotting.

4 Enzyme-Linked Immunosorbent Assay Analysis

The concentration of PRP and PPP of gelsolin, plasma F-actin, VDBP, CK-MB, cTnI, TXB, COX-1 were determined by enzyme-linked immunoadsorbent assay (ELISA), as per the manufacturer's instructions. The absorbance was measured at 450nm in an ELISA reader.

5 Western Blotting Analysis

The level of gelsolin in ischemic heart tissues was determined by Western blot analysis according to the standard procedure as described previously[19]. β-actin was used as a loading control.

6 Detection of MFI of Platelet Calcium Ion

Platelet-rich plasma was prepared and incubated with 4 mol/L Fluo-3-AM (Sigma, Saint Louis, MO, USA) at 37 ℃for 40 min. The calcium concentration of platelets was determined using flow cytometry to measure the mean fluorescence intensity (MFI), as previously described[20].

7 Statistical Analysis

Data are presented as mean SD. The SPSS Statistics 11.0 package was utilized to analyze the data. Differences among groups were analyzed using the one-way analysis of variance (ANOVA), followed by multiple comparisons by Least-Significant Difference (LSD)test. Spearman's correlation coefficients were calculated to study the relations between gelsolin concentration in PRP and plasma P-selectin level. Differences between groups were at $P < 0.05$.

RESULTS

1 General Condition

All the rats in the different groups survived and exhibited normal physical appearance and behavior during the gavage period of different drugs. The outcome among the different groups after ligation of LAD is presented in Table 1.

Table 1　The Outcome among the Different Groups after Ligation of LAD

Group	*N*	Dead rats (*n*)	Surviving rats (*n*)
Sham	15	6	9
Model	15	6	9
Aspirin	15	5	10
Xscd	15	6	9
Xscx	15	7	8
Verapamil	15	7	8

2 XSC Reduces the Concentration of Myocardial Injury Markers

We chose CK-MB and cTnI as the myocardial injury markers in rats with acute myocardial infarction (AMI). Compared with the Sham group, the concentration of CK-MB and cTnI of Model group increased significantly after ligation of LAD for 3 hours ($P < 0.01$). The high dose of XSC (390 mg/kg/day)can reduce the concentration of CK-MB and cTnI markedly ($P < 0.05$); this has similar effect withaspirin in vivo (see Table 2).

Table 2　Effect of Xiongshao Capsule (XSC)on the Concentration of Myocardial Injury Markers of AMI Rats

Group	*N*	CK-MB (ng/mL)	cTnI (pg/mL)
Sham	9	0.279 ± 0.074	9.81 ± 2.62
Model	9	0.386 ± 0.043**	15.18 ± 4.3**
Aspirin	10	0.340 ± 0.024†	12.04 ± 1.19†
Xscd	9	0.336 ± 0.027†	12.23 ± 1.41†
Xscx	8	0.351 ± 0.013	13.85 ± 3.02
Verapamil	8	0.358 ± 0.017	14.43 ± 2.98

Notes: **$P < 0.01$ compared to Sham group and †$P < 0.05$ compared to Model group.

3 XSC Inhibits the Platelet Activation Level

We choose the plasma P-selectin as the marker of platelet activation level. Compared with Sham group, the plasma P-selectin concentration of the Model group increased significantly after ligation of LAD for 3 hours ($P < 0.01$). The high dose of XSC can inhibit P-selection level markedly ($P < 0.05$), this has similar effect with the Aspirin group (see Figure 1).

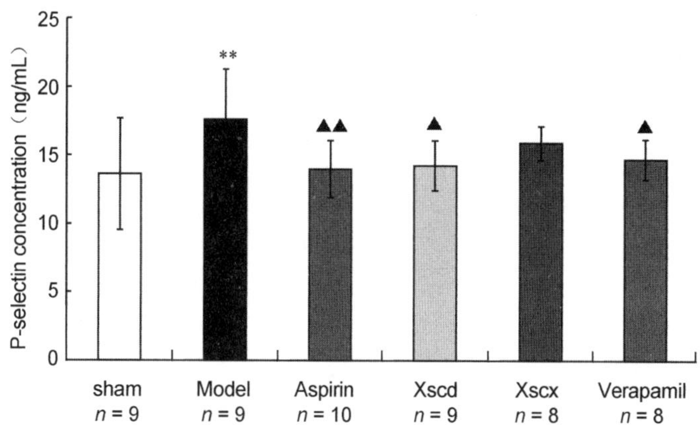

Figure 1 Effect of Xiongshao Capsule (XSC)on P-selectin Concentration of AMI Rats

Notes: $^{**}P < 0.01$ compared to Sham group, and $^{▲}P < 0.05$ or $^{▲▲}P < 0.01$ compared to Model group.

4 XSC Reduces the Platelet Gelsolin Level and Enhances the Activity of Extracellular Actin-Scavenger System (EASS)

Plasma gelsolin and VDBP are the main components of the EASS which undertake the responsibility as scavenger of the abnormal increased extracellular filament actin (F-actin). Compared with the Sham group, the plasma gelsolin and VDBP of the Model group was reduced significantly ($P < 0.05$)and F-actin increased markedly ($P < 0.01$), while platelet gelsolin it increased markedly ($P < 0.01$). High dose of XSC can reduce platelet gelsolin and F-actin level ($P < 0.05$), while it increased plasma gelsolin and VDBPsignificantly ($P < 0.05$) (see Figures 2, 3, and 4).

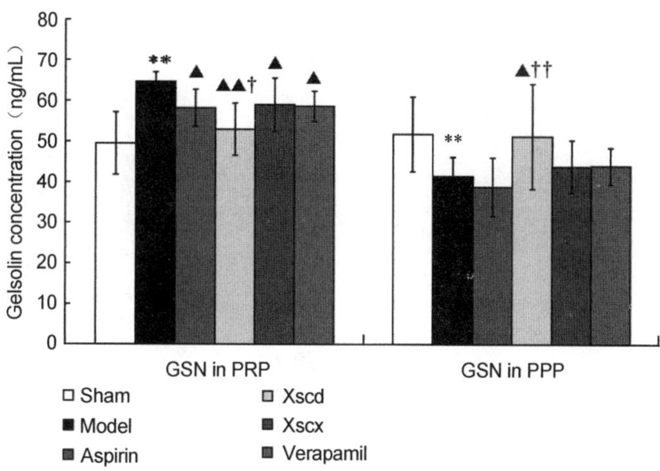

Figure 2 Effect of Xiongshao Capsule (XSC)on Gelsolin Concentration among PRP and PPP of AMI Rats

Notes: $^{**}P < 0.01$ compared to Sham group, $^{▲}P < 0.05$ or $^{▲▲}P < 0.01$ compared to Model group, and $†P < 0.05$ or $^{††}P < 0.01$ compared to Aspirin group.

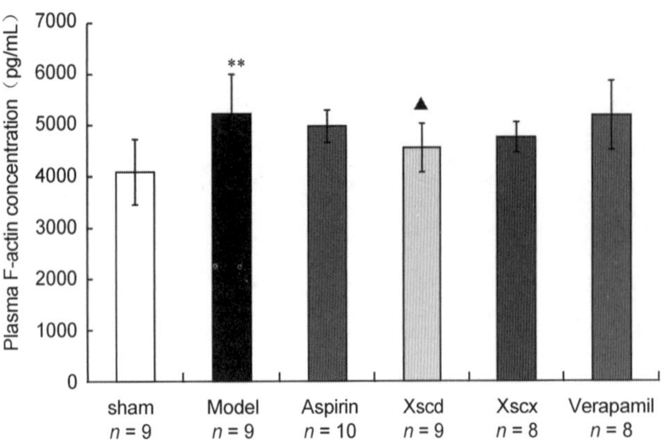

Figure 3 Effect of Xiongshao Capsule (XSC)on Plasma F-actin Concentration of AMI Rats

Notes: $^{**}P < 0.01$ compared to Sham group, and $^{▲}P < 0.05$ compared to Model group.

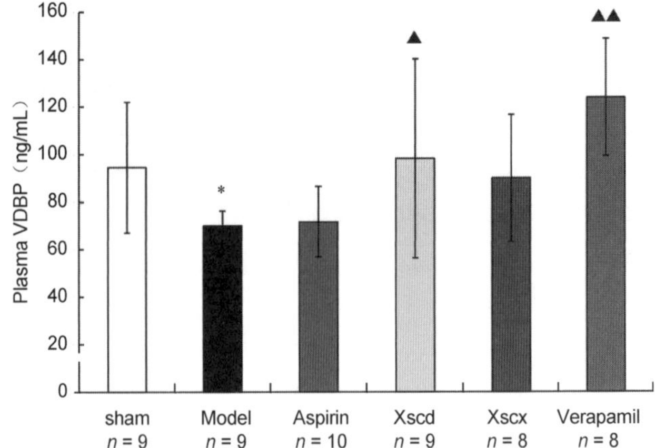

Figure 4 Effect of Xiongshao Capsule (XSC)on Plasma VDBP Concentration of AMI Rats

Notes: $^{*}P < 0.05$ compared to Sham group, and $^{▲}P < 0.05$ or $^{▲▲}P < 0.01$ compared to Model group.

5 XSC Inhibits the Activation of TXB2 and COX-1

Compared with Sham group, the concentration of TXB2 and COX-1 of Model group increased significantly after ligation of LAD for 3 hours ($P < 0.01$). High dose of XSC can reduce COX-1 and TXB2 level significantly ($P < 0.05$); this has similar effect with the Aspirin group (see Figure 5).

6 XSC Inhibits the MFI of Calcium

Compared with Sham group, the MFI of calcium of the Model group increased markedly ($P < 0.01$), High dose of XSC can inhibit platelet calcium increase ($P < 0.05$). This has similar effect to the Verapamil group ($P < 0.05$) (Figure 6).

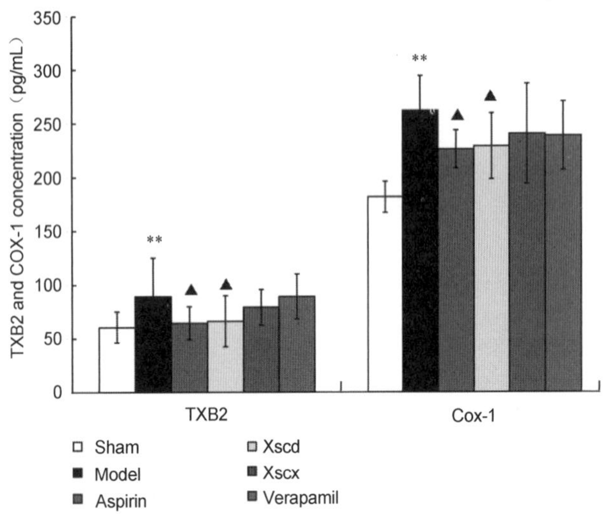

Figure 5 Effect of Xiongshao Capsule (XSC)on Plasma TXB2 and COX-1 Concentration of AMI Rats

Notes: $^{**}P < 0.01$ compared to Sham group, and $^{▲}P < 0.05$ compared to Model group.

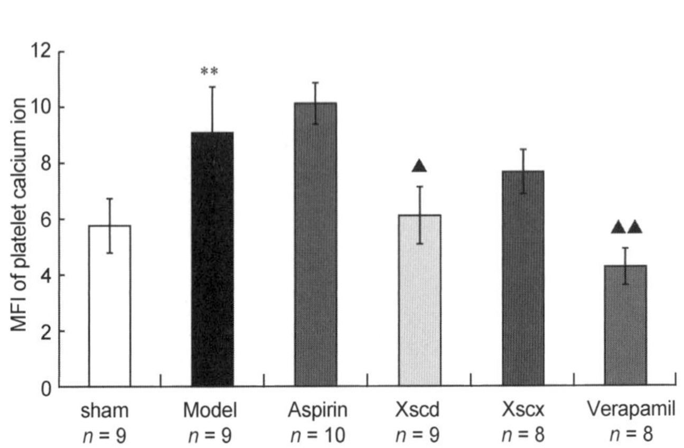

Figure 6 Effect of Xiongshao Capsule (XSC)on MFI of Platelet Calcium Ion Concentration of AMI Rats

Notes: $^{**}P < 0.01$ compared to Sham group, and $^{▲}P < 0.05$ or $^{▲▲}P < 0.01$ compared to Modelgroup.

7 XSC Attenuates the Expression of Gelsolin in Infarcted Myocardium

Compared with Sham group, the gelsolin expression of infarcted myocardium of Model group increased markedly, and XSC can inhibit gelsolin expression of infarcted myocardium, but verapamil has no such effect (see Figure 7).

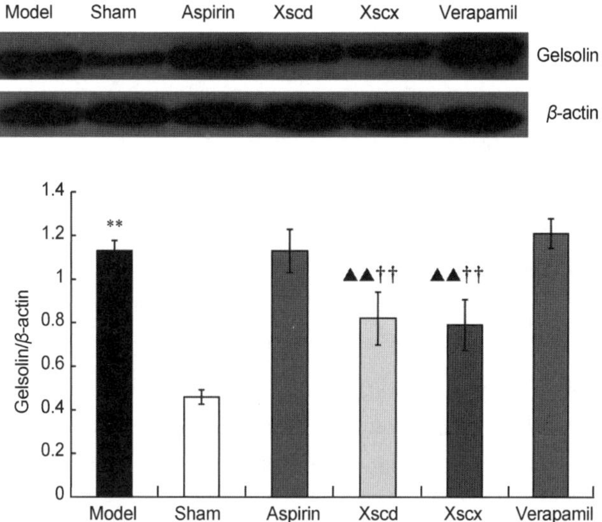

Figure 7 Effect of Xiongshao Capsule (XSC)on Protein Level of Gelsolin in Ischemic Heart Tissue of AMI Rats

Notes: $^{**}P < 0.01$ compared to Sham group, and $^{▲▲}P < 0.01$ compared to Model group, $^{††}P < 0.01$ compared to Aspirin group.

8 Analyses of Correlation between Platelet Gelsolin Concentration and Plasma P-Selectin Level

Next we investigated any potential correlation between the platelet gelsolin concentration and plasma P-selectin levels that may exist in the Model group and Xscd group. Correlation analysis showed that platelet gelsolin concentrations were high positively correlated with plasma P-selectin levels in the Model group (see Figure 8 (a))and Xscd group (see Figure 8 (b)).

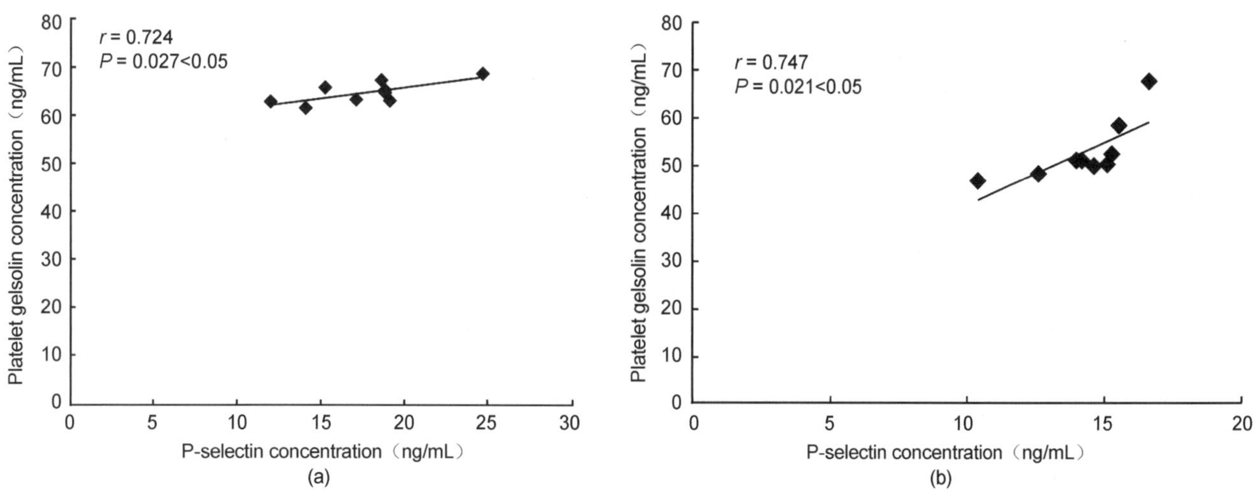

Figure 8 Correlation between Gelsolin Concentration in PRP and Plasma P-selectin Level of Model Group and XSCD Group

Notes: (a)Model group and (b)Xscd group.

DISCUSSION

Gelsolin is a calcium-regulated actin filament (F-actin)severing and capping protein, which is expressed as both cytoplasmic and plasma isoforms. The functions of extracellular gelsolin are less well defined. Gelsolin is also an important cytoskeletal protein, which is a key actin binding protein (ABPs)as well. Increasingly evidence has shown that gelsolin has close relationship with many diseases and pathological processes, such as cancer, apoptosis, infection and inflammation, pulmonary diseases, and aging[21]. During the past 5 years, many scholars began to focus on gelsolin's possible role in the development of cardiovascular diseases[22].

Activated platelets play a pivotal role in the formation of arterial thrombi, and antiplatelet drugs become the core in the prevention and treatment of CVD. Platelet activation not only causes the changes of membrane protein, but also a series of morphological changes, from inviscid, discotic circulating platelets to a paste-like, protruding platelet jelly, that affects the regulation of platelet cytoskeletal proteins. Using differential proteomics of platelet, our previous study[9] indicated that platelet gelsolin was the main platelet differential functional proteins between patients with coronary heart disease and healthy people. In addition, data from our previous clinical studies demonstrated that[10,11] platelet gelsolin was highly expressed in patients with acute coronary syndrome (ACS)and the blood stasis syndrome (BSS)of traditional Chinese medicine. Meanwhile, based on the Chinese medicine principle of "prescription to syndrome." Platelet gelsolin may be viewed as a new target for ABC herbs. In this study, we evaluated the biological role of platelet gelsolin in the development of platelet activation in a rat model of AMI and the potential contribution of XSC prophylaxis in this progress in vivo.

As we know, P-selectin is a 140 kD glycoprotein that is presented in the granules of platelets and translocates rapidly to the cell surface after platelet activation; it is generally considered as the gold marker of platelet activation[23]. In this study, after ligation of LAD for 3 hours, the concentration of CK-MB and cTnI and the P-selectin level of the Model rats increased significantly compared with Sham rats, which indicated that the model rats had myocardial injury and platelet activation.

The actin cytoskeleton plays a central role in many fundamental cellular processes involving the generation of force and facilitation of movement, which are enabled by the assembly of actin monomers into filaments and cooperation with a wide variety of ABPs[21], including gelsolin. Actin monomers (G-actin) spontaneously associates to form F-actin under physiological conditions and vice versa. This dynamic progress keeps in balance all the time. In the presence of tissue injury or cell death, G-actin is released into the circulation where it can interact with components of the haemostatic and fibrinolytic systems, or polymerize and form F-actin excessively. Studies[24] have suggested that F-actin can lead to platelet aggregation directly in vitro, and the presence of excessive F-actin in blood vessels, which can plug smaller vessels and decrease blood flow to promote the formation of blood clots, can be fatal. Infusion of high doses of G-actin in rabbits caused the rapid and fatal formation of massive F-actin-containing thrombi in arterioles and capillaries of pulmonary veins[25]. An extracellular actin-scavenger system (EASS)[12] was therefore likely to exist.

Plasma gelsolin, together with vitamin D binding protein (VDBP), another extracellular ABPs, were regarded as potentially important components of this system. They are capable of removing F-actin from the circulation and inhibiting F-actin elongation to alleviate the vascular toxicity of excessive F-actin. In this study, the concentration of gelsolin in PRP of AMI rats increased accompanied by the high platelet activation and increased level of F-actin while gelsolin in PPP decreased which indicates the EASS of AMI rats was suppressed. Correlation analysis showed that platelet gelsolin concentrations were high, positively correlated with plasma P-selectin levels in the Model group.

Xiongshao capsule (XSC)is a patent drug developed from Xue Fu Zhu Yu Decoction. It is the classic formula used for activating blood circulation (ABC)in China for hundreds of years. Clinical studies have shown that XSC can effectively prevent restenosis after percutaneous coronary intervention (PCI)[17]. XSC was shown to enhance the protective effect of ischemic postconditioning on rat with myocardial ischemic reperfusion injury[26]. It was also shown to stabilize atherosclerotic plaque by suppressing inflammation and the expression of Fcγ RIIIA[27]. But the potential antiplatelet mechanism of XSC prophylaxis is unclear. In this study, we found that high dose of XSC prophylaxis could decrease the concentration of myocardial injury markers, CK-MB and cTnI, and reduce the plasma P-selectin level of AMI rats as well. The antiplatelet mechanism of aspirin involves the inhibition of COX-1 and TXA2, our study shows that high dosage of XSC can inhibit the activation of TXB2 and COX-1 in vivo, which has similar cardio-protection effect with aspirin in vivo. Meanwhile, high dosage of XSC prophylaxis inhibited the expression of platelet gelsolin in AMI rats by inhibiting the platelet calcium influx, but increased the concentration of plasma gelsolin and plasma VDBP simultaneously, so the EASS was activated, and the concentration of F-actin in AMI rats decreased which indicated that the F-actin was being removed from the circulation. Calcium ions not only promote gelsolin secretion but also play a vital role in the development of platelet activation. Studies have shown increased platelet Ca2+ in patients with CVD[28], and that calcium channel platelet aggregation[29]. Verapamil is a classic CCB agent and a previous study *in vivo*[30] shows that verapamil exhibits a dose-dependent inhibitory effect on platelet aggregation and thrombus formation in rats. In this study, our results show that high dosage of XSC can mimic the calcium channel antagonist effect. We have also investigated the expression of the gelsolin in infarcted myocardium of AMI rats. The results indicate that the gelsolin expression of infarcted myocardium of the Model group increased markedly; while XSC can inhibit gelsolin expression of infarcted myocardium significantly, verapamil or aspirin has no such effect, holding that other pathway existed in the regulation of gelsolin as well. Heart failure (HF)is the end stage of CVD (including after AMI). It is of great importance to know the effects and mechanism of XSC on cardioprotection at earlier stages of CVD. Ventricular remodeling after AMI is the main pathological change of HF. A previous study[31] has showed that gelsolin is an important contributor to heart failure progression through novel mech-and DNaseI activation and downregulation of antiapoptotic survival factors. Based on these results and our study, we propose that gelsolin inhibition is a promising target for CVD therapy besides antiplatelet agent.

CONCLUSION

We have provided experimental evidence supporting our conclusion that high correlation between platelet gelsolin and platelet activation level in AMI rats, the aspirin-like cardio-protection, and antiplatelet effects of XSC are related to its inhibition on platelet gelsolin, platelet calcium influx and activated the EASS. Taken together, our results suggest that platelet gelsolin is a potential antiplatelet target and XSC is a promising lead compound for antiplatelet and cardiovascular therapy.

REFERENCES

[1] J. Choi and J. C. Kermode. New therapeutic approaches to combat arterial thrombosis[J]. Molecular Interventions, 2011, 11 (2): 111-123,

[2] Tseeng S, Arora R. Reviews: aspirin resistance: biological and clinical implications[J]. Journal of Cardiovascular Pharmacology and Therapeutics. 2008, 13 (1): 5-12.

[3] Michelson AD. Antiplatelet therapies for the treatment of cardiovascular disease[J]. Nature Reviews Drug Discovery, 2010, 9 (2): 154-169.

[4] Baigent C, Blackwell C, Collins R, et al. Aspirin in the primary and secondary prevention of vascular disease: collaborative meta-analysis of individual participant data from randomised trials[J]. The Lancet, 2009: 373 (9678): 1849-1860.

[5] Juurlink DN, Gomes T, Ko DT et al. A population-based study of the drug interaction between proton pump inhibitors and clopidogrel[J]. Canadian Medical Association Journal, 2009, 180 (7): 713-718.

[6] J. L. Mega, S. L. Close, S. D. Wiviott et al.Cytochrome P-450polymorphisms and response to clopidogrel[J]. N Engl J Med, 2009，360（4）：354-362.

[7] Seshasai SR, Wijesuriya S, Sivakumaran R, et al. Effect of aspirin on vascular and nonvascular outcomes: meta-analysis of randomized controlled trials[J]. Archives of Internal Medicine, 2012, 172 (3): 209-216.

[8] Garc'ıa A. Clinical proteomics in platelet research: challenges ahead[J]. Journal of Thrombosis and Haemostasis, 2010, 8 (8): 1784-1785.

[9] Li XF, Jiang YR, Wu CF, et al. Study on the correlation between platelet function proteins and symptom complex in coronary heart disease[J]. Zhongguo Fen Zi Xin Zang Bing Xue Za Zhi, 2009, 9 (6): 326-331.

[10] Liu Y, Yin HJ, Chen KJ. Research on the correlation between platelet gelsolin and blood-stasis syndrome of coronary heart disease[J]. Chinese Journal of Integrative Medicine, 2011, 17 (8): 587-592.

[11] Liu Y, Yin HJ, Jiang YR, et al. Correlation between platelet gelsolin level and different types of coronary heart disease[J]. Chinese Science Bulletin, 2012, 57 (6): 631-638.

[12] Lee WM, Galbraith RM. The extracellular actin-scavenger system and actin toxicity[J]. New England Journal of Medicine, 1992, 326 (20): 1335-

1341.

[13] Chen KJ. Explore the possibilities of Chinese herb and formulas for promoting blood circulation and removing blood stasis on reducing the cardiovascular risk[J]. Zhongguo Zhong Xi Yi Jie He Za Zhi, 2008, 28 (5): 389.

[14] Liu Y, Yin HJ, Shi DZ, et al. Chinese herb and formulas for promoting blood circulation and removing blood stasis and antiplatelet therapies[J]. Evidence-Based Complementary and Alternative Medicine, 2012: 8.

[15] Zhang Z, Qing LM, and Chen KJ. Study on the pharma-cokinetics of paeoniflorin contained in Xiongshao capsule in canine[J]. Zhongguo Shi Yan Fang Ji Xue Za Zhi, 2000, 6 (6): 21-24.

[16] Zhang Z, Yan YF, Chen KJ. Study on the pharmacokinetics of ferulic acid in canine serum after giving an intragastrical single dose of Xiongshao capsules to a dog[J]. Beijing Zhong Yi Yao Da Xue Xue Bao, 2001, 24 (1): 25-28.

[17] Chen KJ, Shi DZ, Xu H, et al. XS0601 reduces the incidence of restenosis: a prospective study of 335 patients undergoing percutaneous coronary intervention in China[J]. Chinese Medical Journal, 2006, 119 (1): 6-13.

[18] Sun M, Dawood F, Wen WH, et al. Excessive tumor necrosis factor activation after infarction contributes to susceptibility of myocardial rupture and left ventricular dysfunction[J]. Circulation, 2004, 110 (20): 3221-3228.

[19] Li GH, Shi Y, Chen Y, et al. Gelsolin regulates cardiac remodeling after myocardial infarction through DNase I-mediated apoptosis[J]. Circulation Research, 2009, 104 (7): 896-904.

[20] Zhuang MM, Wen YX, Liu SL, et al. Determination of the level of cytopplasmic free calcium in human platelets with flow cytometry[J]. Xi An Jiao Tong Da Xue Xue Bao, 2005, 26 (5): 508-510.

[21] Li GH, Arora PD, Chen Y, et al. Multifunctional roles of gelsolin in health and diseases[J]. Medicinal Research Reviews, 2012, 32 (5): 999-1025.

[22] Liu Y, Jiang YR, Yin HJ, et al. Gelsolin and cardiovascular diseases[J]. Zhongguo Fen Zi Xin Zang Bing Xue Za Zhi, 2011, 11 (1): 50-53.

[23] Michelson AD， Furman MI.Laboratory markers ofplatelet activation and their clinical significance[j]. Curr Opin Hematol,1999,6(5): 342-348.

[24] C. A. Vasconcellos and S. E. Lind. Coordinated inhibition of actin-induced platelet aggregation by plasma gelsolin and vita-min D-binding protein[J]. *Blood*, 1993, 82 (12): 3648-3657.

[25] J. G. Haddad, K. D. Harper, M. Guoth et al. Angiopathic consequences of saturating the plasma scavenger system for actin, *Proceedings of the National Academy of Sciences of the* [J]. *United States of America*, 1990, 87 (4): 1381-1385.

[26] D. W. Zhang, L. Zhang, J. G. Liu et al. Effects of Xiongshao capsule combined with ischemic postconditioning on mono-cyte chemoattractant protein-1 and tumor necrosis factor-in rat myocardium with ischemic reperfusion injury[J]. *Zhongguo Zhong Xi Yi Jie He Za Zhi*, 2010, 30 (12): 1279-1283.

[27] Huang Y, Yin HJ, Ma XJ, et al. Correlation between RIIIA and aortic atherosclerotic plaque destabilization in ApoE knockout mice and intervention effects of effective components of Chuanxiong Rhizome and Red Peony Root. Chinese Journal of Integrative Medicine, 2011, 17 (5): 355-360.

[28] Yoshimura M, Oshima T, Hiraga H, et al. Increased cytosolic free Mg and Ca in platelets of patients with vasospastic angina[J]. American Journal of Physiology, 1998, 274 (2): R548-R554.

[29] Fujinishi A, Takahara K, Ohba C, et al. Effects of nisoldipine on cytosolic calcium, platelet aggregation, and coagulation/fibrinolysis in patients with coronary artery disease[J]. Angiology, 1997, 48 (6): 515-521.

[30] Li W, Liu Y, Huang Y, et al. Effect of verapamil on the thrombogenes is and nitric oxide level in the serum of rats[J]. Nanjing Yi Ke Da Xue Xue Bao, 2007, 27 (10): 1080-1083.

[31] Li GH, Shi Y, Chen Y, et al. Gelsolin regulates cardiac remod-eling after myocardial infarction through DNase I-mediated apoptosis[J]. Circulation Research, 2009, 104 (7): 896-904.

First published: LIU Yue, YIN Hui-jun, JIANG Yue-rong, XUE Mei, GUO Chun-yu, SHI Da-zhuo, CHEN Ke-ji. Correlation between platelet gelsolin and platelet activation level in acute myocardial infarction rats and intervention effect of Effective components of Chuanxiong rhizome and red peony root[J] . Evid Based Complement Alternat Med, 2013, 2013: 985746.

ITIH4: A New Potential Biomarker of "Toxin Syndrome" in Coronary Heart Disease Patient Identified with Proteomic Method

XU Hao, SHANG Qing-hua, CHEN Hao, DU Jian-peng, WEN Jian-yan
LI Geng, SHI Da-zhuo, and CHEN Ke-ji

Syndrome differentiation is a unique diagnostic method of traditional Chinese medicine (TCM)[1-2]. "Blood stasis syndrome" (BSS)is considered as a major and key syndrome in the process of coronary heart disease (CHD)in TCM[3,4], and activating blood circulation and dissolving stasis has been a mainstream treatment for CHD. However, some stable CHD patients develop acute cardiovascular events (ACEs), while others do not, why? Based on this question, we proposed a hypothesis of "blood stasis and toxin" considering blood stasis was a constant pathogenesis in CHD, while "toxin" was the trigger in transforming to ACEs[5].

The original meaning of "toxin" is a kind of poisonous herb but it has been considered as a pathogenic factor in a narrow sense and pathogenesis, medicine, and syndrome in a broad sense. It is often seen in the fields of epidemic febrile diseases and surgical diseases (such as carbuncle, abscess, hard furuncle, and sore). Zhang et al. [6]presented a theory of "artery carbuncle" according to previous studies that arteriosclerosis plaque has the characteristics such as redness, swelling, and being hot on the local scale, just like the traditional "toxin syndrome." Heat-clearing and detoxifying treatment has been widely used in CHD, especially acute coronary syndrome patients[7–9]. Previous studies showed that Rhizoma Coptidis, Cyrtomium Rhizome, compound simiao yongan decoction, and Huanglian Jiedu decoction could improve clinical symptoms by multiple mechanisms such as anti-inflammatory action, lipid regulation, and AS plaque reduction[10–19]. Furthermore, a lot of researches indicated that drugs for activating blood circulation and detoxifying had a better effect on relieving angina than drugs for activating blood circulation only; it might be related to the effect of anti-inflammatory action[20–27].

Changes in macroscopic manifestation certainly have the corresponding microscopic biological basis. Inflammation has been proved to be a biomarker for CHD/ACS, and the proteome supported us with a new technology for studying it further. The proteome is a subject studying all the proteins in a cell, a kind of tissue, or an organism in specific conditions or at specific times and has been one of the most potential and effective approaches for decoding and revealing the biological foundation and essence of syndromes. Different syndromes consequentially have relevant differential protein expressions; meanwhile, one syndrome also has different protein expressions after treatment of different medicines. Therefore, the protein's characteristics of a specific syndrome can be reflected by the effectiveness of prescriptions corresponding to syndromes.

Berberine extracted from Rhizoma Coptidis, a representative herb of clearing heat and detoxifying, could inhibit the expressions of inflammatory factors such as thromboxane A2 and prostaglandin I2 after the injury of blood vessels[10]. Xiongshao capsule, consisting of active ingredients (Chuanxiongol and paeoniflorin), has shown beneficial effect in atherosclerosis or CHD in clinical and experimental studies[28–34]. Therefore, it was served as a representative Chinese medicine for activating blood circulation.

The aim of this study was to look for the protein biomarker of "toxin syndrome" of CHD patients, which is anticipated to help early identification of high-risk CHD patients in stable period.

DESIGN AND ETHICS STATEMENT

There are two parts in this paper (Figure 1). The first one was a randomized controlled trial (RCT)with 2 study groups conducted at 2 cooperating hospitals (Anzhen Hospital and Tongren Hospital)to look for biomarkers for "toxin syndrome" of TCM. The other was a nested case-control study with a follow-up for ACEs conducted at 5 cooperating hospitals (China Academy of Chinese Medical Sciences Xiyuan Hospital, China-Japan friendship Hospital, Anzhen Hospital, Tongren Hospital, and Fujian Integrative Medicine Clinic) to verify the biomarker found in RCT. The trials were carried out according to the Declaration of Helsinki, and the protocols were approved by the institutional review boards and ethics committees at each center. All the patients provided written informed consent.

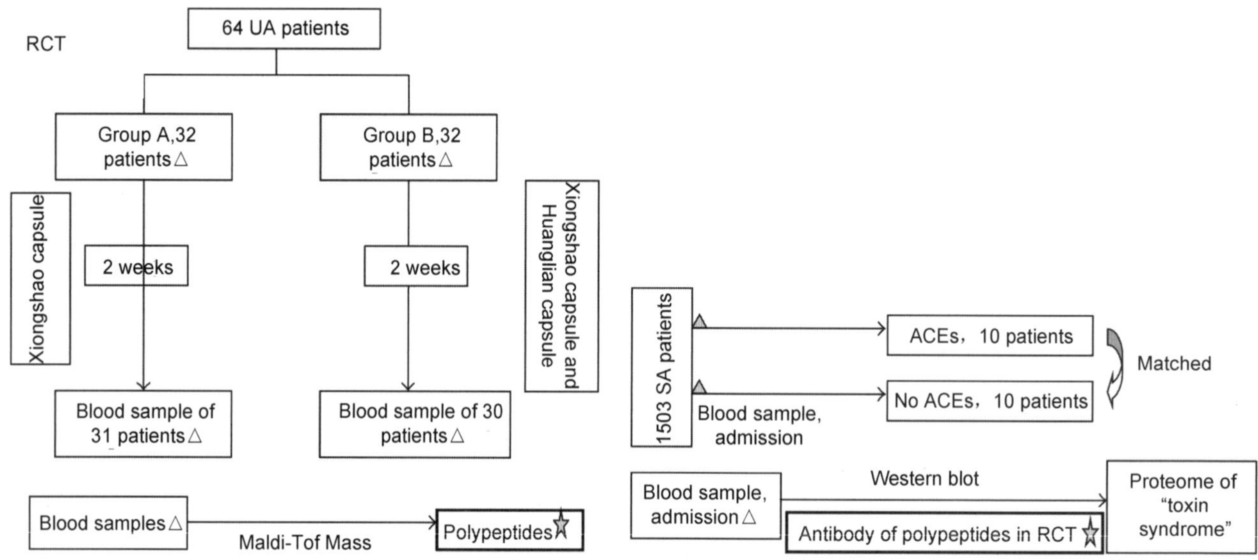

Figure 1　Flow Chart of the Study

Notes: UA: unstable angina pectoris; SA: stable angina pectoris; RCT: randomized controlled trial; ACEs: acute cardiovascular disease.

MATERIALS AND METHODS

1 Randomized Controlled Trial

1.1 Patients

Fasting serum samples were obtained from 64 patients with UA (ICD-10: I20.0/20.1/20.9)[35,36]aged between 40 and 75 years old. All of the patients who were admitted into the 2 cooperating hospitals were enrolled in the study. The inclusion criteria were successful PCI in 48 hours after the first severe angina and BSS of TCM (including Qi-stagnation-blood-stasis syndrome and Qi-deficiency blood-stasis syndrome)[37–39]. Patients were excluded if they met any of the following criteria: presence of (1)stable angina or acute myocardial infarction; (2)inflammation, fever, trauma, bure, or surgery in one recent month; (3)active tuberculosis or rheumatic autoimmune disease; (4)known renal insufficiency and serum creatinine＞2.5 mg/dL in male and＞2.0 mg/dL in female; (5)known hepatic insufficiency and alanine transaminase (ALT)＞three times value of the normal level; (6)severe heart failure (EF＜35%); (7)complication by severe primary disease such as hematologic systems and psychological abnormalities; (8)malignancies; (9) organ transplantation; (10)participants of other clinical trials; (11)taking other Chinese patent drugs; (12) pregnancy or breast-feeding. Patients were removed from analysis if they could not estimate the efficacy for they did not take any medicine or did not participate reexamination as proposal.

1.2 Groups and Drugs

64 eligible patients were randomly assigned in a 1∶1 ratio to group of activating blood circulation (Xiongshao capsule, Z20053499, Hospital preparation approved by Beijing drug administration, group A) or group of activating blood circulation and detoxification (Huanglian capsule, Z19983042, Hubei Xianglian Pharmaceutical Co., Ltd and Xiongshao capsule, group B). Randomization table was performed centrally with the use of SAS software and reserved by a specific person who did not participate this clinic research. Randomized number was obtained by telephone if any patient was eligible.

In the group of activating blood circulation, Xiongshao capsule was taken as 500 mg (2 capsules)3 times per day for 2 weeks. In the group of activating blood circulation and detoxification, Huanglian capsule was taken as 500 mg (2 capsules)3 times perday, and Xiongshao capsule was taken as 500 mg (2 capsules)3 times per day for 2 weeks.

All patients received western standardized medication including antiplatelet drugs (aspirin and/or clopidogrel hydrogen sulfate), anticoagulant drugs (heparin or low molecular weight heparin), anti-ischemic drugs (nitrates, β-blocker, calcium channel blocker, and angiotensin converting enzyme inhibitors), and statins.

1.3 Data Collection

At the beginning of the trial, all patients filled out a standardized questionnaire containing general information, past history, risk stratification of UA[40], angina score, primary symptom score of TCM[41], BSS score[42], medical treatment, and PCI surgery. In addition, to obtain the serum, at the beginning and the end of the trial, 2 ml of blood from each patient with an empty stomach was drawn into common coagulation-promoting tubes, centrifuged at 3000 r for 10 min at room temperature to remove insoluble materials, cells, and debris, and supernatants were kept at –80 ℃ until use.

1.4 Reagents and Instruments

The WCX magnetic bead kit (Bruker Daltonics Tech, Beijing, China), alpha-cyano-4-hydroxycinnamic acid (HCCA), MALDI-TOF MS (type: microflex, Bruker Daltonics Biosciences, Bremen, Germany), 100% ethanol (chromatographic grade), and 100% acetone (chromatographic grade)were freshly prepared (sigma).

1.5 WCX Fractionation and MALDI-TOFMS Analysis

The suspension in the WCX magnetic bead kit was mixed by shaking. After eluting and beating, the magnetic beads were separated from the protein, and the eluted peptide samples were transferred to a 0.5 mL clean sample tube for further MS analysis. Five microliters of HCCA substrate solution (0.4 g/L, dissolved in acetone and ethanol)and 0.8–1.2 μL of elution were mixed. Then, 0.8–1.2 μL of this mixture was applied to a metal target plate and dried at room temperature. Finally, the prepared sample was analyzed by MALDI-TOFMS. A range of 1000–10, 000Da peptide molecular weights was collected, and 400 shots of laser energy were used. Peptide mass fingerprints were obtained by accumulating 50 single MS signal scans.

1.6 Peptide Sequence

Experiment for 4280.13 m/z peptide identification was performed using a nano-liquid chromatography-electrospray ionization-tandem mass spectrometry (nano-LC/ESI-mass spectrometry/mass spectrometry) system consisting of an Acquity UPLC system (Waters)and an LTQ Orbitrap XL mass spectrometer (Thermo Fisher)equipped with a nano-ESI source. The peptide solutions were loaded to a C18 trap column (nano-Acquity) (180 μm × 20 mm × 5 μm (symmetry)). The flow rate was 15 μL/min. Then the desalted peptides were analyzed by C18 analytical column (nano-Acquity) (75 μm × 150 mm × 3.5 μm (symmetry))at a flow rate of 400nL/min. The mobile phases A (5% acetonitrile, 0.1% formic acid)and B (95% acetonitrile, 0.1% formic acid)were used for analytical columns. The gradient elution profile was as follows: 5%B–50%B–80%B-80% B–50%B–5%B in 100 min. The MS instrument was operated in a data-dependent model. The range of full scan was 400–2000 m/z with a mass resolution of 100, 000 (m/z 400). The eight most intense monoisotope ions were the precursors for collision induced dissociation. Mass spectrometry was limited to two consecutive scans per precursor ion followed by 60s of dynamic exclusion.

1.7 Statistical Analysis

ClinProTools (ClinProt software version 2.1, Bruker Daltonics)was used to subtract baseline, normalize spectra (using total ion current), and determine peak m/z values and intensities in the mass range of 1000 to 10, 000Da. The signal-to-noise (S/N)ratio should be higher than five. To align the spectra, a mass shift of no more than 0.1% was determined. The peak area was used as quantitative standardization. Student's *t*-test was used for analysis of normally distributed continuous data, while Wilcoxon test for non-normally distributed continuous data. Chi-square test was used for categorical data analysis. A P value＜0.05 was considered significant.

2 Nested Case-Control Study

2.1 Patients

1503 patients with stable CHD (old myocardial infarction or at least one significant (＞50%)stenosis that was documented on a recent coronary angiogram and WHO[35])younger than 80 years old were enrolled from 5 cooper-ating hospitals. Stable CHD was defined as no symptoms or stable exertional angina or patients in stable condition after ACS for at least 1 month. Patients were excluded if they met any of the following criteria: presence of (1)inflammation, fever, trauma, bure, or surgery in one recent month；(2)active tuberculosis or rheumatic autoimmune disease；(3)severe heart failure (EF＜35%)；(4)complication by severe valvular heart disease, or myocardiopathy；(5)complication by severe chronic obstructive pulmonary disease (COPD), pulmonary heart disease or respiratory failure；(6)known renal insufficiency and serum creatinine＞2.5 mg/dL in male and＞2.0 mg/dL in female；(7)known hepatic insufficiency and alanine transaminase (ALT)＞three times value of the normal level；(8)complication by severe primary disease such as hematologic systems；(9)severe psychological abnormalities；(10)malignancies；(11)viscera transplantation；(12)life expectancy less than 3 years. Patients were removed from analysis if a mistaken inclusion or lack of necessary record for analysis or failure to follow up for ACEs because of missing contact information took place.

2.2 Data Collection

In all patients, follow-up was scheduled at 0.5 and 1 year after inclusion of the trial. At every visit of the trial, information was obtained from each patient by use of a standardized questionnaire, the information regarding general information, past history, and the secondary cardiovascular events in follow-up. Physicians collecting information were unaware of the purpose of the study. Secondary cardiovascular events were defined as death from heart disease, nonfatal myocardial infarction (MI), or ischemic cerebrovascular events (stroke or transient ischemic attack). All the cardiovascular events were estimated by consulting medical records. In addition, the serum also was collected at every visit, and the method of blood collection, centrifugation, and storage was the same as that of RCT.

Twenty three patients were confirmed as ACEs during one-year follow-up, and 10 patients were selected for their well preserved serum sample. Another 10 patients with no follow-up ACEs were matched in a 1∶1 ratio by sex, age (±5 years), hypertension history, diabetes history, and myocardial infarction history. All the sera at the admission of these 20 patients were adopted for verifying the differential protein of "toxin syndrome" obtained from RCT by Western blot method.

2.3 Western Blot

To detect the inter-alpha-trypsin inhibitor heavy chain H4 (ITIH4)obtained from RCT (see results section), blood serum stored in −80 ℃ refrigerator was assayed using Western blot as described before[43]. Additionally, ITIH4 antibody (1: 2500, Sigma, USA)was used for detection of ITIH4. The horseradish peroxidase (HRP) conjugated anti-mouse IgG (0.1 mL/cm^2, Santa Cruz Biotechnology, UAS)was used as the secondary antibody, and signals were visualized using the enhanced chemiluminescence system (ECL, Pierce, USA).

3 Statistical Analysis

Statistical analysis was performed by a statistician in a blind fashion. Statistical analysis was performed with SPSS15.0 software. All tests were two tailed, and a statistical probability of < 0.05 was considered significant. Normality test and homogeneity test of variances were conducted. Frequency table, percentage or constituent ratio for describing enumeration data; $\bar{x} \pm s$ for describing measurement data. χ^2 test or Fisher exact test if necessary was used for comparison of enumeration data, *t*-test was used for comparison of measurement data (corrected *t* test was used if variant heterogeneity), and *Wilcoxon* tests were used for abnormal distribution.

RESULTS

1 Patients' Characteristics in RCT

64 participants with UA were enrolled in 5 centers and were randomized into two groups: 32 to receive Xiongshao capsule (group A)and 32 to receive Xiongshao capsule and Huanglian capsule (group B). During the course of the study, one patient was excluded in group A due to incomplete follow-up, while two patients were excluded in group B with 1 incomplete follow-up, and 1 noncompliance with medications. They were removed from statistics as the stated protocol. Thus finally, the populationin analysis consisted of 61 patients, with 31 patients in group A and 30 patients in group B. The baseline characteristics of the UA patients were summarized in Table 1. The two groups were well matched with regard to baseline clinical and angiographic characteristics ($P > 0.05$).

Table 1 Baseline Information of Two Groups in RCT

Groups	Group A	Group B
Age		
Minimum value (years)	48	42
Maximum value (years)	74	75
Mean value (years)	61.94 ± 8.41	61.24 ± 9.86
Sex		
Male (proportion)	22 (71%)	25 (86.2%)
Female (proportion)	9 (29%)	5 (13.8%)
Angina score 1	14.42 ± 4.86	14.89 ± 4.63
Primary symptom score of TCM	17.97 ± 6.74	18.94 ± 5.64
BSS score	10.89 ± 4.62	10.59 ± 3.38
Past history		
Hypertension (*N*)	18	16
Diabetes (*N*)	7	9
Dislipidemia (*N*)	11	12
Stroke (*N*)	2	4
Peripheral vascular atherosclerosis (*N*)	5	3

Continued

Groups	Group A	Group B
Old myocardial infarction (*N*)	4	1
Western medicine		
Aspirin (*N*)	31	30
Clopidogrel hydrogen sulfate (*N*)	31	30
Nitrates (*N*)	21	16
β-blocker (*N*)	28	30
ACEI/ARB (*N*)	19	17
CCB (*N*)	3	9
Low molecular weight heparin (*N*)	16	19
Statins (*N*)	30	29
UA risk stratification		
Low risk (*N*)	0	0
Mediate risk (*N*)	26	24
High risk (*N*)	5	6
Number of stenosed coronary vessel		
1 vessel (*N*)	8	12
2 vessels (*N*)	12	7
3 vessels (*N*)	11	11
Lesions nature		
De novo (*N*)	28	26
Restenosis (*N*)	3	4
Stent type		
Sirolimus-eluting stent (*N*)	21	21
paclitaxel-eluting stent (*N*)	8	6
Mixed drug-eluting stents (*N*)	2	3
Total length of stents	22.94 ± 7.23	21.67 ± 9.69

Note: group A patients have taken the Xiongshao capsule ; group B patients have taken the Xiongshao capsule and Huanglian capsule.

2 Sample Processing in RCT

During the course of the protein analysis, five blood samples were excluded from group A due to bad peptide mass spectrometry; thus, the population in differential protein analysis consisted of 56patients, with 26 patients in group A and 30 patients in group B. Acquisition mass range 500–10000Da (low-to-medium molecular mass range)would be studied in bioinformatics analysis.

3 MALDI-TOF Mass Spectrometry Analysis of Peptides in Serum of RCT

Statistical analysis of the data revealed that the expression of 24 spots was altered after treatment as compared with that at admission in group A (7 of them upregulated and 17 downregulated, Table 2, Figure 2). The expression of 15 spots was altered after treatment as compared with that at admission in group B (8 of them upregulated and17 downregulated, Table 3, Figure 3), and 4 of the 15 spots were the same as group A. Twelve protein spots were found (Table 4)to be the differential protein for the significant differences between the difference of before-after treatment in group A and group B; 2 of them (3207.37Da and 4279.95Da)were considered to be unique to "toxin syndrome" for being differential proteins of group B but not group A. These 2 spots were identified by mass spectrometry (Figures 4 and 5).

Table 2 Comparison of before and after Treatment in Group A ($\bar{x} \pm s$)

Mass (Da)	Ave ± StdDev (A-Q)	Ave ± StdDev (A-H)	*P*
1076.12	3.77 ± 2.35	2.54 ± 1.24	0.016099
1136.37	7.25 ± 3.12	5.42 ± 2.08	0.008065
1205.62	9 ± 3.32	6.92 ± 4.43	0.018784
1329.42	14.44 ± 7.31	10.26 ± 4.92	0.000268
1348.81	10.41 ± 4.08	7.09 ± 2.89	0.000806
1464.89	24.93 ± 13.64	13.52 ± 6.44	0.000293
1519.06	18.49 ± 8.17	11.39 ± 5.92	0.000111
1544.61	30.66 ± 17.33	19.41 ± 16.3	0.011662
1616.74	33.35 ± 22.17	18.7 ± 9.09	0.002143
2209.31	37.24 ± 18.84	25.45 ± 17.84	0.01935
2279.51	50.15 ± 17.26	40.99 ± 14.08	0.018232
2644.01	30.08 ± 20.39	22.42 ± 14.8	0.000347
2660.01	288.15 ± 231.67	206.03 ± 161.86	0.003587
2862.02	77.55 ± 78.74	45.15 ± 29.33	0.00951
3261.7	125.1 ± 63.45	159.89 ± 62.44	0.043161
3277.49	45.57 ± 23.64	59.7 ± 29.1	0.015557
4053.87	71.26 ± 38.16	95.63 ± 53.55	0.047052
4710.25	15.53 ± 5.5	12.84 ± 4.04	0.028146
4936.1	17.25 ± 15.28	9.77 ± 2.99	0.015955
4964.02	147.4 ± 184.34	59.95 ± 34.25	0.019728
5807.76	52.08 ± 23.63	70.92 ± 24.68	0.010841
5822.51	22.33 ± 13.95	31.77 ± 10.34	0.007368
5904.69	881.7 ± 598.83	1266.04 ± 415.59	0.00471
6049.22	27.36 ± 10.77	32.41 ± 10.1	0.023583

Note: paired sample *t* test was used, 2-tailed, and $P < 0.05$ was considered significant ; Ave: peak area/intensity average ; StdDev: standard deviation of the peak area/intensity average ; A-Q: before treatment in group A ; A-H: after treatment in group A.

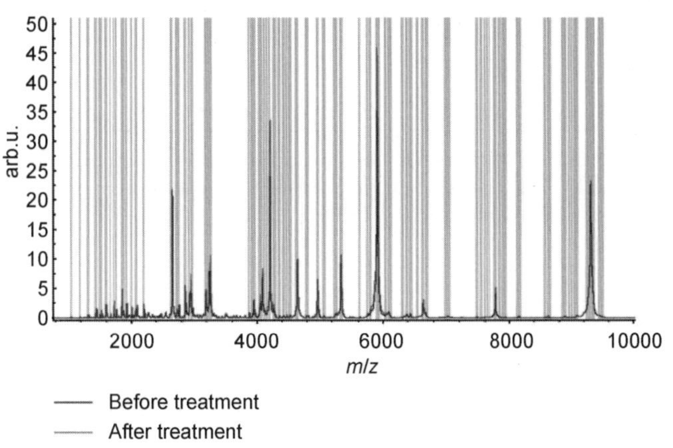

Figure 2 Peptide Mass Spectrometry before and after Treatment in Group A

Table 3　Comparison of before and after treatment in Group B ($\bar{x} \pm s$)

Mass (Da)	Ave±StdDev (B_Q)	Ave±StdDev (B_H)	*P*
1616.74	32.83 ± 18.26	23.95 ± 12.74	0.033415
2209.31	29.04 ± 14.35	21.23 ± 10.27	0.022373
2881.04	49.8 ± 18.98	38.19 ± 10.15	0.010917
3207.37	56.15 ± 17.06	47.84 ± 12.01	0.023899
4053.87	60.23 ± 22.82	83.04 ± 42.14	0.010323
4266.31	35.94 ± 19.99	45.73 ± 19.4	0.020676
4279.95	18.9 ± 8.79	27.23 ± 23.79	0.025866
4817.85	20.34 ± 17.41	11.15 ± 7.93	0.012491
4936.10	21.91 ± 27.22	10.29 ± 3.94	0.02628
5066.25	25.87 ± 7.61	32.1 ± 11.2	0.019568
5248.63	21.01 ± 5.89	25.23 ± 8.04	0.025751
6378.01	47.98 ± 47.92	28.92 ± 10.34	0.045958
7833.86	10.85 ± 2.21	12.97 ± 4.82	0.040051
9064.40	30.36 ± 8.86	35.83 ± 10.12	0.012614
9290.26	907.98 ± 442.14	1126.48 ± 455.76	0.023601

Note: paired sample *t*-test was used, 2-tailed, and $P < 0.05$ was considered significant；Ave: peak area/intensity average；StdDev: standard deviation of the peak area/intensity average；B-Q: before treatment in group B；B-H: after treatment in group B；overstriking mass: unique to group B.

Table 4　Comparison of Difference between before and after Treatment in the Two Groups

Mass (Da)	Ave ± StdDev (A_H-A_Q)	Ave ± StdDev (B_H-B_Q)	*P*
1329.42	-4.18 ± 5.02	0.4 ± 6.86	0.005918
1519.06	-7.1 ± 7.9	-2.47 ± 9.08	0.046435
2660.01	-82.12 ± 130.27	3.85 ± 184.48	0.047102
2881.04	4.86 ± 16.64	-11.62 ± 23.4	0.003442
3207.37	6.56 ± 21.34	-8.31 ± 19.09	0.008696
3277.49	14.13 ± 27.75	-9.87 ± 33.72	0.005087
3972.15	-8.69 ± 22.59	3.47 ± 15.5	0.02561
4279.95	-2.49 ± 14.27	8.32 ± 19.41	0.020196
5066.25	-0.43 ± 10.97	6.23 ± 13.8	0.049446
5807.76	18.84 ± 34.89	-2.2 ± 36.2	0.031283
5822.51	9.44 ± 16.49	-7.75 ± 32.03	0.013558
6088.68	8 ± 28.11	-8.21 ± 25.58	0.029233

Note: paired sample *t*-test was used, 2-tailed, and $P < 0.05$ was considered significant；Ave: peak area/intensity average；StdDev: standard deviation of the peak area/intensity average；"A_H-A_Q"：subtraction between after and before treatment in group A；"B_H-B_Q"：subtraction between after and before treatment in group B；overstriking mass: unique to "Toxin".

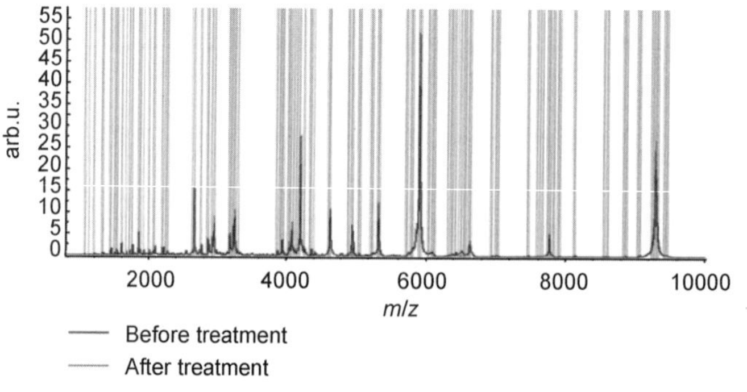

Figure 3　Peptide mass spectrometry before and after treatment in group B

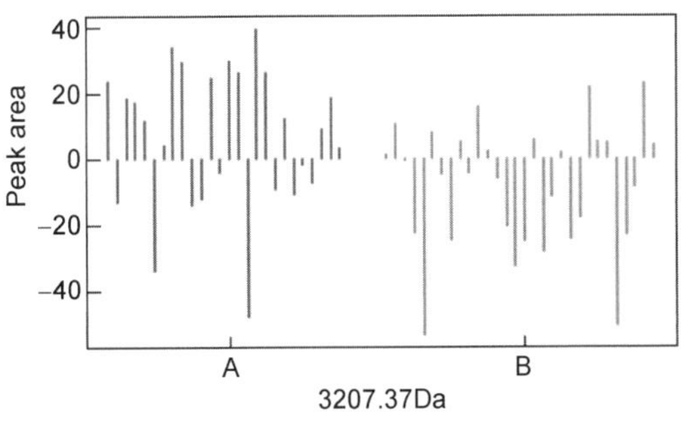

Figure 4 Difference of 3207Da Protein Peak between Group A and Group B

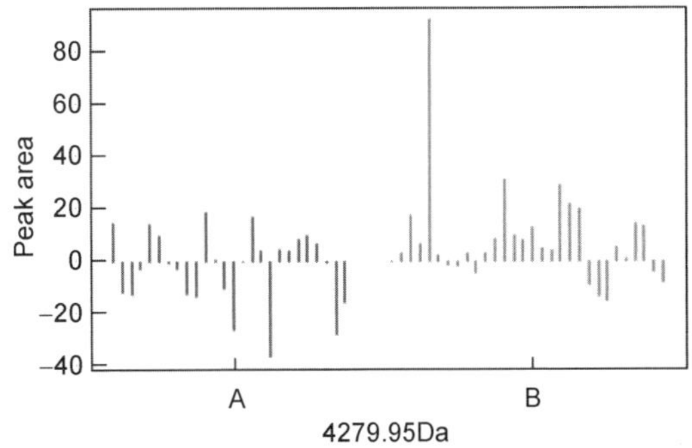

Figure 5 Difference of 4279.95Da Protein Peak between Group A and Group B

4 Identification of Protein Fragments by Proteome Analysis in RCT

Isoform 2 of inter-alpha-trypsin inhibitor heavy chain H4 (ITIH4)and Isoform 1 of Fibrinogen alpha chain precursor (FGA)were identified in different spots by proteome analysis which can be served as biomarkers of "toxin syndrome" in CHD patients (Table 5).

Table 5 Peptides Identification Unique to "Toxin"

MASS	IPI	Gene Symbol	Amino acid sequence
ACEs group	IPI00218192.3	ITIH4 Isoform 2 of inter-alpha-trypsininhibitor heavy chain H4	R. NVHSAGAAGSRMNFRPGVLSSRQLGLPGPPDVPDHAAYHPF. R
Matched group	IPI00021885.1	FGA Isoform 1 of Fibrinogen alpha chain precursor	K. SSSYSKQFTSSTSYNRGDSTFESKSYKM＊. A

5 Western Blot

A large multicenter nested case control study was conducted for verifying the unique protein biomarker to "toxin syndrome" of TCM obtained from RCT. The admission blood samples of 20 patients were collected for Western blot (10 patients, resp. in the ACEs group and the matched group). We assay the serum protein concentrations and based on the readings load the same amount of protein. In the posttranslational process, the protein ITIH4 was modified and cleaved by plasma kallikrein to yield 100kDa and 35kDa fragments. Statistics indicated that protein expression of ITIH4 in the ACEs group was significantly lower than that in the matched group (P=0.027) (Table 6, Figure 6).

Therefore, the results of nested case-control study further demonstrated the biomarker identified in the RCT, which indicated that the reduced ITIH4 might be a unique protein biomarker/bioinformation of "toxin syndrome" in CHD patients.

Table 6 ITIH4 Expression between ACEs Group and Matched Group

Groups	Patients	MOD	P
ACEs group	10	8.41 ± 4.04	0.027
Matched group	10	11.57 ± 5.34	

Note: paired sample t-test was used, 2-tailed, and $P < 0.05$ was considered significant; MOD: mean optical density.

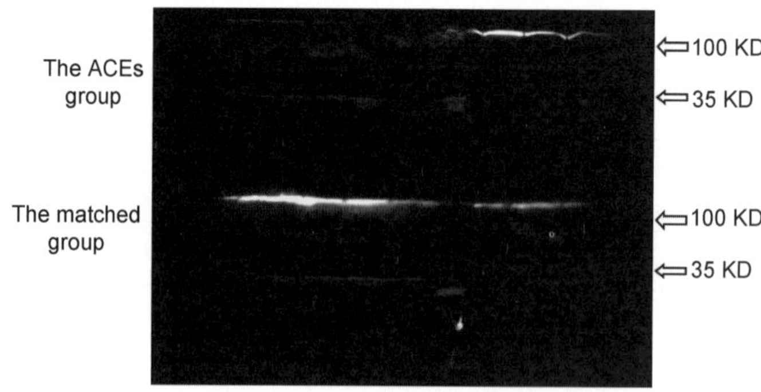

Figure 6 ITIH4 Expression between the ACEs Group and the Matched Group
Note: KD: unit of ITIH4 molecular weight.

DISCUSSION

As the development of systems biology and the advancement of the human genome project increased, more and more attention has been paid on the importance of proteome. In this study, we identified 2 peptides (FGA and ITIH4)related to CHD "toxin syndrome" by "taking special drugs to ascertain syndromes" in RCT using MOLDI-TOF MS. Since fibrinogen has been proven to bea risk factor for ACEs in many previous studies[44-46], we only verified another differential protein, ITIH4, by Western blot in a subsequent nested case-control study. Finally, ITIH4 was ascertained to be a new biomarker for CHD "toxin syndrome", which can also be served as a new risk predictor for ACEs in stable CHD patients.

BSS is one of the basic syndromes in CHD, and "toxin syndrome" is the key in pathogenesis of disease progression. BSS and "toxin syndrome" can coexist or transform to each other, which make up the whole pathological process of CHD[5]. From the macroscopic point of view, Xu et al. [47,48]enrolled 254 stable CHD patients, collected the clinical information and ACEs in follow-up, and thus concluded a series of clinical manifestations for "toxin syndrome" in stable CHD patients including pain in substernal, headache, uneven or irregular pulse, frequent pharyngalgia, and increased high-sensitivity C-reactive protein (hs-CRP). Other scholars[49] collected clinical information and then summarized a differentiation standard for "toxin-stasis syndrome" of ACS in Chinese medicine. From the microcosmic point of view, "inflammatory reaction" is always a research focus for CHD "toxin syndrome." Wen et al. [23]investigated the effect on plaque stabilization among herbs regulating blood circulation (*Salvia Miltiorrhiza*, *Radix Paeoniae Rubra*), activating blood circulation (Szechuan Lovage Rhizome, Panax Notoginseng), and breaking blood stasis (Peach Seed, Rhubarb Root Parched in Wine)from inflammation, pathomorphology, cellular composition, and so on; indicated Rhubarb root parched in wine was the best for its effect of breaking blood stasis and detoxification. Zhou et al. [26]proposed the hypothesis of "activating blood circulation and detoxification—inflammatory reaction inhibition—plaque stabilization," then compared the effect on plaque stabilization among herbs activating blood circulation (Panax Notoginsenosides), herbs for detoxification (Goldthread Rhizome extract) and herbs activating blood circulation and detoxification (Rhubarb alcohol extract and Polygonum Cuspidatum extract). The results indicated the superior effect of Rhubarb alcohol extract and Polygonum Cuspidatum extract on stabilizing vulnerable plaque, showing the "class effect" of herbs activating blood circulation and detoxification in inhibiting inflammatory reaction and stabilizing plaque.

The function of ITIH4 in European Molecular Biology Laboratory-The European Bioinformatics Institute (EMBLEBI)showed that ITIH4 is a type II acute-phase protein (APP)involved in inflammatory responses to trauma. And it may also play a role in liver development and regeneration[50]. Inter-alpha-trypsin inhibitor (ITI) family proteins are all composed by light chain (bikunin)and at least 6 heavy chains. Lots of researches have proved that bikunin could inhibit the activity of protease, but little studies have paid attention to heavy chains of ITI. In 2000, Japanese scholar Choi-Miura et al. found that inter-alpha-trypsin inhibitor family heavy chain-related protein (IHRP)could inhibit the aggregation and phagocytosis of actins in polymorphonuclear leukocyte, implying that IHRP might be a new APP involved in inflammatory responses[51]. In 2004, Fujita et al. showed that genetic locus mutation of ITIH4 might be one of possible factors for dyslipidemia[52]. Then, Piñeiro et al. proved that ITIH4 was a new APP isolated from cattle during experimental infection[53]. Recently, Kashyap et al. found that ITIH4 showed high expression in normal subjects but no expression or little expression in patients with acute ischemic stroke (AIS), and this protein could return to normal level in blood serum gradually as the patients were getting better. The scholars considered that ITIH4 was a novel biomarker in inflammatory responses for AIS due to its close relationship with S-100 β-β, neuron specific enolase (NSE), interleukin-2 (IL-2), and interleukin-10 (IL-10)expression[54].

Results in this study showed that the group of activating blood circulation and detoxification could significantly increase ITIH4 expression and decrease FGA expression compared with the group of activating blood circulation and indicated that ITIH4 and FGA might be potential protein biomarkers for "toxin syndrome" of CHD. ITIH4 was further demonstrated in a nested case-control study, indicating its potential role as a new prewarning biomarker in stable CHD patients.

Before recommending the conclusion of this study to clinical practice, we have to consider the following weaknesses. We cannot ascertain whether the tendency of these two polypeptides is always the same in the process of "toxin syndrome" development. Therefore, a large prospective cohort study collecting information in more time points is necessary.

CONCLUSION

ITIH4 might be a new potential biomarker of CHD "toxin syndrome" in TCM, indicating the potential role as a prewarning biomarker in stable CHD patients.

REFERENCES

[1] A. S. Ferreira, A. J. Lopes. Chinese medicine pattern differentiation and its implications for clinical practice[J]. Chinese Journal of Integrative Medicine, 2011, 17 (11): 818-823.

[2] M. F. Mei. A systematic analysis of the theory and practice of syndrome differentiation[J]. Chinese Journal of Integrative Medicine, 2011, 17 (11): 803-810.

[3] O. Li, H. Xu. The occurrence of cardiovascular events of coronary heart disease inpatients and study on Chinese medicine syndrome distribution laws[J]. Chinese Journal of Integrated Traditional and Western Medicine, 2012, 32 (5): 603-606.

[4] Z. Y. Gao, J. C. Zhang, H. Xu et al. Analysis of relationships among syndrome, therapeutic treatment, and Chinese herbal medicine in patients with coronary artery disease based on complex networks[J]. Chinese Journal of Integrated Traditional and Western Medicine, 2010, 8 (3): 238-243.

[5] H. Xu, D. Z. Shi, H. J. Yin, J. C. Zhang, K. J. Chen. Blood-stasis and toxin causing catastrophe hypothesis and acute cardiovascular events: proposal of the hypothesis and its clinical significance[J]. Chinese Journal of Integrated Traditional and Western Medicine, 2008, 28 (10): 934-938.

[6] Z. Zhang, G. L. Yang, H. Y. Zhang, M. Chen, Y. Chen, Z. B. Luo. A hypothesis of atherosclerosis plaque from the surgical carbuncle theory[J]. Liaoning Journal of Traditional Chinese Medicine, 2008, 35 (2): 201-202.

[7] L. Wang, L. B. Wei, X. F. Liu, S. W. Ding, M. Peng. Toxin theory and acute coronary syndrome[J]. Chinese Journal of Integrative Medicine on Cardio-/Cerebrovascular Disease, 2005, 3 (12): 1080-1081.

[8] W. X. Du, C. Y. Liu, H. X. Zhang, M. Zhang, H. W. Song. Acutemyocardial infarction and TCMtheory[J]. Chinese Journal of Integrative Medicine on Cardio-/Cerebrovascular Disease, 2006, 4 (5): 434-436.

[9] W. Wu, R. Peng. Progress of heat & toxin pathogenesis in coronary heart disease[J]. Journal of New Chinese Medicine, 2007, 39 (6): 3-4.

[10] H. Duan, H. K. Zhang, J. J. Liu, W. J. Nie, Y. Ma, Y. Q. Ga. Effect of berberine on IL-6 of carotid artery after ballon injury in rabbits[J]. Journal of Medical Forum, 2006, 27 (10): 6-9.

[11] M. Wu, J. Wang. Advance on study in anti-atherosclerosis mechanism of berberine[J]. China Journal of Chinese Materia Medica, 2008, 33 (18): 2013-2016.

[12] Z. Q. Lei, S. Y. Chen, X. M. Gao. Traditional Chinese Pharmacology[J]. Shanghai Science and Technology Press, 1995, 1st edition.

[13] S. W. He, R. H. Zhao, H. J. Wu, A. H. Guo. Effect of wild purslane on atherosclerosis formation in rabbit[J]. ChineseJournal of Preventive Medicine, 1997, 31 (2): 91.

[14] H. B. Tan. Study of gynostemma pentaphylla on atherosclerosis in rabbit[J]. Chinese Journal of Gerontology, 2007, 27 (6): 519-521.

[15] L. D. Xie, L. X. Chen, S. X. Wu, B. Nie. Overview of clinical and basic research of Simiao Yong'an decoction in the treatment of coronary heart disease[J]. Global Traditional Chinese Medicine, 2012, 5 (8): 629-633.

[16] N. Zhu, X. M. Cao, Y. X. Cai, Y. Wu, B. B. Wang. Effect of huanglian jiedu decoction on CRP and TNF-α in coronary heart disease[J]. Journal of Emergency in Traditional Chinese Medicine, 2012, 21 (4): 542-543.

[17] G. Q. Li, P. Huang, H. M. Cheng et al. Effect of huanglian jiedu decoction on T cell expression regulated by $CD4^+$ $CD25^+$ in rats with atherosclerosis[J]. Guangdong Medical Journal, 2010, 31 (3): 329-331.

[18] Z. Y. Guo, P. Huang, G. Q. Li. Effect of huanglian jiedu decoction on the expression of MCP-1/CCR2 mRNA in atherosclerosis rats[J]. Traditional Chinese Drug Research and Clinical Pharmacology, 2010, 21 (6): 583-586.

[19] F. Zheng, M. X. Zhou, H. Xu, K. J. Chen. Effects of herbs with function of activating blood circulation and detoxication on serum infl ammatory markers and blood lipids in stable patients with coronary heart disease[J]. China Journal of Traditional Chinese Medicine and Pharmacy, 2009, 24 (9): 1153-1156.

[20] X. H. Lu, S. W. Ding. Clinical effect and mechanism on treating unstable angina pectoris by huanglian jiedu capsule[J]. Journal of Shandong University of Traditional Chinese Medicine, 2005, 29 (6): 457-460.

[21] R. Yu, S. X. He, X. L. Ye, X. C. Wang. The effect of therapeutic method of blood-activating and detoxifying of TCM on serumlevel of sCD40L in the patientswith acute coronary syndrome[J]. Journal of Emergency in Traditional Chinese Medicine, 2008, 17 (11): 1500-1501.

[22] R. Yu, X. S. Hu, S. X. He, X. L. Ye, X. X. Zhang. The effect of huoxuejiedu decoction on serum level of MMP-1, MMP-9, TIMP-1 in the patients with acute coronary syndrome[J]. Journal of Emergency in Traditional Chinese Medicine, 2008, 17 (10): 1337-1346.

[23] C. Wen, H. Xu, Q. F. Chen, P. Li, X. Sheng. Effects of herbs of activation blood on atherosclerotic plaque morphology in ApoE gene-deficient mice[J]. Chinese Journal of Pathophysiology, 2005, 21 (5): 864-867.

[24] C. Wen, H. Xu, Q. F. Huang, K. J. Chen. Effect of drugs for promoting blood circulation on blood lipids and inflammatory reaction of atherosclerotic plaques in ApoE gene deficiency mice[J]. Chinese Journal of Integrated Traditional and Western Medicine, 2005, 25 (4): 345-349.

[25] M. X. Zhou, H. Xu, K. J. Chen, L. Pan, C. Wen, J. G. Liu. Effects of some active ingredients of Chinese drugs for activating blood circulation and detoxicating on blood lipids and atherosclerotic plaque inflammatory reaction in ApoEgene knockout mice[J]. Chinese Journal of Integrated Traditional and Western Medicine, 2008, 28 (2): 126-130.

[26] M. X. Zhou, H. Xu, K. J. Chen, L. Pan, C. Wen, Y. R. Guo. Effects of several herbal extractives with the effect of promoting blood flow and detoxication on atherosclerotic plaque stability in aorta of apoE-gene knockout mice[J]. Chinese Journal of Pathophysiology, 2008, 24 (11): 2097-2102.

[27] J. C. Zhang, K. J. Chen, G. J. Zheng et al. Regulatory effect of Chinese herbal compound for detoxifying and activating blood circulation on expression of NF-kappaB and MMP-9 in aorta of apolipoprotein E gene knocked-out mice[J]. Chinese Journal of Integrated Traditional and Western Medicine, 2007, 21 (1): 40-44.

[28] K. J. Chen, D. Z. Shi, H. Xuet al. XS0601 reduces the incidence of restenosis: a prospective study of 335 patients undergoing percutaneous coronary intervention in China[J]. Chinese Medical Journal, 2006, 119 (1): 6-13.

[29] H. Xu, K. J. Chen, D. Z. Shi, X. C. Ma, S. Z. lv, J. M. Mao. Clinical study of Xiongshao capsule in preventing resterosis after coronary interventional treatment[J]. Chinese Journal of Integrative Medicine, 2002, 8 (3): 162-166.

[30] Q. H. Shang, H. Xu, X. Y. Lu, C. Wen, D. Z. Shi, K. J. Chen. A multi-center randomized double-blind placebocontrolled trial of Xiongshao capsule in preventing restenosis after percutaneous coronary intervention: a subgroup analysis of senile patients[J]. Chinese Journal of Integrative Medicine, 2011, 17 (9): 669-674.

[31] H. Xu, D. Z. Shi, K. J. Chenet al. Effect ofXiongshaocapsule on vascular remodeling in porcine coronary balloon injurymodel[J]. Chinese Journal of Integrative Medicine, 2000, 6 (4): 278-282.

[32] L. Z. Li, J. G. Liu, L. B. Ma et al. Effect of Xiongshao capsule on lipid metabolism and platelet aggregation in experimental atherosclerosis rabbits[J]. Chinese Journal of Integrated Traditional and Western Medicine, 2008, 28 (12): 1100-1103.

[33] D. W. Zhang, L. Zhang, J. G. Liu, C. L. Wang, D. Z. Shi, K. J. Chen. Effects of Xiongshao capsule combined with ischemic postconditioning on monocyte chemoattractant protein-1 and tumor necrosis factor-α in rat myocardium with ischemic reperfusion injury[J]. Chinese Journal of Integrated Traditional And Western Medicine, 2010, 30 (12): 1279-1283.

[34] F. Q. Xu, H. Xu, J. G. Liu, K. J. Chen. Effects of Xiongshao capsule on the proliferation of vascular smooth muscle cells in rabbits with atherosclerosis[J]. Chinese Journal of Integrated Traditional and Western Medicine, 2008, 28 (10): 912-916.

[35] Report of the Joint International Society and Federation of Cardiology/World Health Organization Task Force on Standardization of Clinical NomenclatureS. Nomenclature and criteria for diagnosis of ischemic heart disease[J]. Circulation, 1979, 59 (3): 607-609.

[36] Chinese Society of Cardiology. Guideline for diagnosis and treatment of patients with unstable angina and non-ST segment elevation myocardial

infarction[J]. Chinese Journal of Cardiology, 2007, 35 (4): 295-304.

[37] Subcommittee of Cardiovascular Diseases of China Society of Integrated Traditional Chinese and Western Medicine. Criteria for TCM syndrome differentiation of patients with coronary heart disease[J]. Chinese Journal of Integrated Traditional and Western Medicine, 1991, 11 (5): 257-258.

[38] Professional Committee of Activating Blood Circulation in Chinese Association of the Integration of Traditional and Western Medicine. Criteria for diagnosis of blood stasis syndrome[J]. Chinese Journal of Integrated Traditional and Western Medicine, 1987, 7 (3): 129.

[39] C. G. Fu, Z. Y. Gao, P. L. Wang et al. Study on the diagnostic criteria for coronary heart disease patients of blood stasis syndrome[J]. Chinese Journal of Integrated Traditional and Western Medicine, 2012, 32 (9): 1285-1286.

[40] Chinese Society of Cardiology. Guildline on diagnosis and treatment of unstable angina pectoris and non-ST elecated myocardial infarcion[J]. Chinese Journal of Cardiology, 2007, 35 (4): 295-304.

[41] Y. Y. Zheng. Chinese Herbal Medicine Clinical Research Guilding Principles (for Trial Implementation)[J]. Chinese Medicine and Technology Publishing House, 2002.

[42] K. J. Chen. Study on Activating Blood Circulation and Cllinical Application[J]. Peking Union Medical College Press, 1993.

[43] Y. Gong, X. Wang, J. Liu et al. NSPc1, a mainly nuclear localized protein of novel PcG family members, has a transcription repression activity related to its PKC phosphorylation site at S183[J]. FEBS Letters, 2005, 579 (1): 115-121.

[44] M. C. Tataru, H. Schulte, E. A. Von, J. Heinrich, G. Assmann, E. Koehler. Plasma fibrinogen in relation to the severity of arteriosclerosis in patients with stable angina pectoris after myocardial infarction[J]. Coronary Artery Disease, 2001, 12 (3): 157-165.

[45] M. Naito. Effects of fibrinogen, fibrin and their degradation products on the behavior of vascular smooth muscle cells[J]. Nippon Ronen Igakkai Zasshi, 2000, 37 (6): 458-463.

[46] H. L. Ma, X. Lu, H. J. Yang et al. Fibrinogen is the one of risk factors of coronary heart disease[J]. Chinese Journal ofThrombosis and Hemostasis, 2008, 14 (1): 8-11.

[47] H. Xu, D. Qu, F. Zheng, D. Z. Shi, K. J. Chen. Clinical manifestations of "Blood-stasis and Toxin" in patients with stable coronary heart disease[J]. Chinese Journal of Integrated Traditional and Western Medicine, 2010, 30 (2): 125-129.

[48] Y. Feng, H. Xu, D. Qu, F. Zheng, D. Z. Shi, K. J. Chen. Study on the tongue manifestations for the blood-stasis and toxin syndrome in the stable patients of coronary heart disease[J]. Chinese Journal of Integrative Medicine, 2011, 17 (5): 333-338.

[49] H. Chen. The clinical research on differentiation standard for toxin-stasis syndrome of ACS in Chinese medicine[Doctoral dissertation] [J]. China Academy of Chinese Medical Sciences, 2009.

[50] http: //www. uniprot. org/uniprot/Q14624.

[51] N. H. Choi-Miura, K. Takahashi, M. Yoda et al. The novel acute phase protein, IHRP, inhibits actin polymerization and phagocytosis of polymorphonuclear cells [J]. Inflammation Research, 2000, 49 (6): 305-310.

[52] Y. Fujita, Y. Ezura, M. Emi et al. Hypercholesterolemia associated with splice-junction variation of inter-α-trypsin inhibitor heavy chain 4 (ITIH4) gene [J]. Journal of Human Genetics, 2004, 49 (1): 24-28.

[53] M. Pineiro, M. Andr'es, M. Iturralde et al. ITIH4 (inter-alphatrypsin inhibitor heavy chain 4)is a new acute-phase protein isolated from cattle during experimental infection [J]. Infection and Immunity, 2004, 72 (7): 3777-3782.

[54] R. S. Kashyap, A. R. Nayak, P. S. Deshpande et al. Inter-α-trypsin inhibitor heavy chain 4 is a novel marker of acute ischemic stroke [J]. Clinica Chimica Acta, 2009, 402 (1-2): 160-163.

First published: XU Hao, SHANG Qing-hua, CHEN Hao, DU Jian-peng, WEN Jian-yan, LI Geng, SHI Da-zhuo, CHEN Ke-ji. ITIH4: a new potential biomarker of "Toxin Syndrome" in coronary heart disease patient identified with proteomic method. [J] . Evid Based Complement Alternat Med, 2013, 2013: 360149.

Atherosclerosis: An Integrative East-West Medicine Perspective

XU Hao, SHI Da-zhuo, and CHEN Ke-ji

Recent understanding of atherosclerosis and coronary heart disease has shifted the focus from lumen stenosis to vulnerable plaque, from lipid deposit to inflammatory reaction, and from vulnerable plaque to vulnerable patient. This has led to a new direction of treatment consisting of intervening the inflammatory reaction, stabilizing the vulnerable plaque, inhibiting thrombosis after plaque rupture, and treating the vulnerable patient instead of treating lumen stenosis. This seems to mirror the traditional Chinese medicine (TCM)focus on prevention and on the vulnerable patient with treatment matched to the pattern dysfunction and dysregulation using the Chinese herbal medicine multitargeted approach. Given the convergence of both the East and the West conceptualization of atherosclerosis, it is hopeful that the integrative East-West approach will facilitate early detection and more effective treatment of the vulnerable patients with coronary heart disease.

1 Introduction

Atherosclerosis (AS)is the most common type of arteriosclerosis. It mainly involves the large and middle muscular arteries, especially aorta, coronary and cerebral arteries, which often leads to serious outcomes such as sudden cardiac death, unstable angina pectoris, acute myocardial infarction, stroke, and intermittent claudication due to vessel obliteration or plaque rupture and subsequent thrombosis. In the beginning of the 21st century, we are facing serious challenges of cardiovascular disease (CVD). Although it is becoming less lethal, CVD prevalence is incessantly increasing, and it is still the most common cause of death. How to prevent AS and reduce the incidence and mortality of CVD have been one of the most important health-related issues all the time.

However, biomedicine is at its limits nowadays when confronting degenerative diseases, stress-related diseases, and most chronic diseases. It lacks reference to the self-healing capacity of the human mind and body and focuses on parts rather than the whole, treatment rather than prevention, the suffering disease rather than the diseased person. Confronted with these problems, more and more far-sighted Western scholars began to lay their eyes on traditional Chinese medicine (TCM)[1-3]. Drugs with Chinese herbal medicines as raw materials are increasingly favored by people all over the world for their unique advantages in preventing and curing diseases, rehabilitation, and health care. The benefit of TCM in CVD was also demonstrated in several multicenter clinical trials in recent years[4-7]. More importantly, the unique theory of TCM might also have some implications for the renewal of thinking in fighting against CVD[8]. Therefore, we reviewed traditional understanding and shifted concepts on AS pathophysiology along the track of previous studies and read these transitions taking full advantage of TCM theory together with our experimental and clinical studies in recent years, so as to provide an integrative East-West medicine perspective for future AS prevention and treatment.

2 Updated Concept of Atherosclerosis

2.1 From Emphasizing "Luminal Stenosis" to Highlighting "Vulnerable Plaques"

With the deep understanding and active control of AS risk factors, dramatic advances have been made in primary prevention of chronic cardiovascular diseases since 1990s. However, there is still lack of effective measure to prevent acute cardiovascular events (ACEs), which cause 20 million deaths worldwide per year. Most of the victims die suddenly without any prior symptoms.

The previous studies focused on the severity of coronary stenosis, taking coronary heart disease (CHD) as an example of AS, and highlighted detection of severe luminal stenosis and subsequent treatment of percutaneous coronary intervention (PCI). The development or improvement of coronary stenosis is also regarded as an important indicator to evaluate the state of illness or therapeutic effect. However, angiographic studies on patients before myocardial infarction showed that the majority of subsequent events involved sites with less than 70% obstruction. It indicated that the severity of stenosis was not the main cause of ACEs[9].

In 1989, Muller and his colleagues used the word "vulnerable" to describe rupture-prone plaques, with characteristics of a large lipid pool, a thin cap, and macrophage-dense inflammation on or beneath its surface[10], as the underlying cause of most clinical coronary events. More and more studies suggested that ACEs were triggered by thrombosis associated with rupture of vulnerable atherosclerotic plaques[11]. The change of plaque from its stable state to an unstable one was not related to the plaque size, quantity, or position or the severity of stenosis. Although PCI improves significant stenosis, it cannot influence the biological course of vulnerable plaque, thus the problem of "unstable" plaque is still unresolved.

In recent years, many clinical trials showed that statins could reduce ACEs significantly yet only improve the luminal size slightly[12]. Experimental researches have proved that statins have potential effects on stability of AS plaques[13]. Stenting (including drug-eluting stents)reduces restenosis and repeated intervention, but does not reduce mortality or myocardial infarction[14]. Therefore, it is necessary for us to reevaluate the benefits of active medicinal treatment and invasive PCI treatment in chronic myocardial ischemia. Based on in-depth understanding of AS pathogenesis, the vascular pathophysiological research has turned to new direction of stabilizing vulnerable plaque and inhibiting thrombosis after plaques rupture. The secondary prevention of CHD also focused on intervention of vulnerable plaque instead of treating luminal stenosis of coronary artery[15,16].

2.2 From Predominant Theory of "Lipid Deposit" to General Acknowledgment of "Inflammatory Reaction" Theory

"Lipids deposit" theory of AS has been put forward for over 100 years based on the causal relation between hyperlipidemia and AS[17]. This theory holds that lipids deposition on the artery wall leads to the AS plaques and has played a very important role in AS pathogenesis for a long period.

In recent years, some researches indicated that AS had the basic manifestation of inflammation: degeneration, exu-dation, and proliferation. The cell-cell interaction is similar to other chronic inflammation diseases such as rheumatoid arthritis, chronic pancreatitis, and hepatic cirrhosis. With continuous detection of inflammatory cells and mediators, AS was no longer regarded as a simple disease of lipid deposition on vessel wall but also an advancing inflammatory reaction. Recent advances in basic science have established a fundamental role for inflammation in mediating all stages of this diseases from initiation through progression and, ultimately, the thrombotic complications of AS.

In 1999, based on his famous "injury reaction" theory, Ross declared that AS is one of the inflammatory disease[18]. AS is a process of active inflammatory reaction inside the vessel wall rather than a process of passive lipid deposit onto the vessel wall. This theory initiates a new epoch of AS treatment and it leads to deep understanding of cardiovascular diseases: inflammation fuels the development and progression of atherosclerosis as well as causes certain plaques to rupture and subsequent thrombosis, leading to such atherosclerotic complications as heart attack and stroke. High-sensitivity C-reactive protein (hs-CRP)and other blood inflammatory markers may be useful in the estimation of prognosis, risk level in AS patients, and even be a potential target of AS treatment and prevention[19]. Despite regulating blood lipids metabolism, statins should be recommended for their anti-inflammation and other protective effects on cardiovascular diseases. Aspirin can not only inhibit platelet aggregation but also prevent the malfunction of endothelial cells through its anti-inflammation effects[16]. Anti-inflammation has been one of the most important issues of AS research and several strategies that intervene with inflammation reaction are under study.

2.3 New Concept from "Vulnerable Plaque" to "Vulnerable Patient"

Plaque rupture is the most common type of plaque complication, accounting for nearly 70% of fatal acute myocardial infarctions and/or sudden coronary deaths. Vulnerable plaque is the main, but not the unique, cause for ACEs. The position of plaque rupture, the size and amount of plaques, coronary spasm, hypercoagulable state, collateral circulation, and the degree of myocardial damage should also be considered. In 2003, an article named "From vulnerable plaque to vulnerable patient: a call for new definitions and risk assessment strategies" was published on *Circulation* written by over fifty of the most famous cardiovascular experts of the world[20,21]. The new concept of "vulnerable plaque" to "vulnerable patients" has led in a new direction to the prevention of ACEs.

The term "vulnerable patient" is proposed to define subjects susceptible to an acute coronary syndrome or sudden cardiac death based on plaque, blood, or myocardial vulnerability (1-year risk ⩾ 5%). Extensive efforts are needed to quantify an individual's risk of an event according to each component of vulnerability (plaque, blood, and myocardium). Such a comprehensive risk-stratification tool capable of predicting acute coronary syndromes as well as sudden cardiac death would be very useful for preventive cardiology. The new concept of "vulnerable plaque" to "vulnerable patients" stresses evaluating patients as a whole and thus further optimizes overall assessment of cardiovascular risks, and prevents ACEs by early intervention of vulnerable patients.

3 An Integrative East-West Medicine Perspective for Future AS Management

The transitions in understanding AS, from local plaques to entire coronary tree and patient as a whole, from passive lipid deposit process to an active inflammatory reaction and cell interaction process, innovate strategies of prevention and treatment for AS and CHD from coronary stenosis-targeted invasive PCI treatment to vulnerable patient-targeted comprehensive assessment, early-detection and preventive medication strategies, happen to mirror "holism concept" "living in harmony with the environment" "preventive treatment of disease" and "treatment based on syndrome differentiation or pattern diagnosis" advocated by TCM. They can also help us fully understand the two different medical systems, Western medicine (WM) and TCM, as well as make the best of the advantages of both of them.

The previous researches have shown that Chinese medicines of activating blood circulation (ABC) could treat AS by multiple ways such as lowering blood lipid, inhibiting platelet adhesion and aggregation, and improving blood viscosity and inhibiting SMC proliferation. In 2003, based on AS models of ApoE-deficient mice, we studied the effects of six ABC herbs (Radix Salviae Miltiorrhizae, *Radix Paeoniae Rubra*, Rhizoma Chuanxiong, Radix Notoginseng, Semen Persicae, Wine steamed Radix, and Rhizoma Rhei)and a compound preparation (consisting of Chuanxingol and Paeoniflorin)on stabilizing AS plaque and their potential mechanisms. The results indicated that most ABC herbs showed multiple effects on different links of AS, such as regulating blood lipids, influencing collagen metabolism, and anti-inflammatory reaction, thus had potential effect on stabilizing AS plaque[22,23]. Although the final effect of ABC herbs on stabilizing plaque was slightly less than that of simvastatin, they showed better effects on certain links such as increasing high-density lipoprotein cholesterol (HDL-C), which exhibited the superiorities of Chinese medicine in overall regulation by influencing multiple targets[8]. The superior effect of the compound preparation to either herbal extractive component[24] indicated the synergetic effect based on TCM compatibility theory. Therefore, Chinese herbal medicines, especially compound prescriptions, warrant further investigation and might be an complementary or alternative therapy to statins in stabilizing vulnerable plaque through a synergistic and multitargeted effect.

The new concept of "vulnerable patient" also provides TCM with new opportunity in detecting high-risk CHD patients and further reducing ACEs by early intervention. Under the guidance of TCM holism concept and thought of treatment based on syndrome differentiation, we conducted a multicenter cohort study, enrolling stable CHD patients and documenting one-year follow-up cardiovascular end-point events. Prognosis-related factors, including past medical history, symptoms, body signs, biochemical indicators, and tongue manifestations, were identified to establish an integrative risk-assessment system for detecting high-risk CHD patients[25–27]. A large-scale randomized controlled trial aiming at early intervening high-risk CHD patients based on this integrative risk assessment system is about to start soon. Given the convergence of both the East and the West conceptualization of AS, it is hopeful that this integrative East-West strategy will facilitate early detection and more effective treatment for the vulnerable patients with CHD and other AS-related diseases.

REFERENCES

[1] Dobos G, Tao I. The model of Western integrative medicine: the role of Chinese medicine[J]. Chin J Integr Med, 2011, 17 (1): 11-20.

[2] Robinson N. Integrative medicine-traditional Chinese medicine, a model? [J]. Chin J Integr Med, 2011, 17 (1): 21-25.

[3] Xu H, Chen KJ. Integrating traditional medicine with biomedicine towards a patient-centered healthcare system. [J] Chin J Integr Med, 2011, 17 (2): 83-84.

[4] Chen KJ, Shi DZ, Xu H et al. XS0601 reduces the incidence of restenosis: a prospective study of 335 patients undergoing percutaneous coronary intervention in China[J]. Chinese Medical Journal, 2006, 119 (1): 6-13.

[5] Shang QH, Xu H, Lu XY, et al. A multi-center randomized double-blind placebo-controlled trial of Xiongshao Capsule in preventing restenosis after percutaneous coronary intervention: a subgroup analysis of senile patients[J]. Chin J Integr Med, 2011, 17 (9): 669-674.

[6] Gao ZY, Xu H, Shi DZ, et al. Liu. Analysis on outcome of 5284 patients with coronary artery disease: the role of integrative medicine[J]. Journal of Ethnopharmacology, In press.

[7] Lu Z, Kou W, Du B et al. Effect of Xuezhikang, an extract from red yeast Chinese rice, on coronary events in a Chinese population with previous myocardial infarction[J]. American Journal of Cardiology, 2008, 101 (12): 1689-1693.

[8] Wen C and Xu H. The new strategy for modulating dyslipidemia: consideration from updated understanding on high-density lipoprotein[J]. Chin J Integr Med, 2011, 17 (6): 467-470.

[9] Smith SC. Risk-reduction therapy: the challenge to change[J]. Circulation, 1996, 93 (12): 2205-2211.

[10] Muller JE, Tofler GH, and Stone PH. Circadian variation and triggers of onset of acute cardiovascular disease[J]. Circulation, 1989, 79 (4): 733-743.

[11] Conti CR. Updated pathophysiologic concepts in unstable coronary artery disease[J]. American Heart Journal, 2001, 141 (2): S12-S14.

[12] Dupuis J. Mechanisms of acute coronary syndromes and the potential role of statins[J]. Atherosclerosis Supplements, 2001, 2 (1): 9-14.

[13] Koh KK. Effects of statins on vascular wall: vasomotor function, inflammation, and plaque stability[J]. Cardiovascular Research, 2000, 47, (4): 648-657.

[14] P. W. Serruys, M. J. B. Kutryk, A. T. L. Ong. Coronary-artery stents[J]. New England Journal of Medicine, 2006, 354 (5): 483-495.

[15] I. J. Kullo, W. D. Edwards, R. S. Schwartz. Vulnerable plaque: Pathobiology and clinical implications[J]. Annals of Internal Medicine, 1998, 129 (12): 1050-1060.

[16] K. Ozer, M. Cilingiroglu. Vulnerable plaque: Definition, detection, treatment, and future implications[J]. Current Atherosclerosis Reports, 2005, 7 (2): 121-126.

[17] D. Steinberg, L. Joseph, J. L. Witztum. Lipoproteins and atherogenesis. Current concepts[J]. Journal of the American Medical Association, 1990, 264 (23): 3047-3052.

[18] R. Ross. Atherosclerosis—an inflammatory disease[J]. New England Journal of Medicine, 1999, 340 (2): 115-126.

[19] A. M. Wilson, M. C. Ryan, A. J. Boyle. The novel role of C-reactive protein in cardiovascular disease: Risk marker or pathogen[J]. International Journal of Cardiology, 2006, 106 (3): 291-297.

[20] M. Naghavi, P. Libby, E. Falk, et al. From vulnerable plaque to vulnerable patient: a call for new definitions and risk assessment strategies: Part I[J]. Circulation, 2003, 108 (14): 1664-1672.

[21] M. Naghavi, P. Libby, E. Falk, et al. From vulnerable plaque to vulnerable patient: a call for new definitions and risk assessment strategies: part II[J]. Circulation, 2003, 108 (15): 1772-1778.

[22] C. Wen, H. Xu, Q. F. Huang, K. J. Chen. Effect of drugs for promoting blood circulation on blood lipids and inflammatory reaction of atherosclerotic plaques in ApoE gene deficiency mice[J]. Chinese Journal of Integrated Traditional and Western Medicine, 2005, 25 (4): 345-349.

[23] C. Wen, H. Xu, Q. F. Huang, K. J. Chen. Effects of herbs for promoting blood circulation and Xiongshao Capsule on collagen deposition and metabolism of atherosclerotic plaques in ApoE gene deficient mice[J]. Chinese Journal of Pathophysiology, 2005, 21 (8): 1640.

[24] H. Xu, C. Wen, K. J. Chen, D. Z. Shi, J. G. Liu. Study on the effect of rhizoma Chuanxiong, radix paeoniae rubra and the compound of their active ingredients, Xiongshao Capsule, on stability of atherosclerotic plaque in ApoE (-/-)mice[J]. Chinese Journal of Integrated Traditional and Western Medicine, 2007, 27 (6): 513-518.

[25] H. Xu, D. Qu, F. Zheng, D. Z. Shi, K. J. Chen. Clinical manifestations of "blood-stasis and toxin" in patients with stable coronary heart

disease[J]. Chinese Journal of Integrated Traditional and Western Medicine, 2010, 30 (2): 125-129.
[26] Y. Feng, H. Xu, D. Qu, F. Zheng, D. Z. Shi, K. J. Chen. Study on the tongue manifestations for the blood-stasis and toxin syndrome in the stable patients of coronary heart disease[J]. Chinese Journal of Integrative Medicine, 2011, 17 (5): 333-338.
[27] K. J. Chen, D. Z. Shi, H. Xu, H. J. Yin, J. C. Zhang. The criterion of syndrome differentiation and quantification for stable coronary heart disease caused by etiological toxin of Chinese medicine[J]. Chinese Journal of Integrated Traditional and Western Medicine, 2011, 31 (3): 313-314.

First published: XU Hao, SHI Da-zhuo, CHEN Ke-ji. Atherosclerosis: an integrative East-west medicine perspective[J] . Evid Based Complement Alternat Med, 2012, 2012: 148413.

Chinese Herb and Formulas for Promoting Blood Circulation and Removing Blood Stasis and Antiplatelet Therapies

LIU Yue, YIN Hui-Jun, SHI Da-zhuo, and CHEN Ke-ji

Cardiovascular and cerebrovascular events have become the major killer of people's health and life all over the world. Rupture of atherosclerotic plaque in an artery wall and the ensuing thrombotic events are the triggers for acute ischemic injury. Activated platelets play a pivotal role in the formation of pathogenic thrombi underlying acute clinical manifestations of vascular atherothrombotic disease. Oral antiplatelet drugs are a milestone in the therapy of cardiovascular atherothrombotic diseases and provide the primary and secondary prevention strategy to combat these diseases. Effcient antiplatelet therapy can make the death rates of heart disease and stroke decline by about 25%[1,2]. Commonly used oral antiplatelet drugs include cyclooxygenase inhibitor aspirin, the glycoprotein IIb/IIIa inhibitor ReoPro, and the P_2Y_{12} inhibitor clopidogrel, et al. Many clinical studies show that dual antiplatelet therapy with aspirin and clopidogrel is currently the standard of drugs for prevention of adverse cardiovascular events in most patients at high risk owing to acute coronary syndromes or recent placement of a stent.

But along with prolonging of treatment by dual or triple antiplatelet drugs, the effectiveness and security have garnered particular attention in clinic. Despite their proven benefit, recurrent cardiovascular events still occur in those taking antiplatelet drugs. This has led to the concept of antiplatelet resistance[3], most commonly aspirin resistance as this drug is the cornerstone of most regimens. Although there are some debates on definition and mechanism of antiplatelet resistance[4,5], it cannot be denied that it has important clinical significance. At the same time, numerous adverse reactions including serious bleeding risk (digestive and nervous systems)and combination with PPIs and statin[6,7], which limit the clinical practice of antiplatelet drugs. So developed novel classes of antiplatelet agents possess high effciency, and fewer adverse effects have been always the research focus for prevention of cardiovascular disease. Modern medicine and pharmacology has done a lot of valuable exploration, newer agents are in development recent years that include prasugrel, cangrelor, ticagrelor, and vorapaxar, et al. [8]

Study on the blood stasis syndrome (BSS)and promoting blood circulation and removing blood stasis (PBCRBS)is the most active field of research of integration of traditional and western medicine in China. During the past 50 years, much significant progress has been made from theory, experiments to clinic fields based on the inherit, and innovation of thoughts in traditional Chinese medicine[9], to clarify the treatment regulations and principles of PBCRBS, which has already got consensus in medical community in China. A lot of formulas for PBCRBS (see Table 1)have showed great antiplatelet effect in clinic, and most of them are the Chinese patent drugs. On the prevention of atherosclerosis or vulnerable plaque, Chinese and Western medicine have the consensus that stabling plaque and promoting blood circulation. Based on the agreed thoughts of the Eastern and Western worlds, the application of Chinese herb and formulas for PBCRBS has valuable significance in the exploration of reducing the risk of cardiovascular event[10].

Blood-stasis syndrome has the status of platelet activation, and it has high correlation[11,12]. As early as the last century of 1970s, there were scholars who had made pilot study to observe the mechanism of Chinese herb and formulas for PBCRBS on platelet function[13]. BSS has the definite diagnostic criteria[14] from 1991 in China, and during the past 5 years, diagnosis criteria have improved by scholars and keep pace with the development of TCM. There is a special focus on natural compounds present in dietary and medicinal plants exhibiting antiplatelet/thrombotic properties. Now we know that platelet mainly was regulated by three kinds of substance, one kind is generated out of platelet such as catecholamine, collagen, thrombin, and prostacyclin; the second kind is generated from platelet and acts on the platelet membrane glycoproteins such as ADP, PGD_2, PGE_2, and 5-HT; the last kind is generated from platelet and acts on the platelet such as TXA2, cAMP, cGMP, and Ca^{2+}, et al. Some of these substances have been identified as effective target of antiplatelet. Owing to the many problems of effectiveness and security of current antiplatelet drugs, a great need now arises to develop both effcacious and pharmaceutical medicines to combat these diseases. Screening the highly effciency and fewer adverse effects of antiplatelet drugs from Chinese herb and formulas for PBCRBS attracts great attention of researchers, and the study of target or mechanism of Chinese herb and formulas for PBCRBS to be the hot topic of research and development of antiplatelet drugs. It had been approved that antiplatelet mechanism of Chinese herb and formulas for PBCRBS involves the following aspects.

Table 1 The Ingredient of Frequently Used Formulas for Promoting Blood Circulation and Removing Blood Stasis

Names of formulas	Ingredients of formulas Label	Label
Xiongshao capsule	*Szechuan Lovage Rhizome*, *Red Paeony Root*	Chinese patent drug
Compound danshen dripping pills	*The root of red-rooted salvia*, *Panax notoginseng, Borneol*	Chinese patent drug
Buyanghuanwu decoction	*Radix Astragali Bunge*, *Peach Seed*, *Saffower*, *Szechuan Lovage Rhizome*, *Angelica sinensis*, *Red Paeony Root*, *earthworm*	
Xuesaitong capsule	*Panax Notoginsenosides*	Chinese patent drug
Tongxinluo capsule	*Sanguisuge*, *Scorpio*, *centipede*, *ground beeltle*, *cicada slough*, et al.	Chinese patent drug
Danhong injection	*The root of red-rooted salvia*, *saffower*	Chinese patent drug
Taohongsiwu decoction	*Peach Seed*, *Saffower*, *Szechuan Lovage Rhizome*, *Angelica sinensis*, *white paeony root*, *Radix Rehmanniae Praeparata*	
Xue Fu Zhu Yu decoction	*hovenia dulcis*, *radix achyranthis bidentatae*, *peach seed*, *saffower, Szechuan Lovage Rhizome*, *Angelica sinensis*, *white paeony root*, *Radix Rehmanniae Praeparata*, *radix bupleuri*, *Platycodon grandiflorum*, et al.	

1 Antiplatelet Mechanism of Chinese Herb and Formulas of Promoting Blood Circulation and Removing Blood Stasis

1.1 Inhibition of Platelet Aggregation

Platelet aggregation means the clumping together of platelets in the blood, which is the main function of platelet and has key role in the physiological hemostasia and pathogenesis of atherothrombosis. Platelet activates when it adheres to breakage of vessel or has been induced by activator. Activated platelet membrane glycoprotein (GP)IIb/IIIa exposes its fibrinogen receptor with the participation of Ca^{2+}, one fibrinogen can bind to at least two GP IIb/IIIa at the same time, and platelet clump together with fibrinogen by GP IIb/IIIa. The typical aggregation is induced by different activators, which included the following two aspects, one is chemical agents such as ADP, collagen, thrombin, AA, and PAF, et al. ; the other is shear stress. It is now taken that platelet aggregation rate (PAR)is the evaluation criterion of the intensity. Born designed the platelet aggregation analyzer in 1962 by the turbidimetry principle which to accelerate the understanding of platelet aggregation. Now PAR was considered as the marker of antiplatelet effcacy evaluation and was used intensively in medical research of platelet. Studies show that the vast majority of Chinese herb and formulas for PBCRBS such as Xiongshao Capsule[17], Compound Danshen dripping pills[18], Buyanghuanwu Decoction[19], Xuesaitong Capsule[20], Da Huang Zhe Chong pill[21], and Tongxingluo Capsule[22], et al. can reduce the PAR of patients or animal model of thromboembolic diseases significantly. Active principles such as ferulic acid[23], ligustrazine[24], propyl gallate[25], resveratrol[26], curdione[27], Total flavone in Sanguis Draconis[28],

Salvianolic acid B[29], Hirulog[30], and Saffower flavin[31] et al. can inhibit the platelet aggregation induced by AA, ADP, PAF, collagen, and thrombin to some extent, bringing out the superior antiplatelet effect.

1.2 Inhibition of Platelet Release Reaction

Platelet release reaction means that many substances stored in α-granules, dense granule, and lysosome in platelet are released out of platelet upon different activator. These substances including CD62p (P-selection), GPIIb/IIIa compound, PKC, β-TG, PF-4, and Ca^{2+}, which has been considered as the usual evaluation indicator of screening the effective antiplatelet drug from Chinese herb and formulas for PBCRBS.

1.2.1 CD62p

CD62p (P-selection)is a 140 kD glycoprotein which is present in the granules of platelets and translocates rapidly to the cell surface after platelet activation and is generally considered to be the gold marker of platelet activation[32,33]. Clinical research indicates that the expression of CD62p increases markedly in the different types of cardiovascular patients (including patients with stable angina and ACS)[34-36] and has found high positive correlation between CD62p level and blood stasis syndrome (BSS)[37]. So making the increased expression of CD62p after platelet activation dropped is taken for the one of the antiplatelet mechanisms and scientific measurements of Chinese herb and formulas for PBCRBS. According to the current studies, Danhong injection[38], Ligustrazine injection[39], Compound Danshen dripping pills[40], Taohongsiwu Decoction[41], and Tongxinluo capsule[42] can reduce the CD62p expression after platelet activation significantly and inhibit platelet activation in vivo, to show satisfactory effect of antiplatelet.

1.2.2 GPII b/III a Compound

The detection of PAC-1 is considered as the sensitive and important marker of platelet acti-vation[43], PAC-1 is the specific monoclonal IgMK, which only binds to activating platelet GPIIb/IIIa compound, while it has no recognition capability for resting one. The activation of GPIIb/IIIa depends on the platelet activation which makes the former change its configuration to have strong affnity with receptors. Using the flow cytometry to detect PAC-1 which has the characteristic of specific fast sensitive, and has splendid future in the study on screening antiplatelet drugs from Chinese herb and formulas for PBCRBS.

Da Huang Zhe Chong pill is the earliest formula of PBCRBS and is widely used for atherothrombotic disease treatment. Research shows that it has better antiplatelet aggregation ability than aspirin[44], the further study indicates that it can reduce the level of PAC-1 after ADP-induced platelet activation and of patients with coronary heart disease and cerebral infarction in clinic, which also has superior antiplatelet activation than aspirin[21] and is an ideal antithrombotic drug. Other study[45] found that Xue Fu Zhu Yu decoction can inhibit the ADP-induced expression of GPIIb/IIIa compound significantly and restrain the ADP-induced platelet activation, which provides experimental evidence to long-term treatment of coronary heart disease, and no symptoms of myocardial ischemia, et al.

1.2.3 PKC

protein kinase C (PKC), a ubiquitous protein kinase found in a variety of animal tissues, has been implicated in the regulation of many cellular processes and plays a central role in signal transduction. In platelets, the PKC is an important signaling mediator required for activation, secretion of granule contents, and aggregation[46]. During the process of platelet activation, close relationship between translocation of PKC in platelet and platelet function has been found. PKC has both cytosolic and plasma membrane-bound forms, and the former is the most abundant under resting conditions. The cytosolic form can translocate to the plasma membrane upon cell stimulation and elevation of cellular Ca^{2+} one particular and important aspect of PKC activation is the intracellular redistribution of the enzyme from the cytosol to the cell membrane[44]. Now translocation or redistribution of PKC from the cytosolic form to the plasma membrane can be taken for an indicator of PKC activation[47].

Resveratrol (RESV), a well-known polyphenolic compound of, was extracted from Polygonum

Cuspidatum, which was a Chinese herb for PBCRBS and has been effcaciously used in traditional Chinese medicine to treat several diseases, including thromboembolic diseases for over hundreds of years. In recent years, pharmacological studies have found that RESV possesses multifaceted cardiovascular benefits, but the mechanism is not clear. Recent research[48] shows that PKC distributed mostly across the cytosol of platelets in resting platelets and redistributed to the membrane later to be activated by ADP. If pretreated by RESV, PKC translocation to the membrane was partially inhibited in the platelets activated by ADP. These results suggested that RESV inhibited the PKC-mediated signal transduction pathway in platelets, and it might act as an inhibitor on PKC activity in platelets and serve as a novel antithrombotic agent.

1.2.4 PF-4 and β-TG

It is thought that PF-4 and β-TG are the specific indicators of platelet release reaction[49]. Both increases of PF-4 and β-TG indicate the height of platelet release reaction, which is common in thromboembolic disease and prethrombotic state. On the contrary, both decreases of PF-4 and β-TG indicate the suppression of plate-let release reaction. β-TG can make the PGI2 concentration and adenylate cyclase activity reduction, and then make cAMP decrease which bring about weak inhibition and enhance the aggregation of platelet[50,51]. PF-4 can reduce the anticoagulation of heparan sulphate in endothelial cell and enhance the metabolism of membrane phospholipid and AA, to produce TXA2, also PF-4 can promote precipitation and polymerization of fibrin monomer and accelerate platelet aggregation[52]. Research has found that *Salvia miltiorrhiza Bunge injection*[53] can reduce the PF-4 and β-TG concentration markedly to inhibit platelet aggregation.

1.2.5 Ca^{2+}

Calcium ion plays a vital role in the development of platelet activation. The transformation, aggregation, and release reaction of platelet are triggered by the increase of free calcium ion concentration of platelet ($[Ca^{2+}]_i$), which is the essential mechanism of thrombosis[54]. Studies have found that the increase of$[Ca^{2+}]_i$ in patient with CHD, meanwhile calcium antagonist can reduce$[Ca^{2+}]_i$ of platelet accompanied by inhibiting platelet aggregation[55].

Studies[56] have indicated that some Chinese herbs, such as *Salvia Miltiorrhiza*, *Ligusticum wallichii Franch*, *Carthamus tinctorius*, *Radix Paeoniae Rubra*, and some active constituents as *Ligustrazine* (see Figure 1), Tanshinone IIA (see Figure 2), et al. have the certain effect of calcium channel antagonists and have good results of inhibit platelet aggregation and activation. Another research[57] shows that Saffor yellow (a kind of soluble natural pigment of *Carthamus tinctorius*)can inhibit platelet release of 5-HT and Ca^{2+}, which has similar effect to Ginkgolides (admitted PAF receptor antagonist), which means that Saffor yellow might suppress the platelet activation via inhibition of PAF and calcium influx.

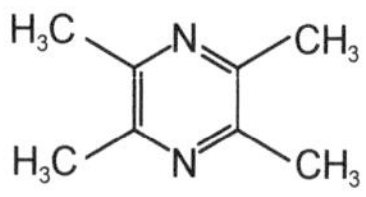

Figure 1 Chemical Structures of Ligustrazine

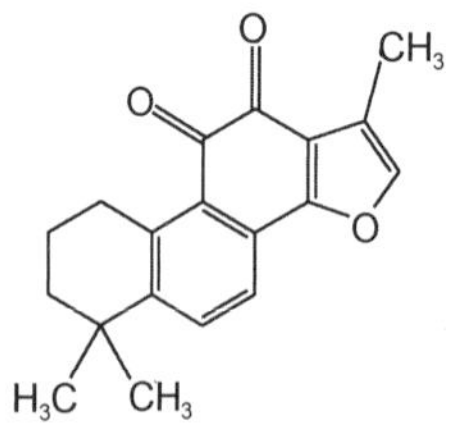

Figure 2 Chemical Structures of Tanshinone IIA

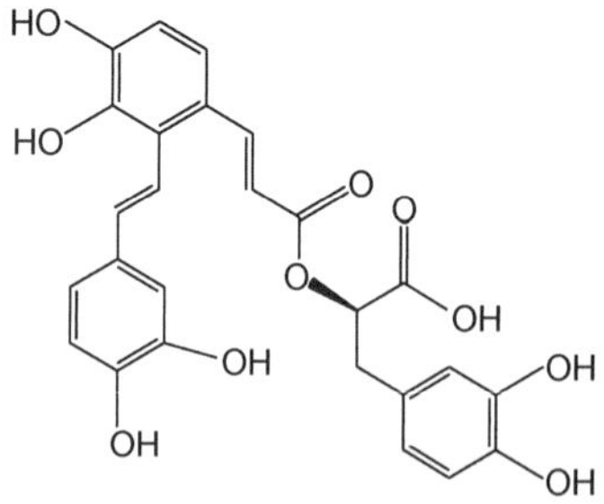

Figure 3 Chemical Structures of Salvianolic Acid A

1.3 Influence of the Process of Platelet Metabolism

1.3.1 Influence of the Metabolic System of Arachidonic Acid (AA)

TXA2 and PGI2 are the metabolites of AA, which have the strong bioactivity of PG, and have a short half-life, quickly degrade to the TXB2 and 6-keto-PGF1α, the latter make further metabolizes to the 6-keto-PGE.

It is now thought that many cardiovascular diseases such as atherosclerosis, thrombosis, coronary spasm, acute myocardial infarction, and hypertension have close relationship with the disequilibrium of TXA2/PGI2[58]. TXA2, which is synthesized and released by platelet microsome and has the function of promoting platelet aggregation and thrombosis, is one of the strong inducers of platelet aggregation and vasoconstrictor. TXA2 promotes the Ca^{2+} of density tube system free to make dense bodies contracting and releasing ADP and 5-HT, which result in platelet aggregation. PGI2 is the main metabolite of AA and is the strong endogenous inhibitor of platelet aggregation; it has the function of antiplatelet aggregation and vasorelaxant and is considered as the vascular protection factor. Under normal physiological state, TXA2 and PGI2 have the balance condition and keep the platelet internal environment stable. Out of balance of TXA2 and PGI2 in plasma or tissue is one of the reasons of platelet aggregation, vasospasm, and thrombosis. Studies show that influence of TXA2/PGI2 has been closely related to antiplatelet mechanism of Chinese herb and formulas for PBCRBS, such as Total saponins of paeonia[59] can reduce the ADP-induced platelet maximum aggregation rate and plasma TXB2 concentration, meanwhile, increase the plasma 6-keto-PGF1α concentration, which means it can promote the release of PGI2, inhibit the produce of TXA2, improve the balance of TXA2/PGI2, and reach the aim of antithrombotic therapy. The same results have been found in the following drugs: *Guanxin II*[60], *Taohongsiwu Decoction*[61], *Notoginsenoside*[62], *salvianolic acid A*[63], *Honghua injection*[64], et al.

1.3.2 Influence of the Metabolic System of cAMP and cGMP

cAMP and cGMP in platelet are the second messengers of signal transmission, which make the different platelet activators acting on the specific receptor, then resulting in platelet aggregation and activation. Studies[65,66] show that drugs which make the level of cAMP and cGMP increase can inhibit platelet aggregation owing to promoting the intake of calcium ions, lowering the level of Ca^{2+}, and having close relation with the phosphorylation of myglobulin. So whether can affect the metabolic system of cAMP and cGMP has been taken as the main point of antiplatelet mechanism of Chinese herb and formulas for PBCRBS. Research[19] shows that BuYang HuanWu decoction can inhibit the ADP-induced platelet aggregation and the decrease of cAMP and cGMP after the platelet aggregation, which suggested that its antiplatelet aggregation may be related to inhibiting the decrease of cyclic nucleotide in platelets after the aggregation. Compound Danshen dripping pills[67] and pseudoginseng[68] have the same mechanism of antiplatelet.

1.4 Influence of the Signal Transduction in Platelet

There is a series of signal transductions in platelet, which has close relationship with platelet activation. Upon agonist stimulation, specific receptor of membrane binds to the ligand to make the conformational changes and to activate the key enzymes action, which produces or releases the signal molecules and led to adhesion, aggregation, and reaction release to form thrombus at last. The mechanism of transmembrane signal transduction in platelet is unclear owing to more than one receptor bound by platelet agonist and the activated platelet release α-granules as secondary agonist to bring about amplification effect[69]. Platelet signal transduction pathway usually includes several aspects[70]: PI3-K pathway, PLC-β pathway, PTK pathway, MARK pathway, cAMP-PKA pathway, and PLA2 pathway. At present, most researches are about Phosphoinositide 3-kinase (PI3K). PI3K is a critical transmitter of intracellular signaling during platelet activation. The PI3K family is divided into three classes (I, II, and III). Depending on differences in the heterodimerization of catalytic subunits and regulatory subunits, class I is further divided into IA (PI3Kα, PI3Kβ, and PI3Kγ)and IB (PI3Kδ), PI3Kβ and PI3Kγ are crucial in platelet signaling[71]. Akt phosphorylation can be used as an indicator of PI3K pathway activation[72,73].

In recent years, with the further study of antiplatelet mechanism of Chinese herb and formulas for PBCRBS, there are studies involving signal transduction in platelet to investigate the mechanism. Salvianolic acid A (SAA, Figure 3)is a water-soluble component from the root of *Salvia miltiorrhiza* Bunge, a herb that is widely used for atherothrombotic disease treatment in China. New study[74] shows that SAA could inhibit platelet spreading on fibrinogen, a process mediated by outside-in signaling. Western blot analysis showed that SAA, like the PI3K inhibitors LY294002 and TGX-221, potently inhibited PI3K, as shown by reduced akt phosphorylation, which indicates that the target spot may be the PI3Kβ. The in vitro findings were further evaluated in the mouse model of arterial thrombosis, in which SAA prolonged the mesenteric arterial occlusion time in wild-type mice. Interestingly, SAA could even counteract the shortened arterial occlusion time in LdlrtmlHer mutant mice. And for the first defined the fact[74] that SAA inhibits platelet activation via the inhibition of PI3K and attenuates arterial thrombus formation in vivo. The results suggest that SAA may be developed as a novel therapeutic agent for the prevention of thrombotic disorders.

2 Discussion and Perspective

From above mentioned, during the past 30 years, research of antiplatelet and antithrombotic therapy of Chinese herb and formulas for PBCRBS has made rapid progress, but there are still some problems existing. In the clinical research, at present many studies limited to small sample of curative effects, lack of multicenter, prospective, large sample, and control study which made the clinical practice of Chinese herb and formulas for PBCRBS be short of definite clinical evidence. And Chinese scholars has begun to attempt to study like above and got to some good results[75]. But those which deserve attention are, in the practical use of clinical medicine, we should comply with the principle of differentiation of symptoms and signs, minimize the potential abuse, and improve on the clinical practical effects. In the experimental research, many studies mainly focused on the mechanism on one aspect of a certain Chinese herb and formulas for PBCRBS, the experimental design owes rigor, and only a few studies were equipped with in vitro and in vivo at the same design. It is generally known that platelet activation is a complex, multifactor process, which involves adhesion, aggregation, and reaction release, for example, there are different platelet activation stimulators, which have the different mechanism of platelet aggregation and signal transduction, it is necessary to take a systematic study on the mechanism of Chinese herb and formulas for PBCRBS inhibiting platelet aggregation by different stimulators in the future and making further study on the signal transduction in platelet, now Chinese scholars[74] have made good study and publish the paper on the well-famous journal.

Proteomics technology has been successfully applied to platelet research, contributing to the emerging field of platelet proteomics which led to the identification of a considerable amount of novel platelet proteins, many of which have been further studied at functional level[76]. During the last 3 years, a rapid development of two-dimensional gel electrophoresis and mass spectrometry-based proteomic approaches has been used to profile alterations in platelet proteins[77-79]. Using differential proteomics of platelet, our previous studies found many different platelet proteins[37,80] between CHD patients of blood stasis syndrome (BSS)and non-BSS patients, and healthy controls, which indicate that the platelet cytoskeleton may play an important role in the development in BSS of CHD. Based on the Chinese medicine principle of "prescription and syndrome are corresponding", these platelet differential proteins may be the new target spots or target group. Getting intensive study on it, we believe that we can develop many new anti-platelet and antithrombolytic drugs possess definite curative effect and target, clear mechanism.

REFERENCES

[1] Antiplatelet Trialists' Collaboration. Collaborative overview of randomised trials of antiplatelet therapy—I: prevention of death, myocardial infarction, and stroke by prolonged antiplatelet therapy in various categories of patients "[J]. British Medical Journal, 1994, 308 (6921): 81-106, .

[2] Antithrombotic Trialists' Collaboration. Collaborate meta-analysis of randomized trials of antiplatelet therapy for prevention of death, myocardial infarction, and stroke in high-risk patien [J]. British Medical Journal, 2002, 324 (7329): 71-86.

[3] Rafferty M, Walters MR, Dawson J. Anti-platelet therapy and aspirin resistance Clinically and chemically relevant? " [J]. Current Medicinal Chemistry, 2010, 17 (36): 4578-4586.

[4] Pena A, Collet JP, Hulot JS, et al. Can we override clopidogrel resistance? [J]. Circulation, 2009, 119 (21): 2854-2857.

[5] Gorog DA, Sweeny JM, Fuster V. Antiplatelet drug 'resistance'. Part 2: laboratory resistance to antiplatelet drugs fact or artifact? [J]. Nature Reviews. Cardiology, 2009, 6 (5): 365-373.

[6] Juurlink DN, Gomes T, Ko DT, et al. A population-based study of the drug interaction between proton pump inhibitors and clopidogrel[J]. Canadian Medical Association Journal, 2009, 180 (7): 713-718.

[7] Mega JL, Close SL, Wiviott SD, et al. Cytochrome P-450 polymorphisms and response to clopidogrel[J]. New England Journal of Medicine, 2009, 360 (4): 354-362.

[8] Choi J, Kermode JC. New therapeutic approaches to combat arterial thrombosis: better drugs for old targets, novel targets, and future prospects[J]. Molecular Interventions, 2011, 11 (27): 111-123.

[9] Chen KJ, Li LD, Weng WL, et al. Blood stasis and research of activating blood circulation and eliminating stasis[J]. Zhong Xi Yi Jie He Xin Nao Xue Guan Bing Za Zhi, 2005, 3 (1): 1-2.

[10] Chen KJ. Exploration on the possibility of reducing cardiovascular risk by treatment with Chinese medicine recipes for promoting blood-circulation and relieving blood-stasis[J]. Zhong Xi Yi Jie He Xin Nao Xue Guan Bing Za Zhi, 2008, 28 (5): 389.

[11] Chen KJ, Xue M, Yin HJ. The relationship between platelet activation related factors and polymorphism of related genes in patients with coronary heart disease of blood-stasis syndrome[J]. Shoudu Yi Ke Da Xue Xue Bao, 2008, 29 (3): 266-269.

[12] Xue M, Chen KJ, Yin HJ. Relationship between platelet activation related factors and polymorphism of related genes in patients with coronary heart disease of blood-stasis syndrome[J]. Chinese Journal of Integrative Medicine, 2008, 14 (4): 267-273.

[13] Wang Z. Mechanism on modulating platelet function of activating blood circulation and removing stasis herbs[J]. Zhong Xi Yi Jie He Xin Nao Xue Guan Bing Za Zhi, 1992, 12 (9): 567-570.

[14] Society of Cardiology and Chinese Association of the Integration of Traditional and Western Medicine. The diagnostic criteria of TCM in coronary heart disease[J]. Chinese Journal of Integrated Traditional and Western Medicine, 1991, 11 (5): 257.

[15] Fu CG, The study of diagnostic criterion on blood stasis for patients with coronary heart disease, Doctor Dissertation, Beijing University of Chinese Medicine, Beijing, China, 2011.

[16] Li JZ, He SL, Wang HL, Thrombosis Epidemiology, Science Press, Beijing, China, 1998.

[17] Xu FQ, Chen KY, Ma XC et al. Clinical observation on effect of xiongshao capsule on coronary heart disease with angina pectoris[J]. Zhongguo Zhong Xi Yi Jie He Za Zhi, 2003, 23 (1): 16-18.

[18] Feng J, Wang SL. Effect of Fufang Danshen Diwan to Platelet Aggregation Function[J]. Chinese Journal of Misdiagnostics, 2006, 6 (12): 2261-2263.

[19] Jiang JB, Yang J, Deng CQ. Effect of Buyang huanwu decoction and its active fraction alkaloid and glycoside on platelet aggregation and cyclic nucleotide in rats[J]. Zhong Nan Yao Xue, 2008, 6 (4): 388-391.

[20] Wang J. Xu J, Zhong JB. Effect of Radix notoginseng saponins on platelet activating molecule expression and aggregation in patients with blood hyperviscosity syndrome[J]. Zhong Xi Yi Jie He Xin Nao Xue Guan Bing Za Zhi, 2004, 24 (4): 312-316.

[21] Wang DS, Chen FP, He SL, et al. Mechanism study on Dahuangzhechong pill anti-platelet activation[J]. Zhonghua Zhong Yi Yao Za Zhi, 2008, 23 (9): 818-821.

[22] Liu F, Li J, Wang XD. Effect of tongxinluo capsule on platelet aggregation in patients with cerebral infarction[J]. Zhongguo Zhong Xi Yi Jie He Za Zhi, 2008, 28 (4): 304-306.

[23] Li JM, Zhao YH, Zhong GC, et al. Synthesis of ferulic acid derivatives and their inhibitory effect on platelet aggregation[J]. Yao Xue Xue Bao, 2011, 46 (3): 305-310.

[24] Shu B, Zhou CJ, Ma YH, et al. Research progress on pharmacological activities of the available compositions in Chinese medicinal herb Ligusticum chuanxiong[J]. Chinese Pharmacological Bulletin, 2006, 22 (9): 1043-1047.

[25] Jiang YR, Yin HJ, Li LZ. Treatment of non-ST-elevation acute coronary syndrome with propyl gallate[J]. Zhongguo Zhong Xi Yi Jie He Za Zhi, 2008, 28 (9): 839-842.

[26] Chen P, Yang LC, Lei WY, et al. Effects of polydatin on platelet aggregation and platelet cytosolic calcium[J]. Tianran Chan Wu Yan Jiu Yu Kai Fa, 1005, 17 (1): 21-25.

[27] Xia Q, Dong TX, Zhan HQ, et al. Inhibition effect of curdione on platelet aggregation induced by ADP in rabbits[J]. Chinese Pharmacological Bulletin, 2006, 22 (9): 1151-1152.

[28] Ma JJ, Song Y, Jia M, et al. Effect of total flavone in sanguis draconis on platelet aggregation, thrombus formation and myocardial ischemia[J]. Zhong Cao Yao, 2002, 33 (11): 1008-1010.

[29] Yao Y, Wu WY, Liu AH, et al. Interaction of salvianolic acids and notoginsengnosides in inhibition of ADP-induced platelet aggregation[J]. American Journal of Chinese Medicine, 2998, 36 (2): 313-328.

[30] Jiang ZW, Zhao LJ, Zhang H, et al. Effect of hirudin injecton on antithrombosis in rats[J]. Ji Lin Da Xue Xue Bao (Yi Xue Ban), 2003, 29 (4): 417-418.

[31] Guo ZQ, Chen Z, Li L, et al. Effect of administration of Saffower yellow injection on the platelet aggregate rate and transforming growth factor-β1 in patients without ST elevation acute myocardial infarction[J]. Journal of Clinical Cardiology, 2010, 26 (8): 591-593.

[32] Hsu-Lin SC, Berman CL, Furie BC. A platelet membrane protein expressed during platelet activation and secretion. Studies using a monoclonal antibody specific for thrombin-activated platelets[J]. Journal of Biological Chemistry, 1984, 259 (14): 9121-9126.

[33] Michelson AD, Furman MI. Laboratory markers of platelet activation and their clinical significance[J]. Current Opinion in Hematology, 1999, 6 (5): 342-348.

[34] Ikeda H, Takajo Y, Ichiki K, et al. . Increased soluble form of P-selectin in patients with unstable angina[J]. Circulation, 1995, 92 (7): 1693-1696.

[35] Shimomura H, Ogawa H, Arai H, et al. Serial changes in plasma levels of soluble P-selectin in patients with acute myocardial infarction[J]. American Journal of Cardiology, 1998, 81 (4): 397-400.

[36] Furman MI, Benoit SE, Barnard MR, et al. Increased platelet reactivity and circulating monocyte-platelet aggregates in patients with stable coronary artery disease[J]. Journal of the American College of Cardiology, 1998, 31 (2): 352-358.

[37] Liu Y, Yin HJ, Jiang YR, et al. Research on the correlation between platelet gelsolin and blood-stasis syndrome of coronary heart disease[J]. Chinese Journal of Integrative Medicine, 2011, 17 (8): 587-592.

[38] Chen ZQ, Hong L, Wang H. Effect of danhong injection on platelet activation andinflammatory factors in patients of acute coronary syndrome after intervention therapy[J]. Zhongguo Zhong Xi Yi Jie He Za Zhi, 2009, 29 (8): 692-694.

[39] Chen ZQ, Hong L, Wang H. Effect of tetramethylpyrazine on platelet activation and vascular endothelial function in patients with acute coronary syndrome undergoing percutaneous coronary intervention[J]. Zhongguo Zhong Xi Yi Jie He Za Zhi, 2007, 27 (12): 1078-1081.

[40] Xiong P, Zhou L. Effect of compound danshen droplet pill on plasma endothelin and platelet α-granuleMembrane protein-140 in patients with unstable angina pectoris[J]. Zhong Xi Yi Jie He Xin Nao Xue Guan Bing Za Zhi, 2009, 7 (5): 510-511.

[41] Han L, Peng DY, Xu F, et al. Studies on anti-platelet activation effect and partial mechanisms of Taohong Siwu decoction[J]. Zhongguo Zhong Yao Za Zhi, 2010, 35 (19): 2609-2612.

[42] Luo HM, Fu DY, Ren MZ, et al. Clinical study on tongxinluo capsule affecting activity of platelet's GP IIb/IIIa receptor in patients with coronary heart disease[J]. Zhong Cheng Yao, 2007, 27 (2): 181-183.

[43] Kasirer-Friede A, Cozzi MR, Mazzucato M, et al. Signaling through GP Ib-IX-V activates αIIbβ3 independently of other receptors[J]. Blood, 2004, 103 (9): 3403-3411.

[44] Wang DS, Chen FP, He SL et al. Comparative research between plasma pharmacology and serum pharmacology of dahuang zhe chong pill[J]. Xue Shuan Yu Zhi Xue Xue, 2005, 11 (1): 5-8.

[45] Li YL. Research progress in the treatment of cardiovascular diseases by Xue Fu Zhu Yu Tang[J]. Beijing Zhong Yi Yao, 2008, 27 (3): 228-230.

[46] Yacoub D, Théorêt JF, Villeneuve L, et al. Essential role of protein kinase C δ in platelet signaling, αIIbβ3 activation, and thromboxane A 2 release[J]. Journal of Biological Chemistry, 2006.281 (40): 30024-30035.

[47] Nishizuka Y. Intracellular signaling by hydrolysis of phospholipids and activation of protein kinase C[J]. Science, 1992, 258 (5082): 607-614.

[48] Yang YM, Wang XX, Chen JZ, et al. Resveratrol attenuates adenosine diphosphate-induced platelet activation by reducing protein kinase C activity[J]. American Journal of Chinese Medicine, 2008, 36 (3): 603-613.

[49] Kaplan KL, Owen J. Plasma levels of β-thromboglobulin and platelet factor 4 as indices of platelet activation in vivo[J]. Blood, 1981, 57 (2): 199-202.

[50] Pumphrey CW, Dawes J. Plasma beta-thromboglobulin as a measure of platelet activity. Effect of risk factors and findings in ischemic heart disease and after acute myocardial infarction[J]. American Journal of Cardiology, 1982, 50 (6): 1258-1261.

[51] Slungaard A. Platelet factor 4: a chemokine enigma[J]. International Journal of Biochemistry and Cell Biology, 2005, 37 (6): 1162-1167.

[52] Hope W, Martin TJ, Chesterman CN, et al. Morgan. Human β-thromboglobulin inhibits PGI2 production and binds to a specific site in bovine aortic endothelial cells[J]. Nature, 1979, 282 (5735): 210-212.

[53] Kong YQ, Yao Z, Yun ML, et al. Effect of danshen on angina pectoris and platlet function[J]. Gao Xue Ya Za Zhi, 2002, 10 (5): 451-453.

[54] Yoshimura M, Oshima T, Hiraga H, et al. Increased cytosolic free Mg^{2+} and Ca^{2+} in platelets of patients with vasospastic angina[J]. American Journal of Physiology, 1998, 274 (2): R548-R554.

[55] Fujinishi A, Takahara K, Ohba C, et al. Effects of nisoldipine on cytosolic calcium, platelet aggregation, and coagulation/fibrinolysis in patients with coronary artery disease[J]. Angiology, 1997, 48 (6): 515-521.

[56] Zhang RX, Lian XF, Lian N. study progress of calcium antagonist of Chinese medicine on cardiovascular diseases[J]. Shanxi Zhong Yi Xue Yuan Xue Bao, 1999, 22 (4): 52-54.

[57] Chen WM, Jin M, Wu W. study of Saffor yellow inhibit the PAF-induced platelet activation[J]. Zhongguo Yao Xue Za Zhi, 2000, 35 (11): 741.

[58] Chen C, Yang TL. TXA2/PGI2 and cardiovascular diseases[J]. Xian Dai Sheng Wu Yi Xue Jin Zhan, 2008, 8 (11): 2166-2172.

[59] Xu HM, Liu QY, Dai M, et al. Effect of total glucosides of radix paeoniae rubra on platelet function of rats[J]. Hefei Gong Ye Da Xue Xue Bao (Zi Ran Ke Xue Ban), 2003, 26 (1): 141-144.

[60] Gao HL, Li YK, Tong Y, et al. Comparative study on the protective effects of different Guanxin II formula on acute myocardial ischemia in dogs[J]. Zhong Yao Yao Li Yu Lin Chuang, 2007, 23 (5): 1-4.

[61] Lan ZX, Wang WZ, Ma YN, et al. Experimental research on the influence of Taohong Siwu decoction on the TXB2, 6-keto-PGF1α in the blood stasis syndrom of rats[J]. Hua Xi Yao Xue Za Zhi, 2008, 23 (6): 687-688.

[62] Wu Y, Guo HB, Wang TJ, et al. Comparative study on effects of active ingredients of several traditional Chinese medicines on rabbit platelet aggregation in vitro[J]. Zhong Yao Lin Chuang Yao Li Xue Yu Zhi Liao Xue, 2007, 12 (9): 1047-1051.

[63] Yu WG, Xu LN. Effects of acetylsalvianolic acid A on arachidonic acid metabolism in platelets[J]. Yao Xue Xue Bao, 1998, 33 (1): 62-63.

[64] Yuan SJ, Zhang ZW, Gao TH, ct al. Mcchanism rcscarch of IIonghua injection antithrombotic function[J]. Zhongguo Zhong Yao Za Zhi, 2011, 36 (11): 1528-1529.

[65] Wang ZY, Li JZ, Ruan CG. Basic Theory and Clinical of Thrombosis and Hemostasis, Shanghai Scientific and Technical Publishers, Shanghai, China, 2004.

[66] Xu SH. Cyclic nucleotides and blood platelet function[J]. Sheng li Ke Xue Jin Zhan, 1992, 23 (4): 318-322.

[67] Zhu GG, Luo RZ, Guo ZX. Advance of cardiotonic pill on inhibiting platelet activation and aggregation[J]. Zhong guo Xin Xue Guan Za Zhi, 2007, 12 (2): 149-151.

[68] Yan J, Qin CL. Brief review on effects of Fufangdanshen prescription, Dan-shen and San-qi on the platelet functions[J]. Zhongguo Shi Yan Fangji Xue Za Zhi, 2003, 9 (2): 59-62.

[69] Pei HY, Han Y. Platelet activation through signal transduction-review[J]. Zhongguo Shi Yan Xue Ye Xue Za Zhi, 2004, 12 (5): 704-707.

[70] Lu J, Yu YN, Xu RB, Receptor Signaling System and Diseases, Shandong Science and Technology Press, Shandong, China, 1999.

[71] Cosemans JMEM, Munnix ICA, Wetzker R, et al. Continuous signaling via PI3K isoforms β and γ is required for platelet ADP receptor function in dynamic thrombus stabilization[J]. Blood, 2006, 108 (9): 3045-3052.

[72] Li Z, Zhang G, Le GC, et al. Two waves of platelet secretion induced by thromboxane A2 receptor and a critical role for phosphoinositide 3-kinases[J]. Journal of Biological Chemistry, 2003, 278 (33): 30725-30731.

[73] Kroner C, Eybrechts K, Akkerman JWN. Dual regulation of platelet protein kinase B[J]. Journal of Biological Chemistry, 2000, 275 (36): 27790-27798.

[74] Huang ZS, Zeng CL, Zhu LJ, et al. Salvianolic acid A inhibits platelet activation and arterial thrombosis via inhibition of phosphoinositide 3-kinase[J]. Journal of Thrombosis and Haemostasis, 2010, 8 (6): 1383-1393.

[75] Chen KJ, Shi DZ, Xu H et al. XS0601 reduces the incidence of restenosis: a prospective study of 335 patients undergoing percutaneous coronary intervention in China[J]. Chinese Medical Journal, 2006, 119 (1): 6-13.

[76] Garćıa A. Clinical proteomics in platelet research: challenges ahead[J]. Journal of Thrombosis and Haemostasis, 2010, 8 (8): 1784-1785.

[77] Thiele T, Steil L, Gebhard S, et al. Profiling of alterations in platelet proteins during storage of platelet concentrates[J]. Transfusion, 2007, 47 (7): 221-1233.

[78] Banfi C, Brioschi M, Marenzi G, et al. Proteome of platelets in patients with coronary artery disease[J]. Experimental Hematology, 2010, 38 (5): 341-350.

[79] Senzel L, Gnatenko DV, Bahou WF. The platelet proteome[J]. Current Opinion in Hematology, 2009, 16 (5): 329-333.

[80] Li XF, Jiang YR, Wu CF, et al. Study on the correlation between platelet function proteins and symptom complex in coronary heart disease[J]. Zhongguo Fen Zi Xin Zang Bing Xue Za Zhi, 2009, 9 (6): 362-366.

First published: LIU Yue, YIN Hui-jun, SHI Da-zhuo, CHEN Ke-ji. Chinese herb and formulas for promoting blood circulation and removing blood stasis and antiplatelet therapies[J]. Evid Based Complement Alternat Med, 2012, 2012: 184503.

Atherosclerosis, Vascular Aging and Therapeutic Strategies

LIU Yue and CHEN Ke-ji

Lifespan is the maximum amount of time an organism has been observed to survive from birth to death. It is typically measured by age. The maximum lifespan in humans is believed to be between 100 and 120 years. Of the recognized factors that affect health and lifespan, personal health and heredity only account for 15% of lifespan, while factors such as social economic environment, lifestyle, mental state, and access to medical care account for 60%. Unlike premature aging and lifespan shortening caused by genetic diseases, such as Werner syndrome and Hutchinson-Gilford progeria syndrome, where no treatment is currently available, diseases that are significantly influenced by lifestyle, such as coronary artery disease and type Ⅱ diabetes mellitus, have a much brighter outlook in terms of disease prevention and disease control.

1 Cardiovascular Diseases and Atherosclerosis

Cardiovascular diseases (CVD)is the number one killer in China with annual deaths of more than 3 000 000 from 1990 to 2010. [1] China also has a high incidence of sudden cardiac death (SCD). A survey across four major regions in China (Beijing, Guangzhou, Kelamayi, and Yuxian)showed a SCD incidence of 41.8 per 100 000 per year. [2] This would translate to an estimated annual incidence of 500 000 SCD in China based on a population of 1.33 billion. China is also one of the countries with more prevalent ischemic stroke with an incidence well above that of the developed countries. At the same time, the age-adjusted prevalence of total diabetes and pre-diabetes are 9.7% and 15.5%, respectively, accounting for 92.4 million adult Chinese with diabetes and 148.2 million with pre-diabetes. [3] Diabetes is recognized as a major risk factor for CVD, and those diagnosed with diabetes or pre-diabetes will contributed to the prevalence of CVD in the next 10 to 20 years.

Atherosclerosis is the common pathological mechanism of coronary artery diseases, stroke, and peripheral vascular disease, and it mostly affects the medium and large arteries. The elasticity and flexibility of healthy arteries are fundamental to the delivery of oxygen and nutrients to the body. Over time, however, the thickening of arterial walls and stiffness of arteries may occur and may sometimes restrict blood supply to organs and tissues. This process is called arteriosclerosis or the hardening of the arteries. Atherosclerosis occurs when fat, cholesterol, and other substances build up inside the arteries and leads to the formation of plaques, narrowing of the lumen, hardening of the arterial walls, and ultimately blockade of the blood flow. Clinically, occlusion of the coronary arteries due to atherosclerosis manifests as chest pain, shortness of breath, and other serious symptoms, indicating the acute onset of cardiovascular events. [4] Atherosclerotic plaques are classified into stable and unstable (also called vulnerable)plaques. Stable atherosclerotic plaques, which tend to be asymptomatic, are rich in extracellular matrix and smooth muscle cells. Unstable or vulnerable plaques are rich in macrophages and foam cells, and the fibrous cap separated from the wall by a large lipid pool is particularly unstable and prone to rupture. Ruptured plaques induce thrombus formation and thromboembolism, both leading to cardiocerebrovascular events.

2 From Treating Risk Factors to Treating Arteries

CVD is typically preventable and controllable. The Framingham Heart Study was the first prospective study with the objective of identifying the common risk factors or characteristics that contribute to CVD by following its development over a long period of time in a large group of participants who have not yet developed overt symptoms of CVD or suffered from a heart attack or stroke. [5] A risk factor is defined as a measurable characteristic that is causally associated with increased disease frequency and is a significant independent predictor of an increased risk presenting with the disease. [6] Risk factors are either modifiable (e.g., obesity, hypertension, dyslipidemia, and smoking)or unmodifiable (e.g., age, gender, race, and family history). In the past 50 years, active control of the risk factors has been the focus of CVD prevention and treatment. Both Finland and USA, which were once high CVD risk countries, have demonstrated a sharp decrease in CVD incidence in recent years, indicating the essential role of primary CVD prevention. [7,8] Experiences from other countries have also consistently confirmed that risk factor control could dramatically cut down the mortality of coronary disease. [8]

Although reduction in CVD incidence was demonstrated, the effectiveness of risk factor control has been limited. Virtually all positive randomized trials of cardiovascular prevention in high-risk patients showed relative risk reductions in the range of 9% to 30%, which means that 70% to 80% of events are not prevented by guideline-advocated therapies. [9] In a long-term, intensive, multi-factorial intervention study in diabetic subjects, only 50% of cardiovascular events were prevented during a follow-up of 14 years. [10] Efforts have been made to identify other parameters that can better predict and treat CVD. For instance, the area of carotid plaque was used in identifying and managing the high-risk vascular patients. [11] While cardiovascular events were reported in 30% of subjects with a high Framingham risk score, 70% of those with the events were in the top quartile of total plaque area (TPA). [11] TPA strongly predicted cardiovascular risk, and plaque progression despite treatment according to guidelines further predicted cardiovascular risk. [12] The recognition that treatment according to consensus guidelines was failing half of the patients necessitates a shift in the strategy for patient management from treating risk factors to treating arteries. [9,13]

3 Atherosclerosis and Vascular Aging

Vascular aging is different from atherosclerosis. As Sir William Osler (1849-1919), a legendary physician and one of the founders of Johns Hopkins University, stated in his textbook, “A man is as old as his arteries” . Vascular aging has become a focus for prevention and treatment of CVD in recent years. Vascular aging and atherosclerosis are distinct pathological processes but are often mistakenly used interchangeably. The large-and medium-sized arteries in elderly people show varying degrees of intimal and medial changes, which are known as vascular aging or age-related intima-medial degeneration and sclerosis. [14] Clinically, the assessments of vascular aging include carotid intima-media thickness (cIMT), pulse wave velocity (PWV), and ankle-brachial index (ABI). The detrimental effect of aging on the vascular system is considered in terms of potential mechanisms involved in endothelial dysfunction and age-related atherosclerosis. [15] The cellular and molecular basis of vascular aging is unclear but is shown to be related with oxidative stress and endothelial dysfunction, [15,16] vascular inflammation, [17,18] increased arterial stiffness, [19] impaired angiogenesis, [20] defective vascular repair, [21] endothelial replicative senescence, [22] and impaired endothelial progenitor cell recruitment. [23] Understanding the mechanisms underlying the age-induced vascular pathophysiological alterations[24] may shed light on therapeutic strategies for reducing cardiovascular mortality in an aging population.

4 Therapeutic Strategies to Treat Atherosclerosis and Delay Vascular Aging

Therapeutic strategies to treat atherosclerosis and delay vascular aging include regular exercise, [25,26] caloric restriction, [27] lowering cholesterol, [28] anti-inflammation, [29,30] and Growth Hormone (GH)/ Insulinlike Growth Factor-1 (IGF-1)supplementation. [31]

Progress has been made in the research and development of Chinese medicine (CM)for the treatment of atherosclerosis and delaying vascular aging. According to the CM theory, qi deficiency and blood stasis are the basic characteristics in the pathogenesis of CVD. Tonifying deficiency and removing stasis are the fundamental treatment principle for selection of herbal medications. Ginseng, Notoginseng, and Ligusticum Rhizoma are the main CMs used for anti-aging treatment and have been shown to delay vascular aging in experimental studies. [32,33] Xiongshao Capsule (芎芍胶囊, XSC)is developed from Xuefu Zhuyu Decoction (血府逐瘀汤), which is the classic formula used for promoting blood circulation and removing blood stasis. Clinical studies showed that XSC could effectively prevent restenosis after percutaneous coronary intervention (PCI). [34,35] XSC was shown to enhance the protective effect of ischemic post-conditioning on rats with myocardial ischemic reperfusion injury, and this action may be related to its inhibition of monocyte chemotactic protein-1 (MCP-1)and tumor necrosis factor α (TNF-α)expression as well as inflammatory cell infiltration. [36] XSC was also shown to stabilize atherosclerotic plaque by suppressing inflammation and the expression of FcγRⅢA. [37] These findings indicate that XSC may affect multiple molecular targets and possibly multiple signaling cascades. It is likely that these effects act together to exert clinical benefit of anti-restenosis. The study of XSC exemplifies the multi-component, multi-pathway, and multiple-target characteristics of Chinese herbal medicine, and such treatment strategy may have great advantage over conventional single-target approach in treating the complex processes of atherosclerosis and vascular aging.

5 Conclusion

According to the latest report, [38] the global population is expected to hit 7 billion later in 2011. People over the age of 60 accounts for a big proportion of the total population and the aged population is growing. Population aging is taking place globally, and further acceleration of the process is anticipated for this century. Increase in longevity and decline in fertility are the two main demographic effects that result in population aging. An increase in longevity raises the average age of the population by increasing the number of surviving older people. With the extended lifespan, it is important to ensure that the growing older population living the extra years of life in a good health among other social and economic issues. Atherosclerosis and vascular aging are the key influencing factor of lifespan. Vascular aging, which proceeds atherosclerosis, marks the first sign of cardiovascular system degeneration. [39] Despite some progress in preventing atherosclerosis and vascular aging, the mechanism of pathogenesis requires further investigation and effective therapeutic interventions await to be developed. Therapeutic strategies focused on comprehensive, multi-target interventions rather than the single-target therapy may hold great potential. The holistic approach and long history of human use make Chinese herbs and formulae the ideal candidates for the development of therapeutic interventions for this purpose.

REFERENCES

[1] National Center for Cardiovascular Diseases of China. Report on cardiovascular diseases in China (2010)[M]. Beijing: Encyclopedia of China Publishing House, 2011: 1.

[2] Hua W, Zhang LF, Wu YF, et al. Incidence of sudden cardiac death in China: analysis of 4 regional populations[J]. J Am Coll Cardiol, 2009, 54 (2): 1110-1118.

[3] Yang WY, Lu JM, Weng JP, et al. Prevalence of diabetes among men and women in China[J]. N Engl J Med, 2010, 362 (25): 1090-1101.

[4] Fuster V. Atherosclerosis, thrombosis, and vascular biology. In: Goldman L, Ausiello D, eds. Cecil medicine. 23rd ed. Philadelphia, Pa: Saunders Elsevier, 2007: 69: 383-385.

[5] Kannel WB, Dawber TR, Kagana, et al. Factors of risk in the development of coronary heart disease-six-year follow-up experience. The Framingham Study[J]. Ann Intern Med, 1961, 55: 33-50.

[6] O'Donnell CJ, Elosua R. Cardiovascular risk factors. Insights from Framingham Heart Study[J]. Rev Esp Cardiol, 2008, 61 (3): 299-310.

[7] Laatikainen T, Critchley J, Vartiainen E, et al. Explaining the decline in coronary heart disease mortality in Finland between 1982 and 1997[J]. Am J Epidemiol, 2005, 162 (8): 764 -773.

[8] Ford ES, Ajani UA, Croft JB, et al. Explaining the decrease in U. S. deaths from coronary disease, 1980-2000[J]. N Engl J Med, 2007, 56 (23): 2388-2398.

[9] Spence JD, Hackam DG. Treating arteries instead of risk factors: a paradigm change in management of atherosclerosis[J]. Stroke, 2010, 41 (6): 1193-1199.

[10] Gaede P, Lund-Andersen H, Parving HH, et al. Effect of a multifactorial intervention on mortality in type 2 diabetes[J]. N Engl J Med, 2008, 358 (6): 580-591.

[11] Spence JD. Point: uses of carotid plaque measurement as a predictor of cardiovascular events[J]. Prev Cardiol, 2005, 8 (2): 118-121.

[12] Spence JD, Eliasziw M, DiCicco M, et al. Carotid plaque area: a tool for targeting and evaluating vascular preventive therapy[J]. Stroke, 2002, 33 (12): 2916-2922.

[13] Spence JD. Technology insight: ultrasound measurement of carotid plaque—patient management, genetic research, and therapy evaluation[J]. Nat Clin Pract Neurol, 2006, 2 (11): 611-619.

[14] Sawabe M. Vascular aging: from molecular mechanism to clinical significance[J]. Geriatr Gerontol Int, 2010, 10 (Suppl): S213-S220.

[15] Donato AJ, Eskurza I, Silver AE, et al. Direct evidence of endothelial oxidative stress with aging in humans: relation to impaired endothelium dependent dilation and upregulation of nuclear factor-kappaB[J]. Circ Res, 2007, 100 (11): 1659-1666.

[16] Csiszar A, Wang M, Lakatta EG, et al. Inflammation and endothelial dysfunction during aging: role of NF-kappa B[J]. J Appl Physiol, 2008, 105: 1333-1341.

[17] Franceschi C, Bonafè M, Valensin S, et al. Inflamm-aging. An evolutionary perspective on immunosenescence[J]. Ann N Y Acad Sci 2000, 7 (908): 244-254.

[18] Wang M, Zhang J, Jiang LQ, et al. Proinflammatory profile within the grossly normal aged human aortic wall[J]. Hypertension, 2007, 50 (1): 219-227.

[19] Jiang L, Wang M, Zhang J, et al. Increased aortic calpain-1 activity mediates age-associated angiotensin Ⅱ signaling of vascular smooth muscle cells[J]. PLoS One, 2008, 3 (5): e2231.

[20] Rivard A, Fabre JE, Silver M, et al. Age-dependent impairment of angiogenesis[J]. Circulation, 1999, 99: 111-120.

[21] Weinsaft JW, Edelberg JM. Aging-associated changes in vascular activity: a potential link to geriatric cardiovascular disease[J]. Am J Geriatr Cardiol, 2001, 10 (6): 348-354.

[22] Erusalimsky JD. Vascular endothelial senescence: from mechanisms to pathophysiology[J]. J Appl Physiol, 2009, 106 (1): 326-332.

[23] Chang EI, Loh SA, Ceradini DJ, et al. Age decreases endothelial progenitor cell recruitment through decreases in hypoxia-inducible factor 1alpha stabilization during ischemia[J]. Circulation, 2007, 116 (24): 2818-2829.

[24] Ungvari Z, Kaley G, de Cabo R, et al. Mechanisms of vascular aging: new perspectives[J]. J Gerontol A Biol Sci Med Sci, 2010, 65 (10): 1028-1041.

[25] Sindler AL, Delp MD, Reyes R, et al. Effects of aging and exercise training on eNOS uncoupling in skeletal muscle resistance arterioles[J]. J Physiol 2009, 587 (15): 3885-3897.

[26] Taddei S, Galetta F, Virdis A, et al. Physical activity prevents age related impairment in nitric oxide availability in elderly athletes[J]. Circulation, 2000, 101 (25): 2896-2901.

[27] Ungvari Z, Parrado-Fernandez C, Csiszar A, et al. Mechanisms underlying caloric restriction and lifespan regulation: implications for vascular aging[J]. Circ Res, 2008, 102 (5): 519-528.

[28] Okazaki S, Yokoyama T, Miyauchi K, et al. Early statin treatment in patients with acute coronary syndrome: demonstration of the beneficial effect on atherosclerotic lesions by serial volumetric intravascular ultrasound analysis during half a year after coronary event: the ESTABLISH Study[J]. Circulation, 2004, 110 (9): 1061-1068.

[29] Csiszar A, Ungvari Z, Edwards JG, et al. Aging-induced phenotypic changes and oxidative stress impair coronary arteriolar function[J]. Circ Res, 2002, 90 (11): 1159-1166.

[30] Bruunsgaard H, Skinhoj P, Pedersen AN, et al. Ageing, tumour necrosis factor-alpha (TNF-alpha)and atherosclerosis[J]. Clin Exp Immunol, 2000, 121 (2): 255-260.

[31] Sonntag WE, Ramsey M, Carter CS. Growth hormone and insulinlike growth factor-1 (IGF-1)and their influence on cognitive aging[J]. Ageing Res Rev, 2005, 4 (2): 195-212.

[32] Lei Y, Yang J, Zhao H, et al. Experimental study on extracts from Ginseng, Notoginseng and Chuanxiong for delaying vascular aging in senescent Mice[J]. Chin J Integr Tradit West Med (Chin), 2010, 30 (9): 946-951.

[33] Yang J, Lei Y, Fang SP, et al. Study on acting mechanism of extracts from Ginseng, Notoginseng and Chuanxiong for delaying the aging of endothelial cells induced by angiotensin Ⅱ [J]. Chin J Integr Tradit West Med (Chin), 2009, 29 (6): 524-528.

[34] Lu XY, Shi DZ, Xu H, et al. Clinical study on effect of Xiongshao Capsule on restenosis after percutaneous coronary intervention[J]. Chin J Integr Tradit West Med (Chin), 2006, 26 (1): 13-17.

[35] Chen KJ, Shi DZ, Xu H, et al. XS0601 reduces the incidence of restenosis: a prospective study of 335 patients undergoing percutaneous coronary intervention in China[J]. Chin Med J, 2006, 119 (1): 6-13.

[36] Zhang DW, Zhang L, Liu JG, et al. Effects of Xiongshao Capsule combined with ischemic postconditioning on monocyte chemoattractant protein-1 and tumor necrosis factor-α in rat myocardium with ischemic reperfusion injury[J]. Chin J Integr Tradit West Med (Chin), 2010, 30 (12): 1279-1283.

[37] Huang Y, Yin HJ, Ma XJ, et al. Correlation between Fc γ RⅢA and aortic atherosclerotic plaque destabilization in apoE knockout mice and intervention effects of effective components of Chuanxiong rhizome and red peony root[J]. Chin J Integr Med, 2011, 17 (5): 355-360.

[38] David E. Bloom. 7 billion and counting[J]. Science, 2011, 333 (6042): 562-569.

[39] Boos CJ, Goon PK, Lip GY. Endothelial progenitor cells in the vascular pathophysiology of hypertension: arterial stiffness, ageing and more[J]. J Hum Hypertens, 2006, 20 (7): 475-477.

First published: LIU Yue, CHEN Ke-ji. Atherosclerosis, vascular aging and therapeutic strategies. [J] . Chin J Integr Med, 2012, 18 (2): 83-87.

Correlation between Platelet Gelsolin Levels and Different Types of Coronary Heart Disease

LIU Yue, YIN Hui-jun, JIANG Yue-rong, XUE Mei, and CHEN Ke-ji

Coronary heart disease (CHD)remains a major global public health problem. Platelets play an important role in hemostasis but are also responsible for the formation of pathogenic thrombi underlying acute clinical manifestations of vascular atherothrombotic disease. Multiple pathways, including adenosine diphosphate (ADP), thromboxane A_2 (TXA_2), and thrombin are capable of activating platelets. Deregulated platelet activation can lead to the formation of platelet-rich thrombi that occlude the arterial lumen and are capable of causing ischemia and cardiovascular events. Oral antiplatelet drugs are a milestone in the therapy of cardio-vascular atherothrombotic diseases. The efficacy of antiplatelet drugs, such as aspirin and clopidogrel, in decreasing the risk of adverse events in CHD patients has been well studied in the past 20 years. Despite oral antiplatelet therapy, a number of adverse CHD events continue to occur. In re-cent years, many reports have shown a possible relationship between residual platelet activity, as measured by a variety of laboratory tests, and clinical outcomes; raising the possibility that "resistance" to oral antiplatelet drugs may underlie many such adverse events [1]. These phenomena suggest that other pathways capable of stimulating platelet activation may exist. It is therefore meaningful to identify new therapeutic targets for anti-platelet therapy for CHD.

Using differential proteomics in platelets, our previous studies [2] found that gelsolin protein levels show the highest difference between the platelets of CHD patients and healthy controls. This suggests that the platelet cytoskeleton may play an important role in CHD development. Based on previous results, this paper further studied the distribution of gelsolin in human platelets and plasma, and studied any potential correlation with different types of CHD to verify the role of platelet gelsolin in CHD development.

METHODS

1 Diagnostic Criteria

Patient diagnosis meet the standards established under the ACC/AHA/ACP-ASIM Guidelines (1999)[3] for the management of patients with chronic stable angina, and the ACC/AHA Guidelines (2002)[4] for the management of patients with unstable angina and non-ST-segment elevation myocardial infarction. We selected those patients having symptoms of angina and/or objective evidence of myocardial ischemia and those with at least one marked coronary stenosis (>50%)shown by coronary arteriography examination.

2 Inclusion and Exclusion Criteria

The inclusion standard required that patients must meet all the following criteria, namely, (1)falls under one of the various classifications of ischemic heart diseases; (2)suffering from angina pectoris symptoms and/or showing signs of myocardial ischemia; (3)latest coronary arteriography examination showing significant stenosis (>50%); and, (4)age between 35 to 75 years.

Patients who met any one of the following conditions were excluded: severe valvuloplasty, diabetes mellitus type I, presence of severe primary diseases of the liver, kidney, hemopoietic system, presence of malignant tumors, calcium channel blockers (CCB)administration in the last two weeks, inability to obtain informed consent or deemed poor compliance case, participation in other clinical trials, and pregnant or lactating women.

Subjects enrolled in the healthy control group (31 cases)were identified as healthy by history and physical examination. Tests included routine blood count, liver function, chest X-ray, and electrocardiograph (ECG), no history of prior administration of drugs affecting atherosclerotic or thrombotic processes in the last two weeks, no history of significant mental or physical diseases nor history of familiar or self-psychiatric illnesses. This study is in accordance with the Helsinki Declaration[5], with no contravention to medical ethics.

3 Blood Preparation

Fresh blood (12 mL)was drawn from an antecubital vein and collected into vacutainer tubes containing acid-citrate-dextrose (ACD)9% v/v (trisodium citrate 22.0 g/L, citric acid 8.0 g/L, dextrose 24.5 g/L)as anticoagulant, and the initial 2 mL of blood discarded to avoid spontaneous plate-let activation. We collected the blood of patients before antithrombotic therapy and angiography examination. The blood was centrifuged for 10 min at $150 \times g$ at room temperature to obtain platelet-rich plasma (PRP)and the remaining blood centrifuged for 20 min at $800 \times g$ to obtain platelet poor plasma (PPP).

4 Determination of CD62p Expression in Platelets

We determined the level of platelet activation, as represented by the fluorescent intensity of platelet glycoprotein CD62p, by flow cytometry (EPICS Elite, Beckman Coulter Inc., Fullerton, CA, USA). We mixed the blood evenly and completed the following procedures within 4 h. Control and test tubes containing 50 mL of blood had 20 mL of homotype control CD61-FITC/CD62p-PE (CD61-FITC, Anti-GPIIIa, Cat: 348093; CD62p-PE, Anti-GMP-140, Cat: 348107; Becton Dickinson Co., Franklin Lakes, NJ, USA)added. Samples were mixed evenly by light shaking, and incubated in darkness at room temperature for 20 min. One milliliter of cold (2–8 ℃)fixative liquid was added into each tube, mixed well and incubated again in darkness at 2–8 ℃ for 30 min. Samples were then analyzed by flow cytometry to measure the mean fluorescence intensity (MFI)of CD62p. We used multi-parameter and multi-fluorescent flow cytometry with standard fluorescent micro-balloon adopted to correct the beam path and stream. Test data was obtained by Forward Scatter (FSC) vs. Side Scattering (SSC)gate, flow cytometry special software (Expo32, Beckman Coulter Inc.).

5 Determination of Platelet Aggregation Rate (PAR)

We determined the PAR among different patient groups using turbidimetry (Platelet Aggregation Instrument, LBY-NJ2, Beijing Lipusheng Co., China). The inducer of platelet aggregation is arachidonic acid (AA, Helena Biosciences Co., Sunderland, Tyne and Wear, UK).

6 Determination of $[Ca^{2+}]_i$ in Platelets

Platelet-rich plasma was prepared and incubated with 4 mol/L Fluo-3-AM (Sigma, Saint Louis, MO, USA) at 37 ℃ for 40 min. The Ca^{2+} concentration of platelets was determined using flow cytometry to measure their MFI, as previously described [6]. The platelet Ca^{2+} concentration (nmol/L)is calculated as $[Ca^{2+}]_i = K_d \times (F - F_{min})/ (F_{max} - F)$[7].

7 Determination of Gelsolin, F-actin and Gc-globulin

The plasma concentration (PRP and PPP)of gelsolin (Cat: E0372h, R&D Co., Minneapolis, MN, USA), F-actin (Cat: E1876h, R&D Co.)and Gc-globulin (Cat: E1910h, R&D Co.)were determined by enzyme-linked immunoadsorbent assay (ELISA), as per the manufacturer's instructions.

8 Statistical Analysis

Statistical analysis was conducted using SPSS 13.0 software package. Data are expressed as mean ± standard deviation ($\bar{x} \pm s$)or counts (percentage), unless otherwise specified. We used Chi-square or rank sum test to evaluate enumeration data. For measurement data, we used variance analysis or *t*-tests. We assessed correlations of platelet gelsolin with other variables by Spearman correlation coefficient and unitary linear regression. A *P*-value of < 0.05 was considered statistically significant.

RESULTS

1 General Clinical Materials

All CHD patients enrolled were in-patients admitted from August 2010 to February 2011 in Beijing Anzhen Hospital of Capital Medical University and were diagnosed and as-signed to the SAP (33 cases), UAP (39 cases)and AMI (42 cases)groups accordingly.

There was no statistical difference among the three groups in age, sex and platelet count ($P > 0.05$). The risk factors (smoking, hypertension, dyslipidemia and diabetes history), location of affected coronary artery and medication history (statins and aspirin)was comparable among the three groups ($P > 0.05$) (Table 1).

Table 1 Clinical features of Each Study Groups

Parameter	CHD patients			Control group
	SAP group (33 cases)	UAP group (39 cases)	AMI group (42 cases)	(31 cases)
Age (years, $x \pm s$)	54.0 ± 6.5	52.5 ± 5.5	51.5 ± 7.5	50.5 ± 8.0
Male/females (case)	26/7	30/9	35/7	23/8
Risk factor [case (%)]				
Hypertension	15 (45.5)	17 (43.6)	20 (47.6)	0
Dyslipidemia	14 (42.4)	17 (43.6)	19 (45.2)	0
Diabetes	4 (12.1)	4 (10.3)	5 (11.9)	0
Current smokers	22 (66.7)	25 (64.1)	29 (69.05)	0
Medication [case (%)]				
Aspirin	20 (60.6)	24 (61.5)	26 (61.9)	0
Statins	13 (39.4)	15 (38.5)	17 (40.5)	0
Single-vessel disease [case (%)]	12 (36.4)	15 (38.5)	16 (38.1)	0
Multi-vessel disease [case (%)]	21 (63.6)	24 (61.5)	26 (61.9)	0
Platelet count ($\times 10^3$/L)	214 ± 56.9	215 ± 38.8	216 ± 22.8	210.9 ± 42.7

2 Comparison of Plasma Gelsolin Concentration of CHD Patients among Each Patient Group

Compared with the control group, the gelsolin concentration in the PRP of the UAP and AMI groups was significantly higher ($P < 0.01$), while that in the PPP of the three patient groups decreased markedly ($P < 0.01$). Compared with the SAP group, the gelsolin concentration in the PRP of the UAP and AMI groups was significantly higher ($P < 0.01$) (Table 2).

Table 2 Comparison of Plasma Gelsolin Concentration among Different Patient Groups ($\bar{x} \pm s$, g/m)

Group	Case	PRP	PPP
SAP	33	$105.13 \pm 15.27^{**}$	$109.17 \pm 18.12^{**}$
UAP	39	$128.23 \pm 17.55^{**\dagger\dagger}$	$112.58 \pm 11.47^{**}$
AMI	42	$162.16 \pm 21.07^{**\dagger\dagger}$	$112.40 \pm 8.66^{**}$
Control	31	117.55 ± 9.91	121.44 ± 6.77

Notes: **, $P < 0.01$, compared with the control group ; ††, $P < 0.01$, compared with the SAP group.

3 Comparison of CD62p and $[Ca^{2+}]_i$ of Platelets for CHD Patients among Each Patient Group

Compared with healthy controls, the CD62p and $[Ca^{2+}]_i$ of platelets was significantly higher ($P < 0.01$) among the three patient groups. Compared with the SAP group, the CD62p and $[Ca^{2+}]_i$ of platelets among the UAP and AMI groups was significantly higher ($P < 0.01$)again (Figures 1 and 2).

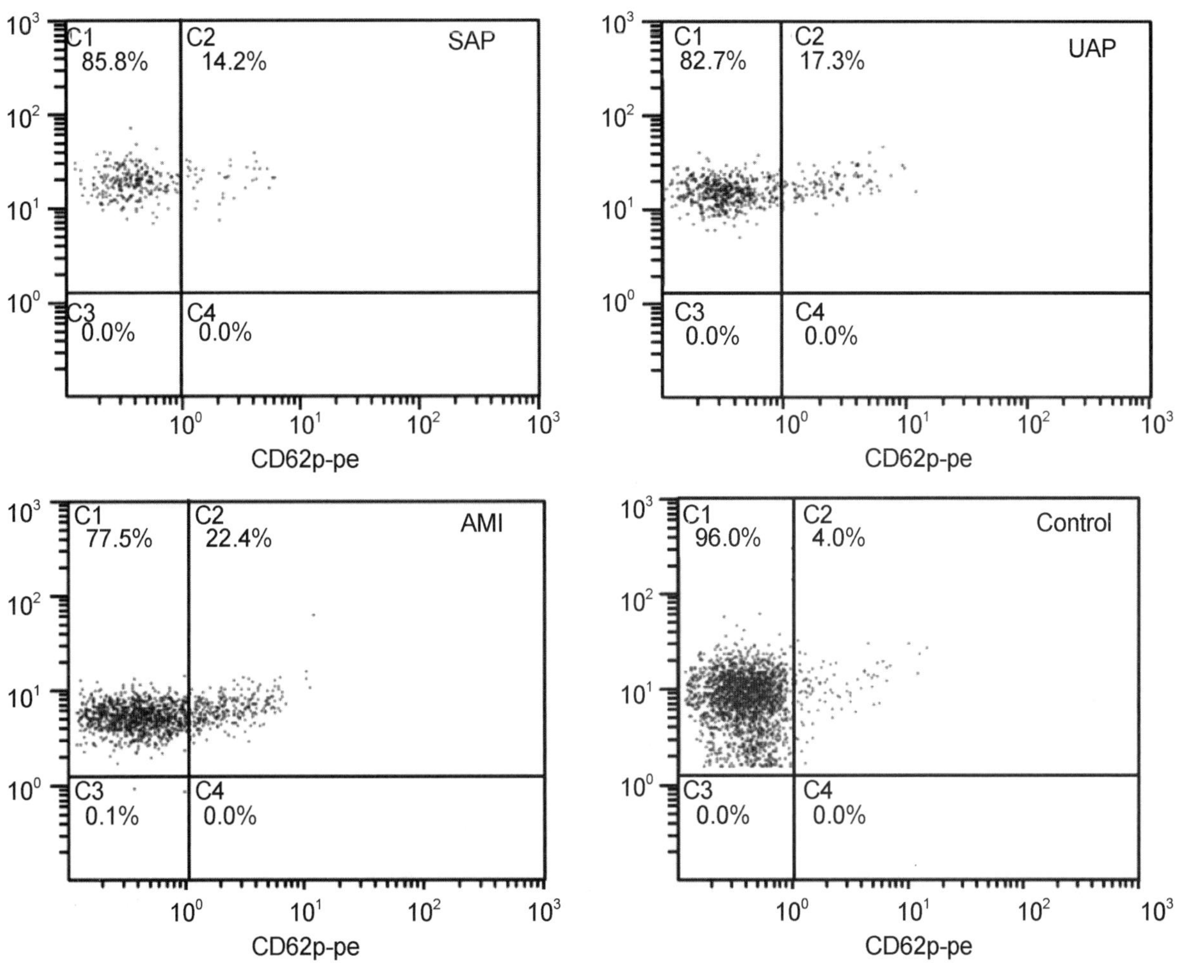

Figure 1 Comparison of CD62p of Platelet for CHD Patients among Different Groups (mean ± standard deviation)

Notes: SAP group, 12.97%±4.01%; UAP group, 18.62%±4.05%; AMI group, 20.54%±6.75%; Control group, 5.55% ±2.20%. **, $P < 0.01$, compared with the control group; ††, $P < 0.01$, compared with the SAP group.

4 Comparison of PAR for CHD Patients among Each Patient Group

Compared with healthy controls, the PAR of the three patient groups was markedly increased ($P < 0.01$). Compared with the SAP group, the PAR of the UAP and AMI groups was significantly increased ($P < 0.01$) again (Figure 3).

5 Comparison of F-actin and Gc-globulin Concentration for CHD Patients among Each Patient Group

Compared with healthy controls, the F-actin of the UAP and AMI groups was significantly increased ($P < 0.05$ and $P < 0.01$ respectively). The Gc-globulin of the three CHD groups was also significantly higher ($P < 0.01$). Compared with the SAP group, the F-actin of the AMI group was significantly increased ($P < 0.01$). However, the Gc-globulin of the other two groups was not statistically different ($P > 0.05$) (Figure 4).

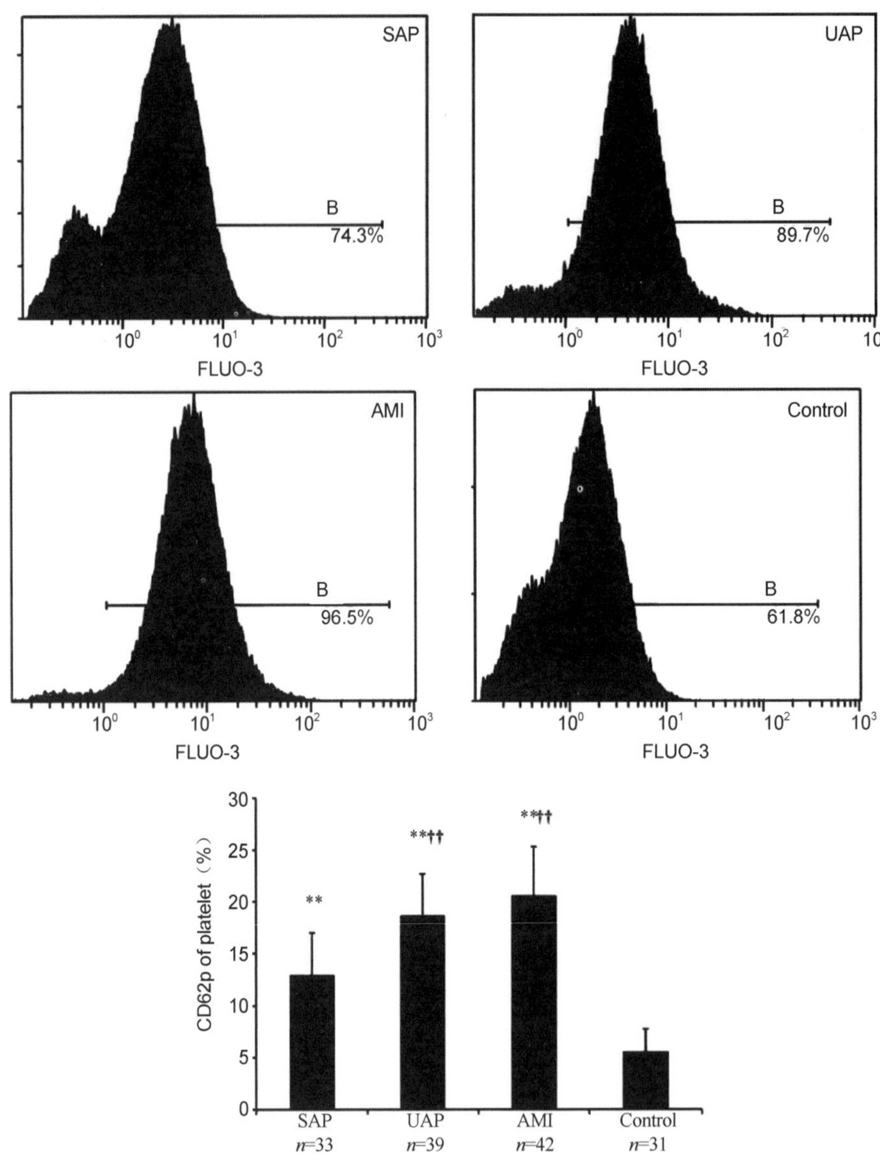

Figure 2　Comparison of $[Ca^{2+}]_i$ of Platelet for CHD Patients among Different Groups (mean ± standard deviation)

Notes: SAP group, 258.22±30.19 nmol/L；UAP group, 315.98±28.88 nmol/L；AMI group, 352.51±32.51 nmol/L；Control group, 109.62±9.84 nmol/L. **, $P < 0.01$, compared with the control group；††, $P < 0.01$, compared with the SAP group.

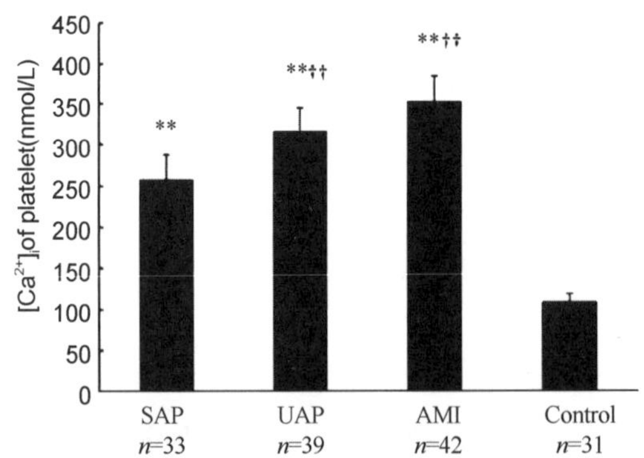

Figure 3　Comparison of Platelet Aggregation Rate (PAR)for CHD Patients among Different Groups (mean ± standard deviation).

Notes: SAP group, 30.18%±2.6%；UAP group, 39.07%±3.41%；AMI group, 64.29%±5.67%；Control group, 20%±2.93%. **, $P < 0.01$, compared with the control group；††, $P < 0.01$, compared with the SAP group.

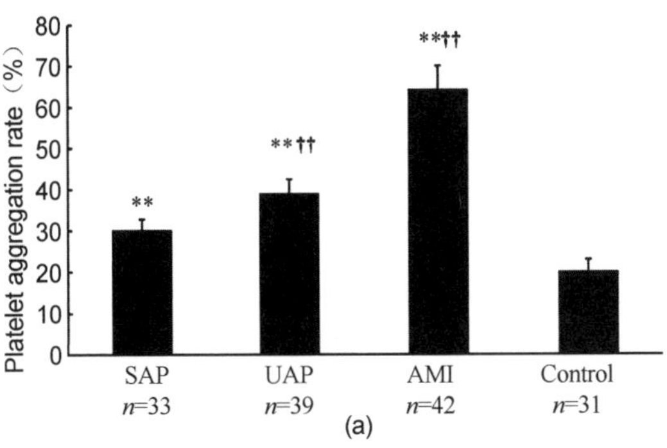

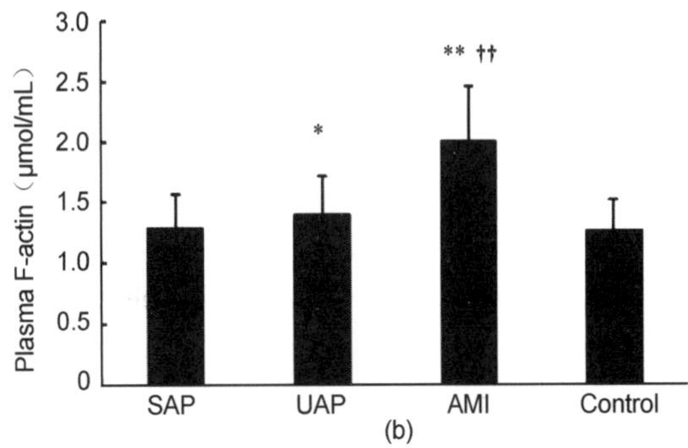

Figure 4 Comparison of F-actin and Gc-globulin Concentration for CHD Patients among Different Groups (mean ± standard deviation)

Notes: (a)Plasma F-actin concentration for CHD patients among different groups. SAP group, 1.29±0.29 mol/mL; UAP group, 1.41±0.31 mol/mL; AMI group, 2.01±0.46 mol/mL; CONTROL group, 1.27±0.25 mol/mL. (b)Plasma Gc-globulin concentration for CHD patients among different groups. SAP group, 220±26.78 g/mL; UAP group, 218.27±27.30 g/mL; AMI group, 224.49±32.73 g/mL; CONTROL group, 181.81±37.67 g/mL. $^{*}P < 0.05$, $^{**}P < 0.01$, compared with control group; ††, $P < 0.01$, compared with SAP group.

6 Analyses of Correlations between Platelet Gelsolin Concentration and CD62p or Plasma F-actin Levels among Each Patient Group

Next, we investigated any potential correlation between the platelet gelsolin concentration and CD62p or plasma F-actin levels that may exist between the SAP, UAP and AMI groups. Correlation analysis showed that platelet gelsolin concentrations were high positively correlated with CD62p or plasma F-actin levels in each of the three patient groups (Figure 5).

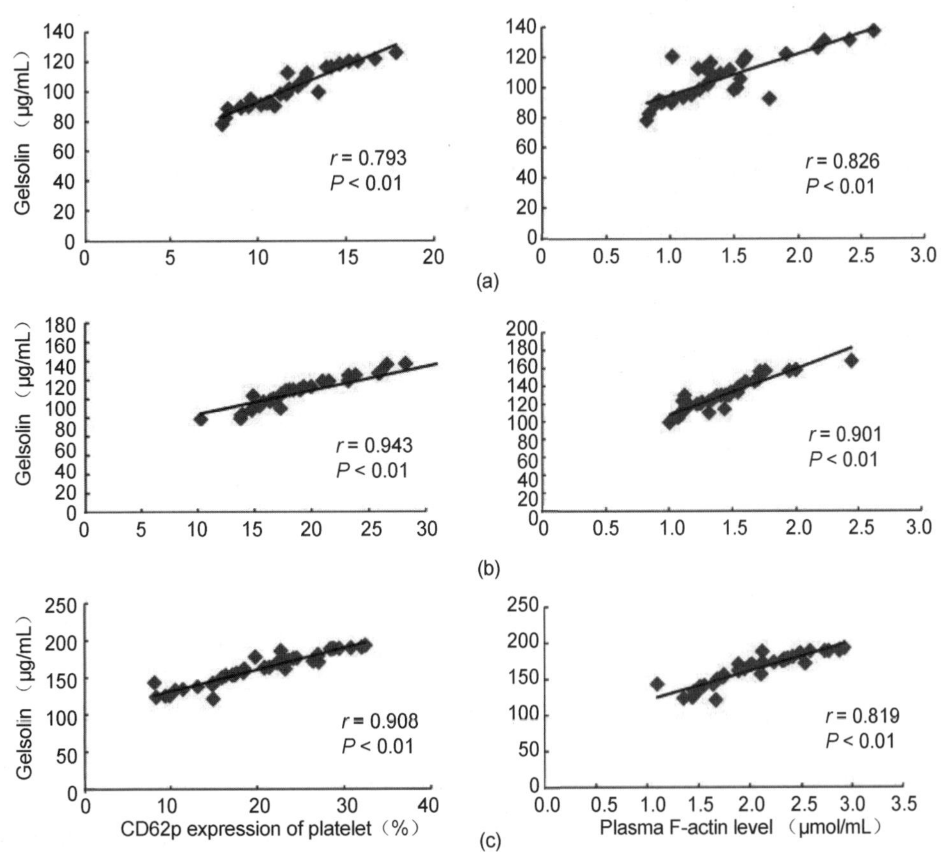

Figure 5 Analysis of Correlations between Platelet Gelsolin Concentration and CD62p or Plasma F-actin Level among Different Groups.

Notes: (a)SAP group (n=33); (b)UAP group (n=39); (c)AMI group (n=42).

DISCUSSION

CHD is a leading cause of death in many developed countries. It is increasingly clear that cardiovascular outcomes depend on an understanding of the biology of CHD, which may involve vascular inflammation, endothelial dysfunction, and plaque instability [8], among others. Activated platelets play a pivotal role in the formation of arterial thrombi [9]. CD62p (P-selection)is a 140 kD glycoprotein that is present in the granules of platelets and translocates rapidly to the cell surface after platelet activation, and is generally considered to be the gold marker of platelet activation [10, 11]. There is evidence that patients with various types of CHD, including stable [12] and unstable [13] angina and acute myocardial infarction [14] have increased CD62p levels. Among all types of CHD, symptomatic stable angina is a clinical expression of myocardial ischemia associated with fixed atherosclerotic coronary stenosis; however, patients with acute coronary syndrome (ACS)constitute the major proportion of persons who require admission to cardiac units for urgent care, including invasive treatment and aggregate anticoagulant and antiplaque drug therapy [15]. In this study, our results were consistent with these observations, indicating that varying degrees of platelet activation appear in all types of CHD and that ACS (including unstable angina and non-ST elevation MI)has a higher level of platelet activation and PAR compared with that of stable angina. These findings suggest an important role for CD62p in the arterial thrombosis of ACS.

Platelet activation not only causes membrane protein change, but also a series of morphological changes, from inviscid, discotic circulating platelets into a paste-like, protruding platelet jelly, that depends on the regulation of platelet cytoskeletal proteins.

Over the past ten years, laboratories have successfully applied proteomics technology to platelet research, contributing to the emerging field of platelet proteomics. Those studies led to the identification of a considerable number of novel platelet proteins, many of which have been studied further at a functional level [16]. Our previous study [2] had identified gelsolin as having the greatest difference in ex-pression levels between the platelets of CHD patients and healthy subjects. However, the role of platelet gelsolin in the development of CHD is unclear.

Gelsolin is a calcium-activated F-actin severing and capping protein found in many cell types and that is expressed as both cytoplasmic and plasma isoforms, and is an important cytoskeletal protein [17]. Two regulatory mechanisms are thought to modulate gelsolin activity *in vivo*. Calcium activates gelsolin to allow capping and severing of F-actin, while phosphatidylinositol-4, 5-bisphosphate (PIP_2)at the cell membrane keeps gelsolin sequestered in an inactive state. Upon hydrolysis of PIP_2, gelsolin is released into the cytoplasm and Ca^{2+} dependent activation can occur [18]. Previous work on gelsolin has mainly focused on the calcium regulated remodeling of F-actin, while more recent data has begun to elucidate the importance of gelsolin-mediated function in pathological conditions, including cardiovascular disease [19].

During tissue injury and cell death, actin is released into the circulation where it can interact with components of the haemostatic and fibrinolytic systems, or polymerize and form F-actin. *In vitro* studies [20] have suggested that F-actin can lead to platelet aggregation directly, and the presence of F-actin in blood vessels, which can plug smaller vessels and decrease blood flow to promote the formation of blood clots, can be fatal. Infusion of high doses of G-actin in rabbits caused the rapid and fatal formation of massive actin filament-containing thrombi in arterioles and capillaries of pulmonary veins, as well as endothelial injury [21]. An ac-tin scavenger system [22] is therefore likely to exist, plasma gelsolin, together with Gc-globulin, another extracellular actin-binding protein, were regarded as potentially important components of this system: capable of removing F-actin from the circulation and inhibiting F-actin elongation.

Our results were consistent with previous studies and showed that the gelsolin concentration of PPP decreased in SAP and ACS patients [23]. ACS is often associated with the rupture of vulnerable atherosclerotic plaques and coronary thrombus formation, leading to adverse outcomes. The results of this study clearly demonstrated that actin is re-leased into the bloodstream, leading to accumulation of F-actin at the higher level of platelet activation of ACS, and that circulating actin concentrations in excess of plasma gelsolin or Gc-globulin have prothrombotic or cytotoxic activities resulting in the severe depletion of plasma gelsolin. Gc-globulin (vitamin D binding protein)is a multifunctional protein [24]; its main physiological importance is probably the binding of actin, or binding and transportation of vita-min D analogous. Interestingly, in this study we observed that the plasma of CHD patients contains greater amounts of Gc-globulin compared with healthy subjects. Previous studies[25] demonstrated that three vitamin D binding protein isotypes were increased in asprin-resistant CHD patients and this could reduce the inhibitory effect of asprin on thromboxane A_2 production. Thus, this may suggest that the increased Gc-globulin level in this study may be associated with a large number of asprin-resistant patients included in our study or with increased reactively due to sudden severe depletion.

Another finding from our present study is the different levels of gelsolin in human platelet and plasma. Namely, an increase in platelet gelsolin levels, which was in agreement with our findings from a study of platelet proteomics [2], and a decrease in plasma gelsolin levels in ACS patients, compared to healthy subjects and stable angina patients. An analysis between platelet gelsolin concentrations and CD62p showed that platelet gelsolin levels have a high positive correlation with the level of platelet activation in ACS. Calcium ions not only promote gelsolin secretion but also play a vital role in the development of platelet activation. Studies have shown increased platelet $[Ca^{2+}]_i$ in patients with CHD [26], and that calcium chelators can reduce platelet $[Ca^{2+}]_i$ and inhibit platelet aggregation [27]. Our results showed an increased platelet $[Ca^{2+}]_i$ in ACS com-pared with healthy subjects and stable angina patients. The increased calcium influx in platelets could be one of the main mechanisms causing the abnormally increased platelet gelsolin levels observed in ACS.

Previous research has focused on gelsolin's possible role in cardiovascular diseases; several directions are currently being explored to test whether gelsolin itself can be used as a therapeutic molecule [28]. Our findings provide further insight into the important role of platelet gelsolin in the process of platelet activation in ACS. In this study, we have shown that platelet cytoskeletal proteins vary between different types of CHD, manifested mainly in gelsolin and F-actin. It is likely that plasma gelsolin clears away a great deal of F-actin released into circulation, and this is consistent with a role as an actin scavenger. At the onset of ACS, plasma gelsolin levels diminish significantly, while platelet gelsolin level increased abnormally, accompanied by an increased level of platelet activation and calcium in-flux. Platelet gelsolin levels are more highly correlated with ACS, compared to SAP. Therefore, does platelet gelsolin represent a novel therapeutic target of anti-platelet activation in ACS? We believe this is a significant area of further study, and it will be our research direction in the future.

REFERENCES

[1] Gergely F, Andrea F, Gabriella P, et al. Clinical importance of aspirin and clopidogrel resistance[J]. World J Cardiol, 2010, 2 (7): 171-186.

[2] Li X F, Jiang Y R, Wu C F, et al. Study on the correlation between platelet function proteins and symptom complex in coronary heart disease (in Chinese)[J]. Mol Cardiol China, 2009, 9: 326-331.

[3] Gibbons R J, Chatterjee K, Daley J, et al. ACC/AHA/ACP-ASIM guide-lines for the management of patients with chronic stable angina: A report of the American college of cardiology/American Heart Association task force on practice guidelines (committee on management of patients with chronic stable angina)[J]. J Am Coll Cardio, 1999, 34 (1): 2092-2197.

[4] Braunwald E, Antman E M, Kupersmith J W, et al. ACC/AHA 2002 guideline update for the management of patients with unstable angina and non-ST-segment elevation myocaridal infarction-summary article: A report of the American college of cardiology/American Heart Association task force on practice guidelines (committee on the management of patients with unstable angina)[J]. J Am Coll Cardio, 2002, 40: 1266-1374.

[5] World Medical Association declaration of Helsinki. Recommendations guiding physicians in biomedical research involving human subjects[J]. JAMA, 1997, 35 (1): 925-926.

[6] Zhuang M M, Wen Y X, Liu S L, et al. Determination of the level of cytopplasmic free calcium in human platelets with flow cytometry (in Chinese)[J]. J Xi'an Jiaotong Univ (Med Sci), 2005, 26 (2): 508-510.

[7] Grynkiewicz G, Poenie M, Tsien R Y. A new generation of Ca^{2+} indicators with greatly improved fluorescence properties[J]. J Biol Chem, 1985,

260 (6): 3440-3450.
[8] Libby P. Inflammation and cardiovascular disease mechanisms. Am J Clin Nutr, 2006, 83 (6): 456S-460S.
[9] Brydon L, Magid K, Steptoe A. Platelets, coronary heart disease, and stress[J]. Brain Behav Immun, 2006, 20 (2): 113-119.
[10] Hsu-Lin S, Berman C L, Furie B C, et al. A platelet membrane pro-tein expressed during platelet activation and secretion: Studies using a monoclonal antibody specific for thrombin-activated platelets[J]. J Biol Chem, 1984, 259 (14): 9121-9126.
[11] Michelson A D, Furman M I. Laboratory markers of platelet activation and their clinical significance[J]. Curr Opin Hematol, 1999, 6 (5): 342-348.
[12] Furman M I, Benoit S E, Barnard M R, et al. Increased platelet reactivity and circulating monocyte-platelet aggregates in patients with stable coronary artery disease[J]. J Am Coll Cardiol, 1998, 31 (2): 352-358.
[13] Ikeda H, Takajo Y, Ichiki K, et al. Increased soluble form of P-selectin in patients with unstable angina[J]. Circulation, 1995, 92 (7): 1693-1696.
[14] Shimomura H, Ogawa H, Arai H, et al. Serial changes in plasma levels of soluble P-selectin in patients with acute myocardial infarction[J]. Am J Cardiol, 1998, 81 (4): 397-400.
[15] Lichtman J H, Bigger J T Jr, Blumenthal J A, et al. Depression and coronary heart disease. Recommendations for screening, referral, and treatment: A science advisory from the American Heart Association Prevention Committee of the Council on Cardiovascular Nursing, Council on Clinical Cardiology, Council on Epidemiology and Pre-vention, and Interdisciplinary Council on Quality of Care and Out-comes Research. Endorsed by the American Psychiatric Association[J]. Circulation, 2008, 118 (7): 1768-1775.
[16] García A. Clinical proteomics in platelet research: Challenges ahead[J]. J Thromb Haemost, 2010, 8 (8): 1784-1785.
[17] Kwiatkowski D J, Stossel T P, Orkin S H, et al. Plasma and cytoplasmic gelsolins are encoded by a single gene and contain a duplicated actin-binding domain[J]. Nature, 1986, 323 (6087): 455-458.
[18] Allen, P G. Actin filament uncapping localizes to ruffling lamellae and rocketing vesicles[J]. Nat Cell Biol, 2003, 5 (11): 972-979.
[19] Liu Y, Jiang Y R, Yin H J, et al. Gelsolin and cardiovascular diseases (in Chinese)[J]. Mol Cardiol China, 2011, 11: 50-53.
[20] Vasconcellos C A, Lind S E. Coordinated inhibition of actin-induced platelet aggregation by plasma gelsolin and vitamin D-binding protein[J]. Blood, 1993, 58 (12): 3648-3657.
[21] Haddad J G, Harper K D, Guoth M, et al. Angiopathic consequences of saturating the plasma scavenger system for actin[J]. Proc Natl Acad Sci USA, 1990, 87 (4): 1381-1385.
[22] Lee W M, Galbraith R M. The extracellular actin-scavenger system and actin toxicity[J]. N Engl J Med, 1992, 326 (20): 1335-1341.
[23] Suhler E, Lin W, Yin H L. Decreased plasma gelsolin concentrations in acute liver failure, myocardial infarction, septic shock and myonecrosis[J]. Crit Care Med, 1997, 25 (4): 594-598.
[24] White P, Cooke N. The multifunctional properties and characteristics of vitamin D-binding protein[J]. Trends Endocrinol Metabol, 2000, 11 (8): 320-327.
[25] López-Farré A J, Mateos-Cáceres P J, Sacristán D, et al. Relationship between vitamin D binding protein and aspirin resistance in coronary ischemic patients: A proteomic study[J]. J Proteome Res, 2007, 6 (7): 2481-2487.
[26] Kato M, Kambe M, Kajiyama G. Increased cytosolic free Mg^{2+} and Ca^{2+} in platelets of patients with vasospastic[J]. Am J Physiol, 1998, 274 (2): 548-554.
[27] Fujinishi A, Takahara K, Ohba C, et al. Effects of nisoldipine on cytosolic calcium, platelet aggregation, and coagulation/fibrinolysis in patients with coronary artery disease[J]. Angiology, 1997, 48 (6): 515-521.
[28] Li G H, Shi Y, Chen Y, et al. Gelsolin regulates cardiac remodeling after myocardial infarction through DNase I-mediated apoptosis[J]. Circ Res, 2009, 104 (7): 896-904.

First published: LIU Yue, YIN Hui-jun, JIANG Yue-rong, XUE Mei, CHEN Ke-ji. Correlation between platelet gelsolin levels and different types of coronary heart disease[J]. Chin Sci Bull, 2012, 57 (6): 631-638

Effect of Chinese Herbal Drug-Containing Serum for Activating-Blood and Dispelling-Toxin on ox-LDL-Induced Inflammatory Factors' Expression in Endothelial Cells

JIANG Yue-rong, MIAO Yu, YANG Lin, XUE Mei, GUO Chun-yu, MA Xiao-juan,
YIN Hui-jun, SHI Da-zhuo, and CHEN Ke-ji

Atherosclerosis (AS)is a kind of inflammation injured disease. It has been shown by many researches that the oxidized low-density lipoprotein (ox-LDL)plays an important role in the pathologic process of AS and could activate the vascular endothelial cells to enhance expressions of multiple adhesive factors and cytokines in cells. Our research group has worked in recent years to recognize AS from pathogenetic angle of "stasis-toxin" and discovered that Chinese drugs for activating blood and dispelling toxin are more effective than those for activating-blood to resolve stasis singly in attenuating and stabilizing AS plaque. [1-3]This study was designed to explain the relationship of the two pathogens (stasis and toxin)from cell injury and inflammation response aspects by comparing the difference of acting links and targets between the two kinds of Chinese drugs in ox-LDL injured endothelial model cells through observing the physio-pathologic changes that occurred after endothelial injury in expressions and releasing of factors related to tissue damage and inflammation response.

METHODS

1 Experimental Animal

Wistar rats, weighing 200 ± 20 g, SPF grade, supplied by the Institute of Experimental Animal, Chinese Academy of Medical Sciences, certification No. SCXK (Jing)20050013.

2 Testing Drugs

Xiongshao Capsule (芎芍胶囊, XS), 0.25 g/ capsule, containing drug's markers of paeoniflorin 28 mg, ferulic acid 3.5 mg, and total phenolic acid 34 mg, was provided by Dalian Institute of Physics and Chemistry, China, batch No. 070929.

Huanglian Capsule (黄连胶囊, HL), 0.25 g/capsule, product of Hubei Xianglian Pharmaceutical Co., Ltd., China, batch No. 070502, certification No. Z19983042.

3 Reagents

DMEM culture medium (high-sugar type)and top-grade fetal bovine serum were purchased from Hyclone Co. Epidermal growth factor (EGF), pancreatin, collagenase Ⅰ, L-glutamine, gelatin, HEPES, EDTA, and sodium pyruvate were products of Sigma Co., USA. Penicillin, streptomycin, heparin, and short-acting insulin injection were made in China, analytic pure. Ox-LDL was purchased from the Biochemical Department of Basic Medical Institute, Chinese Academy of Medical Sciences, which showed single protein strip in agarose gel electrophoresis. Kits for enzyme immunoassay testing human interleukin-6 (IL-6), tumor necrosis factor-α (TNF-α), and soluble intercellular adhesion molecule-1 (sICAM-1)were products of R&D Co., sub-packed in China. Healthy human umbilical cord was from Hospital for Mother and Child Health Care of Haidian District, Beijing, China. CD54-FITC antibodies (IgG2α, κ, MEM-111), CD62E-PEantibodies (mouse IgG 2α, κ, Clone

HCD62E), and their homotype controls were purchased from BioLegend Co., USA.

4 Experimental Instruments

Flow cytometer, EPICS Elite, product of Beckman Coulter Co., USA；automatic enzyme-labeled detector, Wellscan type MK3, product of Labsystems Dragon Co., Finland.

5 Drug-Containing Serum Preparation

Thirty-two Wistar rats were divided into four groups equally: the blank group treated with distilled water, the positive control group treated with simvastatin (1.8 mg/kg), the test group Ⅰ treated with Chinese herbal compound for activating blood (XS 0.135 g/kg), and the test group Ⅱ treated with Chinese herbal compound for both activating blood and dispelling toxin (XS 0.135 g/kg and HL 0.135 g/kg). All treatments were administered once a day for 7 successive days by gastric infusion. Blood of rats was collected 1 h after final administration from abdominal aorta under sterilization, kept unchanged for 1 h, and centrifuged at 3 000r/min for 15 min to separate the drug-serum. The drug-sera from rats of the same groups were mixed, subjected o56 ℃ water bath for 30 min to inactivate, filtrated with microporous membrane to eliminate germs, sub-packaged in tubes, and preserved under –70 ℃until ready for testing.

6 Isolation, Cultivation, and Identification of Human Umbilical Vein Endothelial Cells

Referring to Jaffe's method[4] with a little modification, human umbilical cords of newborn collected in aseptic condition from healthy puerperal were processed by collagenase digestive method to separate cells. Human umbilical vein endothelial cells (HUVECs)were cultured with DMEM culture medium containing 20% fetal bovine serum, 10 ng/mL EGF, 40 μU/mL insulin, 40 U/mL heparin, 2 mmol/L glutamine, 50 U/mL penicillin, 50 μg/mL streptomycin, and 1 mmol/L sodium pyruvate. Cells of the third generation were taken for experiment after identification by factor Ⅷ immunochemical test and morphological observation with an inverted phase-contrast microscopy.

7 Cell Grouping and Treatment

HUVECs were divided into five groups: the blank control group, the model group, the positive control group, the test group Ⅰ, and the test group Ⅱ. Cells of each group (1×10^{8}/L)were inoculated in 30 mm culture disc separately, and when grown to confluence condition, they were treated as follows: except those in the blank control group, HUVECs were made into injured model cells by adding ox-LDL of inducing dosage (final concentration of 100 μg/mL, which had been determined in advance)to culture medium. At the same time, 10% drug-serum from corresponding groups of rats was added to the medium of the latter three groups, respectively, while serum from rats of the blank control group was added in medium of the first two groups. Cells werethenincubatedinanincubatorfor24 h.

8 Items and Methods of Detection

Levels of IL-6, TNF-α, and sICAM in the supernatant from centrifugation were detected by enzyme-linked immunosorbent assay (ELISA).

The expressions of ICAM-1 and E-selectin on HUVECs' surface were detected using flow cytometry adopting the following procedures: cells were collected, digested with pancreatin, and washed with PBS to prepare single-cell suspension of 1×10^{6}/mL in concentration. Each sample was divided into two tubes. The corresponding monoclonal antibodies of CD54-FITC and CD62E-PE were added into the first tube, while the corresponding isotype control of mouse IgG2α-FITC and mouse IgG2α-PE were added in the second tube and then were mixed sufficiently, incubated for 30 min at room temperature light protectively, and washed with PBS. The supernatant was discarded, and cells were put in a flow cytometer to detect the respective index by multi-color analysis, adopting FS/SS gate method to sort cells, and the percentage of positive expressed cells was calculated by EXPO32software.

9 Statistical Analysis

Data were expressed by mean ± standard deviation ($\bar{x} \pm s$), managed by software SPSS 13.0. The comparison among multiple groups was managed by single-factor variance analysis, and the paired comparison between groups was managed by *LSD* test.

RESULTS

1 Effects on Levels of IL-6, TNF-α, and sICAM-1 in the Supernatant

Compared with the blank control group, levels of IL-6, TNF-α, and sICAM-1 in the supernatant of the model group were significantly higher ($P < 0.01$), while these abnormal changes, except sICAM level in test group Ⅰ, could be reversed in the three treated groups (positive control, test Ⅰ, and test Ⅱ)significantly, showing statistical differences ($P < 0.01$ or $P < 0.05$). As for comparisons of effects between the two test groups, nosignificantdifferenceonIL-6andTNF-α was found, although the decrease in the test group Ⅱ seemed more significant (Table1).

Table 1 Effects on Levels of IL–6, TNF–α, and sICAM–1 in the Supernatant of HUVEC Culture (pg/ml, $\bar{x} \pm s$, n=8)

Group	IL-6	TNF-α	sICAM-1
Blank	63.38 ± 19.70	82.70 ± 27.14	819.60 ± 75.45
Model	128.18 ± 14.01 **	168.83 ± 18.68 **	1323.75 ± 286.12 **
Test Ⅰ	93.06 ± 28.93 **△△	121.13 ± 38.63 **△△	1144.13 ± 252.65 **
Test Ⅱ	89.80 ± 9.71△△	116.67 ± 12.89 *△△	1003.64 ± 180.37△△
Positive control	88.48 ± 24.97△△	115.67 ± 33.77 *△△	1023.23 ± 175.39△

Notes: * $P < 0.05$, ** $P < 0.01$, compared with the blank control group ; △ $P < 0.05$, △△ $P < 0.01$, compared with the model group.

2 Effect on the Cell Surface Positive Expression Rates of ICAM-1 and E-selectin

Compared with the blank control group, levels of cell surface ICAM-1 (CD54)and E-selectin (CD62E) expression increased significantly in the model group ($P < 0.01$)and were lower in the three treated groups than those in the model group, respectively, showing significant differences ($P < 0.05$). However, insignificant differences among the three groups were found (Table 2).

Table 2 Effects on Cell Surface Positive Expression Rates of CD54 and CD62E (% , $\bar{x} \pm s$, n=3)

Group	CD54 positive rate	CD62E positive rate
Blank	56.27 ± 20.43	18.70 ± 13.66
Model	96.13 ± 1.34**	43.97 ± 12.33**
Test Ⅰ	79.00 ± 8.88*	25.73 ± 9.37△
Test Ⅱ	76.37 ± 10.30△	21.93 ± 3.12△
Positive control	74.73 ± 10.31△	25.93 ± 4.79△

Notes: * $P < 0.05$, ** $P < 0.01$, compared with the blank control group ; △ $P < 0.05$, compared with the model group.

DISCUSSION

AS is a disease manifested mainly by vascular inflammation response, and its pathogenesis involves many factors. Abnormal blood lipid metabolism-induced hyperlipidemia and lipo-peroxidation are the crucial factors for AS genesis and development process. Among them, the effect of ox-LDL in promoting the inflammation response of AS has been assured by many researchers; [5] it could injure vascular endothelium through multiple paths, including advancing the production of inflammation factors and adhesive molecules. The pathogenetic initiating step of AS is the adhesion of monocytes on vascular endothelium, which could be promoted by the adhesive molecules, such as ICAM-1 (CD54), VCAM-1, and E-selectin.

Being a cellular constituent-type expressed adhesive molecule, ICAM-1 plays central actions in the process of leukocyte recruitment to endothelium, [6] and it could mediate adherence and spillage of various types of leukocyte toward endothelium. [7]E-selectin (CD62E)is a functional cell membranous adhesive molecule that belongs to the selectin family, and it is expressed in the very early stage of inflammation course but is limited in the vascular endothelium only.

The adhesive molecules-mediated leukocyte adhesion could enhance the instability of AS plaques and attenuate their fibrous cap, thus accelerate the breakage of plaque and the formation of thrombus, which is manifested in clinics as instable angina and myocardial infarction. [8, 9]

Considering the Chinese medicine (CM)recognition of "stasis and toxin" and combining with the relevant modern medical ideals, our research group suggested that most of the pathologic damages, such as tissue-injured necrosis caused by breakage of AS plaque and thrombosis obstruction, inflammatory cascade reaction, oxidized lipid deposition, calcium overload, and cell apoptosis, are similar to that of CM evil pathogens (stasis and toxin)in specialties such as acute initiation, rapid transmitting and changing, direct attack to internal organs, and great damage to tissues. [1, 8] Therefore, a full-scale Chinese medical explanation on genetic specialty and pathogenesis of vascular thrombotic cardio-cerebral diseases could be made by combining the two pathogens. Many small-sample clinical observations have illustrated the reliable clinical effectiveness of Chinese drugs for clearing heat and dispelling-toxin in preventing and treating instable angina and apoplexy, [9] and a study regarding the intervening effect of Chinese drugs on AS instable plaque in apolipoprotein E gene defect mice has proven that the effect of drugs for activating blood and dispelling toxin is superior to those simply for activating blood to remove stasis, [2] which indicated from an experimental aspect the important role of "toxin" in the pathogenesis of arterial thrombotic diseases.

XS is composed of the effective ingredients of Chinese herbal medicines, total phenols of *Radix Paeoniae rubra*, and total glycosides of Radix Chuanxiong. It was shown by a previous study as being effective as anti-AS. This study was designed to compare the effectiveness of drug-serum of XS+HL (drugs for both activating blood and dispelling toxin)to that of XS alone (drugs for activating blood only)on ox-LDL-stimulated HUVECs. The results showed that ox-LDL stimulation could significantly raise the levels of IL-6, TNF-α, and sICAM in the culture supernatant as well as the expressions of ICAM-1 and E-selectin in cell surface, and these abnormally heightened indices, except sICAM level in the test group Ⅰ, could be reduced to some extent by the test drug-sera, with the effect similar to that of simvastatin (the positive control), suggesting that the combination of XS+HL has definite inhibitory actions on the vascular endothelial inflammation response injured by ox-LDL. However, its concrete mechanism awaits further studies.

REFERENCES

[1] Shi DZ, Xu H, Yin HJ, et al. Combination and transformation of toxin and blood stasis in etiopathogenesis of thrombotic cerebrocardiovascular diseases[J]. J Chin Integr Med (Chin), 2008, 6: 1105-1108.

[2] Wen C, Xu H, Huang QF, et al. Effect of drugs for promoting blood circulation on blood lipids and inflammatory reaction of atherosclerotic plaques in apoE gene deficiency mice[J]. Chin J Integr Tradit West Med (Chin), 2005, 25: 345.

[3] Zhang JC, Chen KJ, Zheng GJ, et al. Regulatory effect of Chinese herbal compound for detoxifying and activating blood circulation on expression of NF-κB and MMP-9 in aorta of apolipoprotein E gene knocked-out mice[J]. Chin J Integr Tradit West Med (Chin), 2007, 27: 40-44.

[4] Jiang YR, Chen KJ, Xu YG, et al. Effects of Propyl Gallate on adhesion of polymorphonuclear leukocytes to human endothelial cells induced by tumor necrosis factor alpha[J]. Chin J Integr Med, 2009, 15: 47-53.

[5] Ou HC, Lee WJ, Lee IT, et al. Ginkgo biloba extract attenuates oxLDL-induced oxidative functional damages in endothelial cells[J]. J Appl Physiol, 2009, 106: 1674-1685.

[6] Landsberger M, Wolff B, Jantzen F, Rosenstengel C, Vogelgesang D, Staudt A, et al. Cerivastatin reduces cytokine-induced surface expression of ICAM-1 via increased shedding in human endothelial cells[J]. Atherosclerosis, 2007, 190: 43-52.

[7] Xenos ES, Stevens SL, Freeman MB, et al. Nitric oxide mediates the effect of fluvastatin onintercellularadhesionmolecule-1andplateletendothelial cell adhesion molecule-1 expression on human endothelial cells[J]. Ann Vasc Surg, 2005, 19: 386-392.

[8] Hopkins AM, Baird AW, NusratA. ICAM-1: targeted docking for exogenous as well as endogenous ligands[J]. Adv Drug Deliv Rev, 2004, 56: 763-778.

[9] Kaski JC, Fernández-Bergés DJ, et al. A comparative study of biomarkers for risk prediction in acute coronary syndrome—results of the SIESTA (Systemic Inflammation Evaluation in non-ST-elevation Acute coronary syndrome)study[J]. Atherosclerosis, 2010, 212: 636-643.

[10] Zhang JC, Chen KJ. Theoretical thinking on relationship between toxic-stasis pathogenicity and atherosclerotic vulnerable plaque[J]. Chin J Integr Tradit Westn Med (Chin), 2008, 28: 366-368.

[11] Lu XH, Ding SW. Clinical effect and mechanism on treating unstable angina pectoris by Huanglian Jiedu Capsule[J]. J Shandong Univ Tradit Chin Med (Chin), 2005, 29: 457-460.

First published: JIANG Yue-rong, MIAO Yu, YANG Lin, XUE Mei, GUO Chun-yu, MA Xiao-juan, YIN Hui-jun, SHI Da-zhuo, and CHEN Ke-ji. Effect of Chinese herbal drug-containing serum for activating-blood and dispelling-toxin on ox-LDL-induced inflammatory factors' expression in endothelial cells[J]. Chin J Integr Med, 2012, 18 (1): 30-33.

Research on the Correlation between Platelet Gelsolin and Blood-Stasis Syndrome of Coronary Heart Disease

LIU Yue, YIN Hui-jun, and CHEN Ke-ji

Atherothrombosis, which directly threatens the public health, is the main cause of morbidity and mortality throughout the world. The underlying mechanism of atherogenesis has generated a lot of research interest. Platelets play a key role in the development of acute coronary syndromes (ACS)and contribute to cardiovascular events. They participate in the process of forming and extending atherosclerotic plaques. [1,2] The activation of platelets may be the critical process of atherothrombosis which is the key point in basic and clinical research of cardiovascular diseases in recent years. Over the last decade, proteomics technology has been successfully applied to platelet research, contributing to the emerging field of platelet proteomics. Those studies led to the identification of a considerable amount of novel platelet proteins, many of which have been further studied at the functional level[3] During the last 3 years a combination of two-dimensional gel electrophoresis and mass spectrometry-based proteomic approaches has been used to profile alterations in platelet proteins. [4-6]

Our previous data demonstrate that coronary heart diseases (CHD), blood-stasis syndrome and platelet activation are closely related. [7, 8] We also studied the correlation between blood stasis syndrome (BSS)/non-BSS and platelet function proteins in CHD by the differential proteomics of platelets and found that gelsolin is the main differential protein of platelets between them, [9] which indicates that the cytoskeleton of platelets may play an important role in the development of BSS in CHD. Based on the above results, this study further addresses the distribution of gelsolin in human platelet and plasma, and the correlation with BSS in CHD, to verify the role of platelet gelsolin in theformation of BSS in CHD.

METHODS

1 Diagnostic Criteria

The diagnoses of the patients were according to criteria of the "Nomenclature and Diagnosis of Ischemic Heart Diseases" reported by the united special group for standardization of clinical nomenclature of the World Health Organization. [10] The patients selected were those having symptoms of angina or/and objective evidence of myocardial ischemia and those with at least one marked coronary stenosis (>50%) shown by coronary arteriography examination. BSS typing was made based on the standard diagnostic criteria established by the Special Committee of Promoting Blood Circulation and Removing Blood Stasis, Chinese Association of Integrative Medicine[11] Those enrolled must be diagnosed blindly and consistently by three Chinese medicine (CM)doctors.

2 Inclusion and Exclusion Criteria

The patients included were required to fit all the following criteria: diagnosed with ischemic heart diseases of any CM syndrome type; having symptoms of angina pectoris and/or objective evidence of myocardial ischemia; latest coronary arteriography examination showing significant stenosis (>50%); age between 35 and 75 years.

The patients were excluded with any one of the following conditions: severe valvulopathy; type 1 diabetes mellitus; complicated with severe primary diseases of the liver, kidney, hemopoietic system, and malignant tumors; medication history of calcium channel blockers in the last 2 weeks; refusing to sign the informed consent or being estimated as with poor compliance; participating in other clinical trials; women in pregnancy or lactation stage.

3 General Clinical Materials

All CHD patients enrolled were the inpatients of Beijing Anzhen Hospital, Capital Medical University, from August 2010 to December 2010, who were diagnosed and assigned to the BSS group (30 cases)and the non-BSS group (30 cases). The subjects recruited as the healthy control group (30 cases)were persons who had been identified as healthy by examination of history, physique, blood routine, hepatic function, chest film, and electrocardiogram (ECG), etc., not taking drugs affecting atherosclerotic or thrombotic processes in the last 2 weeks, with those having mental or significant physical diseases as well as familial or self psychiatric history excluded. The study is in accord with the Helsinki Declaration, with no contravention to the medical ethics.

There was no statistical difference among the 3 groups in age, sex, and platelet count ($P>0.05$). The risk factors (smoking, hypertension, dyslipidemia, and diabetes history), different branches of affected coronary artery, and medication history (statins and aspirin)were comparable between BSS of CHD group and non-BSS of CHD group ($P>0.05$, Table 1).

4 Blood Preparation

Fresh blood (12 mL)was drawn from an antecubital vein and collected into vacutainer tubes containing acid-citrate-dextrose (ACD)9% v/v as anticoagulant, and the initial 2 mL of blood was discarded to avoid spontaneous platelet activation. The blood of the patients was collected before the antithrombotic therapy and angiography examination. The blood was centrifuged for 10 min at 900r/min (150 × g)at room temperature to obtain platelet-rich plasma (PRP)and the rest of the blood were centrifuged for 20 min at 3 000r/min (800 × g) to obtain poor-platelet plasma (PPP).

Table 1 Clinical Features of the Studied Groups

Parameter	CHD patients		Healthy control group (30 cases)
	BSS group (30 cases)	Non-BSS group (30 cases)	
Age (Year, $\bar{x} \pm s$)	53.0 ± 7.5	52.0 ± 8.5	49.5 ± 9.0
Male/female (Case)	21/9	23/7	22/8
Risk factor [Case (%)]			
Hypertension	18 (60.0)	17 (56.7)	0
Dyslipidemia	17 (56.7)	15 (50.0)	0
Diabetes	6 (20.0)	7 (23.3)	0
Current smoker	19 (63.3)	20 (66.7)	0
Medication [Case (%)]			
Aspirin	23 (76.7)	25 (83.3)	0
Statins	8 (26.7)	10 (33.3)	0
Single-vessel disease [Case (%)]	11 (36.7)	12 (40.0)	0
Multi-vessel disease [Case (%)]	19 (63.3)	18 (60.0)	0
Platelet count ($\times 10^3$/μL)	210 ± 45.8	207 ± 47.3	208.9 ± 39.1

5 Determination of CD62p Expression of Platelet

The level of the platelet activation represented by the fluorescent intensity of platelet glycoprotein CD62p was determined by flow cytometry (FCM). The blood was mixed evenly and the following procedures were finished within 4 h. The control and test tubes contained 50 μL of the blood sample, then had homotype control CD61-FITC/CD62p-PE (CD61-FITC, Anti-GP Ⅲ a, Cat: 348093, Lot: 49817, Becton Dickinson Co., USA; CD62P-PE, Anti-GMP-140, Cat: 348107, Lot: 60928, Becton Dickinson Co., USA)added into them respectively, 20 μL in each tube. Then the samples were mixed evenly by light shaking, and incubated in darkness at room temperature for 20 min. One milliliter of cold (2-8 ℃)fixative liquid was added into each tube, mixed well and incubated again in darkness under 2-8 ℃ for 30 min; then the samples were put into the analyzer to measure the mean fluorescence intensity (MFI)of CD62p using multi-parameter and multi-color fluorescent FCM (EPICS Elite, Beckman Coulter Co., USA)and standard fluorescent micro-balloon was adopted to correct the beam path and stream. The test data were obtained by FS vs. SS gate, Expo32 special software.

6 Determination of Cytoplasmic Calcium of Platelet

PRP was prepared and incubated with 4 μmol Fura-3/AM at 37 ℃ for 40 min, the mean fluorescence intensity (F)of $Ca^{2+}$of platelet was determined using FCM as previously described, [12] and the Ca^{2+} level of platelet (μmol/L)is calculated as follows: cytoplasmic calcium ($[Ca^{2+}]_i$)= Kd × (F-Fmin)/ (Fmax-F). [13]

7 Determination of Gelsolin, Filamentous Actin and Group-Specific Component Globulin

The plasma concentration (PRP and PPP)of gelsolin (Cat: E0372h, R&D Co., USA), filamentrus actin (F-actin, Cat: E1876h, R&D Co., USA)and group-specific component (Gc-globulin, Cat: E1910h, R&D Co., USA)were determined by double-antibody sandwich avidin-biotin peroxidase complex enzyme-linked immunosorbent assay (ABC-ELISA), following the instruction of the ELISA-kit respectively.

8 Statistical Analysis

Statistical analysis was performed by SPSS 13.0 software. Chi-square or rank sum test was used to evaluate enumeration data. For measurement data, t-test or variance analysis was used. A P-value of < 0.05 was considered statistically significant.

RESULTS

1 Comparison of Plasma Gelsolin Concentration of CHD Patients among Different Groups

Compared with the control group, the gelsolin concentration in PRP of BSS group increased significantly ($P < 0.01$), while that in PPP of BSS and non-BSS group decreased markedly ($P < 0.05$). Compared with the non-BSS group, the gelsolin concentration in PRP of BSS group increased significantly ($P < 0.01$, Table 2).

Table 2 Comparison of Plasma Gelsolin Concentrations among Different Groups (μg/mL, $\bar{x} \pm s$)

Group	Case	Gelsolin in PRP	Gelsolin in PPP
BSS	30	$155.47 \pm 25.46^{**\triangle}$	$116.04 \pm 9.80^{*}$
Non-BSS	30	118.75 ± 26.48	$115.50 \pm 14.71^{*}$
Control	30	117.48 ± 10.08	121.45 ± 6.89

Notes: $^{*}P < 0.05$, $^{**}P < 0.01$, compared with the control group ; $^{\triangle}P < 0.01$, compared with the non-BSS group.

2 Comparison of CD62p and $[Ca^{2+}]_i$ of Platelet for CHD Patients among Different Groups

Compared with the control group, the CD62p and $[Ca^{2+}]_i$ of platelets of the BSS group and non-BSS group increased significantly ($P < 0.01$). Compared with the non-BSS group, $[Ca^{2+}]_i$ of platelets of the BSS group increased markedly ($P < 0.01$, Table 3 and Figure 1).

Table 3 Comparison of CD62p and $[Ca^{2+}]$ of Platelet for CHD Patients among Different Groups ($\bar{x} \pm s$)

Group	Case	CD62p (%)	$[Ca^{2+}]$ of Platelet (nmol/L)
BSS	30	$19.68 \pm 8.61^{*}$	$366.87 \pm 23.34^{*\triangle}$
Non-BSS	30	$17.68 \pm 7.54^{*}$	$286.49 \pm 41.99^{*}$
Control	30	5.56 ± 2.24	109.39 ± 9.92

Notes: $^{*}P < 0.01$, compared with the control group ; $^{\triangle}P < 0.01$, compared with the non-BSS group.

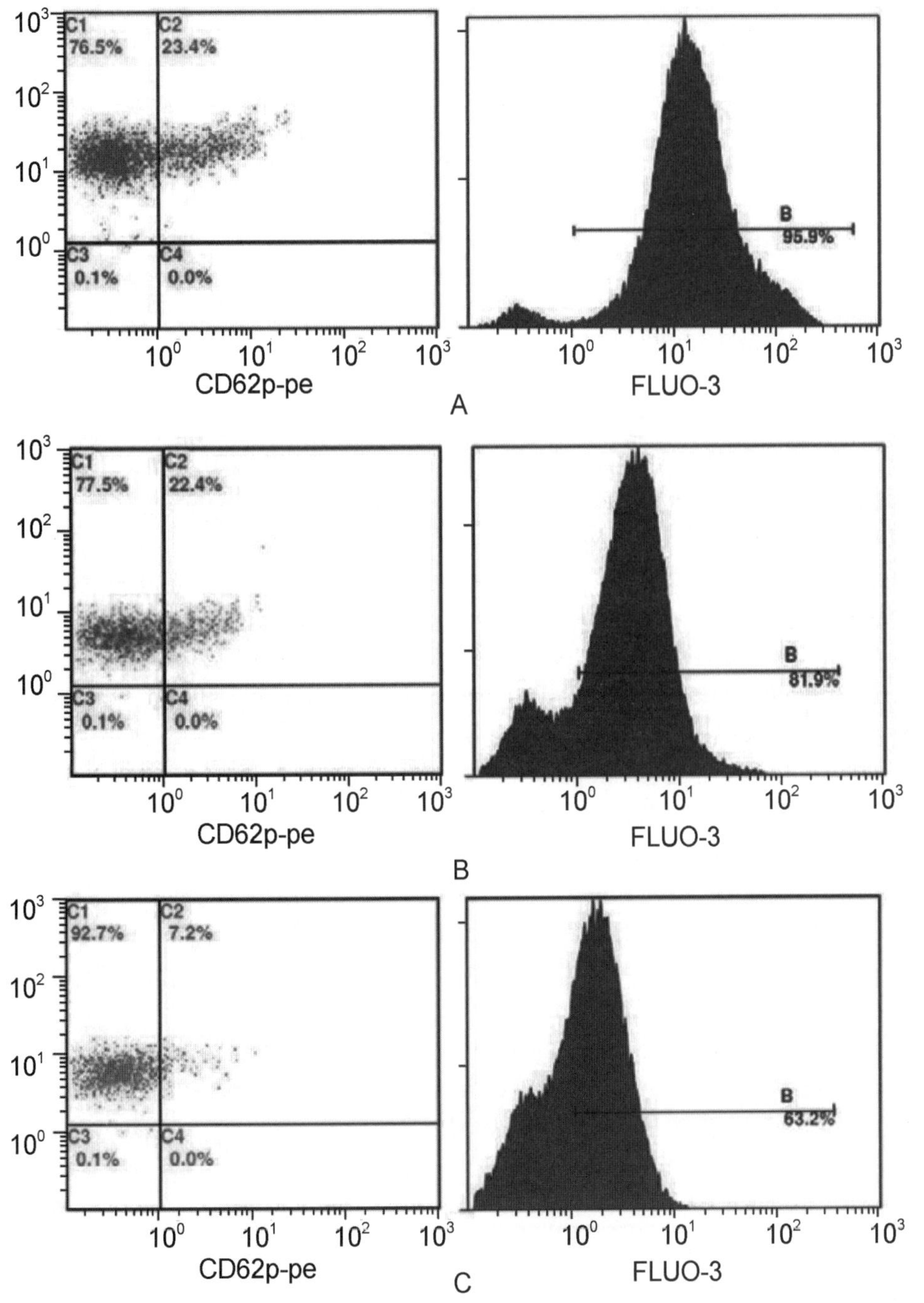

Figure 1 Flow Cytometry Analysis of CD62p-PE and $[Ca^{2+}]_i$ of Platelet

Notes: A: a CHD patient with BSS, B: a CHD patient with non-BSS, C: a healthy control subject.

3 Comparison of F-actin and Gc-globulin Concentrations for CHD Patients among Different Groups

Compared with the control group, the F-actin and Gc-globulin of BSS and non-BSS groups increased significantly ($P < 0.01$). Compared with non-BSS of CHD group, F-actin and Gc-globulin of BSS group have no statistical difference ($P > 0.05$, Table 4).

Table 4 Comparison of F–actin and Gc–globulin Concentrations for CHD Patients among Different Groups (μmol/L, $\bar{x} \pm s$)

Group	Case	F-actin	Gc-globulin
BSS	30	$19.68 \pm 8.61^{*}$	$366.87 \pm 23.34^{*\triangle}$
Non-BSS	30	$17.68 \pm 7.54^{*}$	$286.49 \pm 41.99^{*}$
Control	30	5.56 ± 2.24	109.39 ± 9.92

Notes: $^{*}P < 0.01$, compared with the control group.

DISCUSSION

CHD is the leading cause of death throughout the world, and its development is associated with many pathogenic factors. A common feature of CHD is coronary artery occlusion, whether permanent or intermittent, as a result of the rupture of vulnerable plaque and subsequent thrombosis. Activated platelets play a pivotal role in the formation of arterial thrombi. [14] BSS is the most common CM syndrome type, which is closely related to platelet activation and thrombosis. The integrated research between disease and syndrome of BSS, which involves pathologic and clinical diagnostics of Western and Chinese medicine, will provide a better understanding of the disease and its therapeutic target.

Platelets are anuclear cells derived from megakaryocytes. They are produced in the bone marrow, released in the blood flow and circulate for 7 to 10 days. Under normal conditions platelets are in loose contact with the vascular wall, without adhering to the endothelium. Platelet activation leads to the release of numerous molecules stored in their granules, e.g., adenosine diphosphate (ADP), thromboxane A2 (TXA2), and platelet-activating factor (PAF). [15] CD62p is one of the human platelet membrane glycoproteins and only released on the activated platelet membrane, which is identified as the most specific biomarker of platelet activation so far. Our results showed that the expression of CD62p of CHD increased significantly compared with the healthy group ($P < 0.01$), which indicate that CHD has the status of platelet activation, and is consistent with previous research results. [8]

Platelet activation can not only cause the membrane protein change, but also a series of morphological changes, from inviscid, discotic circulating platelets into a paste, and protruding platelet jelly, which depends on the regulation of platelet cytoskeletal protein.

Our previous study demonstrates that gelsolin is the main differential protein of platelets between BSS of CHD and non-BSS of CHD patients. [9] Gelsolin, discovered in 1979 by Yin and Stossel[16] based on its ability to activate the gel-sol transformation of F-actin in a calcium-dependent manner, is also one of the actin binding proteins (ABPs)that can sever or cap F-actin and is a secreted form in the plasma of vertebrates. The actin cytoskeleton plays a central role in many fundamental cellular processes involving the generation of force and facilitation of movement, which are enabled by the assembly of actin monomers (G-actin)into F-actin and cooperation with a wide variety of ABPs. [17]

Some research suggests that F-actin can lead to platelet aggregation directly, and the presence of F-actin in blood vessels can be fatal, which can plug smaller vessels and decrease blood flow to promote the formation of blood clots. [18] Gelsolin, together with Gc-globulin, another extracellular actin-binding protein, functions as an "extracellular actin scavenger system" (EASS)responsible for the clearing of much more actin released by tissue injury[19] and for holding back the lengthening of F-actin. By severing F-actin, gelsolin reduces blood viscosity by promoting polymer disassembly. Our results showed that F-actin of BSS in CHD increased markedly ($P < 0.01$)while gelsolin in PPP decreased compared with the healthy group ($P < 0.05$), which coincides with the results of a previous study[20] and indicates that F-actin released into the circulation at the status of platelet activation of BSS of CHD, results in the depletion of plasma gelsolin severely. Meanwhile, the plasma Gc-globulin of BSS group increased compared with the healthy control group ($P < 0.01$), which may be associated with elevation of irritability because of severe depletion.

Calcium ion plays a vital role in the development of platelet activation. The transformation, aggregation, and release reaction of platelets are triggered by the increase of free calcium ion concentration of platelet, which is the essential mechanism of thrombosis. Studies have found an increase of [Ca^{2+}] in patients with CHD; [21] meanwhile, calcium antagonist can reduce [Ca^{2+}] of platelets accompanied by inhibiting platelet aggregation. [22] Our results show that [Ca^{2+}] and gelsolin concentration in PRP of BSS increased significantly compared with the non-BSS and control groups ($P < 0.01$), which was in agreement with our previous study of platelet proteomics.[9] Based on the fact that the change of $[Ca^{2+}]_i$ is the promoter of gelsolin secretion, we postulate that platelet gelsolin may be a new potential biomarker and/or therapeutic target of BSS of CHD, and the increased calcium influx of platelets could be one of the main mechanisms.

The study shows that platelet cytoskeleton protein dynamic changes during the development of BSS of CHD, which focus on gelsolin and F-actin. Plasma gelsolin clears F-actin from circulation, and results in depletion of plasma gelsolin significantly, in addition to the increased calcium influx of platelet. This may lead to the gelsolin expression on platelets which increases abnormally during the process of BSS of CHD. However, it is not clear whether the excessive F-actin released by tissue injury at the status of platelet activation stimulates the platelet directly to secrete gelsolin, and if the platelet gelsolin can be therapeutically targeted by the anti-platelet action of Chinese herbs for promoting blood circulation and removing blood stasis. These issues are well worth further investigation.

REFERENCES

[1] Davi G, Patrono C. Platelet activation and atherothrombosis[J]. N Engl J Med, 2007, 357: 2482-2494.

[2] Moliterno DJ. Advances in antiplatelet therapy for ACS and PCI[J]. J Interv Cardiol, 2008, 21 (S11): S18-S24.

[3] García A. Clinical proteomics in platelet research: challenges ahead[J]. J Thromb Haemost, 2010, 8 (8): 1784-1785.

[4] Thiele T, Steil L, Gebhard S, et al. Profiling of alterations in platelet proteins during storage of platelet concentrates[J]. Transfusion, 2007, 47 (7): 1221-1233.

[5] Banfi C, Brioschi M, Marenzi G, et al. Proteome of platelets in patients with coronary artery disease[J]. Exp Hematol, 2010, 38 (7): 341-350.

[6] Senzel L, Gnatenko DV, Bahou WF. The platelet proteome[J]. Curr Opin Hematol, 2009, 16: 329-333.

[7] Chen KJ, Xue M, Yin HJ. The relationship between platelet activation and coronary heart disease and blood-stasis syndrome[J]. J Capital Med Univ (Chin), 2008, 29 (4): 266-269.

[8] Xue M, Chen KJ, Yin HJ. Relationship between platelet activation related factors and polymorphism of related genes in patients with coronary heart disease of blood-stasis syndrome[J]. Chin J Integr Med, 2008, 14 (4): 267-273.

[9] Li XF, Jiang YR, Wu CF, et al. Study on the correlation between platelet function proteins and symptom complex in coronary heart disease[J]. Mol Cardiol China (Chin), 2009, 9: 326-331.

[10] Chen HZ, ed. Practical internal medicine. 12th ed. Beijing: People's Medical Publishing House, 2005: 1472-1473.

[11] Society of Cardiology, Chinese Association of the Integrative Medicine. The diagnostic criteria of Chinese medicine in coronary heart disease[J]. Chin J Integr Tradit West Med (Chin), 1991, 11: 257.

[12] Zhuang MM, Wen YX, Liu SL, Hong XP. Determination of the level of cytopplasmic free calcium in human platelets with flow cytometry[J]. J Xi'an Jiaotong Univ (Med Sci, Chin), 2005, 26: 508-510.

[13] Grynkiewicz G, Poenie M, Tsien RY. A new generation of Ca^{2+} indicators with greatly improved fluorescence properties[J]. J Biol Chem, 1985, 260 (13): 3440-3450.

[14] Brydon L, Magid K, Steptoe A. Platelets, coronary heart disease, and stress[J]. Brain Behav Immun, 2006, 20 (2): 113-119.

[15] Antoniades C, Bakogiannis C, Tousoulis D, et al. Platelet activation in atherogenesis associated with low-grade inflammation[J]. Inflamm Allergy Drug Targets, 2010, 9 (5): 334-345.

[16] Yin HL, Stossel TP. Control of cytop lasmic actin gelsol transformation by gelsolin, a calcium dependent regulatory protein[J]. Nature, 1979, 281 (5732): 583-586.

[17] Spinardi L, Witke W. Gelsolin and diseases[J]. Subcell Biochem 2007, 45: 55-69.

[18] Vasconcellos CA, Lind SE. Coordinated inhibition of actin-induced platelet aggregation by plasma gelsolin and vitamin D-binding protein[J]. Blood, 1997, 82 (12): 3648-3657.

[19] Lee WM, Galbraith RM. The extracellular actin scavenger systern and actin toxicity[J]. N Engl J Med, 1992, 326 (20): 1335-1341.

[20] Suhler E, Lin W, Yin HL. Decreased plasma gelsolin concentrations in acute liver failure, myocardial infarction, septic shock and myonecrosis[J]. Crit Care Med, 1997, 25 (4): 594-598.

[21] Kato M, Kambe M, Kajiyama G. Increased cytosolic free Mg2+ and Ca^{2+} in platelets of patients with vasospastic[J]. Am J Physiol, 1998, 274 (2): 548-554.

[22] Fujinishi A, Takahara K, Ohba C, et al. Effects of nisoldipine on cytosolic calcium, platelet aggregation, and coagulation/fibrinolysis in patients with coronary artery disease[J]. Angiology, 1997, 48 (6): 515-521.

First published: LIU Yue, YIN Hui-jun, CHEN Ke-ji. Research on the correlation between platelet gelsolin and blood-stasis syndrome of coronary heart disease[J]. Chin J Integr Med, 2011, 17 (8): 587-592.

Correlation between FcγRⅢA and Aortic Atherosclerotic Plaque Destabilization in ApoE Knockout Mice and Intervention Effects of Effective Components of Chuanxiong Rhizome and Red Peony Root

HUANG Ye, YIN Hui-jun, Ma Xiao-juan, WANG Jing-shang, LIU Qian, WU Cai-feng, and CHEN Ke-ji

Coronary heart disease (CHD)is a global cardiovascular disease that remains the principal killer all over the world. Blood stasis syndrome (BSS), a major syndrome type of CHD, is a common Chinese medicine pathological characteristic; its development mechanism and progression are complex and different with a common pathological basement. BSS of CHD is a focus in the field of Chinese medicine and integrative medicine. Our previous study investigated the differential gene expression profiles in peripheral leukocytes of patients with CHD of BSS by oligonucleotide microarray technique. Fc receptor γ ⅢA (FcγRⅢA), one of the differential genes[1], is mainly present on monocytes, which plays a key role in pathological conditions, such as autoimmune diseases and infections[2]. The main pathogenesis of CHD is atherosclerosis. Inflammation and immune response are the key factors of local vulnerable plaques, among which monocytes/macrophages are the main origin of inflammatory factors and plasmas[3]. Atherosclerosis (AS)is a critical and major contributor of CHD and inflammation and immune response play a key role in the pathogenesis of atherosclerosis, while FcγRⅢA contributes to the inflammation and immune response. Thus, we hypothesized that FcγRⅢA, as the target molecule of CHD with BSS, might participate in the occurrence and progression of coronary atherosclerotic plaque destabilization by mediating systemic inflammation.

The apoE knockout (apoE KO)murine model of AS is established, which can mimic the features of fatty streak to plaque formation[4] and the characteristics of stable and unstable atherosclerotic plaque during the progression of AS at different stages[5]. In this study, the AS model by apoE KO mice with 10-week high-fat diet was established and the role of FcγRⅢA in the progression of plaque destabilization and the intervention effects of effective components of Chuanxiong Rhizome and Red Peony Root were analyzed in order to provide a new molecular target for protection and prevention of CHD.

METHODS

1 Drugs and Reagents

Xiongshao Capsule (XSC, 芎芍胶囊)was provided by Beijing International Institute of Biological Products (batch No. 200091), which consists of effective components of Chuanxiong Rhizome and Red Peony Root, 0.25 g/capsule. Simvastatin (Sm), 20 mg/tablet, was produced by Hangzhou Moshadong Pharmaceutical Co., Ltd (batch No. 100243). Intraperitoneal immunoglobulin (pH 4, IVIG), 5% 50 mL, 2.5 g/bottle, was produced by Chengdu Rongsheng Pharmaceutical Co., Ltd (batch No. 200911B037).

Monoclonal antibody (mAb)against CD14 directly coupled to fluorescein isothiocyanate (FITC) (Clone Sa14-2), mAb against CD16/32 directly coupled to phycoerythrin (PE) (Clone 93), and PE-conjugated anti-mouse IgG2a, κ, the isotypic control mAb, were from BioLegend (USA). OptiLyse C lysing solution (Lot No. 12)was from Beckman Coulter (USA). TRIzol reagent (Lot No. 15596-018)was from Invitrogen (USA). Reverse transcriptase M-MLV kit (Lot No. D2639A)was from Takara (Japan). Real-time PCR amplification kit (Lot No.

A4011)was from Bio-Rad (USA). Enzyme-linked immunosorbent assay (ELISA)kit of tumor necrosis factor-α (TNF-α, Lot No. 1011126)was from R&D (USA).

2 Animals Grouping and Treatment

Forty 8-week-old male apoE KO mice and eight 18 to 20 g C57BL/6J mice with the same genetic background were obtained from Beijing University Laboratory Animal Center [animal certificate No. SCXK (Jing)2006-0008]. The strain of apoE KO mice was developed in the Jackson Laboratory on a 129/J background. Mice were housed in humidity-controlled 55% ± 5% rooms at 22 ± 2 ℃ with a 12 h on/12 h off light cycle. After 1 week adaptive fed, mice were switched from normal rodent diet to a high-fat diet[6] that contained 21% fat from lard and supplemented with 0.15% (wt/wt)cholesterol (Experimental Animal Center of the Academy of Military Medical Sciences). Mice were put on a high-fat diet for 10 weeks with different interventions. Eight C57BL/6J mice were selected as the control group and forty apoE KO mice were randomly divided into five groups, model group, IVIG group, Sm group, XSCH group, and XSCL group, 8 mice in each group. Mice in the IVIG group received an intraperitoneal injection of 10 mg IVIG daily over a 5-day period before a high-fat diet. Sm (0.026 g/kg)and XSC (0.39 and 0.195 g/kg)were used in each gavage for 10 weeks in the Sm group, XSCH group, and XSCL group, respectively. Mice in the control group and model group only received the same volume of distilled water per gavage for 10 weeks.

3 Sample Preparation

Blood samples from abdominal aorta after anesthesia by intraperitoneal injection of 20% urethane (0.5 mL/100 g)were collected (fasting 24 h before sampling). Monocyte CD16 expression was detected from 0.2 mL ethylenediamine tetraacetate (EDTA)anticoagulant blood by using flow cytometry. Then, the serum was centrifuged 3 000r/min for 15 min and preserved at −20 ℃ for TNF-α level analysis. Aorta tissue was taken and preserved at −80 ℃ for matrix metalloproteinase-9 (MMP-9)mRNA expression analysis.

4 Whole-Blood Flow Cytometry Analysis

Monocyte CD16 expression was analyzed by flow cytometry. A total of 200 μ L EDTA-anticoagulated whole-blood sample of each group was divided into two tubes, the control tube and the detected tube, and incubated either with anti-CD14 mAb directly coupled to FITC and anti-CD16/32 mAb directly coupled to PE or with the corresponding isotypic control at room temperature in the dark for 20 min. For erythrocyte lysis and fixation of leukocytes, 500 μL OptiLyse C 500 solution was added in each tube. After centrifugation of 1 500r/min for 5 min, cells were washed twice in 3 mL phosphate-buffered saline (PBS)and the final pellet was diluted in 500 μL PBS. EPICS Elite (Beckman Coulter, USA)adjusted by Flow-ChecTM Fluorospheres (Beckman Coulter, USA)was used for flow cytometric analysis. Monocytes were gated in a forward scatter/sideward scatter (FSC/SSC)dotplot. Voltage value of fluorescence channel was determined by analyzing isotypic control and the other tube was measured. EXPO32 software was used to analyze the percentage of CD14+/CD16+ monocytes.

5 Real-time Quantitative PCR

Total mRNA was extracted with TRIzol reagent according to the manufacturer's specifications from the aorta. First-strand cDNA was synthesized from 3 μL total RNA samples according to the reverse transcriptase M-MLV manufacturer's specifications. MMP-9 and glyceraldehyde phosphate dehydrogenase (GAPDH)gene sequences from GenBank were synthesized by Shanghai Sangon Biotech Co., Ltd., and were as follows: the primer series for MMP-9: forward 5'-GCGTGTCTGGAGATT CGAC-3' and reverse 5'-CCATGGCAGAAATAGGCT TT-3', length of amplified segment 138 bp; the primer series for GAPDH:

5'-GCACAGTCAAGGCCGAGAA-3'and 5'-CCTCACCCCATTTGATGTTAGTG-3', length of amplified segment 142 bp. PCR amplification of MMP-9 and GAPDH cDNAs was performed according to the real-time PCR amplification kit with 1.5 μL cDNA and same parameters. All reverse transcription-polymerase chain reactions (RT-PCRs)and analysis were performed on the ABI PRISM 7500 sequence detection system (Applied Biosystems). Cycling parameters were both for 94 ℃ for 15 min; 40 cycles at 94 ℃ for 15 s, 60 ℃ for 34 s, and 72 ℃ for 15 s; and 72 ℃ for 10 min. For each series, the threshold cycle (Ct)value recorded indicates the fractional cycle number at which the amount of amplified target reached a fixed threshold. The housekeeping gene GAPDH was used for internal control. The $2^{-\Delta\Delta Ct}$ method is a convenient way to analyze the relative changes in gene expression from real-time quantitative PCR experiments[7]. The mean Ct value from each sample was normalized to the corresponding GAPDH Ct values, calculated as (Ctexperimental gene-CtGAPDH). The relative gene expression in a particular sample was then given as follows: relative quantification for each gene=$2^{-\Delta\Delta Ct}$ value as mentioned before.

6 ELISA Analysis

Serum TNF-α level was determined using a sandwich-type ELISA kit.

7 Statistical Analysis

Statistical analysis was performed using SPSS 13.0 for Windows. *P* values less than 0.05 were considered statistically significant. Data were expressed as the mean ± standard deviation. Differences among groups were tested using one-way ANOVA followed by multiple comparisons by LSD test. Spearman's correlation coefficients were calculated to study the relations between monocyte CD16 expression and aortic MMP-9 mRNA expression or serum TNF-α level.

RESULTS

1 Comparison of Monocyte $CD14^+/CD16^+$ Expression among Groups

Percentage of peripheral monocyte $CD14^+/CD16^+$ in the model group was significantly higher than that in the control group and was decreased obviously in IVIG group than that in the model group ($P < 0.01$). After 10-week medication intervention, percentage of $CD14^+/CD16^+$ decreased in a different degree in each group compared with that in the model group ($P < 0.01$), but there was no significant statistical difference among these three groups ($P > 0.05$, Table 1, Figure 1).

Table 1 Comparison of Percentage of Peripheral Monocyte $CD14^+/CD16^+$ among Groups ($\bar{x} \pm s$)

Group	*n*	Concentration	$CD14^+/CD16^+$ (%)
Control	8	0	18.16 ± 4.70
Model	8	0	62.32 ± 11.79*
IVIG	8	10 mg	22.28 ± 9.56$^\triangle$
Sm 8	8	0.026 g/kg	32.18 ± 8.38$^\triangle$
XSCH	8	0.390 g/kg	35.43 ± 9.83$^\triangle$
XSCL	8	0.195 g/kg	38.12 ± 7.35$^\triangle$

Notes: $^*P < 0.01$, compared with the control group; $^\triangle P < 0.01$, compared with the model group.

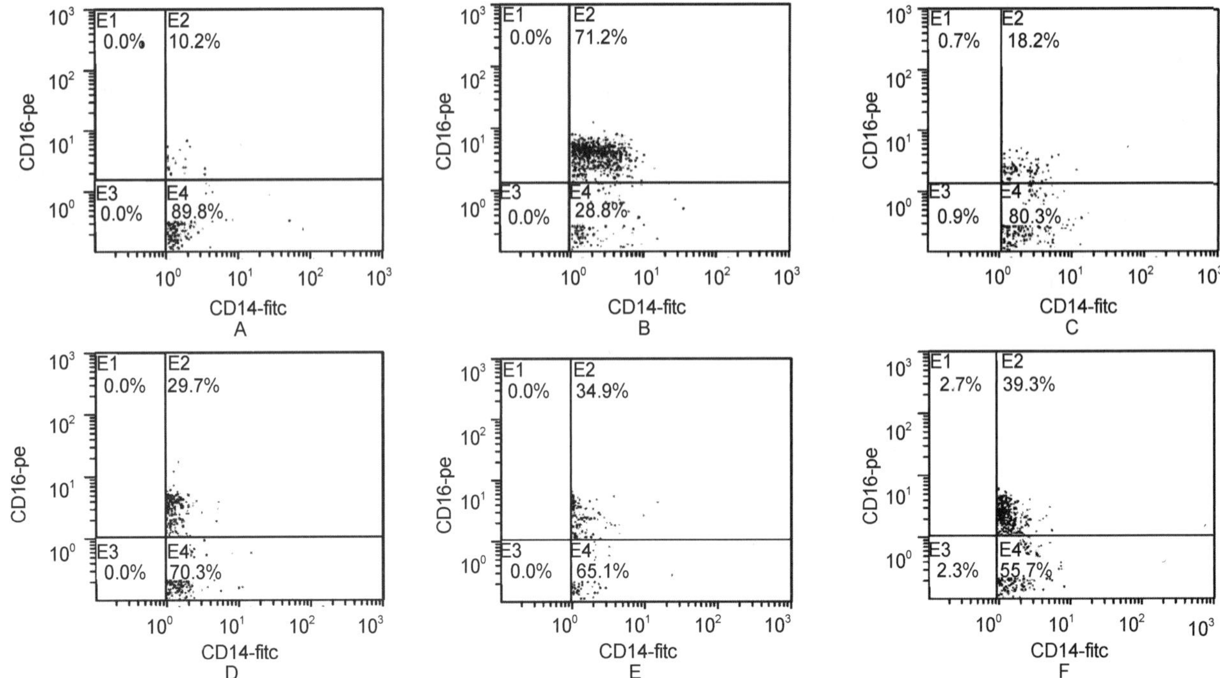

Figure 1 Representative Flow Cytometric Analysis of Monocyte CD16 Expression among Groups

Notes: A: control group; B: model group; C: IVIG group; D: Sm group; E: XSCH group; F: XSCL group.

2 Comparison of Aortic MMP-9 mRNA Expression among Groups

Aortic MMP-9 mRNA expression in the model group was significantly higher than that in the control group and was decreased obviously in the IVIG group compared with the model group ($P < 0.01$). After 10-week medication intervention, aortic MMP-9 mRNA expression decreased in a different degree in each group compared with that in the model group. Aortic MMP-9 mRNA expression in the XSCH group was lowest among these three groups ($P < 0.01$)and this effect was better than that in the Sm group ($P < 0.05$, Table 2).

Table 2 Comparisons of Aortic MMP–9 mRNA Expression and Serum TNF–α Level among Groups ($\bar{x} \pm s$)

Group	n	Concentration	MMP-9 mRNA ($2^{-\Delta\Delta Ct}$)	TNF-α (pg/mL)
Control	8	0	0.930 ± 0.062	16.193 ± 3.942
Model	8	0	$3.968 \pm 0.284^{*}$	$41.758 \pm 9.776^{*}$
IVIG	8	10 mg	$2.539 \pm 0.359^{\triangle\triangle}$	$26.337 \pm 11.855^{\triangle}$
Sm 8	8	0.026 g/kg	$1.991 \pm 0.228^{\triangle\triangle}$	$23.768 \pm 5.268^{\triangle}$
XSCH	8	0.390 g/kg	$1.488 \pm 0.123^{\triangle\triangle\blacktriangle}$	$28.222 \pm 8.484^{\triangle}$
XSCL	8	0.195 g/kg	$2.330 \pm 0.210^{\triangle\triangle}$	35.596 ± 11.180

Notes: $^{*}P < 0.01$, compared with the control group ; $^{\triangle}P < 0.05$, $^{\triangle\triangle}P < 0.01$, compared with the model group ; $^{\blacktriangle}P < 0.05$, compared with the Sm group.

3 Comparison of Serum TNF-α Level among Groups

Serum TNF-α level in the model group was significantly higher than that in the control group ($P < 0.01$) and was decreased in the IVIG group compared with that in the model group ($P < 0.05$). After 10-week medication intervention, TNF-α level decreased in a different degree in each group compared with that in the model group. The TNF-α level was lowest in the XSCH group ($P < 0.05$)and there was no significant statistical difference between XSCH group and Sm group ($P > 0.05$, Table 2).

4 Analyses of Correlation between Monocyte CD16 Expression and Aortic MMP-9 mRNA Expression or Serum TNF-α Level

Correlation analyses showed that monocyte CD16 expression was positively correlated with MMP-9 mRNA expression and serum TNF-α in the IVIG group, XSCH group, and XSCL group (Figure 2).

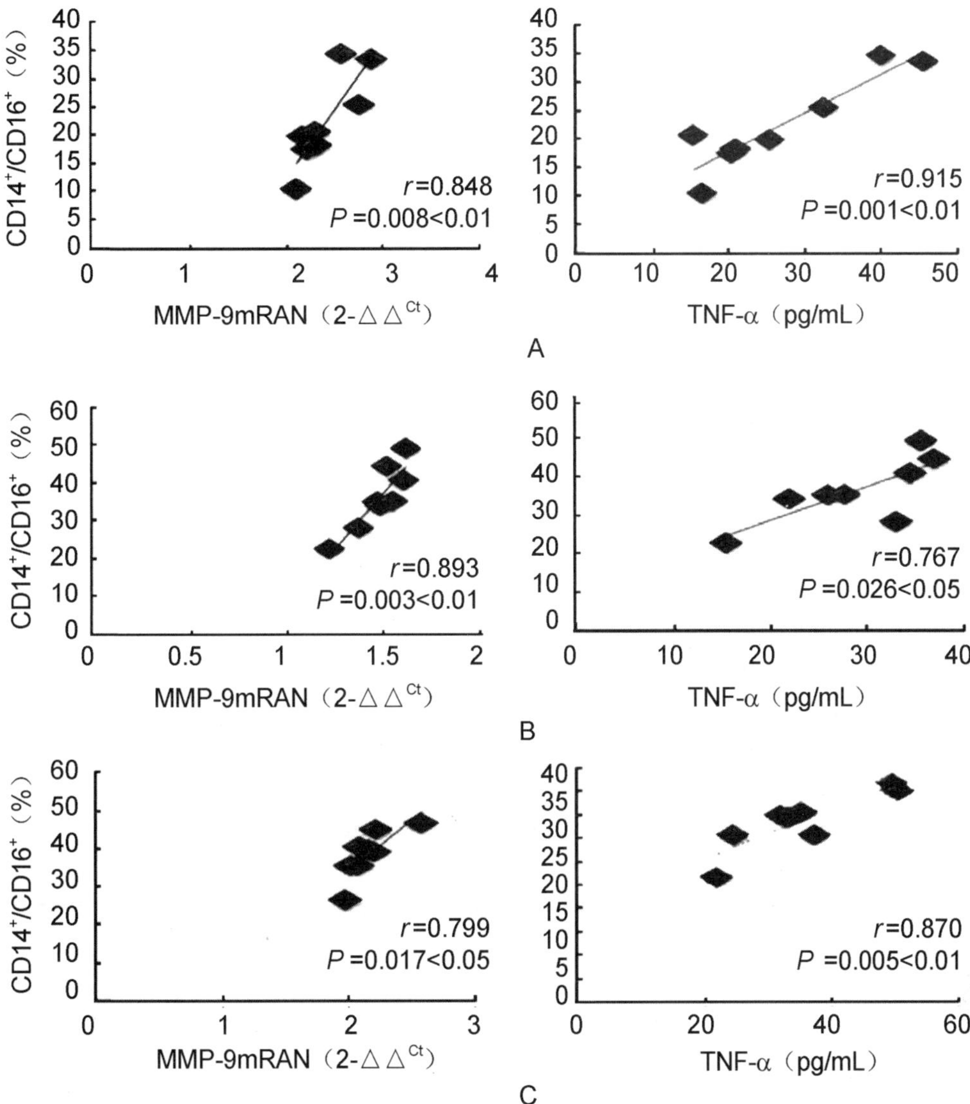

Figure 2 Correlation Analyses between Monocyte CD16 Expression and Aortic MMP-9 mRNA Expression or Serum TNF-α Level

Notes: A: IVIG group; B: XSCH group; C: XSCL group.

DISCUSSION

FcRs, a group of membrane glycoproteins that belongs to the immunoglobulin superfamily, are the specific receptors for the Fc regions of immunoglobulins that are expressed in almost all leukocytes. FcRs are defined by their specificity for immunoglobulin isotypes. Fc γ receptor (FcγR)plays an essential role in the process of immunoinflammatory responses, which is used as an important trigger molecule of inflammation, allergy, and cytophagy. Three different classes of FcγRs have been found on human leukocytes. FcγRⅢ exists in two isoforms, FcγRⅢA and FcγRⅢB. The former is a transmembrane subtype that mainly expresses on monocytes[8]. Researches of FcγR ⅢA mainly focus on the relationship between gene polymorphism or expression level and diseases. The FcγRⅢA F158 allele is reported to be a susceptibility factor for many autoimmune diseases[2], such as rheumatoid arthritis, systemic lupus erythematosus, idiopathic thrombocytic purpura, Wegener's granulomatosis, and CHD[9]. Meanwhile, high levels of FcγRⅢA in a different degree have been observed in patients with coronary bypass operation, Kawasaki disease, and chronic renal failure dialysis[10-12].

AS is a critical and major contributor of CHD. Monocytes play an important role in the early phase of atherogenesis. Recruitment of monocytes from the peripheral blood to the intima of the vessel wall is a primordial event in atherosclerosis[13]. Which role do FcγRⅢA play in the progression of AS? Therefore, we constructed a model by apoE KO mice with high-fat diet to analyze the function of FcγRⅢA in vivo.

IVIG is composed of immunoglobulins, mainly of the IgG isotype. In our study, injections of apoE KO mice with IVIG for 5 days reduced monocyte CD16 expression over the model group. Accordingly, we suggested that IVIG could block FcγRⅢA and suppress its expression and function. This result was consistent with previous study[14].

Inflammation occurs in most vulnerable plaques composed of monocytes, macrophages, and lymphocytes, which is key to plaque rupture. [13] Monocytes themselves produce plenty of MMPs but also release various cytokines, such as TNF-α, which are key players during atherogenesis. MMPs are a family of zinc-dependent enzymes that digest extracellular matrix. Several MMPs are identified in atherosclerotic plaque, playing key roles in vascular remodeling. MMP-9 is essential for plaque destabilization and tissue remodeling and closely related with atherosclerosis[15]. Activation of monocytes and macrophages leads to the release of cytokines, such as TNF-α, which has extensive biological effects. TNF-α, as one of pro-inflammatory cytokines, is also implicated in atherosclerosis[16]. Therefore, we detected MMP-9 and TNF-α as indicators of plaque destabilization and systemic inflammation analyzing by RT-PCR and ELISA, respectively. We found that, after 10-week high-fat diet, these two mediators increased significantly. IVIG and drugs could reduce MMP-9 mRNA expression and serum TNF-α level in order to attenuate atherosclerotic plaque destabilization and suppress systemic inflammation.

Correlation analyses of monocyte CD16 expression, plaque destabilization index, and inflammation factor level in the IVIG group, XSCL group, and XSCH group suggested that IVIG could block FcγRⅢA and reduce monocyte CD16 expression, MMP-9 mRNA expression, and serum TNF-α level. After 10-week intervention, Sm and XSC could reduce monocyte CD16 expression, MMP-9 mRNA expression, and serum TNF-α level. Moreover, there was significantly positive correlation between monocyte CD16 expression and MMP-9 mRNA expression or serum TNF-α level. Thus, we assume that FcγRⅢA may be involved in the progression of CHD by mediating atherosclerotic plaque destabilization and systemic inflammatory. Researches have proven that XSC is suitable for CHD with BSS by preventing AS, stabilizing plaque, and inhibiting restenosis[17]. In our previous study, we constructed the leukocyte gene expression profile of CHD with BSS using entire genome chip. CHD with BSS was found to be related to the inflammatory reaction and immune response at molecular level through gene ontology analysis and pathway analysis. Meanwhile, six differential genes of CHD with BSS were screened and identified. FcγRⅢA was one of them[1]. According to the principle of the corresponding formula and syndrome, whether FcγRⅢA is the target of XSC preventing for CHD with BSS, our research proves that FcγRⅢA may participate in atherosclerotic plaque destabilization by mediating systemic inflammation. XSC can stabilize unstable atherosclerotic plaque by attenuating inflammation and its target was relevant to FcγRⅢA.

REFERENCES

[1] Ma XJ, Yin HJ, Chen KJ. Differential gene expression profiles in coronary heart disease patients of blood stasis syndrome in traditional Chinese medicine and clinical role of target gene[J]. Chin J Integr Med, 2009, 15: 101-106.

[2] Ivan E, Colovai AI. Human Fc receptors: critical targets in the treatment of autoimmune diseases and transplant rejections[J]. Hum Immunol,

2006, 67: 479-491.

[3] Apple FS, Wu AH, Mair J, et al. Future biomarkers for detection of ischemia and risk stratification in acute coronary syndrome[J]. Clin Chem, 2005, 51: 810-824.

[4] Johnson J, Carson K, Williams H, et al. Plaque rupture after short periods of fat feeding in the apolipoprotein E-knockout mouse: model characterization and effects of pravastatin treatment[J]. Circulation, 2005, 111: 1422-1430.

[5] van Bochove GS, Straathof R, Krams R, et al. MRI-determined carotid artery flow velocities and wall shear stress in a mouse model of vulnerable and stable atherosclerotic plaque[J]. MAGMA, 2010, 23: 77-84.

[6] Johnson J, Carson K, Williams H, et al. Plaque rupture after short periods of fat feeding in the apolipoprotein E-knockout mouse: model characterization and effects of pravastatin treatment[J]. Circulation, 2005, 111: 1422-1430.

[7] Livak KJ, Schmittgen TD. Analysis of relative gene expression data using real-time quantitative PCR and the 2-[Delta Delta C (T)] method[J]. Methods, 2001, 25: 402-408.

[8] Masuda A, Yoshida M, Shiomi H, et al. Role of Fc receptors as a therapeutic target. Inflamm Allergy Drug Targets, 2009, 8: 80-86.

[9] Gavasso S, Nygard O, Pedersen ER, et al. Fc gamma receptor ⅢA polymorphism as a risk-factor for coronary artery disease[J]. Atherosclerosis, 2005, 180: 277-282.

[10] Stefanou DC, Asimakopoulos G, Yagnik DR, et al. Monocyte Fc gamma receptor expression in patients undergoing coronary artery bypass grafting[J]. Ann Thorac Surg, 2004, 77: 951-955.

[11] Abe J, Jibiki T, Noma S, et al. Gene expression profiling of the effect of high-dose intravenous Ig in patients with Kawasaki disease[J]. J Immunol, 2005, 174: 5837-5845.

[12] Kawanaka N, NagakeY, Yamamura M, et al. Expression of Fc gamma receptor Ⅲ (CD16)on monocytes during hemodialysis in patients with chronic renal failure[J]. Nephron, 2002, 90: 64-71.

[13] Libby P, Ridker PM, Maseri A. Inflammation and atherosclerosis[J]. Circulation, 2002, 105: 1135-1143.

[14] Samuelsson A, Towers TL, Ravetch JV. Anti-inflammatory activity of IVIG mediated through the inhibitory Fc receptor[J]. Science, 2001, 291: 484-486.

[15] Johnson JL, George SJ, Newby AC, et al. Divergent effects of matrix metalloproteinases 3, 7, 9, and 12 on atherosclerotic plaque stability in mouse brachiocephalic arteries[J]. Proc Natl Acad Sci USA, 2005, 102: 15575-15580.

[16] Stefanadi E, Tousoulis D, Papageorgiou N, et al. Inflammatory biomarkers predicting events in atherosclerosis[J]. Curr Med Chem, 2010, 17: 1690-1707.

[17] Chen KJ, Shi DZ, Xu H, et al. XS0601 reduces the incidence of restenosis: a prospective study of 335 patients undergoing percutaneous coronary intervention in China[J]. Chin Med J, 2006, 119: 6-13.

First published: HUANG Ye, YIN Hui-jun, MA Xiao-juan, WANG Jing-shang, LIU Qian, WU Cai-feng, and CHEN Ke-ji. Correlation between Fc γ R III a and aortic atherosclerotic plaque destabilization in ApoE knockout mice and intervention effects of effective components of chuanxiong rhizome and red peony root[J]. Chin J Integr Med, 2011, 17 (5): 355-360.

Effect of Chinese Herbal Medicine for Activating Blood Circulation and Detoxifying on Expression of Inflammatory Reaction and Tissue Damage Related Factors in Experimental Carotid Artery Thrombosis rats

XUE Mei, ZHANG Lu, YANG Lin, JIANG Yue-rong, GUO Chun-yu, YIN Hui-jun, and CHEN Ke-ji

The lesion of thrombosis in cardio-cerebrovascular diseases is based on atherosclerosis, and many clinical and lab researches have confirmed that thrombosis due to atherosclerosis is closely related to inflammation[1-3]. The etiology and pathogenesis of platelet activation and thrombosis in the process of cardiac and cerebral thrombotic diseases are considered as "blood stasis" in Chinese medicine (CM). A series of therapeutic principles and methods of promoting blood circulation and removing blood stasis was formed under the guidance of this theory, which showed a positive therapeutic effect on the prevention and treatment of cardio-cerebrovascular diseases. However, the pathological changes such as tissue necrosis and inflammation cannot be considered only as CM blood stasis [4]. Based on the combination of the basic theory of blood stasis and pathogenic toxins of CM, experimental carotid artery thrombosis rats model were used in this study. The pathophysiological changes were reflected in thrombosis, inflammatory reaction and tissue damage in three aspects, and the difference of the therapeutic effects of Chinese drugs for activating blood circulation to that of activating blood circulation and detoxifying were compared as well. We then tried to determine the micro-pathological basis of the relationship between blood stasis and the pathogenic toxin, and provide an objective experimental basis for the CM treatment of cardiac and cerebral thrombotic diseases.

METHODS

1 Animals

Fifty SPF Wistar rats, half male and half female, weighing 190 ± 10 g, were provided by Experimental Institute of Chinese Academy of Medical Sciences [Certificate No. SCXK (Beijing)2005-0013].

2 Main Reagents and Instruments

Enzyme-linked immunosorbent assay (ELISA)kit: matrix metalloproteinases (MMP-9, batch number: 20080413), tissue inhibitors to metalloproteinase (TIMP-1, batch number: 20080617), granule membrane protein-140 (GMP-140, batch number: 20080621), tissue-type plasminogen activator (t-PA, batch number: 080523), high-sensitivity C-reactive protein (hs-CRP, batch number: 20080617), interleukin-6 (IL-6, batch number: 20080524), were provided by R & D Systems Inc, USA and were sub-packaged by Shanghai Boatman Biotech Inc., which were detected by micro-plate reader (Thermo MK3, USA).

3 Medication

Simvastatin (Hangzhou MSD Pharmaceutical Co. Ltd., batch number: 07432), 40 mg each tablet, was made into powder in mortar and dissolved into suspension with double-distilled water. Xiongshao Capsule (芎芍胶囊, XSC, Dalian Institute of Chemical Physics, batch number: 070929), 0.25 g each Capsule, contained paeoniflorin (greater than or equal to 28 mg each capsule), ferulate (greater than or equal to 3.5 mg each capsule)and total phenolic acid (greater than or equal to 34 mg each capsule). Huanglian Capsule (黄连胶囊, HLC, Hubei XiangLian Pharmaceutical Co. Ltd., National Medicine Permit No. Z19983042), each Capsule contained 0.25 g Huanglian.

4 Grouping and Methods of Model Establishment

Fifty Wistar rats were randomly divided into the sham operation group, the model group, the Simvastatin group (SG), the activating blood circulation group (ABCG)and the activating blood circulation and detoxifying group (ABCDG), with 10 in each group. The dose was determined by equivalent conversion method according to the animals' body surface area ratio[6]. Simvastatin (1.8 mg/kg), XSC (0.135 g/kg)and Xiongshao Capsule and Huanglian Capsule (XSHLC, 0.135 g/kg)were administered to SG, ABCG and ABCDG by gastrogavage, respectively, once every 24 h for two weeks, and an equal volume of normal saline was given to the sham operation group and the model group. One hour after the last administration, the anesthetized rats (20% urethane solution 0.6 mL/100 g, intraperitoneal injection)were set on the operating table in supine position with head fixed, stretched limbs lashed and neck fully exposed. The right side of the neck was shaved, with local skin sterilized with 75% alcohol and incised. According to Kurz's method[6], the right common carotid artery was separated about 2 cm, a small piece of plastic film was put (4 cm × 1.8 cm)under it to protect surrounding tissues, and then filter paper (1 cm × 1 cm)soaked in 20 μL $FeCl_3$ (70%)was used, which was placed on the vessel to induce the injury. Filter paper soaked in an equal volume of normal saline was used in the sham operation group. Thirty minutes later the filter paper was removed, local tissue was flushed with normal saline and sutured and the rats were put back to the feeding room. After 24 h, the blood samples were collected from the abdominal aorta of rats and kept in a red tube biochemical procoagulant at room temperature for 30 min. The serum was separated by low-speed centrifugation (2 000r/min for 15 min)and then was stored at −20 ℃ for use. Two rats in each group were selected randomly, and about 1.5 cm of the right common carotid artery was cut down and fixed with 10% formaldehyde for the follow-up biopsy.

5 Items of Observation and Methods

The serum level of MMP-9, TIMP-1, GMP-140, t-PA, hs-CRP and IL-6 were detected with enzyme-linked immunosorbent assay. The thrombosis from the common carotid artery was observed by HE staining with an optical microscope (Olympus BX51, Japan).

6 Statistical Analysis

All statistical analyses were performed with SPSS 11.5, and $P < 0.05$ was considered as statistically significant. The t test and analysis of variance (ANOVA)were applied in the intergroup comparison of measurement data, and the χ^2 test was used in the comparison of enumeration data.

RESULTS

1 Pathological Changes of Common Carotid Artery

The histophysiological structure of the sham operation group was clear and complete, arranged in neat rows. The structures of the tunica media and tunica externa were normal, and the tunica intima was smooth and complete without foreign bodies. In the other groups, the vessel wall was thin and a cord-like mixed thrombus was formed, which had a homogeneous red staining region (mainly composed of platelets and fibrin)and a small amount of plasma with some cracks. There were also large stained areas (mainly composed by cracked red blood cells and white blood cells)in the vessel. The tunica intima was damaged, covered with hemosiderin and cracked macrophages, and the basic structure of the tunica media and tunica externa maintained integrity while the elastic layer was thinner. See Figure 1.

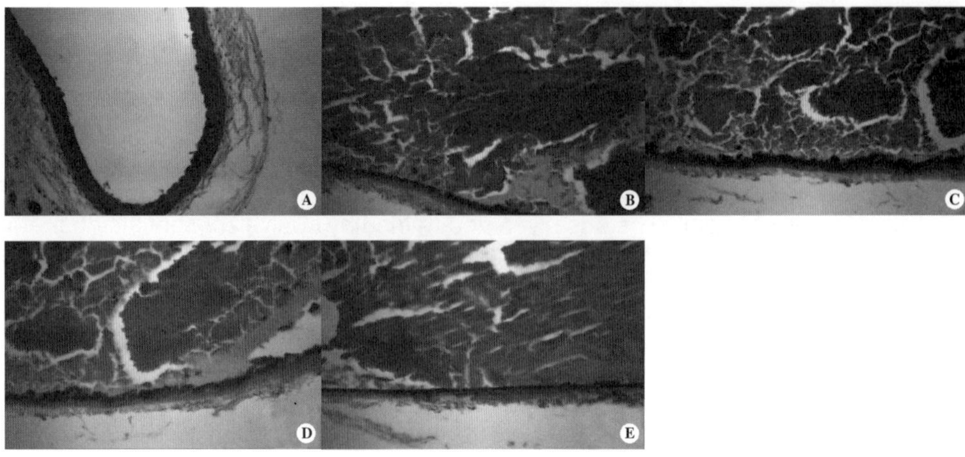

Figure 1　Pathological Changes of Common Carotid Artery in Each Group (HE Staining, ×200)

Notes: A: sham operation group; B: model group; C: Simvastatin group; D: activating blood circulation group; E: activating blood circulation and detoxifying group.

2 Comparison of Thrombosis-related Indicators among Groups

Compared with the sham operation group, the serum level of GMP-140 was significantly increased and the serum level of t-PA was significantly decreased in the model group ($P < 0.01$, $P < 0.05$). The serum level of GMP-140 was significantly decreased and the serum level of t-PA was significantly increased in the SG, ABCG and ABCDG compared with those in the model group ($P < 0.05$, Table 1).

Table 1　Comparison of the Serum Level of GMP–140 and t–PA in Different Groups (pg/mL, $\bar{x} \pm s$)

Group	n	GMP-140	t-PA
Sham operation	10	659.18 ± 247.75**	1089.14 ± 299.19*
Model	10	1319.37 ± 403.94	689.90 ± 292.63
SG	10	946.95 ± 404.67*	1095.38 ± 451.44*
ABCG	10	956.64 ± 366.72*	1055.29 ± 377.24*
ABCDG	10	967.77 ± 432.22*	1130.23 ± 505.08*

Notes: *$P < 0.05$, **$P < 0.01$, compared with the model group.

3 Comparison of Inflammation-related Indicators among Groups

Compared with the sham operation group, the serum levels of hs-CRP and IL-6 were significantly increased in the model group ($P < 0.01$). The serum levels of hs-CRP and IL-6 were significantly decreased in the SG, ABCG and ABCDG compared with those in the model group ($P < 0.05$). The level of serum hs-CRP in ABCDG decreased significantly compared to that in ABCG ($P < 0.05$).

Table 2　Comparison of the Serum Level of hs–CRP and IL–6 among Groups ($\bar{x} \pm s$)

Group	n	hs-CRP (ng/mL)	IL-6 (pg/mL)
Sham operation	10	6.29 ± 2.64**	234.07 ± 99.22**
Model	10	13.55 ± 3.56	433.55 ± 224.34
SG	10	8.96 ± 4.28**	246.23 ± 147.07*
ABCG	10	10.14 ± 3.07*	277.67 ± 152.56*
ABCDG	10	7.17 ± 2.50**△	246.40 ± 161.76*

Notes: *$P < 0.05$, **$P < 0.01$, compared with the model group; △$P < 0.05$, △△$P < 0.01$, compared with the activating blood circulation group.

4 Comparison of Indicators of Tissue Damage among Groups

Compared with the sham operation group, the serum level of MMP-9 was significantly increased in the model group ($P < 0.01$). The serum levels of MMP-9 were significantly decreased in SG, ABCG and ABCDG compared with the model group ($P < 0.05$). There was no significant difference in the levels of serum TIMP-1 among the different groups ($P > 0.05$).

Table 3 Comparison of the Serum Level of MMP–9 and TIMP–1 among Groups (pg/mL, $\bar{x} \pm s$)

Group	n	MMP-9	TIMP-1
Sham operation	10	$228.12 \pm 74.51^{**}$	272.83 ± 55.11
Model	10	466.05 ± 173.15	284.25 ± 78.27
SG	10	$341.17 \pm 123.71^{*}$	305.94 ± 75.20
ABCG	10	$336.84 \pm 88.34^{*}$	328.79 ± 107.78
ABCDG	10	$334.47 \pm 110.16^{*}$	298.07 ± 101.75

Notes: $^{*}P < 0.05$, $^{**}P < 0.01$, compared with the model group.

DISCUSSION

Blood stasis syndrome and its treatment by promoting blood circulation is one of the most active fields in Chinese medicine research, which has made remarkable progress on the pathogenic characteristics, determination of standards, scoring and pathologic changes. This has thus led to the changing of clinical treatment methods and significantly improved the clinical diagnosis and treatment efficacy towards cardiac and cerebral thrombotic diseases. Although there were many discourses about the status of the pathogenic toxin in the pathogenesis of cardio-cerebrovascular diseases, no common understanding with regards to its pathogenic characteristics, whole-and micro-pathological changes, and syndrome and disease differentiation has been up to standard. Especially, there has been inadequate understanding of whether the toxin or the combination and transformation of the toxin and blood stasis of CM are involved in the pathogenesis of cardio-cerebrovascular diseases. This limited the in-depth study and improvement of clinical efficacy of CM in the treatment and prevention of cardio-cerebrovascular diseases.

Modern research has confirmed that modern physics and chemistry-related indicators of cardio-cerebrovascular thrombosis diseases considered to be CM blood stasis syndrome are involved in platelet activation, adhesion, congregation and thrombosis, etc. However, some scholars have made modern biological researches on the toxin and the therapeutic method of detoxifying. The combined use of Chinese herbal medicine for detoxifying and activating blood circulation (giant knotweed rhizome, Latin name XSC) could reduce the expression of nuclear factor-κ B and MMP-9 in the aorta of ApoE (-/-)mice, and the effect of the combination is superior to that of use of either of them alone [7], which could also reduce the serum hs-CRP level[8]. Active ingredients from Chinese drugs for activating blood circulation and detoxifying, including notoginseng saponins, coptis chinensis, giant knotweed rhizome and rhubarb, could lower the blood lipid levels in ApoE knockout mice, and a significant difference was still seen between giant knotweed rhizome and the others. However, a significant decrease in the level of TNF-α was seen only in the rhubarb treated group[9]. But whether toxin and blood stasis are the reciprocal causations involved in the disease process, or which modern pathological and biochemical indicators may be involved, or whether the therapeutic method of activating blood circulation and detoxifying is superior to that of activating blood circulation, or which indexes are sensitive indicators, remain unanswered and there are still no systematic researches about these.

Atherosclerosis is a common basis for thrombosis in cardio-cerebrovascular diseases. According to CM theory, the pathogenetic factors involved in the formation of AS such as platelet aggregation, thrombosis, and vascular endothelial proliferation have an intrinsic relationship with blood stasis, and Chinese drugs for activating blood circulation have shown better efficacy in clinics in the prevention and treatment of AS and its related diseases[10]. Meanwhile, the pathological changes such as inflammatory cell infiltration and increased levels of inflammation markers in the AS process have similar presentations with toxin and blood stasis. According to the CM theory of blood stasis and pathogenic toxins, we made the experimental carotid artery thrombosis rat model using Kurz's method, tried to imitate the pathological process of disease due to blood stasis combined with the etiology and pathogenesis of understanding of blood stasis and the pathogenic toxin of CM, observed its pathophysiological changes in the indexes of thrombosis, inflammatory reaction and tissue damage, and compared the therapeutic effects of Chinese drugs for activating blood circulation to that for activating blood circulation and detoxifying. The results showed that the serum levels of GMP-140, hs-CRP, IL-6, and MMP-9 increased and the serum level of t-PA decreased in the model group compared to those in the sham operation group.

Xiongshao Capsule is, based on experience, an effective prescription for the treatment of coronary heart disease in our hospital, whose composition is based on the classic prescription of Xuefu Zhuyu Decoction (血府逐瘀汤)and its modern pharmacological study. The capsule is composed of the effective part of Chuanxiong total phenols, red peony glycoside. HLC is a heat-clearing and detoxifying herb, so we used the XSC as the therapeutic drug of ABCG and used the XSC and HLC as the therapeutic drugs of ABCDG. Compared with the model group, the levels of serum GMP-140, hs-CRP, IL-6 and MMP-9 in ABCG and ABCDG were significantly reduced ($P < 0.05$), while the level of serum hs-CRP in ABCDG decreased significantly compared to that in ABCG ($P < 0.05$).

GMP-140, a member of the selectin family, can be only expressed on the surface of the platelet after degranulation, which is the specific marker for platelet activation and one of the micro-dialectical indicators for blood stasis syndrome [11]. t-PA is secreted mainly by vascular endothelial cells, which can reflect the state of fibrinolysis and coagulation. Atherosclerosis is a chronic inflammation of the endarterium, and CRP is closely related with cardiovascular diseases such as acute coronary syndrome, while hs-CRP may be a predictor for the risk of cardiovascular disease. IL-6 has extensive biological activities, and plays many biological roles in inflammatory reaction, infection and injury[12]. In our study, the results showed that platelets and the coagulation system could be activated after $FeCl_3$ injured the tunica intima, increased the expression of GMP-140 and formed the obstructive thrombus in the injured local tissue. Thus, the content of t-PA in the blood decreased and the thrombosis model of "blood stasis" was formed, The increase of hs -CRP and IL-6 levels compared to that in the sham-operated group just confirmed an inflammatory response. XSC used alone or combined with HLC can reduce the levels of serum GMP-140, hs-CRP, IL-6 and MMP-9 and increase the serum level of t-PA, so as to inhibit platelet activation and relieve inflammation. XSC combined with HLC could decrease the serum level of hs-CRP than either used alone, which showed that hs-CRP might be one of the sensitive indicators for evaluation of the therapeutic effect of activating blood circulation and detoxifying drugs. The relative balance between MMP and TIMP plays an important role in many physiological and pathological conditions, such as infection, autoimmune reactions and hypoxia/ischemia etc[13]. In this study, the serum level of MMP-9 could be decreased in the SG, ABCG and ABCDG compared to that in the model group, but the level of serum TIMP-1 showed no significant difference among the groups, which maybe related to the time of taking the blood samples after modeling, and should be explored in our follow-up study.

REFERENCES

[1] Paoletti R, Gotto AM Jr, Hajjar DP. Inflammation in atherosclerosis and implications for therapy[J]. Circulation, 2004, 109 (23 SuppI 1): III 20-26.

[2] Zouridakis E, Avanzas P, Arroyo-Espliguero R, Fredericks S, Kaski JC. Markers of inflammation and rapid coronary artery disease progression in patients with stable angina pectoris[J]. Circulation, 2004, 110 (13): 1747-1753.

[3] Nijm J, Wikby A, Tompa A, et al. Circulating levels of proinflammatory cytokines and neutrophil-platelet aggregates in patients with coronary artery disease[J]. Am J Cardiol, 2005, 95 (4): 452-456.

[4] Shi DZ, Xu H, Yin HJ, et al. Combination and transformation of toxin and blood stasis in etiopathogenesis of thrombotic cerebrocardiovascular diseases[J]. Chin J Integr Med (Chin), 2008, 6 (11): 1105-1108.

[5] Chen Q. Technology of research on pharmacology of traditional Chinese medicine[M]. Beijing: People's Medical Publishing House, 1996: 1103-1105.

[6] Kurz KD, Main BW, Sandusky GE. Rat model of arterial thrombosis induced by ferric chloride[J]. Thromb Res, 1990, 60 (4): 269-280.

[7] Zhang JC, Chen KJ, Zheng GJ, et al. Regulatory effect of Chinese herbal compound for detoxifying and activating blood circulation on expression of NF-κ B and MMP-9 in aorta of apolipoprotein E gene knocked-out mice[J]. Chin J Integr Tradit West Med (Chin), 2007, 27 (1): 40-44.

[8] Zhang JC, Chen KJ, Liu JG, et al. Effect of assorted use of Chinese drugs for detoxifying and activating blood circulation on serum high sensitive C-reactive protein in apolipoprotein E gene knock-out mice[J]. Chin J Integr Tradit West Med (Chin), 2008, 28 (4): 330-333.

[9] Zhou MX, Xu H, Chen KJ, et al. Effects of some active ingredients of Chinese drugs for activating blood circulation and detoxicating on blood lipids and atherosclerotic plaque inflammatory reaction in ApoE-gene knockout mice[J]. Chin J Integr Tradit West Med (Chin), 2008, 28 (2): 126-130.

[10] Shi DZ, Ma XC, Gao XA. Research Overview of the prevention and treatment of atherosclerosis by prescriptions for activating blood circulation[J]. Journal of Traditional Chinese Medicine (Chin), 1995, 36 (7)：433-435.

[11] Chen KJ, Xue M, Yin HJ. The relationship between platelet activation and coronary heart disease and blood-stasis syndrome[J]. Journal of Capital Medical University (Chin), 2008, 29 (3): 266-269.

[12] Ma XJ, Yin HJ, Chen KJ. Research progress of correlation between blood-stasis syndrome and inflammation[J]. Chin J Integr Tradit West Med (Chin), 2007, 27 (7): 669-672.

[13] Candelario-Jalil E, Yang Y, Rosenberg GA. Diverse roles of matrix metalloproteinases and tissue inhibitors of metalloproteinases in neuroinflammation and cerebral ischemia[J]. Neuroscience, 2009, 158 (3): 983-994.

First published: XUE Mei， ZHANG Lu，YANG Lin， JIANG Yue-rong，GUO Chun-yu，YIN Hui-jun，and CHEN Ke-ji. Effect of Chinese herbal medicine for activating blood circulation and detoxifying on expression of inflammatory reaction and tissue damage related factors in experimental carotid artery thrombosis rats[J]. Chin J Integr Med, 2010, 16 (3): 247-251.

Effects of Propyl Gallate on Adhesion of Polymorphonuclear Leukocytes to Human Endothelial Cells Induced by Tumor Necrosis Factor Alpha

JIANG Yue-rong,CHEN Ke-ji,XU Yong-gang,YANG Xiao-hong,and YIN Hui-jun

Leukocyte adhesion to the vascular endothelium is a critical initiating step in inflammation and atherosclerosis[1]. Upon exposure to pro-inflammatory cytokines, such as tumor necrosis factor alpha (TNF-α) or interleukin -1β (IL-1β), endothelial cells (ECs)synthesize and express on their surface numerous adhesion molecules and other molecules such as intercellular adhesion molecule-1 (ICAM-1 or CD54), vascular cell adhesion molecule-1 (VCAM-1)and E-selectin (CD62E)[2], which participate in leukocyte and platelet recruitment, coagulation and inflammation.Various drugs, including statins,non-steroidal anti-inflammatory drugs(NSAIDs)and antioxidants, were reported to have the effects of regulating adhesion molecule expression and inhibiting the adhesion of leukocytes to ECs[3].

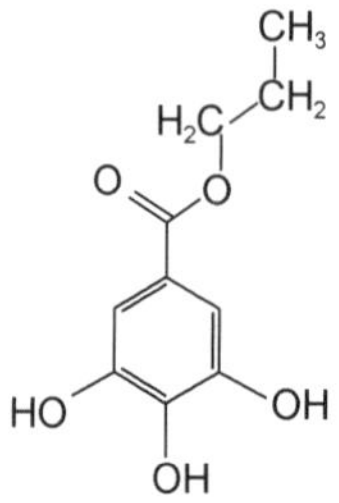

Figure 1 Chemical Structure of Propyl Gallate

Propyl Gallate (PrG, molecular formula: $C_{10}H_{12}O_5$, structure formula: see Figure 1), also named as Radix Paeoniae 801, is an alkyl ester derivative of gallic acid, one of the active ingredients of radix Paeonia rubra. PrG is a strong antioxidant and has various effects such as blocking lipooxygenase and cyclooxygenase activities, scavenging free radicals, inhibiting arachidonic acidinduced platelet aggregation, and anti-inflammation[4-6]. It is clinically used for the treatment of coronary heart disease, cerebral thrombosis, thrombotic phlebitis, dysmenorrhea and so on in China. Several anti-inflammatory effects of PrG have been reported including its inhibitory action on acute inflammatory reactions induced by carragheenin, bradykinin or 5-hydroxytryptamine (5-HT)[7]. However, the effects of PrG on vascular inflammatory responses and underlying cellular mechanisms are still not known. In the present study, we tested the hypothesis that PrG, an inhibitor of lipooxygenase and cyclooxygenase-2[8] with potent antioxidant property, could inhibit TNF-α-induced endothelial adhesion to human polymorphonuclear cells (PMNs), an early sign of vascular inflammatory reaction.

METHODS

1 Reagents

Monoclonal antibody against CD54 directly coupled to FITC (mouse IgG1κ, Clone 84H10)and FITC-conjugated anti-mouse IgG, the isotypic control monoclonal antibody, were from Beckman Coulter (Immunonotech, Mareille, France). The monoclonal antibody against CD62E directly coupled to PE (mouse IgG1, Clone 68-5H11)and PE-conjugated anti-mouse IgG, the isotypic control monoclonal antibody, were from Pharmingen (Becton Dickinson, USA). PrG was provided by Fujian Mindong Rejuvenation Pharmaceutical Co.,

Ltd., China (batch No. 030505). Acetylsalicylic acid (ASA)was from Sigma (Lot No. 033K0026). Stock solutions (0.1 mol/L)of PrG and ASA were made in dimethylsulfoxide (DMSO)and then diluted to proper concentrations just before application. Dulbecco's modified Eagle medium (DMEM, with D-glucose at 4 500 mg/L, Lot No. 1136551) was from GIBCO. Fetal calf serum (FCS, Lot No. ALA 12918)was from Hyclone (USA). Epidermal growth factor (Lot No. 060305H253)and TNF-α (Lot No. 22CY25)were from Perprotech (USA). Human lymphocyte isolation medium was from Tianjin Haoyang Biological Manufacture Co., Ltd., China (Lot No. 060305H253). Collagenase Ⅰ, trypsin, HEPES, L-glutamine, gelatin and sodium pyruvate were from Sigma (USA).

2 Culture of Endothelial Cells and Experimental Conditions

Human umbilical vein endothelial cells (HUVECs)were obtained from newborn infant umbilical cord veins by digestion with 0.1% collagenase according to the method described by Jaffe[9] with some modifications. The resulting cells were cultivated on gelatin and grown to subconfluence in DMEM culture medium containing 20% FCS and supplemented with 40 U/mL heparin, 40 μU/mL insulin, 10 ng/ mL EGF, 2 mmol/L glutamine, 50 U/mL penicillin, 50 μg/mL streptomycin and 1 mmol/L sodium pyruvate at 37 ℃ under 5% CO_2. Cells were judged to be more than 99% endothelial cells by their characteristic cobblestone morphology in an inverted microscope (Leica DMIRB, Germany)and by immunocytochemical demonstration of factor Ⅷ staining. HUVECs were used for experiments at the third to fourth passages of individual preparations. They were seeded in either 96-well plates (0.5 mL/ well)for adhesion experiments, or in 30 mm culture dishes for cytometry analysis.

3 Preparation of Peripheral Blood PMN

Whole blood from normal healthy donors was collected in syringes containing 3.8% sodium citrate (9 : 1 v/v). PMNs were isolated by lymphocyte isolation medium gradient centrifugation (20 ℃, 500×g for 30 min). Mononuclear cells banded on the surface of the upper layer. PMNs banded at the interface of the two density concentrations and erythrocytes banded at the bottom. PMNs were obtained from the interface after gradient centrifugation and erythrocytes were removed from this fraction with hypotonic lysis. PMNs were then washed three times with phosphate-buffered saline (PBS)and placed in DMEM medium with 10% FCS at the concentration of 1×10^6/mL.

4 Analysis of Surface Levels of Adhesion Molecules

Surface adhesion molecules in HUVECs were analyzed by flow cytometry. When HUVECs at the third passage grew to confluence, ECs were pre-incubated with various concentrations of PrG (0.001, 0.01, 0.1, 1, 2, and 5 mmol/L)or 1‰ DMSO (v : v)or 10 mmol/L ASA for 1 h, and then were stimulated with 10 ng/mL TNF-α for 6 h; 1‰ DMSO served as the negative control. The HUVEC monolayer was then washed twice with PBS, detached by trypsin and neutralized by the addition of medium with 10% FBS. Cells were then transferred to flow cytometry tubes, washed three times with PBS and adjusted to be at the concentration of 1×10^6/mL. Each specimen was divided into two tubes and incubated either with anti-CD54 monoclonal antibody (mAb) directly coupled to FITC and anti-CD62E mAb directly coupled to PE or with the corresponding isotypic control at 4 ℃ in the dark for 30 min and then washed twice. EPICS Elite (Beckman Coulter, USA)was used for flow cytometric analysis. Forward light scatter was measured as an index of cell size and fluorescence. The calibration of fluorescence positivity was performed as follows. The negative control was cells incubated with an FITC-labeled mouse IgG and a PE-labeled mouse IgG, and this was set so that the fluorescence-positive rate was inflnitely close to 1%. All cells above this setting were regarded as positive. EXPO32 software was used to analyze the percentage of cells staining positive above the gate and mean fluorescence intensity (MFI)of all cells.

5 PMN Adherence Assays

Rose bengal vital staining was performed to measure PMN adherence to HUVECs according to Gamble[10].

HUVEC cells were plated in DMEM culture medium containing 20% FCS into 96-well plates at approximately 1×10^5/mL and grown to confluence. ECs were pre-incubated with various concentrations of PrG (0.001, 0.01, 0.1, 1, 5 mmol/L)or 1‰ DMSO (v ∶ v)or 10 mmol/L ASA for 1 h, and then were stimulated with 10 ng/mL TNF-α for 6 h. Prior to assay, the medium was removed and the HUVEC monolayer washed once by PBS. PMNs were then added to the HUVEC monolayer in a volume of 200 μL per well at 37 ℃ for 30 min. The non-adherent cells were removed by aspiration and each well washed twice. All medium was removed by aspiration and 100 μL of a 0.25% solution of Rose Bengal in PBS was added to each well for 5 min at room temperature. The stain was then aspirated off, and each well washed twice by PBS. Then 200 μL of a solution of ethanol: PBS (1 ∶ 1)was added. After approximately 30 min, when total release of stain from the cells had occurred, the optical density (OD)at wavelength 570nm was determined for each well using an ELISA reader (Wellscan MK3, Labsystems Dragon, Finland). The OD value of each well was proportional to the number of adherent PMNs

6 Statistics

Five different preparations of HUVECs were tested. Results were expressed as mean ± standard deviation. Differences among groups were tested using One-Way ANOVA, followed by multiple comparisons by LSD test using SPSS 11.0 for Windows and signiflcance was calculated at $P < 0.05$.

RESULTS

1 Effects on Fluorescence-positive Rate and MFI of FITC-CD54

As shown in Table 1, CD54 was constitutively expressed in 32.53 ± 1.98% of HUVECs and the corresponding MFI of CD54 was 2.36 ± 0.72. After 6 h of incubation with 10 ng/mL TNF-α, CD54 was expressed in 95.70 ± 2.52% of HUVECs, while the corresponding MFI was 10.37 ± 3.30 ($P < 0.01$). Compared with basal levels, the percentage of fluorescence-positive cells and MFI of surface FITC-CD54 increased significantly after stimulation by TNF-α for 6 h ($P < 0.01$). PrG at doses ranging from 1 mmol/L to 5 mmol/L decreased CD54 surface expression in a dose-dependent way. PrG at doses ranging from 0.001 mmol/L to 0.1 mmol/L did not alter the TNF-α-mediated increase in CD54 surface expression. ASA at dose of 10 mmol/L could significantly decrease the MFI of CD54 ($P < 0.05$, Figure 2).

Table 1 Effects on Fluorescence–positive Rate and MFI of FITC–CD54 in HUVEC ($\bar{x} \pm s$)

Group	n	Concentration	CD54 positive rate (%)	CD54 MFI
control	5	0	32.53 ± 1.98	2.36 ± 0.72
TNF-α	5	10 ng/mL	95.70 ± 2.52**	10.37 ± 3.30**
TNF-α+ASA	5	10 mmol/L	86.40 ± 2.46	6.27 ± 1.70*
TNF-α+PrG	5	5 mmol/L	16.87 ± 3.77$^{\triangle\triangle}$	2.03 ± 0.41$^{\triangle\triangle}$
TNF-α+PrG	5	2 mmol/L	52.20 ± 20.09$^{\triangle\triangle}$	2.46 ± 0.81$^{\triangle\triangle}$
TNF-α+PrG	5	1 mmol/L	84.30 ± 9.90$^{\triangle\triangle}$	3.67 ± 1.26$^{\triangle\triangle}$
TNF-α+PrG	5	0.1 mmol/L	95.10 ± 3.58	9.48 ± 2.75
TNF-α+PrG	5	0.01 mmol/L	96.00 ± 1.01	10.80 ± 1.15
TNF-α+PrG	5	0.001 mmol/L	98.10 ± 0.97	10.26 ± 2.85

Notes: $^{*}P < 0.05$, $^{**}P < 0.01$, compared with the control ; $^{\triangle}P < 0.05$, $^{\triangle\triangle}P < 0.01$, compared with the TNF-α control.

2 Effects on Fluorescence-positive Rate and MFI of PE-CD62E

Without stimulation, about 9.16 ± 3.43% of HUVECs constitutively expressed CD62E and the corresponding MFI was 1.53 ± 0.58. After 6 h of incubation with 10 ng/mL TNF-α, CD62E was expressed in 42.58 ± 5.91% of HUVECs, while the corresponding MFI was 5.68 ± 1.46. Compared with basal levels, CD62E surface expression increased significantly after stimulation by TNF-α (10 ng/mL)for 6 h ($P < 0.01$). PrG at doses ranging from 1 mmol/L to 5 mmol/L dose-dependently decreased CD62E surface expression ($P < 0.01$). PrG at doses ranging from 0.001 mmol/L to 0.1 mmol/L did not alter the TNF-α-mediated increase in CD62E surface expression. However, PrG at doses lower than 0.1 mmol/L showed a trend of slight increase in CD62E ($P > 0.05$). ASA did not alter the MFI and positive rate of CD62E ($P > 0.05$, Table 2 and Figure 2).

Table 2 Effects on Fluorescence-positive Rate and MFI of PE-CD62E in HUVEC ($\bar{x} \pm s$)

Group	*n*	Concentration	CD62E positive rate (%)	CD62E MFI
control	5	0	9.16 ± 3.43	1.53 ± 0.58
TNF-α	5	10 ng/mL	42.58 ± 5.91*	5.68 ± 1.46*
TNF-α+ASA	5	10 mmol/L	47.25 ± 4.25	4.35 ± 1.85
TNF-α+PrG	5	5 mmol/L	8.99 ± 2.30△	1.53 ± 0.21△
TNF-α+PrG	5	2 mmol/L	13.83 ± 2.23△	1.63 ± 0.06△
TNF-α+PrG	5	1 mmol/L	30.32 ± 5.08	2.67 ± 0.76△
TNF-α+PrG	5	0.1 mmol/L	43.66 ± 9.55	4.82 ± 1.16
TNF-α+PrG	5	0.01 mmol/L	45.20 ± 6.04	5.93 ± 0.47
TNF-α+PrG	5	0.001 mmol/L	50.96 ± 9.77	7.46 ± 0.92

Notes: * $P < 0.01$, compared with the control ; △ $P < 0.01$, compared with the TNF-α control.

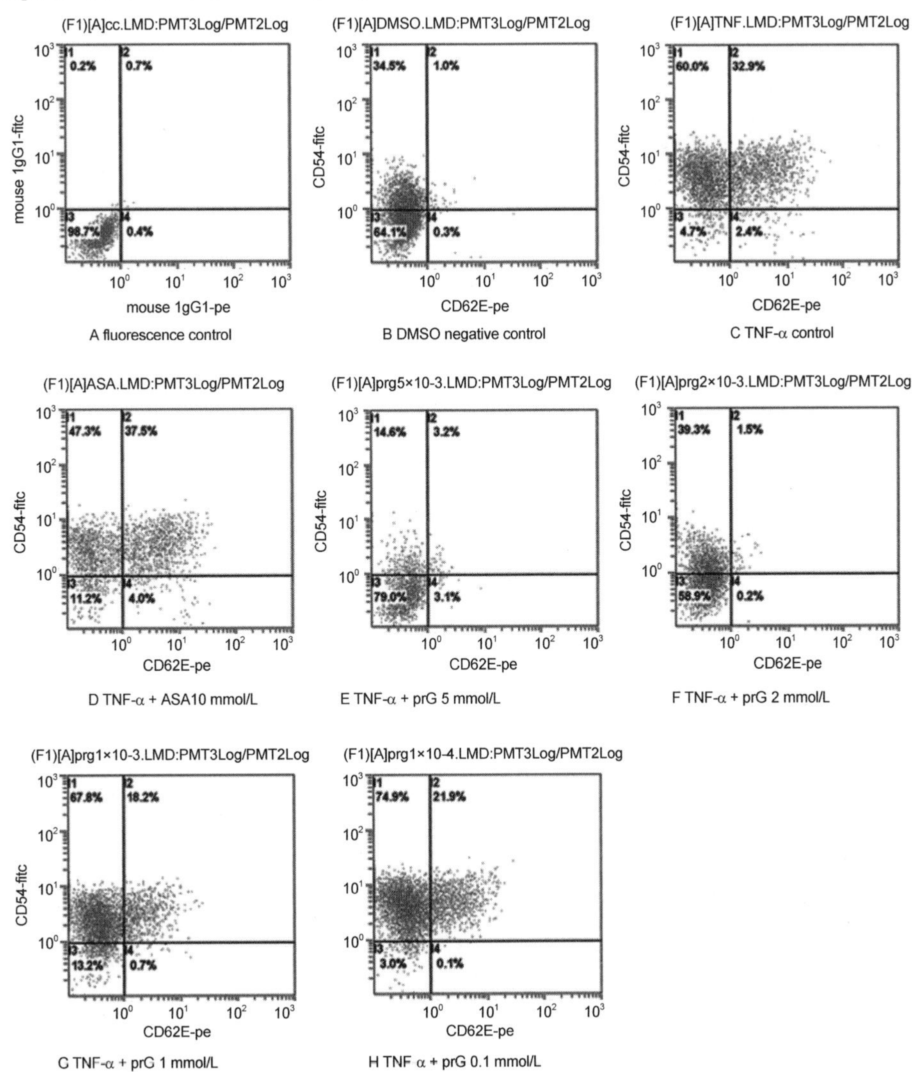

Figure 2 Representative Flow Cytometric Analysis from One of Three Separate Experiments of CD54 and CD62E Surface Expression in TNF-α -activated HUVEC

Notes: A: fluorescence control, B: DMSO negative control,C: TNF-α control, D: TNF-α+ASA 10 mmol/L, E: TNF-α+PrG 5 mmol/L, F: TNF-α+PrG 2 mmol/L, G: TNF-α +PrG 1 mmol/L, H: TNF-α+PrG 0.1 mmol/L, I: TNF-α +PrG 0.01 mmol/L, J: TNF-α+PrG 0.001 mmol/L; the number of positive cells (%) is indicated in the different panels.

3 Effects on Adhesion of PMNs to TNF-α -activated HUVECs

As shown in Figure 3, compared with non stimulated HUVECs, TNF-α enhanced the ability of HUVECs to attach PMN cells (OD values from 0.276 ± 0.023 to 0.357 ± 0.071). At doses ranging from 0.1 mmol/L to 5 mmol/L, PrG significantly reduced the adhesion of PMN induced by TNF-α ($P < 0.01$). ASA did not alter the adhesion of PMN to HUVECs.

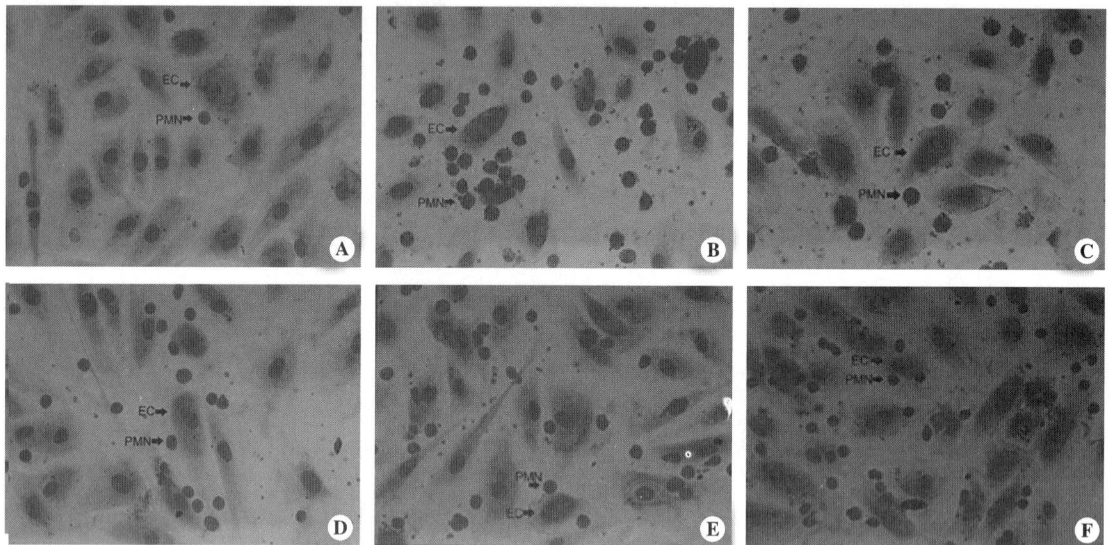

Figure 3　Rose Bengal Staining of PMNs Adhered to HUVECs with Inverted Microscope (×400)

Notes: A: DMSO negative control; B: TNF-α control; C: TNF-α +PrG 1 mmol/L; D: TNF-α +PrG 0.1 mmol/L; E: TNF-α +PrG 0.01 mmol/L; F: TNF-α +ASA 10 mmol/L.

DISCUSSION

Endothelial cells provide a non-thrombogenic and non-adhesive surface, but under pathologic conditions they become pro-adhesive and pro-coagulant. Pro-inflammatory cytokines initiate the vascular inflammatory response via up-regulation of adhesion molecules on the endothelium[11]. Leukocyte and platelet adhesion to endothelial cells, an early step in the pathogenesis of atherosclerosis, is mediated through adhesion molecules[12]. The PMN is one of the vital cell types participate in inflammatory reaction in vivo.

ICAM-1 (CD54), an adhesion molecule constitutively expressed by endothelial cells, is an important member of the immunoglobulin superfamily (IgSF)that is centrally involved in trafficking of leukocytes to endothelial and epithelial barriers[13]. Upon stimulation by cytokines or bacterial lipopolysaccharides (LPS), the increased ICAM-1 expression contributes to the initiation and continuation of the inflammatory reaction. CD54 mediates adhesion and extravasation of all classes of leukocytes to and through the endothelium[14]. The predominant function of CD54 and related cell adhesion molecules, such as VCAM-1 and E-selectin (CD62E), is related to the recruitment and trafficking of leukocytes via interactions with leukocyte-expressed integrins[15]. The leukocyte adhesion mediated by adhesion molecules may promote the instability of atheromatous plaques, and the consequent fissuring or rupture of these plaques and the formation of thrombus, which may play a key role in the pathogenesis of unstable angina and myocardial infarction[16].

The basal expression of CD54 and CD62E, as well as the expression after incubation with TNF-α, are an indication that the cells are in a good condition[17]. In the present study, CD54 and CD62E were constitutively expressed in 32.53 ± 1.98% and 9.16 ± 3.43% of HUVECs, respectively. The corresponding MFIs of CD54 and CD62E were 2.36 ± 0.72 and 1.53 ± 0.58, respectively. After 6 h of incubation with 10 ng/mL TNF-α, CD54 and CD62E were expressed in 95.70 ± 2.52% and 42.58 ± 5.91% of HUVECs respectively, while the corresponding MFIs of CD54 and CD62E were 10.37 ± 3.30 and 5.68 ± 1.46 respectively. These expression levels were in agreement with levels found in other published studies[17], indicating that the cells were in a good condition.

According to Kapiotis[18], ASA at high doses (i. e., 10 mmol/L), by inhibition of NF-κB mobilization, inhibited VCAM-1, but not CD54 expression and adhesion of U937 monocytic cells in HUVECs. The NSAID Ibuprofen was identified as a potent inhibitor of IL-1α and TNFα-induced surface expression of VCAM-1 and a less potent inhibitor of pyrogen-induced expression of ICAM-1, whereas no effect on CD62E was found. Ibuprofen caused a significant ($P < 0.01$ at 2 mmol/L)dose-dependent inhibition of pyrogen-induced expression of VCAM-1 and CD54 on HUVECs (IC50 0.1-0.3 mmol/L). Ibuprofen (at 2 mmol/L)did not affect PMN-adherence to HUVECs.

In the present study, pre-treatment with PrG suppressed TNFα-induced surface expression of CD54 and CD62E ($P < 0.05$ at 1-5 mmol/L). PrG also reduced the adherence of PMNs to TNFα-treated HUVECs at doses ranging from 0.1 mmol/L to 5 mmol/L. Hence, PrG showed the effect of inhibiting TNFα-induced up-regulation of these adhesion molecules, similar to non-selective cyclooxygenase inhibitors ASA and Ibuprofen. With the dose of ASA tested in our study (10 mmol/L), we did not detect a signiflcant inhibitory effect on the expression of CD54or CD62E. Thus the concentrations of ASA needed to affect CD54 expression seem to be higher than those of PrG in the presence of TNF-α. PrG inhibited CD54 and CD62E in endothelial cells, which may indicate an additional anti-inflammatory property of this drug.

On the other hand, PrG at doses lower than 0.1 mmol/L showed a trend of slight increase in CD62E ($P > 0.05$), which was similar to the effect of atorvastatin on potentiating TNF-α-mediated CD62E induction according to Denis Bernot's report, in which atorvastatin (1.0 μmol/L)up-regulated the TNF-α-induced expression of VCAM-1, ICAM-1 and E-selectin at the endothelial cell surface, and also altered the surface distribution of adhesion molecules, which may account for its reduced binding of monocytes[19].

In conclusion, our results show that PrG (0.1-5 mmol/L)decreased adhesion of PMNs to human endothelial cells by regulating the surface expression of adhesion molecules. Although our *in vitro* results cannot be directly extrapolated to the in vivo situation, they suggest a potential therapeutic mechanism of PrG for its intervention in cytokine-mediated vascular inflammatory processes at the endothelial cell level.

REFERENCES

[1] Nomura S. Tandon NN, Nakamura T, et al. High-shear-stress-induced activation of platelets and microparticles enhances expression of cell adhesion molecules in THP-1 and endothelial cells[J]. Atherosclerosis, 2001, 158: 277-287.

[2] Landsberger M, Wolff B, Jantzen F, et al. Cerivastatin reduces cytokine-induced surface expression of ICAM-1 via increased shedding in human endothelial cells[J]. Atherosclerosis, 2007, 190: 43-52.

[3] Desideri G, Croce G, Tucci M, et al. Effects of bezafibrate and simvastatin on endothelial activation and lipid peroxidation in hypercholesterolemia: evidence of different vascular protection by different lipid-lowering treatments[J]. J Clin Endocrinol Metab, 2003, 88: 5341-5347.

[4] Reddan JR, Giblin FJ, Sevilla M, et al. Propyl gallate is a superoxide dismutase mimic and protects cultured lens epithelial cells from H_2O_2 insult[J]. Exp Eye Res, 2003, 76: 49-59.

[5] Huang JD, Song Z, Li J, et al. Study on the therapeutic mechanism of the active principle of the Chinese drug Paeoniae Radix 801 through afflnity biosensors IAsys plus quartz crystal microbalance[J]. Chin J Integr Med, 2005, 11 (1): 37-40.

[6] Franzone JS, Natale T, Cirillo R, et al. Influence of propyl-gallate and 2-mercaptopropionylglycine on the development of acute inflammatory reactions and on biosynthesis of PGE2[J]. Boll Soc Ital Biol Sper, 1980, 56: 2539-2545.

[7] Soares DG, Andreazza AC, Salvador M. Sequestering ability of butylated hydroxytoluene, propyl gallate, resveratrol, and vitamins C and E against ABTS, DPPH, and hydroxyl free radicals in chemical and biological systems[J]. J Agric Food Chem, 2003, 51: 1077-1080.

[8] Yin HJ, Jiang YR, Wu XH, et al. Effect of propyl gallate on activity of cyclooxygenase 1 and 2 in mice's peritoneal macrophages[J]. Chin J Integr Med, 2004, 10 (3): 213-217.

[9] Jaffe EA. Culture of human endothelial cells derived from umbilical veins[J]. Identification by morphologic and immunologic criteria. J Clin Invest, 1973, 52: 2745-2754.

[10] Gamble JR, Vadas MA. A new assay for the measurement of the attachment of neutrophils and other cell types to endothelial cells[J]. J Immunol

Methods, 1988, 109: 175-184.

[11] Jiang MZ, Tsukahara H, Hayakawa K, et al. Effects of antioxidants and NO on TNF-alpha-induced adhesion molecule expression in human pulmonary microvascular endothelial cells[J]. Respir Med, 2005, 99: 580-591.

[12] Xenos ES, Stevens SL, Freeman MB, et al. Nitric oxide mediates the effect of fluvastatin on intercellular adhesion molecule-1 and platelet endothelial cell adhesion molecule-1 expression on human endothelial cells[J]. Ann Vasc Surg, 2005, 19: 386-392.

[13] Hopkins AM, Baird, AW, Nusrat A. ICAM-1: targeted docking for exogenous as well as endogenous ligands[J]. Adv Drug Deliv Rev, 2004, 56: 763-778.

[14] Carlos TM, Harlan JM. Leukocyte-endothelial adhesion molecules[J]. Blood, 1994, 84: 2068-2101.

[15] Springer TA. Adhesion receptors of the immune system[J]. Nature, 1990, 346: 425-434.

[16] Crea F, Biasucci LM, Buffon A, et al. Role of inflammation in the pathogenesis of unstable coronary artery disease[J]. Am J Cardiol., 1997, 80 (5A): 10E-16E.

[17] Lanbeck P, Odenholt I, Riesbeck K. Dicloxacillin and erythromycin at high concentrations increase ICAM-1 expression by endothelial cells: a possible factor in the pathogenesis of infusion phlebitis[J]. J Antimicrob Chemother, 2004, 53: 174-179.

[18] Kapiotis S, Sengoelge G, Sperr WR, et al. Ibuprofen inhibits pyrogen-dependent expression of VCAM-1 and ICAM-1 on human endotheial cells[J]. Life Sci, 1996, 58: 2167-2181.

[19] Bernot D, Benoliel AM, Peiretti F, et al. Effect of atorvastatin on adhesive phenotype of human endothelial cells activated by tumor necrosis factor alpha[J]. J Cardiovasc Pharmacol, 2003, 41: 316-324.

First published: JIANG Yue-rong, CHEN Ke-ji, XU Yong-gang, YANG Xiao-hong, and YIN Hui-jun. Effects of propyl gallate on adhesion of polymorphonuclear leukocytes to human endothelial cells induced by tumor necrosis factor alpha[J] . Chin J Integr Med, 2009, 15 (1): 47-53.

Relationship between the Platelet Activation Related Factors and the Polymorphism of Related Genes in Patients with Coronary Heart Disease of Blood-stasis Syndrome

XUE Mei, CHEN Ke-ji, and YIN Hui-jun

Blood-stasis syndrome (BSS)is all along a hot-spot for studies on TCM syndrome, and the combination of disease diagnosis with syndrome differentiation is the pattern adopted in most present researches. BSS is one of the mostly often encountered syndrome type of CHD. The intensive platelet aggregation on the ruptured atherosclerotic plague constitutes the pathological basis for acute coronary syndrome, cerebral vascular diseases and peripheral vascular ischemic diseases. Since the activation, adhesion and aggregation of platelets is the core in coronary thrombi formation, universal attention is accordingly paid on the relationship between platelet activation and CHD. At present, CHD has been the main killer threatening health of human being. Except the environmental factors, genetic factor also plays important role in the genesis and development of CHD. Previous researches pointed out that CHD is a multiple factors disease, and along with the rapidly advancing in human genome project, the orientation and identification of CHD related gene has become a hot-spot of studies.

Two platelet membrane glycoproteins, GP Ⅱ b- Ⅲ a, the glycoprotein plays crucial action in platelet aggregation and thrombi growing, and GP Ⅰ b, the glycoprotein closely related with platelet adhesive capacity, were selected by the authors in the study as the cut-in point. The expressive levels of platelet activation related factors, GP Ⅰ b, GP Ⅱ b- Ⅲ a and GMP-140, in CHD patients of BSS or non-BSS, and these indexes in healthy subjects were compared, and the relationship between them and gene polymorphisms was analyzed in order to probe in the essential of CHD with BSS from a new viewing angle, and to provide a new thinking path and target in CHD prevention and treatment upon the gene level.

MATERIALS AND METHODS

1 Diagnosis Standard

Patients' diagnosis should be up to the standard of "Nomenclature and diagnosis of ischemic heart diseases" promulgated by the united special group for standardization of clinical nomenclature, WHO[1]. Among them, patients having symptom of angina or/and objective evidence of myocardial ischemia, and with marked coronary stenosis (>50%)showed by coronary contrast examination were selected. The TCM syndrome typing was made in referring to the standard for syndrome differentiation of coronary heart disease issued from the Chinese Association of Integrative Chinese and Western Medicine[2]. The standard for inclusion was patients who met with the all following 4 criteria, i. e. suffered from ischemic heart diseases of various TCM syndrome types without restriction; had symptom of angina or/and objective evidence of myocardial ischemia; latest coronary contrast examination showed significant stenosis (>50%); age between 35-75 years. The standard for exclusion was patients who had any one of the following conditions: severe infection; severe heart failure (EF < 35%); uncontrolled hypertension grade Ⅲ; severe valvulopathy; diabetes mellitus type Ⅰ; complicated with severe primary diseases of liver, kidney, hemopoietic system and nerve system as well as psychiatric diseases and malignant tumor; had taken drugs for anti-platelet or anti-coagulant in the latest 2 weeks; refused to subscribe on the inform consent or being estimated as with poor compliance; participated in other clinical trial; women in pregnancy or lactation stage. The subjects selected into the healthy control group were persons who had been identified healthy by examinations of history, physical, blood routine, liver function, chest film, ECG, etc., and mental or significant physical diseases as well as familial or self psychiatric history in them had been foreclosed.

2 General Clinical Materials

All patients enrolled came from Beijing or Hebei area, Han nationality, with no genetic connection among them, and they visited Xiyuan Hospital or Anzhen Hospital from March 2005 to January 2007. They were assigned, according to the inclusive criteria, into the CHD of BSS group and the CHD of non-BSS group. The subjects selected into the healthy control group were persons who came to the physical checking Center of Xiyuan Hospital for medical examination. All the subjects taking part in the examination voluntarily, were informed with the content of studying, and subscribed on the consent note. In the patients enrolled, the 40 in the group of CHD with BSS (Group A)were 25 males, with mean age of 62.78 ± 10.94 years, body weight index (BWI)of 25.24 ± 2.75 kg/m^2, acute myocardial infarction presented in 4 of them, stable angina in 1, unstable angina pectoris in 35, history of myocardial infarction presented in 11 of them, that of hypertension in 18, hyperlipemia in 10, diabetes mellitus in 5, and smoking in 8; the 37 in the group of CHD with non-BSS (Group B)were 29 males, with mean age of 58.21 ± 10.24 years, BWI of 24.95 ± 2.87 kg/m^2, acute myocardial infarction presented in 3 of them, stable angina in 1, unstable angina pectoris in 33, history of myocardial infarction presented in 10 of them, that of hypertension in 9, hyperlipemia in 8, diabetes mellitus in 8, and smoking in 12. Statistical analysis showed no significant difference between the two groups ($P > 0.05$). The control group consisted of 39 healthy persons showed no statistical difference in age, sex and BWI as compared with the two groups of CHD patient, so they were comparable ($P > 0.05$).

3 Observation Items

3.1 The Activities of GP Ⅰb, GP Ⅱb- Ⅲa and GMP-140

The degree of platelet activation represented by the fluorescent intensity of platelet glycoprotein was determined using whole blood flow cytometry. CTDA vacuum blood taking tube was used to draw out 2 ml of venous blood on an empty stomach in the morning . The blood was mixed evenly for determination within 6 hours. The determination is conducted in the following procedures: The control tube, test tube 1 and 2, contained 5 μl of blood sample, were added respectively with homotype control CD61-FITC (Anti-GP Ⅲa, CAT. NO. 348093, Becton Dickinson, USA)/ IgG1-PE, CD61-FITC/CD62p-PE (Anti-GMP-140, CAT. NO. 348107, Becton Dickinson, USA)andCD42b-FITC (Anti-GP Ⅰb, CAT. NO. 555472, Becton Dickinson, USA), 20 μl in each tube; mixed evenly by light shaking; incubated under light shielding at room temperature for 15-20 min; added in cold (2-8 ℃)fixative liquid 1 ml for each tube, mixed well, incubated again in light protective condition under 2-8 ℃ for 30 min; then the sample was put into the analyzer for measuring the mean fluorescence intensity (MFI)of CD42b, CD61 and CD62p using multi-parameter multi-color fluorescent flow cytometry (EPICS Elite, Beckman Coulter Co, USA)with standard fluorescent micro-balloon collection beam path and stream, and the test data were obtained by FS vs SS access, Expo32 special software.

3.2 Gene Polymorphism of GP Ⅱb- Ⅲa and GP Ⅰb

We selected the HPA-3 polymorphism of GP Ⅱb- Ⅲa and HPA-2 polymorphism of GP Ⅰb as the point of penetration. 2 ml venous blood was collected with EDTA anti-coagulant for DNA extraction on an empty stomach in the morning. We isolated genomic DNA from whole blood according to the direction of the kit (Wizard® Genomic DNA Purification Kit, Promega, USA). The polymorphism of HPA-3 gene was detected by Tapman probe technique (PCR instrument type ABI 9700; fluorescent quantitative PCR instrument type ABI 7700 HT, ABI, USA), and that of HPA-2 gene was determined by gene sequencing (DNA sequencing device type 3700, ABI, USA). Polymorphism of GP Ⅱ b was detected with TaqMan probe technique (PCR instrument type ABI 9700; fluorescent quantitative PCR instrument type ABI 7700 HT, ABI, USA), the direct sequencing was chosen for detecting polymorphism of GP Ⅰ b. The detection on the two loci was processed put in charge of the Shanghai Jikang Ltd. Co. of Bio-products. Agents: Ex Taq DNA polymerase, P/N: DRR100B, Lot: CKA1801A, Dalianbao Bio-engineering Ltd. Co. ; ABI TaqMan 2×PCR Master mix, P/N: 4326614, Lot: G15502, USA; DNA Marker DL2000, Code D501A, Lot: CD3401, Takara, Japan.

4 Statistical Methods

The statistical analysis was carried out with SPSS 11.5 software, $P < 0.05$ was regarded as having statistical significance. The enumeration data was tested by chi-square test, the measurement data tested by *t*-test, and the significance test for average value among multiple groups was analyzed by variance analysis.

RESULTS

1 Spectrum of GP Ⅰ b, GP Ⅱ b- Ⅲ a and GMP-140 Activities See Figure 1-3.

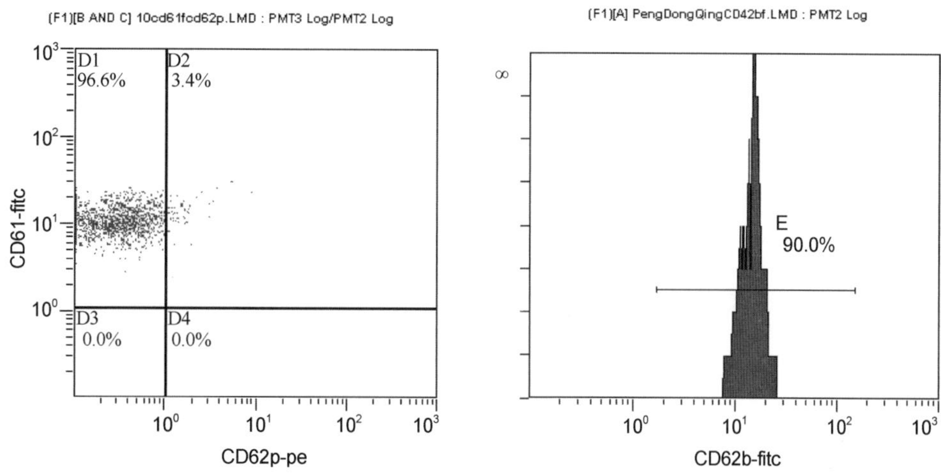

Figure 1　Typical Spectrum of Healthy Subject

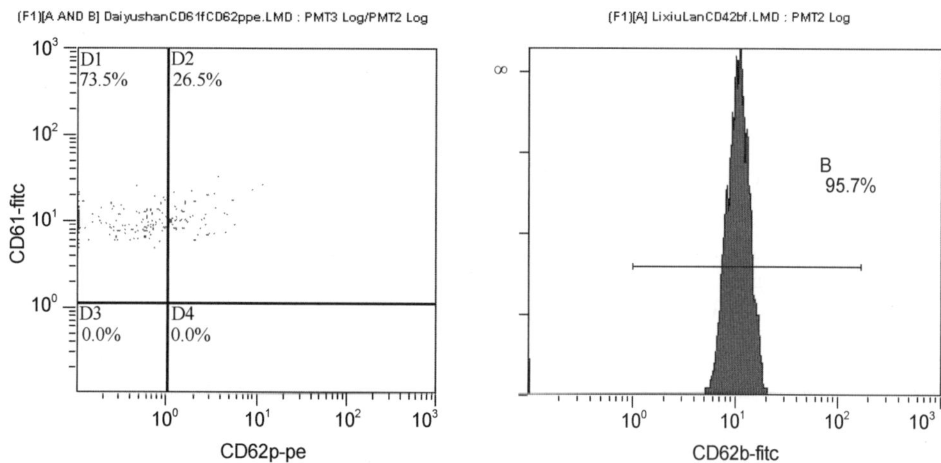

Figure 2　Typical Spectrum of CHD Patients with BSS

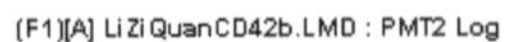

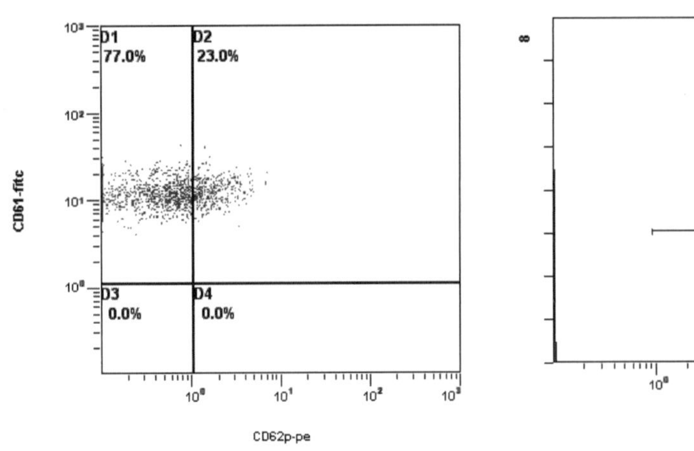

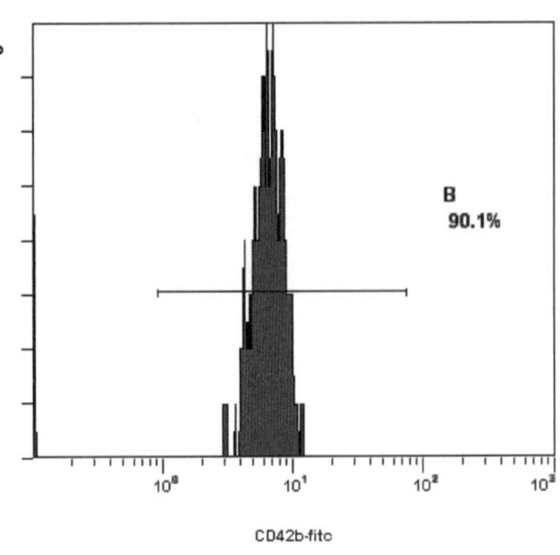

Figure 3 Typical Spectrum of CHD Patients with Non-BSS

Note: Figure 1-3 were typical scatterplots of CD61-FITC、CD62p-PE and histograms of CD42b-FITC in flow cytometry. As compared with the healthy subjects, the MFI of CD61 and CD62p of CHD patients were higher, and the MFI of CD42b was weaker.

2 Comparison of GP Ⅰb, GP Ⅱb-Ⅲa and GMP-140 Activities between Groups

As compared with the control group, the MFI of CD61 and CD62p were higher, the MFI of CD42b was weaker in the two groups of patients ($P < 0.05$). Table 1. As compared with the Group B, the MFI of CD61 and CD62p were higher in Group A ($P < 0.05$), but the MFI of CD42b was insignificantly different between the two groups of patients. Table 2.

Table 1 Comparisons of GP Ⅰ b, GP Ⅱ b- Ⅲ a and GMP-140 Activities between CHD Patients and Healthy Subjects

Group	*n*	CD61 MFI	CD62p MFI	CD42b MFI
Healthy Subjects	39	13.66 ± 4.23	2.26 ± 0.76	14.36 ± 3.11
CHD Patients	77	17.65 ± 4.97*	2.84 ± 0.92*	12.28 ± 2.58*

Notes: * $P < 0.05$, vs Healthy Subjects.

Table 2 Comparison of GP Ⅰ b, GP Ⅱ b- Ⅲ a and GMP-140 Activities between Two Groups of CHD Patients

Group	*n*	CD61 MFI	CD62p MFI	CD42b MFI
Group B	37	15.95 ± 4.37	2.62 ± 0.80	12.83 ± 2.94
Group A	40	19.21 ± 5.02*	3.04 ± 0.98*	11.77 ± 2.10

Notes: * $P < 0.05$, vs Group B.

3 Relationship between the Number of Affected Coronary Branches and the Levels of GP Ⅰb, GP Ⅱb-Ⅲ and GMP-140

As shown in the Table 3, MFI of CD61, CD62p and CD42b in CHD patients with different numbers of affected coronary branches was insignificantly different ($P > 0.05$).

Table 3 Comparison of GP Ⅰ b, GP Ⅱ b- Ⅲ a and GMP-140 Activities in CHD Patients with Different Branches of Affected Coronary Artery

Group	*n*	CD61 MFI	CD62p MFI	CD42b MFI
Single Branch Lesion	28	17.62 ± 5.23	2.96 ± 0.87	12.35 ± 2.95
Bi-branched Lesion	31	17.37 ± 4.55	2.82 ± 1.03	12.56 ± 2.15
Tri-branched Lesion	18	18.16 ± 5.50	2.66 ± 0.80	11.68 ± 2.67

4 Genotype Pattern

Allelic Discrimination Plot of GP Ⅱ b was Figure 4. Sequencing Map of GP Ⅰ b was Figure 5-7.

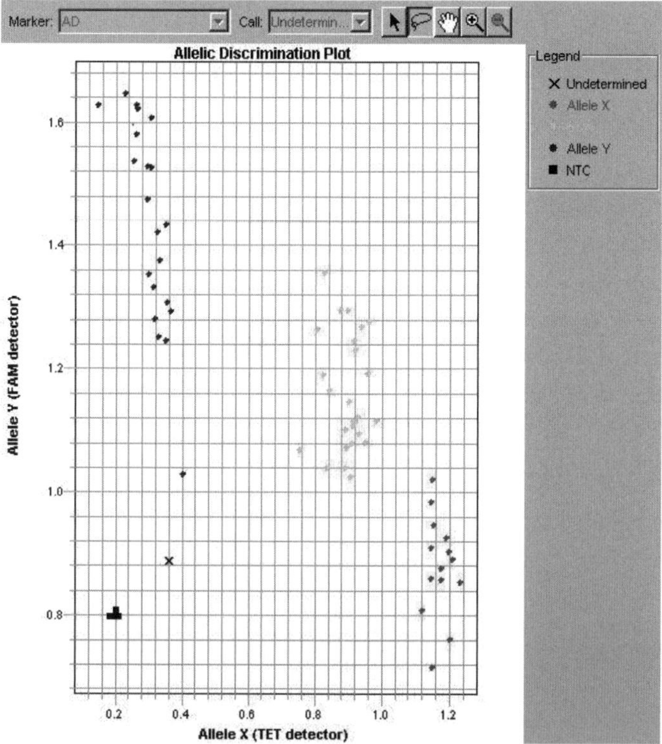

Figure 4 Allelic Discrimination Plot of GP Ⅱ b

Notes: NTC: No Template control; Undetermined; Red spot: Allele C homozygote; Blue spot: Allele A homozygote; Green spot: heterozygote. The genotype of Allele C homozygote was HPA-3b/3b, that of Allele A homozygote was HPA-3a/3a, and that of AC heterozygote was HPA-3a/3b.

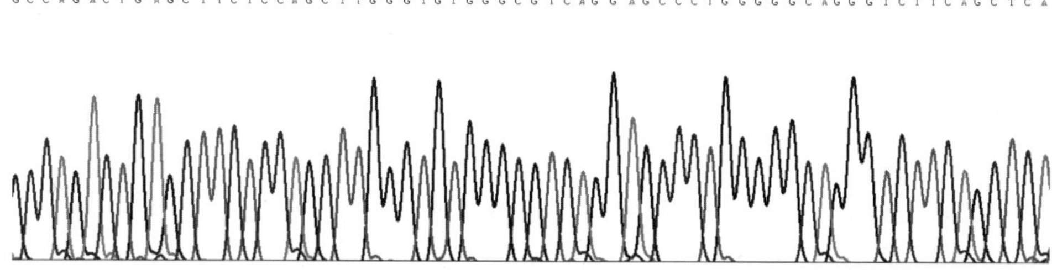

Figure 5 Positive Direction Sequencing Map of Complementary Chain of GP Ⅰ b CC Genotype

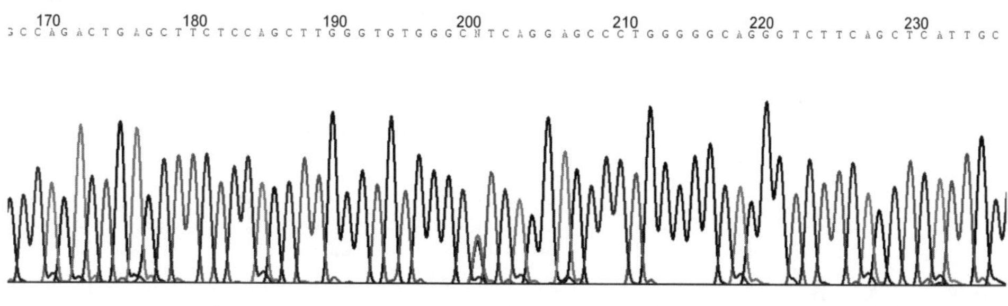

Figure 6 Positive Direction Sequencing Map of Complementary Chain of GP Ⅰ b CT Genotype

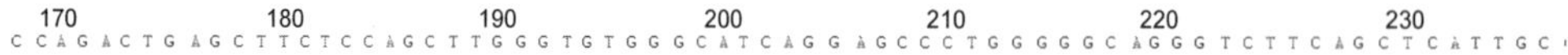
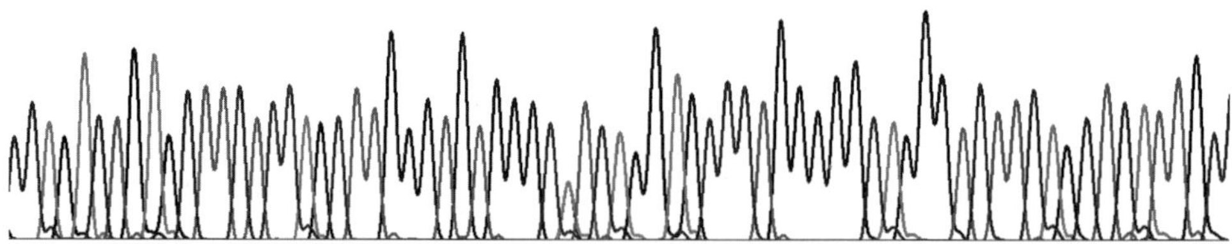

Figure 7 Positive Direction Sequencing Map of Complementary Chain of GP Ⅰ b TT Genotype

Notes: The basic group in the 200th locus was the position for polymorphism detection. The genotype of Allele C homozygote was HPA-2a/2a, that of Allele T homozygote was HPA-2b/2b, and that of CT heterozygote was HPA-2a/2b.

5 Comparisons of GP Ⅰ b, GP Ⅱ b-Ⅲ a and GMP-140 Activities in All the Subjects Enrolled with Different Genotypes

MFI of GP Ⅰ b, GP Ⅱ b- Ⅲ a and GMP-140 were insignificantly different in subjects of HPA-3a/3a genotype as compared with in those of HPA-3a/3b+HPA-3b/3b genotype, also insignificantly different in subjects of HPA-2a/2a genotype as compared with in those of HPA-2a/2b+HPA-2b/2b genotype (all $P>0.05$). See Table 4 and 5.

Table 4 GP Ⅰ b, GP Ⅱ b– Ⅲ a and GMP–140 Activities on HPA–3 Polymorphism Locus

Group	*n*	CD61 MFI	CD62p MFI	CD42b MFI
HPA-3a/3a	31	16.01 ± 5.25	2.41 ± 0.88	13.15 ± 2.36
HPA-3a/3b+ HPA-3b/3b	85	16.41 ± 5.04	2.73 ± 0.91	12.92 ± 3.11

Table 5 GP Ⅰ b, GP Ⅱ b– Ⅲ a and GMP–140 Activities on HPA–2 Polymorphism Locus

Group	*n*	CD61 MFI	CD62p MFI	CD42b MFI
HPA-2a/2a	105	16.17 ± 5.08	2.64 ± 0.89	12.99 ± 2.98
HPA-2a/2b+ HPA-2b/2b	11	17.62 ± 5.12	2.60 ± 1.10	12.86 ± 2.42

6 Comparisons of GP Ⅰ b, GP Ⅱ b-Ⅲ a and GMP-140 Activities in All the CHD Patients Enrolled with Different Genotypes

MFI of GP Ⅰ b, GP Ⅱ b- Ⅲ a and GMP-140 were insignificantly different in patients of HPA-3a/3a genotype as compared with in those of HPA-3a/3b+HPA-3b/3b genotype, also insignificantly different in patients of HPA-2a/2a genotype as compared with in those of HPA-2a/2b+HPA-2b/2b genotype (all $P>0.05$). See Table 6 and 7.

Table 6 GP Ⅰ b, GP Ⅱ b– Ⅲ a and GMP–140 Activities on HPA–3 Polymorphism Locus

Group	*n*	CD61 MFI	CD62p MFI	CD42b MFI
HPA-3a/3a	14	18.64 ± 4.77	2.73 ± 0.96	12.08 ± 2.02
HPA-3a/3b+ HPA-3b/3b	63	17.42 ± 5.03	2.86 ± 0.92	12.33 ± 2.70

Table 7 GP Ⅰ b, GP Ⅱ b– Ⅲ a and GMP–140 Activities on HPA–2 Polymorphism Locus

Group	*n*	CD61 MFI	CD62p MFI	CD42b MFI
HPA-2a/2a	70	17.54 ± 4.92	2.82 ± 0.90	12.26 ± 2.61
HPA-2a/2b+ HPA-2b/2b	7	18.70 ± 5.70	3.01 ± 1.19	12.51 ± 2.58

DISCUSSION

Coronary heart disease is the most commonly seen pattern of atherosclerosis induced organic changes, its main risk factors including smoking, hyperlipidemia, hypertension and diabetes mellitus. The pathogenesis of atherosclerosis is closely related with platelet aggregation and thrombus formation, and the adhesion and aggregation of platelet in the subintima of injured vessels is one of the important initiating factors for thrombus formation[3]. Platelet membranous glycoprotein plays important role in the platelet adhesion, aggregation and releasing reaction, and it is the specific molecular marker of platelet activation.

GP Ⅱ b- Ⅲ a (CD41-CD61)is a member of connexin family, the final common channel for platelet aggregation induced by different stimulants[4], excepting participates the aggregation, it also take part in the platelet adhesion. It is decreased in case of thrombasthenia, platelet deletion and platelet abnormality. Therefore, the platelet activation can be accurately detected by using its fluorescent mono-antibody in rather early stage. GP Ⅰ b (CD42b)is a vWF receptor belongs to the mucoprotein family, and will be absent in giant platelet syndrome. Platelet α-granular membrane protein 140 (GMP-140, CD62p), as a member of lectin family, has the function for intermediating the adhesion of activated platelet with neutrophilic granulocyte and monocyte. It is interiorly located as the platelet in silent state, but when platelet is activated, along with the de-granulating and releasing reaction, it is redistributed to the surface of platelet membrane, therefore, CD62p is regarded as the best marker for platelet activation, a sensitive flag of activated platelet[5-7].

In this study on the relationship of platelet activity with CHD and BSS in CHD, patients receiving no drugs for anti-platelet and anticoagulation in the latest two weeks were selected to avoid the interfering of drugs on platelet activity as possible, and detection on the fluorescence intensity of related glycoprotein at platelet surface is performed for representing the degree of platelet activation. The results showed that the levels of platelet activation markers, GP Ⅱ b- Ⅲ a and GMP-140, were higher in CHD patients than those in healthy persons ($P < 0.05$), also higher in CHD patients with BSS than those in CHD patients with non-BSS ($P < 0.05$); but the level of GP Ⅰ b was significantly lower in CHD patients than that in healthy persons ($P < 0.05$), these results suggested that platelet activation plays important role in the genesis and development process of CHD and BSS in CHD. Thus, the platelet activated molecules, GP Ⅱ b- Ⅲ a and GMP-140, could be taken as objective indexes for microscopic syndrome differentiation of BSS, while the lowering of GP Ⅰ b expression is possibly have respect to the entering of GP Ⅰ b into the open pipe system[8] after platelet activation. There is no report concerning the relation of GP Ⅰ b activity with BSS in CHD so far. In this study, CHD patients with BSS showed no difference in GP Ⅰ b level as compared with CHD patients with non-BS syndrome ($P < 0.05$), suggesting that this glycoprotein is not a sensitive indicator for BSS in CHD.

The results displayed that the MFI of CD61、CD62p及CD42b were not significantly different in CHD patients with various number of affected branches ($P < 0.05$). This outcome is unlike to that reported previously[9], which showed that the positive CD61 receptor expression was higher in unstable patients of angina with complex lesions than in patients with simple lesion. The discrepancy might be due to the difference in some factors as observation indexes, grading of complexion and time of case registration.

No study on the relationship between gene polymorphism and platelet membrane glycoprotein activity was reported previously. In this study, it was found that the MFI of CD61, CD62p and CD42b in the two different polymorphism genotypes, GP Ⅱ b HPA-3 and GP Ⅰ b HPA-2, were insignificantly different ($P > 0.05$), suggesting that the changes of amino acid expressions induced by the two polymorphism loci didn't have significant affection on the activities of GP Ⅰ b and GP Ⅱ b- Ⅲ a. This outcome was somewhat connected with the study recently reported overseas, in which[10], the constitution platelet embolus was compared between populations of Caucasian and Africa origin American (AOA)with different Ko^a expression rates, which was induced by shear force in a platelet aggregation induction test. It was found that the polymorphism of HPA-2 in AOA could not induce changing of platelet function. Whereas, the activities of GP Ⅰb, GP Ⅱb-Ⅲa and GMP-140 were truly different between CHD patients and healthy persons, also between CHD with BSS and CHD with non-BSS, so the existence of other polymorphism loci influencing activity expression in the coded gene of platelet membrane glycoprotein could not be excluded.

REFERENCES

[1] Chen HZ. Practical Internal Medicine[M]. 12th ed. Beijing: People's Medical Publishing House, 2005, 1472-1473.

[2] Society of Cardiology, Chinese Association of the Integration of Traditional and Western Medicine. The diagnostic criteria of TCM in coronary heart disease[J]. J Integr Tradit West Med, 1991, 11 (5): 257.

[3] Jackson SP, Schoenwaelder SM. Antiplatelet therapy: in search of the 'magic bullet' [J]. Nat Rev Drug Discov, 2003, 2 (10): 775-789.

[4] Rauch U, Osende JI, Fuster V, et al. Thrombus formation on atherosclerotic plaques: pathogenesis and clinical consequences[J]. Ann Intern Med, 2001, 134 (3): 224-238.

[5] Michelson AD, Barnard MR, Krueger LA, et al. Circulating monocyte-platelet aggregates are a more sensitive marker of in vivo platelet activation than platelet surface P-selectin: studies in baboons, human coronary intervention, and human acute myocardial infarction[J]. Circulation, 2001, 104 (13): 1533-1537.

[6] Zhang WG, Yan TX, Gao FJ, et al. Study on Effect of Zhixinkang Capsule (脂欣康胶囊)in TreatingUnstable Effort Angina and Hyperlipidemia and Its Function in Vascular Endothelium Protection[J]. Chinese Journal of Integrative Medicine, 2003, 9 (1): 25-30.

[7] Liu ZG, Yu XY. Effects of Xuezhikang Capsule (血脂康胶囊)on Blood Lipids, Platelet Activation and Coagulation-Fibrinolysis Activity in Patients with Hyperlipidemia[J]. Chinese Journal of Integrative Medicine, 2004, 10 (4): 259-262.

[8] Wang JZ. Applications of Flow Cytometry in Clinical Researches[M]. Shanghai: Shanghai Science and Technology Press, 2005: 1.

[9] Tian XY, Liu ZZ, Zhang JL. Relationship between different coronary lesions of unstable angina pectoris and platelet GP Ⅱb-Ⅲa receptor expression[J]. Journal of Cardiovascular & Pulmonary Diseases, 2002, 21 (1): 22-23.

[10] Williams Ms, Ng'alla LS, Vaidya D, et al. Platelet functional implications of glycoprotein Ⅰbalpha polymorphisms in African Americans[J]. Am J Hematol, 2007, 82 (1): 15-22.

First published: XUE Mei, CHEN Ke-ji, YIN Hui-jun. Relationship between platelet activation related factors and polymorphism of related genes in patients with coronary heart disease of blood-stasis syndrome. [J] . Chin J Integr Med, 2008, 14 (4): 267-273.

Effects of Propyl Gallate on Carotid Artery Thrombosis and Coagulation/Fibrinolysis System in Rats

JIANG Yue-rong, YIN Hui-jun, LIU Jian-gang, MA Lu, and CHEN Ke-ji

Propyl gallate (PrG, $C_{10}H_{12}O_5$)is an alkyl ester of gallic acid, an active component from *Radix Paeoniae rubra*. It is reported that PrG has the effect of inhibiting platelet aggregation induced by arachidonic acid and preventing hydroxy radical injury[1,2]. PrG has been clinically used for the treatment of thrombotic diseases such as coronary heart disease, cerebral thrombosis, and thrombophlebitis, etc. Recently, a study reported that PrG is a new inductor of *in vitro* platelet activation[3]. Our previous in vitro studies also show that PrG could activate cyclooxygenase-1 (COX-1)at concentrations lower than 1×10^{-6} mol/L. It was presumed that PrG might have an *in vitro* platelet activating function at lower concentrations, which was not agreeable with its antiplatelet-aggregation and antithrombogenesis functions as seen in *in vivo* studies[4]. Therefore, the effect of PrG on the thrombus formation time as well as coagulation and fibrinolysis system was observed in an experimental carotid artery thrombosis model in rats and changes induced by PrG in the *in vivo* coagulation and fibrolytic pathway were also explored.

METHODS

1 Experimental Animals

Fifty Sprague-Dawley rats, SPF grade, weighing 180-200 g, half females and half males, were provided by Beijing Weitong Lihua Experimental Animal Co., Ltd., China, with a certificate serial number SCXK (Beijing)2003-0003.

2 Drug and Reagents

Propyl gallate injection was provided by Fujian Mindong Rejuvenation Pharmaceutical Co., Ltd., China (batch No. 030505). Heparin sodium injection was provided by Shanghai Biochemistry Pharmaceutical Co., Ltd., China (Lot No. 030112). The tested drugs were prepared with normal saline to the appropriate concentrations.

Enzyme linked immunosorbent assay (ELISA)kits for tissue-type plasminogen activator (t-PA)and plasminogen activator inhibitor-1 (PAI-1)were both purchased from Beijing Laibo Biological Experimental Technique Research Institute (Lot No. M24001), China.

3 Experimental Apparatus

The experimental in vivo thrombosis radiometer (Type BT87-3)was manufactured by Inner Mongolia Medical College, China. The automatic enzyme micro-plate reader (Type Wellscan MK3)was manufactured by Labsystems Dragon Company, Finland.

4 Grouping and Administration

The rats were randomly divided into 5 groups after 1 week of adaptive breeding. There were 10 rats in each group: the normal group (normal saline, 2 mL/kg), the model group (normal saline, 2 mL/kg), the heparin group (1 250 IU/kg), the low dose PrG (30 mg/kg)group and the high dose PrG (60 mg/kg)group. The rats were administered with saline or corresponding drugs by intravenous injection, respectively. Thirty minutes after administration, the carotid artery thrombus was induced by continuous electric stimulation except for those in the normal group.

5 Establishment of Carotid Artery Thrombosis Model

The rats were anaesthetized with 20% ethyl urethane (0.7 mL/100 g body weight)and the skin of neck was routinely sterilized. The right common carotid artery was carefully separated for about 1.5 cm in length and then the stimulating electrode and the temperature feeler of the thrombosis radiometer were linked to the double ends of the artery, respectively. Thirty minutes after intravenous injection of the corresponding drugs into the femoral vein, the arterial endothelium was injured with a galvanic current stimulation of 1.5 mV for 7 min after turning on the switch of the radiometer. With the formation of the thrombus, the arterial blood flow was gradually blocked. When the carotid arterial embolism occurred, the surface temperature of the artery would drop abruptly and the apparatus would automatically trigger an alarm. The surface temperature of the artery was monitored and the duration from the initiation of electric stimulation to the sudden drop of the carotid surface temperature was recorded as the thrombus formation time.

6 Determination of t-PA and PAI-1

Blood samples (2 mL)drawn from abdominal aorta were anticoagulated by natrium citricum and centrifuged at 3 000r/min for 15 min. The plasma was collected and preserved in a refrigerator at −20 ℃. Plasma t-PA and PAI-1 were determined by ELISA according to the manual in the kits.

7 Statistical Analysis

Analysis was performed using SPSS 11.0 software. Data were expressed as mean ± standard deviation. *One-way ANOVA* was used to compare the results among groups and q-test to compare the data between groups. A P value < 0.05 was considered statistically significant.

RESULTS

1 Effect of PrG on Thrombus Formation Time in Rats with Carotid Artery Thrombosis

The thrombus formation time was prolonged in both high and low dose PrG groups as compared with the model group with a significant difference seen only in the high dose group (60 mg/kg, $P < 0.01$), indicating that PrG has a certain effect on preventing arterial thrombosis. Compared with the heparin control group, the thrombus formation time was obviously shortened in both high and low dose PrG groups ($P < 0.05$, $P < 0.01$), indicating that the antithrombotic action of PrG was obviously weaker than that of heparin (Table 1).

Table 1 Effect of PrG on Thrombus Formation Time in Rats with Carotid Artery Thrombosis ($\bar{x} \pm s$)

Group	Dose	n	Thrombus formation time (s)
Model	--	10	742.60 ± 202.89
Heparin control	1250 IU/kg	10	1740.63 ± 379.99*
Low dose PrG	30 mg/kg	10	1111.60 ± 307.05$^{\triangle}$
High dose PrG	60 mg/kg	10	1297.50 ± 131.24$^{*\triangle\triangle}$

Notes: $^{*}P < 0.01$, compared with the model group ; $^{\triangle}P < 0.05$, $^{\triangle\triangle}P < 0.01$, compared with the heparin control group.

2 Effect of PrG on Plasma Levels of t-PA and PAI-1 in Rats with Carotid Arterial Thrombosis

Compared with the normal group, the plasma t-PA was obviously lower and PAI-1 obviously higher in the model group (both $P < 0.05$), indicating the existence of disequilibrium of t-PA and PAI in rats with thrombosis. Compared with the model group, the plasma t-PA and the ratio of t-PA/PAI in the heparin group were significantly raised, while PAI-1 levels were significantly decreased ($P < 0.05$ or $P < 0.01$). The plasma t-PA levels in both high and low dose PrG groups were raised ($P < 0.05$), while the PAI-1 levels were not changed significantly. The ratio of t-PA/PAI in both groups show an increasing tendency but there was no significant difference ($P > 0.05$). Compared with the heparin group, the ratio of t-PA/PAI-1 in both high and low dose PrG groups was significantly lowered ($P < 0.01$), indicating that the effect of PrG in regulating the disequilibrium of t-PA/PAI-1 was weaker than that of heparin (Table 2).

Table 2 Effect of PrG on Plasma Level of t–PA, PAI–1 and t–PA/ PAI–1 in Rats with Carotid Arterial Thrombosis ($\bar{x} \pm s$)

Group	Dose	n	t-PA (μg/L)	PAI-1 (μg/L)	t-PA/PAI-1
Normal	-	10	14.77 ± 2.37	13.94 ± 3.51	1.06 ± 0.18
Model	-	10	$8.91 \pm 2.23^{*}$	$20.49 \pm 8.20^{*}$	$0.59 \pm 0.25^{*}$
Heparin control	1 250 IU/kg	10	$13.88 \pm 5.97^{\triangle}$	$6.00 \pm 5.59^{\triangle\triangle}$	$2.02 \pm 1.09^{\triangle\triangle}$
Low dose PrG	30 mg/kg	10	$13.32 \pm 2.74^{\triangle}$	$19.48 \pm 6.51^{\blacktriangle}$	$0.88 \pm 0.27^{\blacktriangle}$
High dose PrG	60 mg/kg	10	$13.63 \pm 3.99^{\triangle}$	$22.17 \pm 5.87^{\blacktriangle}$	$0.74 \pm 0.25^{\blacktriangle}$

Notes: $^{*}P < 0.05$, compared with the normal group ; $^{\triangle}P < 0.05$, $^{\triangle\triangle}P < 0.01$, compared with the model group ; $^{\blacktriangle}P < 0.01$, compared with the heparin control group.

DISCUSSION

Ninety percent of arterial thromboembolism was accompanied by arterial sclerotic plaques, such as coronary arterial thrombosis. Moreover, arteriole thrombus is also common, mostly seen in lung, liver, brain and kidney, etc. In this study, the common carotid artery was stimulated with a galvanic current to injure the vascular intima and to activate the platelet and blood coagulation system, leading to the injury of vascular endothelial cells, thus decreasing the synthesis and release of prostacyclin (PG Ⅰ 2), and resulting in the gradual formation of intravascular mixed thrombus. When the arterial blood flow was blocked due to the formation of thrombus in the carotid artery, the temperature of the distal end of the artery would abruptly drop. After sensing the decreased surface temperature of the artery, the thermal detector used in this study would automatically trigger an alarm. The duration from the initiation of electric stimulation to the sudden drop of carotid temperature was recorded as the thrombus formation time, i. e. occlusion time, which is used as an indicator to evaluate the drug action[5].

The fibrinolytic pathway and the blood coagulation pathways are kept in an equilibrium state under physiological conditions. The functional disorder of blood coagulation and/or fibrinolysis serves as one of the pathophysiologic mechanisms of cardiovascular and/or cerebrovascular diseases. t-PA and PAI-1, secreted by vascular endothelium cells, co-regulate the plasmin activity and play an important role in the balance of blood coagulation and fibrinolysis. The main function of t-PA is to lower and clear fibrinogen and thus, prevent thrombosis. PAI-1 can deactivate t-PA and is also regarded as an independent risk factor of cardio-and/or cerebrovascular thrombotic diseases[6]. Some research has shown that PAI-1, secreted into plasma in an active form, had an inhibitory effect on t-PA and urokinase type plasminogen activator (u-PA), resulting in a decrease of active fibrinolysin and a disturbance of fibrin degradation, promoting thrombogenesis. Under pathological conditions, the ratio of t-PA/PAI-1 decreases, indicating decreased endogenic fibrinolytic activity.

When the level of t-PA decreases and/or PAI-1 increases, the fibrinolytic pathway cannot timely lyse the intravascular fibrin deposits. Hence a tendency to go into a pre-thrombotic or hypercoagulabale thrombotic state will occur.

This study shows that the arterial thrombus formation time was prolonged in the high dose PrG animals compared with the model group ($P < 0.01$), indicating that PrG had a certain effect of preventing arterial thrombosis. Both high and low dose PrG animals showed a trend in elevating the ratio of t-PA/PAI.

However, no significant difference was noted compared with the model control group. Therefore PrG was believed to have certain anti-arterial thrombosis effects, but the action was obviously weaker than that of heparin. Regulating the t-PA/PAI-1 ratio to an equilibrium may be one of the mechanisms for PrG to inhibit thrombosis.

REFERENCES

[1] Liu J, Lu EW, Li XG, et al. Effect of propyl gallate on thromboxane B2, arachidonic acid metabolism and platelet aggragation in patients with coronary heart disease or cerebral thrombosis[J]. Chin Med J (Chin), 1983, 63 (8): 477-481.

[2] Zheng GY, Chen XC, Du J, et al. Inhibition of neuronal apoptosis induced by cerebral ischemia-reperfusion through down-regulation of nNOS and iNOS expression by propyl gallate[J]. Chin Pharma Bull (Chin), 2006, 22 (8): 992-997.

[3] Xiao H, Kovics R, Jackson V, et al. Effects of platelet inhibitors on propyl gallate-induced platelet aggregation, protein tyrosine phosphorylation, and platelet factor 3 activation[J]. Blood Coagul Fibrinolysis, 2004, 15: 199-206.

[4] Yin HJ, Jiang YR, Wu XH, et al. Effect of propyl gallate on activity of cyclooxygenase 1 and 2 in mice's peritoneal macrophages[J]. Chin J Integr Med, 2004, 10 (3): 213-217.

[5] Qin JM, Li Z, Shi S. Research and application of an experimental in vivo thrombosis measurement apparatus[J]. Chin Pharm Bull (Chin), 1992, 8 (3): 236-237.

[6] Yazici M, Demircan S, Durna K, et al. Relationship between myocardial injury and soluble P-selectin in non-ST elevation acute coronary syndromes[J]. Circ J, 2005, 69: 530-535.

First published: JIANG Yue-rong, YIN Hui-jun, LIU Jian-gang, MA Lu, and CHEN Ke-ji. Effects of propyl gallate on carotid artery thrombosis and coagulation/fibrinolysis system in rats[J]. Chin J Integr Med, 2008, 14 (1): 42-45.

附　　录

附录一　硕士、博士研究生，博士后人员及师承学生名录

姓 名	学 位	学习时间	毕业论文题目	指导老师
何愉生	硕士	1978-1981	赤芍精抗血小板作用的临床和实验研究	
董泉珍	硕士	1978-1981	生脉散注射液治疗急性心肌梗死的血流动力学效应	
刘裕钊	硕士	1978-1981	青心酮对冠心病心绞痛病人运动标测心电图及左心功能的影响	
刘　京	硕士	1979-1982	赤芍 801 对冠心病、脑血栓形成病人血栓素 $β_2$、花生四烯酸代谢及血小板聚集性的影响	
张铁忠	硕士	1979-1982	男性冠心病患者血浆雌激素水平与中医证候类型关系研究	
马胜兴	硕士	1979-1982	延胡索碱抗心律失常作用的实验与临床研究	
梁洪之	硕士	1982-1985	核听诊器 ^{99}TC 评价人参与复方人参注射液对老年心力衰竭影响研究	
余　真	硕士	1983-1986	生脉口服液治疗冠心病的临床与实验研究	
陈　楷	硕士， 博士	1984-1987, 1994-1997	清宫长春丹对老年液化智能影响临床及实验研究； 益智胶囊治疗老年血管性痴呆的临床与实验研究	
张文彭	硕士	1984-1987	老年肾虚证血浆过氧化脂质、高密度脂蛋白胆固醇水平及清宫长春丹治疗作用的临床观察	
陈耀青	硕士	1984-1987	冠心病气阴两虚证心功能特点及生脉注射液的效应观察	
王　阶	博士	1985-1988	血瘀证诊断标准研究	
吴　锦	博士	1985-1988	冠心病血瘀证患者血小板超微结构和功能的研究	
丘万嵩	硕士	1986-1989	消补减肥片对高脂血症影响的临床研究	
卫　明	硕士	1986-1989	长生降压液对中老年肾虚型高血压病及心肌肥厚影响的临床研究	
崔　晶	硕士	1987-1990	复方西洋参口服液延缓衰老作用的临床研究	
史大卓	博士	1990-1993	中医药防治经皮冠状动脉成形术后再狭窄的基础实验与临床研究	陈明哲
李　静	博士	1991-1994	活血化瘀复方（血管通）抗动脉粥样硬化的实验及临床研究	
李艳梅	博士	1992-1995	中药复方血府逐瘀丸抗动脉粥样硬化临床与实验研究	
王　伟	博士	1993-1996	精制血府逐瘀胶囊抗心肌缺血的实验与临床研究	
雷　燕	博士	1993-1996	愈心痛胶囊抗心肌缺血的实验研究及临床观察	
张群豪	博士	1993-1996	血府逐瘀浓缩丸抗 AS 的实验与临床研究	
申铉守（韩国）	博士	1993-1996	中韩医学对缺血性中风的临床比较研究	
夏亦嗣（美国）	博士	1994-1997	高血压病中医证型的临床与实验研究	
秦淑兰	师承	1994-1996	陈可冀临床医疗经验总结	
潘苏燕	师承	1994-1996	陈可冀临床医疗经验总结	
周亚伟	博士	1994-1997	藿酮胶囊抗心肌缺血的实验研究及临床观察	
尹太英（韩国）	博士	1994-1997	抗心肌缺血及冠心病辨证冠脉造影所见研究	
赵英杰 （新加坡）	博士	1994-1997	中西医结合生理学年龄的临床与实验研究	
谢梅林	博士	1995-1998	消瘀片调脂和抗动脉粥样硬化实验与临床研究	顾振纶
柯富扬 （中国台湾）	博士	1995-1998	芎芍制剂对冠心病影响的临床与实验研究	戴锡孟
张　壮	博士	1995-1998	芎芍制剂成分及其血液动力学研究	
于　蓓	硕士	1995-1998	活血化瘀方药防治冠心病介入治疗后再狭窄研究	

续表

姓 名	学 位	学习时间	毕业论文题目	指导老师
黄 熙	博士后	1996-1998	方剂治疗药物监测：理论与方法学初探	
张方直	博士	1996-1999	川芎嗪对血管系统血流动力学影响的实验与临床研究	洪传岳 林昭庚 黄怡超
韩 玲	博士	1997-2000	益心康胶囊抗心肌缺血及再灌注损伤的实验药理学研究	
徐 浩	博士	1997-2000	芎芍胶囊预防冠心病介入治疗后再狭窄的研究	史大卓
马晓昌	师承 博士	1997-2000, 2002-2005	陈可冀老师学术经验总结； 冠心病心绞痛冠脉病变及中医证型与血小板膜糖蛋白、溶血磷脂酸的研究	杜建
徐凤芹	师承 博士	1997-2000, 2000-2003	陈可冀老师学术经验总结； 芎芍胶囊防治动脉粥样硬化血管重构的临床与实验研究	邵念方（博士学位）
张荣华	博士后	1998-2000	益骨胶囊（补肾活血液）治疗骨质疏松症的临床和实验研究	
蔡 晶	博士	1999-2002	康欣胶囊对血管性痴呆影响的实验和临床研究	杜建 林求诚
卢全生	博士	2000-2003	清眩降压胶囊治疗轻中度高血压病的实验和临床研究	
马春涛	博士	2000-2003	老年心肌缺血研究	
王卫霞	硕士	2000-2005 因 SARS 延后	血脂康胶囊治疗高脂血症有效性和安全性的系统评价	
陆 曙	博士后	2001-2005	中药对钙超载心肌损伤的保护作用	
鹿小燕	博士	2001-2004	芎芍胶囊改善血管重构干预冠心病介入治疗后再狭窄的研究	吕树铮
尤士杰	博士	2001-2004	心血管病临床诊断治疗研究	
姚魁武	博士	2001-2004	血瘀证量化诊断及病证结合研究	王阶
徐丽林	博士	2001-2004	冠心病危险因素、冠状动脉病变及支架术后再狭窄与中医证型相关性研究	王阶
刘菊妍	博士后	2002-2004	戒毒中药研究	
赵含森	博士后	2002-2004	中西医结合临床医学发展规律和历史	
张京春	师承 博士 博士后	2002-2005, 2004-2007, 2007-2010	陈可冀老师有关血瘀证及活血化瘀治法临床应用的经验； 解毒活血干预动脉粥样硬化易损斑块的综合研究； 陈可冀学术思想和及临证经验的研究	张文高（博士学位）
李立志	师承 博士	2002-2005 2004-2007	陈可冀老师诊治心力衰竭学术思想及临证经验总结 基于数据挖掘方法冠心病中医辨证相关规律的探索	
宋 军	博士	2002-2005	脑梗死血瘀证的量化研究	杜建
蒋跃绒	博士 博士后	2002-2005, 2007-2010	赤芍 801 调节血管炎症反应和血小板活化的基础与临床研究 陈可冀病证结合学术思想及其在活血化瘀防治心血管病中的应用	
文 川	博士	2002-2005	活血中药对 ApoE 基因缺陷小鼠动脉粥样硬化斑块稳定性影响的研究	黄启福
周佩云	博士	2002-2005	代谢综合征及清脂降糖片治疗作用研究	葛文津
苗 阳	硕士	2002-2005	西苑医院中西医结合诊治急性心肌梗死的系统性回顾与分析	黄尧州 王阶
汪晓芳	硕士	2002-2005	洋参二醇皂苷注射液治疗冠心病心绞痛临床研究	史大卓 魏子孝 李振华
王承龙	博士后	2003-2005	西洋参茎叶总皂苷对急性心肌梗死大鼠心肌血管新生及能量代谢的影响	史大卓
王振瑞	博士后	2003-2005	中国中西医结合史论	李经纬
郭 艳	博士后	2003-2005	蒺藜总皂苷对高脂血症大鼠心肌梗死后心室重构的作用及机制研究	
马 路	博士后	2003-2005	理气活血“药对”组分配伍保护内皮细胞损伤的机理研究	
王文祥	博士后	2003-2005	丹参、赤芍活血化瘀有效部位配伍抗肝纤维化作用的研究	

续表

姓 名	学 位	学习时间	毕业论文题目	指导老师
曾显棠(中国台湾)	博士后	2003-2006	北京地区中医医院急性心肌梗死患者中医证型和生存质量分析	
张　颖	博士	2003-2006	西洋参茎叶总皂苷对冠心病胰岛素敏感性影响及其作用机制研究	
王培利	博士	2003-2006	益气活血治法促缺血心肌血管生成实验研究及其疗效评价	
张红霞	博士	2003-2006	川芎嗪与丹参酚酸B联合干预剪应力诱导血栓形成的研究	廖福龙
梅之南	博士后	2004-2006	臭灵丹化学成分及新剂型研究	史大卓
薛　梅	博士	2004-2007	血小板GP Ⅱ b- Ⅲ a、Ⅰ b基因多态性、活性与冠心病血瘀证的相关性研究	
饶向荣	博士	2004-2007	马兜铃酸中药肾损害的临床研究	戴希文
吴大嵘	博士后	2005-2008	建立以中医理论为基础的健康量表的初步研究	赖世隆 史大卓
毛　炜	博士后	2005-2008	中药肾康注射液防治慢性肾功能衰竭作用机理探讨	
江　巍	博士后	2005-2008	生脉散改善冠状动脉搭桥术后患者生活质量的临床研究	
王宁元	博士后	2005-2007	人参皂甙Rg1促进骨髓干细胞分化及毛细血管新生的机理研究	
郑广娟	博士后	2005-2007	不同解毒活血中药配伍稳定动脉粥样硬化斑块的机理研究	
周明学	博士	2005-2008	活血解毒中药干预动脉粥样硬化易损斑块的作用及机理研究	
马晓娟	博士	2005-2008	冠心病血瘀证差异基因表达谱的构建、目标基因的鉴定及功能分析	
胡雯青(中国台湾)	博士	2005-2008	老年冠心病患者中西医结合诊疗状况的前瞻性研究	
谢元华	博士	2005-2008	清宫医案病证与方药的关联性研究	
李　深	博士	2005-2008	慢性原发性肾小球疾病患者血瘀证临床及病理关系研究	戴希文
衡先培	博士后	2006-2008	丹栝方对高糖性血管内皮细胞损害的保护研究	
杨庆有	博士后	2006-2008	黄芪颗粒剂对慢性心衰干预作用量效关系的临床研究	
刘龙涛	博士后	2006-2008	血栓性疾病“瘀毒”理论的文献与实验研究	
朱　伟	博士后	2006-2008	调脾护心方化学信息学研究	徐筱杰 阮新民
迟东升	博士后	2006-2008	纳豆激酶防治兔动脉粥样硬化的实验研究	阮新民
付肖岩	博士后	2006-2008	大肠癌高危人群的中西医临床研究	
郑　锋	博士	2006-2009	冠心病稳定期“瘀毒致病”假说及临床表征研究	
高铸烨	博士	2006-2009	冠心病通补治法的临床应用研究	
夏城东	博士	2006-2009	血糖相关因素对血管内皮功能的影响及川芎嗪干预研究	
陈　浩	博士	2006-2009	解毒活血法治疗急性冠脉综合征临床研究	史大卓
褚剑锋	博士	2006-2009	老年高血压病动态血压与证候联系及清眩降压汤对SHR血压的研究	
任　毅	博士	2006-2009	冠心病介入治疗前后中医证候特征及与实验室指标相关性研究	
吕渭辉	博士	2006-2009	急性冠脉综合征介入治疗围手术期血瘀证诊断试验相关性研究	陈纪言
徐慧聪	博士	2006-2009	黄芪注射液治疗气虚型慢性心力衰竭急性失代偿患者随机对照临床研究	
吴宗贵	师承	2006-2009	心血管病临床研究	
凌昌全	师承	2006-2009	中西医结合临床研究途径	
冯　妍	硕士，博士	2006-2009，2009-2012	不稳定心绞痛活血解毒干预及稳定心绞痛终点事件分析； 基于证候要素的不稳定心绞痛中西医结合治疗方案优化方法学研究	
郗瑞席	硕士	2006-2009	急性冠脉综合征介入术后中医证型及理化指标的研究	
区文超	博士后	2007-2009	薤白皂甙类新化合物FAC-5β的抗血小板作用研究	姚新生
李雪峰	博士	2007-2010	冠心病血瘀证血小板差异蛋白表达分析及川芎赤芍有效部位干预机制研究	
张大武	博士	2007-2010	急性冠脉综合征血运重建前后中医证候要素衍变规律及中药干预机制研究	

续表

姓 名	学 位	学习时间	毕业论文题目	指导老师
徐　伟	博士	2007-2010	急性冠脉综合征中医瘀毒病因研究	
曲　丹	博士	2007-2010	冠心病患者中医证候特点及其衍变规律研究	
王　磊	博士	2007-2010	冠通胶囊动员内皮细胞修复损伤内皮作用机制研究	张敏州
郑国华	博士后	2008-2011	PAFR 基因多态性与冠心病血瘀证关系的病例对照研究	
杨　琳	博士后	2008-2011	西洋参茎叶总皂苷的体内代谢研究	史大卓
黄　烨	博士	2008-2011	活血化瘀中药抗血小板研究	
李　欧	博士	2008-2011	冠心病中西医结合诊治规律的数据挖掘及验证研究	
陈懿宇	博士	2008-2011	中药对高血压伴睡眠呼吸暂停综合征患者血管内皮功能保护机制研究	
麦舒桃	博士	2008-2011	扶阳法联合无创通气治疗急性心力衰竭临床研究	张敏州
刘　玥	博士	2009-2012	血小板骨架蛋白 Gelsolin 在冠心病血瘀证中的作用及赤芍川芎有效组分的干预效应研究	殷惠军
张　萍	博士	2009-2012	延胡索提取物治疗冠心病室性心律失常的机理研究	徐凤芹 马晓昌
杨叔禹	博士	2009-2012	代谢综合征中医病理特征及泽泻汤加味方的疗效观察和机制研究	李灿东
尚青华	博士	2010-2013	冠心病血瘀证“瘀毒”病机转变的蛋白质组学研究	徐　浩
郗瑞席	博士	2010-2013	冠心病介入治疗后中医证候诊断标准的系统研究	李立志
彭　军	博士后	2011-2014	片仔癀治疗大肠癌的作用机制研究	潘　杰
李思铭	博士	2011-2014	丹参酮Ⅱ A 磺酸钠对冠心病血瘀证炎症反应增强患者的干预作用研究	徐　浩
王景尚	博士	2011-2014	赤芍川芎有效部位对波动性高血糖介导血管内皮损伤过程中血小板活化及 PKCβ1 表达的影响	殷惠军
王　宁	博士	2011-2014	慢性斑块型银屑病“痰瘀互结 营卫不和”证的研究	庄国康
白瑞娜	博士	2012-2015	冠心病瘀毒证差异 ncRNAs 表达谱的构建及赤芍枳壳活性成分干预效应研究	李立志 丛伟红
罗　静	博士	2012-2015	陈可冀血瘀证辨证方法传承研究	徐　浩
张立晶	博士	2013-2016	PCI 术后氯吡格雷抵抗人群证候特点及血府逐瘀胶囊干预的临床评价	
邬春晓	博士	2013-2016	慢性间歇性低氧对高血压血管内皮 P38 MAPK/NF-κB 信号通路的影响及补肾清肝方干预机制的研究	
信琪琪	博士	2013-2016	基于腺苷 A1 受体探讨芍药苷促血管新生作用	丛伟红 李铭源
付长庚	传承博士后	2013-2017	陈可冀教授病证结合活血化瘀学术思想传承研究	
丛伟红	传承博士后	2013-2017	陈可冀院士治疗老年病学术思想传承研究	
施伟丽	博士	2014-2017	葛根素对自发性高血压大鼠血压的干预作用及机制研究	丛伟红 徐　浩
王　燕	博士	2014-2017	基于网络药理学与血管新生探讨川芎赤芍保护缺血性心脑损伤的机制	
于美丽	博士	2015-2018	八段锦应用于冠心病慢性心衰患者Ⅱ期康复的随机对照研究	徐　浩
崔源源	博士	2015-2018	莪术愈创木烷型倍半萜化合物干预介入后再狭窄的机制研究	赵福海
李　力	博士	2015-2018	基于 miRNA 及其相关信号通路调控研究川芎嗪抑制血小板活化的作用机制	
何　飞	博士	2015-2018	清眩降压汤对血压影响的基础与临床药效学研究	彭　军
陈宏伟	博士	2015-2018	精制清眩降压汤改善血管重构抑制高血压的作用机制研究	彭　军
李四维	博士后	2016-2018	坐式八段锦对冠状动脉旁路移植 (CABG) 术后患者早期心肺功能影响的随机对照研究	
杨巧宁	博士后	2016-2018	基于真实世界研究评价辨证应用中成药干预急性冠脉综合征介入后的临床疗效	高　蕊

续表

姓 名	学 位	学习时间	毕业论文题目	指导老师
袁　蓉	博士	2016-2019	基于 circRNAs 探讨川芎 - 赤芍药对活性成分干预 AS 斑块血管新生的分子机制	丛伟红
王安璐	博士	2016-2019	陈可冀院士血瘀证辨治方法的临床评价研究	徐　浩
王松子	博士后	2017-2019	基于瘀毒理论的解毒活血中药组分配伍抗动脉粥样硬化机制研究	刘龙涛
陈盛君	博士后	2017-2019	清达颗粒全过程多成分精准质控的研究	
张　玲	博士	2017-2021	基于 Rab5a 介导的信号通路研究清达颗粒抗高血压的作用机制	彭　军
蔡巧燕	博士	2017-2021	清达颗粒通过自噬调控高血压引起的心脏重构的机制研究	彭　军
于子凯	博士	2017-2020	瓣膜性心脏病预后的影响因素分析及中药联合康复措施对 TAVR 术后患者的疗效评价	吴永健
郑　源	博士	2017-2020	中医药联合血液超滤治疗心力衰竭的临床及代谢组学研究	马晓昌
刘献祥	师承	2018-2020	基于数据挖掘探讨陈可冀之《清宫配方集成》治疗骨关节炎的组方用药规律	
徐丹苹	博士后	2018-2020	宽胸气雾剂临床疗效评价研究	
朱正川	博士	2018-2021	基于 TLR4 通路介导的炎疗反应研究清达颗粒调节血压减轻脑损害作用机制	
孙敬辉	博士	2018-2021	人参皂苷 Re 介导 lnC RNA CHRF 多角度优化心室重构的效应机制研究	
郭丽君	博士	2018-2021	基于网络药理学及代谢组学探讨参附强心丸治疗心力衰竭的机制	
沈志清	博士	2018-2021	RAB22A 敲除对急性心肌梗死后心室重构调控机制及活心丸（浓缩丸）的干预作用	
陈达鑫	博士	2018-2021	待定	
王丽丽	博士	2018-2022	荣筋拈痛方水提物对骨关节炎作用机制的研究	彭军
龙霖梓	博士	2019-2022	待定	
董国菊	师承	2019-2022	临床经验	
刘征堂	师承	2019-2022	临床经验	
姜众会	博士	2019-2022	待定	
王泽平	博士	2019-2022	待定	
黄明艳	博士	2019-2022	待定	
吴宝君	师承	2019-2022	清宫膏方研究	

附录二　主编及参编书目

一、主编书目

[1]　医学科研设计与SCI论文写作, 科学出版社 (2019, 与郭艳共同主编)
[2]　中华茶文化与健康, 人民卫生出版社 (2019)
[3]　片仔癀基础研究与临床应用, 科学出版社 (2018)
[4]　中华文化与中医学丛书, 中国中医药出版社 (2017)
[5]　十年一剑: 福建中西医结合研究院十周年论文集, 科学出版社 (2017)
[6]　My Integrative Medicine Life-Selected Papers by Keji Chen, 科学出版社 (2017)
[7]　陈可冀学术思想与医疗经验选集, 北京科学技术出版社 (2016, 陈可冀编著；付长庚, 丛伟红, 刘龙涛整理)
[8]　师道师说: 中国文化书院八秩导师文集．陈可冀卷, 东方出版社 (2016, 陈可冀著；陈维养, 付长庚编)
[9]　清代御医力钧文集, 国家图书馆出版社 (2016, 力钧著, 陈可冀主编)
[10]　中华老年医学, 江苏凤凰科学技术出版社 (2016, 与曾尔亢、于普林、张存泰、成蓓共同主编)
[11]　中医美容笺谱精选, 人民卫生出版社 (2016, 与李春生共同主编)
[12]　清宫医案精选, 中国中医药出版社 (2016, 与张京春共同主编)
[13]　中医药科研设计与SCI论文写作, 青岛出版社 (2015)
[14]　中医药与中西医结合临床研究方法指南, 人民卫生出版社 (2015, 与刘建平共同主编)
[15]　黄芪的基础与临床, 人民卫生出版社 (2015, 与孙燕共同主编)
[16]　清宫膏方精华, 科学出版社 (2015)
[17]　中医英译思考与实践, 北京大学医学出版社 (2015)
[18]　养老奉亲书订正评注 (第2版), 北京大学医学出版社 (2014, 与李春生共同订正评注)
[19]　冠心病及急性心肌梗死中医临床辨证标准及防治指南, 人民卫生出版社 (2014, 与史大卓共同主编)
[20]　中国传统老年医学文献精华 (第2版), 科学技术文献出版社 (2014, 与周文泉, 李春生共同主编)
[21]　川芎嗪的化学药理与临床应用 (第2版), 人民卫生出版社 (2014)
[22]　中西医结合心血管病基础与临床, 北京大学医学出版社 (2014)
[23]　实用血瘀证学 (第2版), 人民卫生出版社 (2013, 与史载祥共同主编)
[24]　清宫配方集成, 北京大学医学出版社 (2013)
[25]　中西医结合思考与实践, 人民卫生出版社 (2013)
[26]　现代著名老中医名著重刊丛书 (清宫代茶饮精华, 清代宫廷医话, 清代名医医话精华, 清宫外治医方精华, 清宫药引精华), 人民卫生出版社 (2012)
[27]　岳美中全集, 中国中医药出版社 (2012)
[28]　彩图中医学丛书 (中医基础, 中医辨证论治, 中医方药, 中医经络穴位, 中医养生), 江苏科学技术出版社 (2011, 总主编陈可冀)
[29]　慈禧光绪医方选议, 北京大学医学出版社 (2011)
[30]　中国中西医结合学科史, 中国科学技术出版社 (2010, 王振瑞, 李经纬, 陈可冀主编)
[31]　中国宫廷医学 (修订版), 中国青年出版社 (2009, 与李春生共同主编)
[32]　清宫医案集成 (上下册), 科学出版社 (2009)
[33]　心血管病与活血化瘀, 北京科学技术出版社 (2009)
[34]　清宫医案研究, 中医古籍出版社 (2006, 第二版)
[35]　循证医学与中医药, 中医古籍出版社 (2006)
[36]　细说心理——帮你保持心理平衡, 人民军医出版社 (2006)
[37]　结合医学现状与发展趋势, 中国协和医科大学出版社 (2006, 与吕爱平共同主编)
[38]　老年健康新导航, 北京科学技术出版社 (2005, 陈可冀主编；中华人民共和国卫生部疾病控制司, 中华人民共和国卫生部离退休干部局主编)
[39]　季钟朴纪念文集, 中医古籍出版社 (2005, 与姚乃礼共同主编)
[40]　家庭用药必读, 中国妇女出版社 (2005)
[41]　老年健康指导, 北京科学技术出版社 (2004, 中华人民共和国卫生部疾病控制司, 中华人民共和国卫生部离退休干部局主编；陈可冀执行主编)
[42]　中成药家庭用药指南, 人民卫生出版社 (2004)
[43]　中老年人的自我保健, 清华大学出版社 (2003, 与衷敬柏共同主编)
[44]　老龄化中国: 问题与对策, 中国协和医科大学出版社 (2002, 陈可冀主编；中国科学院生物学部专题咨询组编著)
[45]　国学举要・医卷, 湖北教育出版社 (2002, 与林殷合著, 丛书总主编汤一介)
[46]　陈可冀医学选集: 七十初度, 北京大学医学出版社 (2002, 陈维养主编)
[47]　自然疗法丛书, 湖南科学技术出版社 (2001)

[48] 中国养生文献全书, 甘肃人民出版社 (2000)
[49] 中国宫廷医学, 中国青年出版社 (2003, 与李春生合编)
[50] 中医内科学, 中国协和医科大学出版社 (2002)
[51] 岳美中医学文集 (简体字本), 中国中医药出版社 (2000)
[52] 岳美中医学文集 (繁体字本), 台北启业书局 (1999)
[53] 实用血瘀证学, 人民卫生出版社 (1999, 与史载祥共同主编)
[54] 川芎嗪化学、药理与临床应用, 人民卫生出版社 (1999)
[55] 经济实效谈治病丛书 (共40分册), 中国医药科技出版社 (1999)
[56] 实用中西医结合内科学, 中国协和医科大学北京医科大学出版社 (1998, 与袁钟、钱自奋共同主编)
[57] 跨世纪脑科学: 老年性痴呆发病机理与诊治, 中国协和医科大学北京医科大学出版社 (1998)
[58] 新编抗衰老中药学, 人民卫生出版社 (1998, 与李春生共同主编)
[59] 金手杖丛书, 青岛出版社 (1998, 与徐诚共同主编)
[60] Chinese Patent Medicine, Hunan Science &Technology Press (1997)
[61] 中国传统医学发展的理性思考, 人民卫生出版社 (1997)
[62] 中国养生文献全书 (共3卷), 甘肃人民出版社 (1997, 与程士德, 张九超共同主编)
[63] 东西医结合治疗 (韩文版, 张日武等译韩文), SSC出版 (1996)
[64] 清宫外治医方精华, 人民卫生出版社 (1996)
[65] 当代医学难题的中医药对策, 山西高校联合出版社 (1996)
[66] Imperial Medicaments, Foreign Language Press (1996, 尤本林译)
[67] 心脑血管疾病研究, 台北南天书局 (1995, 与廖家桢、肖镇祥共同主编)
[68] 血瘀证与活血化瘀研究, 台湾知音出版社 (1995, 与张之南, 梁子钧, 徐理纳等共同主编)
[69] 自然疗法丛书 (共20册), 湖南科学技术出版社 (1995)
[70] 养老奉亲书订正评注, 上海科学技术出版社 (1995, 与李春生合作)
[71] 活血化瘀药化学、药理与临床, 山东科学技术出版社 (1995)
[72] Traditional Chinese Medicine: Clinical Case Studies, Foreign Language Press and New World Press (1994)
[73] 中医药临床验案范例, 新世界出版社 (1994)
[74] 水蛭的临床及研究进展, 中医古籍出版社 (1994)
[75] 清宫代茶饮精华, 人民卫生出版社 (1994)
[76] 中华文化与中医学丛书 (共16分册), 福建科学技术出版社 (1993)
[77] 中国实用传统养生术, 福建科学技术出版社 (1993)
[78] 实用中西医临床治疗手册, 中国医药科技出版社 (1993, 与府强等合作)
[79] 清宫药引精华, 人民卫生出版社 (1992)
[80] 老年医学研究, 台湾知音出版社 (1992, 与邝安堃等合著)
[81] 迈向21世纪的中西医结合, 中医医药科技出版社 (1991)
[82] 血瘀证与活血化瘀研究, 上海科学技术出版社 (1990, 与张之南, 梁子钧, 徐理纳等共同主编)
[83] 清宫医案研究, 中医古籍出版社 (1990, 与中国第一历史档案馆合作)
[84] 中西医结合防治老年心血管病, 人民卫生出版社 (1990)
[85] 中国传统养生学精华, 香港商务印书馆 (1990, 与周文泉共同主编)
[86] 实用中医内科学, 台北启业书局 (1989, 与方药中, 李克光, 金寿山, 黄星垣, 董建华, 邓铁涛共同主编)
[87] 抗衰老中药学, 中医古籍出版社 (1989)
[88] 老年医学在中国, 湖南科学技术出版社 (1988, 与邝安堃共同主编)
[89] 中国传统康复医学, 人民卫生出版社 (1988)
[90] 心脑血管疾病研究, 上海科学技术出版社 (1987, 与廖家桢、肖镇祥共同主编)
[91]中国传统老年医学文献精华, 科技文献出版社 (1987, 与周文泉合作主编)
[92] 清代宫廷医话, 人民卫生出版社 (1987)
[93] 实用中医内科学, 上海科学技术出版社 (1985, 与方药中, 李克光, 金寿山, 黄星垣, 董建华, 邓铁涛共同主编)
[94] 岳美中医话集 (增订本), 中医古籍出版社 (1984, 与李春生、江幼李、岳沛芬合作)
[95] 慈禧光绪医方选议 (日文版), 东京美术出版社 (1983, 与中国第一历史档案馆合作)
[96] 活血化瘀研究与临床, 中国协和医科大学、北京医科大学出版社 (1983)
[97] 心脏病问答, 科普出版社 (1981, 与邵耕、徐济民、翁维良合作)
[98] 慈禧光绪医方选议, 中华书局 (1981, 与中国第一历史档案馆合作)
[99] 岳美中医话集, 中医古籍出版社 (1981, 与李春生、江幼李、岳沛芬等合作)
[100] 岳美中医案集, 人民卫生出版社 (1978, 与时振声、李祥国、王占玺合作)
[101] 岳美中论医集, 人民卫生出版社 (1978, 与时振声、李祥国、王占玺合作)
[102] 岳美中老中医治疗老年病经验, 科技文献出版社 (1978)

[103] 美国科学家与发明家, 科技文献出版社及中国翻译公司 (1978, 与陈维养合作, 英译中)
[104] 男子性机能障碍, 人民卫生出版社 (1959, 与董征合作, 俄译中)
[105] 胃痛泄泻便秘的中医疗法, 科学普及出版社 (1958)

二、参编书目

[1] 心脏病学实践: 中西医结合卷, 人民卫生出版社 (2013, 王显、刘红旭主编, 陈可冀、胡大一、马长生主审)
[2] 当代名老中医养生宝鉴, 人民卫生出版社 (2013, 卢传坚主编)
[3] 中西医结合导论, 人民卫生出版社 (2010, 陈可冀主审, 赵春妮, 吕志平主编)
[4] 陈可冀学术思想及医案实录, 北京大学医学出版社 (2007, 张京春编著, 陈可冀顾问)
[5] 当代心脏病学, 广东教育出版社 (2000, 冯建章主编, 雷燕、陈可冀编写第19篇)
[6] 现代心脏病学, 人民军医出版社 (1999, 钱学贤、戴玉华、孔华宇主编, 徐凤芹、陈可冀编写第7章)
[7] 中国老年保健全书, 人民卫生出版社 (1997, 耿德章主编, 方圻 、陈可冀副主编)
[8] 艾滋病中西医防治学, 人民卫生出版社 (1994, 吕维柏主编, 谢雁鸣、 陈可冀编写第20 章)
[9] 实用高血压病学, 科学出版社 (1993, 余振球, 洪昭光主编, 衷敬柏、陈可冀编写第39 章)
[10] 中国古代医史图录, 人民卫生出版社 (1992, 李经纬主编, 陈可冀等副主编)
[11] 临床药理学, 人民卫生出版社 (1991及1998, 李家泰主编, 陈可冀、史大卓编写第56章)
[12] 生脉散口服液的综合研究, 中国医药科技出版社 (1990, 严永清主编, 刘国卿、陈可冀、严克东、廖工铁副主编)
[13] 老年心脏病学, 人民卫生出版社 (1987, 王士雯、钱方毅主编, 何愉生、陈可冀编写第3、4章)

附录三　生平备忘录

1930 年 10 月 20 日（马年）

出生于福建省福州市（闽侯），因父陈在梅当年在京津河北新闻界工作，故以“冀”为名。

1936 年 ~1942 年

福州铺前顶小学——闽侯苏坂小学——闽侯南灵小学（因抗日战争变更学校），毕业。

1942 年 9 月

私立三山中学一年级，因抗日战争转内地续学。

1943 年 ~1946 年

福建省立初级中学（后更名福建闽清中学），毕业。

1946 年 ~1949 年

福建省立高级中学（后更名福建省立福州第一中学），毕业。1948 加入中国作家协会。

1949 年 9 月 ~1954 年 9 月

福建医学院（后更名福建医科大学）医疗系，毕业。曾两次获全省诗歌比赛及论文比赛第一名。大学毕业论文为“毛地黄中毒”，发表于《中华医学杂志》。1954 年 9 月留校任福建医学院内科助教，附属医院内科住院医师，主任王中方教授。

1956 年 2 月 4 日

与福建医学院毕业的同学陈维养医师结婚。

1956 年 4 月 6 日

与著名中医冉雪峰同一天到中国中医研究院报到上班，同在高干外宾治疗室；同诊室尚有著名中医王易门大夫。

1957 年 1 月

获北京市人民政府在职西医学习中医一等奖。

1957 年 7 月 31 日

子陈舟出生。

1959 年 3 月

与著名中医赵锡武、郭士魁等和中国医学科学院心脏血管疾病研究所、阜外医院合作研究高血压病的中医药治疗。

1959 年 4 月

参加中国医学科学院心血管病研究所心电图进修班学习，授课老师为黄宛、方圻二医师。

1959 年 12 月

①在第一届全国心血管病大会（西安）作“高血压病的中医分型论治”报告；②与章宗穆医师合作研究以压电晶体酒石酸钾钠为换能元件的脉搏描记器，与心电图、心音图、心冲击图同步描绘 14 种脉搏图象；出席全国群英会；③邝安堃教授到访我院，著名中医王文鼎和我负责接待；④与董征教授合作翻译出版《男子性机能障碍》（俄文版）一书，由吴阶平教授审校（人民卫生出版社）。

1960 年 3 月 8 日

女儿陈丹出生。

1961 年 10 月

在黄宛、张锡钧教授指导下，完成“高血压病弦脉及其机制的研究”，认为弦脉不同等级与儿茶酚胺水平及血管反应性有关，论文发表于《中华内科杂志》。

1961 年 12 月

与岳美中教授、梁漱溟先生同去福建厦门出席“辨证论治学术研讨会”。梁先生和岳美中教授分别作“东西文化之比较”和“辨证论治实质的探讨”报告。

1962 年 3 月

对北京广济寺等各大寺院僧尼长期素食者 260 例血脂水平及心血管病发病情况作调查研究，注意到随增龄其内源性脂质代谢失调同样存在。

1963 年 8 月

任西苑医院内科主治医师。

1964 年 9 月 ~1965 年 7 月

参加中国医学科学院心血管病研究所心血管内科医师进修班进修和临床实践，结业。

1965 年 7 月 ~1966 年 6 月

到山西稷山县农村巡回医疗队工作。

1966 年 6 月

“文革”开始，被召回北京参加“文化大革命”运动。分配在内科临床及心电图室工作。

1971 年

与郭士魁老中医等参加由阜外医院院长吴英恺院士为组长的北京地区防治冠心病协作组。黄宛、陈在嘉教授等也参加。冠心 2 号复方研究工作由此时开始。同时研究宽胸气雾剂的抗心绞痛作用。前者部分工作发表于《中华心血管病杂志》，后者发表于印度 *Indian J of Integrated Medicine*。

1972 年

参加川芎总碱、川芎一号碱（川芎嗪、四甲基吡嗪）、赤芍甙及赤芍 801（没食子酸丙酯改构）等研究工作。首先在电镜下观察了川芎嗪抗血小板作用，获证实发表于《中华内科杂志》，并首先用于治疗缺血性脑血管病。负责组织协作单位，包括北京制药工业研究所及北京地区 10 余所医院等。

1973 年

①与郭士魁老中医等与北京地区几所医院合作研究益气活血复方治疗急性心肌梗死，论文发表于 *Planta Medica*；② 参加由外经贸部长柴树藩为团长的中法首航代表团访问法国约 10 个城市，参加者包括夏菊花、苏河清等；③ 参加卫生部西北医疗队去甘肃武威一年，同队有北京医院钱贻简教授。结束任务后又领队到滩歌公社医疗队。

1974 年 ~1976 年

继续研究冠心 2 号等活血化瘀方药对血栓烷和血小板功能的影响。总结各类治法的异同。

1978 年

①冠心 2 号、抗心梗合剂、活血化瘀治则及宽胸气雾剂等研究获全国科学大会奖，川芎嗪获全国医药卫生科学大会奖。这几项成果分别同时被评为卫生部级科技成果奖，川芎嗪为北京市科技成果奖。② 被聘任国务院学位委员会学科评议组成员，后并任中西医结合学科评议组召集人；③ 被选为中华医学会心血管病学会常委兼秘书，《中华心血管病杂志》第 1~4 届副总编辑。国家科委中医学专业组成员。④与赵锡武、郭士魁同时被任命为西苑医院心血管病研究室主任；⑤世界卫生组织传统医学官员巴拉曼和该组织心血管病官员考察西苑心血管病工作，吴英恺、陶寿淇教授陪同同来；⑥晋升为副研究员，开始招收研究生。

1979 年

①被世界卫生组织聘任为传统医学专家咨询团顾问，并多次续聘。当年 10 月到日内瓦总部参加全球应用传统医学治疗心血管病及糖尿病会议。报告论文后发表于 *Am J of Chinese Medicine*。②主持召开“全国中西医结合冠心病、心律失常座谈会”（上海），会议制定了冠心病诊断及疗效评价标准，被全国引用至今，董承琅、陶寿淇、陶清、邝安堃、黄铭新、邵耕等教授到会。

1980 年

①主要负责整理出版《岳美中论医集》、《岳美中医案集》（获全国优秀科技图书奖）及《岳美中老中医治疗老年病经验》。随后又主要负责整理出版《岳美中医话集》（获卫生部科技成果奖）。② 4 月出席在马尼拉由世界卫生组织召开的传统医学临床科学会议，并作 *The Clinical Efficacy of Chinese Medicine* 报告。③ 11 月倡议整理研究现存故宫博物院的清代宫廷原始医药档案 3 万余件，经中国中医研究院季钟朴院长、西苑医院郑学文院长同意，又经中办和国家档案局同意，与中国第一历史档案馆单士魁、徐艺圃等合作整理研究，并组织清宫医案研究室，任首任主任，周文泉、江幼李、李春生等参加，先后出版《清宫医案研究》、《慈禧光绪医方选议》（中、英、日文版）、《清代宫廷医话》、《清宫药引精华》、《清宫代茶饮精华》及《清宫外治医方精华》等。④与郭士魁老大夫等共同主持召开“全国冠心病辨证论治研讨会”（广东新会），会议制定了冠心病中医诊断分型标准，李介鸣、邓铁涛、任应秋教授等到会。

1981 年

①附子 I 号（去甲乌药碱）与宽胸气雾剂研究分别获得卫生部甲级成果奖；②与陈维养合作翻译《美国科学家和发明家》一书（英文版）由科学技术文献出版社出版；③指导的第一批研究生毕业，迄今共陆续培养博士、硕士及博士后人员 110 名，分别由邝安堃、方圻 、周金黄、祝谌予、顾复生、林传骧、邵耕、谢竹藩、钱贻简、胡旭东、陈明哲等教授主持答辩会。④中国科协批准成立中国中西医结合研究会，季钟朴任会长，陈可冀任秘书长；⑤ 12 月与唐由之、吕维柏、闫润茗教授等访问日本及印度；⑥晋升为研究员。

1982 年

与天津达仁堂、承德制药厂、北京中医药大学陈文为教授等合作研究清宫寿桃丸、清宫长春丹抗自由基作用；与本院消化科合作研究清宫八仙糕改善小肠吸收功能作用，开展清宫仙药茶调脂作用的观察。

1983 年

参加在马尼拉由世界卫生组织召开的西太区医学科学研究会议，方圻、毛守白教授同时与会。

1984 年

① 3 月应香港中文大学中药研究中心之邀与季钟朴、沈自尹教授同到香港讲学。初识名中医学家陈存仁、谢永光。②与张之南教授等合编之《血瘀证与活血化瘀研究》及与廖家桢、肖镇祥合编之《心脑血管疾病研究》先后出版。③与周文泉、张大钊、李春生等合作编纂之《中国传统老年医学文献精华》出版。

1985 年

应香港中国医学促进会之邀，与名中医董建华及王凤玲教授同到香港讲学。

1986 年

①被选为第三届中国科协常委，以后续被选任第四、五届常委；②参加以矢数道明及大塚恭男为首的东京北里研究所被命名为 WHO 传统医学合作中心的学术会议。

1987 年

2~10 月应邀访美，在洛杉矶及圣塔芭芭拉中医药机构及学院作中医药、中西医结合讲学。主持美国第一批中西医结合博士论文答辩会，博士生均为加州大学、加州州立大学西医教授。

1988 年

9 月应邀参加日本富山医科药科大学活血化瘀学术会议并作活血化瘀方药研究进展学术报告。

1989 年

①世界文化理事会授予“爱因斯坦世界科学奖状”；②出席在香港召开的两岸三地中药研究学术会议；③应聘任 *Int. J. of Phytotherapy Research*（UK）编委。

1990 年

①被选为中华医学会老年医学学会副主任委员及《中华老年医学杂志》副主编；② 9 月与中国科学院孙鸿烈副院长等访问日本，参加由孙平化率团出席第五次中日民间友好会议；③ 10 月与辛育龄、刘干中教授同访韩国，做“老年医学在中国”学术报告。

1991 年

①应澳门中医药团体邀请前去讲学；②主编的《清宫医案研究》一书获国务院古籍整理金奖；③主编《中国养生学全书》3 卷；④主编《中华文化与医学丛书》16 册，赵朴初先生题写书名，费孝通、汤一介等任顾问；⑤ 11 月当选中国科学院学部委员（院士）。

1992 年

①出席汉城大学召开韩国传统医学会议，顺访仁川、釜山、大田、汉城各城市医科大学等；② 9 月赴新加坡出席第四届亚细安中医学术会议，应聘为新加坡中医师公会荣誉顾问；③主编的中、英文版 *Clinical Case Studies* 出版；④增补为第七届全国政协委员，以后续任第八、九届委员。

1993 年

①2 月 25 日 ~3 月 12 日，与王佩、李经纬教授应中国医药学院院长陈梅生之邀访台，参加中医教育座谈会，应聘任台湾《中医药杂志》编委。陈立夫先生约见于士林公寓并题赠“中医现代化与中西一元化乃吾人之共同奋斗目标”。台荣民总医院首次邀请中医药界作学术报告，我的报告题目为：“心血管病的中西医结合研究”，著名内科学家姜必宁院长亲自主持会议，被称为“台湾医学史第一笔”。②6 月 15~24 日应台大医学院、台湾医学会之邀，与曹泽毅、顾方舟、王德炳、戴瑞鸿等教授再访台湾；③11 月应朝鲜保健部之邀，偕维养赴平壤访问讲学。

1994 年

①首届立夫中医药学术奖在台北市“中央图书馆”颁奖。陈可冀获中医学奖，李国雄（台“中研院”院士，美北卡天然药研究所所长）获中药学奖，韩济生获针灸学奖。3 月 17~25 日偕维养访台，陈立夫先生在寓所邀见，题“乐善不倦”相赠。②与维养共以客座教授身份在台阳明大学医学院传统医学研究所讲学一周，并应洪传岳教授之邀，到荣民总医院心脏内科会诊 4 个病人；③9 月参加在英伦牛津大学举行的中西医结合学术报告会，拜会李约瑟；顺访剑桥大学及莎士比亚故居等；④11 月 15~22 日参加卫生部张文康部长率团赴日出席中西医结合研讨会，报告了我国中西医结合心血管病研究进展；⑤任《中国中西医结合杂志》主编；⑥应聘任福建中医学院名誉院长，维养为名誉教授；⑦应邀赴美出席由 NIH-FDA 主持召开的“植物药在卫生保健中的作用研讨会”，在大会作了“生脉散综合科学研究报告”；⑧6 月偕维养出席陈丹获美国加州理工学院医学分子生物学博士学位典礼。

1995 年

①3 月 13~20 日应邀出席在越南河内召开的国际传统医学会议，作心血管病医疗研究报告；②4 月 14~16 日与谢竹藩教授应邀去美出席 NIH 召开的“植物药研究方法学会议”；③6 月 22 日 ~7 月 2 日应邀出席在温哥华召开的美洲华人生物科学年会，作心脑血管病研究学术报告；④10 月 16~22 日应邀出席夏威夷医学会召开的传统医学会议，作了“东亚植物药现状”及“中医舌诊”学术报告；⑤主编《活血化瘀药化学、药理与临床》出版；⑥主编《慈禧光绪医方选议》英文版出版；⑦应聘任中国药科大学及天津中医学院名誉教授；⑧出席在马来西亚召开的第五届亚细安中医学术会议，作活血化瘀研究报告；⑨主编《实用中西医结合内科学》启动，第三年由中国协和医科大学出版社出版；⑩出席陈舟获美国德克萨斯州 A&M 大学药理学博士学位典礼。

1996 年

①3 月 21~24 日出席在新加坡召开的传统医学会议；②4 月 19 日 ~5 月偕维养应邀作为客座教授在美国加州大学医学院（洛杉矶）东西方医学中心作关于中西医结合研究报告；③当选中国中西医结合学会第四届会长；④应聘任国家中医药管理局专家咨询委员会委员，中国药典委员，国家新药协调领导小组顾问。国家 OTC 药领导小组成员，国家新药评审委员会委员，国家保健品审评特邀委员，卫生部学位委员会委员；⑤9 月与季钟朴教授担任共同执行主席，主持第 63 次香山科学会议，主题为：“中国传统医学发展的理性思考”；⑥11 月 5~16 日参加在阿姆斯特丹和布鲁塞尔召开的中医药学术会议和天然药会议；⑦应聘任中山医科大学及河北医科大学名誉教授；⑧与王新德教授共同担任执行主席，主持第 91 次香山科学会议，主题为：“老年性痴呆的发病机理与诊治”；⑨“血府逐瘀浓缩丸防治冠心病 PTCA 再狭窄的研究”获国家中医药管理局科技进步一等奖。

1997 年

①首届世界中西医结合大会在北京国际会议中心召开，担任大会主席，包括海外专家 300 人在内的 1100 余名国内外学者参会，被评为当年医药卫生界十大新闻之一；②应台湾中西医整合医学会邀请，率团 9 人赴台，在台湾大学医学院举办中西医结合报告会，该校三任医学院院长及各科主任出席，为台大医学

院举行此类会议的首次，被台大医学院院长誉为“破冰之旅”(ice-breaking journey)；③应聘任山东中医药大学名誉教授；④应邀参加香港浸会大学创办中医学院课程讨论会；⑤再度访问韩国、澳门等地。

1998 年

①应聘任上海中医药大学及伦敦中医学院名誉教授；②应聘任美国旅美中国中医院校同学会名誉会长；③偕维养访问意、法、西班牙及摩洛哥等国；④主编《川芎嗪化学、药理与临床》及 *Chinese Patent Medicine* 出版。

1999 年

①应聘任暨南大学名誉教授；②被选为中华医学会常务理事及老年医学学会主任委员；③应聘任香港特区政府医疗教育委员会成员并出席会议；④ 3 月 14 日在北京友谊宾馆友谊宫举行的北京大学中国文化书院为张岱年、季羡林、侯仁之、何兹全先生 88 龄米寿及王元化先生 80 大寿祝寿会上，由汤一介先生主持，季羡林先生亲自授给聘书，聘任为北京大学中国文化书院导师；⑤与曾毅院士共同担任执行主席，主持第 131 次香山科学会议，主题为：“遏制艾滋病的策略”。

2000 年

①应邀出席在纽约西奈山医疗中心举行的中医及中西医结合报告会，报告“中医药的研究与开发”；②应聘任香港中文大学名誉客座教授；③在香港中大中医学院西医学习中医班作“中西医结合的原则与实践”讲座；④出席在香港召开的国际中医药与丰盛晚年学术会议 (International Conference on Chinese Medicine and Successful Aging)，并在开幕式致辞；⑤纪念岳美中教授百年诞辰座谈会在人民大会堂召开，主编《岳美中医学文集》北京简体字版和台湾繁体字版发行，吴阶平院士和陈立夫先生分别题写书名；⑥被选为《中国老年学杂志》主编；⑦在中国科学院第 9 届院士大会上续被选任生物学部副主任。并任中国科学院咨询评议委员会委员；⑧偕维养及马晓昌医师出席在曼谷召开的第六届亚细安中医药学术会议，作“中医学术的多元化发展”报告，会后顺访新加坡；⑨当年再度访新加坡，出席 ECON 保健中心开幕典礼；⑩被聘为第 5 届北京市中西医结合学会名誉会长；⑪应聘任香港浸会大学中医药学院学术顾问；⑫ 应聘连任北京市人民政府医药专业顾问。

2001 年

① 2 月应聘任北京大学中医药现代研究中心学术委员会主任；② 2 月中央保健委员会授予荣誉证书奖；③ 3 月被推选为中国老年学学会名誉会长；④ 4 月应聘任中国灾害防御协会救援医学学会高级顾问；⑤应聘任中华医学会骨质疏松及骨矿盐病学会名誉顾问；⑥ 4 月末出席在厦门召开的中科院咨询评议委员会会议期间，应聘任厦门市中医院名誉院长；⑦ 5 月份应邀在北京大学作《中医药现代》学术讲座；⑧ 6 月胡锦涛副主席在怀仁堂亲颁给聘书任中央保健委员会专家小组成员；⑨与黄熙教授等合作之“证治药动学研究”被评为国家科技进步奖二等奖公布；⑩出席在波士顿召开的中美医学保健会议，任传统医学、补充医学专题讨论会中方主席；⑪ 在第六届中国科协全国大会期间被选为荣誉委员；⑫ 9 月与另 11 位院士同获 2001 年度求是奖“中医药现代化研究杰出成就集体奖”，由周光召院士颁奖；⑬ 12 月应聘广西中医学院名誉教授。

2002 年

① 1 月受聘为香港大学中医药学院名誉教授；受聘为北京大学医学部兼职教授；② 4 月偕维养出席在首尔召开的 International Symposium of Traditional Korean Medicine；③ 9 月担任在北京召开的第二次世界中西医结合大会主席，并致开幕词；④ 10 月与韩启德院士、邬沧萍教授共同应邀任“中国老年学学术研究重大问题和对策”为主题的第 193 次香山科学会议执行主席并作主评述报告；⑤获本年度何梁何利科技进步奖。

2003 年

① 6 月 4 日应 CCTV 之邀，与钟南山教授共同出席与台湾同行举行的 SARS 视频对谈会；②负责承担国家自然科学基金重点项目“冠心病血瘀证相关因子基因组学研究”。

2004 年

① 1 月 30 日在人民大会堂接受胡锦涛主席亲自颁发“血瘀证与活血化瘀研究”国家科技进步一等奖 (2003 年度) 证书；② 4 月 2 日应邀在澳门“国际传统医学与 *Evidence-based Medicine* 大会”作 *On Evidence-based Medicine* 学术报告；③ 6 月 4 日在中国科学院院士大会被选任中国科学院学部主席团成员；④ 4 月 26 日参观福建永定土楼；⑤ 6 月 26~29 日出席在日本岐阜召开的国际传统医学会议，美国 David Eisenberg 教授等也参会；⑥ 8 月 6~10 日参加在新疆召开的中西医结合会议，访喀纳斯湖；⑦ 10 月 2~4 日应邀在 NCCAM/USA 作 *Anti-platelet therapy and Chinese herbal medicine* 报告，访 NIH 图书馆；⑧ 10 月 4 日应邀在哈佛大学医学院礼堂作“血瘀证与活血化瘀治疗研究”学术报告；⑨ 10 月访问台北 / 台中 / 彰化等医疗机构；⑩ 11 月 15 日 应邀在国际传统医学大会 (北京) 作 *Multiple Patterns for Chinese Medicine R & D* 报告；⑪ 12 月 12 日接受香港浸会大学 (Hong Kong Baptist University) 授予荣誉博士学位并聘为名誉教授；⑫ 12 月 30 日受聘为广东省中医院首席科学家，雷于蓝副省长颁发聘书。

2005 年

① 7 月 3 日福建中西医结合研究院成立并受聘任首任院长；② 7 月 6 日受聘为中央保健委员会专家小组副组长，由中办主任王刚颁发聘书；③ 7 月应聘江西宜春学院名誉院长，抚州高级医专名誉教授；游明月山；7 月出席在吉林延吉召开的全国血瘀证及活血化瘀学术会议，到天池及镜泊湖览胜；④ 7 月 29 日 ~8 月 5 日参加中组部组织的赴北戴河度假活动；⑤ 8 月 30 日受聘解放军总医院名誉教授；⑥ 9 月 1 日作为主编之一参加《季钟朴文集》出版发布会；⑦ 9 月 3 日受聘任福建中西医结合研究院院长，汪毅夫副省长颁发聘书；创立启动陈可冀中西医结合医学基金，资助科学研究项目；⑧ 9 月 11~14 日出席在敦煌召开的全国中西医结合会议，会后访并流连于莫高窟 / 阳关道上；⑨ 10 月 11 日卫生部中日友好医院全国中西医结合心血管病中心成立，受聘担任主任，方圻教授及朱晓东院士参加中心揭牌仪式；⑩ 10 月 16 日世界中医药学会联合会心血管病专业委员会成立，被选任会长；⑪ 12 月中国中医科学院 50 年院庆，被授中药应用奖；在院庆学术报告会作“传统与现代同辉煌”报告。

2006 年

① 3 月在香港大学 / 香港中西医结合学会作“充分应用现代科学技术，促进中西医学的有机结合”报告；② 3 月 17 日游龙虎山与第 65 代天师张金涛主持晤谈，到江西访王安石及汤显祖纪念园；③ 5 月 4 日受聘为南方医科大学名誉教授；④ 承担国家“973”中医药基础创新性病因病机学说研究部分课题；⑤ 8 月在贵阳全国活血化瘀学术会议作循证处方用药报告，并参观黄果树瀑布；⑥ 9 月访日在日本国际中医药学会作活血化瘀研究进展报告 (京都)；⑦ 10 月在中日心血管病学术研讨会作冠心病研究策略学术报告 (神户)；⑧ 10 月 5 日在中国信息研究所 50 周年大会作“充分应用现代科学技术，促进中西医结合发展”学术报告；⑨ 11 月 4~14 日访美出席 UCLA 东西方医学中心年会，参观加州大学动脉粥样硬化研究室，以及衰老及老年医学中心，作“中国中西医结合五十年”报告，在 *Santa Barbara College Hospital* (圣塔芭芭拉医院) 作“冠心病临床研究”学术报告；在南加州八个针灸中医公会会议也作了学术报告，我国驻加州领馆科技参赞出席；加州众议院为陈可冀和 Ka Kit Hui 教授颁发奖状；⑩参加 11 月 21~23 日世界中医药联合会心血管分会学术年会，任主席并作学术报告 (加拿大多伦多)；⑪ 12 月出席两岸四地中医药论坛暨福建中西医结合研究院学术年会；⑫ 12 月 13 日受聘为上海第二军医大学名誉教授，由总后卫生部部长及该校校长共同颁发聘书；⑬ 12 月 14 日为福建中医学院 / 福建中西医结合研究院研究生做“谈谈研究生的日子该怎么过”的学术报告；⑭ 4 月 20 日 全国中西医结合医师会议在北京友谊宾馆召开，被推选为

中国医师协会中国中西医结合医师分会会长，作“现代中西医结合医院及医生的神圣职责”学术报告。

2007 年

①母校福州第一中学九十周年校庆在福州大学城新址举行，代表校友作大会发言；②6月26日应邀赴香港在国际传统医学大会(纪念香港回归十周年，由香港浸会大学举办)作“冠心病治疗策略的衍变”学术报告；③7月首都医科大学老年医学系成立，应聘任该系学术委员会主任，在大会作“老年心血管病临床治疗”学术报告；④8月根据胡锦涛主席批示，由科学出版社组织出版中国科学家传丛书，由钱伟长院士任总主编，刘德培院士任医学卷主编，陈可冀任中医分卷主编；⑤9月21~23日第三届世界中西医结合大会在广州东方宾馆召开，任大会主席，广东省中医院院长吕玉波任执行主席；15个国家计1500专家到会；⑥10月赴井冈山，出席全国中西医结合管理会议；⑦10月末应邀在江西省心血管病学术会议作“中西医结合心血管病进展学术报告”；再上井冈山；⑧11月女儿陈丹回国，应邀陪同她到南方医科大学及广州中医药大学第二临床医学院分别作“新药临床研究”学术报告，并访中山故居及虎门销烟旧址；⑨12月代表校友在福建医科大学七十年校庆大会发言；⑩12月应聘任首都医科大学心血管学系(北京安贞医院)顾问；应聘任杭州中西医结合医院名誉院长；*Chinese Journal of Integrative Medicine*(中国结合医学杂志，英文版)已通过*Scientific Thomson*审评，公布自2008年开始成为SCI-E收录期刊源。

2008 年

①2月22~23日中医药发展创新香山科学会议举行，陈竺、颜德馨、刘德培、陈可冀、王永炎为执行主席，陈可冀作“提倡多元模式，促进中西医结合，发展传统中医药学”主题报告；②4月首都医科大学成立中西医结合学系，受聘为学术委员会主任委员，作“中西医结合发展模式及进展”学术报告；③作为国家级非物质文化遗产传统医学项目代表性传承人之一，参加颁证会；④5月21日 在中国中医科学院主办的中医药发展讲座(第五讲)作“提倡多元模式，促进中西医结合，发展传统医药学：理念决定方法，方法决定结果”报告；⑤6月6日中华医学会全国心血管学术大会在郑州召开，与陈灏珠、陈在嘉、高润霖、胡大一等同被授予专家会员称号；⑥9月出席在上海召开的全国中西医结合心血管病中青年医师论坛，被授予“伯乐奖”；⑦出席在成都召开的中药饮片高峰论坛，再访宝光寺及武侯祠；⑧10月应聘任广东省人民医院(广东省老年医学研究所)名誉教授；⑨10月世界中医药联合会心血管学会第三次大会任大会主席，举行“聚焦冠心病：中西医如何优势互补”沙龙；⑩被第六届全国中西医结合大会推选为中国中西医结合学会名誉会长；⑪10月24~26日，中日友好医院全国心血管病中心学术年会及中日循环器病第三届大会举行，任中方主席；⑫10月出席广东省中医院心脏中心十周年国际心血管病会议；⑬10月在贵阳探访明代理学家王阳明贬居地阳明洞及抗日时期张学良洞顶住地；⑭10月出席在人民大会堂召开的纪念毛泽东西医学习中医批示五十周年大会，大会发言呼吁继续组织西学中，领导要加强支持力度；⑮12月应香港中文大学中医药学院邀请，为该校师生作“铁肩担道义，妙手好中医”报告；为香港医药界作“中医/中西医结合临床服务”学术报告；访香港中央图书馆；受聘任中国药典委员会执行委员。

2009 年

①4月受聘为山西中医学院名誉教授；②3月指导的论文“益骨胶囊治疗绝经后骨质疏松症的临床研究”获2008南粤科技创新优秀学术论文二等奖；③5月受聘为卫生部中日友好医院心血管病中心名誉主任；④9月受聘担任《中国老年学杂志》主编；⑤11月获“吴阶平医学奖”；⑥12月“冠心病血瘀证基因组学研究”获中国中西医结合学会科学技术二等奖；⑦12月“动脉粥样硬化药理评价技术平台及活血化瘀中药干预机理的系统研究”获北京市科学技术奖二等奖。

2010 年

①被聘为中央保健委员会第一届专家顾问委员会成员；②被授予澳门科技大学荣誉博士学位；③3月中国宫廷医学研究获中国中医科学院科学技术奖三等奖；④受聘为中国中医科学院研究道德委员会委员；

⑤任主任的中日血液流变学可视化合作实验室成立；⑥ 8 月受聘担任中国中医科学院医学伦理委员会主任委员；⑦ 10 月担任中国老年学学会名誉会长；⑧受聘任中国健康教育中心咨询委员会专家；⑨ 11 月获“岐黄中医药基金会传承发展奖”；⑩ 12 月受聘任中华中医药学会介入心脏病学专业委员会名誉主任委员；⑪ 被评为广州中医药大学“优秀博士后合作教授”；⑫ 12 月主编的《清宫医案集成》获中国出版政府奖图书奖。

2011 年

① 2 月受聘任国家中医药发展综合改革试验区建设专家指导委员会委员；② 6 月获 2011 年度“科学中国人”终身成就奖；③受聘任中药质量国家重点实验室（澳门大学、澳门科技大学）学术委员会主任；④ 11 月受聘任香港中医学会学术顾问；⑤ 12 月受聘担任上海市中西医结合心血管病研究所专家委员会主任委员；⑥受聘任北京中医药大学心血管病研究所学术指导委员会主任委员；⑦受聘担任《中国真菌学杂志》名誉主编；⑧担任《中国医药科学》杂志顾问。

2012 年

①指导的“心血管血栓性疾病瘀毒病因病机理论创新的系统研究”获中国中西医结合学会科技进步一等奖及北京市科技进步二等奖；②指导的“冠心病血瘀证诊断标准”在《中国中西医结合杂志》发表，是国内首个病证结合血瘀证标准；③受聘为《Evidence-based Complementary and Alternative Medicine》心血管病专栏特邀主编；④获香港浸会大学第一届张安德中医药国际贡献奖；⑤担任中国医师协会常务理事。

2013 年

① 1 月接待澳门大学代表团来访并做学术交流；② 1 月参加中华医学会学术年会；③ 5 月受聘任《世界中医药》杂志顾问委员会主任委员；④ 5 月担任北京中医药学会活血化瘀专业委员会顾问委员；⑤ 5 月在湖北省中医药学术会议上做报告并访问湖北中医学院；⑥ 5 月召开主题为“从宫廷到民间：清代宫廷原始医药档案研究”学术思想座谈会；⑦ 5 月与台湾黄荣村校长、林昭庚教授和北京中医药大学李良松教授参加第三届中国佛医论坛并访问少林寺；⑧ 6 月受聘任北京联科中医肾病医院高级顾问；⑨ 6 月当选为北京中西医结合学会第七届心血管内科专业委员会名誉主任委员；⑩ 7 月与高润霖院士、孙燕院士共同参加《中国医学论坛报》创刊 30 周年会议；⑪ 7 月在贵州召开中国医师协会中西医结合心血管会议；⑫ 8 月主办召开“中国心脏大会 2013・中西医结合论坛”；⑬ 8 月 26 日在湖北恩施召开《中华老年医学》编委会；⑭ 9 月 17 日苏泊尔南洋医药气雾剂研究中心成立，科室组织的宽胸气雾剂多中心 RCT 研究结果发布；⑮ 10 月 17 日参加中药上市后再评价国际大会；陈可冀院士被续聘为国家人口与健康科学数据共享平台专家委员会主任；⑯ 11 月陈可冀院士受聘全国首批传承博士后指导老师；受聘任中国医师协会中西医结合医师分会会长；⑰ 12 月陈可冀院士被什刹海书院院长汤一介教授聘为书院导师。

2014 年

① 1 月指导的“冠心病血瘀证证候实质探索研究”项目获北京市科学技术奖二等奖；② 1 月 22 日受聘任为国家神经系统疾病临床医学研究中心专家委员会委员；③ 3 月 23 日参加诺贝尔奖获得者医学峰会暨院士高峰论坛，应邀做“促进传统医学和现代医学更好融合”学术报告；④ 4 月被授予北京中医药薪火传承贡献奖；⑤ 4 月 10 日在广州参加第十六届中国南方国际心血管病学术会议并做报告“芳香温通方药在心血管病的应用”；⑥ 5 月在中国脑卒中大会上荣获中国脑卒中防治卓越成就奖，同时召开第四次学术思想传承会，会议主题为“老年学与老年医学”；⑦ 6 月访问东阿阿胶老字号，并顺访鱼山曹子建墓；⑧ 8 月 7 日，国家心血管病专家委员会成立，陈可冀受聘任国家心血管病中心第一届专家委员会资深委员；⑨ 9 月 22 日，陈可冀院士被评为全国杰出专业技术人才并在人民大会堂领奖，中国中医科学院西苑医院心血管中心活血化瘀防治心血管病研究团队同时获评专业技术人才先进集体荣誉称号；⑩ 9 月 27 日参加第十二届全国中西医结合心血管病学术会议；10 月 19 日参加第三届广东省中西医结合学会学术年

会；⑪ 10 月 30 日，第二届国医大师表彰大会在人民大会堂举行，陈可冀获评国医大师荣誉称号；⑫ 11 月受聘任中华中医药学会第六届理事会顾问；⑬ 11 月 22 日，中华中医药学会第六次全国代表大会召开，陈可冀院士获中医药终身成就奖；⑭ 11 月 28 日在厦门参加海峡两岸医院卫生交流协会中西医结合论坛；⑮ 12 月续聘任香港大学及香港中文大学中医学院名誉客座教授；⑯ 12 月 27 日当选世中联中医健康管理专业委员会名誉会长。

2015 年

① 1 月 18 日担任中国中医药研究促进会痰瘀同治专业委员会名誉主任委员；② 3 月 20 日受聘任《中国医学人文》杂志顾问；③ 4 月 10 日参加南方国际心血管病会议；4 月 18 日参加中华医学会第十二次全国老年学学术会议；④ 5 月 17 日召开以“行进中的现代活血化瘀学派”为主题的第五次学术思想传承座谈会，会上首次提出现代活血化瘀学派；⑤ 6 月 27 日参加纪念郭士魁先生诞辰 100 周年学术会议；⑥ 7 月 29 日国家“十三五”规划教材开编，人民卫生出版社成立中医药专家委员会，陈可冀获聘任委员；⑦ 8 月 8 日参加中国心脏大会中西医结合论坛并报告；⑧ 10 月 11 日，在邓铁涛国医大师百岁生日当天拜访邓老；10 月 17 日参加第十三次全国中西医结合心血管病学术会议；⑨ 11 月 15 日在纪念耿鉴庭诞辰 100 周年的活动上讲话；11 月 28 日召开庆祝福建中西医结合研究院成立 10 周年学术会议；⑩ 12 月 2 日参加中药质量研究国家重点实验室学术委员会会议；12 月 14 日中华医学会第 25 次全国会员代表大会暨成立 100 周年纪念大会召开，陈可冀获终身成就奖；⑪ 12 月 16 日冠心病“瘀毒”病因病机创新的系统研究获国家科技进步二等奖；“血瘀证与活血化瘀研究”入选中国中医科学院最具影响力优秀论文；⑫ 12 月 22 日参加中国中医科学院成立 60 周年纪念大会，并与诺贝尔奖获得者屠呦呦教授一起受到刘延东副总理接见。⑬ 孙陈安（Andy Chen），马里兰大学医学院毕业，医学博士。现在杜克（Duke）大学医学院，麻醉科医师。孙媳时怡（Melody Shi），杜克（Duke）大学医学院毕业，医学博士。现在杜克医学院工作，儿科内分泌专科医师。

2016 年

① 1 月上旬携陈舟、陈丹两家人游览苏杭并举行结婚 60 周年纪念活动；② 3 月 25 日国家神经系统疾病临床医学研究中心成立，陈可冀受聘任专家委员会委员；③ 4 月担任厦门石室书院专家顾问委员会总顾问；④ 4 月 9 日访问香港浸会大学并参加第三届张安德中医药国际贡献奖颁奖典礼；⑤ 4 月 23 日参加中华医学会第八届全国老年心血管病大会；⑥ 5 月 23 日受聘任广州中医药大学深圳医院学术顾问；5 月 25 日在京召开主题为“中西医结合优势互补”为主题的第六次陈可冀院士学术思想传承座谈会；⑦ 6 月 11 日参加第二届世界黄芪论坛；⑧ 7 月 18 日，陈可冀院士受聘担任 973 计划“中医证候临床辨证的基础研究”特聘顾问；⑨ 8 月受聘任中国中药协会药物经济学专业委员会顾问；受聘任世中联痰证学专业委员会名誉会长；⑩ 8 月 14 日召开中国心脏大会中西医结合论坛；8 月 21 日参加世中联综合医院中医药工作委员会成立大会并做报告，访问哈尔滨医科大学并缅怀季钟朴老院长；⑪ 9 月受聘任青岛市科学顾问；受聘担任复旦大学青岛研究院特聘教授；⑫ 9 月 5 日在马来西亚参加第十一届亚细安中医药学术会议；9 月 6 日受聘担任《中国临床药物大辞典》编委、主审；⑬ 9 月 24 日在世中联老年医学专业委员会学术年会上做报告；9 月 28 日参观青岛国风药业并登琅琊台；⑭ 10 月 3 日受聘任国家卫生计生委科技创新战略顾问；10 月 10 日受聘担任中国教育网络电视台健康台专家委员会首席专家；10 月 20 日受聘担任江阴市政府咨询委员会委员；⑮ 11 月携陈丹登泰山，参访孔孟故里；11 月 5 日在上海主持召开中国医师协会中西医结合医师大会；⑯ 12 月 3 日世中联心脏康复专业委员会成立，陈可冀院士担任名誉会长；12 月 5 日参加新加坡国际中医药高层论坛并发表演讲；12 月 14 日在厦门市首届西学中班开班仪式上授课。⑰孙女陈安妮（Annie Chen）马里兰大学医学院医学生。

2017 年

① 1 月 10 日被中国非处方药协会授予“杰出导师”荣誉称号；1 月 20 日获聘任《中华心血管病杂志》

编辑委员会顾问；②2月24日获评首届岐黄中医药传承发展奖；③3月访问香港中文大学；④3月20日受聘为福建中医药大学中医药学术思想传承工作指导教师；3月25日受聘任《中国药物警戒》编委会顾问；⑤4月24日受聘任中国卫生信息学会健康医疗开放大学理事会院士顾问；5月13日召开主题为"开放包容促进传统医学现代医学更好融合"的第七次学术思想传承座谈会；⑥6月20日受聘担任北京中医药治未病健康促进工程首席顾问；⑦6月23日在徐州参加第六届全国雷公藤学术会议；7月2日参加中国中医药临床价值与评价论坛；8月19日在福州参加第15次全国中西医结合心血管病学术会议。⑧9月9日参加中药上市后再评价国际会议并获特殊贡献奖；9月14日参加第24届世界心身医学大会；9月16日在武夷山召开第一届茶疗健康论坛；⑨10月28日陈可冀院士中西医结合老年医学团队入选深圳市医疗卫生"三名工程"；⑩10月30日在名老中医专家传承团队领军人才队伍建设与能力提升高级研修班讲课；⑪12月6日参加第四届中医科学大会；12月8日参加第五次世界中西医结合大会并被授予中西医结合终身成就奖；⑫12月15日受聘担任国家中医药管理局中医药改革发展专家咨询委员会顾问；12月29日获北京中医药大学岐黄奖提名奖。⑬外孙 Jared Rulison 获加州伯克利大学学士学位。

2018年

①4月8日在厦门参加第二届海峡两岸佛医论坛。②4月10日清华大学中药研究院成立，陈可冀受聘任顾问委员会委员。③5月5日参加中国脑卒中大会；5月18日受聘任国家老年医学中心科学指导委员会委员；5月19日参加首届海峡两岸中医名家名师学术对话；5月26日参加中国脑病大会；5月27日召开主题为"新时代、新作为、中西医结合传承创新转化服务"为主题的第八次学术思想传承座谈会④6月16日参加全国中西医结合心血管病学术会议；6月18日福建省院长专家工作站授牌；6月23日参加世界中医药大会第四届夏季峰会。⑤7月17日国家中医药管理局余艳红书记来办公室看望陈可冀院士并合影。⑥8月4日参加中国心脏大会。⑦8月23日主编的《片仔癀基础研究与临床应用》一书出版。⑧8月31日参加中国医学人文大会。⑨9月1日在大理参加中国中西医结合学会第八届虚证与老年医学学术会议。⑩10月20日，在广州召开第二届南北交融-陈可冀学术思想传承会。⑪10月27日，由澳门中医药学会等六家学会联合颁发中华中医药杰出贡献奖。⑫11月10日受聘福建中医药大学名誉校长。⑬外孙 Jared Rulison 伯克利（Berkely）大学电子工程和计算机科学硕士学位，现在旧金山 Affinity 公司工作。

2019年

①3月29日参加通心络干预颈动脉斑块前瞻性、随机、双盲、安慰剂对照、多中心临床研究成果新闻发布会；②5月17日参加世界高血压日活动，18日参加中国脑卒中大会，19日做客凤凰卫视，参加凤凰大健康节目录制；5月26日召开以"传承中国精神，成就时代篇章"为主题的第九次学术思想传承座谈会；5月31日在上海参加第13届东方心脏病学会议；③6月1日在南京参加中国中西医结合学会第八届虚证与老年医学专业委员会；6月22日广西中医药大学附属瑞康医院成立院士专家工作站并揭牌；6月23日在北京西学中高级研究班总结座谈会上授课；6月29日在福州参加海峡康复产业高峰论坛并演讲；④7月6日参加国医大师王绵之学术思想传承与创新研讨会；7月13日国家中医心血管病临床医学研究中心启动，担任中心主任；7月27日在广东省中医院成立院士专家工作站并揭牌。⑤8月8日参加中国医学科学院首次学部会议并当选学部委员；⑥8月19日，在人民大会堂参加中国医师节先进典型报告会，作为先进典型代表发言并接受孙春兰副总理接见；⑦8月24日召开中国医师协会中西医结合医师大会并担任大会主席。⑧外孙 Noah Rulison 毕业于 Chapman 大学音乐系声乐专业，现在加州州立大学音乐系硕士研究生，攻读合唱指挥。

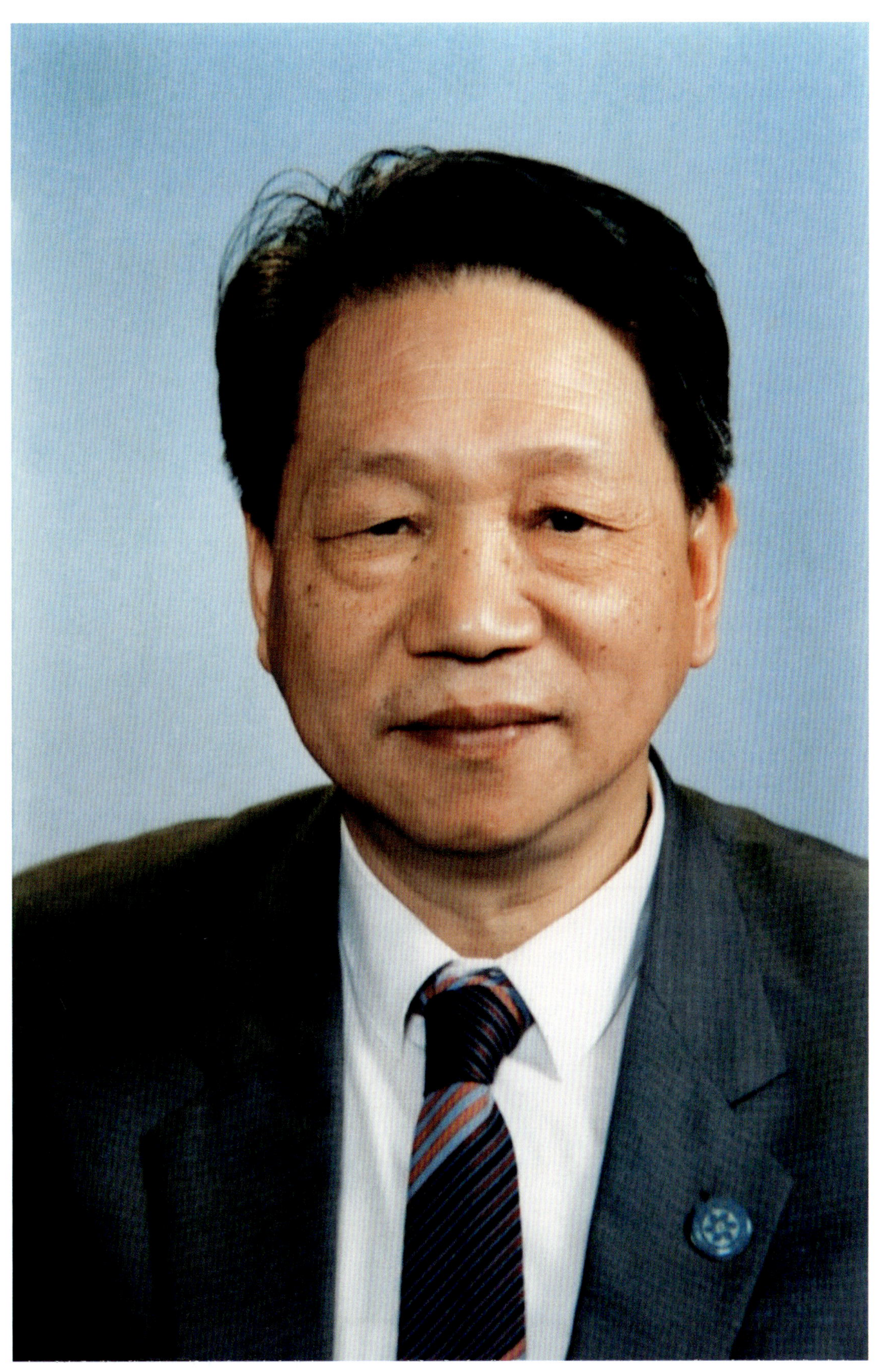

1991 年 11 月当选为中国科学院院士（学部委员）

家庭 / 故土

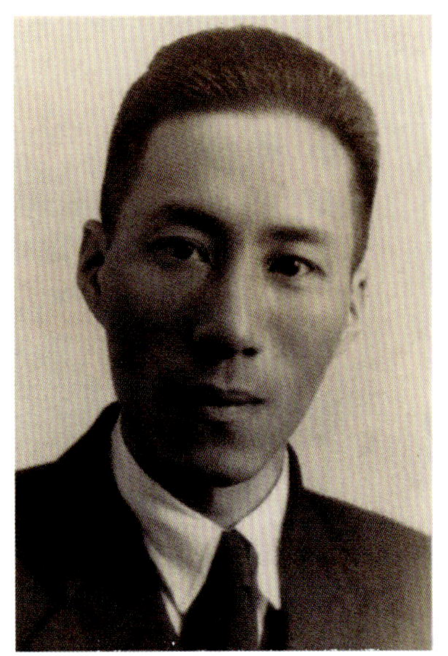

父亲（1947）

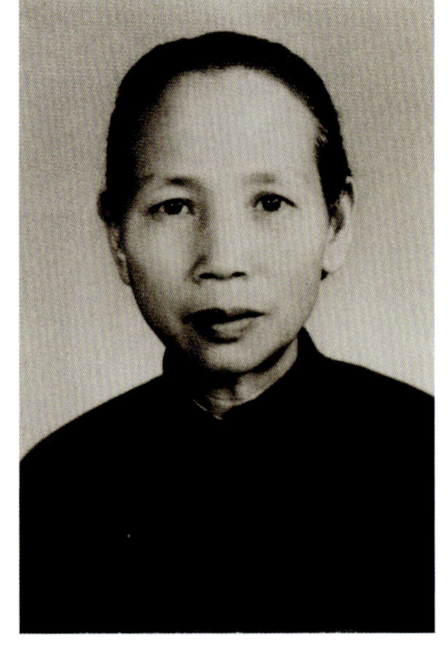

慈母懿容（1964）

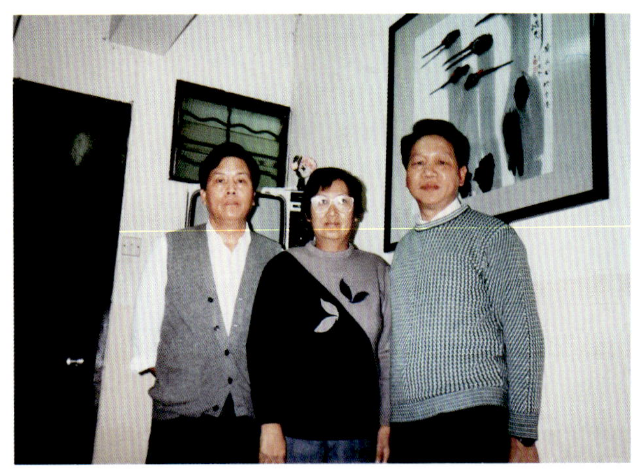

与大哥陈可焜、大嫂蔡若虚（1982，香港大哥家中）

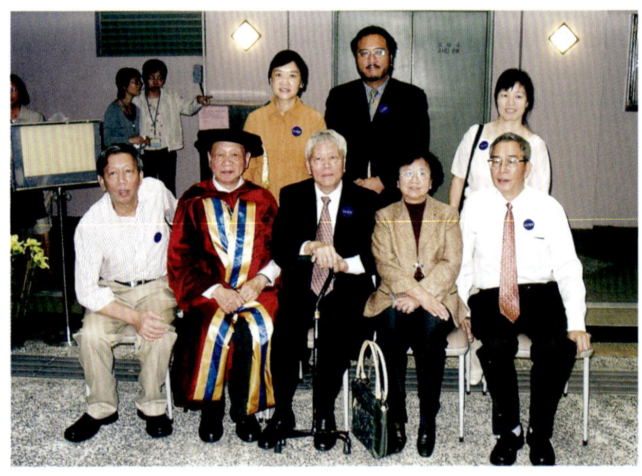

香港浸会大学荣誉博士授予仪式，与家人合影（2004，香港）

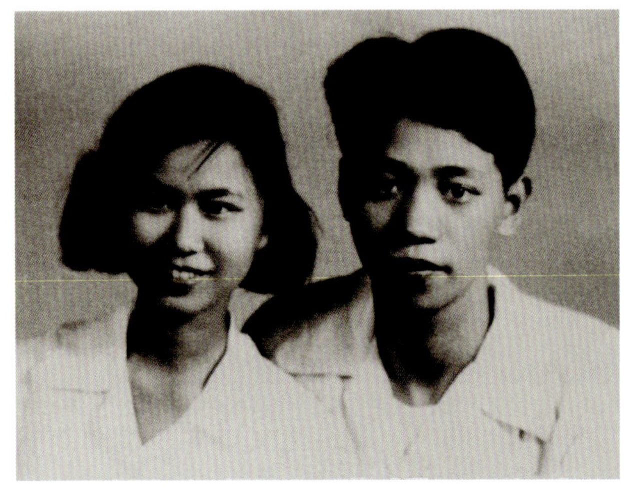

大学时代的陈可冀和同学陈维养（1954，福州）

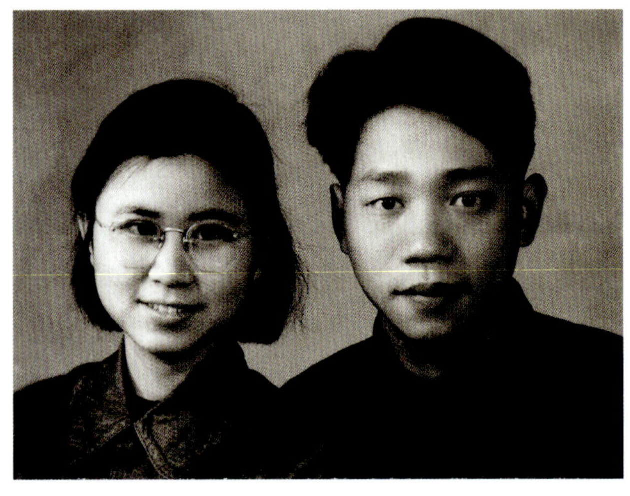

与维养在福州结婚（1956）

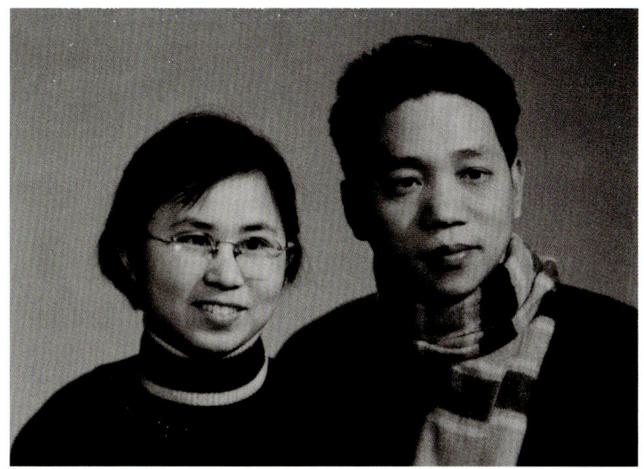
与维养在北京（1965）

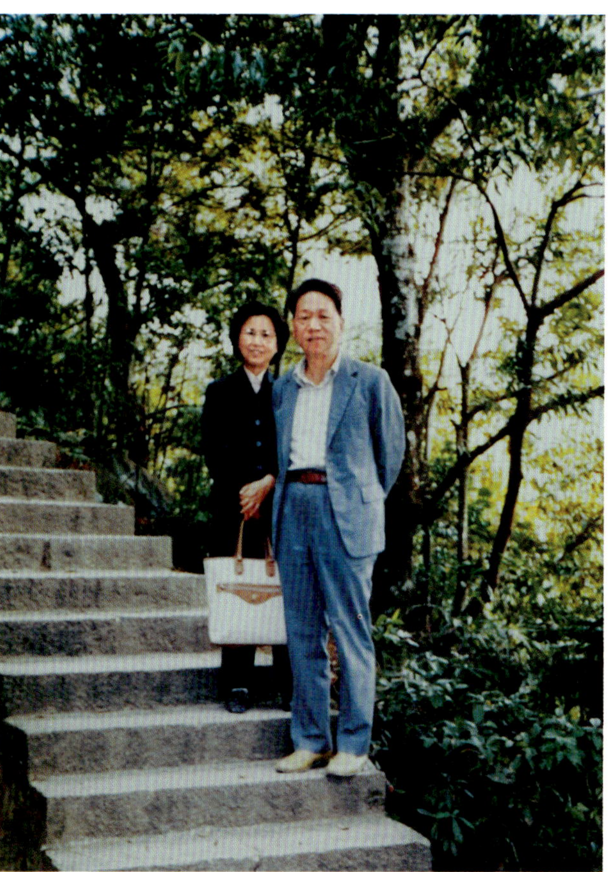
鼓山情思（1984）

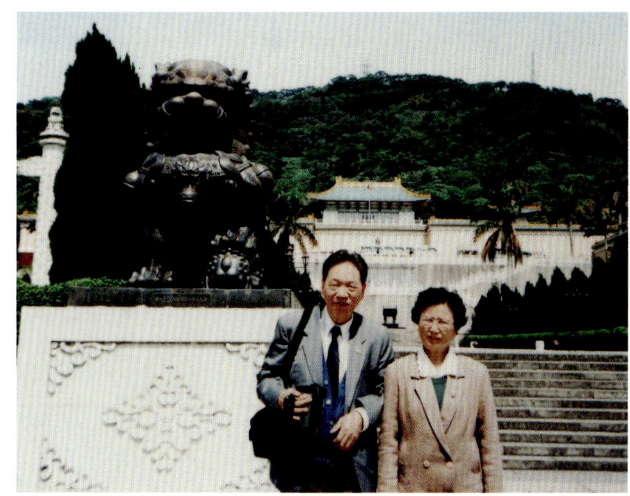
台北故宫博物院前（1994）

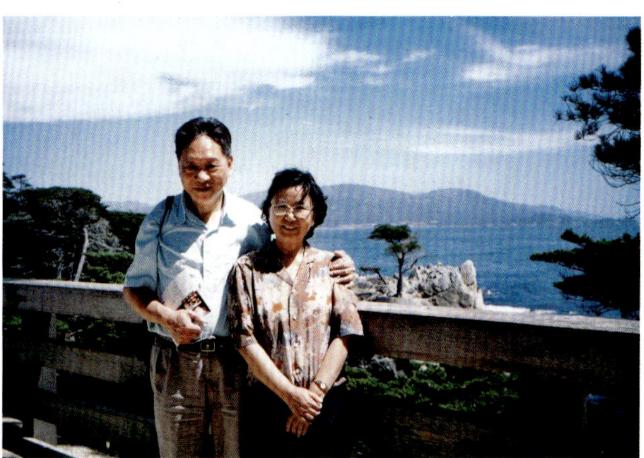
美国旧金山 Seventeen Miles 途中（1994）

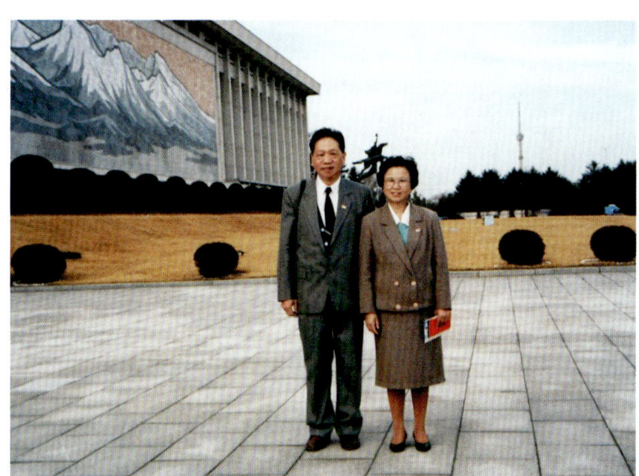
平壤金日成广场（1993）

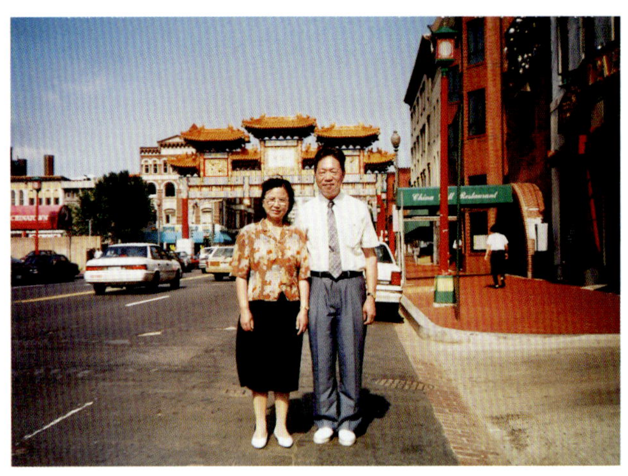

美国华盛顿中国城（1994）

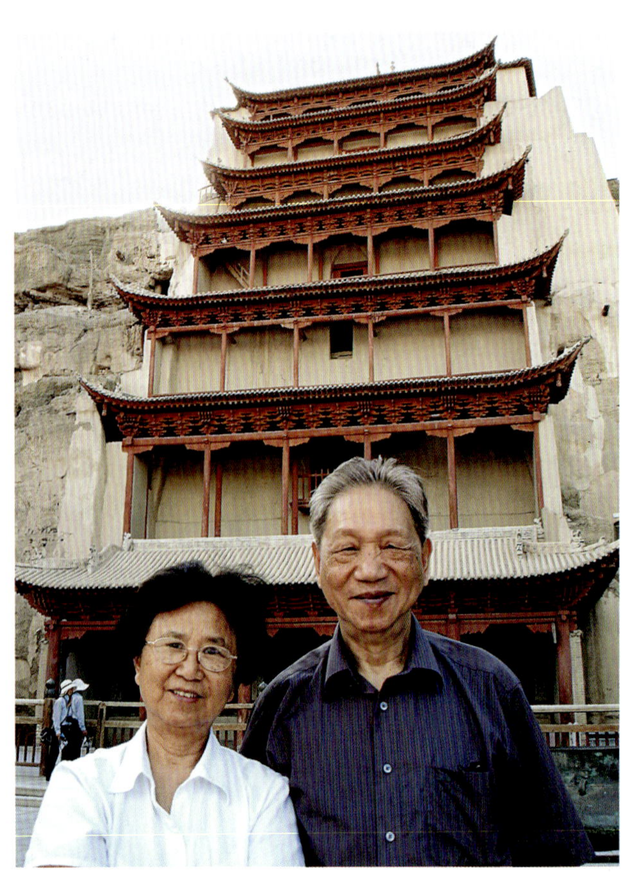

敦煌莫高窟前 (2005)

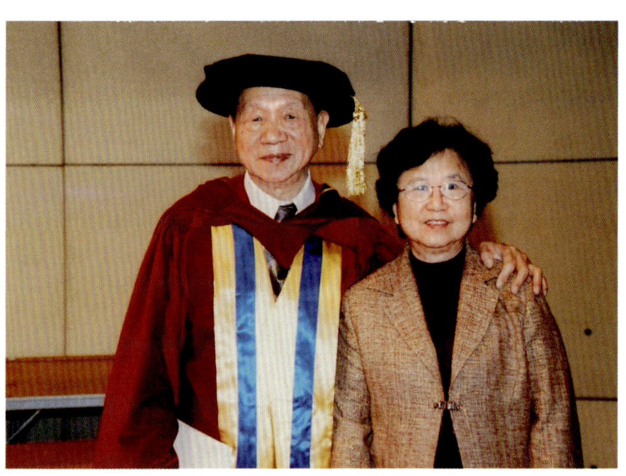

在香港浸会大学（2004）

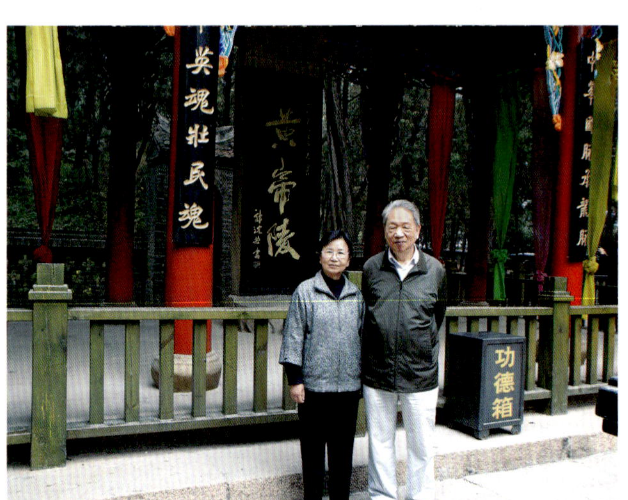

黄帝陵前（2008）

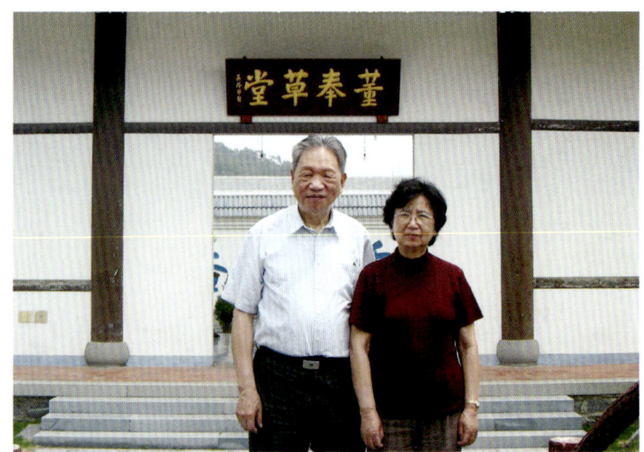

福建长乐董奉草堂（2006）

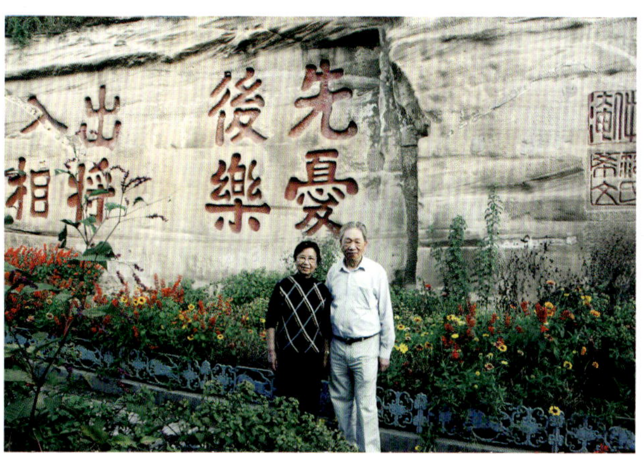

延安宝塔山下范仲淹先忧后乐石碑前（2008）

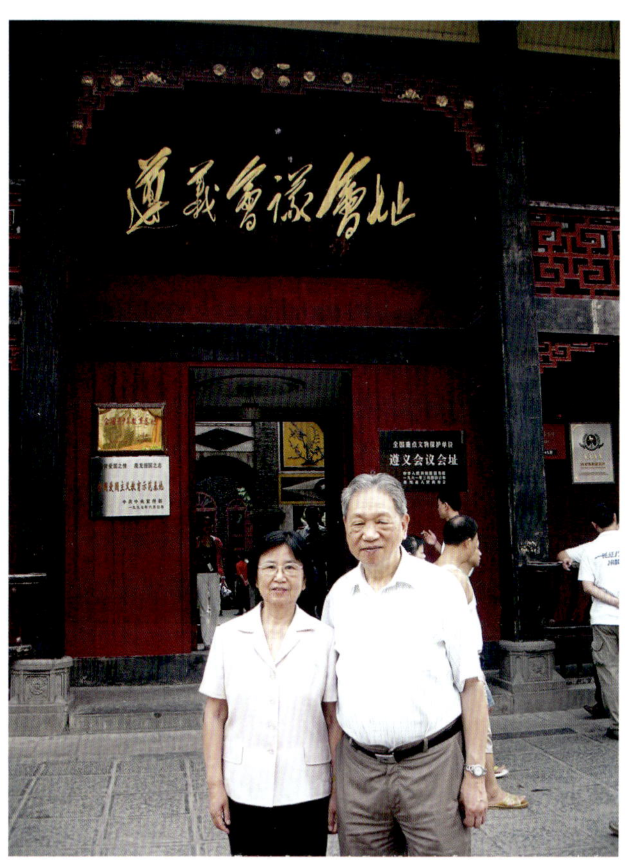

遵义会议会址（2006）

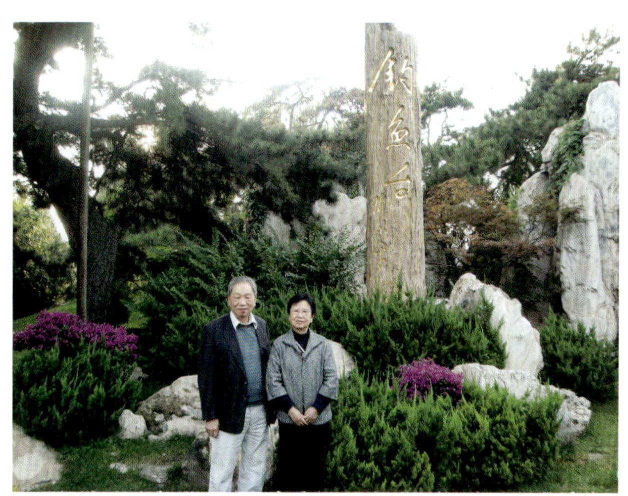

北京钓鱼台（2008)

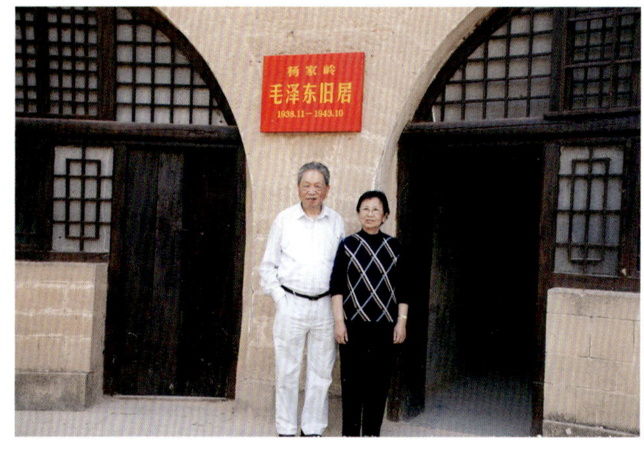

杨家岭毛泽东旧居（2008）

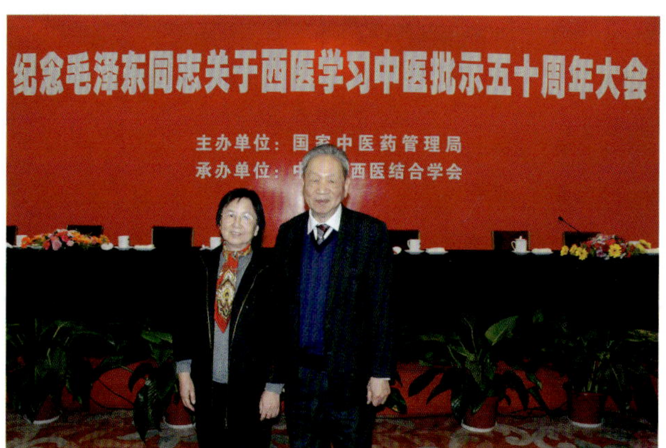

人民大会堂（2008）

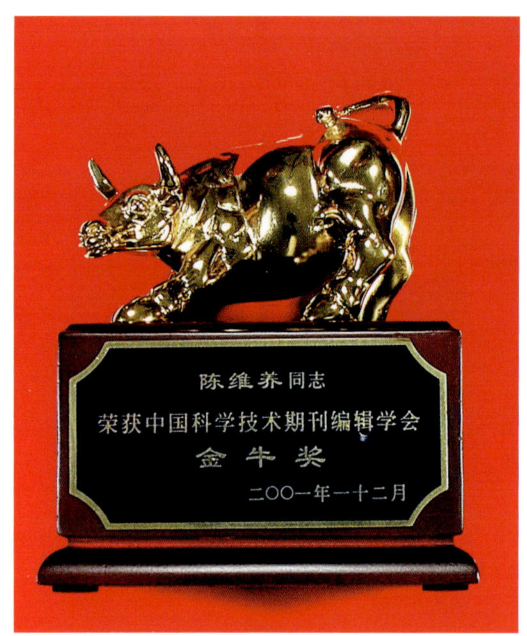

维养获中国科协金牛奖（2001）

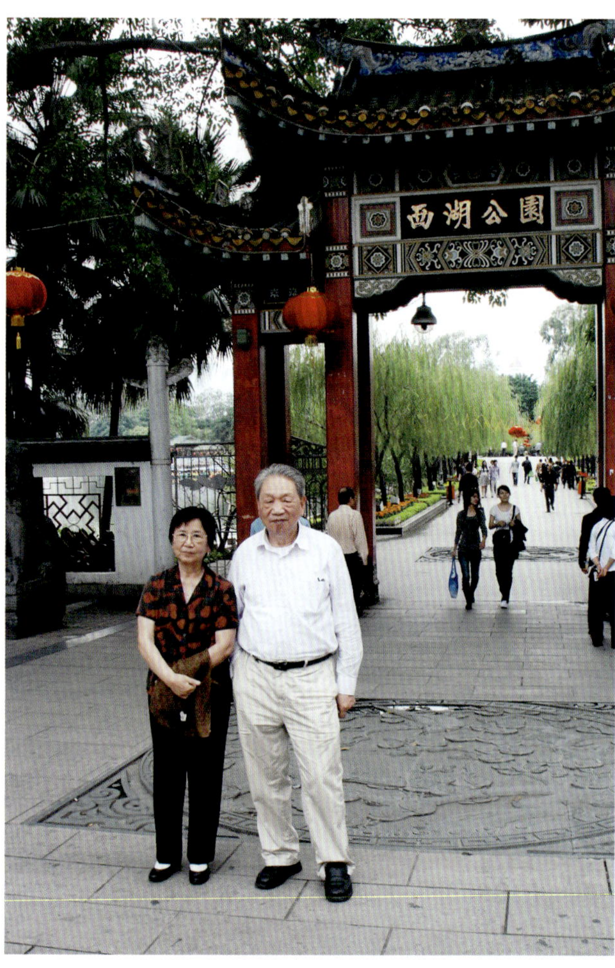

青春的记忆：重游福州西湖公园（2008）

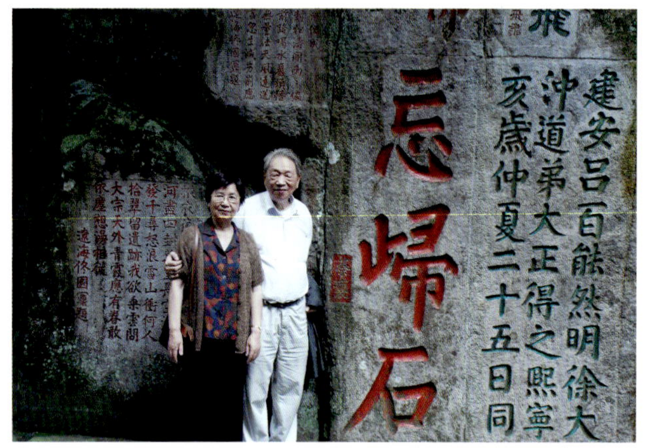

福建鼓山（2008）

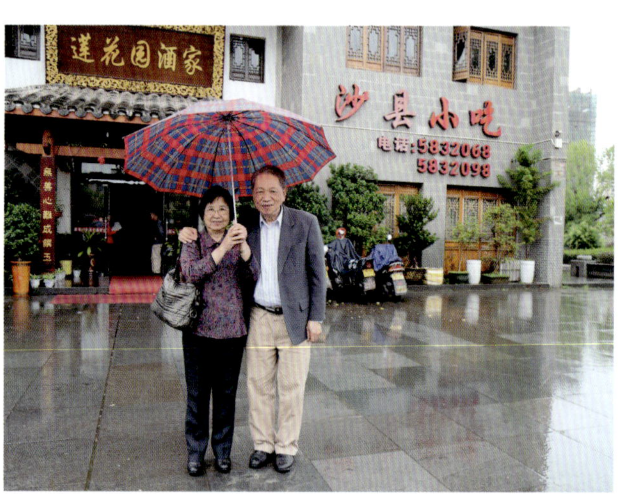

福建沙县（2013）

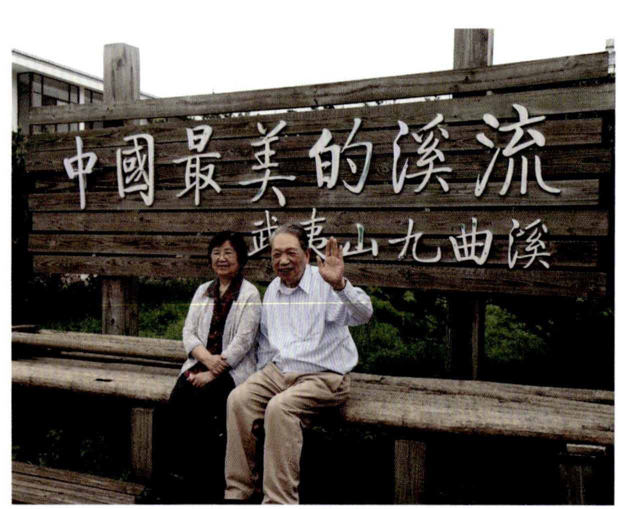

福建武夷山（2014）

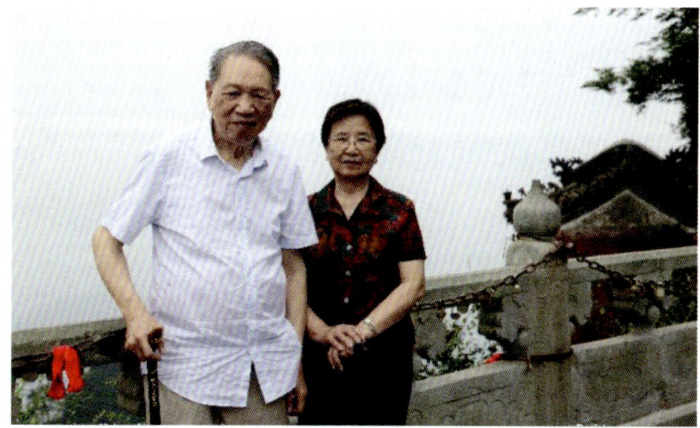
湖北武当山（2015）

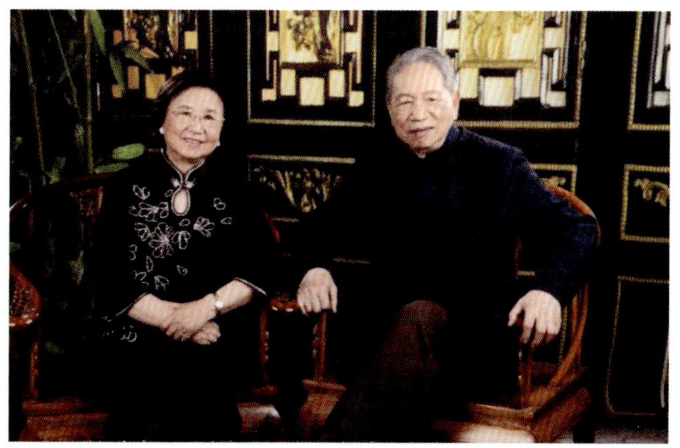
摄于北京照相馆（2015）

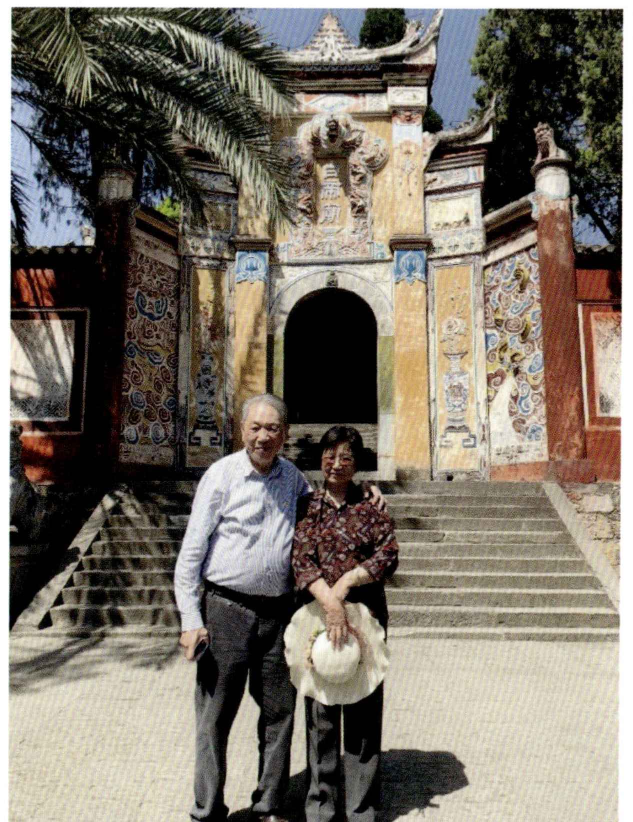
游览白帝城（2018）

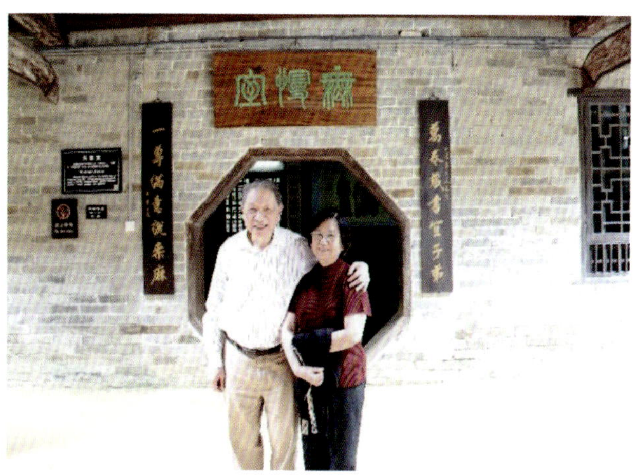
湖南娄底曾国藩故居（2015）

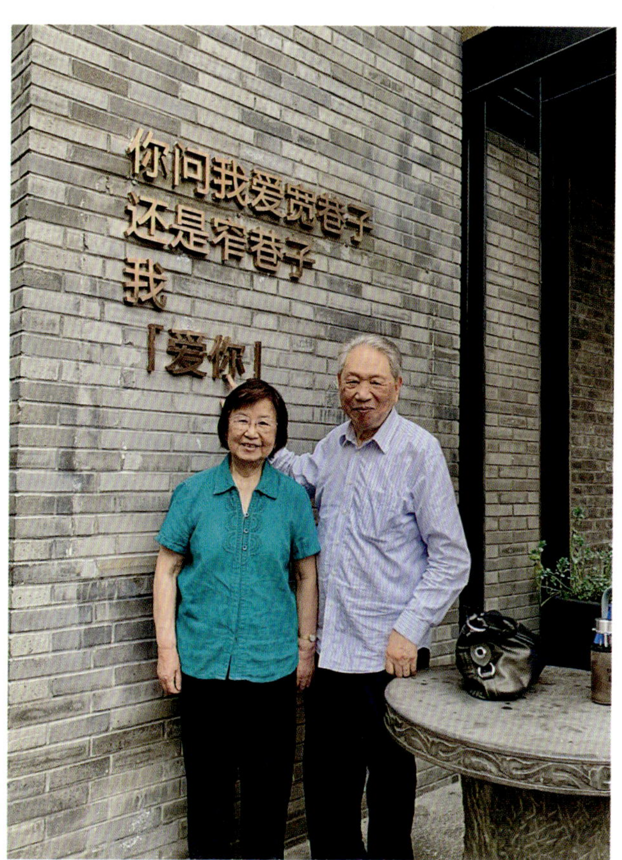

游览成都宽窄巷子（2019）

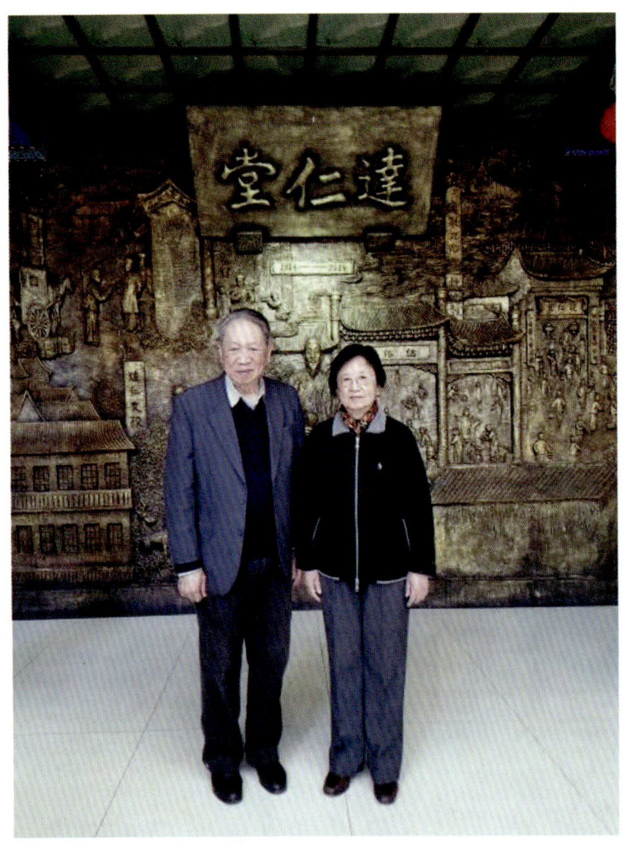

访问天津达仁堂（2018）

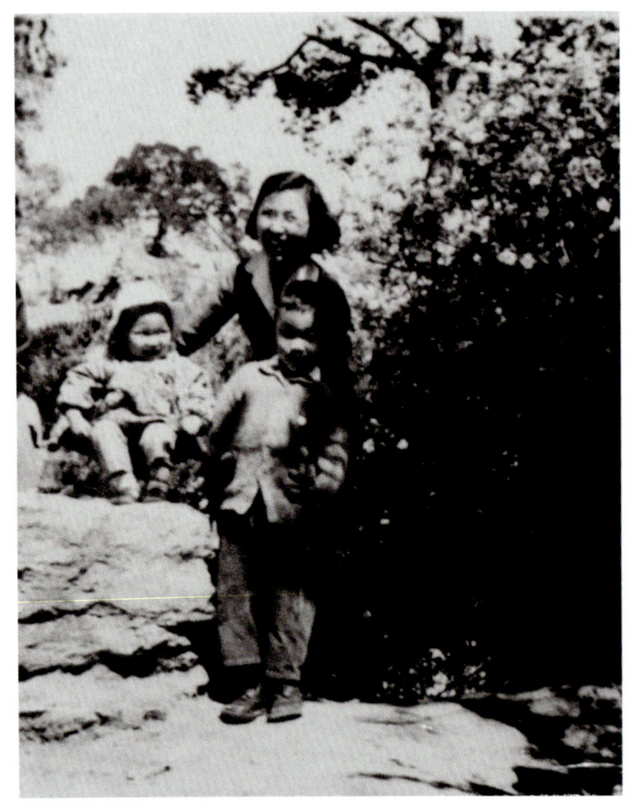

陈舟、陈丹儿时在北海公园（1961）

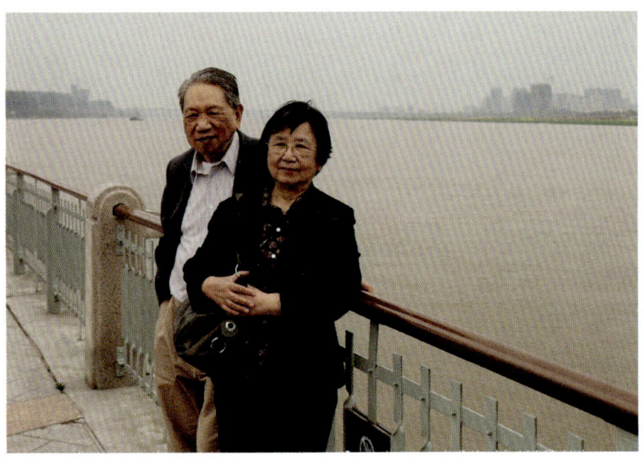

游览湘江橘子洲头（2014）

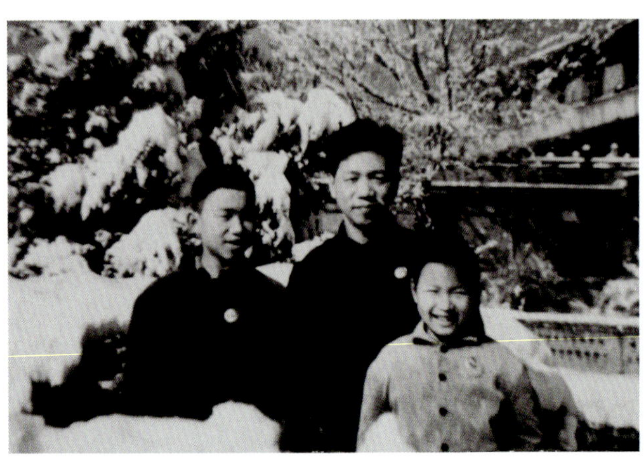

时代的胎记：与儿子陈舟、女儿陈丹在西苑医院（1967）

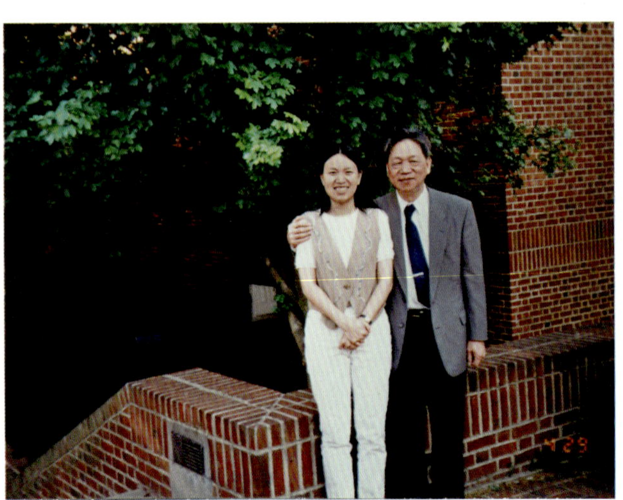

与陈丹在美国 NIH-NIDDK 楼前（1995）

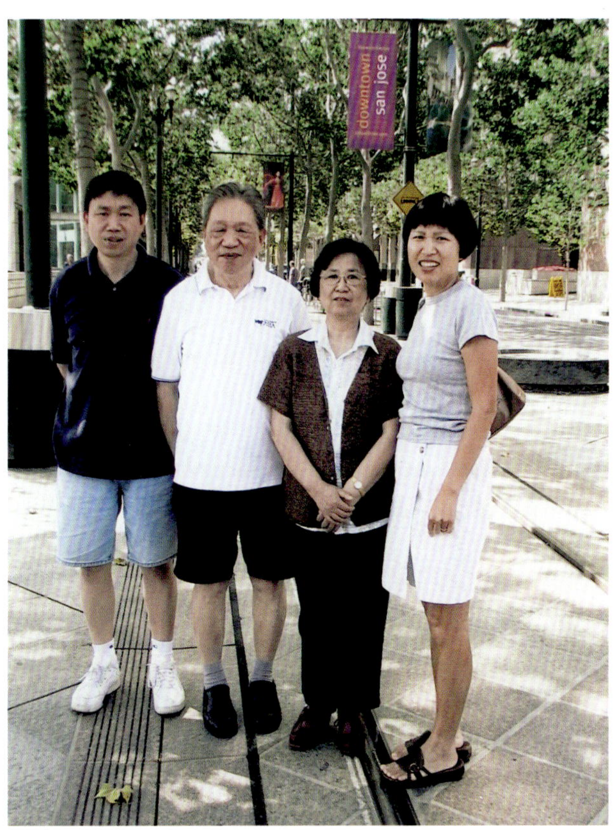

其乐融融：与子女在美国加州 Palo Alto（2004）

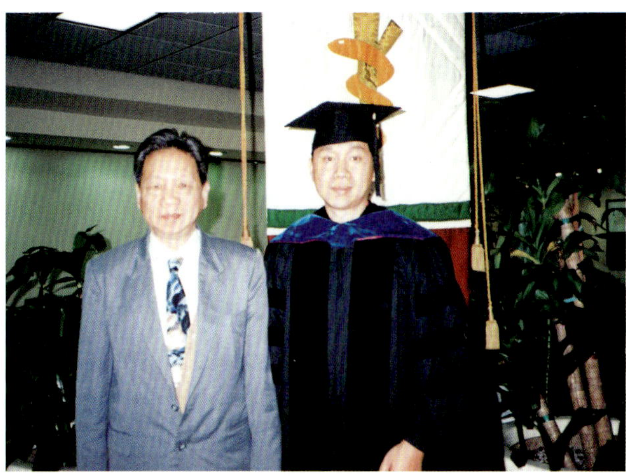
陈舟获德克萨斯州 A&M 大学医学博士学位（1995）

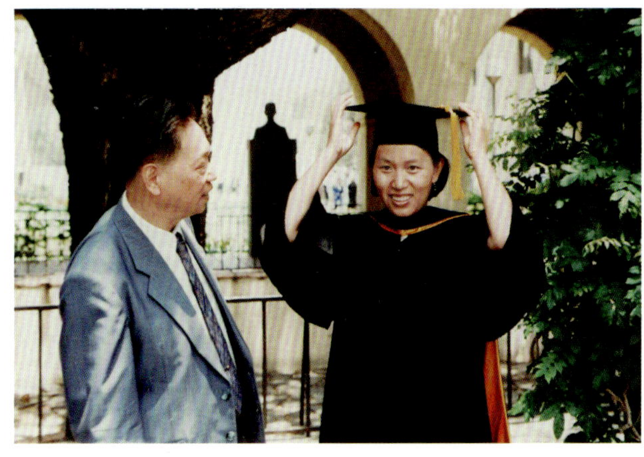
女儿陈丹获加州理工学院博士学位（1994）

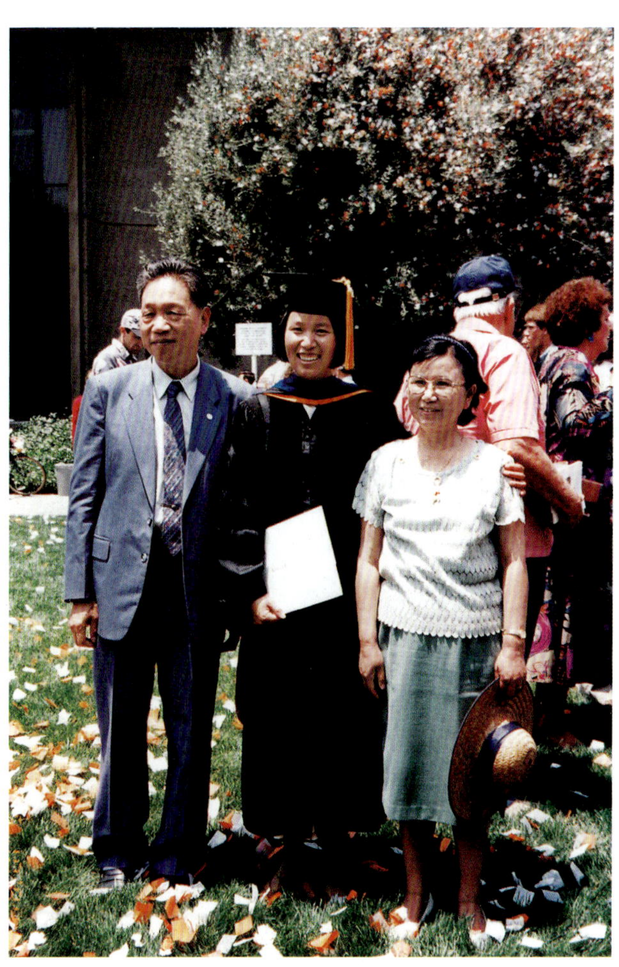
与陈丹同乐（1994）

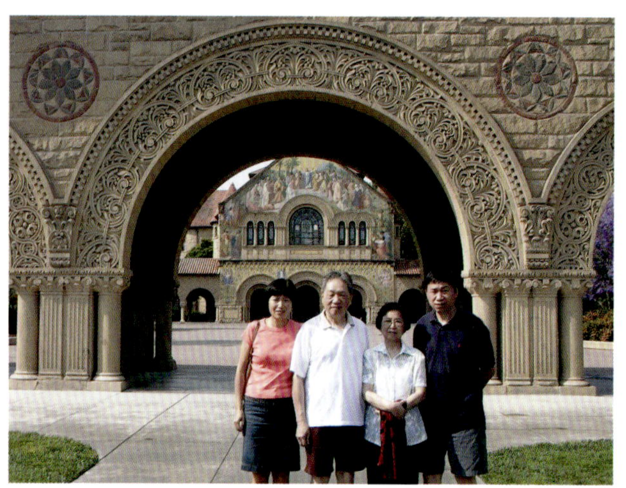

与子女陈舟、陈丹参观斯坦福大学（2004）

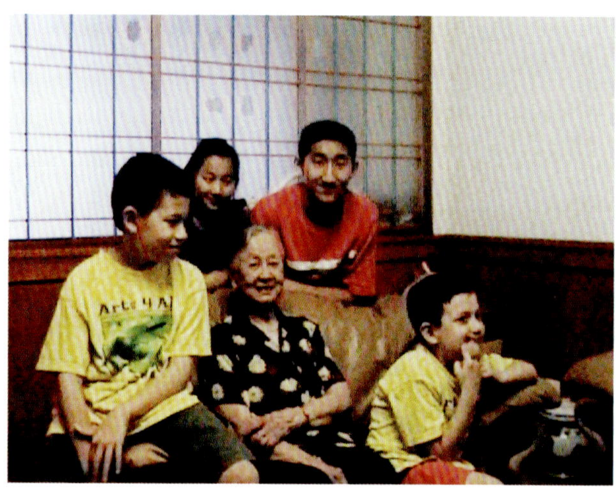

四个孙辈看望 94 岁高龄太姥姥（维养母亲）（2005，福州）

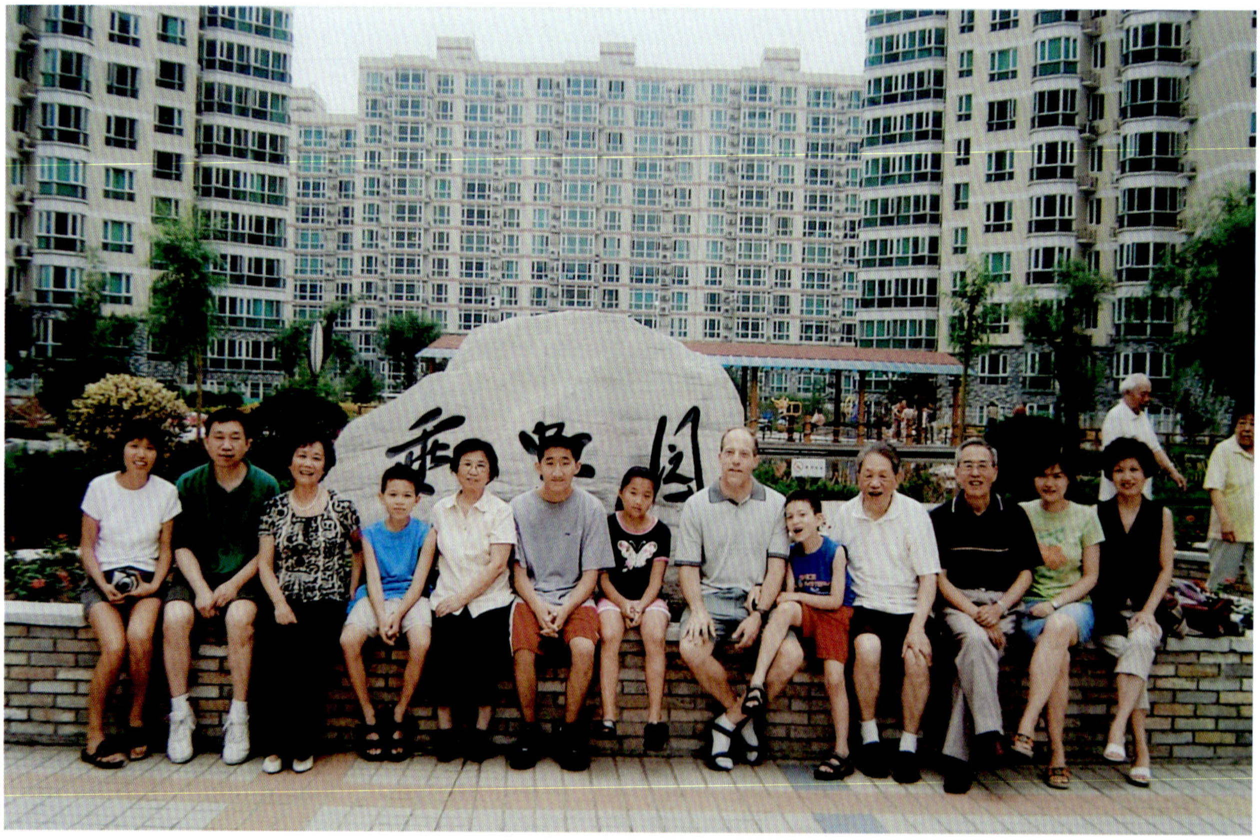

亲情，托起明天的希望：在北京世纪城垂虹园内家人合影（2005）

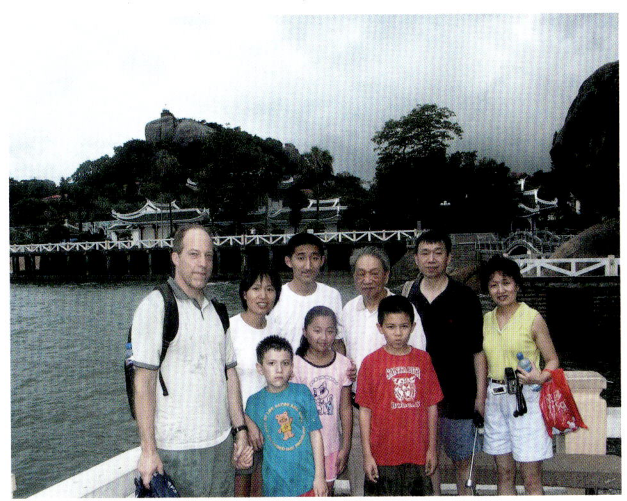

厦门鼓浪屿，维养摄影（2005）

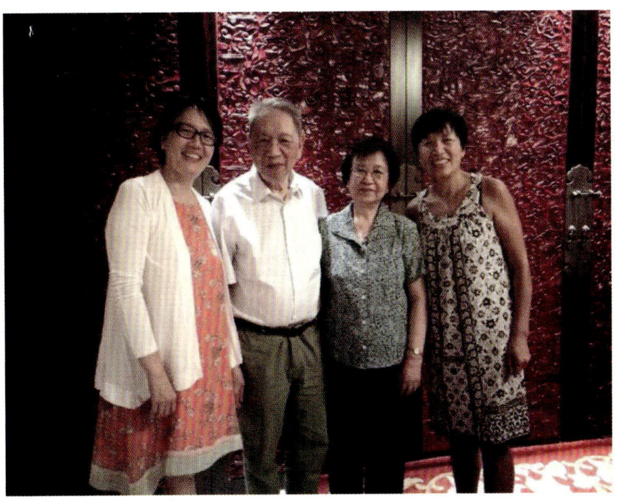

陈丹回国参加北京协和医学院百年校庆，与同学在北京饭店小聚（2017）

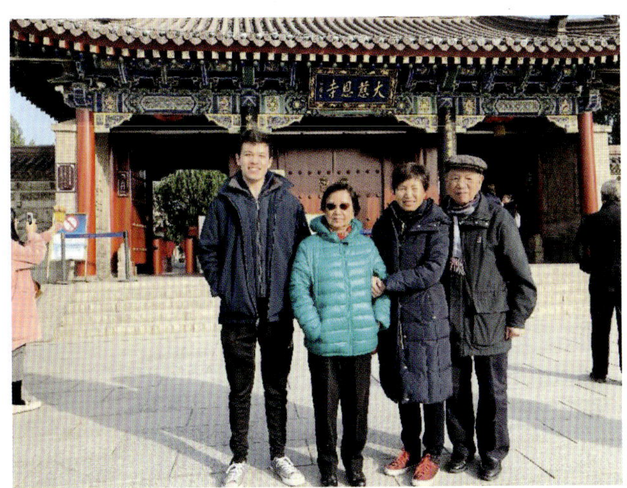

与女儿陈丹、外孙 Jared 游览西安大慈恩寺（2018）

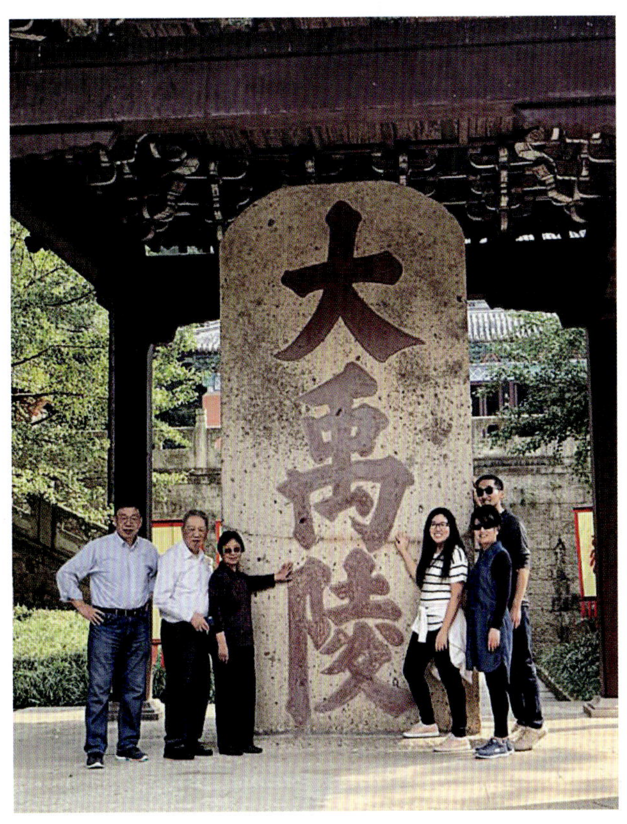

与陈舟一家参观绍兴大禹陵（2018）

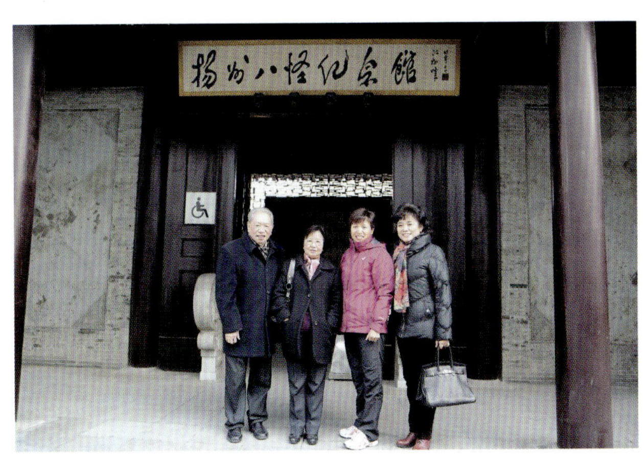

与陈丹游览扬州瘦西湖（2014）

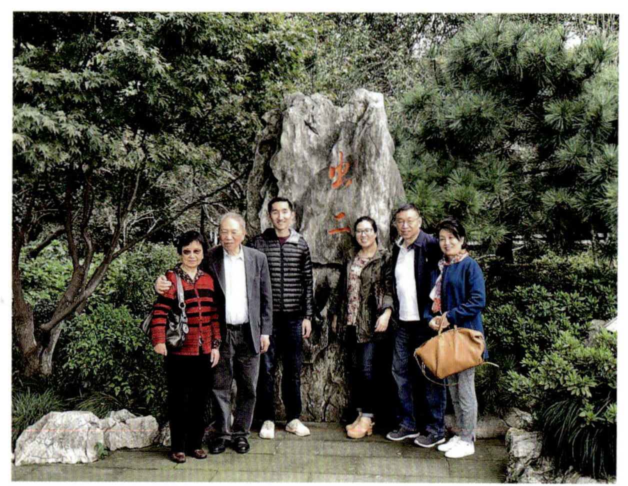
与陈舟一家游览杭州西湖（2018）

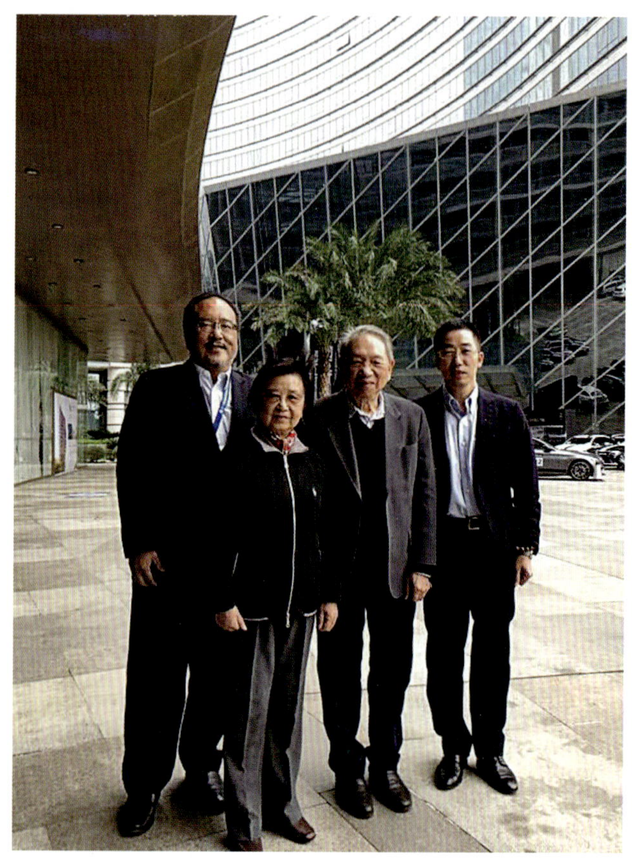
与侄子以三（Nelson Tan）在香港（2017）

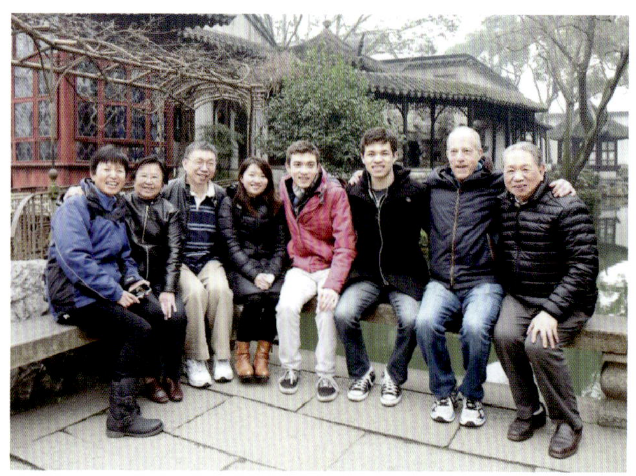
与陈舟、陈丹家人游览苏州拙政园（2016）

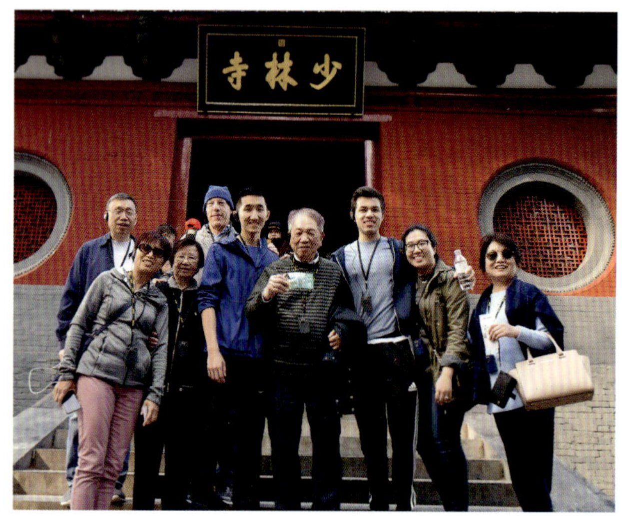

与陈舟、陈丹家人游览河南登封少林寺（2019）

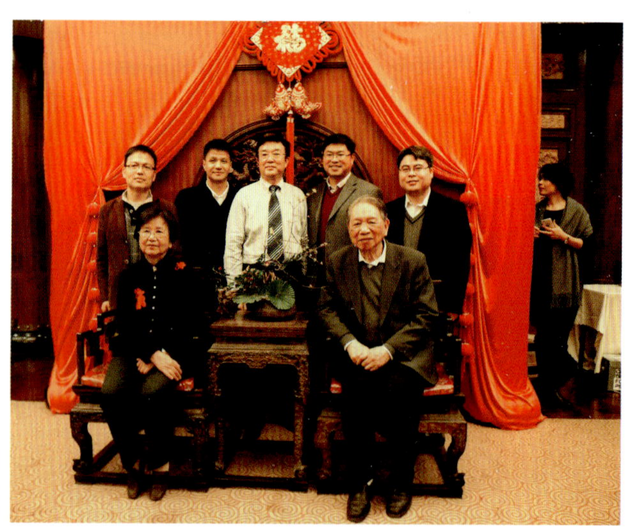
在杭州举办钻石婚纪念活动，吴宗贵（中）、张松富（右 2）、彭军（左 2）等参会（2016）

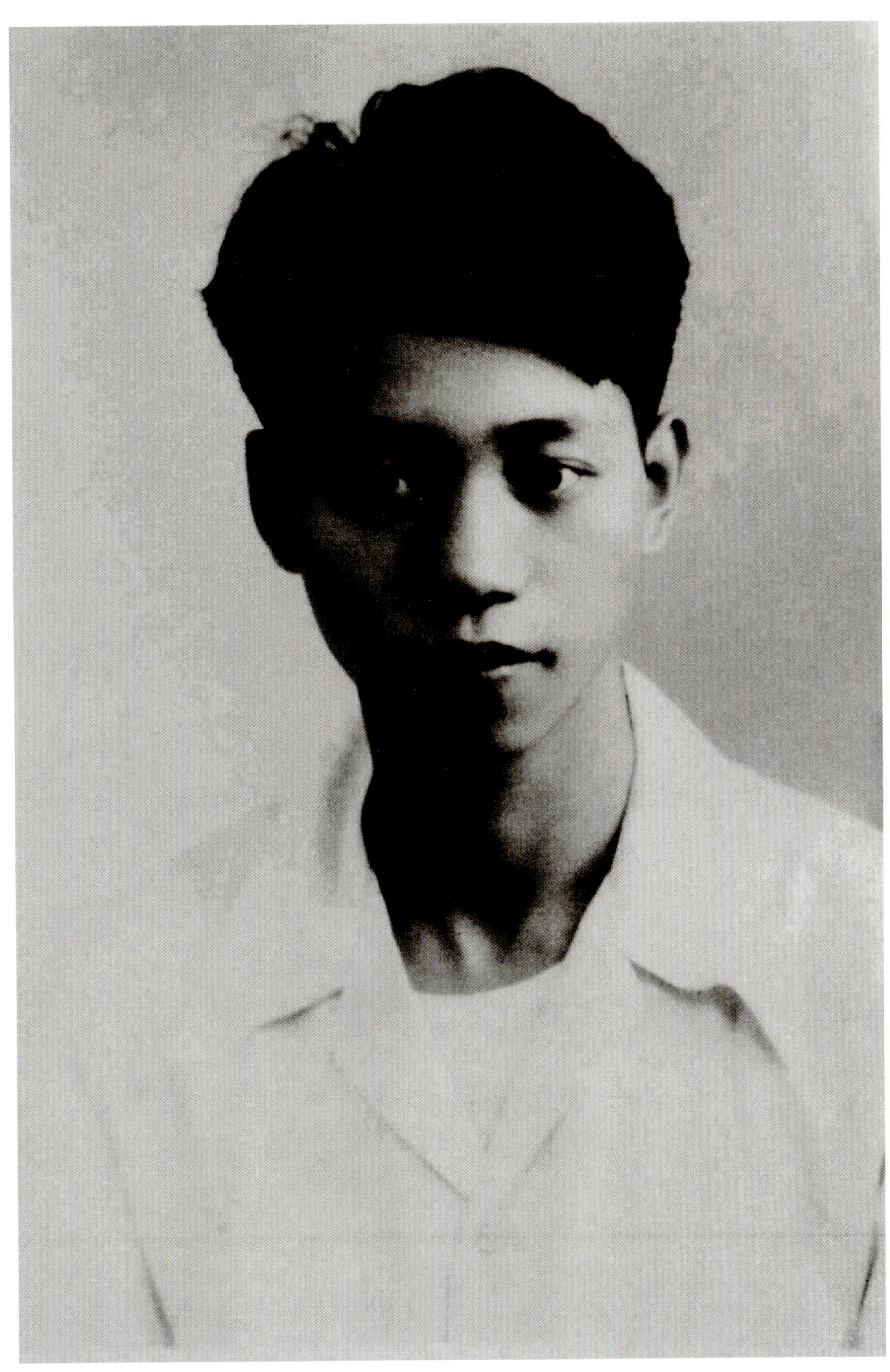

福建医学院（现福建医科大学）毕业照（1954）

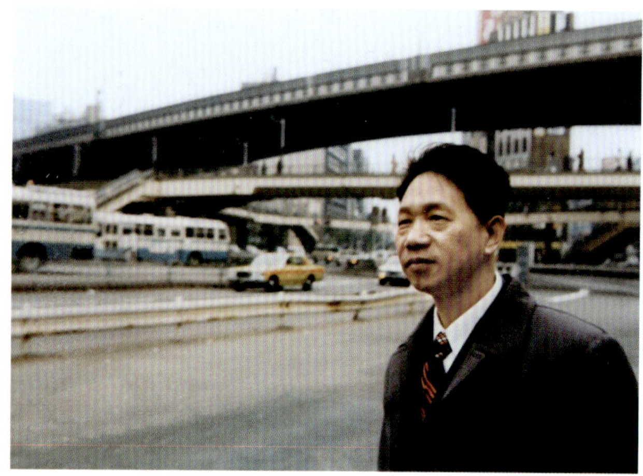

在日本大阪（1981）

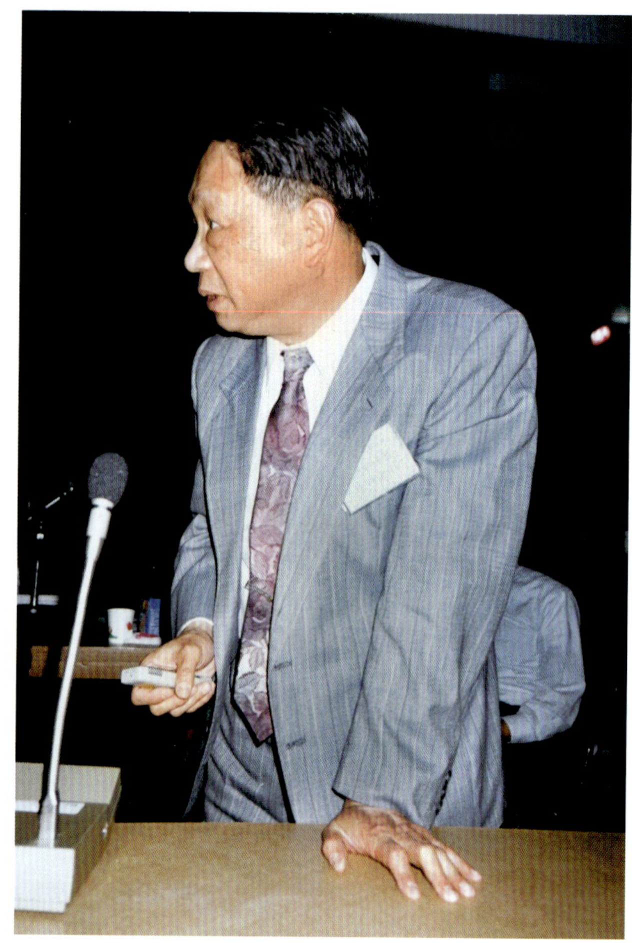

作学术报告（1993，台北）

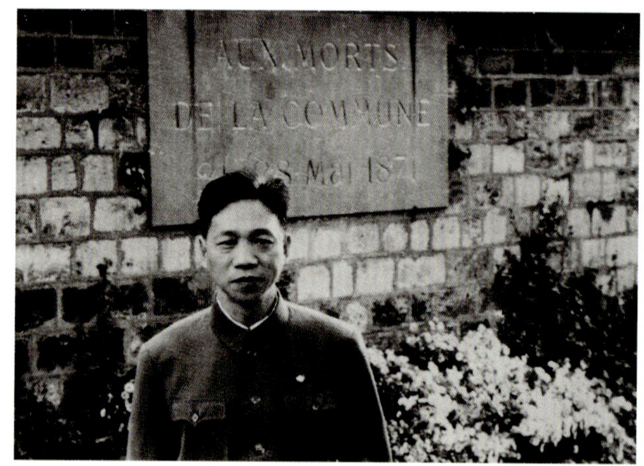

马克思墓前（1973，巴黎）

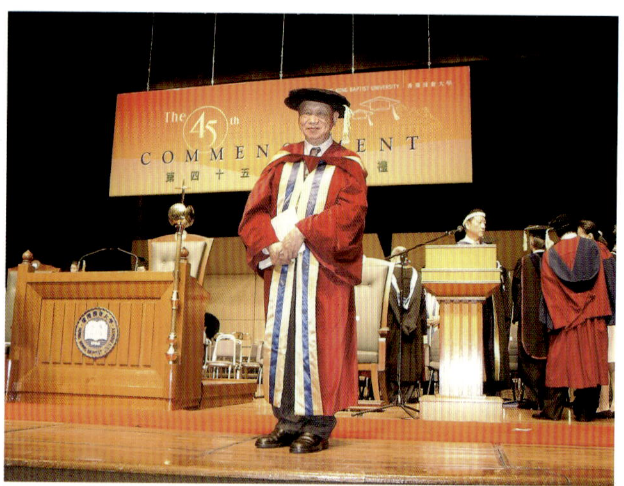

接受香港浸会大学授予荣誉博士学位（2004）

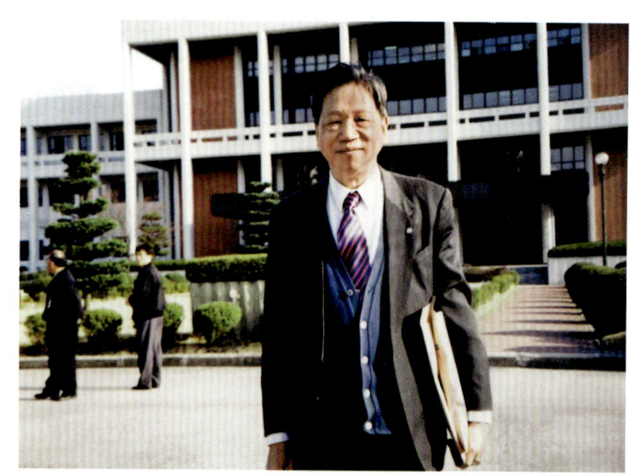

出席全国政协第七次会议（1992）

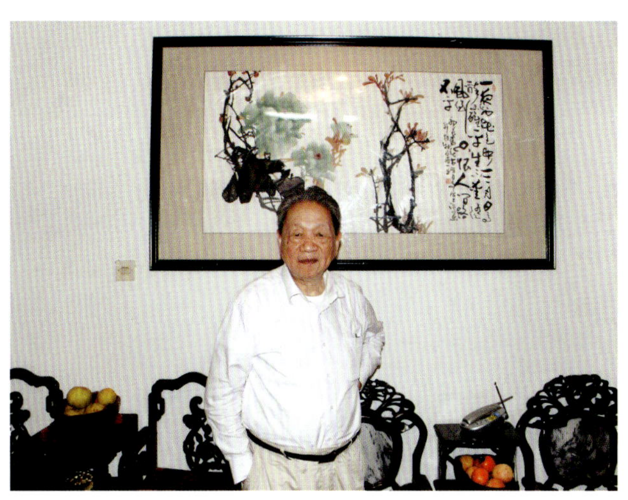

福州父母亲旧居内（2008）

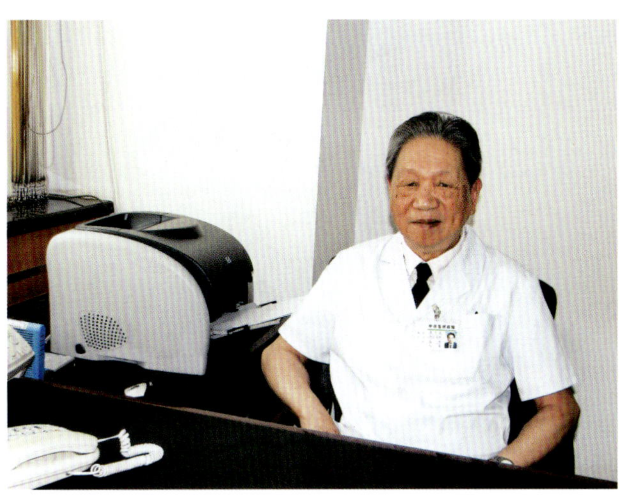

在中日友好医院心血管病中心主任办公室（2008）

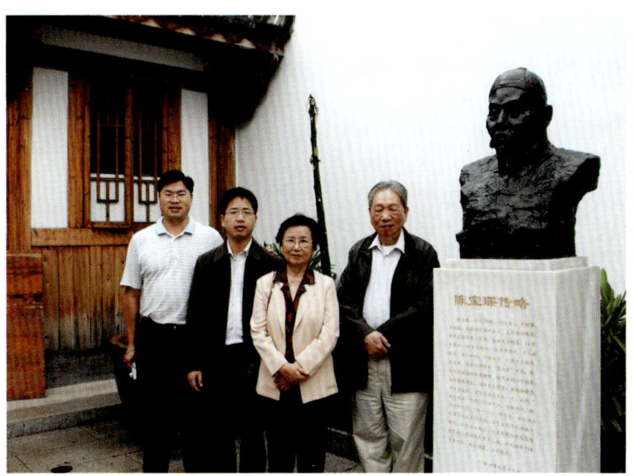

清两朝帝师陈宝琛福州故居沧趣楼（2008）

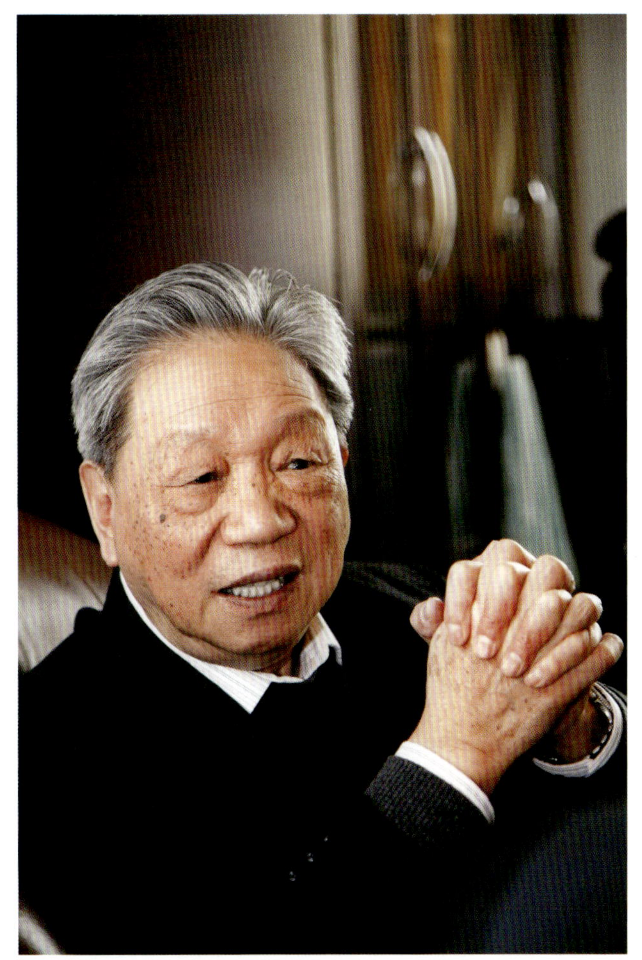

西苑医院院士办公室（2008）

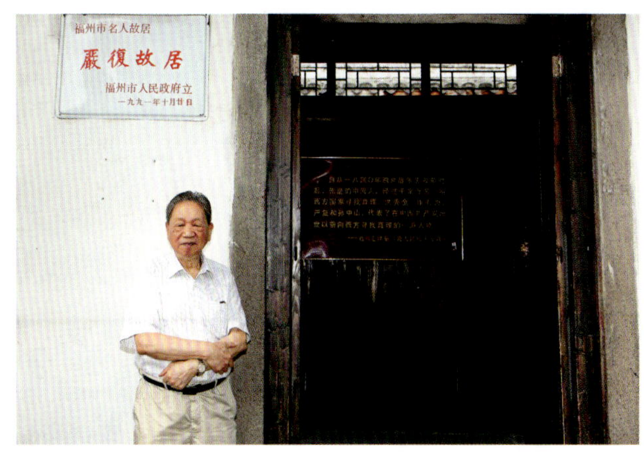

北京大学第一任校长、《天演论》译者严复福州故居（2009）

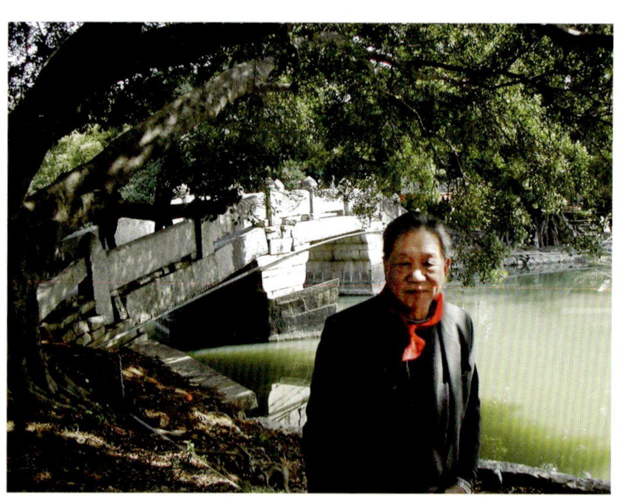

福州苏坂村榕荫桥儿时游泳处（2003）

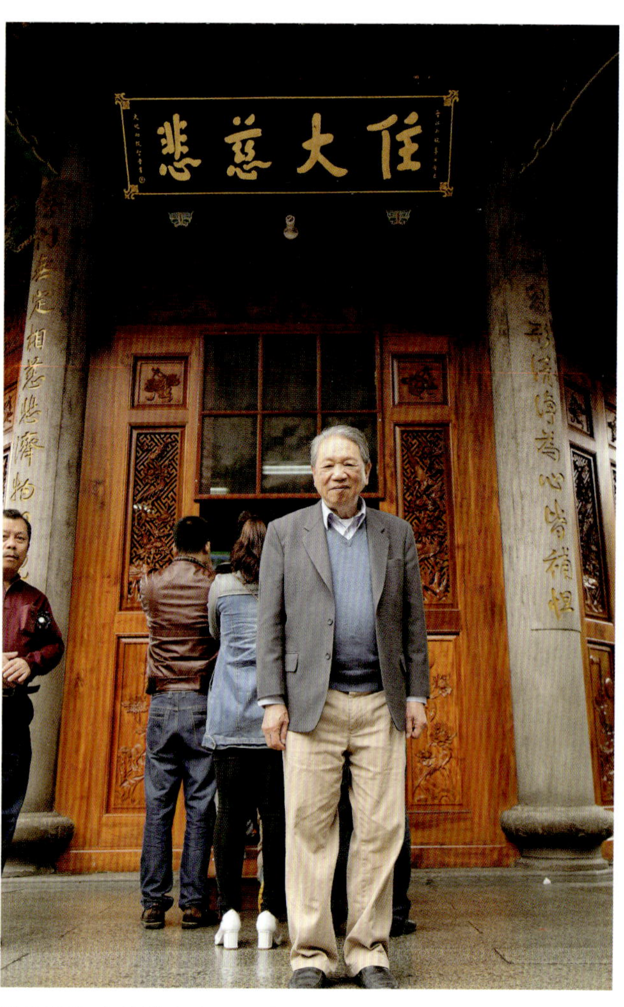

游览厦门南普陀寺（2016）

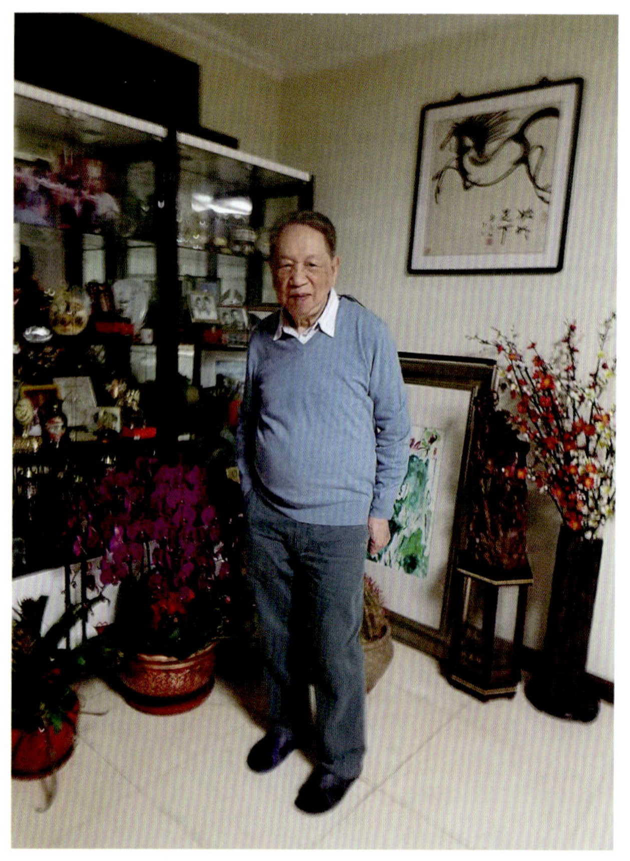

在北京家中（2019）

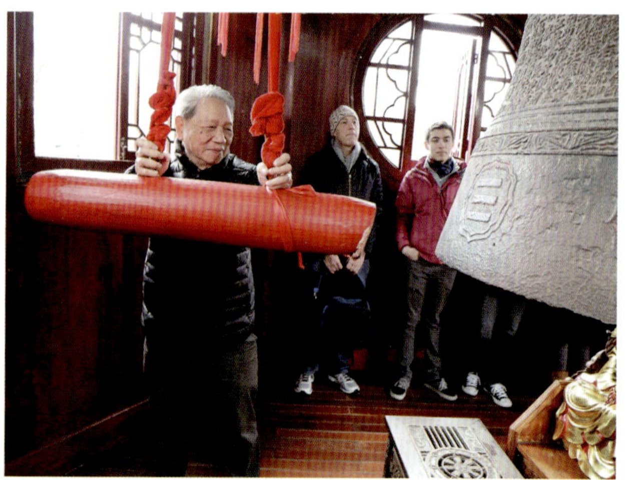

在苏州寒山寺撞钟（2016）

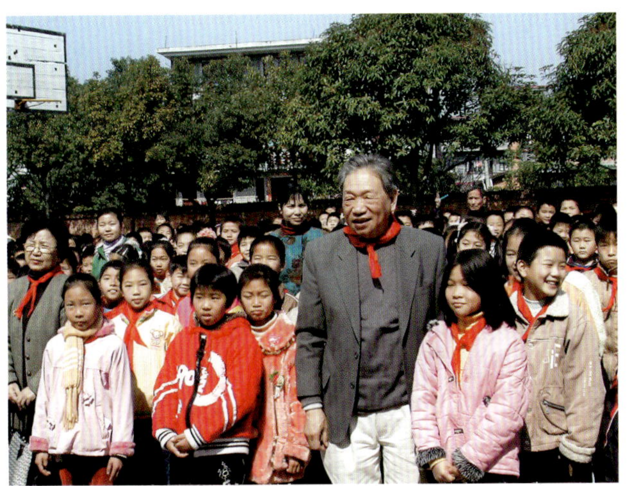
与母校闽侯苏坂小学师生（2003）

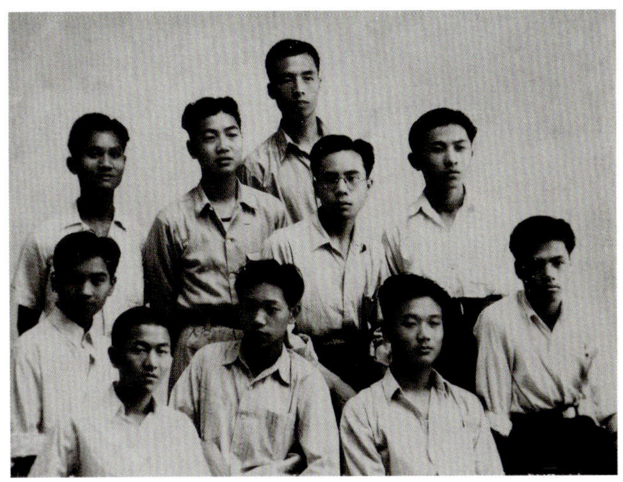
福州第一中学高二舍友（1948）

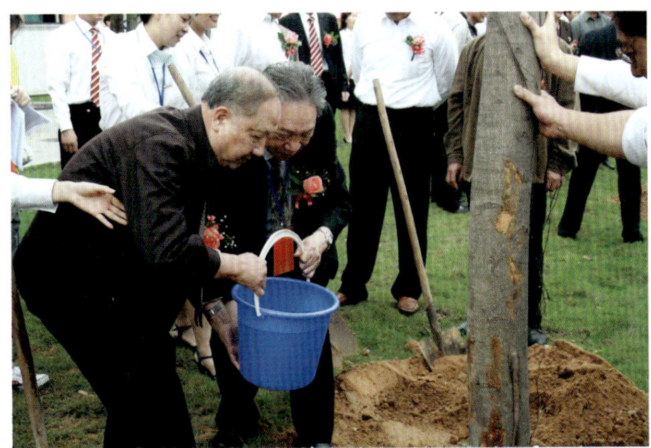
与中学同学原福建省政协游德馨主席（2007）

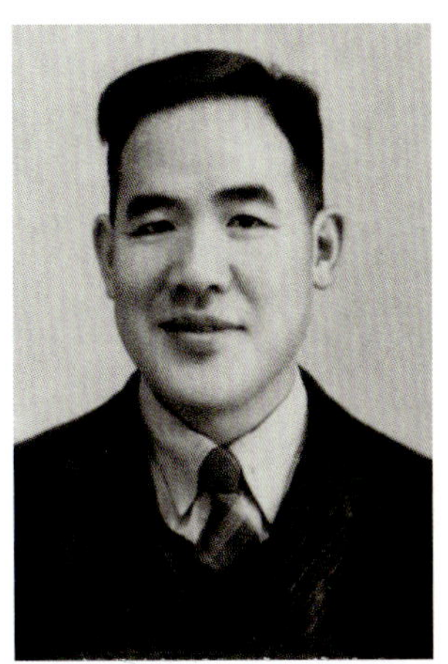
福建医学院附属医院内科主任王中方教授 (1913—1969)

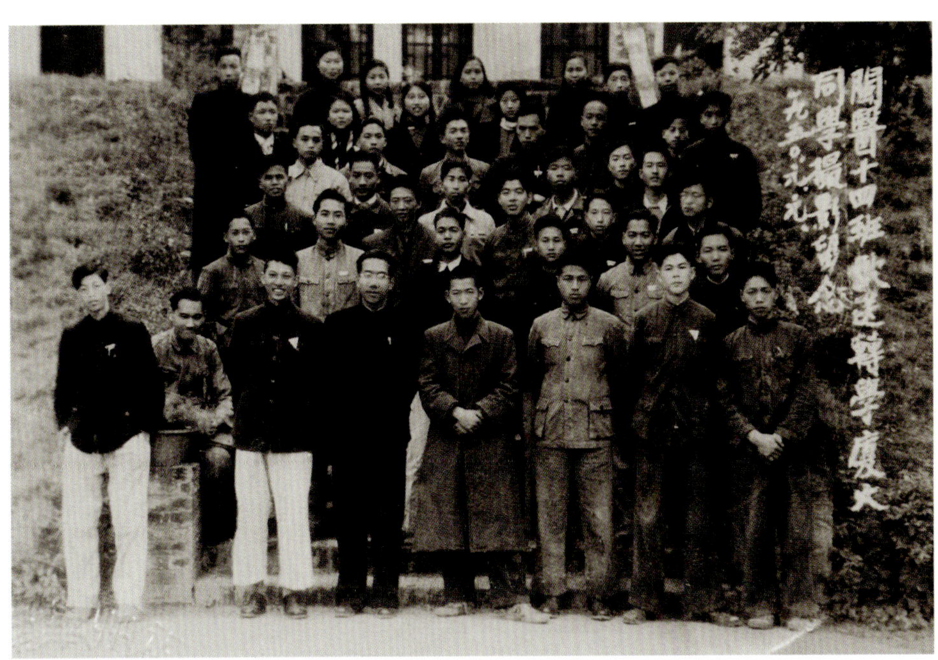

就读福建医学院第一年同学合影（前右 1 陈可冀）（1950）

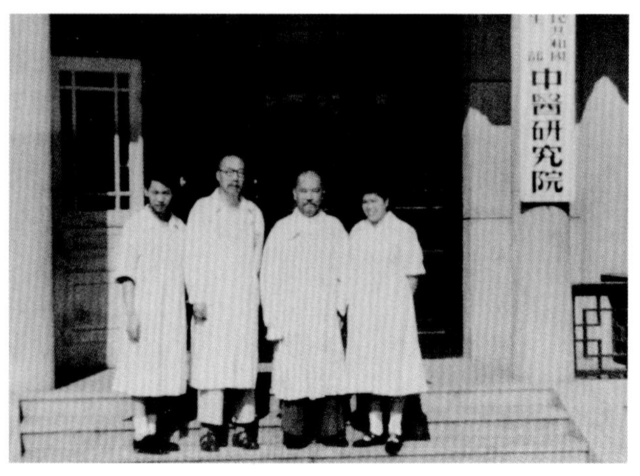

与名中医冉雪峰同一天到中国中医研究院报到工作（左 2 名中医王易门，右 1 陈敏主任医师）（1956）

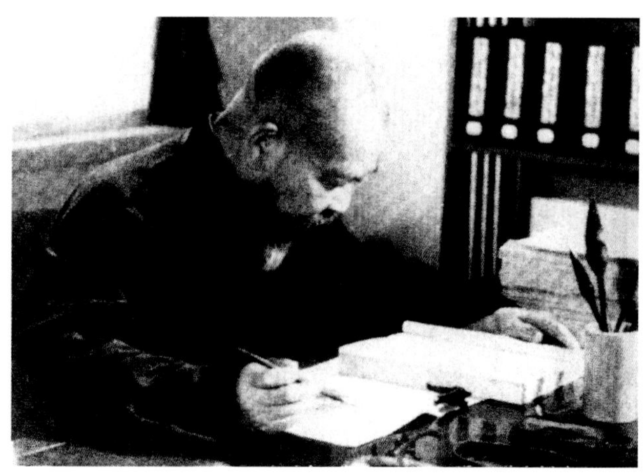

不朽的师魂：业师冉雪峰（1879—1963）

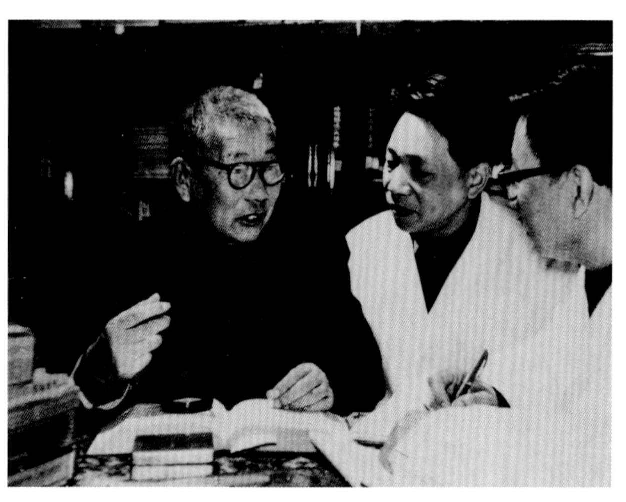

岳美中教授讲授临床经验，右 1 为时振声教授（1978）

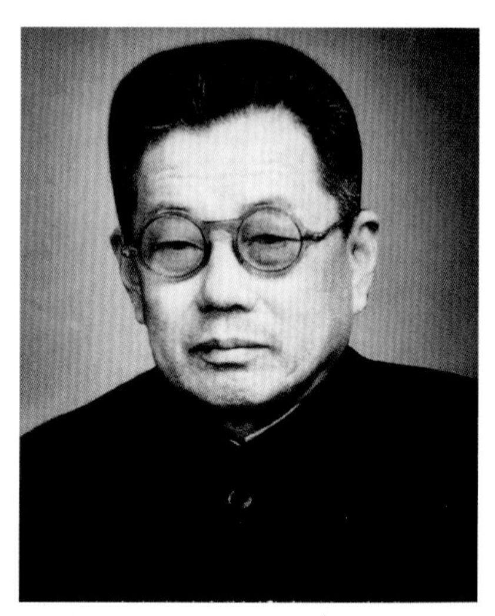

岳美中老师（1900—1982）

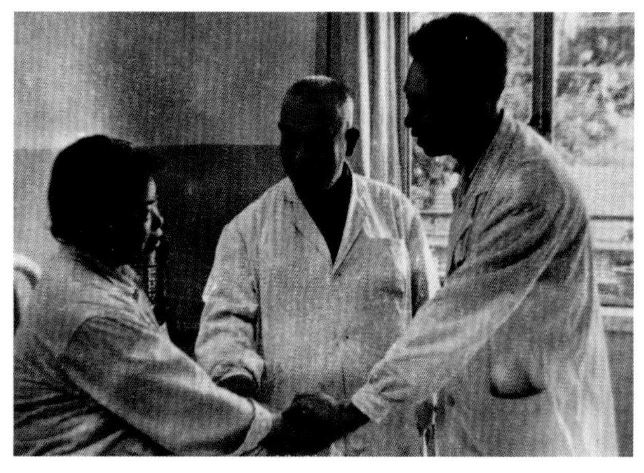

与著名中医郭士魁会诊心脏病病人（1970，西苑医院）

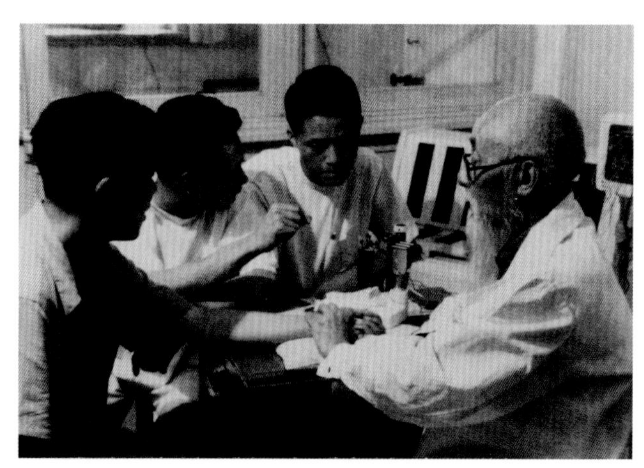

与名医蒲辅周研讨脉诊，右 2 为章宗穆教授（1958）

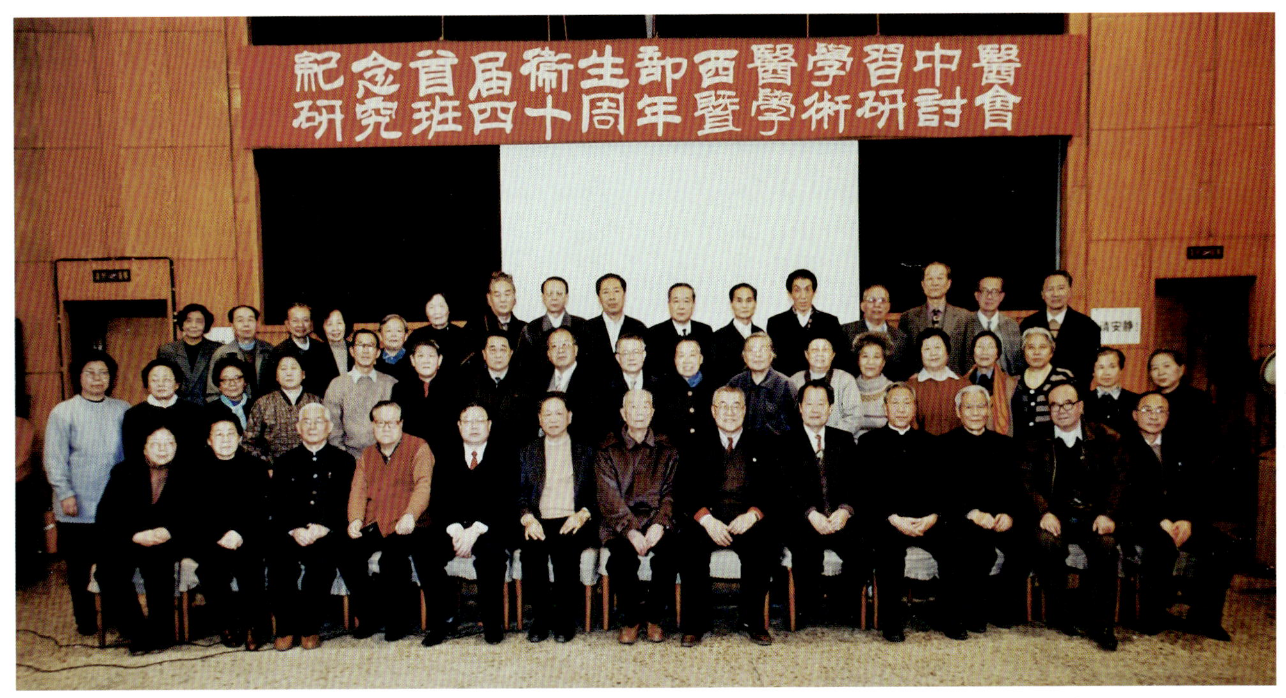

纪念卫生部西医学习中医研究班 40 周年，中为原中医研究院第一任院长鲁之俊（1998）

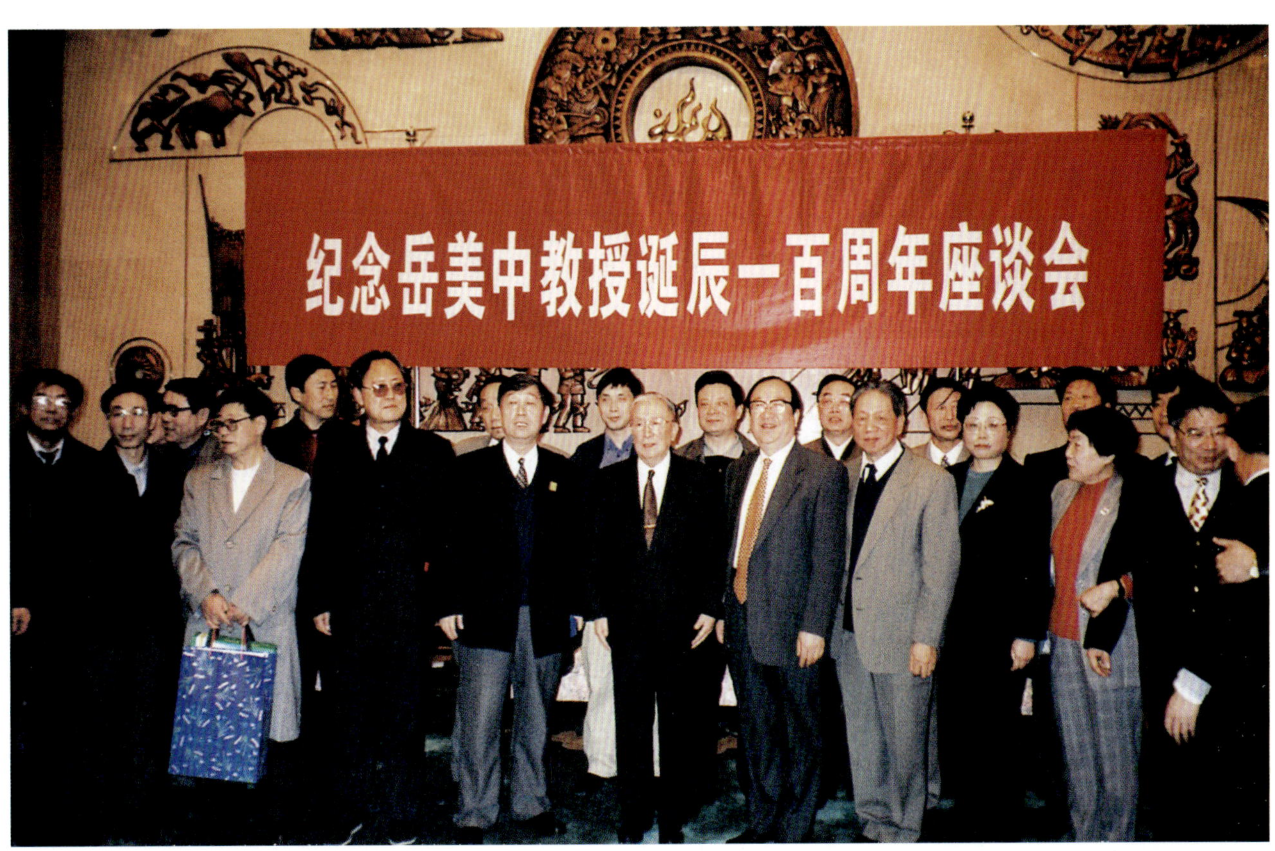

纪念岳美中教授诞辰一百周年座谈会在人民大会堂召开，吴阶平院士（前右 6）、卫生部朱庆生副部长（前右 5）、王永炎院士（前左 5）及陈可冀院士等到会（2000，北京）

岳美中老中医治疗老年病的经验

陈可冀整理

病历续页

姓名　　　　　　　　　　　　病历号　　　　　　第 1 页

岳美中老中医治疗老年病的经验

一、注意结合老年人特点，细观察，勤分析，慎下药，常总结

衰老是人类生命发展中的一种规律性表现。人自出生后，经童年、青年、中年而至老年，至一定年龄时，就出现一系列的衰老征象。当然，这和社会条件、个体条件都有关系。我国解放后，由于人民保健事业的飞速发展，城乡人民的寿命都有普遍的增长，推迟了衰老的年限，这说明人类可以控制生命的发展，达到延年益寿，为社会造福，为后辈谋利益。我们是辩证唯物论者，不同意什么"永生论"，但也不同意那种把衰老看作是注定的、不可改动的、悲观的唯心主义形而上学观点。

根据社会传统概念，认为六十岁就算进入了老年行列，九十岁可以看作是长寿的人。从预防观点上看，把五十岁左右看作是老年前期是必要的。岳老认为，人到六十岁时，脉搏有变化，以粗大为多，血压也常有变化，主气虚。但也有一类人，在六十岁以后多出现一种小脉，主偏寒多寿；曾经验证过，不少是这种情况。关键在于注意日常的较好的体质锻炼和保健，从积极方面着手。历史上不少帝王将相求长生不老，尤其以魏六朝到唐初，风行一时，均以服"金石药"为贵，其结果"疽发于背"、烦躁、中毒致死者甚多，贻害不浅。

欲延寿而反夭折者在老年人的保健医疗工作中，要注意做到："细观察、勤分析、慎用药"，常总结。平时要多留心其脉、舌变化规律，纳食、二便及睡眠情况，知其常才能知其变。例如有的老年人是"六阳脉"，平素就很粗大，临终前还是"六阳脉"，若平时不细观察，下药就会有误。老年人的病证辨可能杂一些，因为生理功能衰减，与青壮体质不同，不像年青人，一、二剂药也许就治好了。有的老年人肠胃素健，大黄用四、五钱不泻，有的用一、二钱就泻得不得了。了解素质寒热虚实之偏，饮食喜暖喜凉、喜酸喜咸，对于施治均有参考价值。有的老年人大便二天一次，俗谓"后门紧"，主多寿；食多便少，主运化功能旺盛，也要了解。

继承整理岳美中治疗老年病学术经验原稿（红字为岳老亲笔修改处）

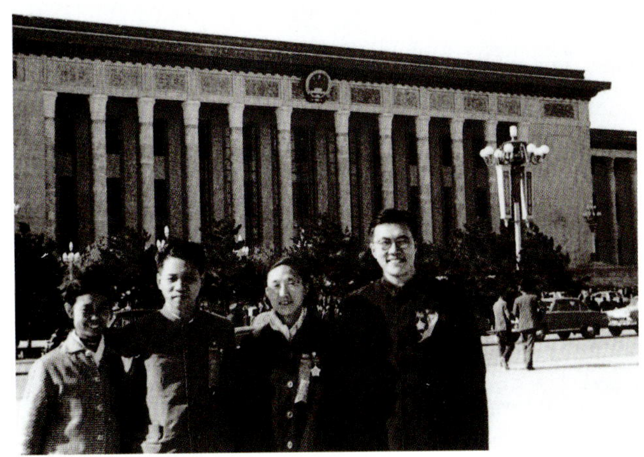

出席全国群英会的中国中医研究院医护人员，左起常立身、陈可冀、王荣和、吕维柏（1959，北京）

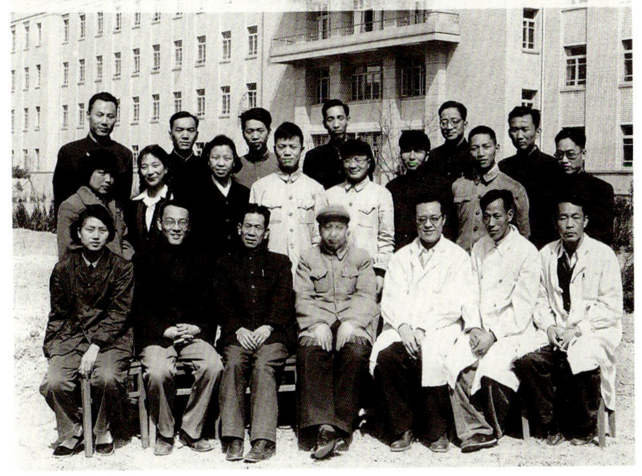

中国医学科学院阜外医院心电图进修班结业合影。黄宛（前左2）、方圻（前右3）教授授课。陈可冀（三排左3）与徐涛医师（三排左1）等参加学习（1959）

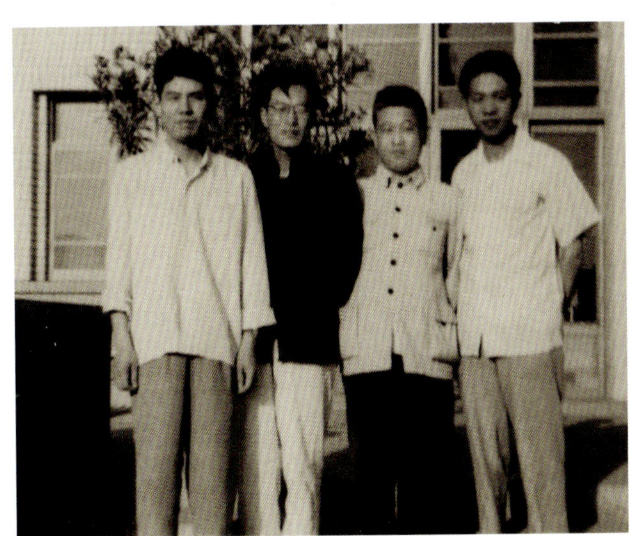

在阜外医院协作期间与名中医郭士魁（右2），张家鹏（左1）、王占玺（左2）等留影（1959，北京阜外医院）

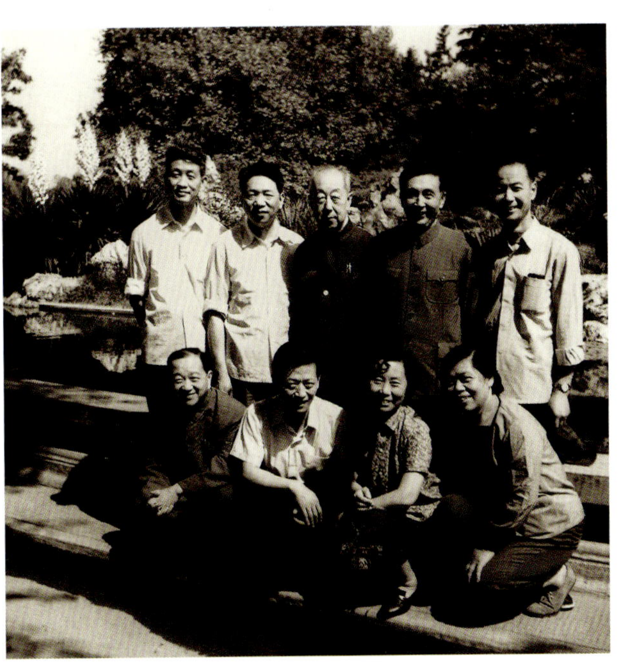

前左起翁心植、陈新、顾复生、戴玉华，后左起陈尚恭、陈可冀、吴英恺、胡旭东、孙瑞龙（1980，南京玄武湖畔）

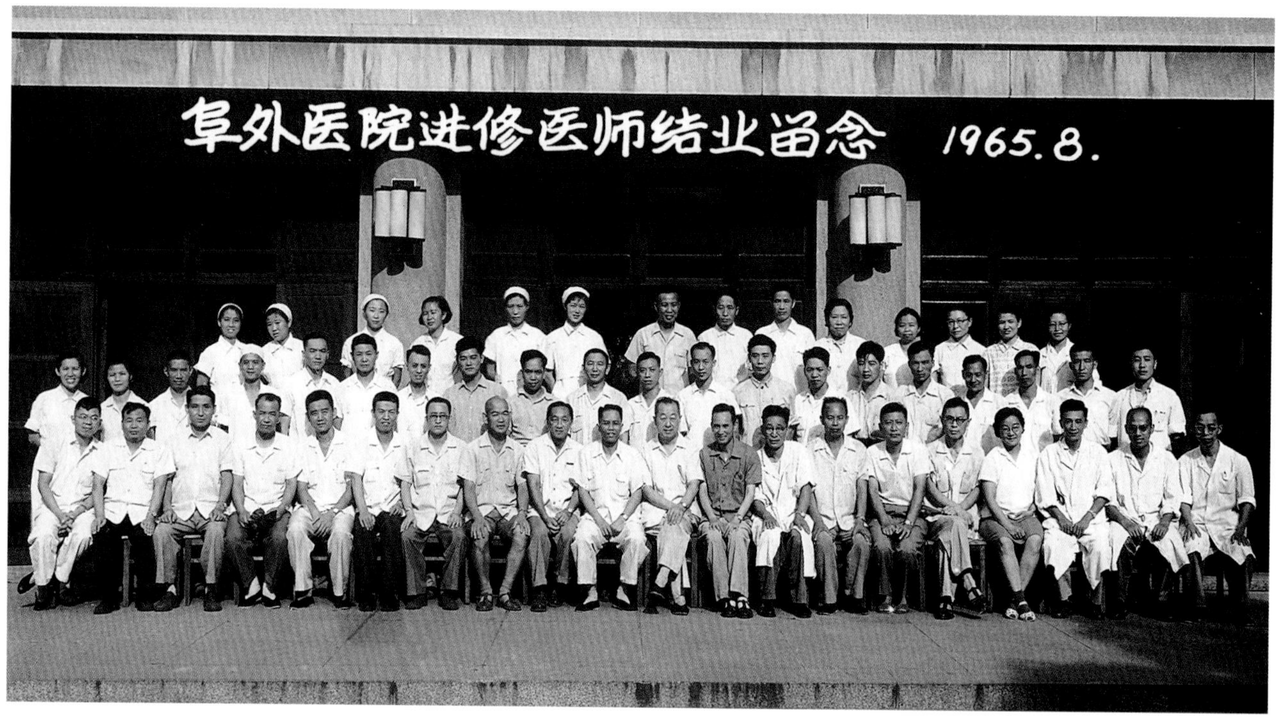

1964 年 9 月至 1965 年 8 月在阜外医院进修，二排右 7 为陈可冀，前排右 10 为吴英恺院士，右 9 为蔡如升副院长、右 5 为刘玉清院士

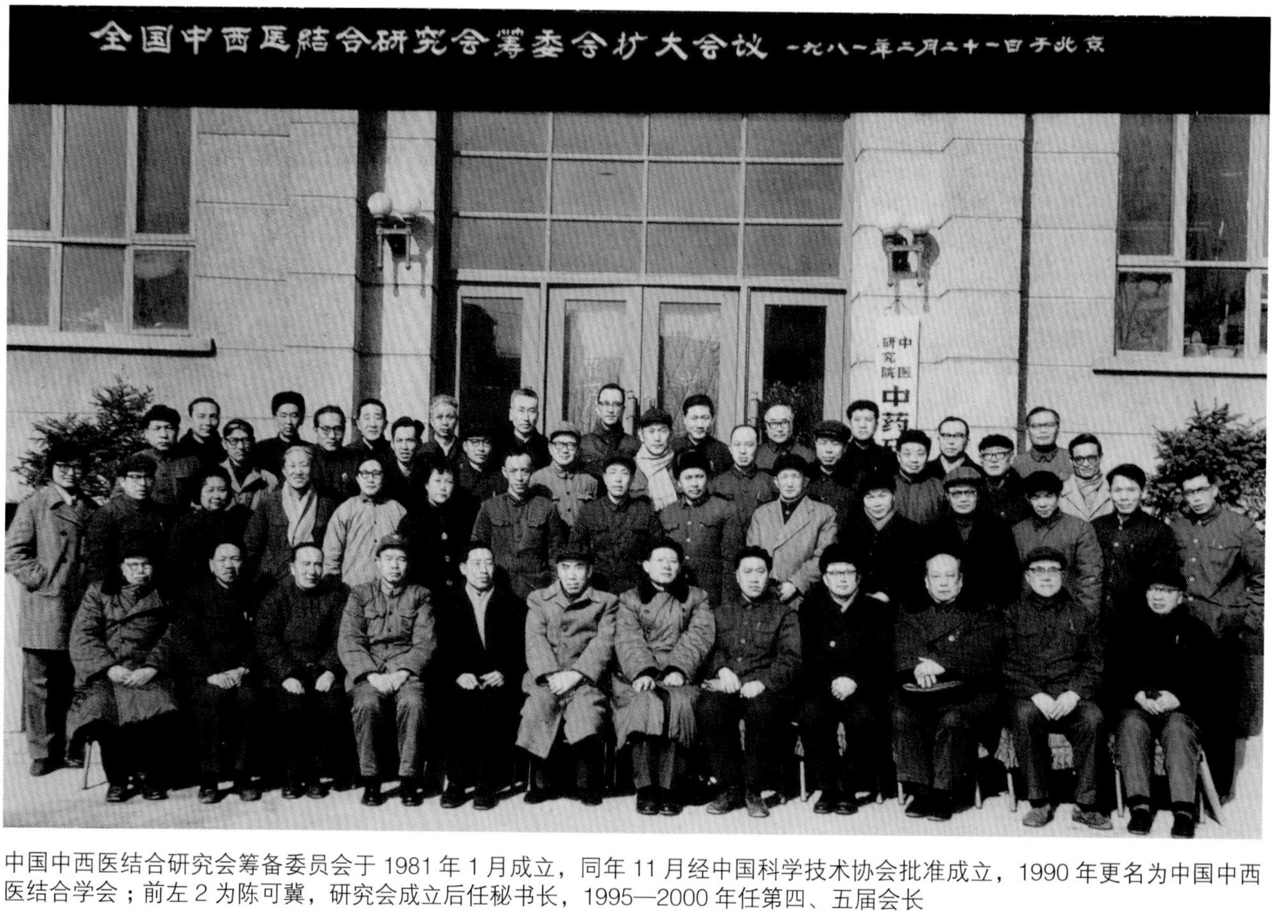

全国中西医結合研究会筹委会扩大会议 一九八一年二月二十一日于北京

中国中西医结合研究会筹备委员会于 1981 年 1 月成立，同年 11 月经中国科学技术协会批准成立，1990 年更名为中国中西医结合学会；前左 2 为陈可冀，研究会成立后任秘书长，1995—2000 年任第四、五届会长

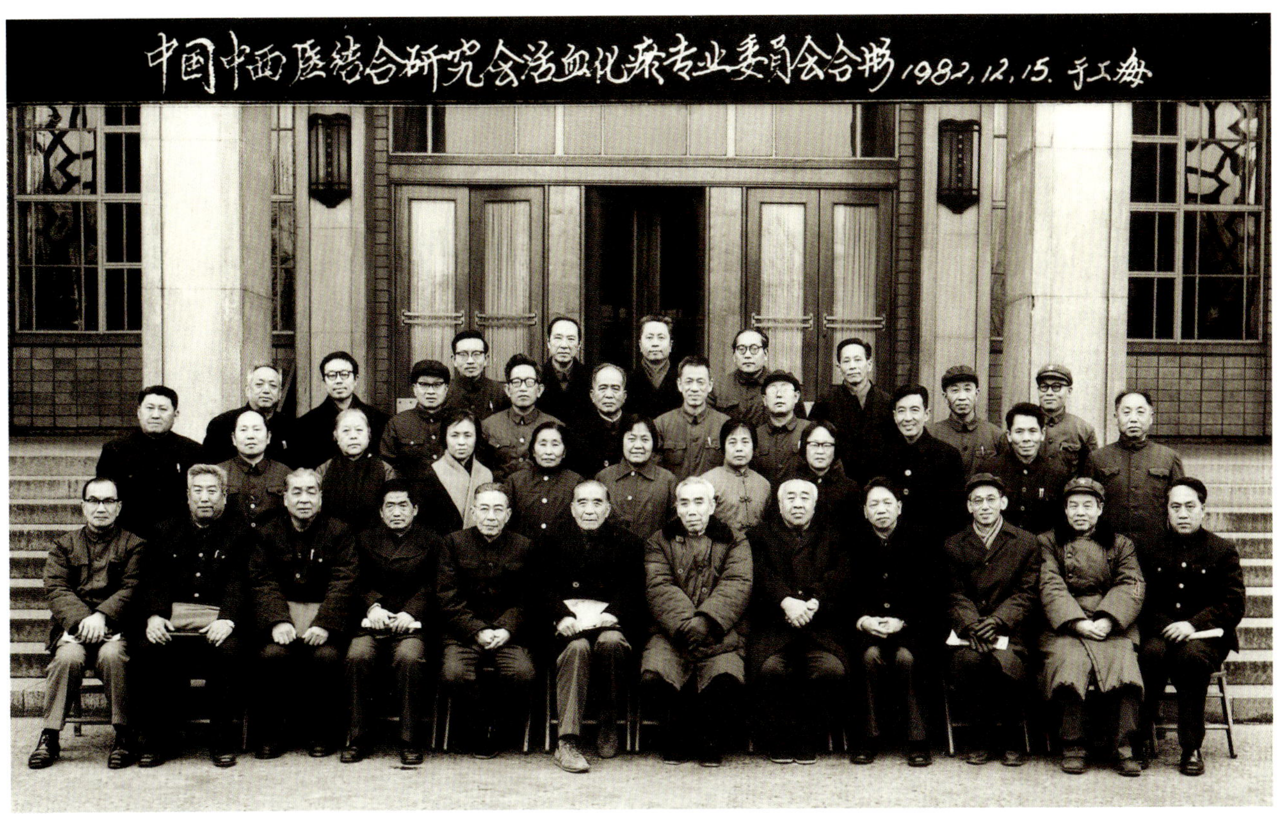

中国中西医结合学会活血化瘀专业委员会成立，陈可冀被选为主任委员，前左 5、6、7、8、10、11 祝谌予、邝安堃、季钟朴、陈文杰、张之南、高辉远教授（1982，上海）

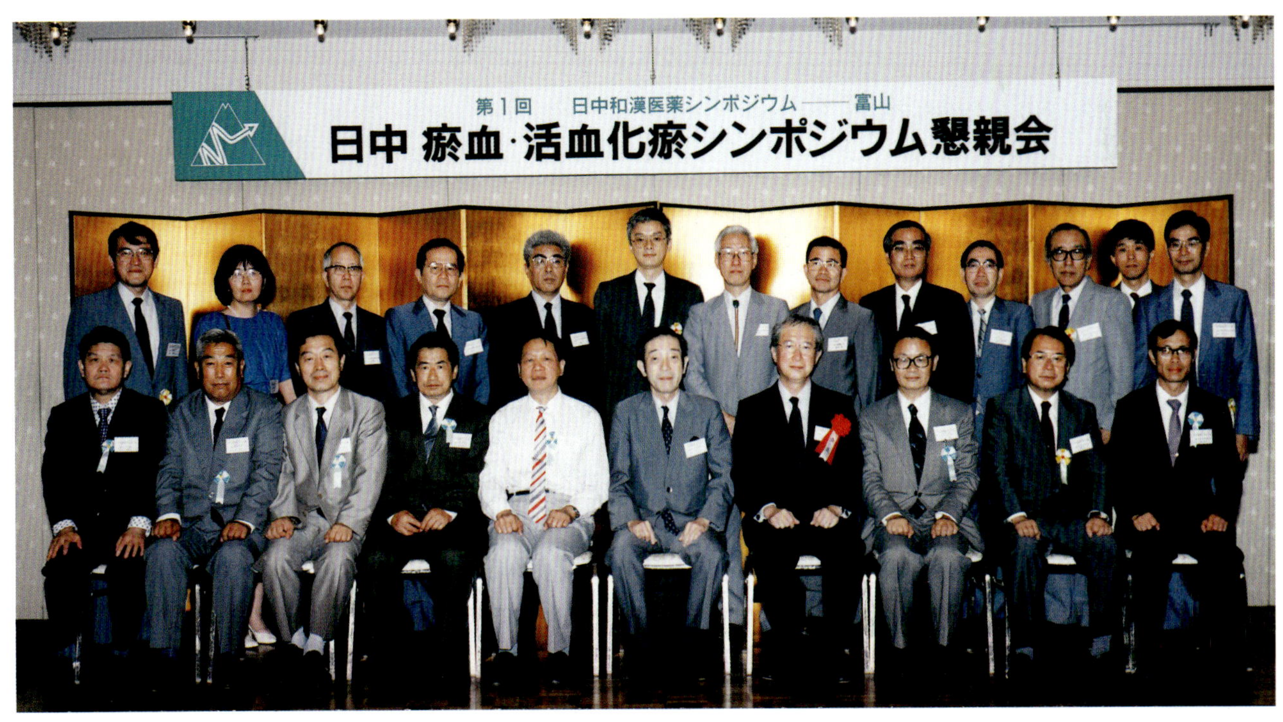

日中瘀血与活血化瘀研讨会与寺泽捷年（后左 1）、横泽隆子（后左 2）、津谷喜一郎（后左 6）、难波恒雄（后左 7）、大浦彦吉（右 5）、熊谷朗（右 4）（1988，日本富山）

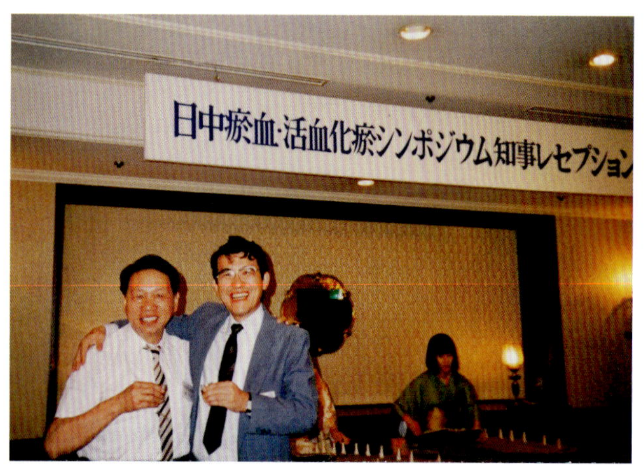

在日本富山参加血瘀证会议，与寺泽捷年教授合影（1988）

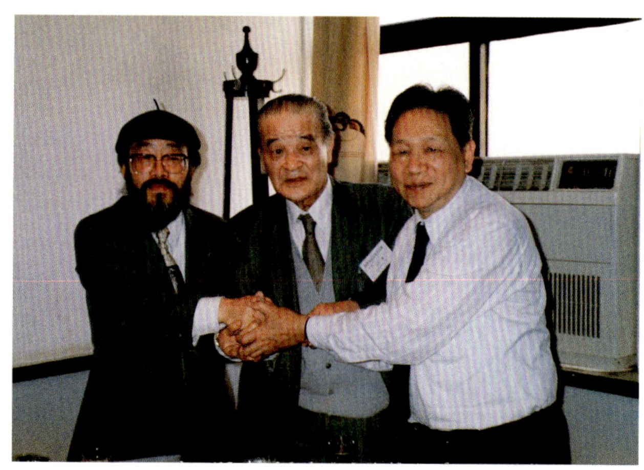

中日韩血瘀证会议上与日本小川新教授（中），韩国郑遇悦教授（左 1）（1995，北京）

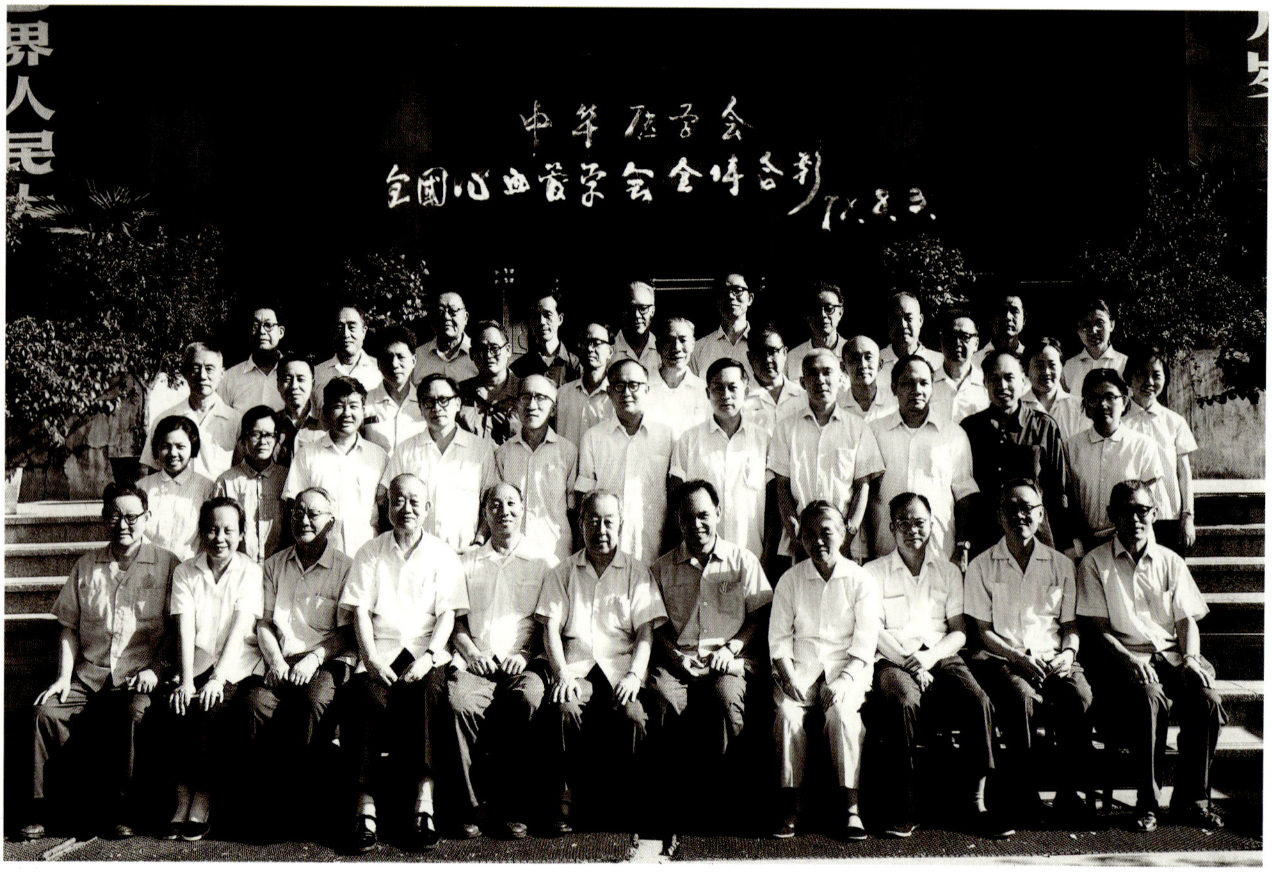

中华医学会心血管病学会第一届理事会合影，中为会长吴英恺院士，右 1—3 为苏鸿熙、黄宛、石美鑫教授，四排左 5 方圻教授，三排左 3 陈可冀院士（1978，太原）

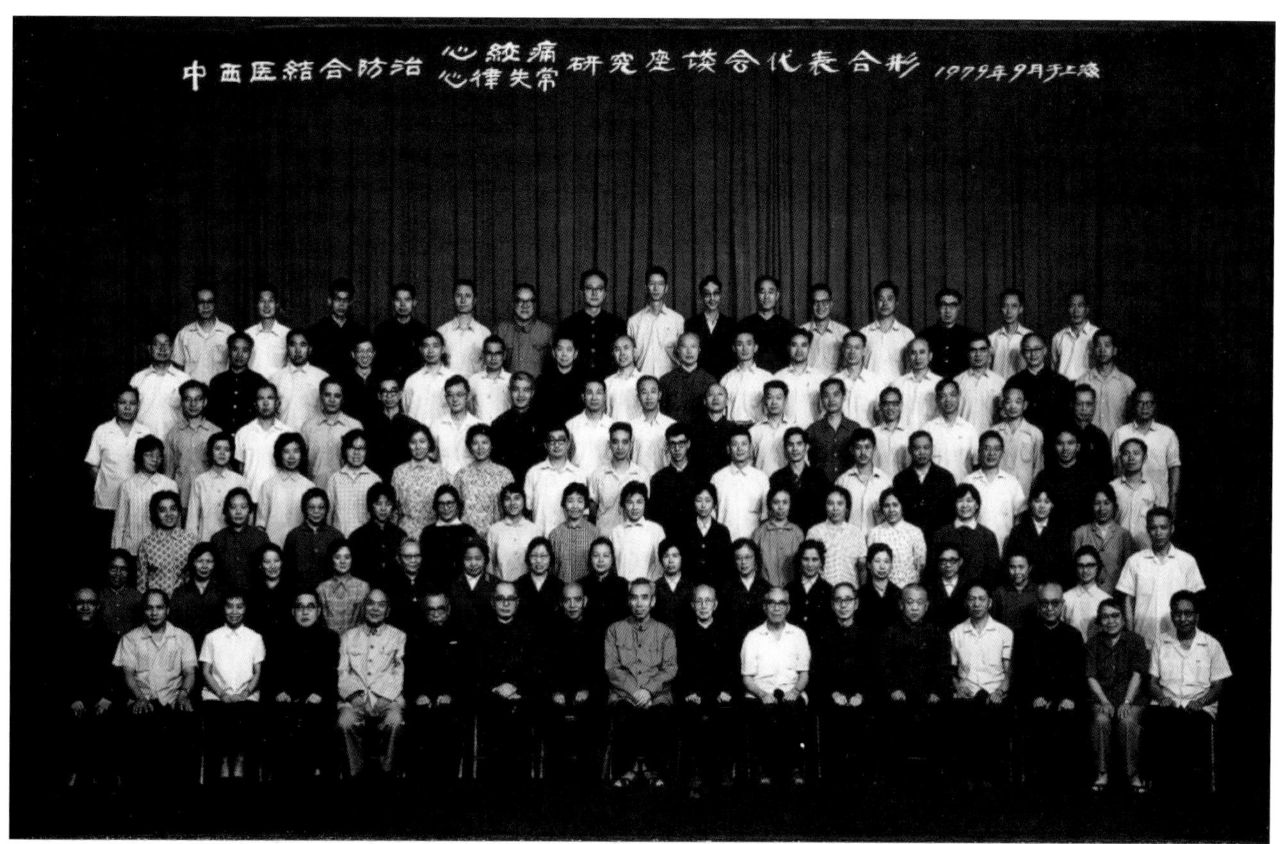

全国中西医结合防治心绞痛、心律失常研究座谈会，季钟朴（前中）、董承琅（前右8）、邝安堃（前右7）、郭士魁（前右5）、陶寿淇（前右6）、黄铭新（前左7）、陶清（前左6）、俞国瑞（前右1）、禤湘耀（前左2）、顾复生（前左3）、佘国膺（2排左2）、陈在嘉（3排左3）、李连达（后左5）、钱振淮（3排右5）、翁维良（4排右1）及陈可冀（前右4）（1979，上海）

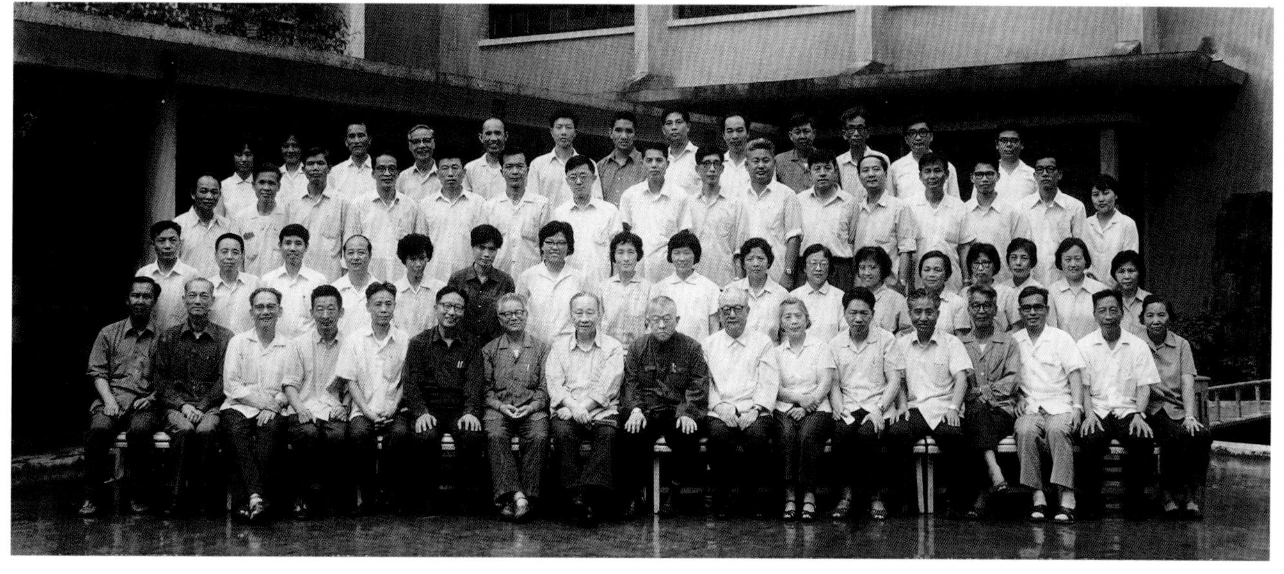

在制定冠心病中医辨证标准的全国冠心病辨证论治研究座谈会上，邓铁涛（前左7），任应秋（前左8）、郭士魁（前中）、郑学文（前右7）、李介鸣（前右8）、陈可冀（前右6）、邵耕（前右5）（1980，广东新会）

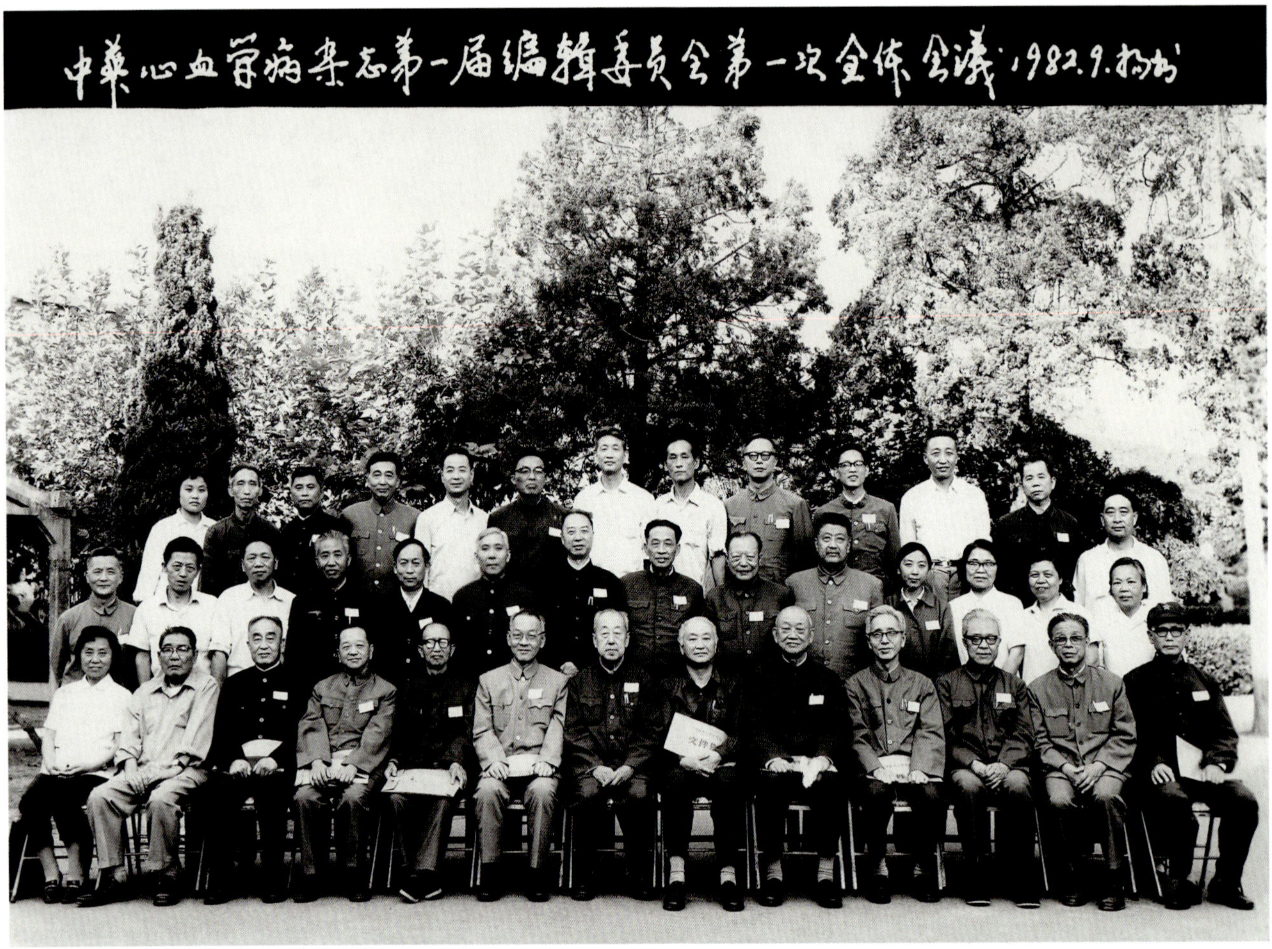

中華心血管病杂志第一届编辑委员会第一次全体会議 1982.9.扬州

陈可冀（2 排左 3）担任《中华心血管病杂志》第 1—4 届副总编，第 1 届总编吴英恺院士（前左 7），副总编黄宛（前左 6），陶寿淇（前右 4），方圻（前右 3），翁心植（前左 4）（1982，扬州）

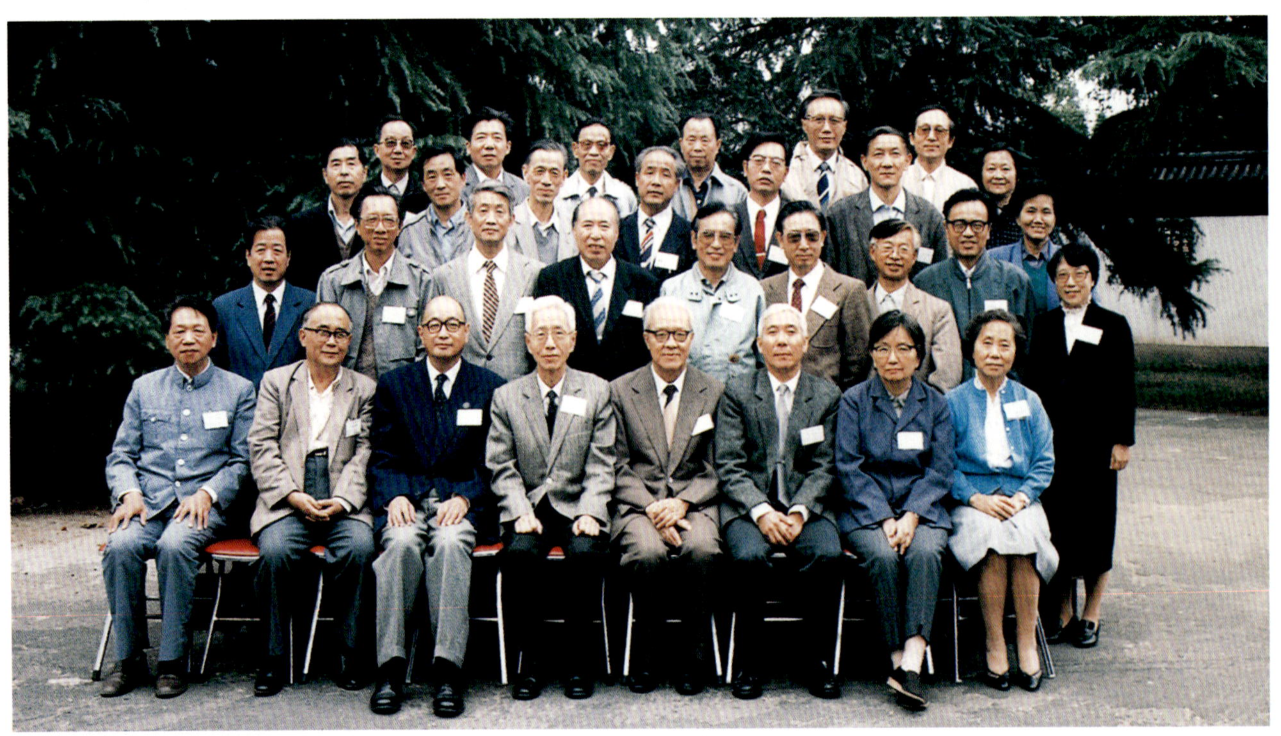

中华心血管病杂志编委会会议，前右起顾复生、刘力生、陈灏珠、方圻、陶寿淇、钱贻简、高德恩、陈可冀（1988，杭州）

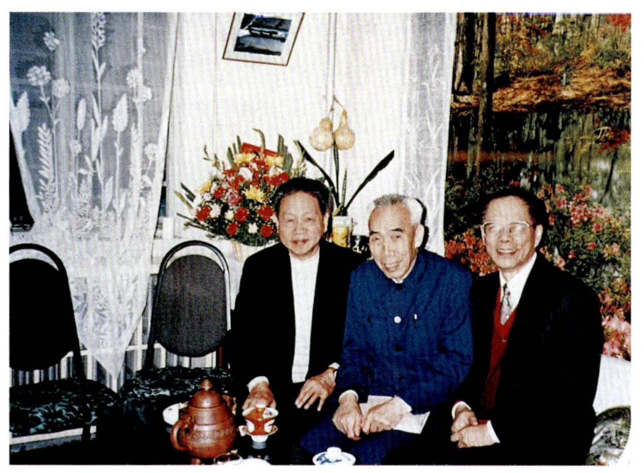

1994 年春节与韩济生院士（右）共同向在学术进步过程中给予有力支持的老院长季钟朴教授（中）拜年（1994，北京）

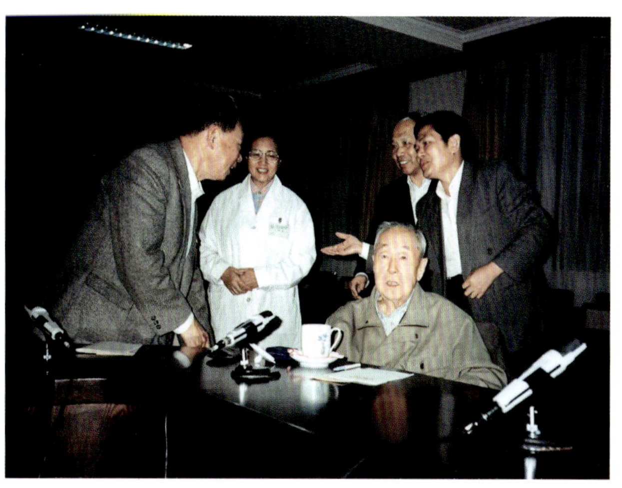

与吴英恺院士（坐）在第 7 次中国科学院院士大会期间一起作心血管病保健问题讲座（1997，京西宾馆）

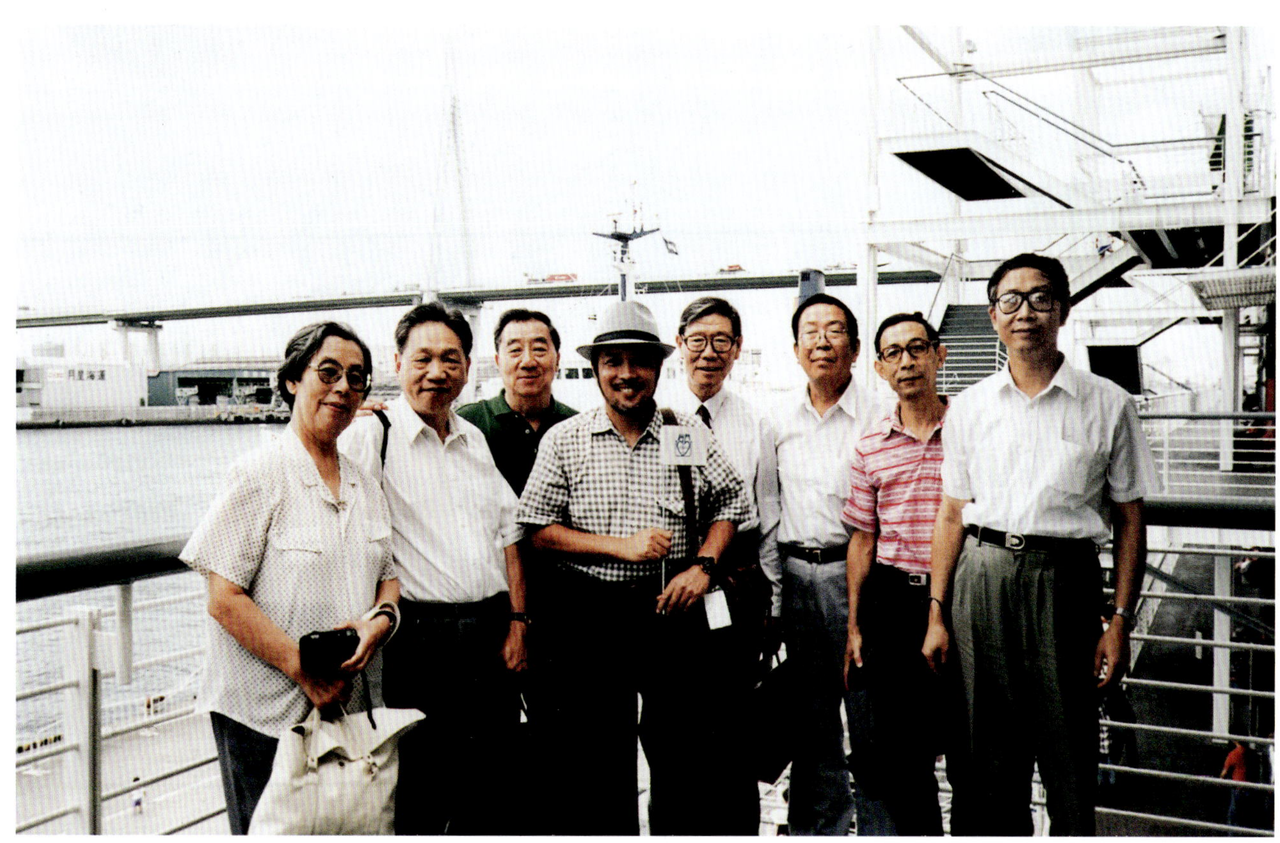

在大阪出席中日动脉粥样硬化学术会议，右起柯元南、周爱儒、齐治家、李顺成、日本朋友、佘铭鹏、陈可冀、崔吉君（1997）

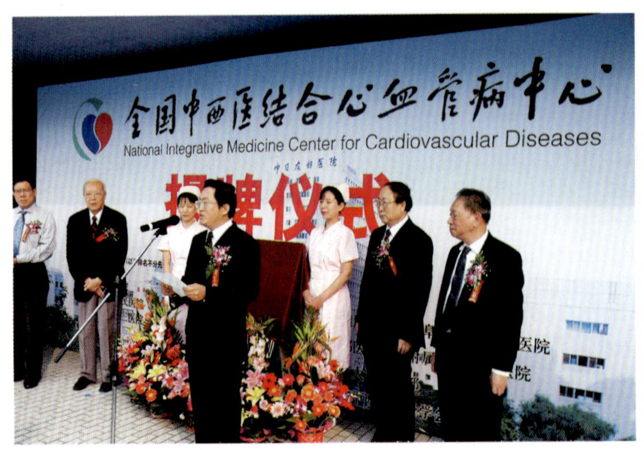

卫生部中日友好医院全国中西医结合心血管病中心成立揭牌仪式并任中心主任，左 2 为方圻教授，右 2 为朱晓东院士，前致词者为许树强院长（2005）

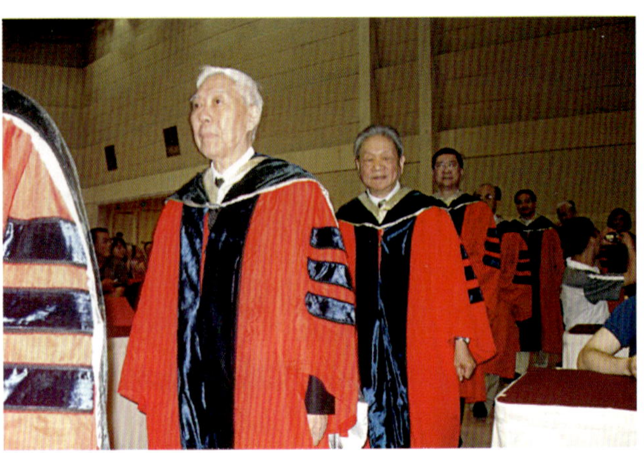

中华医学会心血管病学会专家会员授予仪式，前陈灏珠，第 3 林曙光（2008，郑州）

中华医学会老年医学分会第五届委员会委员合影，陈可冀（中）被选为主任委员（1999，无锡）

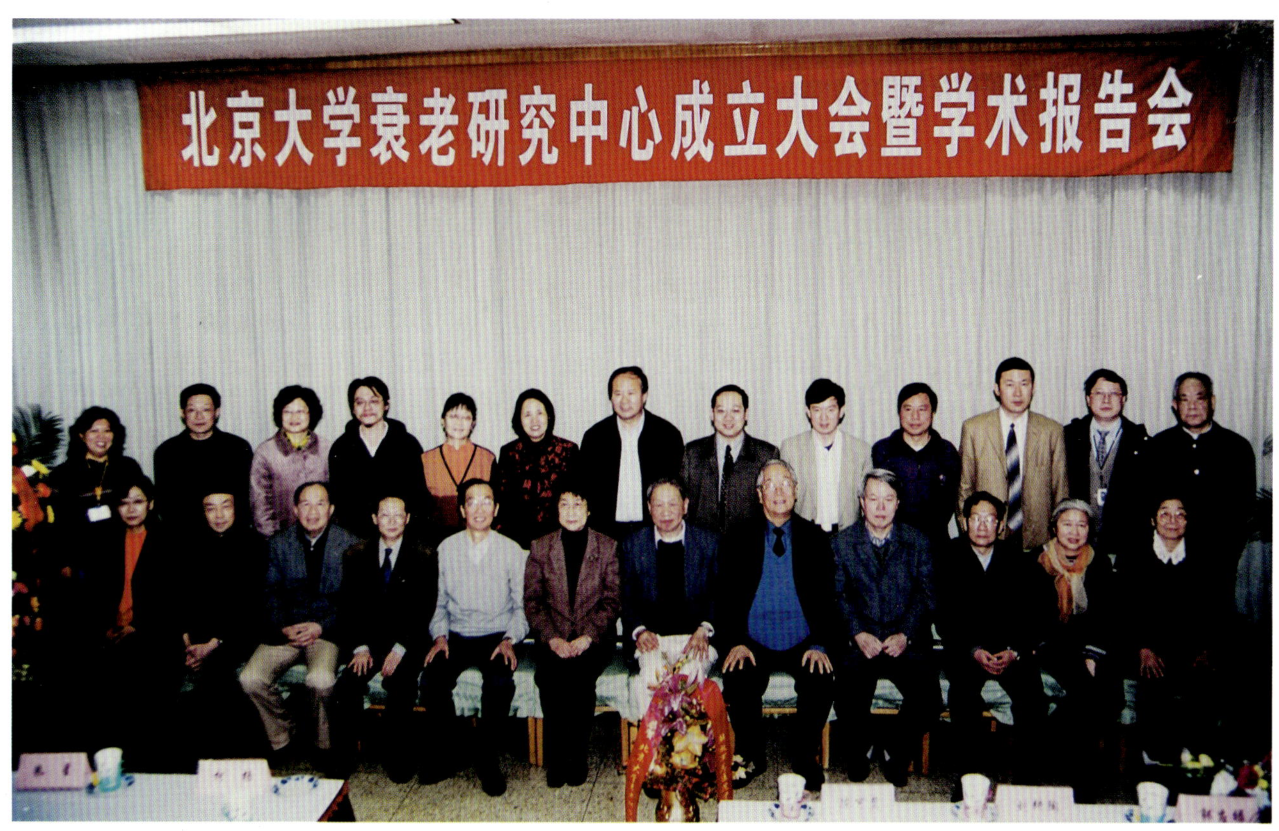

北京大学衰老研究中心成立，受聘为学术委员会主任委员，前左 4 童坦君院士，前左 6 王琳芳院士，前右 4、5 刘耕陶、郭应禄院士，前右 1 张宗玉教授（2006）

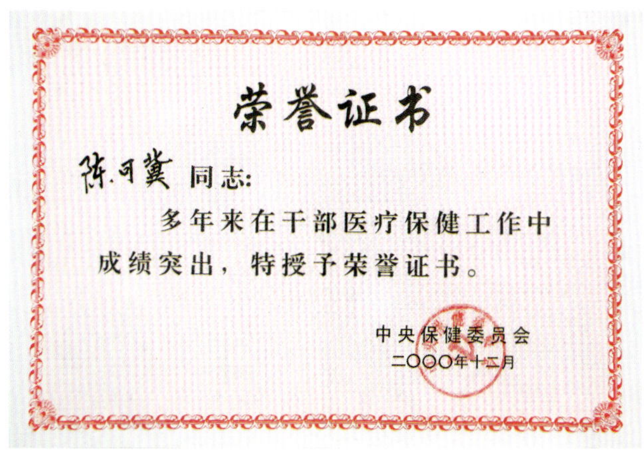

荣誉证书

陈可冀 同志:

多年来在干部医疗保健工作中成绩突出，特授予荣誉证书。

中央保健委员会
二〇〇〇年十二月

授予干部医疗保健工作荣誉证书（2000）

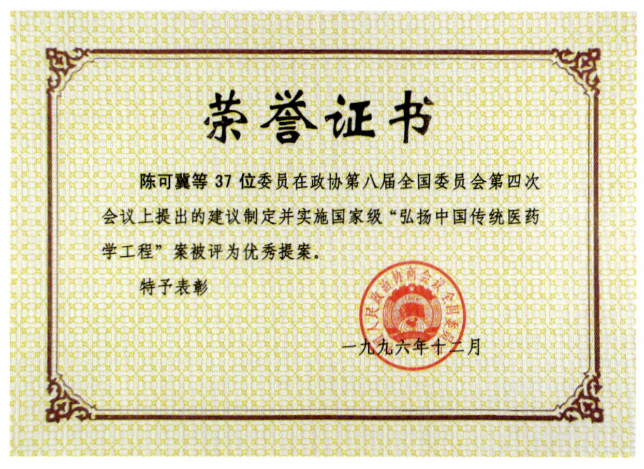

荣誉证书

陈可冀等 37 位委员在政协第八届全国委员会第四次会议上提出的建议制定并实施国家级“弘扬中国传统医药学工程”案被评为优秀提案。

特予表彰

一九九六年十二月

“弘扬中国传统医药学工程”提案被评为优秀提案（1996）

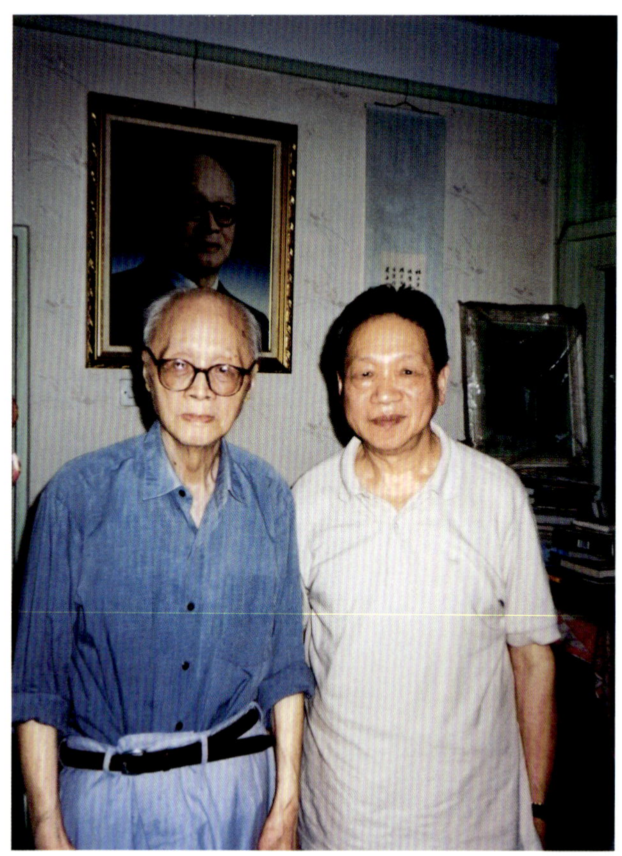

为核物理学家王淦昌院士会诊（1997，北京）

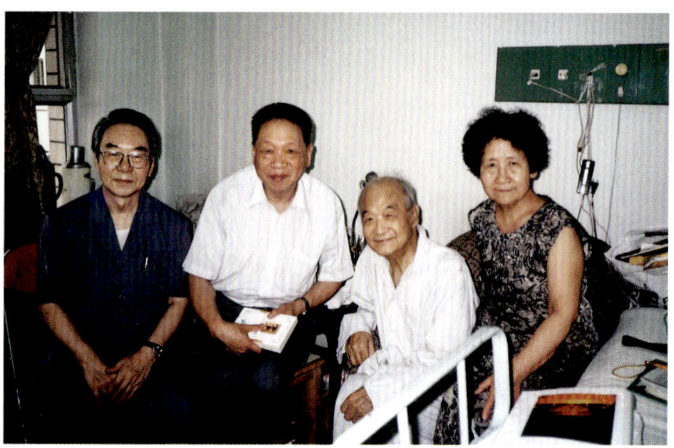

在北京医院为肖乾先生会诊后，右起肖乾夫人文洁若、肖乾、陈可冀、民盟中央副主席吴修平（1996，北京医院病房）

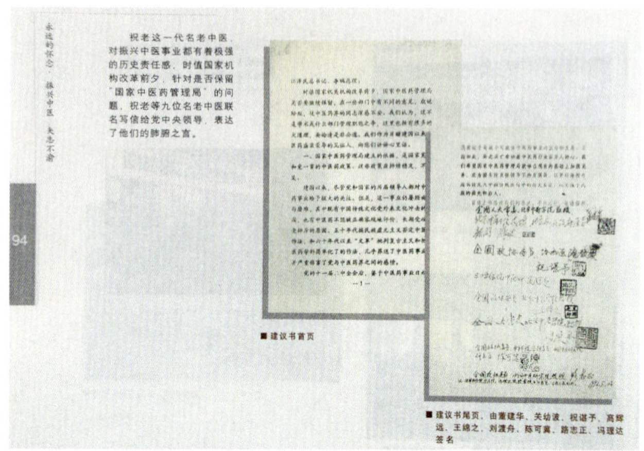

永远的怀念 · 振兴中医 矢志不渝

94

祝老这一代名老中医，对振兴中医事业都有着极强的历史责任感，时值国家机构改革前夕，针对是否保留"国家中医药管理局"的问题，祝老等九位名老中医联名写信给党中央领导，表达了他们的肺腑之言。

■ 建议书首页

■ 建议书尾页，由董建华、关幼波、祝谌予、高辉远、王绵之、刘渡舟、陈可冀、路志正、冯理达签名

1992 年为保留“国家中医药管理局”的问题，陈可冀院士等九位专家联名写信给党中央领导（引自“纪念祝谌予教授诞辰九十周年”画册）

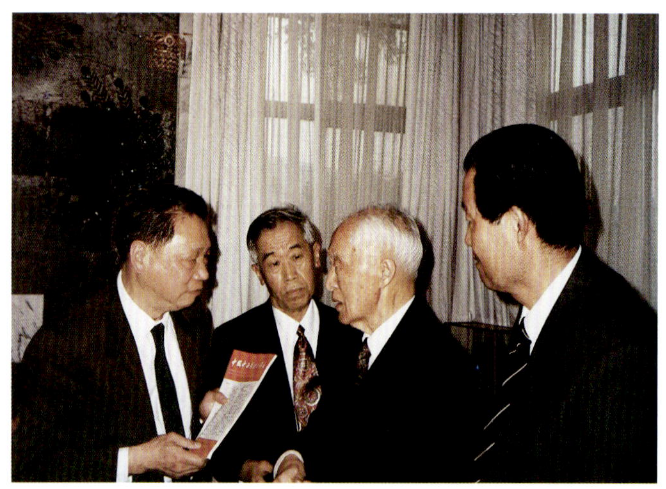

向陈立夫先生赠送《中国中西医结合杂志》，左 2 王佩教授，右 1 李经纬教授（1993）

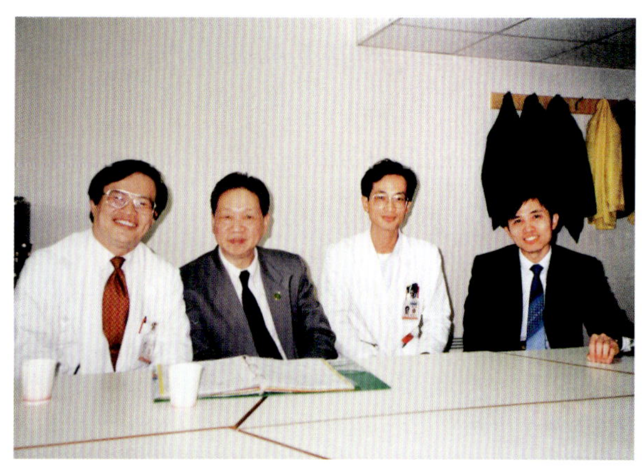

台北荣民总医院心脏科病房会诊并讨论治疗方案，左 1 洪传岳教授、右 1 黄怡超教授（1994）

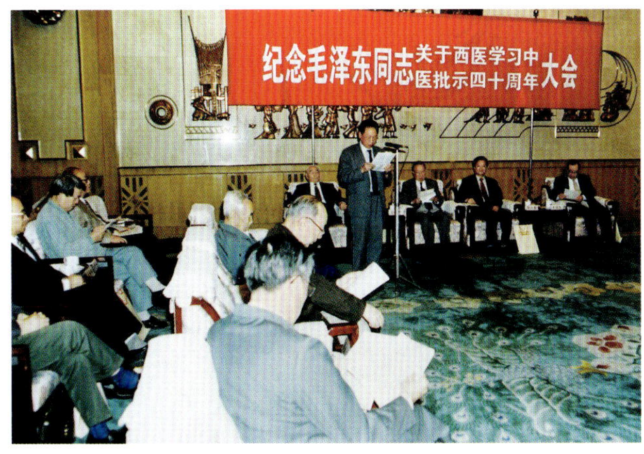

在纪念毛泽东关于西医学习中医批示 40 周年大会上发言。在座的有钱信忠、吴阶平、张文康、朱庆生、季钟朴、吴咸中、沈自尹等（1998）

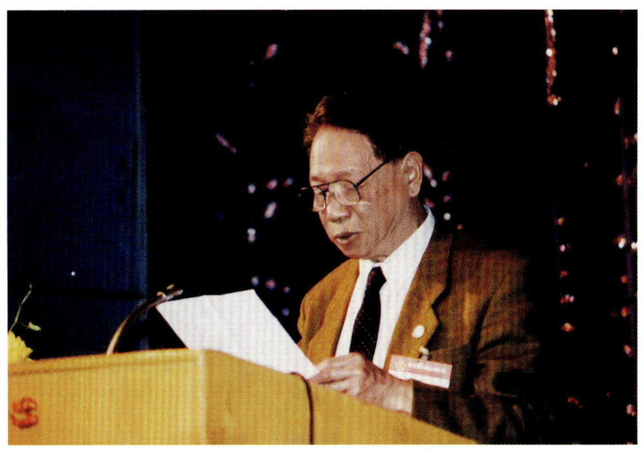

作为当年我国中医药界十大新闻之一的第一次世界中西医结合大会召开，任大会主席致开幕词（1997，北京）

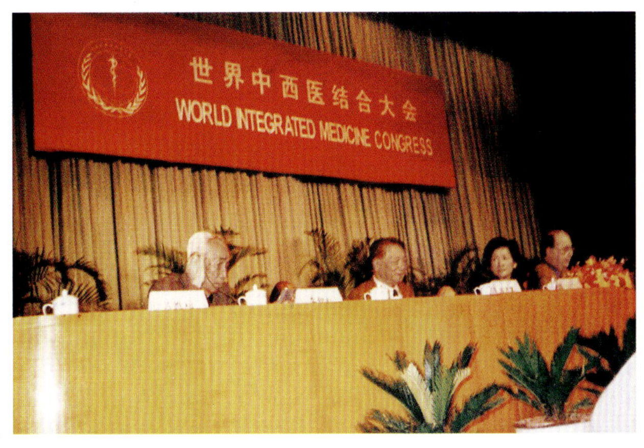

在第一次世界中西医结合大会上。自左至右为季钟朴、陈可冀、Yuan-Yuan Chiu、James Gordon（1997，北京）

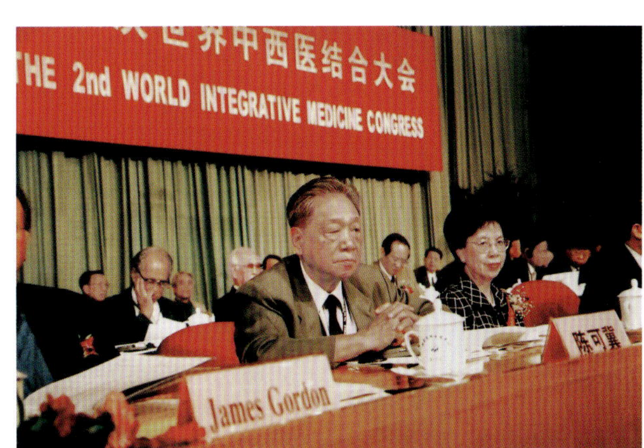

第二次世界中西医结合大会担任大会主席，右为世界卫生组织总干事的陈冯富珍（2002，北京）

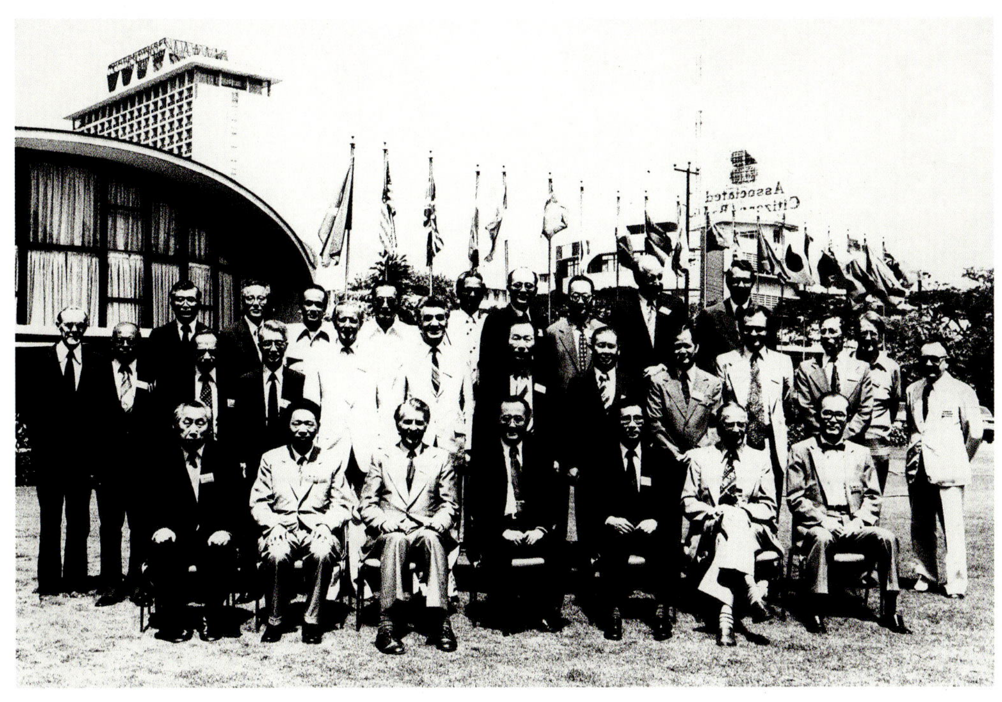

出席世界卫生组织医学研究会议，前排中为中岛宏博士，后排右 3 为毛守白教授（1980，马尼拉）

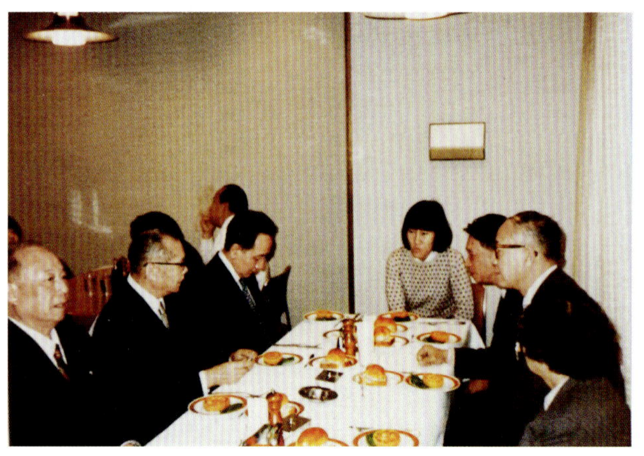

访问日本北里大学汉方医学研究所，前左 2、3 矢数道明、大塚恭男（1981，东京）

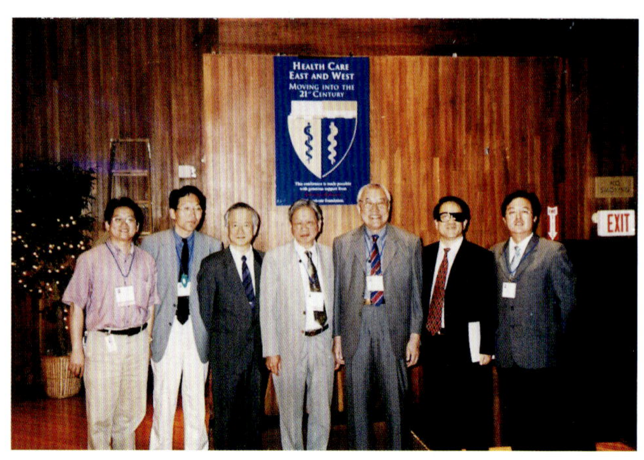

哈佛大学与中华医学会联合召开东西方医学会议（1988，波士顿）

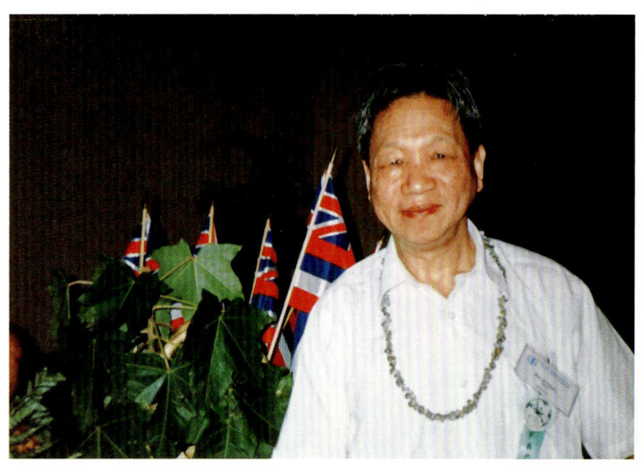

出席夏威夷国际草药会议（1995）

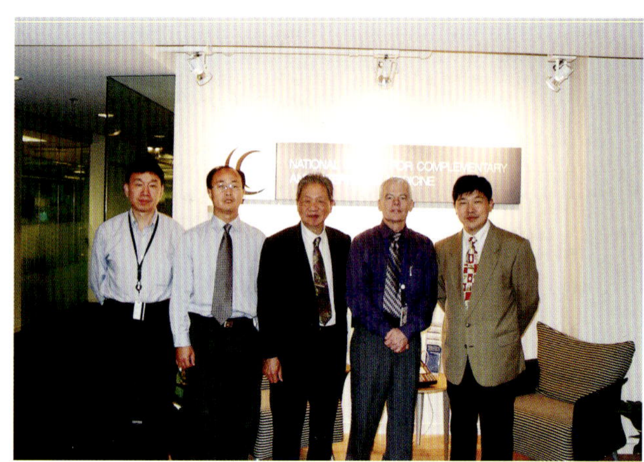

应邀访问 NIH-NCCAM，右 2 为 Dr. Killen，左 1 陈舟，右 1 宋军（2004）

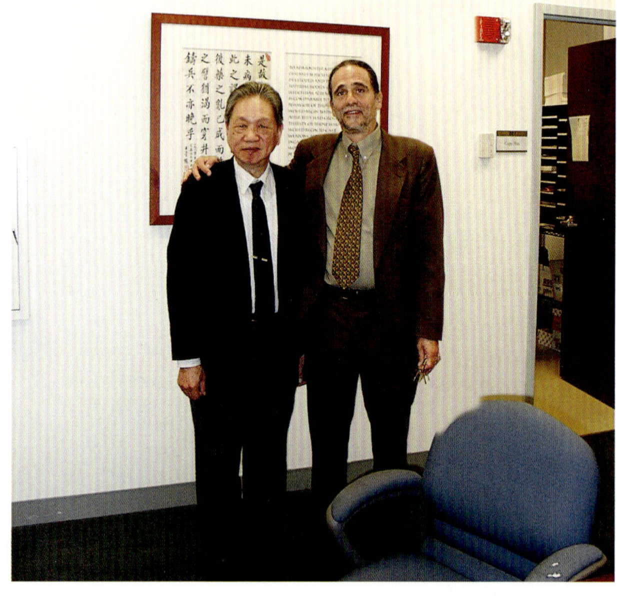

在哈佛大学医学院与著名中医药针灸专家、NIH-NCCAM 顾问 Ted Kapchuck 教授（2004）

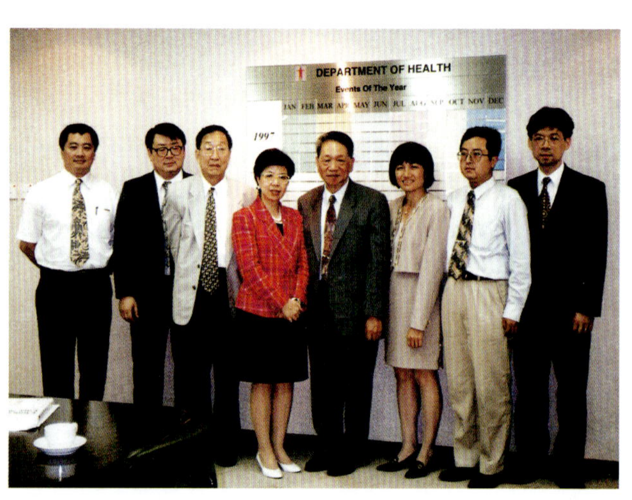

应邀访问香港卫生署，左 4 陈冯富珍署长，左 2、3 林炳恩副署长、张大钊教授，右 1 梁挺雄副署长，右 2 马晓昌医师（1997，香港）

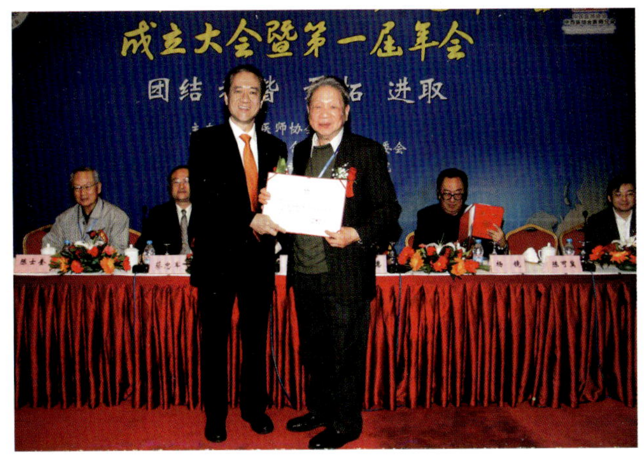

韩启德院士授予中国医师协会中西医结合医师分会会长当选证书（2007，北京）

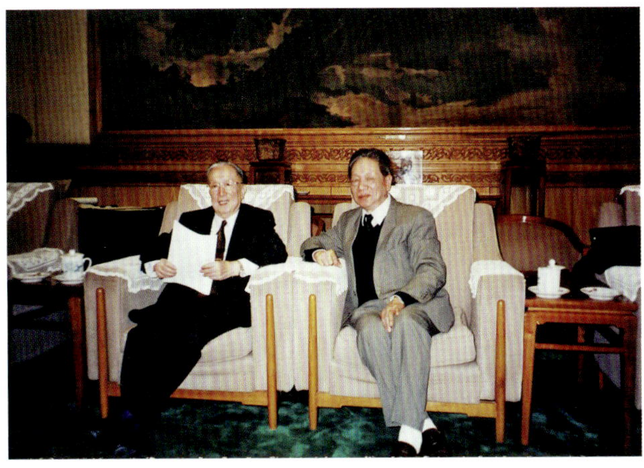

与全国人大副委员长吴阶平院士（2000，北京人民大会堂）

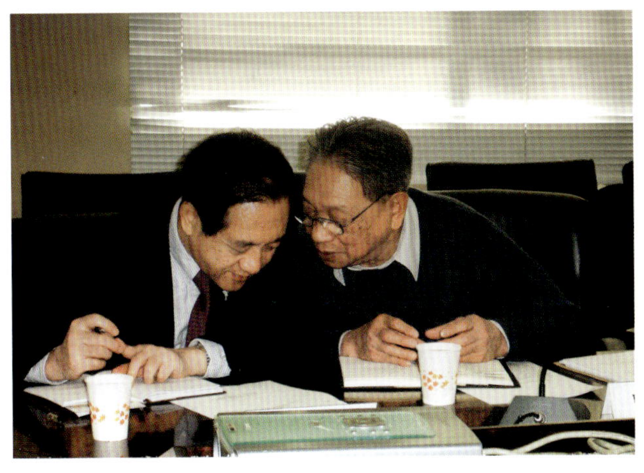

与全国人大副委员长、中国科协主席韩启德院士讨论两人共同主持的中国科学院中西医结合咨询课题（2005）

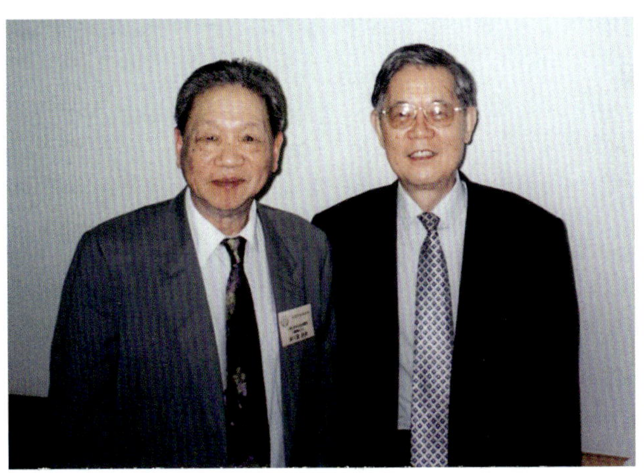

2001 年中国科协年会与中国科协主席周光召院士（2001，长春）

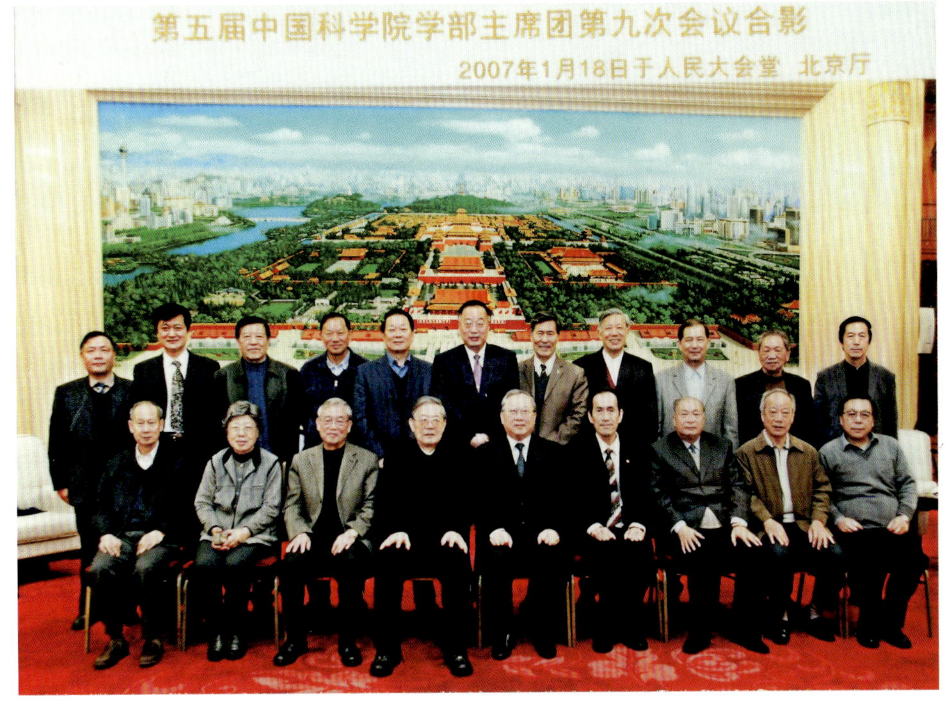

第五届中国科学院学部主席团会议，前排左 4、5、6 为周光召、路甬祥、陈宜瑜院士（2007）

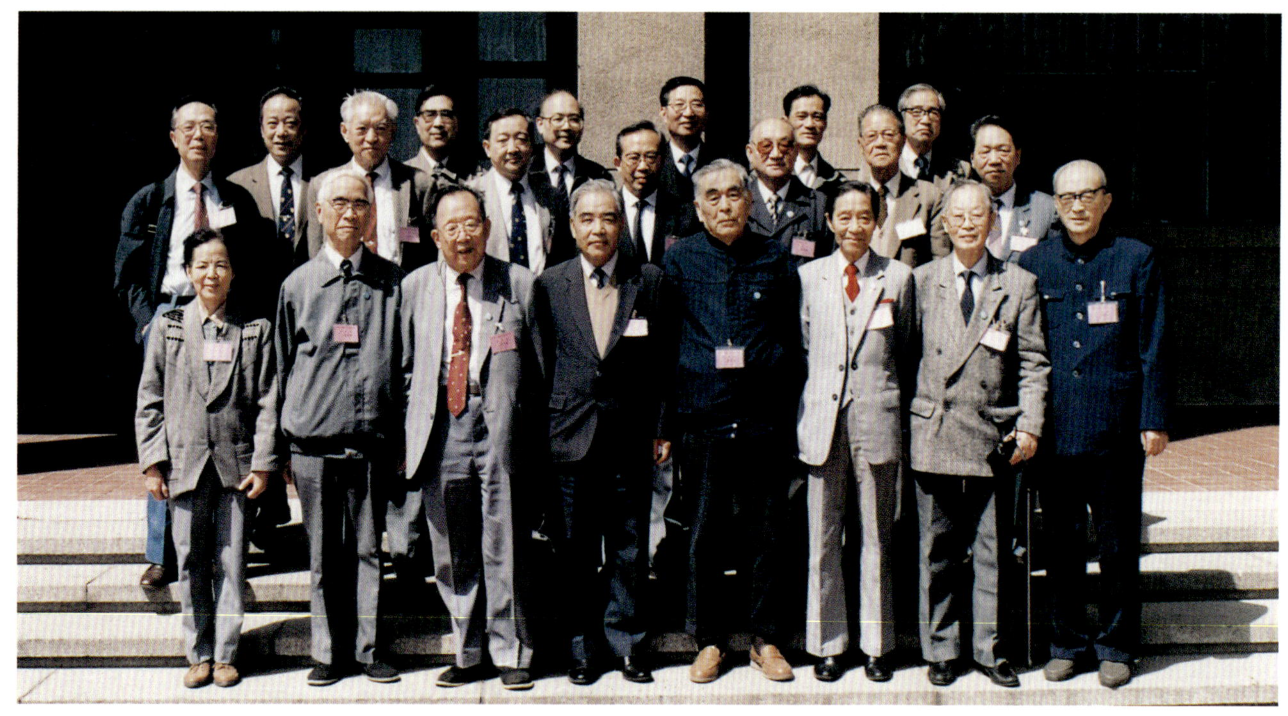

中国科学院生物学部部分院士合影，前左 2、3 冯德培、吴征镒院士，二排左 2、3 邹承鲁、吴旻院士，三排左 4 李振声院士（1992）

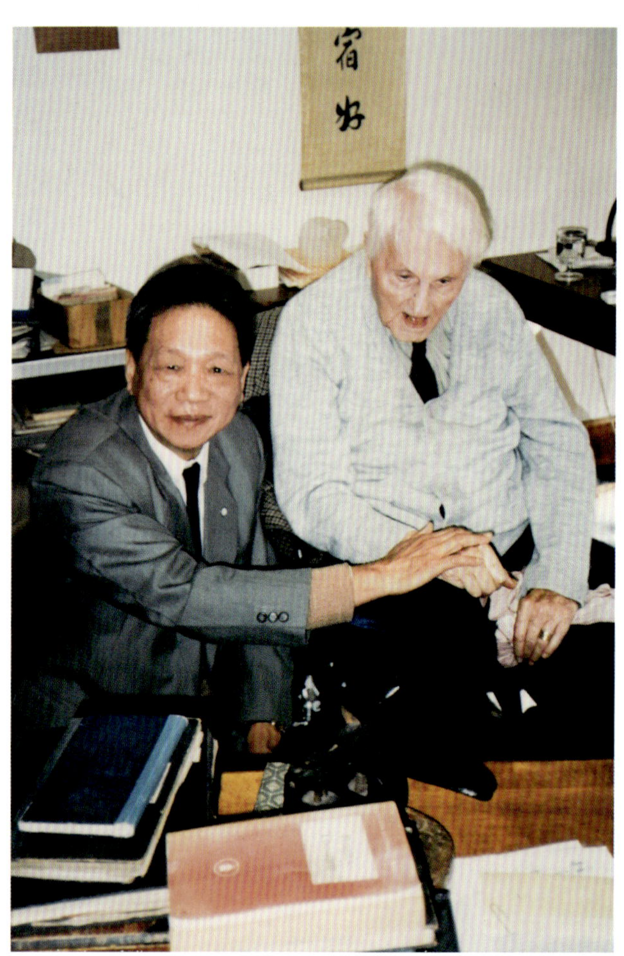

在英国讲学时访晤病中的中国科学院外籍院士李约瑟博士（1994）

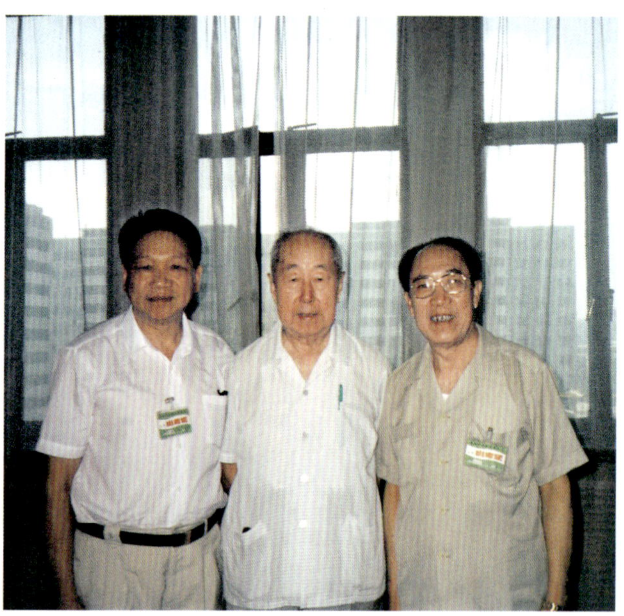

青山依旧在：与吴英恺院士（中）、吴孟超院士（右）在中国科学院院士大会上（1993）

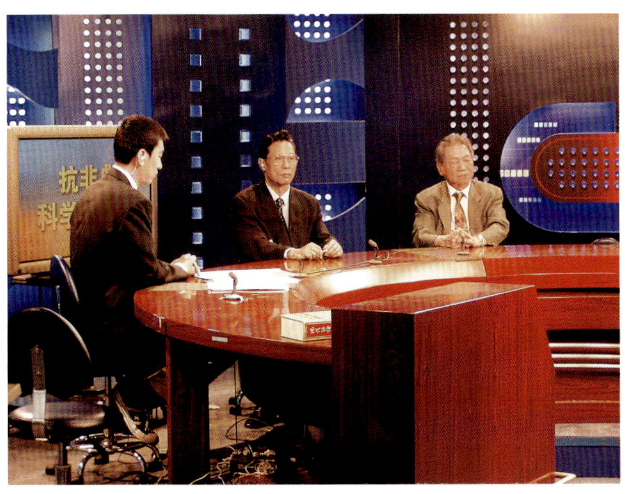

与中国工程院钟南山院士和中国台北学者通过 CCTV 视频进行“非典”学术对话（2003 年 6 月 8 日）

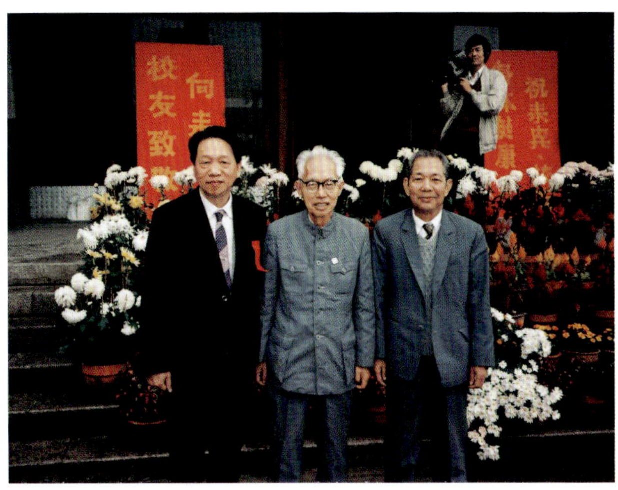

受聘为福建中医学院名誉院长，与福建著名中医专家俞长荣（右 1）、俞慎初（中）教授（1988，福州）

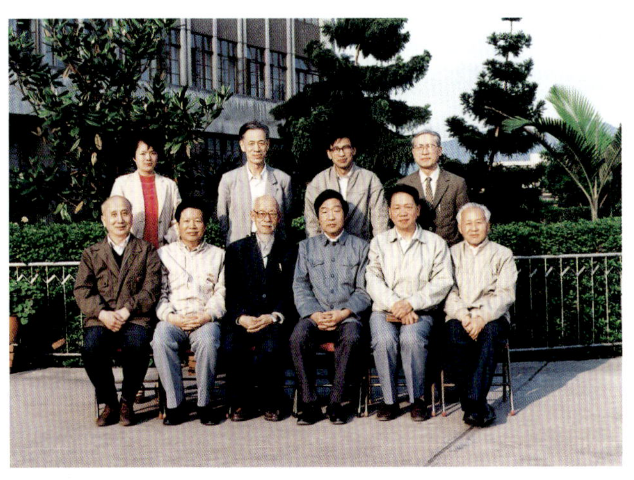

福建医科大学博士点论证会，前排左起郑道声教授、黄春源副厅长、侯宗濂教授、殷凤峙教授，后排左 2 吕俊升教授，左 3 阮长耿院士（1990，福州）

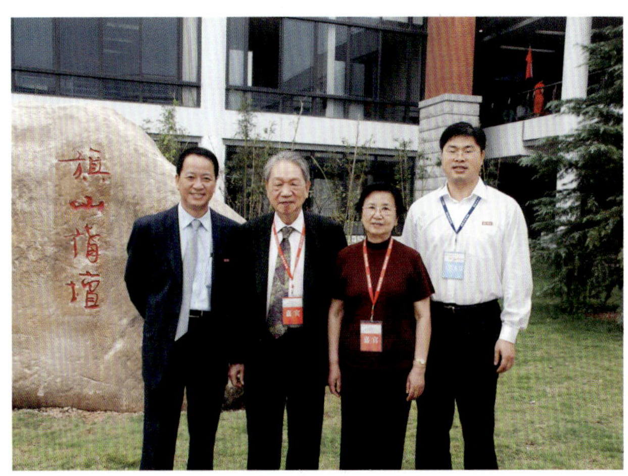

福建中西医结合研究院旗山论坛，左 1 福建中医学院党委书记罗萤，右 1 研究院张松富主任（2008，福州）

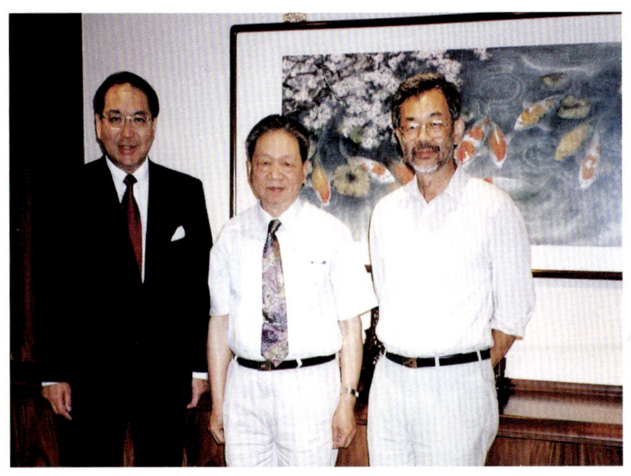

应聘香港中文大学名誉客座教授与校长李国章（左 1），中医药学院江润祥院长（右）合影（2000，香港）

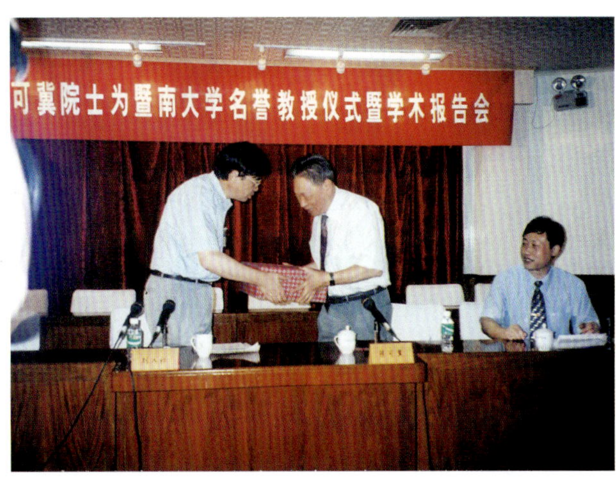

应聘为暨南大学名誉教授，左为校长刘人怀院士（1996，广州）

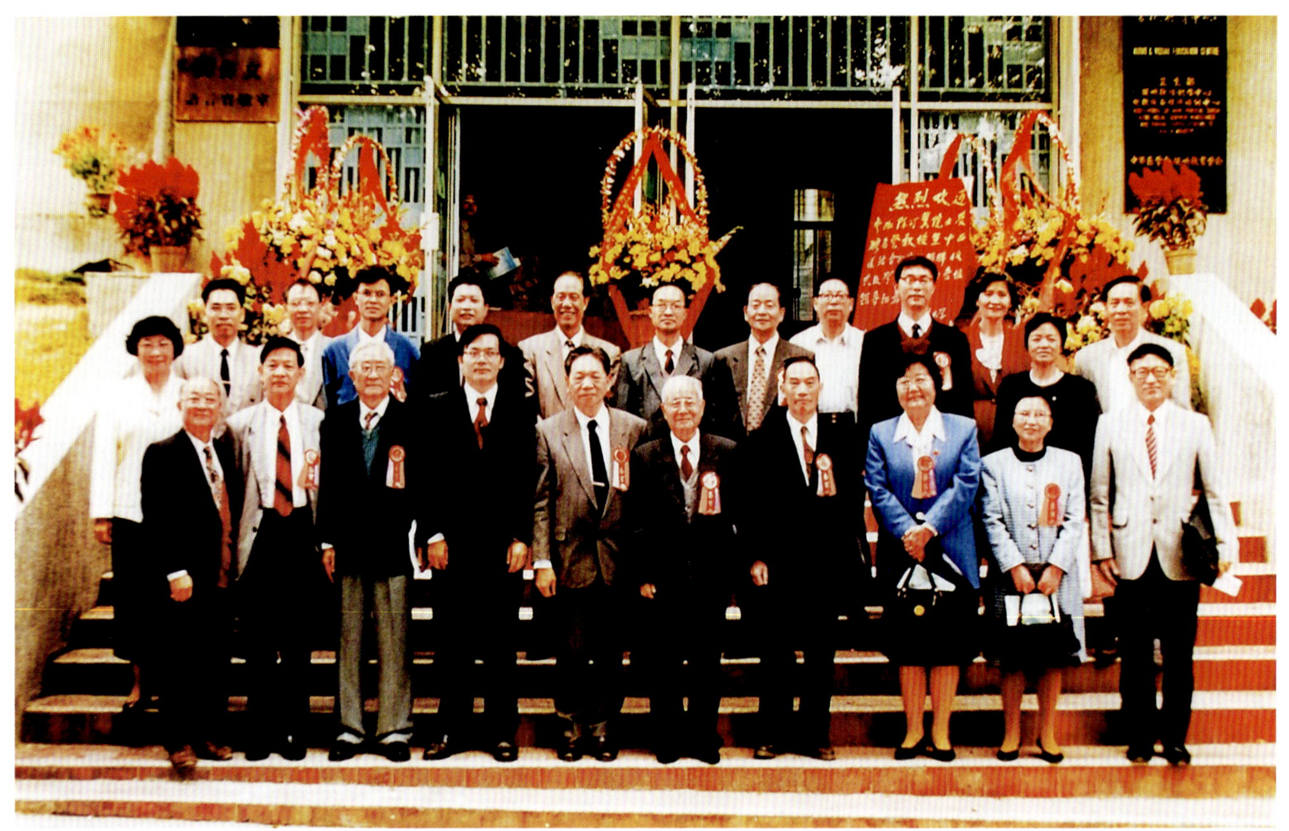

陈可冀受聘为中山医科大学名誉教授（1996，广州）

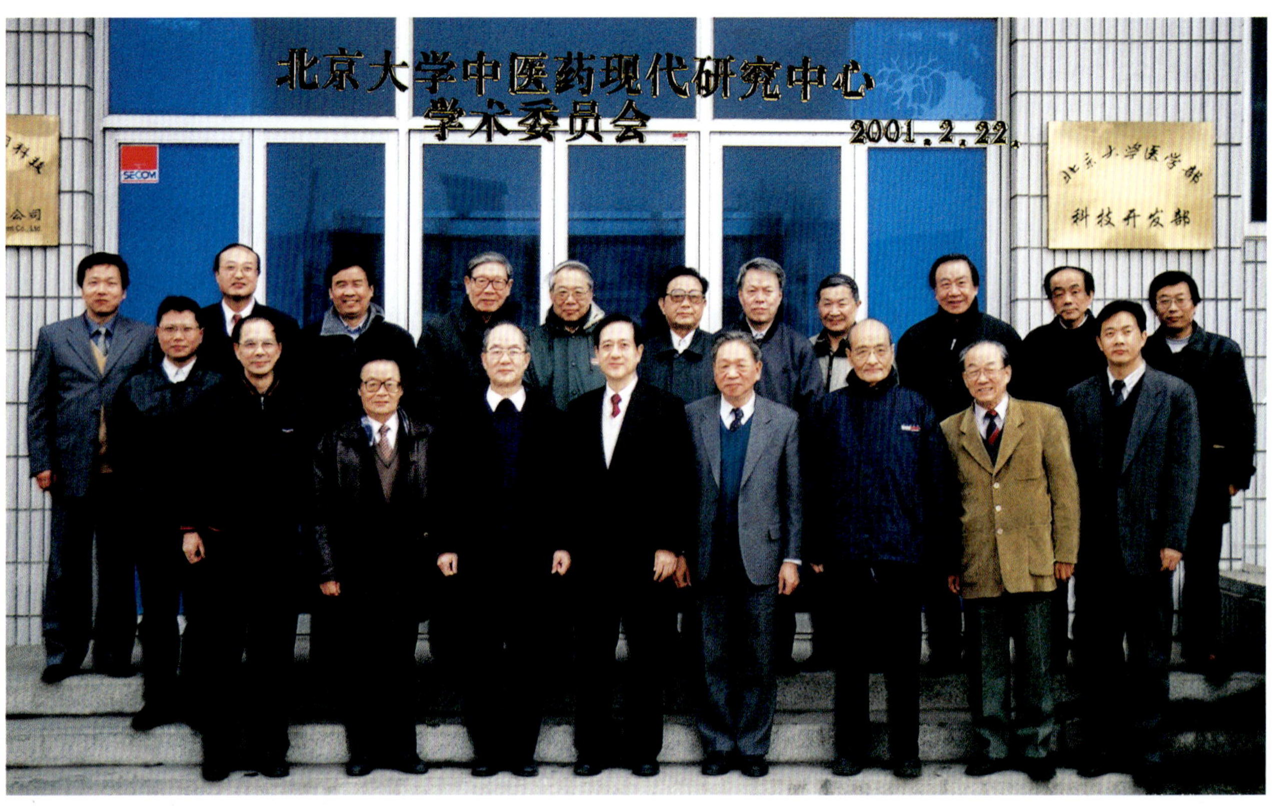

陈可冀受聘为北京大学中医药现代研究中心学术委员会主任。前排自左至右：韩济生院士、谢竹藩教授、秦伯益院士、韩启德院士、陈可冀院士、王夔院士、于德泉院士、果德安教授。后排自左至右：黄熙教授、王剑波教授、屠鹏飞教授、姚新生院士、李顺成教授、陈冀胜院士、龙致贤教授、刘耕陶院士、姜廷良教授、张礼和院士、徐筱杰教授、王传社教授（2001，北京）

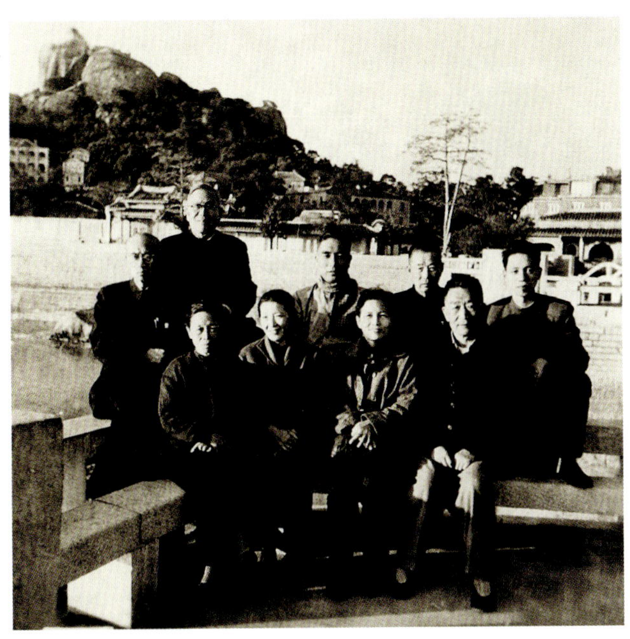

梁漱溟先生（后左 1）、福建卫生厅厅长王灼祖（后左 2）、陈锡谋教授（后右 3）、岳美中教授（后右 2）与陈可冀（后右 1）在厦门鼓浪屿菽庄花园（1961）

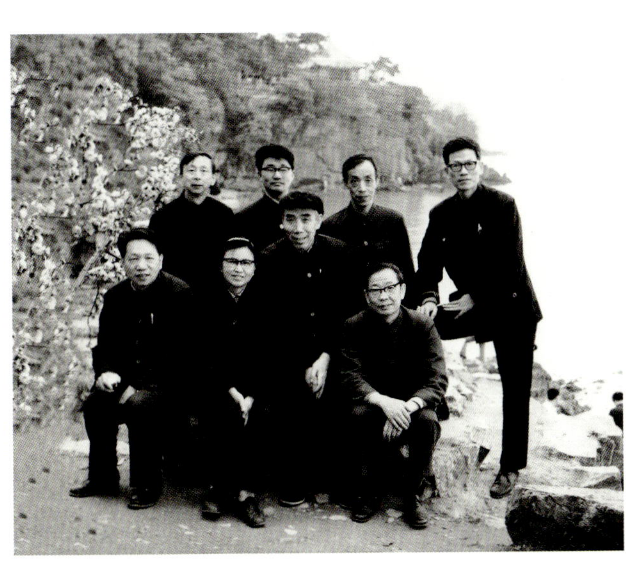

在无锡太湖，前排右起廖家桢、季钟朴、陈维养、陈可冀；后排右起陈士奎、危北海、尹光耀、付湘琦（1983）

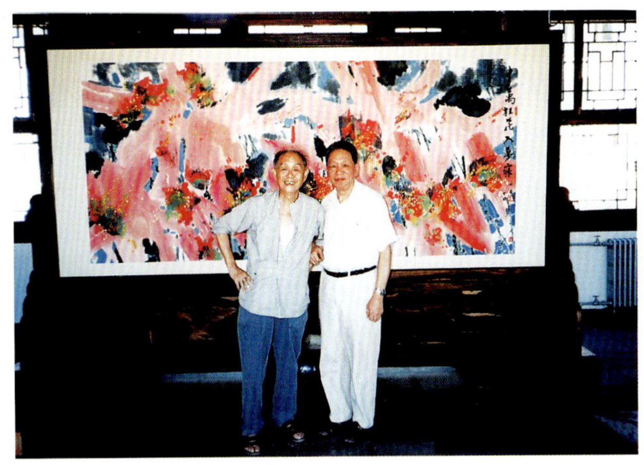

与著名画家黄永玉先生：十万狂花入梦寐（1997）

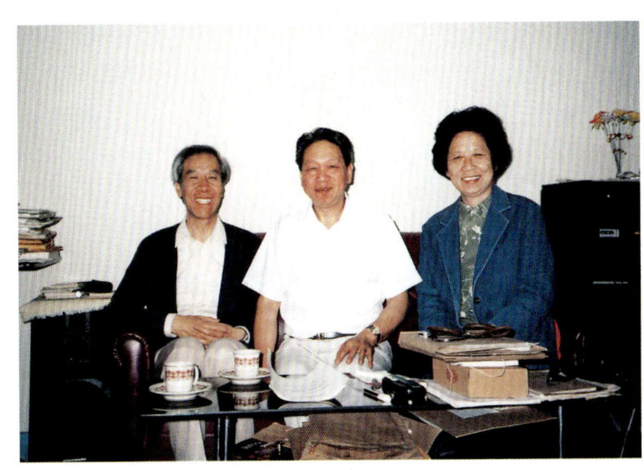

北京大学著名中国文学史、唐诗研究专家袁行霈教授夫妇前来家访（1992）

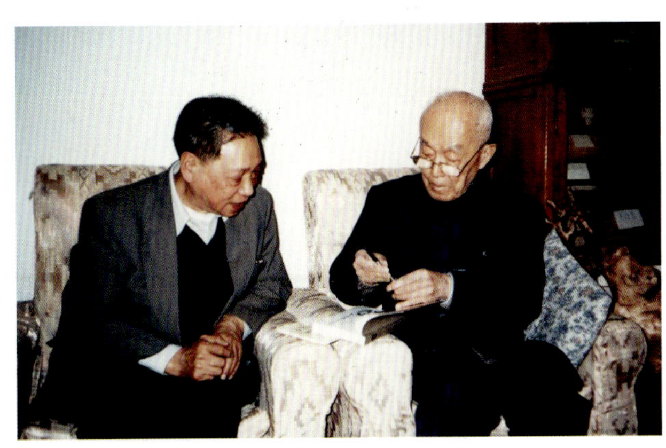

季羡林教授赠书（1999，北京季教授家中）

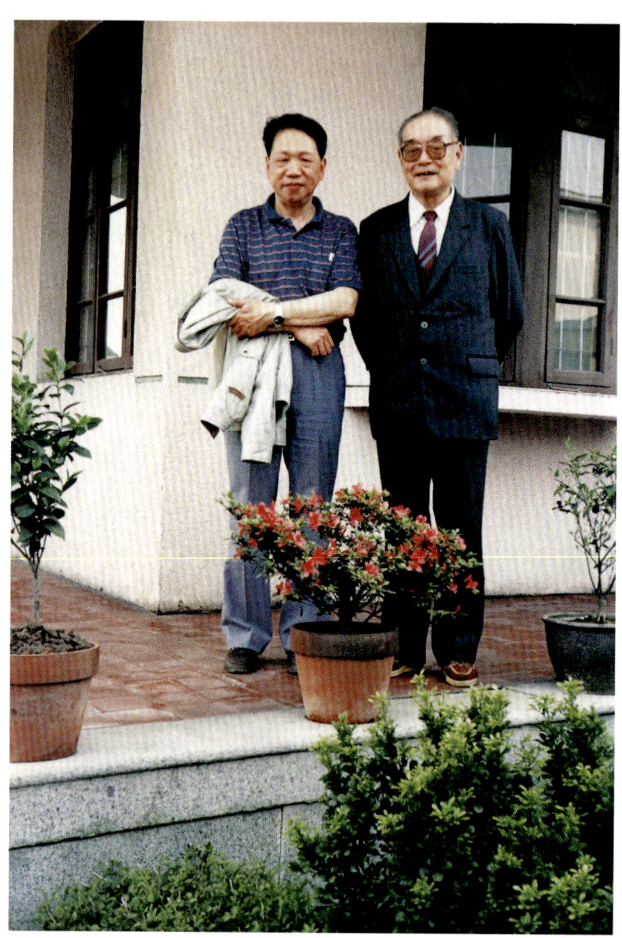

邀著名中医耿鉴庭教授到福州家中（1990）

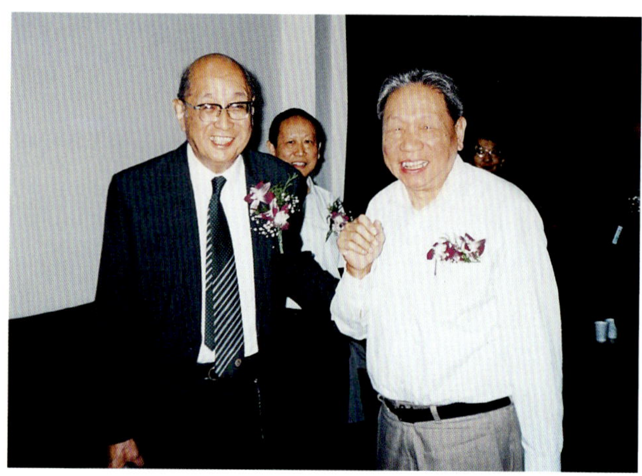

与北京医院名誉院长，心血管病专家钱贻简教授，1973—1974年甘肃武威北京医疗队队友（2005）

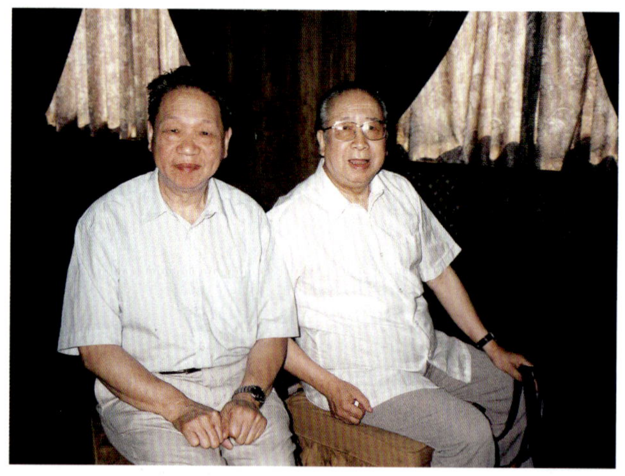

与著名老年人口学家、中国老年学学会名誉会长邬沧萍教授（1997，北京）

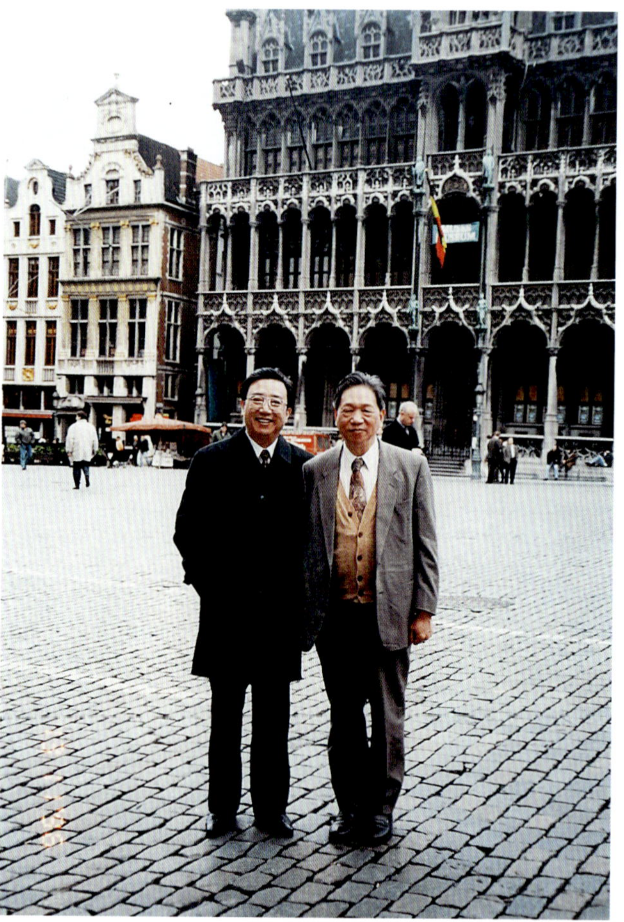

与中国中医研究院原院长陈绍武在比利时布鲁塞尔（1996）

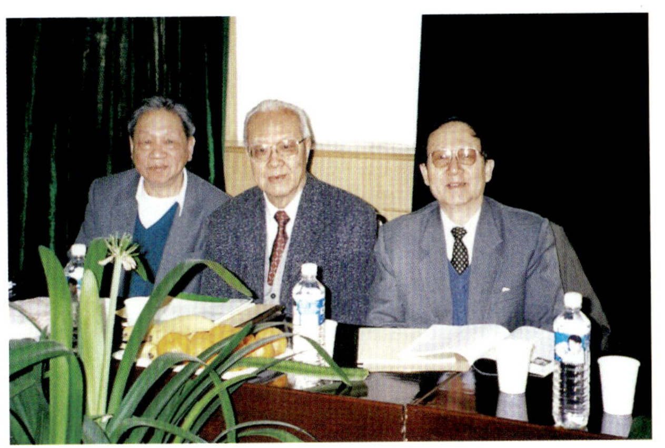

与著名心血管病学家方圻（中）、洪昭光（右）教授在西苑医院（2001）

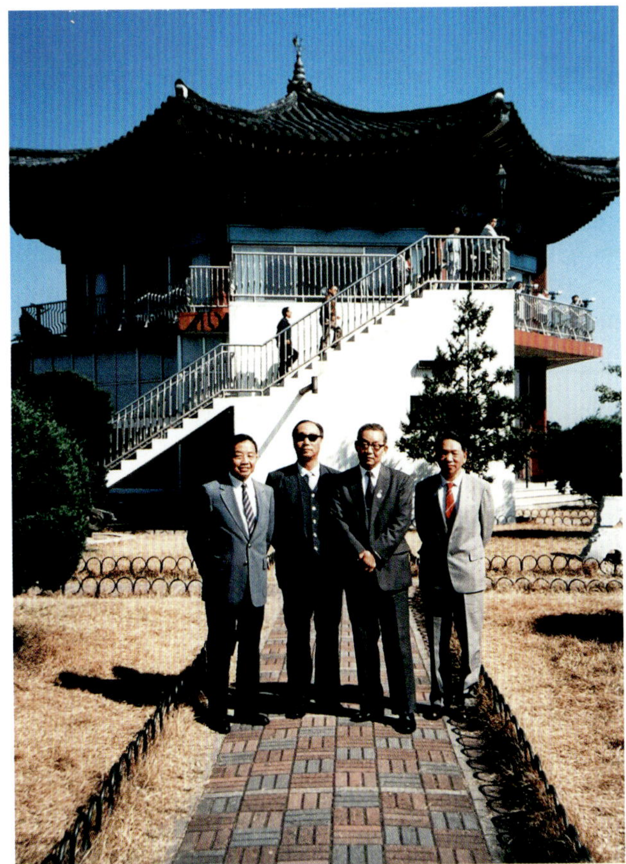

与著名胸外科专家辛育龄（右 2）、药理学家刘干中（左 1）（1990，韩国）

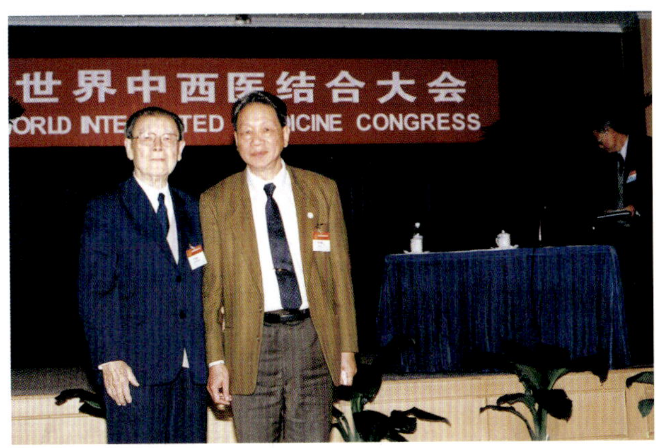

与著名药理学家周金黄教授在首届世界中西医结合大会（1997，北京）

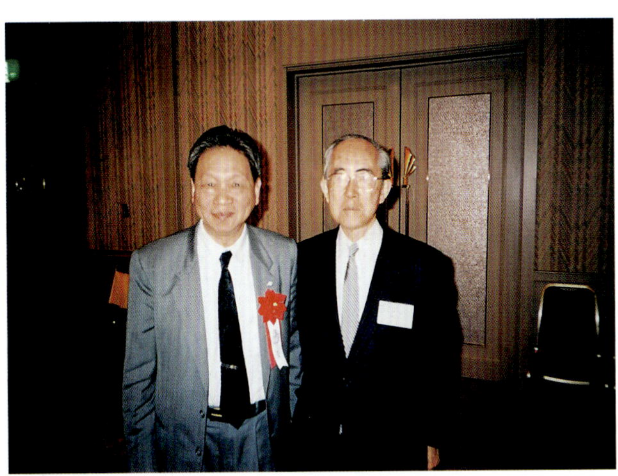

出席在东京召开的中西医结合学术会议时与日本东京大学名誉教授、著名人参研究专家柴田承二（1994）

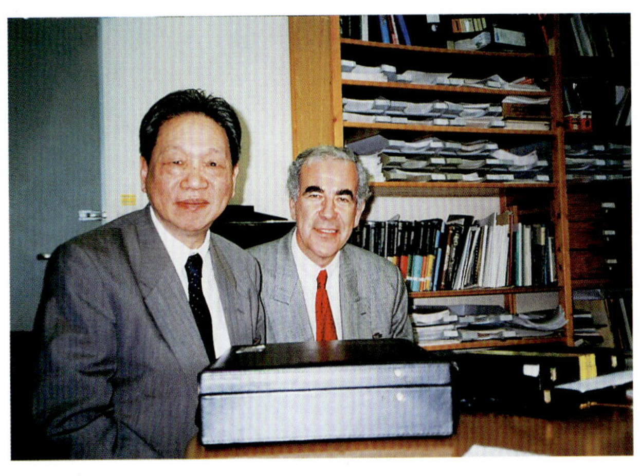

在荷兰脑研究所作学术讲演后，与国际老年痴呆学会会长、荷兰脑研究所所长 Dick Swabb 教授（1996，阿姆斯特丹）

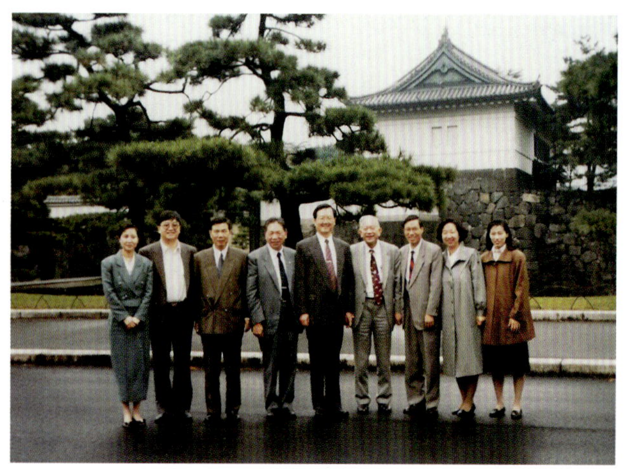

中国医学代表团访日于日本皇宫前，中为团长卫生部部长张文康，右 1 为李静博士（1994）

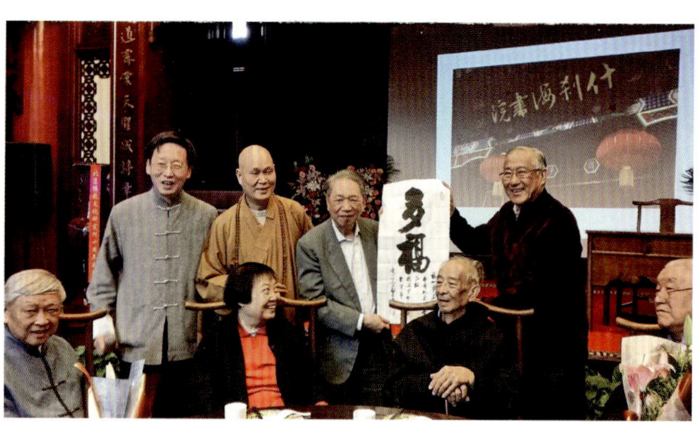

85 周岁时启骧教授（后右 1）赠“多福”题词，前排右 1 汤一介教授、右 2 乐黛云教授、右 3 钱逊教授（2014，什刹海书院）

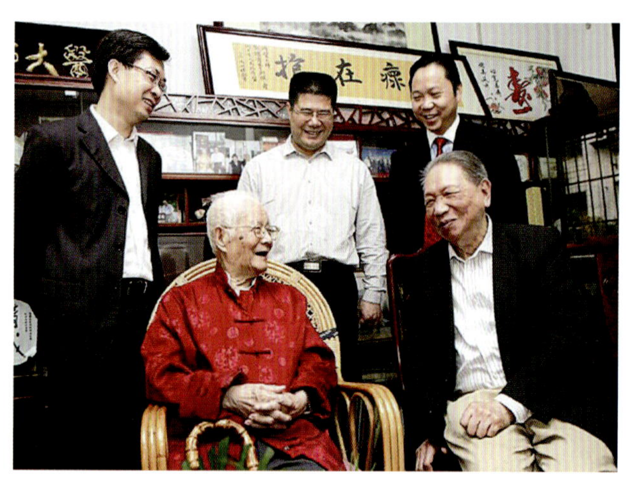

祝贺邓铁涛教授百岁生日（2016，广州）

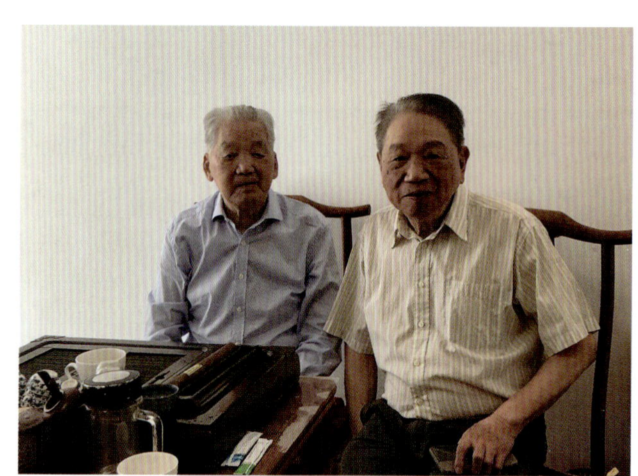

与百岁国医大师路志正教授（2019，北京）

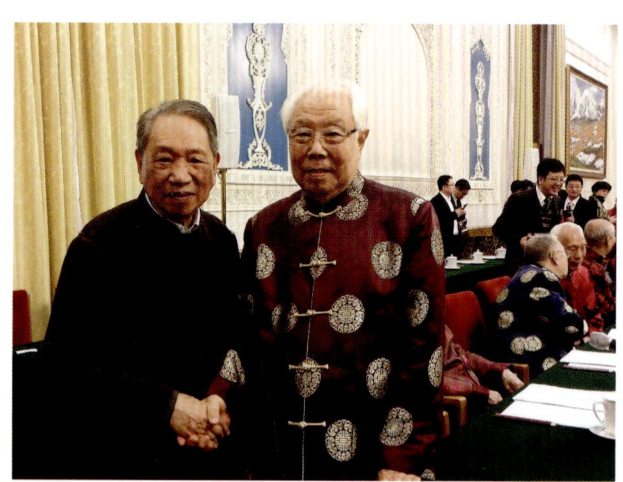

与国医大师李辅仁教授（2014，人民大会堂）

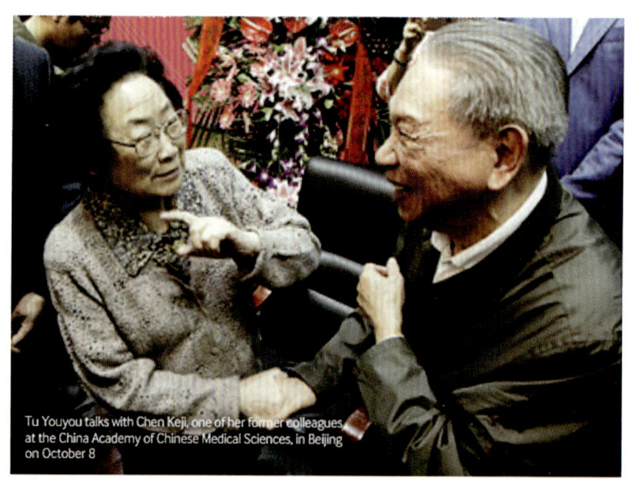

与诺贝尔奖获得者屠呦呦教授会面（2015，北京）

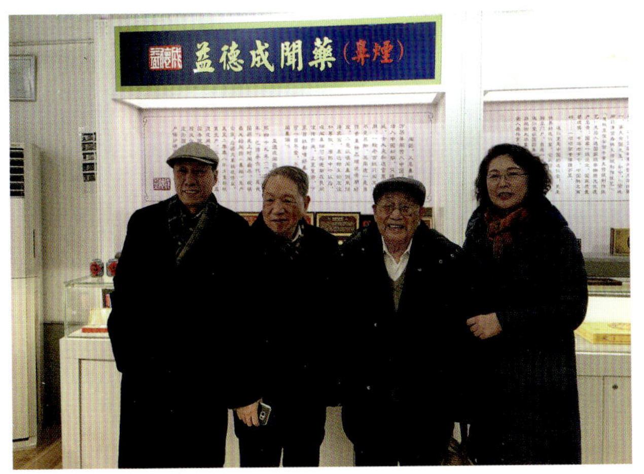

与国医大师金世元教授（右 2）在故宫博物院（2017，北京）

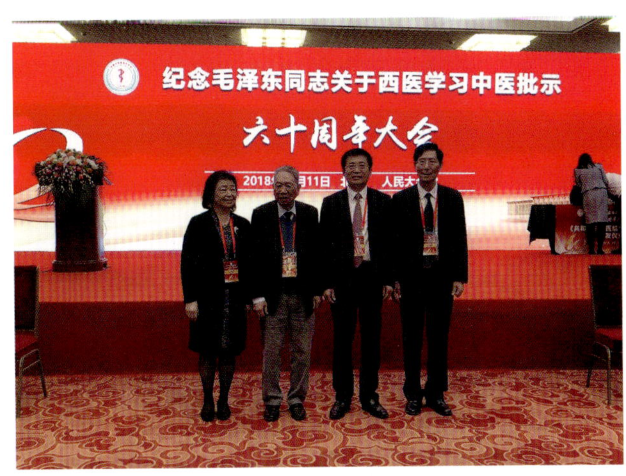

纪念毛泽东同志关于西医学习中医批示六十周年大会，左 1 陈香美院士、右 2 国家中医药管理局于文明局长、右 1 陈凯先院士（2018，人民大会堂）

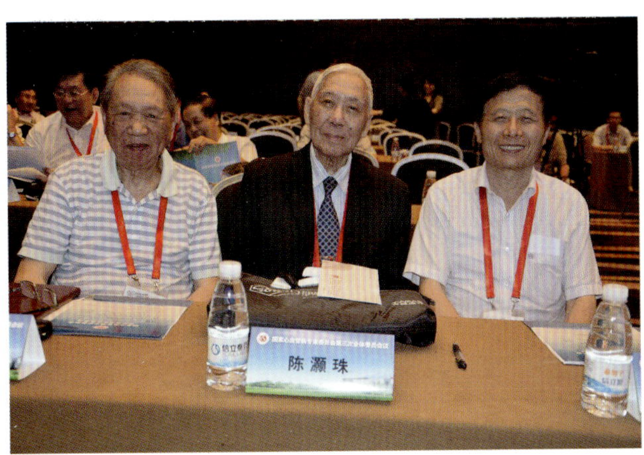

与陈灏珠院士（中）、刘德培院士（右）（2016）

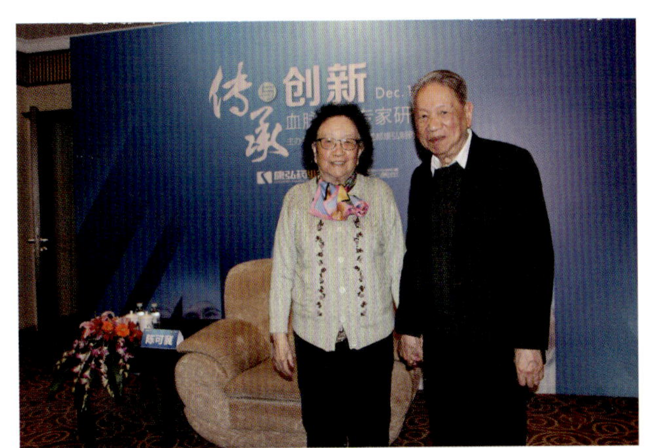

与世界高血压联盟前主席刘力生教授（2016）

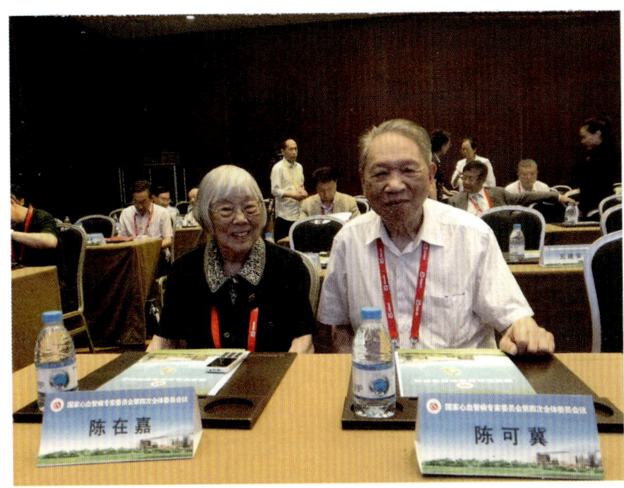

与阜外医院陈在嘉教授（2017）

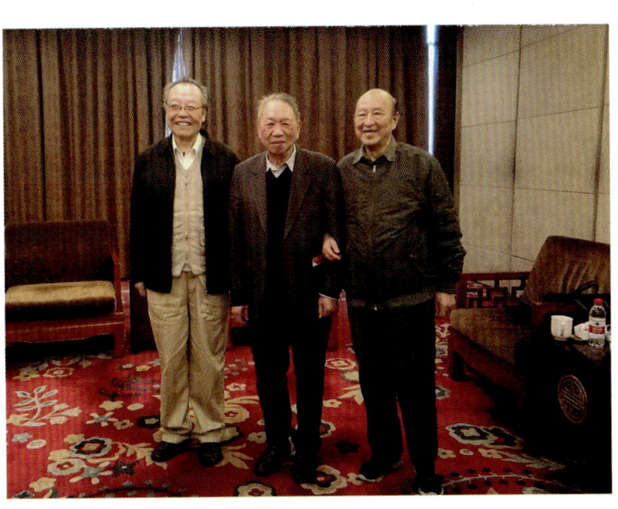

与肖培根院士（右 1）、张世臣教授（2017）

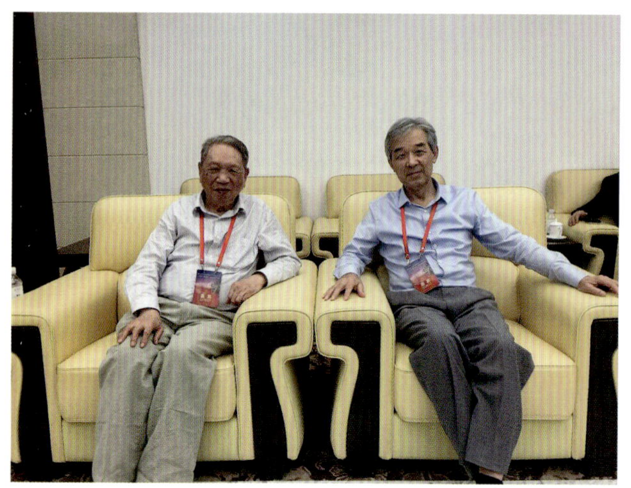

与中国预防医学会会长王陇德院士（2018）

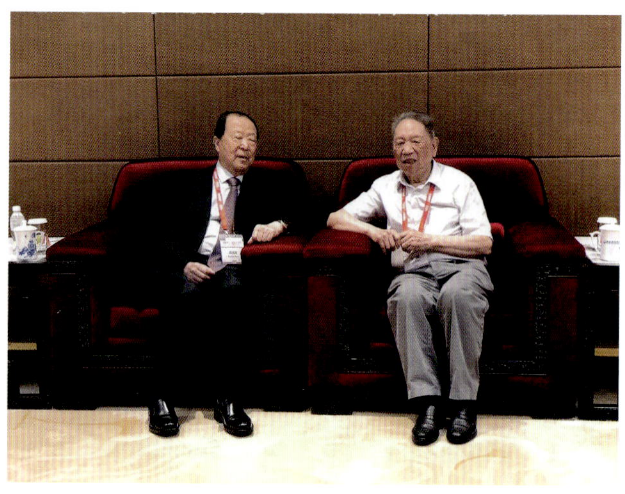

与高润霖院士在中国心脏大会上（2018）

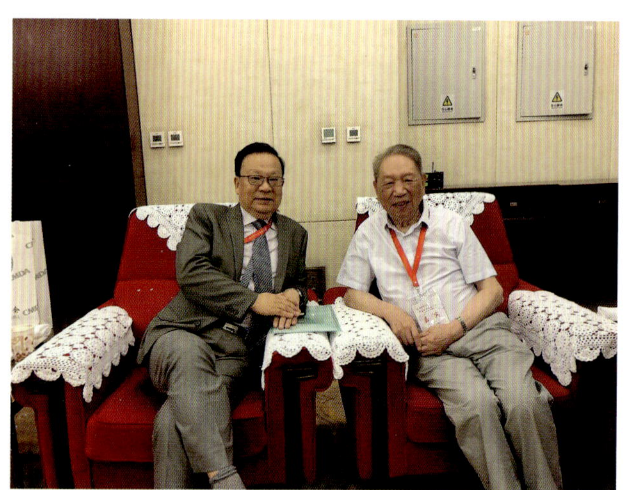

与郎景和院士在中国医学人文大会上（2018）

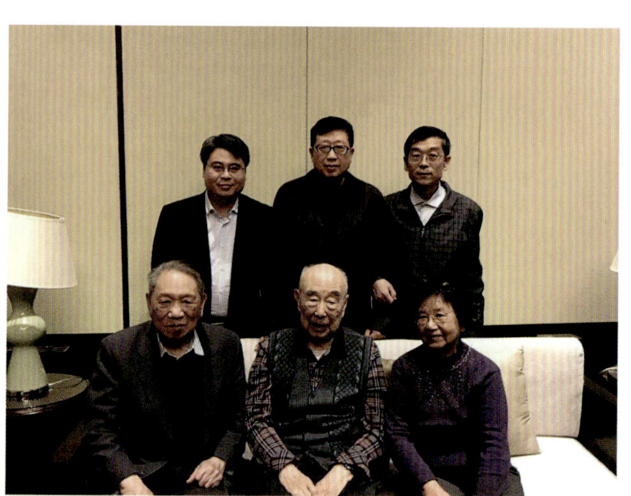

与吴咸中院士在天津（2018）

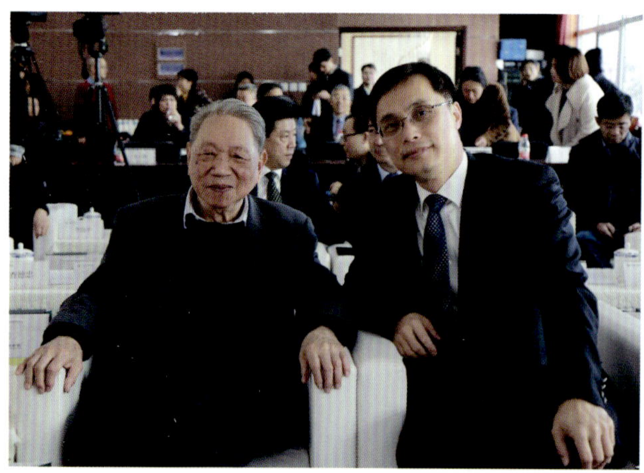

与中国中医科学院院长黄璐琦院士（2019）

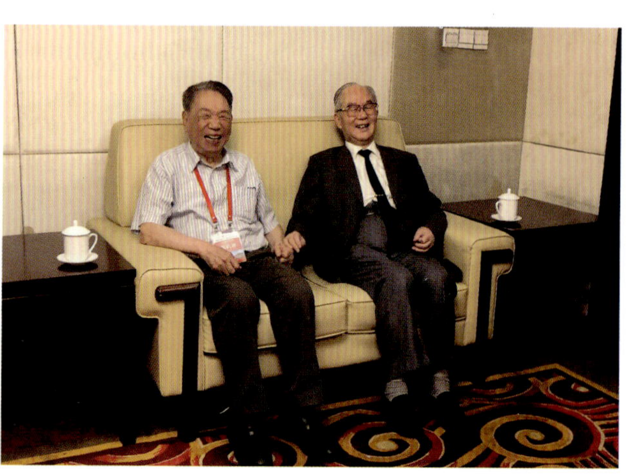

与秦伯益院士（2019）

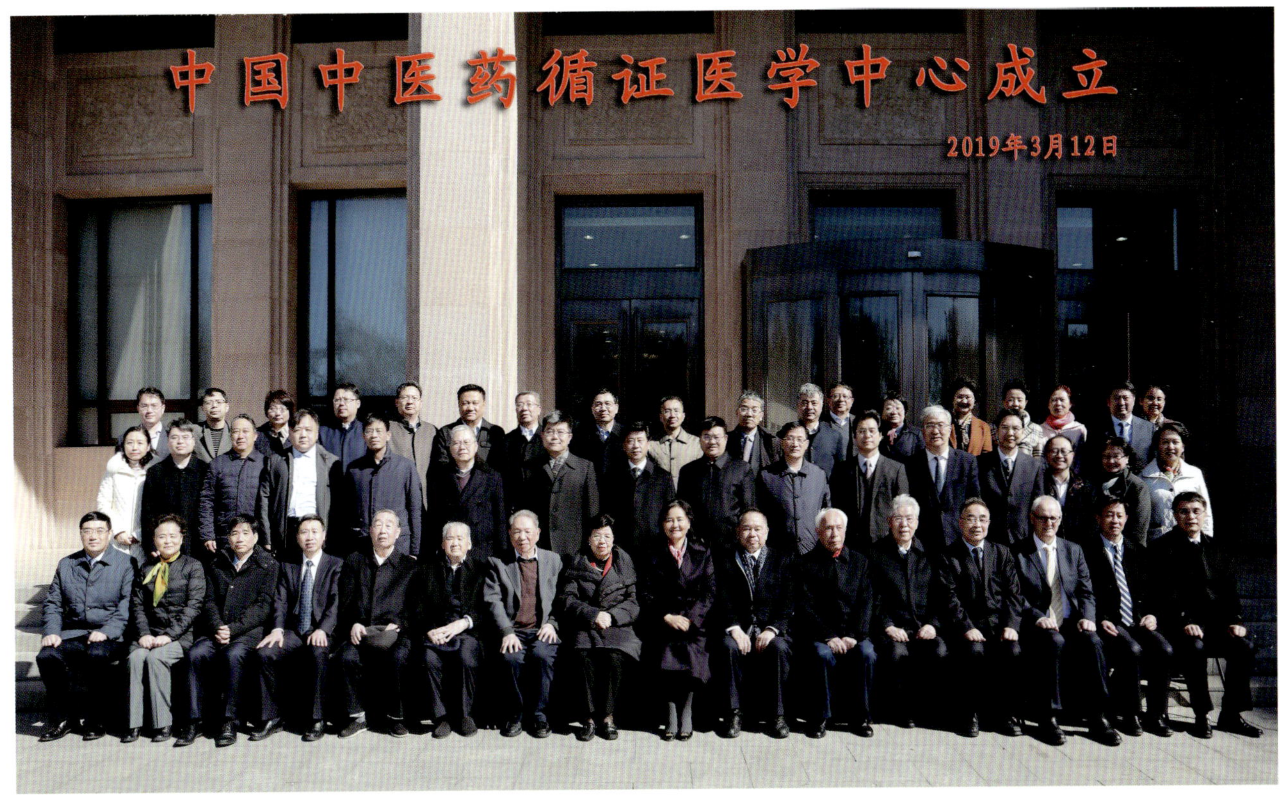

中国中医药循证医学研究中心成立大会，国家中医药管理局党组书记余艳红（前排右 8）、世界卫生组织前总干事陈冯富珍（前排右 9）、中国中医科学院院长、循证医学中心主任黄璐琦院士（前排右 1）等（2019，北京）

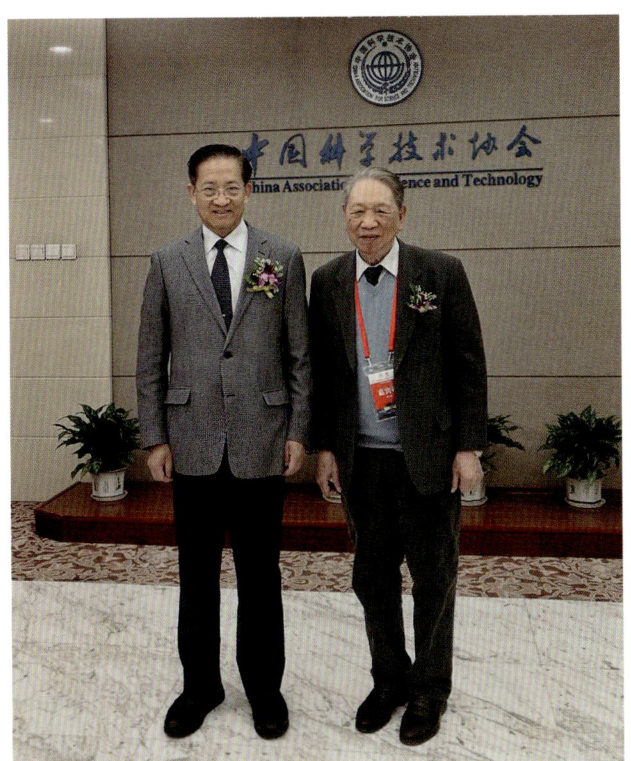

与中国医师协会张雁灵会长（2017）

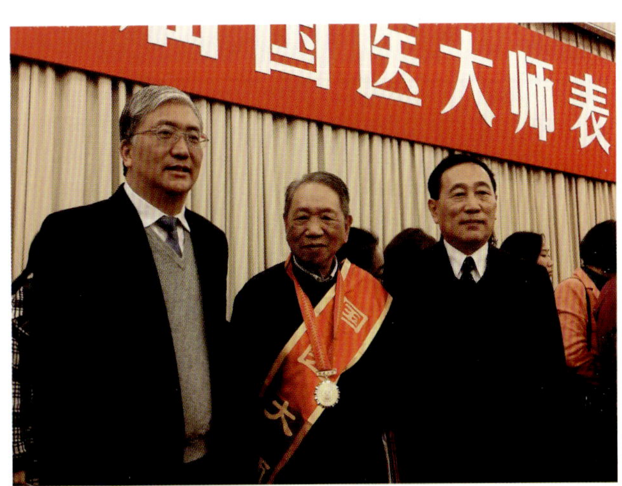

获评第二届国医大师，左 1 唐旭东教授，右 1 何军书记(2014，北京）

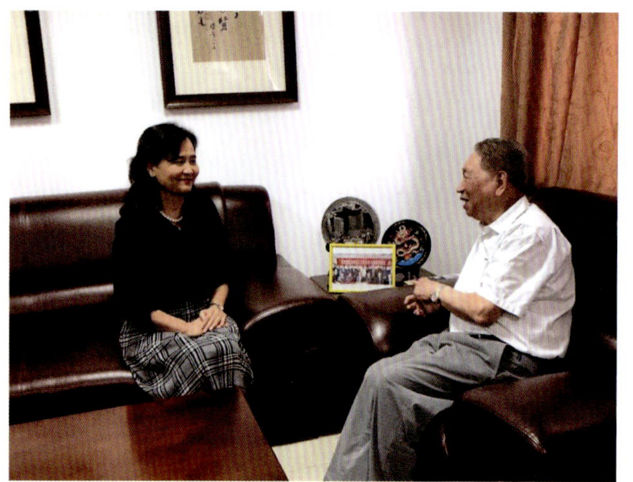

国家中医药管理局余艳红书记看望陈可冀院士（2018）

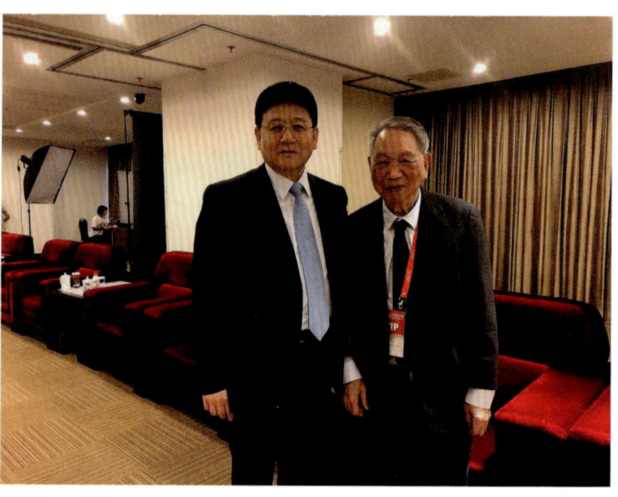

与国家卫健委副主任王贺胜（左 1）参加中国脑卒中大会（2019）

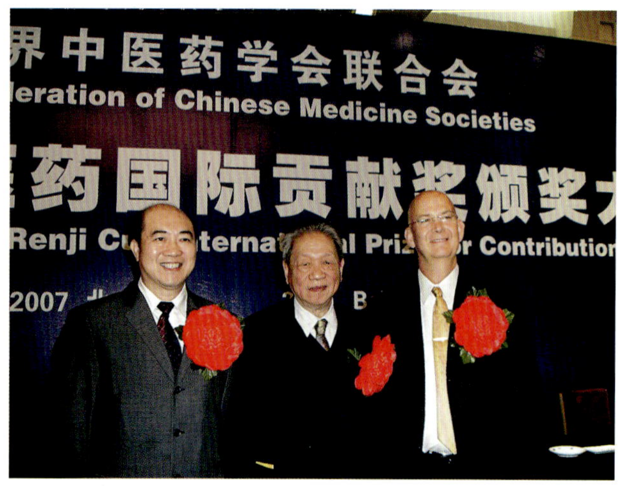

世界中医药联合会授予首届中医药国际贡献奖（2007）

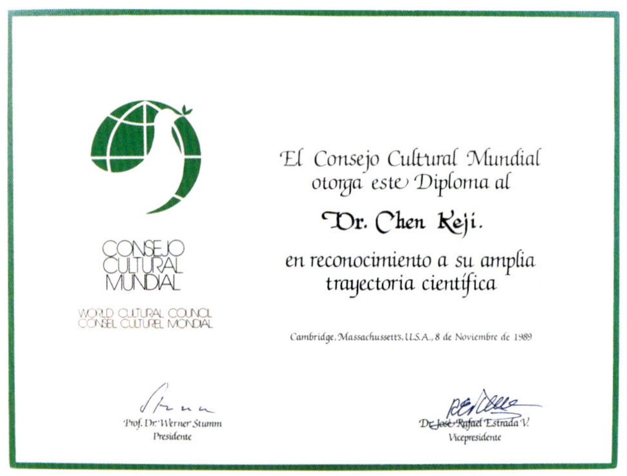

CONSEJO CULTURAL MUNDIAL

WORLD CULTURAL COUNCIL
CONSEIL CULTUREL MONDIAL

El Consejo Cultural Mundial
otorga este Diploma al

Dr. Chen Keji.

en reconocimiento a su amplia
trayectoria científica

Cambridge, Massachussetts, U.S.A., 8 de Noviembre de 1989

Prof. Dr. Werner Stumm
Presidente

Dr. José Rafael Estrada V.
Vicepresidente

世界文化理事会授予爱因斯坦奖状（1989）

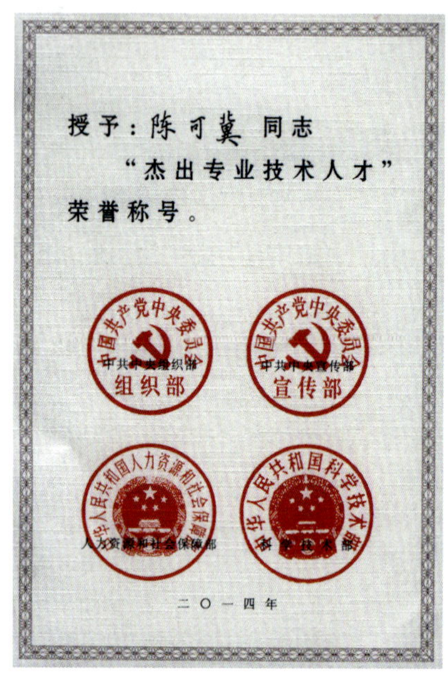

授予：陈可冀 同志

“杰出专业技术人才”

荣誉称号。

中共中央组织部　中共中央宣传部

人力资源和社会保障部　科学技术部

二〇一四年

杰出专业技术人才荣誉称号证书（2014）

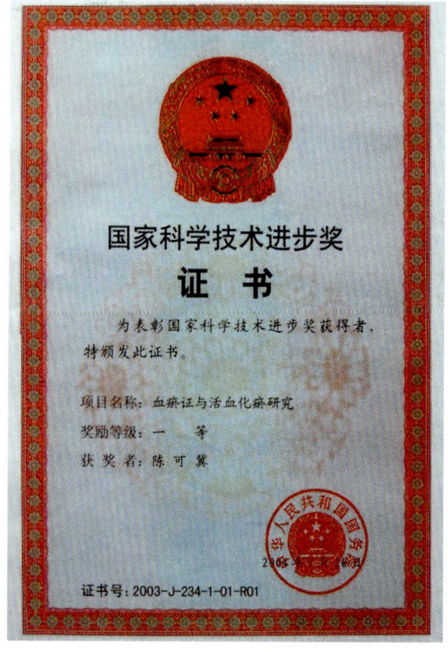

国家科学技术进步奖

证　书

为表彰国家科学技术进步奖获得者，特颁发此证书。

项目名称：血瘀证与活血化瘀研究

奖励等级：一　等

获 奖 者：陈 可 冀

证书号：2003-J-234-1-01-R01

国家科学技术奖一等奖（2003）

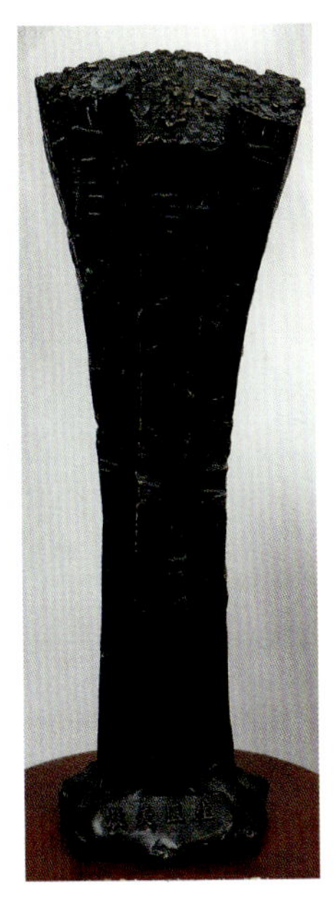

国家卫生健康委员会评选为最美医生（2018）

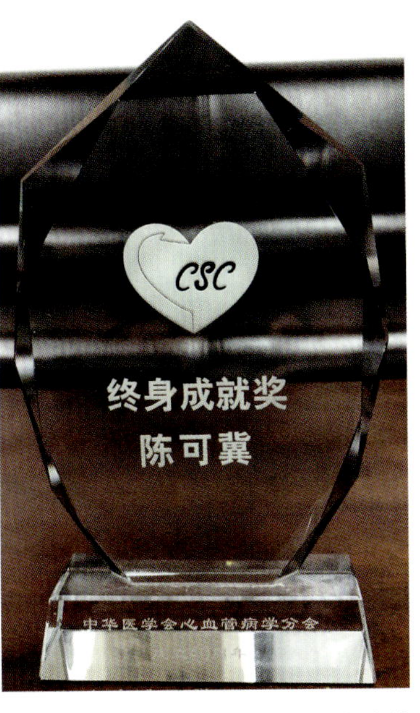

中华医学会心血管病分会终身成就奖（2014）

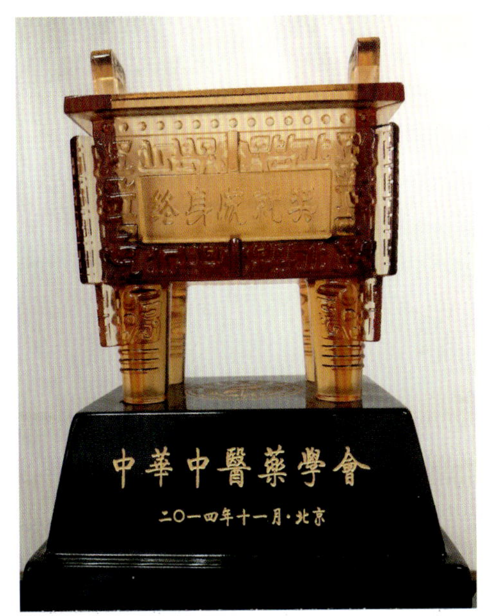

中华中医药学会终身成就奖（2014）

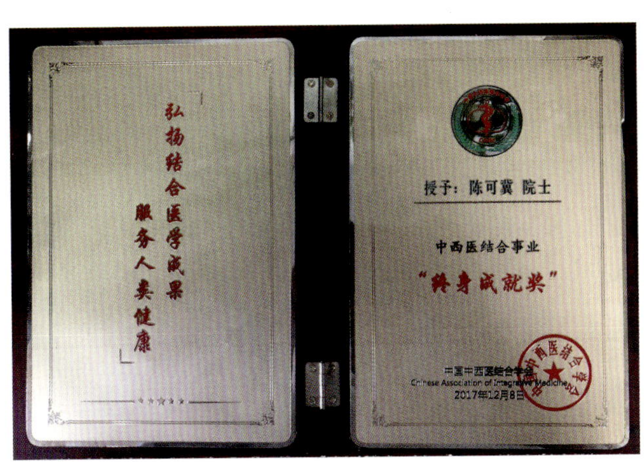

中国中西医结合学会终身成就奖（2017）

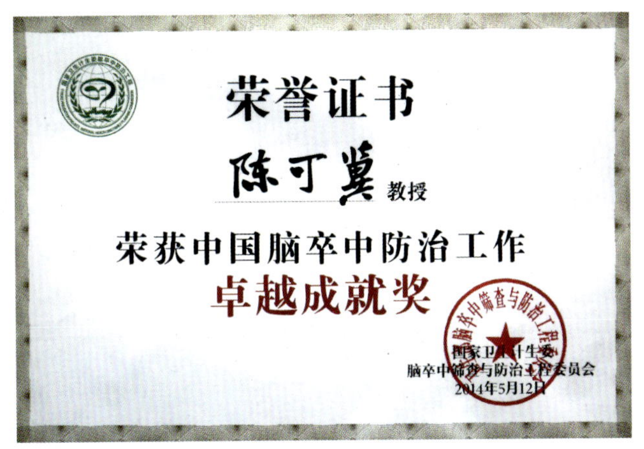

中国脑卒中防治工作卓越成就奖证书（2014）

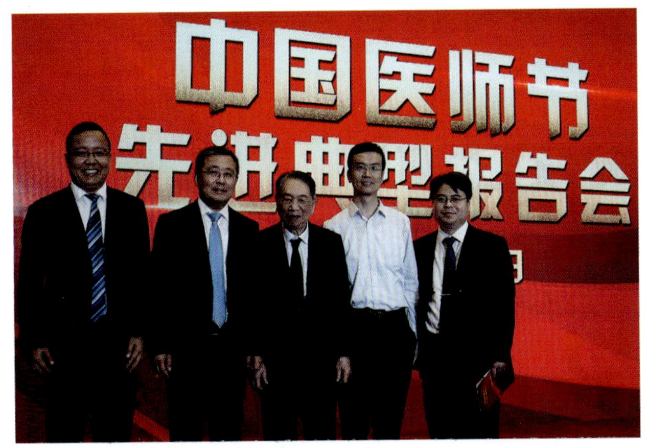

第二届中国医师节先进典型报告会，左 2 为中国中医科学院西苑医院党委书记张允岭教授（2019，人民大会堂）

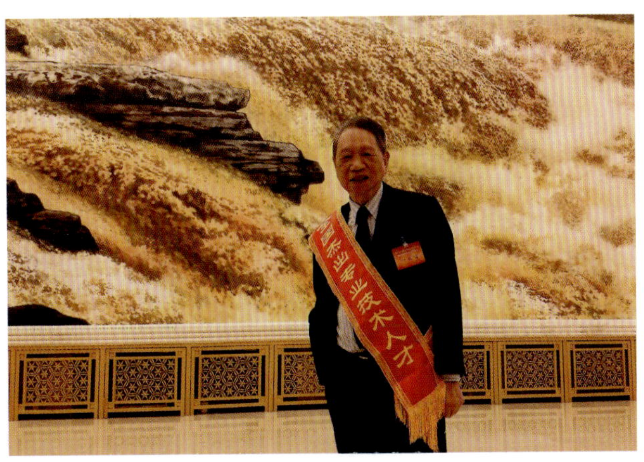

中组部、中宣部、人社部、科技部联合评选为全国杰出专业技术人才（2014，人民大会堂）

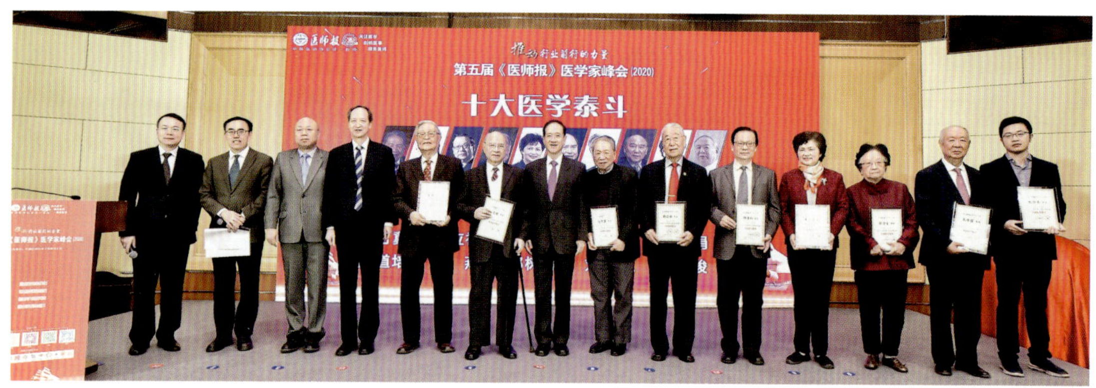

《医师报》评选为十大医学泰斗（2019）

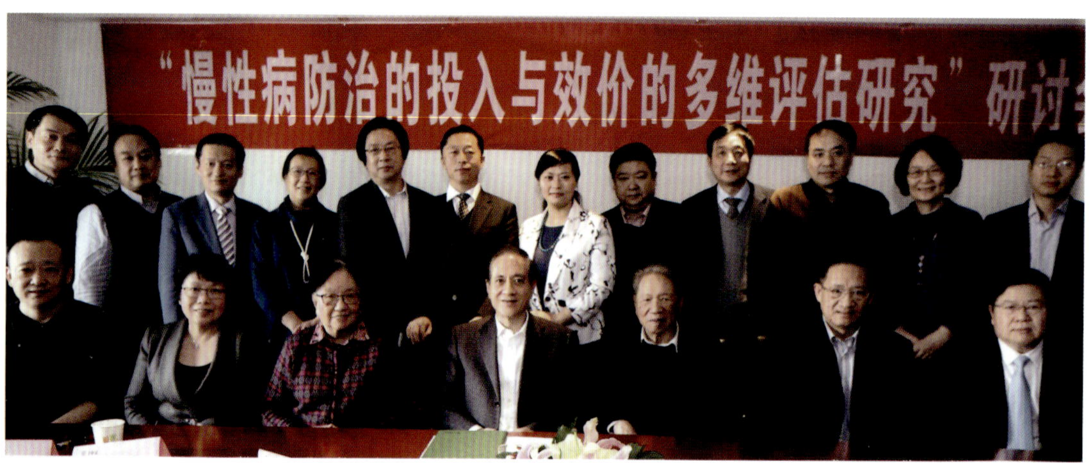

与韩启德院士（前排左 4）、刘力生教授（前排左 3）参加慢病防治座谈会（2017，北京）

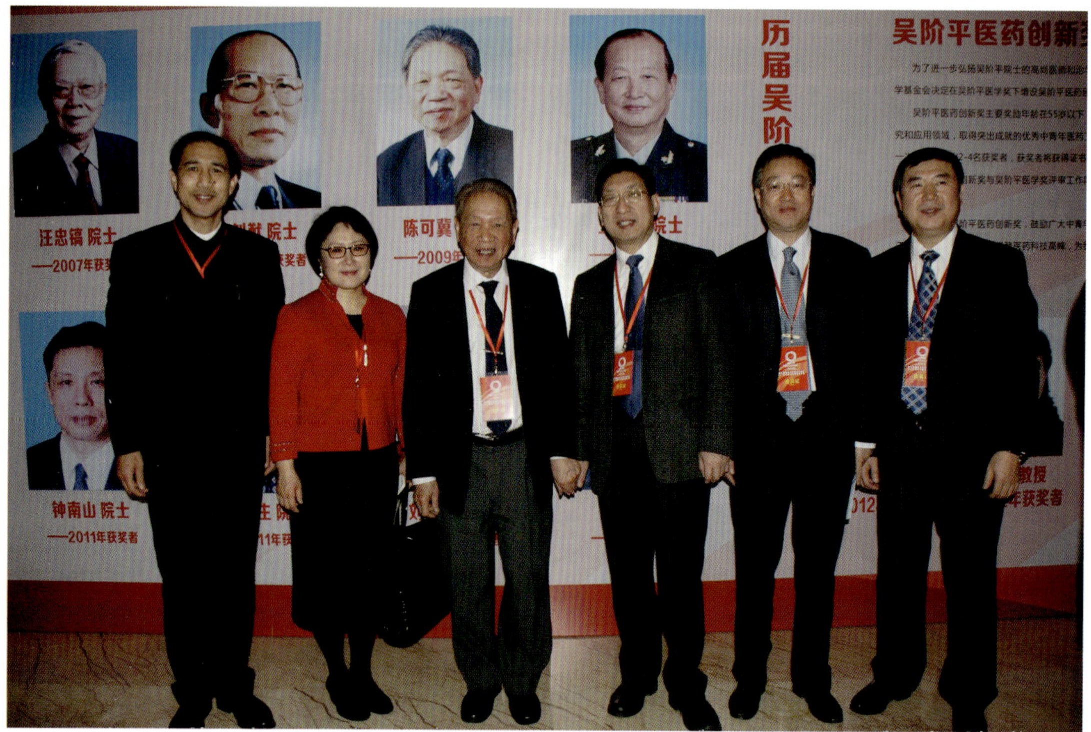

参加吴阶平医学奖颁奖大会，右 3 曾益新院士（2013，广东中山）

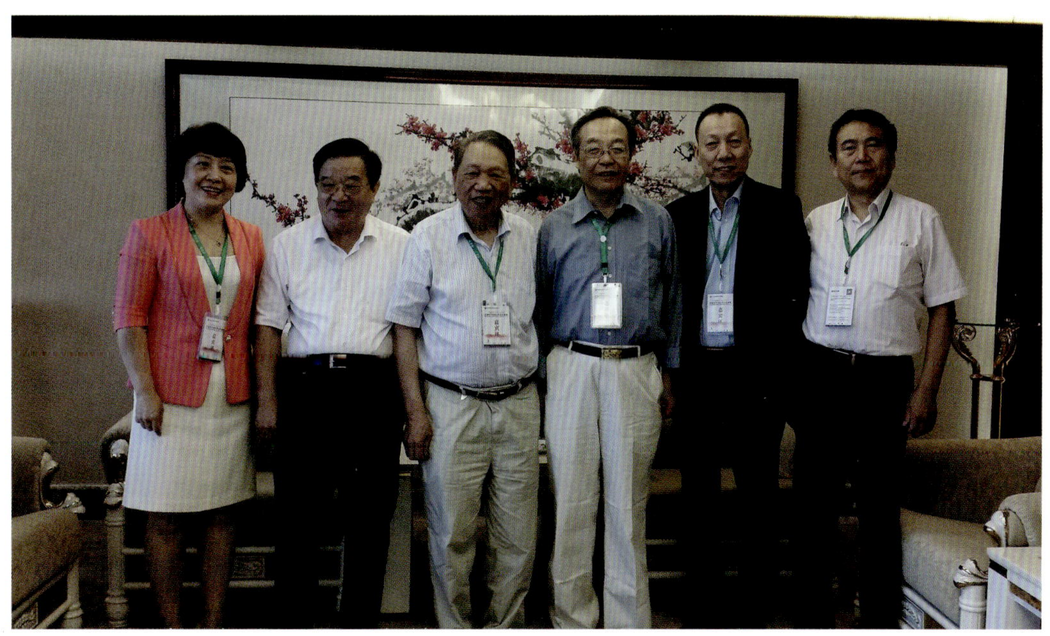

中国中药协会首届中医文化大典，左 2 房书亭会长（2014）

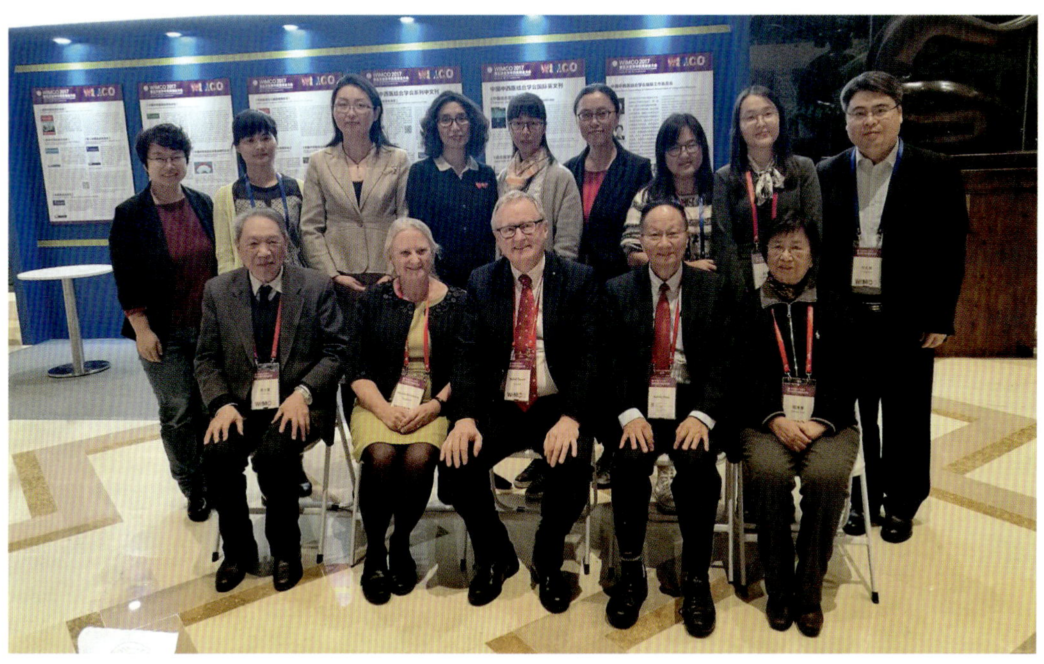

中国中西医结合杂志社编辑在第五届世界中西医结合大会上与部分外籍编委合影（2017）

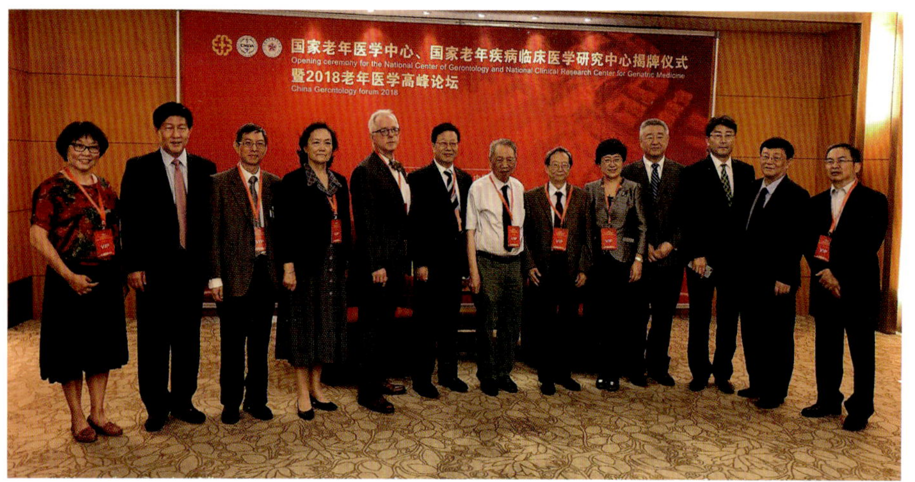

国家老年医学研究中心成立大会，右 6 童坦君院士，左 4 李小鹰教授（2018）

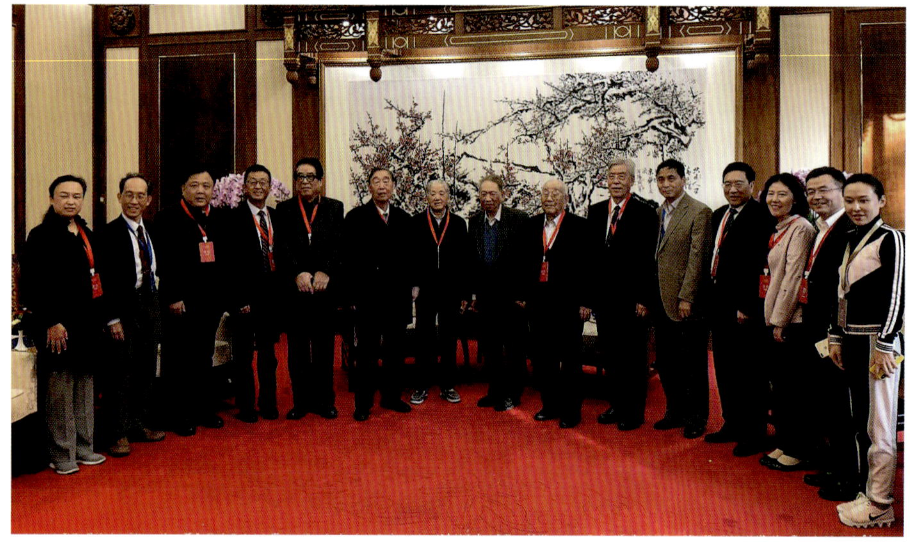

中医药文化发展高峰论坛，左 4—7 曹洪欣教授、张大宁国医大师、王永炎院士、路志正国医大师；右 5—7 吕爱平教授、晁恩祥国医大师、金世元国医大师（2018，钓鱼台国宾馆）

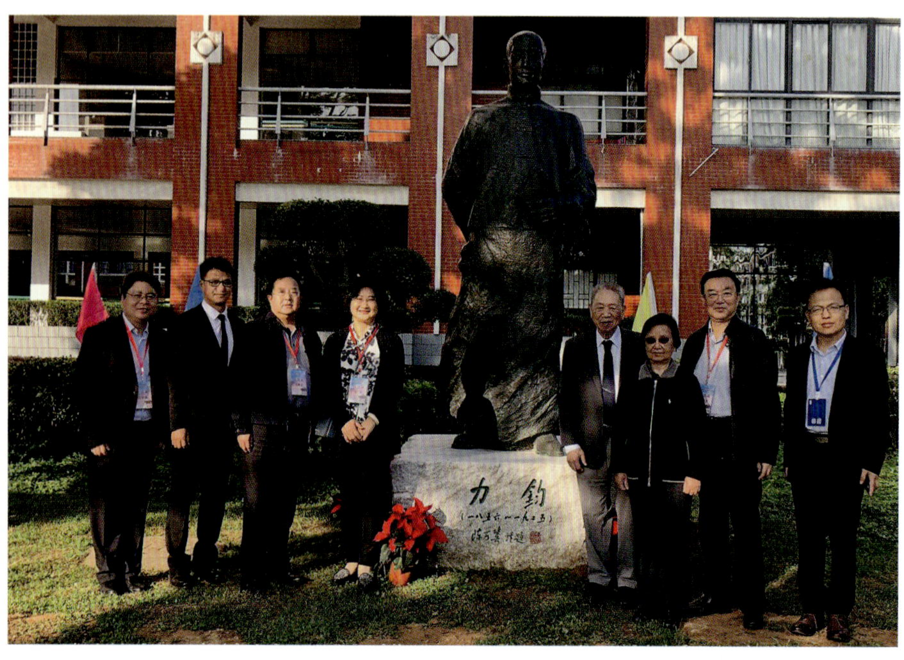

清代中西医汇通派著名医家、御医力钧铜像前（2018，福建中医药大学）

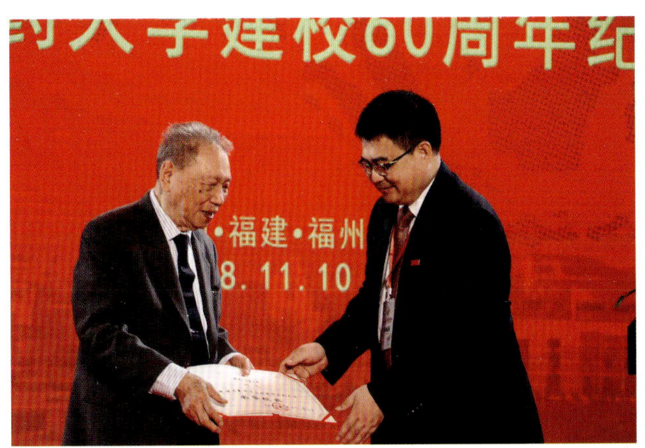

被聘为福建中医药大学名誉校长（2018，福州）

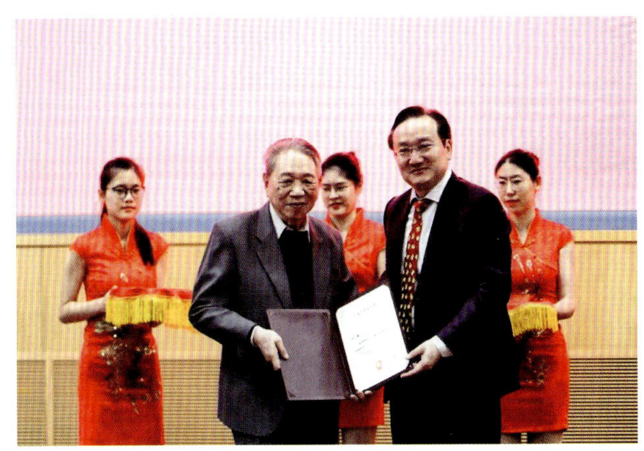
被聘为上海中医药大学名誉教授（2019，上海）

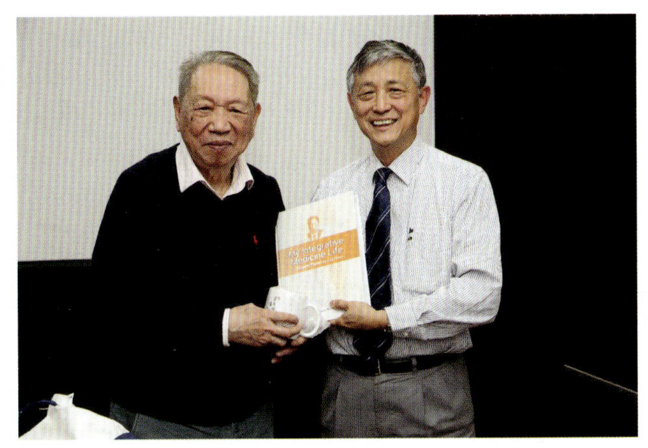
与美国加州大学洛杉矶分校许家杰教授（2017，北京）

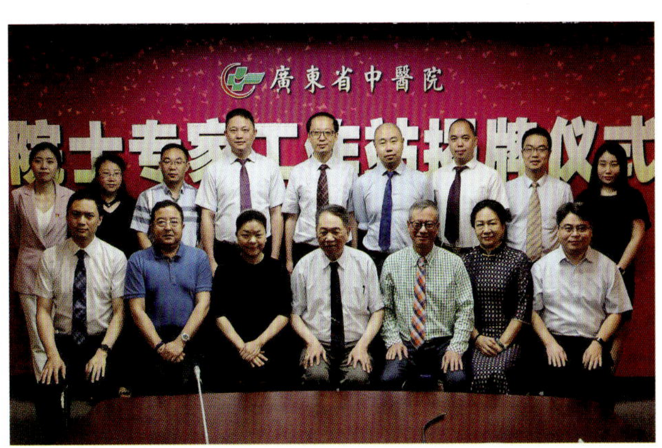

广东省中医院院士专家工作站成立，前排左 3 卢传坚教授、前排右 3 陈秋雄教授（2019）

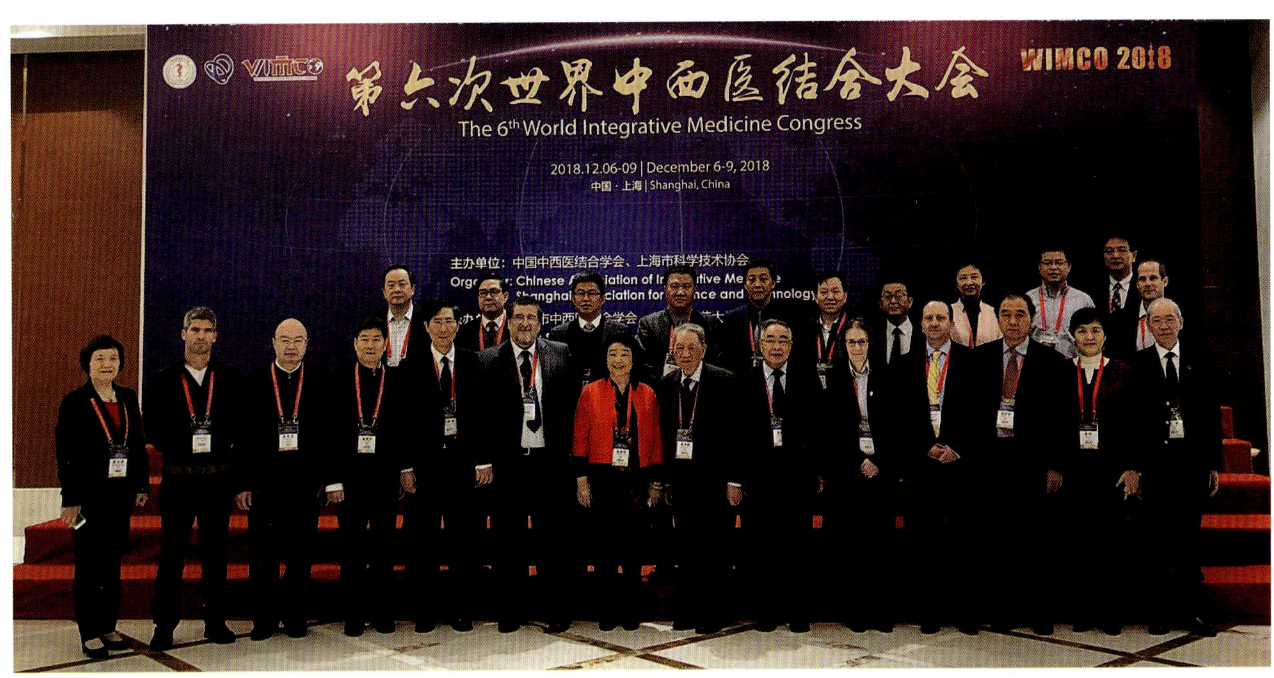

第六次世界中西医结合大会（2018，上海）

国家中医心血管病临床医学研究中心启动会合影留念

2019.07.13

国家中医心血管病临床医学研究中心启动会，陈可冀院士任中心主任（前排左 11），国家中医药管理局王志勇副局长（前排左 10）、中国中医科学院黄璐琦院长（前排左 13）参会（2019，北京）

中国医学科学院首次学部委员会议合影 2019年8月8日

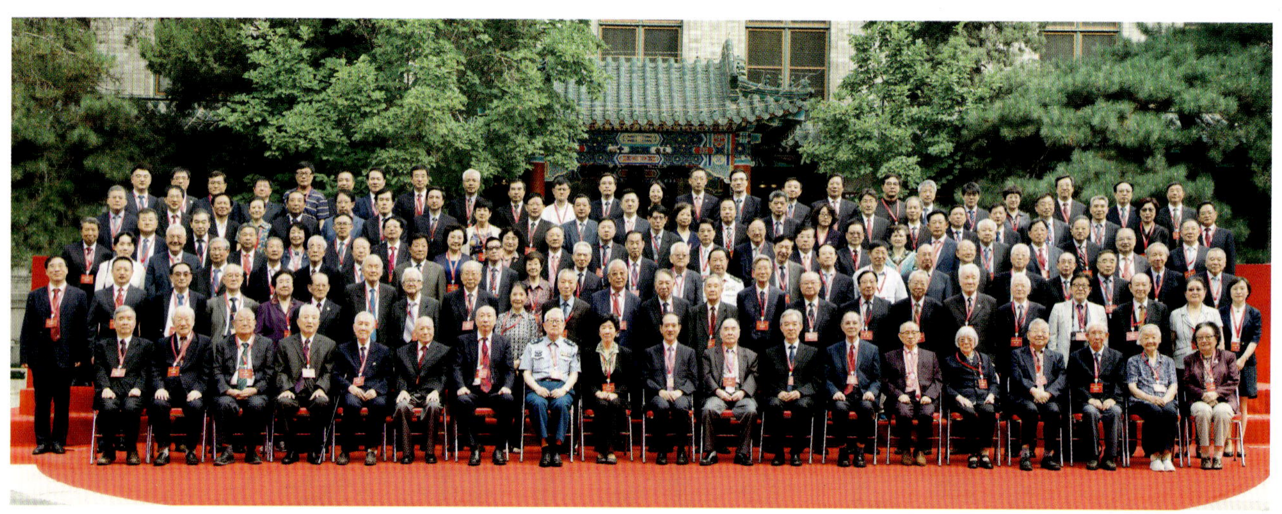

中国医学科学院首届学部委员会议（2019，北京）

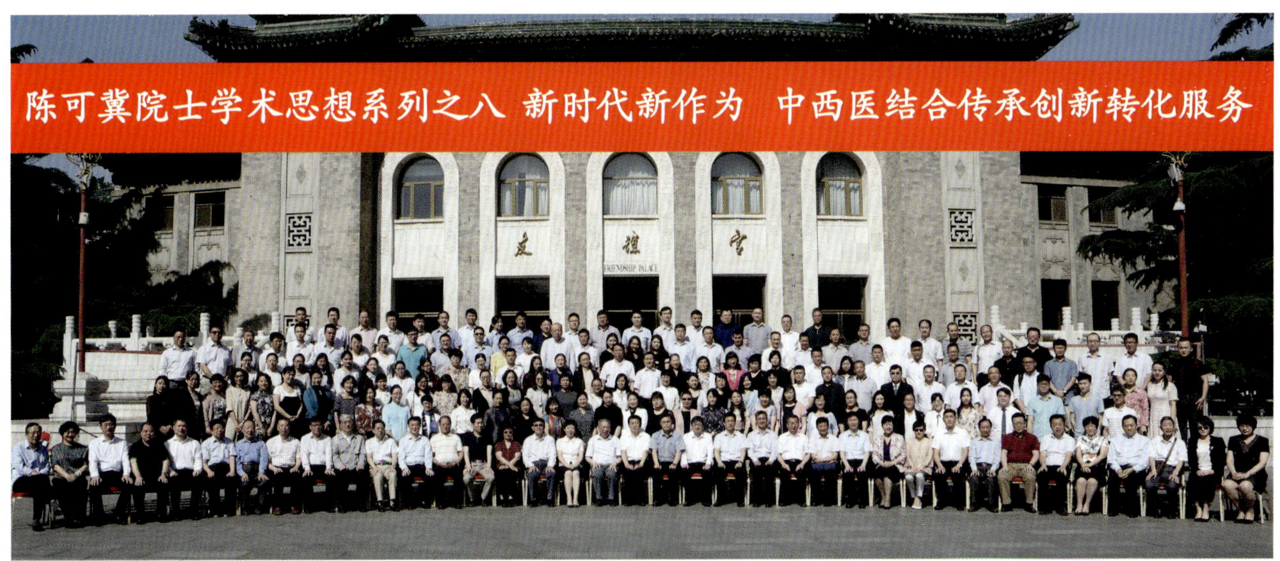

第八次陈可冀院士学术思想传承座谈会，国家中医药管理局于文明局长（前排右 19）参会（2018）

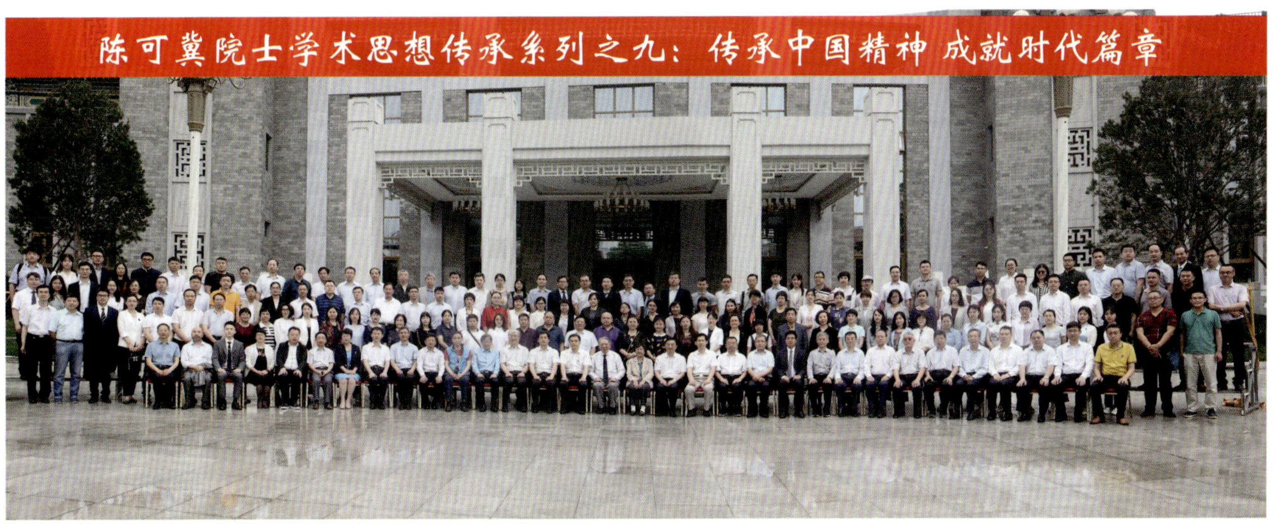

第九次陈可冀院士学术思想传承座谈会合影（2019）

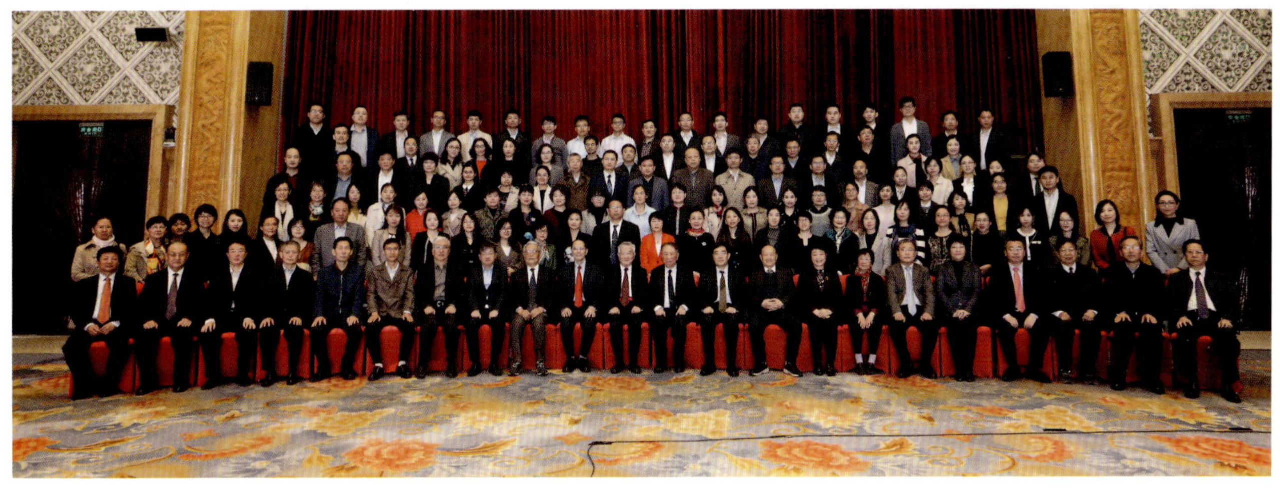

与新中国同行：陈可冀从医七十周年学术座谈会在北京召开，孙燕院士（前排左 9）、韩济生院士（前排左 10）、肖培根院士（前排右 9）、陈香美院士（前排右 8）参会（2019）

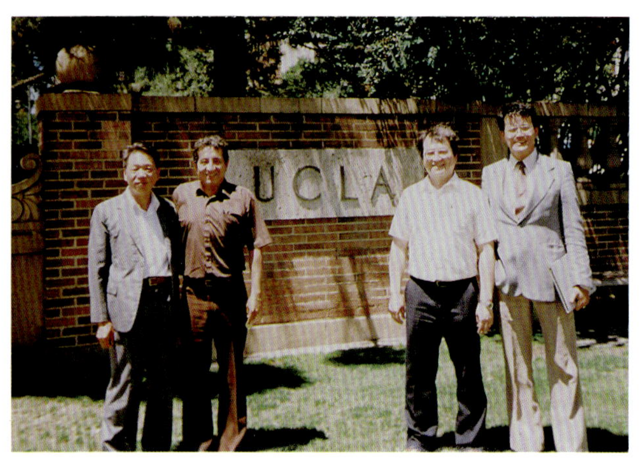

美国三位中西医结合博士答辩会后留影（1987，UCLA）

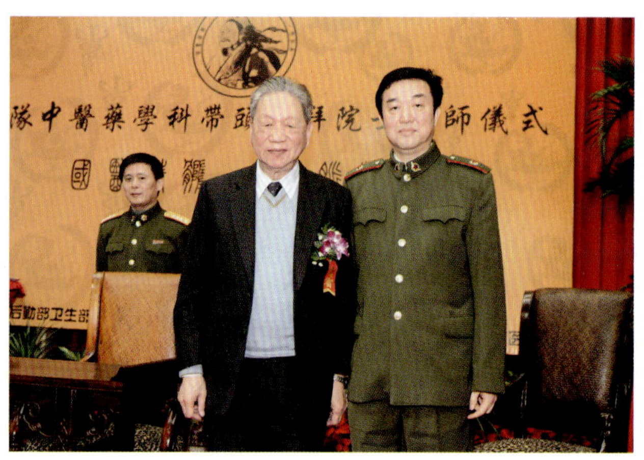

总后卫生部举行中西医结合学科带头人拜师仪式，右 1 吴宗贵教授，右 3 凌昌全教授（2006，上海第二军医大学）

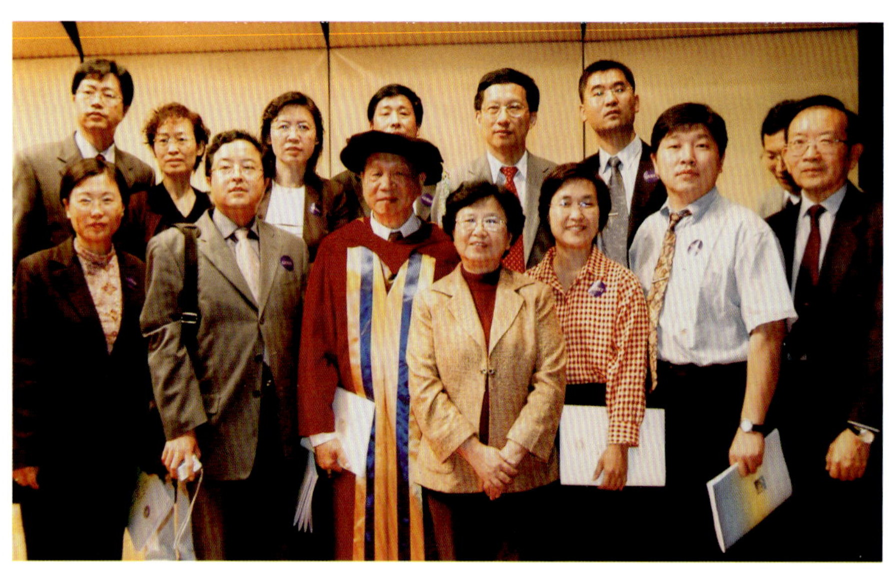

参加浸会大学授予荣誉博士活动师生合影（2004）

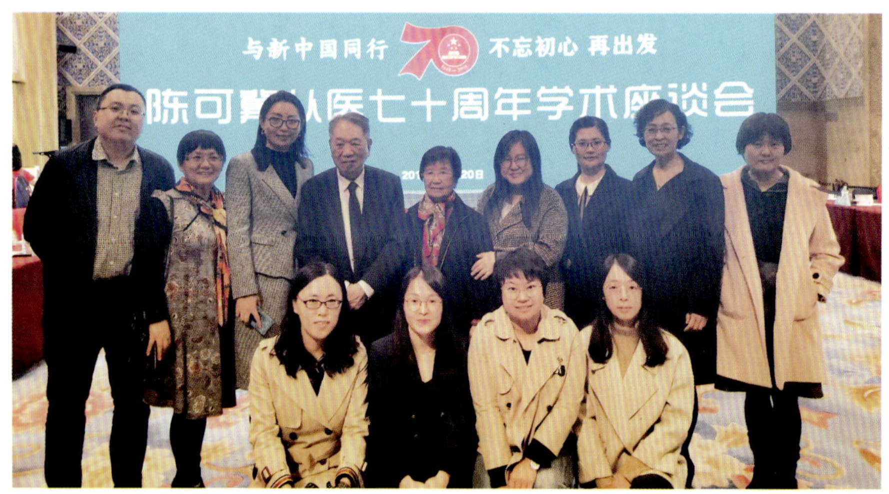

中国中西医结合杂志社编辑在陈可冀从医七十周年学术座谈会合影，前排左起：田琳、赵芳芳、袁琳、于明珠，后排左起：邱禹、段碧芳、郭艳、陈可冀、陈维养、汤静、白霞、王卫霞、张晶晶（2019，北京）

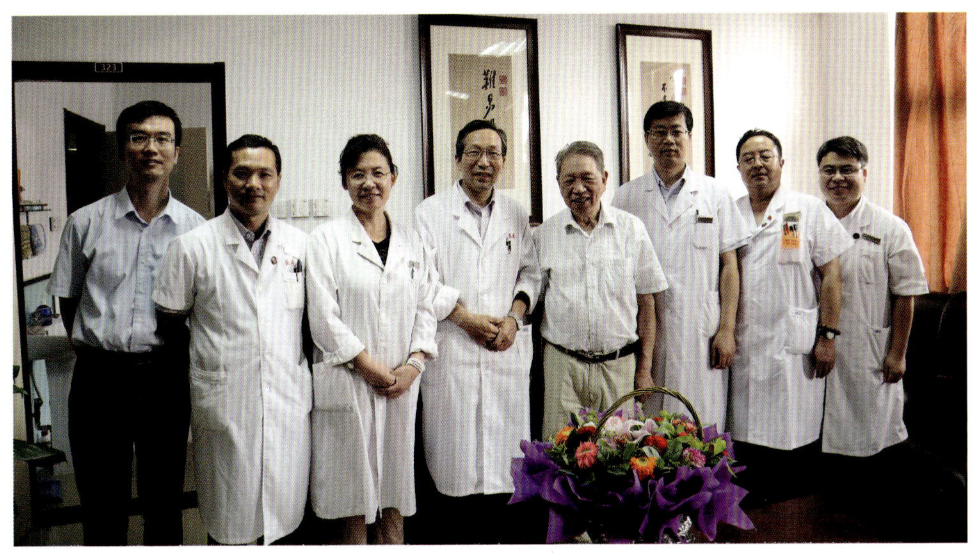

教师节与弟子合影，左起：刘龙涛、李立志、张京春、史大卓、陈可冀、徐浩、马晓昌、付长庚（2014）

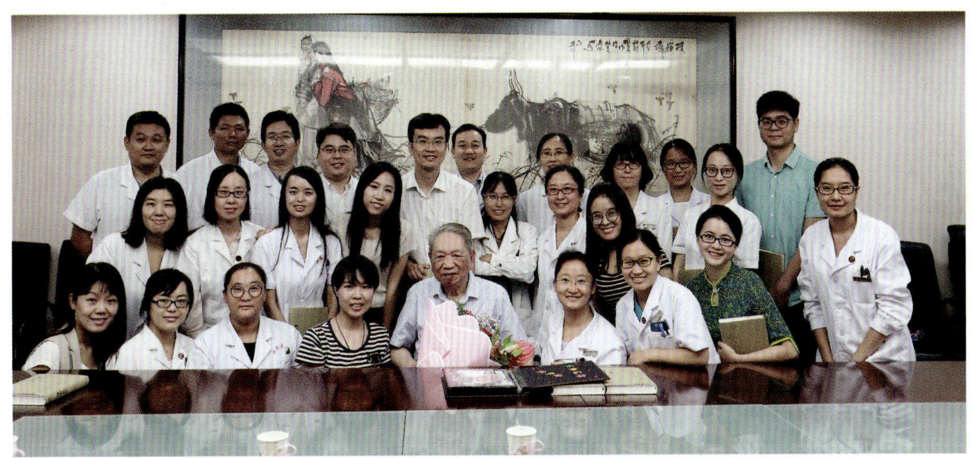

教师节与众弟子合影（2017）

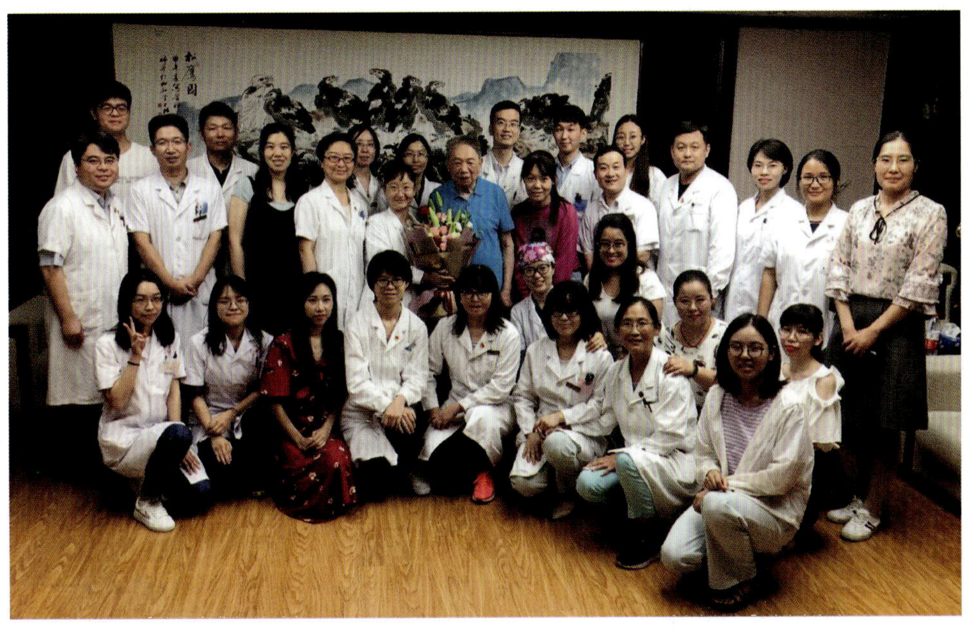

教师节与学生合影（2019）

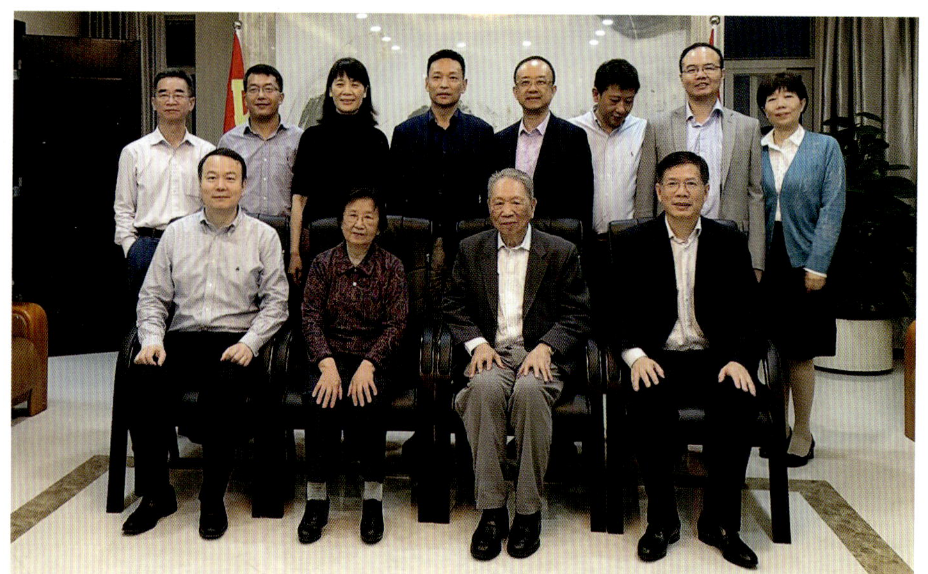

访问母校福建医科大学，前排左1陈晓春校长，右1何明华书记（2018）

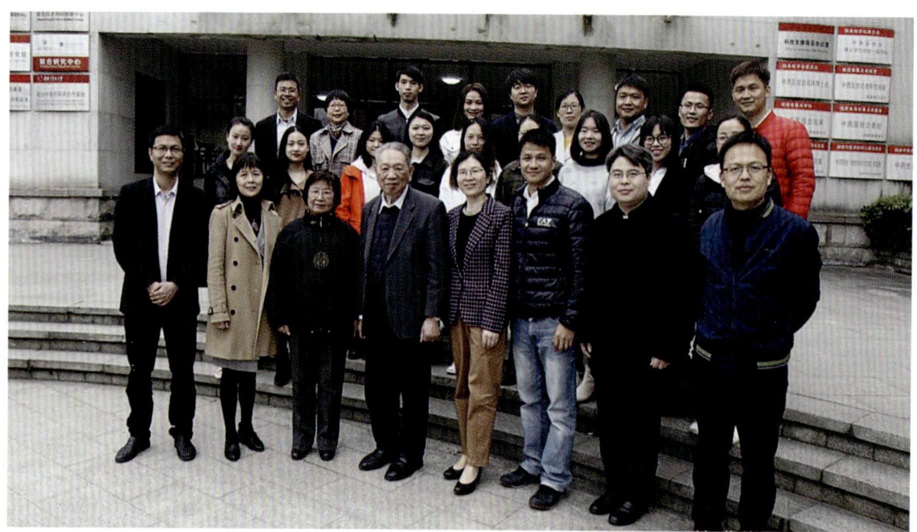

与福建中西医结合研究院同事合影，前排右3彭军副院长，左1龚冰海副院长，右1褚剑锋副院长、右4天江药业陈盛君副总经理（2019）

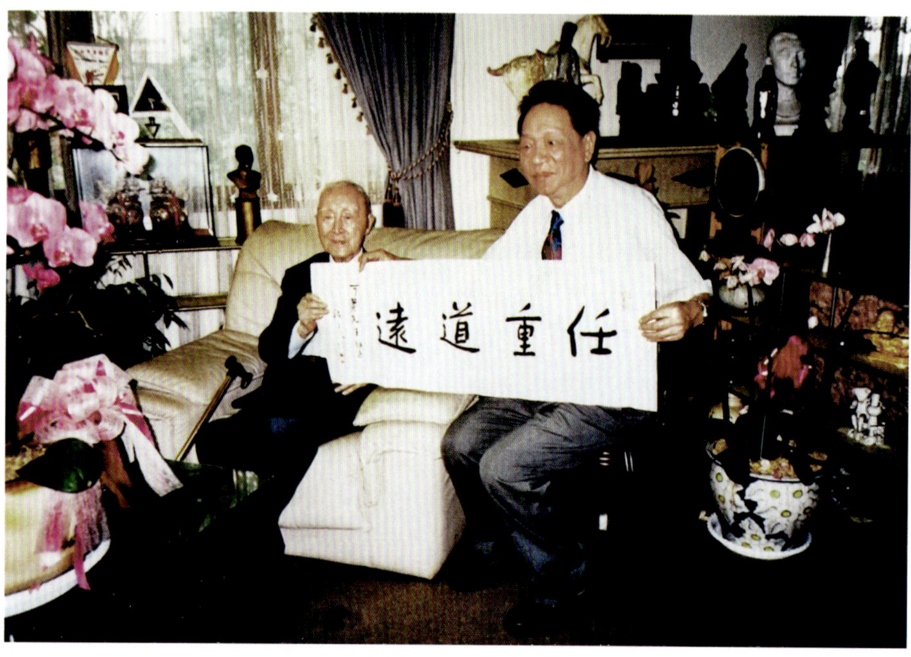

陈立夫先生题赠（1993，台北陈立夫寓所）

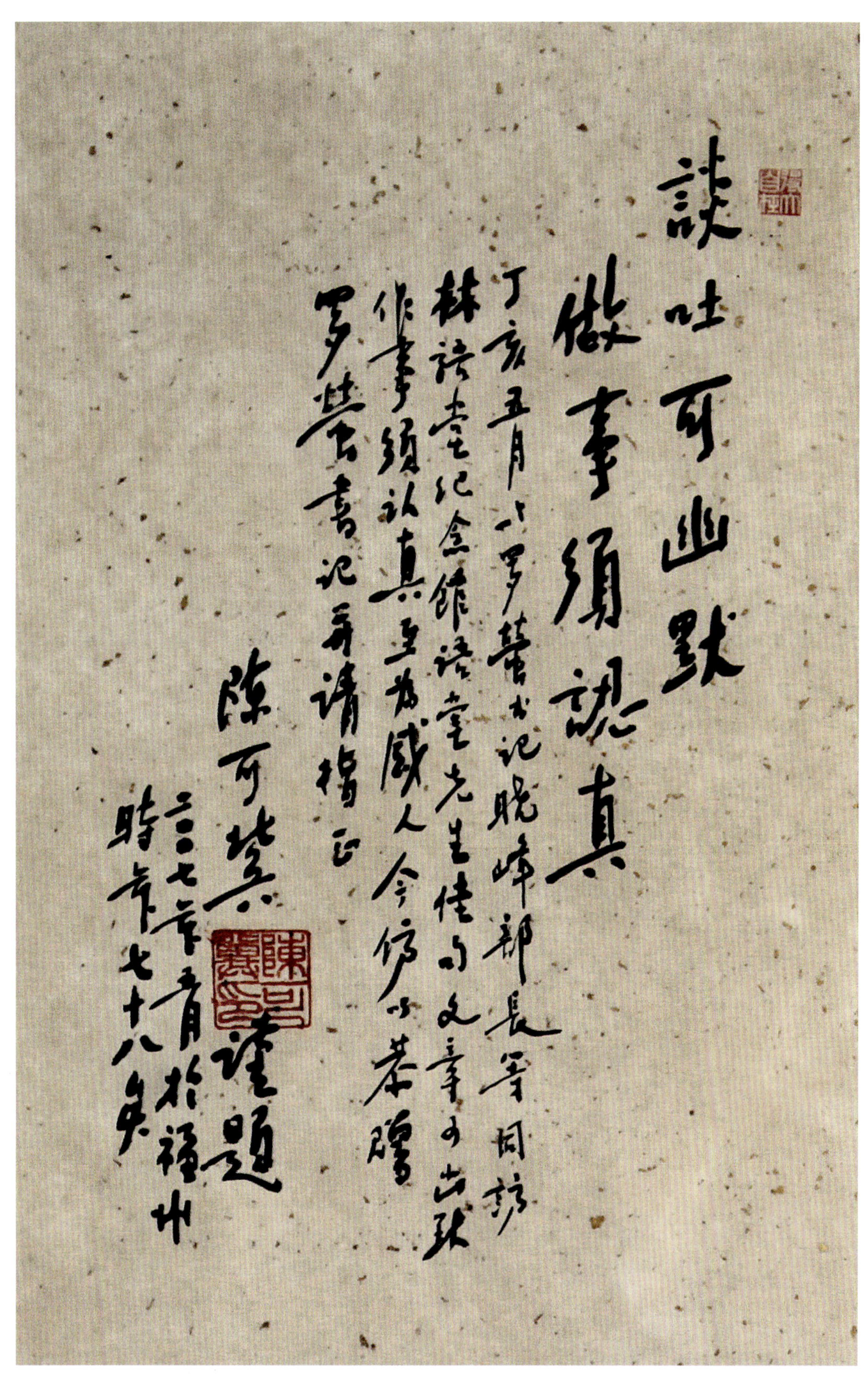

题赠福建中医药大学罗萤书记（2007）

萬物逢搖落
姮娥耐九秌
縞衣人不見
獨上寺南樓
蘇曼殊句书应
可冀先生属
俞平伯

著名红学家俞平伯赠字（1989）

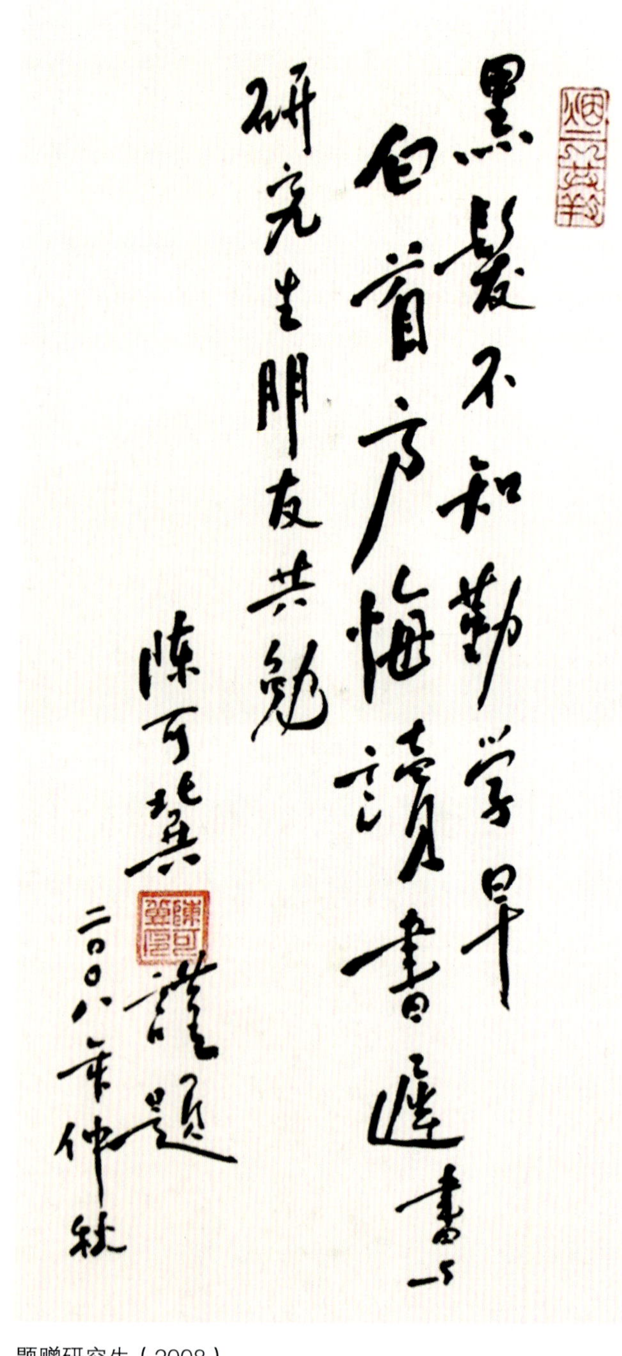

题赠研究生（2008）